VOLCANOGENIC MASSIVE SULPHIDE DEPOSITS OF LATIN AMERICA

EDITORS

ROSS L. SHERLOCK
SRK Consulting,
Vancouver

M. AMELIA V. LOGAN
National Museum of Natural History,
Smithsonian Institution

DESIGN & LAYOUT

RACHEL BROWNE
SRK Consulting,
Vancouver

CONTRIBUTING AUTHORS

G. Alfaro
Anglo American Brasil
F.J. Baars
M. Boudrie
M. Canela-Barboza
R.J. Cathro
M. Chiaradia
F.F. Cortina
H. Echeveste
L. Fontboté
M. Godeas
B.V. Hall
J. Jiménez
M. Klohn
L.M. Lobato
M. Michaud
J. Oliver
K.S. Raman
J. Ruiz
I.B. Schalamuk
K. Steinmüller
E.O. Zappettini

G. Allen
S.M. Araujo
C. Bertoni
J.P. Bout
G.G. Carlson
E. Centeno-García
F. Childe
D. Costelloe
S.G. Enns
J. Franklin
P.P. Gómez-Torres
R.W. Hodder
B.J. Johnson
J.F. Lewis
M.A.V. Logan
L. Millo
J. Payne
M. Rebagliati
N. Russell
R.L. Sherlock
P. Tegart
M. Zubia

S. Ametrano
O. Arce-Burgoa
M. Biste
M.K. de Brodtkorb
A. Carstensen
N. Chacón Abad
R. Cluff
J.C. Cunha
J. Espaillat
J. García F.
A.W. Gourlay
P.M. Holbek
H. Jost
P.D. Lewis
P. Ly Zevallos
J.A. Montante-Martínez
E.U. Petersen
D.A. Rhys
R. Sánchez
M.G. da Silva
H. Uribe-Zeballos

P.F.N. Anderson
V.A. Astacio
T.J. Bottrill
C. Broili
S.G. Carvalho
D.M. DeR. Channer
S. Collao
P.H. Daubney
R. Etcheverry
D.A. Giles
B. Grant
L. Jaramillo Cortés
D. Kerr
F. Lillié
M. Menacho-León
J. Moreira
M. Polliand
K.V. Ross
J.F. Sauvage
C.F. Staargaard
W. Vivallo

Geological Association of Canada
Mineral Deposits Division

Smithsonian Institution

SRK Consulting
Engineers and Scientists

Canadian Cataloguing in Publication Data

VMS Deposits of Latin America

"Geological Association of Canada, Mineral Deposits Divsion - Association géologique du Canada, Division des gîtes minéraux"

Includes bibliographical references.
ISBN 0-919216-72-2

1. Sulphides-Latin America. 2. Geology-Latin America.
I. Sherlock, Ross Lawrence, 1963. II. Logan, Amelia. III. Geological Association of Canada. Mineral Deposits Division.
TN27.5.V57 2000 553.6'68'098 C00-910822-X

The GEOLOGICAL ASSOCIATION OF CANADA is Canada's national society for the geosciences. It was established in 1947 to advance geology and its understanding among both professionals and the general public. The GAC membership of 3000 includes representatives of all geological disciplines from across Canada and many parts of the world employed in government, industry and academia. There are specialist divisions for environmental earth sciences, geophysics, marine geosciences, mineral deposits, paleontology, Precambrian geology, sedimentology, tectonics, volcanology and igneous petrology. Regional sections of GAC have been set up in Victoria, Vancouver, Edmonton, Winnipeg and St. John's, and there are affiliated groups in Toronto and the Maritimes.

GAC activities include the organization and sponsorship of conferences, seminars, short courses, field trips, lecture tours, and student and professional awards and grants. The Association publishes the quarterly journal Geoscience Canada and the quarterly newsletter Geolog , a Special Paper series, Short Course Notes, and several continuing series. GAC also maintains liaison with other earth science societies and provides advice to government and the public on geologic issues. The Association was incorporated under the Canada Corporation Act in January 1984.

L'ASSOCIATION GEOLOGIQUE DU CANADA est la société nationale canadienne pour les sciences de la Terre. Créée en 1947, elle a comme double objectif de faire progresser la géologie et de sensibiliser les spécialistes et les membres du grand public aux sciences de la Terre. Ses trois mille membres représentent toutes les disciplines géologiques; ils viennent de toutes les régions du Canada et de nombreux autres pays; ils oeuvrent dans le secteur public, dans le secteur industriel et dans le monde universitaire. L'Association comprend des divisions de spécialistes en géophysique, en géosciences marins, en gisements minéraux, en paléontologie, en géologie Précambrien, en sédimentologie, en tectonique, en volcanologie, en pétrologie igné et en sciences de la Terre touchant à l'environnement. Des sections régionales existent à Victoria, Vancouver, Edmonton, Winnipeg et St. John's, et des groupes affiliés se sont constitués à Toronto et dans les provinces maritimes.

Les activités de l'Association géologique du Canada comprennent l'organisation et le parrainage de conférences, de colloques, de cours de formation, de courte durée, de visites sure le terrain et de tournées de conférences. Elle décerne des octrois et des bourses aux étudiants et aux personnes qui traivallent dans le domaine des sciences de la Terre. L'Association publie un journal trimestriel, Geoscience Canada, et un bulletin trimestriel d'information, Geolog, une série de mémoires, des notes de cours et diverses autres séries de publications. Elle assure en outre la liaison avec d'autres sociétés en sciences de la Terre et fournit des conseils au gouvernement et au grand public sur des questions géologiques. L'Association a été constituée en corporation en janvier 1984, en vertu de la Loi dur les corporations canadiennes.

Desktop layout: Rachel Browne, SRK Consulting (Vancouver)
Graphic Design: Brad Oltholf, Public Art & Design, Victoria, B.C.
Cover design by Rachel Browne, SRK Consulting (Vancouver)
Front cover image by Geomatics International Inc. - Shaded image based on digital elevation model.
Printed and bound in Canada by Friesens.

Mineral Deposits Division, Geological Association of Canada
Department of Earth Sciences, Memorial University of Newfoundland
St. John's, Newfoundland, A1B 3X5 Canada
Tel: (709) 737-7660, Fax: (709) 737-2532

PREFACE

The purpose of this project has been to provide a venue for publications on VMS deposits in Latin America. The objective was to bring together many disparate sources to contribute manuscripts that include district synthesis and deposit specific studies. These range geographically from Tierra del Fuego through to Mexico and the Caribbean, and geologically from the Archean through to the Tertiary. The manuscripts include initial ideas and thoughts based on exploration and development of deposits through to fully developed and researched papers. In many cases, as projects mature and thinking evolves some of the concepts and models presented will invariably change; however, the basic geologic data will remain. The objective was not to be the final word on Latin American VMS deposits, rather to be the initial word. With this in mind it became important to produce the volume in a timely manner.

The idea from this volume was born in the fall of 1997, in discussion between Bob Cathro (MDD Treasurer) and Dirk Tempelman-Kluit (MDD publications chair). Given the interest among Canadian geologists and their leading role in Latin American exploration this concept was a natural for MDD. The project was approved in principle in January 1998 and James Macdonald approached Roland Bartsch and myself to edit the volume. We later asked Amelia Logan (Smithsonian Institution) to participate, capitalizing on her local knowledge and fluent Spanish. After everything got rolling, Roland left for warmer climes and Amelia and myself finished the project.

To plan the scope of the volume a steering committee was formed with Robert Cathro, David Jennings, Tom Schroeter, Art Soregaroli, Peter Tegart, Dirk Tempelman-Kluit and John Thompson. Robert Cathro and Dirk Tempelman-Kluit played a critical role in providing direction and encouragement. Time and resources for this project were provided by SRK Consulting of Vancouver, the Canada-Nunavut Geoscience Office and the Smithsonian Institute. Geomatics International kindly supplied the satellite imagery used on the cover.

Amelia and I would like to thank the following for thorough reviews of the papers in this volume: David Adamson, Marc Bardoux, Timothy Barrett, Eric Braun, Nate Brewer, Ron Britten, Robert Carmichael, Terry Chandler, Fiona Childe, Garnet Dawson, Jim Franklin, Michael Gray, Charley Greig, Mark Hannington, Dorthy Hosler, Stephen Juras, Chris Lee, John Lewis, Peter Lewis, Robert Macdonald, Mark O'Dea, David Rhys, David Terry, Tina Roth, Norman Russell, Anne Sasso, Chris Sebert, Hugh Squair, Ian Thomson and Richard Tosdal.

Many papers in the volume were presented at an international symposium titled "Volcanogenic massive sulfide deposits of Latin America". The symposium was held in conjunction with GeoCanada 2000, The Millennium Geoscience Summit in Calgary, Alberta, Canada, on May 29- June 2, 2000. The symposium was convened by Andrew Conly (University of Toronto) with the support of the Mineral Deposit Division of the Geological Association of Canada.

This volume would not have been possible without the sustained efforts of our colleague Rachel Browne (SRK Consulting). Her considerable efforts and talents in organizing manuscripts as well as personally typesetting the volume has been key to the timely completion of this volume.

Ross Sherlock
Iqaluit, Nunavut
November, 2000

SRK Consulting
Engineers and Scientists

CANADA-NUNAVUT GEOSCIENCE OFFICE

DEDICATION

On March 24, 1994, three long-time, well-respected members of the Vancouver exploration community, geologists Robert S. Hewton and Christopher Westerman and geophysicist Robert Rivera, died in a helicopter crash near La Tigrera, Ecuador while engaged in mineral exploration. Born and educated in Canada, the United Kingdom and the United States, respectively, they typified the international nature of the profession.

Bob Hewton played an important early role in the creation ot the Mineral Deposits Division of the Geological Assciation of Canada, serving as its Secretary in 1982-1983, as its sixth President in 1984-1985 and as a Director in 1988-1991.

It is our hope that this volume on Volcanogenic Massive Sulfide Deposits in Latin America will contribute to greater international cooperation in the study of mineral deposits. It is dedicated to the memory of our former colleagues and all geologists, prospectors, gambusinos and faiscadores who have died while exploring for minerals in the Americas.

CONTENTS

THE HISTORY OF MINING AND METALLURGY IN LATIN AMERICA, 1500 BC – 1600 AD

ROBERT J. CATHRO
Consulting Geological Engineer, Bowen Island, British Columbia, Canada

ABSTRACT

The Pre-Hispanic period in Latin America was a time of outstanding technical and artistic achievement by indigenous people who were members of one of the few societies on earth that advanced independently to the Bronze Age (the use of metals as tools and jewelry in place of rocks and bones). Turning a hard rock into a softer and more useful metal was a unique step in human development that was only achieved earlier in the Middle East and in Asia. This paper traces the various steps leading from the heating, shaping, annealing and casting of native copper to the roasting of oxidized ores in gossans with carbon to produce metals, the smelting of sulphides, the production of alloys such as gold-copper, gold-silver, arsenic bronze and tin bronze, and electrochemical replacement and depletion gilding to enhance the surface of the alloys.

Recent archaeological studies of metal artifacts and the metallurgical residue from mining activities has shown that the earliest metalworking in Latin America took place in the Andean highlands of southern Peru and Bolivia, commencing about 1500 BC. This technology gradually expanded northward to southern Ecuador and south to northern Chile and Argentina. At least 1000 years before the rise of the Inca empire in 1474 AD, metalsmiths had developed sophisticated techniques of electrochemical replacement to bring gold and silver to the surface of copper-rich alloys. Arsenic bronze was discovered about the same time, and sulphide smelting was achieved about 1200 AD. One of the world's earliest gold placer camps was developed on the Tipuani River in eastern Bolivia.

A separate gold-based metallurgical centre was developed about 200 BC in southwest Colombia and northern Ecuador, which gradually spread north through Panama into Nicaragua. The indigenous people along the Pacific coast of Colombia even learned how to fabricate with placer platinum about 1000 years before it was recognized as a separate metal in Europe.

The final stage of pre-Hispanic mining and metallurgy was the transfer of this technology into western Mexico using watercraft from the coast of Ecuador and Peru about 650 AD. The transmitted metallurgical skills flourished in Mexico using local ores.

After the Spanish Conquest had virtually destroyed the indigenous cultures, European prospectors and miners began to follow up on the known distribution of mineral deposits. This resulted in the most ambitious and successful program of exploration and mining development that the world had ever seen. Most of the giant silver camps of Mexico were discovered between 1546 and 1591, while the great silver lode at Potosi, Bolivia, was found in 1545.

"The tumbaga (copper-gold) alloys, with their inherent gold enrichment properties, swept through the Americas from Peru to Mexico and were in common use in that entire region when the Spaniards invaded Mexico, Central America and South America in the sixteenth century. They constitute the most significant contribution of the New World to the repertoire of alloy systems developed among ancient societies."
(Lechtman, 1988)

INTRODUCTION

The story of Latin American mining prior to 1600 AD consists of two parts, the Pre-Hispanic period prior to 1492 AD and the subsequent Colonial period. The history of Latin America recorded by early European writers generally dismissed the cultural achievements in the former period, which was largely obliterated, as primitive, and stressed the glorious accomplishments in the latter. Recent archaeological studies of metal artifacts and the metallurgical residue from mining activity have shown that the Pre-Hispanic period was actually a time of outstanding technical and artistic achievement by indigenous people who were members of one of the few societies on earth that advanced independently to the Bronze Age. This term refers to the use of metals as tools and jewelry in place of rocks and bones (the Stone Age).

Copper-based alloys were common in Europe and it never occurred to Columbus and the Spanish explorers who followed him that the metallurgical skill required to produce these alloys was clear evidence that they had encountered a remarkable culture.

Throughout this paper, the people who lived in Latin America before the European contact, and their descendants, are referred to as indigenous people rather than as Indians, the name given to them by the Spanish. In Canada, citizens who were previously called indigenous, aboriginal, native or indian now prefer to be called First Nations People.

Space does not permit the inclusion of enough maps to show the location of all the smelting and mining sites mentioned in the text. For more details, the reader should consult the list of references at the end of this paper.

The Bronze Age

Because archaeology is so dependent upon the random preservation and discovery of artifacts, and so much of the record from earlier cultures has been lost because of human scavenging and erosion, scientists are still unsure of how many ancient cultures evolved as far as the ancient Americas. Although several cultures assimilated Bronze Age technology through trade, independent discovery may only have occurred in the Middle East, in China and/or Southeast Asia and in South America. Turning a hard rock into a softer and more useful metal was a unique step in human development (Muhly, 1988). In the words of Wertime (1964), "*one must doubt that the tangled web of discovery, comprehending the art of reducing oxide and then sulphide ores, the recognition of silver, lead, iron, tin, and possibly arsenic and antimony as distinctive new metallic substances, and the technique of alloying tin with bronze, could have been spun twice in human history*".

Archaeologists generally agree that the Bronze Age began in the mountainous region that extends from southeast Turkey through northern Iraq and Iran and east through Armenia to the Caucasus Mountains in Azerbaijan. This region was referred to by Europeans as the Near East, the Middle East or Asia Minor. Much of it now coincides with the ancestral homeland of the Kurdish people.

Charles (1980) has presented a simple summary of the sequential steps of discovery required to produce copper, copper-based alloys and iron. Unless otherwise noted, most of this section is based on his research. These same steps appear to have been followed in all Bronze Age cultures, including Latin America, but since they have been studied most thoroughly in Europe and the Middle East, a brief review of the archaeological history from that region will be helpful here.

There is strong evidence that native copper was the first metal used by man and that this use occurred over a long part of the Neolithic period, starting about 7000 BC. It appears that native copper was used for tools and ornaments in almost every part of the world where it occurs, although only a few cultures advanced to the Bronze Age. In the Middle East, Asia and Latin America, most native copper was formed by the weathering of copper-iron sulphide deposits. In the first stage, oxidation resulted in the formation of sulphuric acid, ferric sulphate and finally copper sulphate. These percolated downward to form copper-carbonate minerals (such as malachite and azurite) and copper-silicate minerals (such as chrysocolla) in the leached cap and gossan zones near surface, and secondary copper sulphide minerals (such as chalcocite, covellite and bornite) in the zone of supergene enrichment below the water table.

The second stage in the formation of native copper depended on the arid conditions associated with the advance of the last glaciation, which lowered the water table and resulted in the oxidation of the low-iron copper minerals in the supergene zone to form cuprite and native copper. Subsequent erosion exposed the native copper at surface and revealed the association between it and the colourful copper oxide, carbonate and silicate minerals in the gossan. Early prospectors soon became adept at recognizing those gossans that contained native copper.

Early metalsmiths discovered that native copper could be shaped by cold-hammering and that this could be accomplished more easily after the object was heated periodically to a temperature of about 330°C. This was sufficient to cause recrystallization, a process that is called annealing. Native copper has a hardness of about 50 on the Vickers scale, whereas repeated cold-working and annealing could raise this to 115, which is even harder than pure iron or low-carbon steel.

As the native copper that could be recovered by primitive shallow trenching or mining became depleted, new raw material had to be found. The smiths then discovered that copper could be produced from the associated carbonate- and oxide-copper minerals in the gossan if these minerals were melted at much higher temperatures in the presence of carbon. This new metallurgy required the same sophisticated pyrotechnological skills and equipment, such as kilns, furnaces, fuel and forced air, that were used in the production of pottery and bricks. By studying the slag produced by the smiths, potters learned which impurities to add to their glazes to produce desired colours.

After the smiths learned how to improve their furnaces enough to produce temperatures above 1083°C, copper could be melted and poured into molds to make castings. When the easily treated copper minerals in the weathered zone had been depleted, further furnace improvements were required to reach the next stage of development, called smelting. Whereas weathering had already removed most of the gangue minerals from the oxidized ores, smelting of sulphide minerals such as chalcopyrite required direct contact with charcoal to produce reducing conditions, and the addition of a flux to lower the melting temperature of the gangue and permit the separation of the liquid metal from the liquid gangue. An abundant supply of trees that would produce good charcoal became essential near the metallurgical centres, so some mining districts could not be exploited until better transportation methods were developed. Luckily, the most useful fluxes were iron oxide minerals such as hematite that occurred naturally with the copper minerals in the gossans. The melting point of these slags was usually about 1400°C, which could be attained in the furnaces by using bellows to produce forced air. All of these discoveries were achieved slowly by trial and error, without any knowledge of the chemistry involved. It is most interesting that modern experiments to produce metals with these techniques have proven extremely difficult (Wertime, 1968; Shimada and Merkel, 1991).

The final metallurgical step was the production of alloys of different metals, of which arsenic bronze and tin bronze were the most useful because of their superior hardness, workability, durability and appearance. Just as impurities in native copper lowered its melting point, metalsmiths later realized that copper alloys also had lower melting points than pure copper, which made them easier to work. Arsenic bronze was apparently the first type to be produced because arsenic minerals and copper minerals commonly occur together in mineral deposits. Tin, on the other hand, seldom occurs with copper and was relatively rare in Europe and the Middle East until large deposits were discovered in Cornwall about 2000 BC. Many arsenic oxide minerals are green and closely resemble oxide copper minerals in gossans, which suggests that the first bronze may have been produced accidentally by the inadvertent contamination of oxide copper ores. The arsenic oxide minerals are derived from the weathering of arsenic-copper sulphides such as enargite and tennantite or the iron-arsenic sulphide arsenopyrite. Bronze Age miners soon learned how to recognize these sulphides because of the distinctive garlic smell they emit when struck with a hammer.

Although arsenic and tin bronzes have similar properties, tin bronze was easier to produce because it only required the mixing of copper and tin, which was easily produced from the common tin oxide mineral cassiterite by roasting with carbon and a flux. By comparison, combining impure mixtures of copper, arsenic and gangue minerals to produce arsenic bronze gave more unpredictable results. The main reason that tin gradually replaced arsenic in bronze production was probably the health of the workers. Roasting arsenic minerals in a furnace produced toxic fumes that would have shortened the lives of the smiths, who held an important position in Bronze Age society. Ownership of mines and metals meant wealth and power and the desire for raw material could lead to war. Owners could not afford to lose such vital workers.

THE USE OF BRONZE IN LATIN AMERICA

For a long time, there was a tendency for historians and miners to ignore the pre-Hispanic achievements in mining and metallurgy. For example, Kemp (1972) stated, "*Tales of 'Indian mines' existing prior to the conquest of Mexico is largely a myth . . . Indians confined themselves to working metals which occurred in the native state.*" Similarly, Prieto (1973) gave almost no credit to pre-Hispanic miners. This was partly because the historic mine workings were often obliterated by subsequent exploitation or erosion and because so much of the metalwork had been melted down, but also because some chroniclers were loath to give credit to people they regarded as too unsophisticated for these achievements.

New facts have begun to emerge during the past 40 to 50 years through the work of archaeologists, mostly from the United States. Using modern analytical and dating techniques and correlation with pottery, they have been able to trace the development of highly sophisticated chemical and metallurgical techniques, identify the centres and societies where the skills were developed and trace the spread of the technology. A large amount of information has now been collected from library research and field studies to show that the first Spanish miners were led to existing mining districts by indigenous miners and prospectors. The investigations have indicated that mining practices were rudimentary, probably because there was no need to develop deeper mining techniques since all metals except gold were in abundant supply. Metallurgical techniques, on the other hand, were relatively advanced and complex. The record shows that sophisticated metalworking first developed in Andean South America and that metallurgical knowledge spread northward as far as Mexico (West, 1994).

Because metals were mainly objects of utility in the Old World, copper, bronze and iron were valued for their hardness, sharpness and strength and were used for warfare, agricultural tools and transportation. In the New World, by comparison, the emphasis was on gold and silver, which were valued for symbolic and religious reasons that imparted political power and social status. Gold was equated with the sweat of the sun while silver was regarded as the tears of the moon (Lechtman, 1984, 1994).

When the Spanish began to melt gold and silver objects into bullion for shipment, they discovered to their surprise that many were actually copper alloys containing a high precious metal content. At least 1000 years before the rise of the Inca empire about 1474 AD, Andean metalsmiths had developed sophisticated techniques of electrochemical replacement, as distinct from electroplating, and depletion gilding or silvering that brought the gold and silver to the surface of the alloy. This was perhaps the greatest achievement of Andean metallurgy (Lechtman, 1984).

Laboratory experiments suggest that the Andean smiths achieved their plating by dissolving silver and gold in aqueous solutions of corrosive minerals common in the desert climate along the Peruvian coast. These include potassium aluminum sulphate, potassium nitrate and sodium chloride. This mixture contains ions present in aqua regia. When added to copper plate, silver and gold are precipitated electrochemically. The smiths probably discovered that hammering and annealing at dull red temperatures produced a copper oxide scale. Removing the scale with stale urine or the acidic juices of certain native plants, a process called pickling, resulted in a surface enriched in silver or gold. After several such cycles, the surface appeared to be pure silver or gold. The smiths also learned how to remove silver from a gold-rich surface using an aqueous paste made from iron sulphate and salt. By selectively treating certain areas, different surfaces could be produced on the same object (Lechtman, 1984). Whereas metallurgical systems elsewhere in the world covered and hid the underlying base metal, the Andean approach of developing and enhancing the surface of the alloy is a striking contrast (Lechtman, 1994).

Copper-gold and copper-silver alloys had three important advantages over pure metals: toughness, enriched gold and silver surfaces when hammered and annealed, and lower melting temperatures. The flexibility and toughness of copper alloy sheet allowed it to be shaped easily and retain its shape better than pure gold or silver. Using an alloy with a high copper content reduced the amount of gold and silver that was needed (Lechtman, 1980). Lowering the melting point was equally important, however, because one of the most difficult problems in the development of metallurgy was attaining sufficiently high temperatures in the reduction process to smelt metals and their ores. The melting point of copper is 1083°C, that of silver is 960°C and that of gold is 1064°C, but that of a copper-silver alloy is only 779°C (West, 1994) and that of a copper-gold alloy only 911°C (Bray, 1985).

Latin American metallurgy never developed the bellows that was used in the Old World for producing a forced air draft and relied instead on the less efficient ceramic tuyere, or blowing tube.

SOUTH AND CENTRAL AMERICA

Although native copper was dug from shallow pits and hammered for use in the Lake Superior region as early as 4000 BC (Easby, 1966), the first pyrometallurgy in the Western Hemisphere involving smelting and the controlled production of alloys was developed by indigenous people in the central Andean highlands of South America about 1500 BC (West, 1994). The oldest artifacts appear to be tiny pieces of hammered gold foil that were found with lapis lazuli beads and a complete gold worker's tool kit (stone hammers and anvil in a bowl) in a grave at Waywa, Peru (Grossman, 1972). There is evidence that by about 500 BC, emphasis had changed from the use of mainly placer gold to a gold-oriented metallurgy that also involved the use of copper and silver, and that copper smelting was underway. This gradually evolved into a copper-based metallurgy and the metalsmiths had learned, by about 200 BC, how to control heat well enough to solder and weld three-dimensional forms by joining pieces of pre-shaped metal sheet. Increased sophistication led to the production of gold-copper and silver-copper alloys and to skills in hammering, annealing and gilding, mainly along the coastal plain in northern Peru. Arsenic bronze was discovered about 200-600 AD and sulphide smelting had been achieved about 1200 AD (Lechtman, 1980, 1984, 1988, 1994; Shimada and Griffin, 1994; West, 1994).

In spite of the arid climate, native copper rarely occurs at surface in the Andes (Georg Peterson, 1970, reported in Lechtman, 1980), which is a region with one of the fastest rates of uplift and erosion in the world. As a result, there is little evidence to suggest that a melting stage preceded smelting. A large variety of complex copper-silver oxide ores were available, however, and a highly sophisticated technical level was achieved much more quickly in South America than in the Old World. Andean metallurgy developed in several distinctive directions because of local variations in mineralogy and the cultural importance assigned to gold and silver. Because of the rugged terrain, ores and metals were traded from the highlands down river valleys to the narrow coastal strip and technology then spread north and south along the coast (Lechtman, 1980).

Three regions emerged as preeminent centres of South American metallurgy. The first was in the northern and north-central highlands of Peru and Bolivia, and adjacent Pacific coast, with extensions into northwest Argentina and northern Chile. This is an arid region with deep oxidation and abundant copper and silver ores. Arsenic ores are common in the north but are not abundant in the southern Andes, although they do exist and were used. The arsenic occurs mainly as copper-arsenic sulphide and sulfosalt minerals (such as domeykite, enargite and tetrahedrite/tennantite) or oxide minerals (such as olivenite and chenevixite), while the copper is present as oxide, carbonate and sulphate minerals (such as malachite, azurite, atacamite, chrysocolla, chalcanthite, brochantite and antlerite) (Lechtman, 1980). Early silver and copper mining was most active in the area between Quiruvilca and Hualcayuc, in northern Peru. Arsenic bronze was probably first produced there through the inadvertent smelting of mixed ores. Later, it was produced at many scattered sites such as the Las Capillitas mines, 50 km from Hualfín, Argentina (Lechtman, 1980). One of the principal silver mines dating to Inca or earlier times was located at Porco, Bolivia (Bakewell, 1997). According to de Lucio (1997), another was situated at Cailloma, Peru and primitive mining tools have been found at Nazca and Cusco.

Although it is widely believed that the lead mineral galena, which is common in this region, was used to smelt silver ores, no undisturbed ancient sites have ever been found. The best evidence has been found as manufacturing debris near the town of Jauju in the Peruvian highlands (Howe and Petersen, 1994).

It may seem surprising that few ancient mines have been found but, as suggested earlier, mine production expanded significantly after the Conquest and most of the evidence of earlier activity was likely obliterated by subsequent mining or erosion, or simply ignored. One interesting example of the type of evidence that was probably quite common has been documented at Chuquicamata, Chile, the site of one of the world's largest porphyry copper mines. It is located

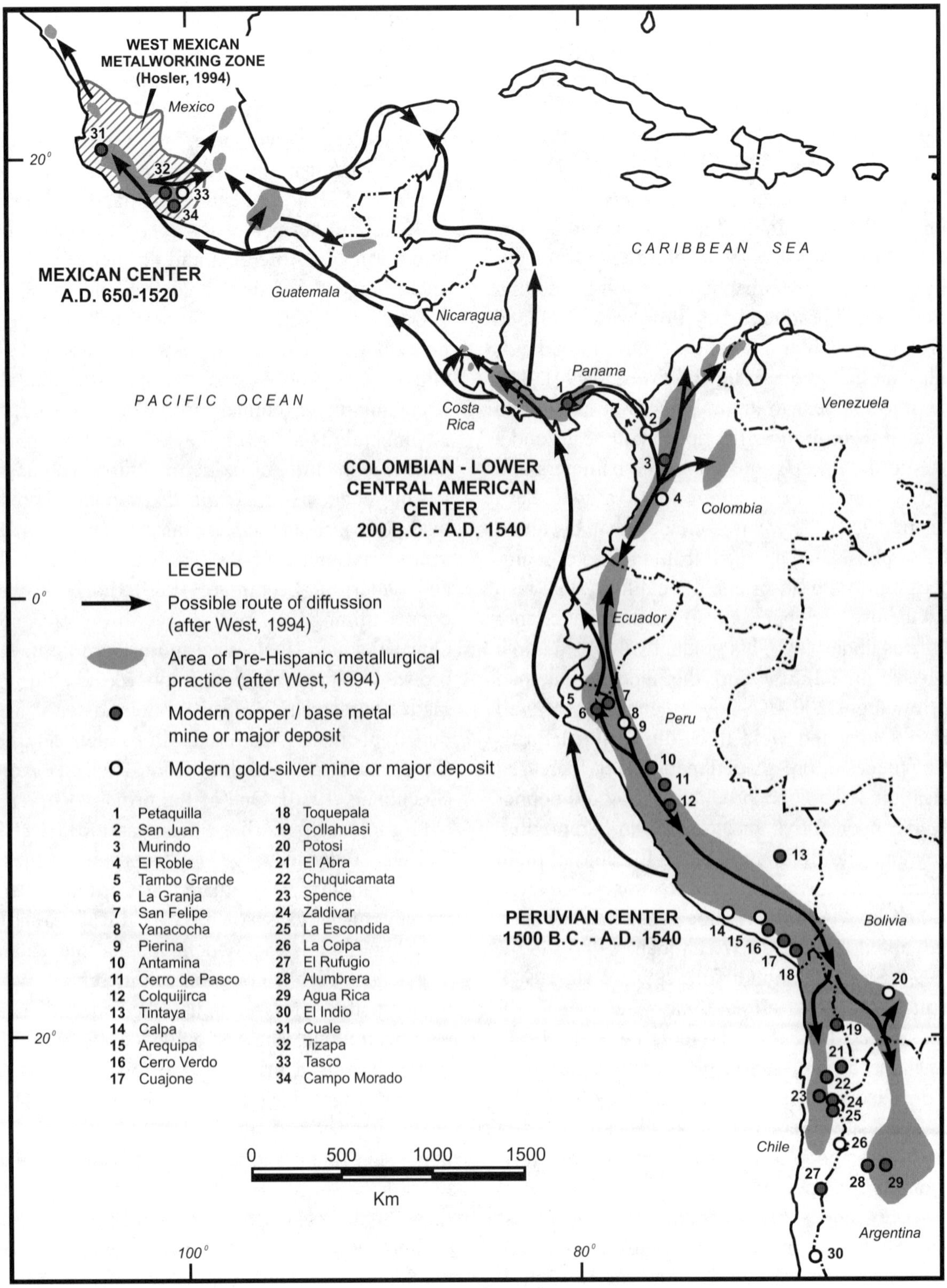

Figure 1. Pre-Hispanic (Bronze Age) mining and metallurgy in Latin America

at an elevation of about 2700 m in the Atacama desert, one of the driest areas on earth, and is about 18 km from the nearest water source. In 1899, long before large-scale surface mining began, the remarkably preserved body of a miner was found in a shallow, collapsed shaft in the Restauradora Mine. The body had become desiccated in the dry, cold air and impregnated in part with copper, imparting a greenish tone. He became know as the "*Copper Man*" (Bird, 1979).

The site was not professionally studied at the time and few details exist about the mine or tools found with the body. He was mining veins of the copper chloride mineral atacamite, which would have been an easy ore to smelt. It was assumed initially that he must have died at about the time of the Conquest. Fortunately, the body and some stone tools from the vicinity were donated to the American Museum of Natural History in New York in 1905. When the body was radiocarbon-dated in about 1979, the date of death was determined to be about 484 AD (Bird, 1979). A similar find has been reported from the Huantajaya Mine in Chile (West, 1994).

Although the metallurgy in the Peruvian-Bolivian highlands was originally gold-based, little information appears in the archaeological literature about the source of the gold. Most of the gold looted from the Incas probably came from the Tipuani region of Bolivia, located about 110 km north of La Paz on the eastern flank of the Andes. Linked to the capital at Cusco by trails and roads long before the conquest was completed in Bolivia in 1548, this is one of the oldest and most poorly documented gold fields in the world. All the easterly flowing tributaries of the Rio Beni that drain the Cordillera Real, such as Mapiri, Kaka, Challana, Zongo and Coroico, were auriferous, but Tipuani was the most important. The Rio Beni flows into the Rio Madeira on its way to the Amazon. One of the principal sites of ancient mining on the Rio Tipuani, known as the Roman playa (riverbank), contained crude tools of stone, wood and copper as well as charms and perfectly rounded beads of gold pierced for a string. According to Woodbridge (1927) and Stoll (1961), the Incas concealed the location of the Tipuani placer deposits from the Spanish until 1562.

Because information on the gold placer is hard to find, a brief description of the geology is included here. The main part of the gold field occurs where the steep gradient of the streams down the mountain front flattens into wider valleys. The richest paystreak occurs in a channel 500 to 2500 m wide of naturally cemented conglomerate within the oldest gravels, although gold is also found in younger beds. The gold tends to occur as flattened grains the shape and size of oatmeal, and is associated with minor amounts of tin and iron minerals. The gold is quite pure, ranging from 915 to 960 fine. It is derived from widely scattered gold veinlets that occur throughout the Cordillera Real in the Yani and Polo Sur areas. Other, less important sources of placer gold exploited in the Pre-Hispanic period are situated in the Suches-Antaquilla area of Bolivia, 230 km northwest of La Paz (Herail, 1991; Herail and Viscarra, 1991; Stoll, 1961) and in the Madre de Dios river system (Ross Beaty, personal communication) and Santa and Marañon river basins (de Lucio, 1997) of Peru.

Rich vein and placer deposits of the oxide tin mineral cassiterite were found in southern Peru and Bolivia about 1000 AD and tin bronze was soon produced in an area centred at Machu Picchu, Peru. As mentioned earlier, tin bronze was easier to produce than arsenic bronze. The new tin district and the arsenic-rich district in northern Peru produced their own distinctive varieties of bronze from their local ores until the formation of the Inca state about 1474 AD. Tin bronze became the standard after political unification because the Incas controlled the supply of tin. Tin bronze became a "*peoples alloy*", while gold and silver were produced by a state monopoly and reserved for royal use. Under the Incas, the best metalsmiths in the empire were brought to the capital at Cusco and metal production was substantially increased (Lechtman, 1980).

The second metallurgical district in South America was situated farther north, along the coastal plain near the present border between Peru and Ecuador. It was centred on the Moche Valley and Lambayeque-Vicus area, where gold is rare but copper is locally available. By about 1250 AD, complex sulphide ores containing arsenic were being transported from the highlands. In addition, recent studies have identified ancient shallow copper-arsenic mines and smelting sites near Batán Grande, Peru (Shimada,

1994; Shimada et al, 1991,1994). Both sources were used in the production of arsenic bronze.

Metallurgy in the third region, which was located in southwest Colombia and extended into northern Ecuador, was based on abundant gold in the mountains and platinum in placer deposits along the Pacific coast. The discovery and utilization of native platinum by the indigenous people living in the Choco area of Colombia and along the Colombia-Ecuador border was a unique development in metalworking. Platinum was not recognized as a separate metal in Europe until the early decades of the 18th Century (Bray, 1974b). In fact, the Spanish placer miners in Colombia considered the dull gray metal to be a useless impurity and threw it back into the river (Scott and Bray, 1994). Because of its high melting point (about 1750°C), it could not be melted with available technology but the smiths learned how to sinter it with gold by heating on a bed of charcoal. This melted the gold, causing it to flow and bind with the platinum.

The platinum occurred with gold in placer deposits in rivers that drain ultramafic intrusions occurring along the coastal plain. True platinum metallurgy, as opposed to the use of gold with accidental platinum inclusions, was confined to the coastal Tumaco-Esmeraldas belt that straddles the border. Extensive studies of a major site at La Tolita, Ecuador showed that this metalwork originated about 300 BC and was fully developed about five centuries later. Technologically, it was characterized by the use of sheet and pieces assembled by means of soldering, welding or filigree and included objects made of native platinum, sintered gold-platinum alloys and gold objects coated with platinum on one side. The pronounced differences from Peruvian metallurgy argue against transfer of technology from there (Bray, 1974; Scott and Bray, 1994).

Before the 10th century AD, southwest Colombia hosted a separate metallurgical tradition that contrasted with those of the central and northern Andes (Plazas and Falchetti, 1985). Placer gold was abundant in the tropical lowland valleys between the northern Andean ranges of Colombia. Mining started about the 4th century BC from tributaries of the Cauca and lower Magdalena rivers, as well as from ancient lode gold mines located at Los Remedios and Cerro de Buriticá in Antioquia and at Mariquita near the Magdalena valley (West, 1994). Although some of this gold was traded southward, most was sent to the Gulf of Uraba on the Caribbean coast through a jewelry and trading centre at Dabeiba. The Colombians perfected the lost-wax process of casting finely fashioned figurines and ornaments and worked extensively with the gold-copper alloy known as tumbaga. The period from 400 to 700 AD is considered by some to have been the classical period in Colombian metallurgy when the best goldwork was produced (Bray, 1974a; West, 1994). Madrid's Museo de America holds one of the most elegant collections of ancient gold objects that has survived. It was collected from two ancient tombs at La Soledad, near the town of Filandia in Quimbaya (Jones, 1974b).

Colombia, Panama and Costa Rica formed a single metallurgical province characterized by a preference for lost-wax casting and by the use of gold-copper alloys, depletion gilding and false filigree. Metallurgy reached Panama, where gold and copper are quite abundant, by 200-300 AD and Costa Rica by at least 700 AD. Metal objects were traded as far north as Mayan Mexico. Much later, Nicaragua became famed for its exquisite goldsmithing (West, 1994). Since 1930, a large cemetery has been excavated at Sitio Conte, Panama, on the Gulf of Panama. This cemetery, which was abandoned around 900 AD, has yielded a major collection of gold jewelry and revealed that a complex society lived there (Bray, 1974a, 1992; Cooke and Bray, 1985; Hearne, 1992).

MEXICO

Metal artifacts first appeared in the central part of the Pacific coast around 650 AD after metallurgy was introduced from South America via a maritime route. This region, called West Mexico by archaeologists, contains a varied array of ore minerals, including copper carbonates and sulphides, arsenopyrite, argentite, silver sulfosalts and cassiterite. West Mexican metalworkers produced mainly ritual and sacred objects throughout the 900-year history of this technology (Hosler, 1994).

Before 1200 AD, copper was used mainly for bells but also for small cold-worked implements. After 1200 to 1300 AD, the smiths began to produce arsenic bronze, tin bronze and copper-silver alloys, not only for their golden and silvery colours but also to optimize the design and function of objects previously made of copper. After 900 AD, metallurgical knowledge spread into parts of northern and central Mesoamerica and copperware from Mexico was being traded into the Hohokam culture in the United States southwest by 1100 AD (Hosler, 1988a).

Lead isotope analyses have been used to demonstrate that many of the artifacts found in other parts of Mesoamerica were produced in West Mexico (Hosler and Macfarlane, 1996). This isotopic study was stimulated by Cumming et al (1979), who found that there is a trend in West Mexican ores toward higher lead isotope ratios with increasing distance from the Middle American Trench, which they attributed to increasing concentrations of crustal lead.

Strong archeological evidence exists to support the theory that metal objects and metallurgical ideas were introduced into West Mexico from Peru and Ecuador by traders using watercraft capable of long distance voyages. The evidence includes pottery styles, an unusual type of tomb (called a shaft tomb) that dates to 200-400 AD, and the copper-based metallurgy. These traits do not appear in other parts of Mexico, or farther to the south in Central America (Hosler, 1988b). At least two coastal groups of indigenous people were noted for their expertise in navigation, one that lived along the Manabi coast of Ecuador and the other around the Bay of Sechura in northern Peru. Both had developed balsa log sailing rafts with a centreboard and large dugout canoes equipped with a sail (Murra, 1975; West, 1994).

Merrill (1906) and Jennison (1924) were among the first geologists or engineers writing in English who acknowledged the important Pre-Hispanic accomplishments in mining. Documents dating from the early years of the Conquest, in the 1520's, indicate that the Spanish conquerors and early settlers, who were mostly soldiers and adventurers, were abysmally ignorant of mining and ore reduction (West, 1997).

Fortunately, there are better records from the early years of the conquest in Mexico than there are from South America. The following evidence of Pre-Hispanic mines has been derived from West (1997), Hosler (1994), Prieto (1973), Merrill (1906), Kemp (1972), and the monograph on Jalisco State by the Consejo de Recursos Minerales (1992). Sites mined by the Spanish prior to about 1540 were probably known to the indigenous people whereas sites that were not mined until later are probably Spanish discoveries. Copper-silver mining districts that are definitely Pre-Hispanic are Zumpango del Rio and Tasco in Guerrero State; Temascaltepec, Sultepec, Zacualtipán and Amatapec in Mexico State; and Tamazula, Talpa de Allende, Espíritu Santo, Ayutla, Zapotlan and Purificación in Jalisco State. Tamazula may be the Morcillo Mine acquired by Hernán Cortés. Of special interest, according to West (1994), are mercury mines in the Sierra Gorda of Querétaro State, which date from the time of Christ, and turquoise mines at Chalchihuites in Zacatecas state, which have been dated from 200 to 900 AD. Archaeological evidence has also been reported for Pre-Hispanic mercury mining in the Guadalcazar area of San Luis Potosi State. According to Merrill (1906), mercury was mined by indigenous people at Chilapan and tin was recovered at Tasco and Izmiquilpan.

THE SPANISH CONQUEST

As every student knows, Christopher Columbus "*discovered*" America in 1492. Discovery, in this case, means the bringing of newly found lands within the habitual knowledge of the society from which the discoverer came. By this definition, the Europeans discovered the rest of the world between about 1430 and 1600 (Palmer and Colton, 1995).

During the fifteenth century, trade expanded steadily and merchants and traders began to rely more on ships rather than caravans to transport their goods. At the same time, gold currency was becoming increasingly important to settle accounts. Columbus, who was born in Genoa, received much of his training and was first exposed to the gold trade while working for the merchants of Portugal, which was home to the finest mariners and navigators of the day. Gold had been transported by caravan across the Sahara from West Africa to the Mediterranean coast since the 10th Century (Boyle, 1979) and up to 1350, at least two thirds of the European supply had come from West Africa (Barraclough, 1978). About 1430, Portuguese mariners began to extend their trade for slaves and gold farther south along the coast of West Africa. In 1471, they established a medieval stone castle called São Jorge da Mina (St. George of the Mine) at Elmina on the Gold Coast of Ghana. Columbus made at least one trip there in a Portuguese ship about 1483. In contrast to the later conquest of Latin America, the European gold trade with Africa was accomplished without occupying the continent (Wilks, 1997).

By this time, most educated men knew that the world is a sphere (Morison, 1974). Inspired by Marco Polo's grand and romantic tales of the exotic mineral- and spice-opulent Indies, Christopher Columbus longed for a seagoing mission west to Asia. Between 1483 and 1492, he sought financial backing from various royal patrons but his plan was rejected as too costly and impractical. Spain was the logical supporter because it was restricted from eastward exploration around Africa toward Asia by a papal decree that had awarded that part of the world to Portugal. However, Spain was preoccupied until 1492 with a war against the Moors.

It was the practice of the day for explorers to negotiate concessions for their discoveries: rights, property, titles and so forth. In spite of poverty and discouragement, Columbus had continued to demand extensive privileges and when royal backing was finally obtained, he negotiated a lavish concession that included a tax-free income of ten percent of all revenues - gold, silver, gems, and spices – obtained in the new lands. He was also granted the right to invest in one-eighth of any subsequent voyage and the hereditary titles of Admiral of the Ocean Sea and Viceroy or Governor of any lands that he might discover (Morison, 1974; Rachlin, 1996). In modern mining terms, Columbus had negotiated an incredibly rich "*finders fee*".

Throughout the years, Columbus collected more rights and privileges and these were recorded in documents signed by King Ferdinand, Queen Isabella and royal officials. Columbus had several copies of the documents, called the Books of Privileges, prepared for safekeeping in various locations. Four sets have been preserved, none of which is complete. They are located at Genoa, Paris, Seville, and the Library of Congress in Washington (Rachlin, 1996).

The timing of this first voyage across the Atlantic was closely linked to other momentous events that were occurring in Europe at the time. The Middle Ages were giving way to the Renaissance and Columbus was lucky to be seeking financial support at a time when new ideas in fine arts, literature, science, philosophy, politics and religion were being accepted. This was the age of Leonardo da Vinci, Erasmus, Gutenburg, Machiavelli, Copernicus, Martin Luther, Raphael, Paracelsus, Rabelais, Titian, Galileo and Michelangelo.

Christopher Columbus was a devout man, whose journals indicate that his main motivations were adventure, glory and the desire to enlarge the Kingdom of the Cross rather than the lust for gold. However, he and his crew became understandably excited when the first people they encountered in America, on the Bahamian island of San Salvador, were found to wear small gold pendants suspended from the nose. Columbus noted in his diary how peaceful they appeared and how easily they could be converted to Christianity and enslaved. The expedition then sailed south to Cuba, where more evidence of gold was found, and finally to Haiti, where gold jewelry was more abundant and nuggets were panned from the Rio Yaque del Norte on the north coast. He returned to Spain with glowing accounts of gold, naked natives and the potential to convert them. Pope Alexander VI responded by awarding the lands west of Longitude 45°30'W to Spain in 1494 (Morison, 1974). That meridian was later found to cross South America between Rio de Janeiro and Sao Paulo, which explains why Portugal was able to lay claim to Brazil.

For the second voyage, which involved twelve hundred men and seventeen ships compared with the original three, Columbus warned that there should be strict controls on gold trading to prevent the colonists and priests from neglecting their other duties. By the time of his third voyage in 1498, royal consent was required for prospecting and mining (Jones, 1974). During this voyage, Columbus became aware that the indigenous people living on the Paria Peninsula of Venezuela, opposite Trinidad, possessed ornaments made of an alloy of copper and gold (later named tumbaga), which they valued more highly than local gold because it had to be imported from Central America (Morison, 1974).

By the time of his fourth and final voyage, Spain had introduced a system of mining claims and taxes (royalties) (Jones, 1974). In October 1502, Columbus encountered indigenous people on the coast of Costa Rica wearing disks of gold and later traded for gold on the north coast of Panama. When he died in Spain in May 1506, a disappointed man, Columbus did not realize the he had set in motion the Spanish Conquest and the Spanish Colonial Period in the New World. The few royalty payments he had received had been reduced to one tenth of the Royal Fifth (2 per cent) and everything else that he had been promised except the titles was ignored. No court officials or bishops attended his modest funeral (Morison, 1974).

The voyages of Columbus created fantastic new trade and revenue opportunities for Spain and many converts for the Catholic Church. However, it was gold rather than land or a desire to convert the indigenous people that attracted a new breed of settler. These were mercenaries and footloose gentry of warlike habits called "*conquistadores*", who had been left idle after the Moors were finally driven out of Spain in 1492. The Moorish Wars had taught them that no atrocity was too horrible to commit against the infidels they found at the end of their heroic quest (Palmer and Colton, 1995). The conquistadores created the world's first gold rush but they also established a pattern of mindless, ruthless greed that would be linked with the search for gold to the present day.

The Spanish Empire was a remarkable creation. Whereas the Roman and British Empires took centuries to build, Spain was in possession of a major portion of the Western Hemisphere within a few years after Columbus's voyages. With Spain, the colonial idea took explicit form. Land, mines and inhabitants were to be worked exclusively to enrich their Spanish masters although rescuing souls was a strongly avowed purpose. A clever reconciliation was found between these two conflicting objectives. In the words of Prescott (1886), "*the Indians would not labor without compulsion, and unless they labored they could not be brought into communication with the whites nor be converted to Christianity*". By this means, Christianity became the sanction for slavery (Galbraith, 1977). In his classic contemporary history of the conquest of Mexico, Bernal Díaz del Castillo recalled "*we came here to serve God, and also to get rich*" (quoted in Morison, 1974).

The voyages of Columbus were soon followed by the conquest of the Aztecs and Mayas in Mexico in 1519 and of the Incas, centred in Peru, a little over a decade later. By the middle of the 16th century, the major gold-producing regions were in Spanish hands and huge quantities of Indian artifacts had been melted down into bullion for shipment to Europe (Bray, 1985). In an unsuccessful attempt to save his life, the Inca ruler at Cajamarca agreed in November 1532 to pay a ransom of gold objects that filled a room about 6.7 m long and 4.9 m wide to a depth of about 2.3 m, plus twice as much silver (Jones, 1974). This was melted down to produce 6.1 tonnes of 22-carat gold and 11.8 tonnes of silver, enough to give each infrantryman a booty of 20.5 kg of gold and 41 kg of silver. The plunder from Cusco was even greater (Burkholder and Johnson, 1994). Shimada and Merkel (1991) estimated the total as 10 tonnes of 22 carat gold and 70 tonnes of fine silver.

Having stripped the living Indians of their wealth, the conquistadores next turned their attention to the tombs and monuments of the dead. Before the end of the 16th century, "*mining companies*" were carrying out this work on a large scale. Sacred gravesites were ransacked for gold, initiating a sad tale of destruction that has continued until the present. For example, the great Pyramid of the Sun at Chan Chan in northern Peru was divided into 23 parts and sold to treasure hunters in the late 1500's. Each part came with a grant of Indian laborers to do the heavy work. In 1602, another consortium of looters diverted the Moche River against the pyramid to destroy nearly two-thirds of it and recover 2.79 tonnes of gold (Bray, 1985).

At the ancient mining and metallurgical centre of Batán Grande in the Leche River valley, northern Peru, Shimada and Griffin (1994) counted over 100,000 looter's holes and hundreds of long bulldozer trenches on air photos in 1978. The magnitude of the treasure looted from individual tombs became clear when a ruling-class gravesite that had been overlooked by the looters was professionally excavated there by archaeologists in 1991-1992. It yielded 1.1 tonnes of jewelry and grave goods, of which 75 per cent consisted of metal objects and scrap, mostly 14 to 18 carat gold, as well as 3 kg of cinnabar.

Other examples of looting have also been documented. In Panama, a single cemetery at Bugaba yielded over 300 kg of gold between 1858 and 1860 (Bray, 1992). In Colombia, 300 kg of fine gold and 100 kg of base gold were recovered from the Sinú region, the main centre for early grave robbing, between 1533 and 1537. A single tomb produced 85 kg of gold. Grave robbing became a specialized field in Colombia with its own language and skills that were handed down from one generation to the next (Bray, 1974a).

The destruction of the Indian treasures by the Spanish not only deprived the world of some of the most exquisite metallic objects ever produced, it destroyed most of the evidence of the Pre-Colombian mining and metallurgical skills that had been used to produce the objects. Most of the gold that was looted had been painstakingly collected by indigenous placer miners over three millennia.

There were two reasons why the conquistadores were in such a hurry to melt these objects into bullion. First, the objects were considered to be heathen idols that offended the Christian sensitivity and did not appeal to European tastes (Bray, 1985; Muller, 1985). Second, financing the rapid expansion of the Spanish Empire required all the gold and silver that looting and mining could supply. This enormous treasure established the realm of the Hapsburg monarch Charles V, King of Spain, Catholic ruler of the Holy Roman Empire and Emperor of the Indies. Part of it was used to create the largest fleet in the world and to influence the European power structure for centuries (Jones, 1974).

Notwithstanding the brutality that the conquistadores and settlers inflicted on the indigenous people, an even worse cruelty was the European and, later, African diseases that decimated the population. On the island of Hispaniola (Dominican Republic and Haiti), for example, it has been estimated that forced labor and disease exterminated almost the entire population, from 250,000 in 1492 to 500 in 1538 (Morison, 1974). In New Spain (Latin America north of the Isthmus of Panama), there was a catastrophic decline in the Indian population between 1520 and 1620, from an estimated twenty-two million to one million (Gerhard, 1993; Burkholder and Johnson, 1994).

SPANISH COLONIAL MINING

After the initial flurry of activity in which Spanish explorers and investors acquired and evaluated the Pre-Hispanic mines, Spain embarked on the most aggressive and successful program of mining exploration and development that the world had ever seen. The leading mining region in Europe at the time was centred in Saxony and the Spanish quickly took advantage of the expertise that was available there. By a fortunate accident of timing, Georgius Agricola (whose real name was Georg Bauer) published a definitive study of geology and mining practice in Latin in 1556 (Hoover and Hoover, 1950). This textbook was not superceded for 180 years. The recently invented printing press enabled Agricola's ideas to be rapidly disseminated throughout the world. Within a year, King Philip II had obtained a copy, as well as a set of German mining ordinances, to aid Spanish miners. Within ten years, a Spanish edition that also incorporated information from a 1540 mining text by an Italian author, Vannoccio Biringuccio, had been published by Bernado Pérez de Vargas (Kemp, 1972).

Agricola had received a classical education before becoming town physician in the Erzgebirge district of Bohemia, then the most prolific mining region in Europe. His spare time was spent visiting mines and studying Greek and Latin literature, which contained much information about mining that had been forgotten during the Dark Ages. In 1533, he began to write his masterpiece, which gave the first explanation of the effects of erosion, described 20 new minerals in addition to the 60 previously known, and explained for the first time scores of methods and processes used in mining and metallurgy. According to Hoover and Hoover (1950), Agricola's main contributions were his ideas on the origin of mineral deposits, the circulation of groundwater and the filling of veins by circulating solutions. "*He was the first to found any of the natural sciences upon research and observation as opposed to previous fruitless speculation*".

Within a few short years, Spanish miners, aided by German experts, had discovered almost all of the great Mexican silver districts, such as Zacatecas in 1546, Guanajuato and Santa Bárbara in 1548, Velardena about 1550, Pachuca in 1552, Fresnillo in 1554, San Martin, Sombrerete and Chalchihuites in

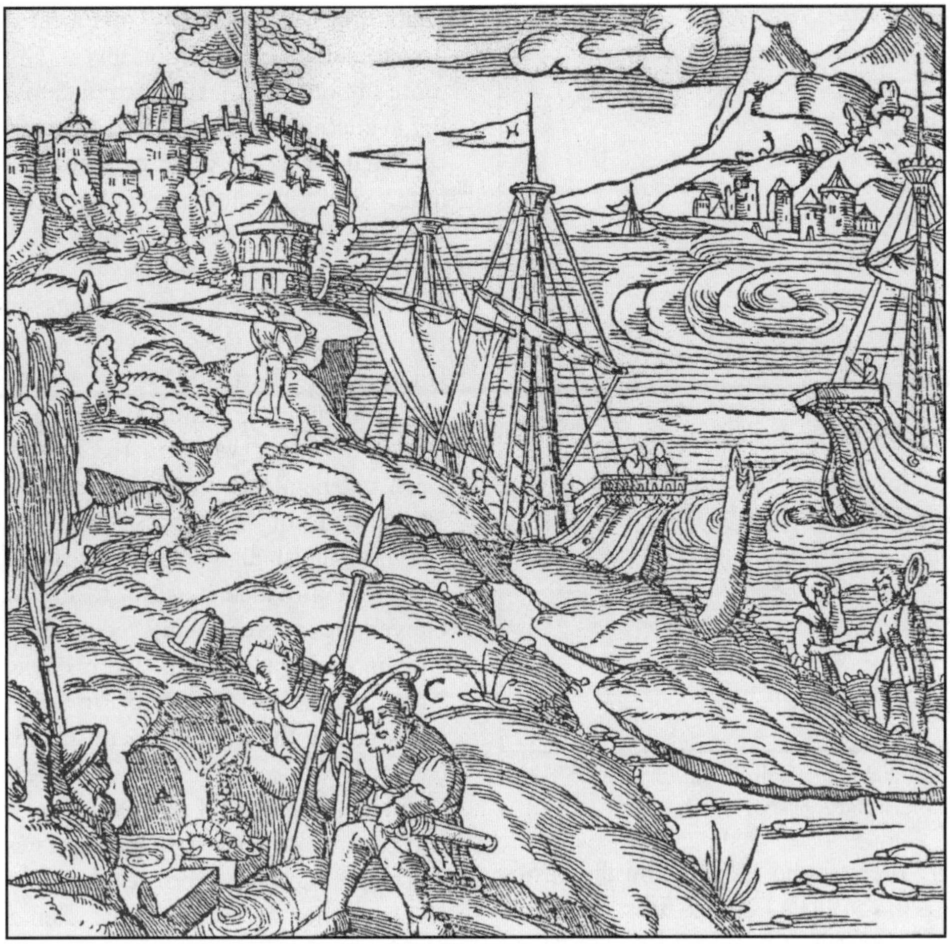

A-SPRING. B-SKIN. C-ARGONAUTS

Figure 2. A well equipped prospecting expedition in the 16th Century (from Agricola's De Re Metallica, 1556

1555, San Francisco del Oro in 1567, Charcas in 1570, and Santa Eulalia and Real de Angeles in 1591. Meanwhile, the great silver lode at Potosí, Bolivia was discovered in 1545. The geographical boundaries of Spanish colonial mining were thus identified between the mid-1540's and 1600 (Bakewell,1997).

Most of these new discoveries consisted of oxidized silver minerals, which were highly weathered and friable, making them easy to mine. Although these new silver discoveries were huge, many of them had relatively low silver contents and contained too little lead to be profitably exploited with the available smelting techniques. Silver grades of less than about 6000 grams/tonne (200 ozs/ton) could not be profitably treated at the time. The answer to this problem, called the patio process, was introduced in 1554 by Bartolomé de Medina,. It was a simple system based on mercury amalgamation of silver ore in place of the former method of smelting it with a lead oxide flux and charcoal. Mexico became the greatest silver-producing nation in the world and the patio process was used with little change for 350 years (Probert, 1997). From the middle of the 16th century until the end of the colonial era, about 1810, Spanish America produced between 3 and 3.5 billion ounces, or about one hundred thousand tonnes of silver (Garner, 1997).

Medina was an unlikely person to make such an important discovery. He was a prosperous textile trader in Seville when he developed an interest in silver smelting at the age of 50. Medina apparently met a

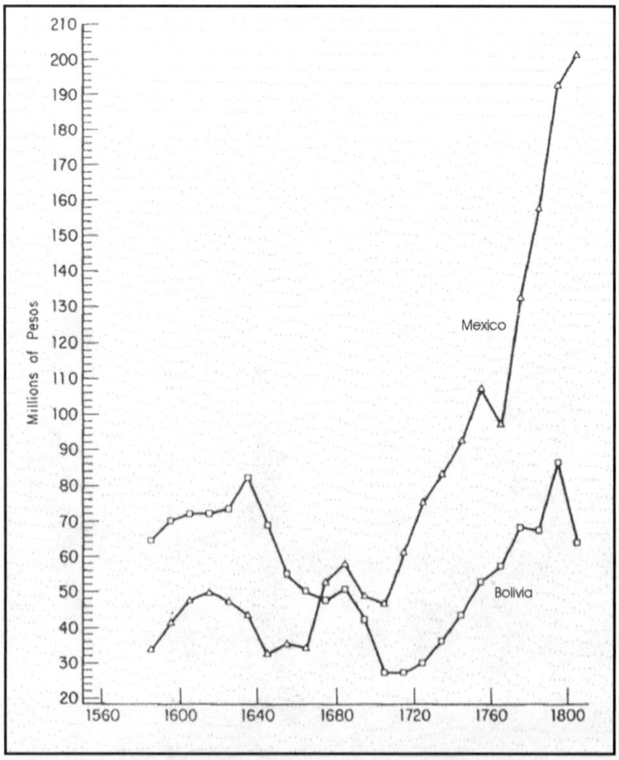

Figure 3. Silver production in Bolivia and Mexico, 1581 to 1810 (after Burkholder and Johnson, 1994)

German named Lorenzo who showed him the basics of the patio process. When Lorenzo was unable to obtain a Spanish visa, Medina went to Mexico alone in 1553 and settled in Pachuca, where he demonstrated the process and was awarded a royalty for its use.

Medina's process involved mixing finely crushed ores of silver oxide, chloride and sulphide with mercury and the catalysts salt, lime and majistral (copper sulphate). Workers spread the resulting paste on the stone floor of a large patio, where it was mixed by animals or bare-legged laborers. After the mixture had 'cooked' for six to eight weeks, the workers washed it, removed the silver amalgam and heated it over a fire to remove the mercury, which was saved for the next batch. The effect on the workers was to substitute the hazard of mercury vapor for the toxic fumes produced by silver-lead smelting. The patio process was also introduced in 1571 at Potosí, where the mixture was cooked in large stone tanks rather than on a patio because of colder temperatures at high altitude (Burkholder and Johnson, 1994).

Because mercury (quicksilver) was essential in the patio process, its supply and cost became crucial determinants of production levels. Crown policy was more important than supply and demand in determining availability and price. The Crown eventually realized that when the price of mercury was raised too high, silver production declined (Burkholder and johnson, 1994). The royal mine at Almadén, Spain (which is still an important world source), supplied all the Latin America requirements until the Santa Barbara mine was opened by the Crown at Huancavelica, Peru, in 1571. The discovery was made by indigenous people, who either showed the Spaniards 'silver water' in 1532 or cinnabar in 1564. Unitl Independence in 1821, the mine produced over 50,000 tones of mercury (Strauss, 1909).

The Spanish also made other substantial contributions that provided benefits to the mining industry. Universities were established at Lima and Mexico City in 1551 and others were opened at Cordoba, Argentina in 1614 and Potosí in 1624, which was 12 years before the establishment of the first college at Harvard, Massachusetts. One of the most important Spanish legacies in Latin America was the mining code, which was based on mining laws used in Spain, that were derived from German practice (Prieto, 1973). Many of the principal elements of modern international mining law can be traced to the act that was proclaimed in Mexico in 1584. For instance, deposits of gold and silver, whether situated on public or private land, were the property of the Crown and open for staking. Both the Crown and local governments imposed numerous taxes, including a royal monopoly levy on mercury (and later on gunpowder), and a royal tax (royalty) against the gross output of metals. Mining rights were acquired as rectangular concessions (claims), regulations were written to prevent careless working of mines, and concessions reverted to the Crown if they were not worked (Jenison, 1923).

One unfortunate legacy of the Spanish Empire was bureaucracy. The files of the colonial department, which have been preserved in Seville, reveal that some 400,000 regulations had been issued by 1700. An effort to consolidate and codify these in 1681 produced 11,000 laws. The Spanish Empire may have worked only because its regulations were so numerous that no one imagined that they would be enforced (Galbraith, 1977).

Much has been written about the cruel working conditions in the Spanish Colonial mines and patios. Although slavery was widely practiced at first, it is important to remember that slavery and forced labor were widely practiced at that time in much of the world. Each of the prominent miners in Tasco and Sultepec owned between 100 and 150 slaves. A new law issued in 1542 formally abolished indigenous slavery but the regulations could not be enforced (West, 1997). By 1600, 60 to 70 per cent of the indigenous workers were wage laborers, partly because epidemics had created a labor shortage (Bakewell, 1997). Conditions had been even harsher in the early years after the Conquest but that, too, has to be viewed in context. Indigenous people at the bottom of the social structure had not enjoyed any freedom under their tribal chiefs before the Spanish arrived and faced the risk of being killed in daily ritual sacrifices to ensure that the sun rose each day. In the words of Burkholder and Johnson (1994) "*war captives, criminals, slaves and persons supplied by subject peoples as tribute fell victim to the obsidian sacrificial blade atop the great pyramids. After a victory ceremony, warriors often provided a feast for friends and relatives, in which the sacrificed captives' flesh was served in a stew . . . In 1487, the Mexicas dedicated the new temple of Huitzilopochtli in Tenochtitlán by sacrificing more (some sources say many more) than twenty thousand persons*"!

The attempts by the church to protect its indigenous converts, restrictions set by the crown on their exploitation, and epidemics led almost immediately to the importation of African slaves. It has been estimated that 100,000 had been brought to America by 1560. However, African slavery was never as important in most of Spanish America as it later became in some of the Dutch, French and English colonies or in Portuguese Brazil (Palmer and Colton, 1995).

EPILOGUE

Mining and metallurgy in the western hemisphere, which was mainly directed and financed from the United States and Canada during the twentieth century, started in the Peruvian Andes about 1500 BC. Our current knowledge of the technical evolution and its spread throughout the Andes and into Central America and western Mexico by 650 AD has resulted from an intensive investigation by archaeologists during the past 40 to 50 years. These studies have shown that Latin America had reached a sophisticated stage in metal production at a time when no mining activity whatsoever was taking place north of Mexico. Because the knowledge required for a culture to advance from the Stone Age to the Bronze Age is so profound, some people have suggested that the Andean metallurgical centre might have developed from information transmitted via trans-Pacific contact from Asia. However, the long interval between parallel metallurgical discoveries in Europe/Asia and South America is considered strong evidence against that theory.

By coincidence, there is an interesting symmetry between the Latin American archaeological research and the advances made by geologists in the study of volcanogenic massive sulphide (VMS) deposits, the subject of this volume, during the same 40 to 50 year time frame. These polymetallic deposits of copper, zinc, lead, silver and gold were previously thought to have formed by injection from great depths along structural pathways. Metals were believed to have differentiated during magmatic recrystallization from the nearest granitic intrusion. Despite the inadequate understanding of the genesis of these deposits, many were discovered by prospecting, geophysics and geochemistry. Canada is richly endowed with VMS deposits and it is natural that Canadian geologists have taken a prominent role in studying and searching for them.

Our understanding of ancient, land-based VMS deposits has benefited from the recent discovery and study of active, sulphide-producing hydrothermal vents on modern seafloor spreading ridges. VMS deposits are now known to be predominantly stratiform accumulations of sulphide minerals that have precipitated from hydrothermal fluids at or just below the seafloor, and are associated with volcanic rocks in a wide range of ancient and modern geological settings (Barrie and Hannington, 1997).

Latin America is currently undergoing vigorous exploration for VMS and other types of mineral deposits. This is providing new opportunities for geologists to contribute to the archeological research by identifying ancient mine workings and metallurgical sites that contain slag and other artifacts. By ensuring that these sites are protected for professional study by archeologists and contributing lead isotope and other data, geologists and miners can provide invaluable assistance to this incredible study.

ACKNOWLEDGEMENTS

This paper has benefited from suggestions provided by many colleagues and family members. Special thanks are due to Profesor Dorothy Hosler of MIT, who kindly reviewed an earlier draft.

REFERENCES

Barraclough, G., Editor. 1978. The Times Atlas of World History. Times Books Limited, London.

Bakewell, P., 1997. Introduction. in Mines of Silver and Gold in the Americas. Edited by Peter Bakewell. Variorum-Ashgate Publishing Ltd., Aldershot, UK.

Barrie, C.T., and Hannington, M.D., 1997. Introduction: Classification of VMS Deposits Based on Host Rock Composition. in Volcanic-Associated Massive Sulfide Deposits: Processes and Examples in Modern and Ancient Settings. Notes from a Short Course Sponsored by the Geological Association of Canada, Mineral Deposits Division and the Society of Economic Geologists, Ottawa. Edited by C.T. Barrie and M.D. Harrington.

Bird, J. B., 1979. The "*Copper Man*": A Prehistoric Miner and his Tools from Northern Chile. in Pre-Columbian Metallurgy of South America. Edited by E. P. Benson. Dumbarton Oaks, Washington.

Boyle, R.W., 1979. The Geochemistry of Gold and its Deposits. Geological Survey of Canada, Bulletin 280, Ottawa.

Bray, W., 1974. a) The Organization of the Metal Trade; and b) Gold Working in Ancient America. in El Dorado, the Gold of Ancient Colombia (exhibition catalogue). Edited by Julie Jones. Center for Inter-American Relations and the American Federation of Arts, New York.

Bray, W., 1985. Ancient American Metallurgy: Five Hundred Years of Study. in The Art of Precolumbian Gold: The Jan Mitchell Collection. Edited by Julie Jones. Little, Brown and Company, Boston.

Bray, W., 1992. Sitio Conte Metalwork in Its Pan-American Context. in River of Gold: Precolumbian Treasurers from Sitio Conte. Edited by Pamela Hearne and Robert J. Sharer. University of Pennsylvania, Philadelphia.

Burkholder, M. A. and Johnson, L. L., 1994. Colonial Latin America. Second Edition. Oxford University Press, New York.

Charles, J. A., 1980. The Coming of Copper and Copper-Base Alloys and Iron, in The Coming of the Age of Iron. Edited by Theodore A. Wertime and James D. Muhly. Yale University Press, New Haven.

Consejo de Recursos Minerales. 1992. Geological-Mining Monograph of the State of Jalisco. Edited by José Cárdenas Vargas. Mexico City.

Cooke, R. G. and Bray, W. The Goldwork of Panama: An Iconographic and Chronological Perspective. in The Art of Precolumbian Gold: The Jan Mitchell Collection. Edited by Julie Jones. Little, Brown and Company, Boston.

Cumming, G.L., Kesler, S.E. and Kristic, D., 1979. Isotopic Composition of Lead in Mexican Mineral Deposits. Economic Geology, 74: 1395-1407.

De Lucio, F., 1997. A History of Mining Technology in Peru. in The Silver and Silversmiths of Peru. Edited by Jose Torres Della Pina and Victoria Mujica. Patronata Plata del Peru, Lima.

Easby, D. T. Jr., 1966. Early Metallurgy in the New World. Scientific American, 214(4): 73-81.

Galbraith, J. K., 1977. The Age of Uncertainty. Houghton Mifflin Company, Boston.

Garner, R. L., 1997. Long-Term Silver Mining trends in Spanish America: A Comparative Analysis of Peru and Mexico. in Mines of Silver and Gold in the Americas. Edited by Peter Bakewell. Variorum-Ashgate Publishing Ltd., Aldershot, UK.

Geological Society of America. 1991. The Geology of North America, Volume P-3, Economic Geology, Mexico. Edited by Guillermo P. Salas.

Gerhard, P., 1993. A Guide to the Historical Geography of New Spain. University of Oklahoma Press, Norman.

Grossman, Joel W. 1972. An Ancient Gold Worker's Tool Kit: The Earliest Metal Technology in Peru. Archaeology, 25: 270-275.

Hearne, P., 1992. The Story of the River of Gold. in River of Gold: Precolumbian Treasures from Sitio Conte. Edited by Pamela Hearne and Robert J. Sharer. University of Pennsylvania, Philadelphia.

Herail, G., 1991. The Glacial Gold Placer of Suches Antaquilla and its Exploration. Field Guidebook, International Symposium on Alluvial Gold Placers, La Paz.

Herail, G., and Viscarra, G., 1991. The Gold Placer of Tipuani. Field Guidebook, International Symposium on Alluvial Gold Placers, La Paz.

Hoover, H. C. and Hoover, L. H., 1950. De Re Metallica by Georgius Agricola. Translated from the First Latin Edition of 1556. Dover Publications, Inc., New York.

Hosler, D., 1988a. Ancient West Mexican Metallurgy: A Technological Chronology. Journal of Field Archaeology, 15: 191-217.

Hosler, D., 1988b. Ancient West Mexican Metallurgy: South American Origins and West Mexican Transformations. American Anthropologist. 90: 832-855.

Hosler, D., 1988c. The Metallurgy of Ancient West Mexico. in The Beginning of the Use of Metals and Alloys. Edited by Robert Maddin. MIT Press, Cambridge, Massachusetts.

Hosler, D., 1994. The Sounds and Colors of Power. MIT Press, Cambridge, Massachusetts.

Hosler, D. and Macfarlane, A., 1996. Copper Sources, Metal

Production, and Metals Trade in Late Postclassic Mesoamerica. Science, 273: 1819-1824.

Howe, E. G. and Petersen, U., 1994. Silver and Lead in the Late Prehistory of the Mantaro Valley, Peru. in Archaeometry of Pre-Columbian Sites and Artifacts. Edited by David A. Scott and Pieter Meyers. The Getty Conservation Institute, Marina del Rey, CA.

Jennison, H.A.C., 1923. Mining History of Mexico. Engineering and Mining Journal-Press, 115: 364-368; 401-403.

Jones, J., 1974. a) Gold and the New World; b) Precolumbian Gold. in El Dorado, The Gold of Ancient Colombia (exhibition catalogue). Edited by Julie Jones. Center for Inter-American Relations and the American Federation of Arts, New York.

Kemp, D. C., 1972. Quicksilver to Bar Silver: Tales of Mexico's Silver Bonanza. Socio-Technical Publications, Pasadena.

Lechtman, H., 1980. The Central Andes: Metallurgy Without Iron. in The Coming of the Age of Iron. Edited by Theodore A. Wertime and James D. Muhly. Yale University Press, New Haven.

Lechtman, H., 1984. Pre-Columbian Surface Metallurgy. Scientific American, 250(6): 56-63.

Lechtman, H., 1988. Traditions and Styles in Central Andean Metalworking. in The Beginning of the Use of Metals and Alloys. Edited by Robert Maddin. MIT Press, Cambridge, Massachusetts.

Lechtman, H., 1994. The Materials Science of Material Culture: Examples from the Andean Past. in Archaeometry of Pre-Columbian Sites and Artifacts. Edited by David A. Scott and Pieter Meyers. The Getty Conservation Institute, Marina del Rey, CA.

Merkel, J.F., Shimada I., Swann, C.P. and Doonan, R., 1994. Pre-Hispanic Copper Alloy Production at Batan Grande, Peru: Interpretation of the Analytical Data for Ore Samples. in Archaeometry of Pre-Columbian Sites and Artifacts. Edited by David A. Scott and Pieter Meyers. The Getty Conservation Institute, Marina del Rey, CA.

Merrill, F.J.H., 1906. Aboriginal Mining in Mexico. The Engineering and Mining Journal, 82: 822-823.

Morison, S. E., 1974. The European Discovery of America : The Southern Voyages, 1492-1616. Oxford University Press, New York.

Muhly, J. D., 1988. The Beginnings of Metallurgy in the Old World. in The Beginning of the Use of Metals and Alloys. Edited by Robert Maddin. MIT Press, Cambridge.

Muller, P. E., 1985. The Old World and Gold from the New. in The Art of Precolumbian Gold: The Jan Mitchell Collection. Edited by Julie Jones. Little, Brown and Company, Boston.

Murra, J., 1975. Formaciones Economicas y Politicas del Mundo Andino. Instituto de Estuddios Peruanos: 255-267.

Palmer, R.R. and Colton, J., 1995. A History of the Modern World to 1815. Eighth Edition. McGraw-Hill, Inc, New York.

Plazas, C. and Falchetti, A. Cultural Patterns in the Prehistoric Goldwork of Colombia. in The Art of Precolumbian Gold: The Jan Mitchell Collection. Edited by Julie Jones. Little, Brown and Company, Boston.

Prescott, W. H., 1886. History of the Conquest of Mexico, Volume 1. John B Alden, New York.

Prieto, C., 1973. Mining in the New World. The Spanish Institute, Inc. McGraw-Hill Book Company, New York.

Probert, A., 1997. Bartolomé de Medina: The Patio Process and the Sixteenth Century Silver Crisis. in Mines of Silver and Gold in the Americas. Edited by Peter Bakewell. Variorum-Ashgate Publishing Ltd., Aldershot, UK.

Rachlin, H., 1996. Columbus's Book of Privileges. in Lucy's Bones, Sacred Stones and Einstein's Brain. Henry Holt and Company, New York: 115-125.

Scott, D. A. and Bray, W., 1994. Pre-Hispanic Platinum Alloys and Their Composition and Use in Ecuador and Colombia. in Archaeometry of Pre-Columbian Sites and Artifacts. Edited by D.A. Scott and Pieter Meyers. The Getty Conservation Institute, Marina del Rey, CA.

Shimada, I., 1994. Pre-Hispanic Metallurgy and Mining in the Andes: Recent Advances and Future Tasks. in In Quest of Mineral Wealth: Aboriginal and Colonial Mining and Metallurgy in Spanish America. Edited by Alan K. Craig and Robert C. West. Louisiana State University, Baton Rouge.

Shimada, Izumi and Griffin, Jo Ann. 1994. Precious Metal Objects of the Middle Sican. Scientific American, 270(4): 82-89.

Shimada, I. and Merkel, J. F., 1991. Copper Alloy Metallurgy in Ancient Peru. Scientific American, 265(1): 80-86.

Stoll, W.C., 1961. Tertiary Channel Gold Deposits at Tipuani, Bolivia. Economic Geology, 56: 1258-1264.

Strauss, L. W., 1909. Quicksilver at Huancavelica, Peru. Mining and Scientific Press, 49: 561-566.

Wertime, T. A., 1964. Man's First Encounter with Metallurgy. Science, 146: 1257-1267.

Wertime, T. A., 1968, A Metallurgical Expedition through the Persian Desert. Science, 159: 927-935.

West, R. C., 1994. Aboriginal Metallurgy and Metalworking in Spanish America: A Brief Overview. in In Quest of Mineral Wealth: Aboriginal and Colonial Mining and Metallurgy in Spanish America. Edited by Alan K. Craig and Robert C. West. Louisiana State University, Baton Rouge.

West, R. C., 1997. Early Silver Mining in New Spain, 1531-1555. in Mines of Silver and Gold in the Americas. Edited by Peter Bakewell. Variorum-Ashgate Publishing Ltd, Aldershot, UK.

Wilks, I., 1997. Wangara, Akan and Portuguese in the Fifteenth and Sixteenth Centuries. in Mines of Silver and Gold in the Americas. Edited by Peter Bakewell. Variorum–Ashgate Publishing Ltd, Aldershot, UK.

Woodbridge, D. E., 1927. Rejuvenating a Bolivian Placer: Rio Tipuani Region Once Source of Inca Wealth. Engineering and Mining Journal, 124: 87-90.

VOLCANOGENIC MASSIVE SULPHIDE DEPOSITS OF LATIN AMERICA; AN OVERVIEW

ROSS SHERLOCK † AND MICHAEL MICHAUD
SRK Consulting, 800-580 Hornby Street, Vancouver, B.C. V6C 3B6

† Current address
Canada-Nunavut Geoscience Office, P.O. Box 2319, Iqaluit, Nunavut X0A 0H0
sherlock@nrcan.gc.ca

ABSTRACT

Volcanogenic massive sulphides are found in a wide variety of geologic environments spanning geologic time. By far the largest number of deposits are found in the Jurassic and Lower Cretaceous volcanic arcs throughout Latin America, both in terms of average size and contained metals. The disparity in terms of numbers of deposits seen in Mesozoic versus Precambrian rocks as well as the apparent metal content and size is likely a reflection of the high prospectivity of the younger arc rocks as well as a general lack of exploration in the Precambrian terranes for base metal deposits. The Jurassic and Lower Cretaceous volcanic arcs are very prospective for VMS deposits, they tend to consist of local accumulations of felsic volcanic rocks in submarine environments which are favourable localities to form polymetallic deposits. These deposits represent obvious exploration targets and have a relatively long history of exploration and development particularly in the Caribbean and Mexico. As a result there are many VMS occurrences in these young rocks and the average size tends to be rather small despite the inclusion of some very large deposits such as Tambo Grande and San Nicolás.

The Precambrian Terranes of South America do not have a long history of base metal exploration due to the relatively remote locations and poor infrastructure. These areas have generally been the focus of gold exploration. As a result few VMS deposits are known from these areas and the ones that are known tend to be larger, as needed to justify development. It is likely with continued exploration and improved infrastructure that there will continue to be new discoveries of VMS deposits in the Precambrian terranes of South America.

INTRODUCTION

Exploration for volcanogenic massive sulphide deposits over the 1990's has taken on an unprecedented international scope. Exploration and mining companies, mainly Canadian, have been exploring for, and developing VMS deposits in Latin America. In addition to the development of previously known districts, recent work has resulted in discoveries of areas that were not previously recognized as having significant VMS potential.

Deposits are known from rocks that range from Precambrian to Tertiary in age. Given the geologic and geographic variability in Latin America it is no surprise that deposits vary greatly in terms of their mineralogy and host lithologies. The bulk of the deposits however occur in Lower Cretaceous volcanic strata.

The scope of this volume is to provide a venue for recent developments in VMS geology of Latin America. The following sections describe the various formations that host volcanic associated base metal mineralization; organized according to age and country. Also described are individual deposits along with the local stratigraphy and geochemical affinities.

ARCHEAN

Venezuela

The Archean supracrustal rocks of the Guayana Shield dominate the southern portion of Venezuela (Fig. 1; Table 1) and extend into Brazil, Guyana, Surinam and French Guyana (Gibbs and Barron,

1983; 1993; Sidder and Mendoza, 1995). These rocks represent a tholeiitic to calc-alkaline sequence, likely formed in an island arc to back arc setting. Although considered to be highly prospective, to date, no VMS deposits, or even showings, have been identified in Venezuela (Gibbs and Barron, 1993; Sidder et al., 1991; Sidder, 1995).

The Pastoria Province shows a general evolution from mafic to felsic volcanic rocks and sedimentary lithologies (Channer and Anderson, 2000). It has a long history of gold production from shear zone hosted-quartz vein deposits and has excellent potential for hosting a VMS deposit. Both tholeiitic and calc-alkaline differentiation trends have been found, representing the evolution from immature island arcs to back arcs and marginal basin settings.

A number of massive sulphide showings have been identified in Guyana, consisting of disseminated

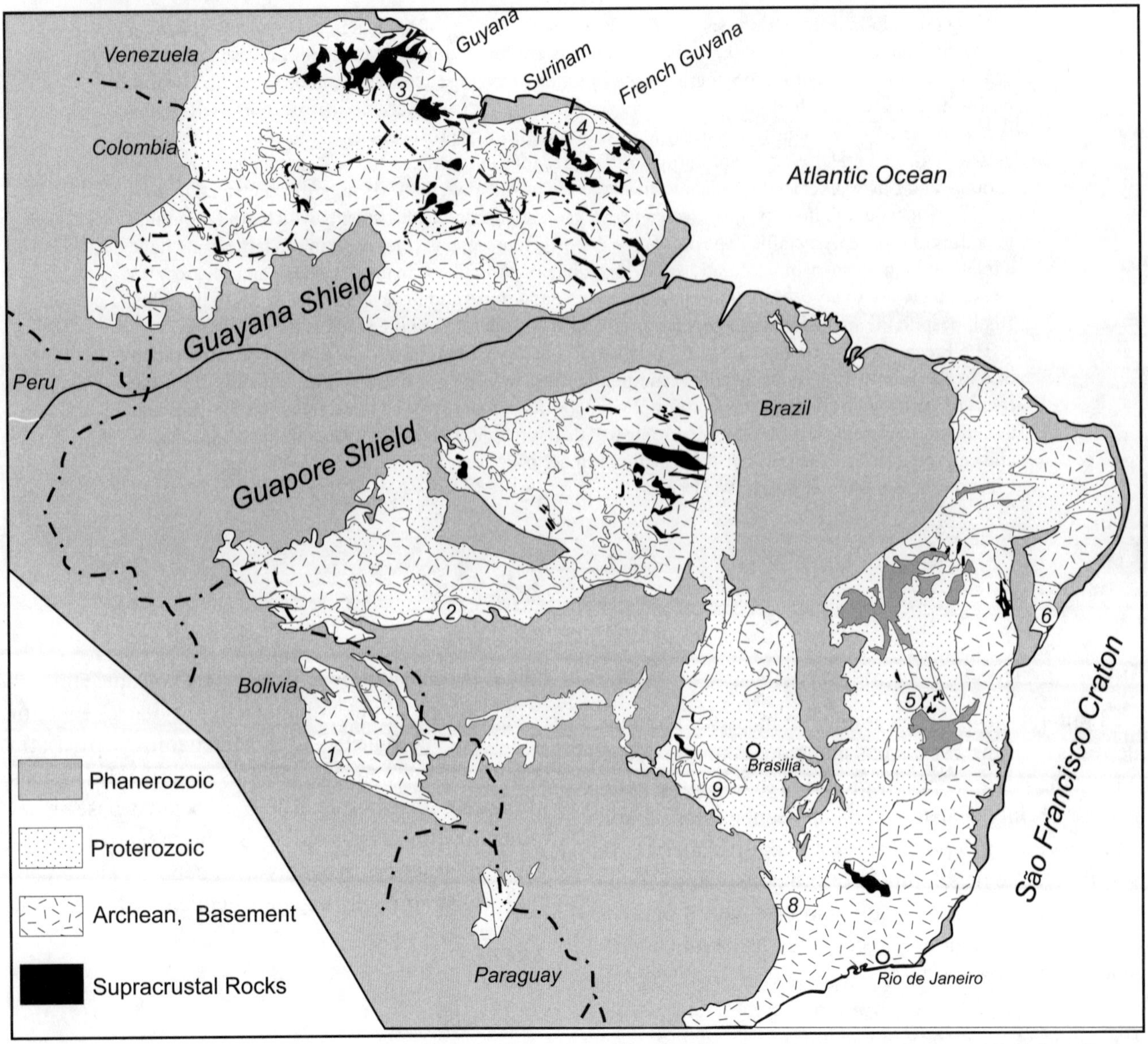

Figure 1. Geologic map of the Archean-Proterozoic rocks of South America showing the location of various VMS deposits. After Araújo (2000), Biste and Gourlay (2000), Channer and Anderson (2000), Franklin et al. (2000), Kerr et al. (2000), Lobato et al. (2000). 1. Miguela, 2. Aripuanã, 3. Groete Creek, 4. Paul Isnard, 5. Boquira Lead, 6. Salobro, 7. Bico de Padra, 8. Alpinópolis 9. Palmeirópolis.

pyrite and chalcopyrite associated with felsic and intermediate volcanic rocks (Ally, 1985). The Barama-Mazaruni greenstone belt in Guayana, which hosts VMS deposits, is directly correlated with the rocks of the Pastora supergroup, indicating this belts prospectivity for VMS mineralization (Channer and Anderson, 2000).

The Cuchivero Province consists of predominantly felsic intrusive and extrusive rocks. Within the Caicara formation, the rocks consist of primarily rhyolites, dacites and associated volcaniclastic rocks. The felsic rocks of the Cuchivero province are not considered to have a high potential for hosting massive sulphide mineralization since the majority of volcanism is subaerial (Channer and Anderson, 2000).

Guyana

Limited exploration has identified a number of massive sulphide showings within the Guayana Shield in Guyana, consisting of disseminated pyrite and chalcopyrite (Ally, 1985). Mineralization is generally spatially related to intermediate to felsic subaqueous volcanism associated with clastic rocks.

The most prominent massive sulphide occurrence in Guayana is within the Barama-Mazaruni greenstone belts and includes the Groete Creek (Fig. 1; Table 1) deposit. This occurrence extends 1,525 metres along strike, 410 m down dip, and has a width of 10 m at an average grade of 0.6 % copper (Channer and Anderson, 2000; Walrond, 1985). Sulphides are associated with a subvolcanic porphyry, coarse breccia and volcanic tuffs.

Brazil

Although few VMS deposits have been discovered in Brazil, there remains good potential for VMS deposits within greenstone belts and volcano-sedimentary sequences of the São Francisco Craton (Lobato et al., 2000; Figure 1; Table 1). Numerous workers have described the belts, including Almeida and Hasui (1984), Mascarenhas et al. (1984), Schrank and da Silva (1993), Pedrosa-Soares et al. (1992), and Baars (1997).

In the region around the town of Mundo Nova, sulphides have been identified in drill holes (Lobato et al., 2000). Drill intersections include zinc grades up to 15 % with low values of Cu, Pb, Ag and Au. The area is dominated by low-grade metamorphosed basalt lava flows and andesitic to dacitic pyroclastic rocks, associated with metagreywackes and chert (Mascarenhas and da Silva, 1994).

Within the Cuieté Velho metavolcano-sedimentary sequence, part of the Mantiqueira Province in Eastern Gerais, massive sulphide layers have been identified (Paes et al., 1998). The VMS occurrences are associated with biotite schists, amphibolite and talc schists, interpreted as metamorphosed tholeiitic volcanic rocks, thought to represent an Archean greenstone belt fragment (Lobato et al., 2000).

The gold-bearing massive sulphide Mina III deposit, located within the Crixás greenstone belt along the southern margin of the São Francisco Craton, may represent a distal, gold-dominated VMS deposit (Jost et al., 1996; Lobato et al., 2000). The deposit consists of an array of massive pyrite lenses up to 2.5 m thick. The country rocks, host to the massive sulphide deposits, consist of carbonaeous schists, oolitic, laminated and massive marble belonging to the Ribeirão das Antas formation and metabasalts of the Rio Vermelho formation. A back-arc environment is interpreted for the origin of these rocks (Jost et al., 1996; Resende, 1998; Resende et al., 1998).

The Quadrilátero Ferrífero (Rio das Velhas) greenstone belt is composed of ultramafic to mafic and intermediate metavolcanic rocks at the base overlain by iron formation, metagreywackes, metaturbidites and felsic to intermediate pyroclastic rocks (Lobato et al., 2000; Baltazar and Pedreira, 1998; Zucchetti et al., 1988). The Bico de Padre Deposit is located within sheared trondjemite and mafic rocks of the Nova Lima Group. Mineralization consists of pyrite, sphalerite, galena and chalcopyrite in centimetre to decimetre veins (Borba, 1998).

The Alpinópolis greenstone belt (Fig. 1; Table 1) hosts up to 16 sub-economic sulphide deposits, containing up to 0.4 % Zn, 0.3 % Cu and 0.15 % Ni (Carvalho, 1990). VMS mineralization is associated with predominantly tholeiitic to calc-alkaline metavolcanic and metasedimentary rocks, consisting of garnet-chlorite and sillimanite-biotite schists (Carvalho, 1990; Carvalho et al., 1992).

The Gavião block contains some of the oldest

Table 1. Summary of Latin American VMS Deposits.

Country	Deposit	Formation	Age	Host Rocks	Size	Grade	References
Archean-Proterozoic							
Guayana	Groete Creek	Barama-Mazaruni	Archean	felsic/intermediate volc .		1,525m (strike) x 410m (dip) x 10m wide @ 0.6% Cu	39
Brazil	Valley Deposit	Guapore Craton	Archean	felsic lavas, pyroclastics	12Mt	6.3 % Zn, 2.2% Pb	37
	Arex Deposit	Guapore Craton	Archean	felsic lavas, pyroclastics	12Mt	6.3 % Zn, 2.2% Pb	37
	Bico de Pedra	Quadrilatero Ferrifero GB	Archean	mafic to int volcanics flows and pyroclastics	0.03Mt	0.36% Cu, 1.53% Zn, 0.52% Pb, 44g/t Ag, 1.45g/t Au	38
	Boquira Lead mine	Boquira formation	Archean	amphibolitic , siliceous magnetite	5.6 Mt	8.9% Pb, 1.4% Zn	42, 43, 44
	Alpinopolis greenstone	Alpinopolis greenstone belt	Archean	metasedimentary		0.4% Zn, 0.3% Cu, 0.15% Ni	45
	Salobro	Riacho dos Machados	unknown	metavolcano-sedimentary N/A		3.9% Zn, 1.1% Pb	46
	Palmeiropolis	Palmeiropolis Sequence	Proterozoic	felsic volcanics, amphibolite	7Mt	3.5% Zn, 0.9% Pb, 1.2% Cu	40, 41
French Guyana	Paul Isnard		Proterozoic	Felsic volcanics	34.7Mt	1.4 g/t Au	48,49
Bolivia	Miguela A-Zone	La Pastora	Proterozoic	intermediate to rhyolite	1.62Mt	3.76%Cu, 1.26g/t Au, 11.3g/t Ag, 0.33% Zn	36
Arizona	Jerome District	Yavapai Series	Proterozoic	Felsic volcanics	42.3Mt	4.16% Cu, 0.31% Pb, 1.46% Zn, 1.73g/t Au, 59.3 g/t Ag	50
	United Verde	Cleopatra Formation	Proterozoic	Felsic volcanics	33.7Mt	4.89% Cu, 0.13% Zn, 1.46g/t Au, 53.0g/t Ag	50
Paleozoic							
Argentina	Santa Elena	Alcaparrosa Fm.	Lr.Paleozoic, Ordovician ?	mafic volcanics-sediments		0.08% Cu, 1.84% Pb, 2.51% Zn, 83g/t Ag 4.52g/t Au	35
	Aguilar	Padrioc Fm.	Lr.Paleozoic	shales	25 Mt	15-18 % Zn, 5-15 % Pb and 134-370 g/t Ag.	58
Venezuela	Bailadores	Mucuchachí	Devonian-Pennsylvanian	felsic tuffs-sediments	1.45Mt	26% Zn, 7% Pb, 1.5% Cu	27
	Aroa District		Paleozoic		1.5Mt	8% Cu	47
	Santa Isabel		Paleozoic	mafic-felsic volcanics			47
Chile	Tirúa		Paleozoic ?	sediments-mafic volcanics	small		53,54
	Pirén		Paleozoic ?	sediments-mafic volcanics	small		55,53
	La Serena		Paleozoic ?	basalts	small		56,53

[continued on following page]

Country	Deposit	Formation	Age	Host Rocks	Size	Grade	References
Mesozoic							
Mexico	Francisco I Madero	Zacatecas subterrane	Ur. Triassic	metamorphosed sediments	36.28Mt	4.7% Zn, 0.8% Pb, 36g/t Ag	20
	Los Gavilanes	Esperanza formation	Triassic ?	Felsic volcanics-sediments			24
	El Gordo	Esperanza Formation	Triassic ?	Felsic volcanics-sediments			
	San Nicolas	Chilitos Formation	Ur. Jurassic-Lr.Cretaceous	bimodal volcanics	75Mt	1.40% Cu, 2.11% Zn, 0.53 g/t Au and 30 g/t Ag	17
					21.8Mt	1.29% Cu.	17
	Campo Morado Group	Campo Morado Felsic	145 Ma	Felsic	29.34Mt	1.57g/t Au, 89g/t Ag, 0.69% Cu, 0.6% Pb, 2.1% Zn	16
	Cuale District	Zihuatanejo subterrane	Lr.Cretaceous	Felsic-sediments	2.24Mt	0.23% Cu, 1.03% Pb, 3.22% Zn, 0.83g/t Au, 103g/t Ag	18
	Rey de Plata	Teoloapan subterrane	Lr.Cretaceous	flesic volcanics -sediments	3.0Mt	0.5% Cu, 2.1% Pb, 8.7% Zn, 240g/t Ag, 1.4g/t Au	20
	Azulaquez	Teoloapan subterrane	Lr.Cretaceous	felsic volcanincs-sediments	<0.3Mt	0.8% Cu, 5% Pb, 14% Zn, 600g/t Ag, 2g/t Au	19,21
	Suriana	Teoloapan subterrane	Lr.Cretaceous	sediments-mafic and felsic volcanics	6Mt	7.7g/t Au, 603g/t Ag, 4.5% Pb, 0.4% Cu	20
	Tizapa	Teoloapan subterrane	Lr.Cretaceous	felsic volcanincs-sediments	4.08Mt	0.7% Cu, 1.8% Pb, 7.9% Zn, 1.9g/t Au, 325g/t Ag	20,23
	La Esmeralda	Teoloapan subterrane	Lr.Cretaceous	felsic volcanincs-sediments	0.38Mt	1.25% Pb, 2.25% Zn	19,23
	La América Mine	Zihuatanejo subterrane	Lr.Cretaceous	felsic volcanics-sediments	0.14Mt	0.2%Cu, 1.25%Pb, 7.5% Zn, 310 g/t Ag and 1 g/t Au.	19
	La Minta	Zihuatanejo subterrane	Lr.Cretaceous	Felsic volcanics-sediments	6Mt	0.3% Pb, 3.0% Zn, 60 g/t Ag and 34% barite	20,22
Cuba	Carlota		Jur.-Lr. Cret.	Peridotite, calc. schists	2.35Mt	1.13% Cu, 0.28% Pb+Zn	1
	Guachinango		Jur.-Lr. Cret.	Peridotite, calc. schists	5.00Mt	0.81% Cu	1
	La Victoria		Jur.-Lr. Cret.	Peridotite, calc. schists	0.54Mt	0.86% Cu, 0.30% Pb+Zn	1
	Hierro Mantua	Esperanza	Ur. Jur.-Lr. Cret.	Porphyritic basalt	11.39Mt	1.76% Cu	1
	Hierro Mantua	Esperanza	Ur. Jur.-Lr. Cret.	Porphyritic basalt	2.04Mt	1.44g/t Au, 11.65g/t Ag	1
	Unión	Esperanza	Ur. Jur.-Lr. Cret.	Diabase		<0.5% Cu	1
	Juan Manuel	Esperanza	Ur. Jur. -Lr. Cret.	Diabase		<0.5% Cu	1

[continued on following page]

Country	Deposit	Formation	Age	Host Rocks	Size	Grade	References
	Júcaro	Encrucijada	Lr.Cretaceous	Tholeitic basalt	0.59Mt	1.38% Cu, 0.31% Pb+Zn	1
	Cacarajícara	Encrucijada	Lr.Cretaceous	Tholeitic basalt	0.62Mt	1.2% Cu	1
	Mendieta	Encrucijada	Lr. Cretaceous	Tholeitic basalt			1
	Buenavista	Encrucijada	Lr. Cretaceous	Tholeitic basalt	0.11Mt	2.58% Cu	1
	Yagruma	Encrucijada	Lr.Cretaceous	Tholeitic basalt		0.72% Cu, 0.9% Pb+Zn	1
	Margot	Margot	Lr.Cretaceous	Tholeitic basalt		<1.55% Cu, <1.17 g/t Au, < 4.4 g/t Ag	1
	América	Margot	Lr.Cretaceous	Serp. Breccia, basalt		<0.52% Cu	1
	Monte Rojo		Lr.Cretaceous	Serp., gabbro			1
	Cuba Libre		Lr.Cretaceous	Serp., basalt, gabbro	1.00Mt	1% Cu	1
	Ventura		Lr.Cretaceous	Serp.		<0.4% Cu, <1.0g/t Au	1
	El Hoyo		Lr.Cretaceous	Serp.		0.5-7.12% Cu, 0.1-11.75% Pb+Zn	1
	Antonio	Los Pasos	Lr.Cretaceous	Dacite breccia	1.67Mt	0.52% Cu	1,7
	San Fernando	Los Pasos	Lr.Cretaceous	Felsic lapilli tuff	2.00Mt	1.84% Cu, 3.35% Pb+Zn	2,1
	Los Cerros	Los Pasos	Lr.Cretaceous	Felsic pyroclastics		0.38% Cu, 0.58% Pb+Zn	1
	Minas	Bahia Honda equivalent	Cretaceous(?)	ophiolite			3,5,6
Domincan Republic	Cerro de Maimon	Maimon	Lr.Cretaceous	bimodal volcanic	3.5Mt	3.77% Cu, 2.04% Zn, 0.62g/t Au, 46.36g/t Ag in sulphides	3,8,9
			Lr.Cretaceous		0.3Mt	3.10g/t Au, 59.9 g/t Ag in oxides	3,8,9
	San Antonio	Maimon	Lr.Cretaceous	bimodal volcanic			3,10
	Loma La Mina	Maimon	Lr.Cretaceous	bimodal volcanic			3,11,12,13
	Loma Pesada	Maimon	Lr.Cretaceous	bimodal volcanic	1.11Mt	2.13% Cu, 0.77% Zn, 4.37g/t Ag, 0.16g/t Au	3,9
	Loma Barbuito	Maimon	Lr.Cretaceous	bimodal volcanic			3,9,14
	El Altar	Maimon	Lr.Cretaceous	bimodal volcanic			3,14
	El Anon	Amina	Lr. Cretaceous	bimodal volcanic	0.3Mt	1.58g/t Au, oxide cap	3,15
	Sabana Potrero	Peralvillo	Ur.Cretaceous	basalt flows			3,5
Guatemala	Oxec	Sierra de Santa Cruz Ophiolite	Cretaceous	mafic	0.91Mt	3% Cu	26
Peru	María Teresa	Huarmey Basin, Casma Fm.	Lr.Cretaceous	mafic volcanics	1.0Mt	4.0% Zn, 1.3% Pb, 0.3% Cu, 100 g/t Ag	31
	Aurora Augusta	Cañete Basin, Casma Fm.	Lr.Cretaceous	mafic volcanics		87% Barite	31
	Perubar	Cañete Basin, Casma Fm.	Lr.Cretaceous	mafic volcanics	2.5Mt	12% Zn, 0.7% Pb, 30g/t Ag & (4.0Mt) 80% Barite	31,32
	Palma	Cañete Basin, Casma Fm.	Lr.Cretaceous	mafic volcanics		12% Zn, 3.8% Pb, 45g/t Ag	31,32
	Balducho	Cañete Basin, Casma Fm.	Lr.Cretaceous	mafic volcanics			31,32
	Cerro Lindo	Cañete Basin, Casma Fm.	Lr.Cretaceous	mafic volcanics	75Mt	0.87% Cu, 3.28% Zn, 50.7g/t Ag	33,32,31

[continued on following page]

Country	Deposit	Formation	Age	Host Rocks	Size	Grade	References
	Tambo GrandeTG-1	Ereo Fm	pre-mid -Cretaceous	felsic-mafic bimodal	64Mt	1.7% Cu, 1.4% Zn, 31 g/t Ag and 0.7 g/t Au	30
	Tambo GrandeTG-1 oxide cap	Ereo Fm	pre-mid -Cretaceous	felsic-mafic bimodal	8.2Mt	5.2 g/t Au, 48 g/t Ag oxide cap	30
	Tambo Grande TG-3	Ereo Fm	pre-mid -Cretaceous	felsic-mafic bimodal	110Mt	0.7% Cu, 1.0% Zn, 19 g/t Ag and 0.7g/t Au	30
Equador	La Plata	Macuchi Fm.	Ur.Cretaceous	felsic footwall - Mafic hangingwall	0.84Mt	4.06% Cu, 4.2% Zn, 4.84 g/t Au and 54.4 g/t Ag	29
	Mercedes (Macuchi)	Macuchi Fm.	Ur.Cretaceous	felsic footwall - Mafic hangingwall	1.95Mt	0.75% Cu, 15 g/t Ag, 3.8 g/t Ag	29
					0.4Mt	4.5% Cu, 68 g/t Ag, 12 g/t Au	
Colombia	El Alacran	Calima Terrane	Ur.Cretaceous	mafic associated	4.8Mt	1.4% Cu, 0.83g/t Au	34
				oxide	0.5Mt	2.5g/t Au in oxides	34
	Guadalupe	Calima Terrane	Ur.Cretaceous	mafic associated	28Mt	1.88% Cu (eq)	34
	El Roble	Calima Terrane	Ur.Cretaceous	mafic associated	1.2Mt	4.7% Cu, 3.1g/t Au, 9.8g/t Ag	34
	Santa Anita	Calima Terrane	Ur.Cretaceous	mafic associated	0.5Mt	2.8% Cu, <1.0g/t Au, 1-2g/t Ag	34
	La Equis	Calima Terrane	Ur.Cretaceous	mafic associated		1-10% Zn, <10g/t Au, 12g/t Ag	34
	Sababablanca	Calima Terrane	Ur.Cretaceous	mafic associated	0.1Mt	4-6% Cu, 10-12g/t Au	34
Argentina	Arroyo Rojo	Lemaire	Ur.Jurassic	felsic footwall, mafic hangingwall			28
Chile	Punta del Cobre		Jurassic- Lr.Cretaceous	Andesita, Dacita	> 40Mt	1-2% Cu, 0.2-0.5g/t Au, 7g/t Ag	51,52,53
	Cutter Cove		Jurassic	basalts	small		57,53
Cenozoic							
Cuba	El Cobre	Hongolosongo Fm.	Lr. Pal.- Ur. Eoc	Andesite lavas, tuffs	8.44Mt	1.83% Cu	1
	La Cristina	El Cobre Group	Lr. Pal.- Ur. Eoc.	Andesite tuff		0.8-8.0% Cu, 0.5-3.0% Pb+Zn, 1.0-6.0g/t Au	1
	Infierno	El Cobre Group	Lr. Eocene	Andesite-dacite tuff		0.6-1.41% Cu, 0.3-38.2% Pb+Zn, 0.5-4.19g/t Au, 10-121g/t Ag	1
	Eureca	El Cobre	Eocene	andesite	0.06Mt	7-9% Cu	3
Jamaica	Hope	Wagwater	Eocene	andesite & volcanic-derived sediments			3,4

(see following page for footnotes)

Footnotes

1. Russell et al. (2000) 2. Bottrill et al. (2000) 3. Childe (2000) 4. Carby (1985) 5. Kesler et al. (1990) 6. Feoktisov et al. (1983) 6. Feoktisov et al. (1983) 7. Bogdanov et al. (1966) 8. Lewis et al. (1989) 9. Lewis et al. (2 000) 10. Holbek and Daubeny (2000) 11. "Energold Mining Ltd. & Atna Resources Inc. News Release, March 12, 1999" 12. Vaughan et al. (1921) 13. Koschmann and Gordon (1950) 14. Espaillat (1995) 15. Espaillat et al. (1989) 16. Oliver et al. (2000) 17. Johnson et al. (2000) 18. Hall and Gomez-Torres (2000a) 19. Miranda-Gasca (1995) 20. Giles and García (2000) 21. Rhys et al. (2000) 22. Ortigoza (1988) 23. Lewis and Rhys (2000) 24. Hall and Gomez-Torres (2000b) 25. Hall and Gomez-torres (2000c) 26. Petersen (2000) 27. Carlson and Staargaard (2000) 28. Broili et al. (2000) 29. O'Dowd (1999) 30. Tegart et al. (2000) 31. Steinmüller et al (2000) 32. Vidal (2000) 33. Ly (2000) 34. Jaramillo Cortes (2000) 35. Zappettini and Brodtkorb (2000) 36. McNamee (1977) 37. Kerr et al. (2000) 38. Borba (1988) 39. Ally (1985) 40. Araujo (1986) 41. Araujo and Nilson (1988) 42. Cassedane (1972) 43. Rocha (1985) 44. Fleischer and Espourteille (1998) 45. Carvalho (1990) 46. De Abreau and Belo de Oliveira (1998) 47. Channer and Anderson (2000) 48. Info-Mine Golden Star Database 49. Franklin et al. (2000) 50. Lindberg (1989) 51. Camus (1980) 52. Marschik (1996) 53. Vivallo (2000) 54. Collao y Alfaro (1982) 55. Schira et al. (1990) 56. Ruiz y Peebles (1988) 57. Thomas (1973) 58. Logan et al., (2000).

rocks in Brazil, 3.35 Ga (Barbosa, 1996). These rocks consist of primarily komatiites and ultramafic volcanic rocks and tholeiitic basalts and dacites (Cunha and Froes, 1994). Within the Gaviao block, the Umburunas, Ibitira-Ubiraçaba, Brumado, Bate-Pé and Guajeru greenstone belts contain numerous Cu-Zn massive sulphide occurrences, often associated with ultramafic and calc-silicate rocks (Lobato et al., 2000).

The Boquira greenstone belt is host to stratabound Pb-Zn deposit at the past producing Boquira Lead mine (Fig. 1; Table 1; Lobato et al., 2000) where in excess of 5.6 Mt of ore grading 8.9 % Pb and 1.4 % Zn were mined. Mineralization is closely associated with amphibolitic, siliceous, magnetite bearing iron formation within dolomitic carbonates (Cassedane, 1972; Fleischer and Espourteille, 1998). These rocks are interpreted as forming in a shallow water marginal basin (Rocha, 1985).

Within the Guaporé craton, recent exploration has identified significant sulphide deposits in the Aripuanã district (Fig. 1; Table 1). These Archean to mid-Proterozoic supercrustal rocks are divided into a southern felsic volcanic sedimentary sequence dominated by tuffaceous rocks, and a northerly basalt-rhyolite package, which have been intruded by granite plutons diorite-gabbro intrusions (Kerr et al., 2000). Two significant sulphide deposits are identified in Aripuanã; the Arex and Valley deposits. The deposits are hosted within felsic lavas, autoclastic breccias and epiclastic and pyroclastic tuffs and are highly altered to sericite and chlorite in the vicinity of the deposits (Kerr et al., 2000). The sulphides are massive to disseminated consisting of pyrite, sphalerite, galena and chalcopyrite.

PROTEROZOIC

Bolivia

The Precambrian rocks of eastern Bolivia consist of three well defined Proterozoic tectonic belts. VMS deposits have recently been discovered in the Miguela and El Porvenir concessions within the Proterozoic Guarayos greenstone belt (Fig. 1; Table 1). The area is underlain by amphibolite grade volcanic sedimentary rocks (Biste and Gourlay, 2000). The rocks of the Guarayos greenstone belt range from tholeiitic to calc-alkaline in geochemical affinity.

The most significant deposit is at the Miguela A-Zone, which is massive to disseminated pyrite, sphalerite, galena and chalcopyrite and is hosted in the La Pastora formation. Sulphides are confined to a 400 m thick sequence of intermediate to rhyolitic volcanic rocks, quartz-muscovite-rich sediments with thin layers of mafic material. The hangingwall and footwall rocks to the felsic unit consist of fine-grained amphibolite. These rocks are overlain by silica, and iron-rich metamorphosed mudstone and siltstone, thin layers of felsic tuff and magnetite or pyrrhotite-rich banded iron formation (Biste and Gourlay, 2000).

Brazil

The Rio Itapicuru greenstone belt is comprised of a lowermost mafic volcanic unit, intermediate felsic unit and uppermost sedimentary unit (Kishida, 1979; da Silva, 1987; Baars, 1997). These rocks have undergone greenschist to amphibolite grade metamorphism. The mafic rocks are ocean-floor tholeiites, which are overlain by compositionally variable calc-alkaline volcanic sequences. Regional thrust and shear structures are known to host significant mesothermal lode-gold mineralization (Santos et al., 1993; Vieira et al., 1998). Base metal occurrences are associated with pelite- and albitic chert-dominated rocks (da Rocha Neto and Pedrieira, 1994).

The Rio Capim greenstone belt, consisting of a lower unit of tholeiitic basalts and an upper unit of calc-alkaline felsic volcanic rocks (Winge and Danni, 1980), represents a remnant of ensialic, back-arc basin fill, metamorphosed to amphibolite facies with local retrograde to greenschist facies (Winge, 1984). A number of pyrite-dominated Cu-Zn showings occur in the felsic intervals.

The Rio Salitre volcano-sedimentary sequence, including the Rio Salitre, Barreiro, Colomi and Casa Nova greenstone belts, consist of tholeiitic to komatiitic ocean-floor basalts, associated with felsic volcanic rocks (Ribeiro and Silva, 1998). These belts are host to numerous massive sulphide deposits.

The Palmeirópolis sequence (Fig. 1; Table 1) consists of a lower unit of banded amphibolites and felsic pyroclastic rocks and greywackes (Ribeiro and Teixeira, 1981; Leão Neto and Olivatti, 1983; Araújo, 1986; 2000). The amphibolites are interpreted to represent basalts which host the sulphide deposits (Araújo, 1986; 2000; Araújo et al., 1996). The intermediate unit consists of felsic metavolcanic rocks and minor metapelite, while the upper unit consists of metapelite with metachert and banded iron formation.

The Salobro Zn-Pb massive sulphide deposit (Fig. 1; Table 1) is hosted by a ferruginous, siliceous horizon of the Salobro sequence, possible correlate of the Riacho dos Machados Group (Mourão et al., 1997). The sulphide mineralization occurs within amphibolite schists, most likely of magmatic origin, with grades of 3.9 % Zn and 1.1 % Pb (de Abreu and Belo de Oliveira, 1998).

Argentina

The Proterozoic ophiolites of the Sierras Pampeanas hosts mafic associated Cu-Co and Ni deposits (Tío, Tacurú, Estrella Gaucha and Las Cuevas; Table 1; Logan et al., 2000). The deposits are hosted in the igneous-metamorphic basement of Precambrian to Lower Paleozoic age (Gordillo and Lencinas, 1979). They are generally small, hosted by gneisses, schists, amphibolites, marbles and consist of massive to disseminated magnetite, ilmenite, pyrite, chalcopyrite and hematite; in addition, carrolite and pyrrhotite occur in the Tío mine (Logan et al., 2000).

Arizona

Although not in Latin America the Jerome district is one of the most significant Proterozoic VMS districts in the world. The outcrop distribution of Proterozoic rocks in Arizona is irregular and limited due to more recent cover rocks; it does however, locally extend into northern Mexico, providing limited potential for VMS deposits in this area. The Jerome district (Table 1) has produced in excess of 42 million tonnes of massive sulphide with an average grade in excess of 4.0 % Cu, the bulk of which was from the United Verde deposit (Lindberg, 1989). Massive sulphide mineralization at United Verde is located near the top of a thick section of rhyolite at the stratigraphic contact between felsic units of the Cleopatra member of the Deception Rhyolite (Lindberg, 1989; Gustin, 1990).

ORDOVICIAN

Argentina

The Ordovician basin of northwestern Argentina forms part of the intracratonic extensional basin extending from Peru to northern Argentina (Logan et al., 2000). The sedimentary sequence begins with conglomerates and sandstones of the Middle Cambrian Mesón Group, which lie discordantly on basement and grade upward into pelitic facies. During the Tremadocian, more than 3,200 m of shales were deposited. Sedimentary exhalitive deposits of Pb-Zn-Ag with the proximal sectors rich in Cu (Aguilar, Jujuy, La Colorada, Salta; Table 1) occur in sedimentary rocks of lower Tremadocian age (Logan et al., 2000; Sureda and Martín, 1990).

The Santa Elena deposit (Table 1) is located in San Juan province, Argentina, on the western side of the Precordillera. The region is underlain by clastic sediments and locally mafic volcanic rocks of Ordovician age. The orebodies are related to the basaltic sequence hosted at the sediment-igneous contact (Zappettini and Brodtkorb, 2000). Kay et al. (1984), based on trace element analyses of the basalts, suggest formation in a back arc basin setting. Mineralization consists of pyrite, marcasite, pyrrhotite, sphalerite, chalcopyrite, arsenopyrite and galena with sulfosalts. The deposit was operated historically in the oxide zone for iron sulphates.

DEVONIAN-PENNSYLVANIAN

Venezuela

The Phanerozoic lithologies of northern Venezuela (Fig. 2) host several massive sulphide prospects in the Cordillera de Mérida a northeast trending mountain range, a continuation of the main Andean chain (Channer and Anderson, 2000). These include the Santa Isabel deposit (Table 1) which is a past-producer and associated with mafic and felsic volcanic rocks. The deposits in the Aroa district (Table 1) which occur as veins and lenses in mafic volcanics, interpreted to be VMS in origin. The deposits in the Aroa district were operated between 1609 and 1963 producing about 1.5 million tonnes of high grade (+8 %) copper ore (Channer and Anderson, 2000).

The Bailadores deposit, the best known of the Phanerozoic VMS deposits of Venezuela, is located in the Cordillera de Mérida and hosted by the Devonian-Pennsylvanian aged Mucuchachí Formation. The Mucuchachí formation unconformably overlies the Sierra Nevada Formation a metamorphosed basement sequence and is in-turn overlain by Pennsylvanian to Permian sequence of continental sediments. The Mucuchachí formation is up to 5,000 m thick consisting of fine grained slates and phyllites with local lenses of limestone and in the Bailadores area a sequence of felsic pyroclastic rocks, up to 2,000 m thick that hosts the deposit (Staargaard and Carlson, 2000).

The immediate footwall to the Bailadores deposit is felsic crystal and lithic tuffs and the hangingwall consists of felsic tuffs overlain by black phyllite (Carlson, 1977). The massive sulphide is defined in two zones with mainly sphalerite-pyrrhotite-galena and chalcopyrite with minor pyrite and arsenopyrite. The resource estimate quoted is 1.45 million tonnes grading 26 % Zn, 7 % Pb, and 1.5 % Cu (Staargaard and Carlson, 2000) making this deposit unusual in terms of its metal content and mineralogy.

TRIASSIC

Mexico

The Fresnillo-Guanajuato Subterrane

The Guerrero Terrane in Mexico (Fig. 3) is subdivided into a series of subterranes Campa and Coney (1983). The bulk of the volcanic associated deposits in Mexico are within Cretaceous arc volcanics built on older basement, generally on the Teloloapan and the Huetamo-Zihuatenejo subterranes. However, some deposits in the Fresnillo-Guanajuato subterranes are interpreted to be hosted in Triassic rocks and may represent older VMS-style mineralization. The oldest unit recognized in the Fresnillo-Guanajuato subterrane is the Late Triassic Zacatecas, Esperanza, Aperos, and El Maguey Formations, all of which likely represent the basement assemblages, upon which the arc sequences were built (Ruiz and Centeno-Garcia, 2000). The Zacatacas Formation consists of shale, sandstone with volcanic tuffs, breccias, pillow lavas and minor limestone, which was deformed and metamorphosed prior to the development of the Cretaceous arc assemblage (Centeno-Garcia et al., 1993; Ruiz and Centeno-Garcia, 2000). Deposits hosted in the basement may include the Fancisco I Madero, which is not obviously VMS related and deposits of the Los Gavilanes area which is inferred to be hosted in Zacatecas Formation equivalent rocks based on similar lithologies.

Francisco I Madero

The Francisco I Madero deposit is located about 15 km northwest of Zacatecas city, and is presently the subject of a feasibility study by Servicios Industriales Peñoles S.A. de C.V. (Giles and García, 2000). Mineralized intervals are enigmatic and at

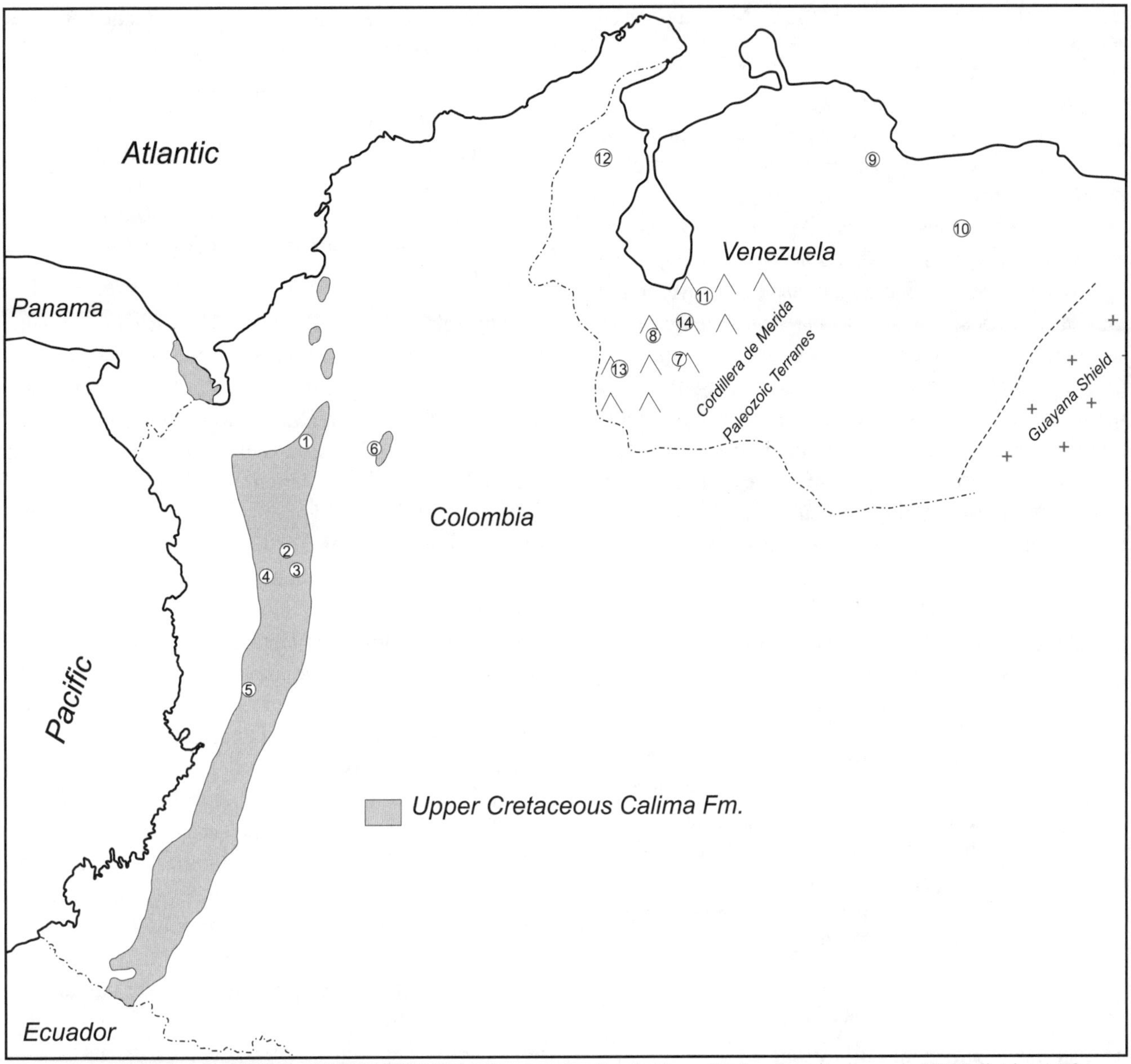

Figure 2. Geologic map of Colombia and Venezuela showing the distribution of Paleozoic and mesozoic VMS districts. After and Channer and Anderson (2000), Jaramilo (2000), Staargarrd and Carlson (2000). 1. El Alacran, 2. El Roble, 3. Santa Anita, 4. La Equis, 5. Sabanablanca, 6. Guadalupe, 7. Bailadores, 8. De Lima II, 9. Aroa, 10. Santa Isabel, 11. Timotes, 12. La Villa, 13. Seboroco, 14. Toronduy.

least partially replacement and partially stratabound in a limestone-shale sequence overlying andesitic marine volcanics, inferred to be Triassic in age (Miranda-Gasca, 1995; Giles and García, 2000). The lower, and largest, manto body is hosted in black slates with abundant graphite and reaches thicknesses of about 200 m. The mineralogy consists of pyrrhotite, galena, chalcopyrite, galena bismuthinite and native bismuth (Miranda-Gasca, 1995). Stratabound mineralization is hosted in graphitic metasediments with banded pyrite and chalcopyrite, galena and sphalerite. The stratigraphic sequence that hosts Francisco I Madero is tentatively correlated, based on lithologic similarities, with the Triassic portions of the Zacatecas Formation (Miranda-Gasca, 1995).

Los Gavilanes / Guanajuato

This district is underlain by the Triassic Esperanza Formation. The age of the Esperanza Formation is poorly constrained and controversial. Based upon regional correlations with the Aperos, Zacatecas, El Maguey and Taray Formations an Upper Triassic age may be appropriate (Sedlock, et al., 1993). At the Los Gavilanes deposit the lowermost stratigraphic unit is a limestone overlain by black argillite and fine grained siliciclastic sediments. Overlying the sediments are a 20 to 80 m thick sequence of felsic-intermediate volcanic rock of calc-alkaline affinity (Hall and Gomez-Torres, 2000a). Massive sulphides are hosted in and overly these volcanic rocks. Overlying the volcanics and sulphide mineralization are additional argillites and fine-grained siliciclastic rocks (Hall and Gomez-Torres, 2000a). The sulphides are polymetallic and are generally typical of felsic volcanic associated mineralization.

El Gordo

The El Gordo deposit is similar to the Los Gavilanes in that it is hosted in the inferred Esperanza Formation. The stratigraphy consists of micritic limestones and argillaceous sediments that are overlain by a 100 m thick sequence of felsic flows and pyroclastics, which host the massive sulphide mineralization (Hall and Gomez-Torres, 2000b).

JURASSIC

Tierra del Fuego Argentina-Chile

The Tierra del Fuego district (Fig. 4) in Argentina is hosted by Jurassic aged rhyolites, part of the Lemaire Formation (Ametrano et al., 2000; Broili et al., 2000). The metamorphic basement in the region is the Upper Paleozoic to Lower Mesozoic Lapataia Formation which consists of amphibolite grade schists and gneisses. Unconformabley overlying the basement rocks is the Lemaire Formation, an Upper Jurassic aged volcano-sedimentary sequence. This sequence is contemporaneous with the subaerial equivalents in Patagonia, host of epithermal precious metal systems (Broili et al., 2000).

Within the Lemaire Formation sequence 5 units are recognized (Broili et al., 2000)

- Stratigraphically lower most shale (~3,000 m)
- Lower basaltic andesite (~500 m)
- Volcaniclastic reworked felsic epiclastic rocks (~500 m)
- Felsic flow dome complexes (~1,000 m)
- Straigraphically upper most andesite flow breccias (200-500 m)

The felsic flow dome complexes of the Lemaire Formation host massive sulphide deposits. The Lemaire Formation is interpreted to have formed in a back-arc environment (Macellari, 1988) and the geochemistry of the volcanic rocks is consistent with an evolved arc signature (Ametrano et al., 2000).

Arroyo Rojo (Fig. 5; Table 1) is the main massive sulphide deposit within the Lemaire Formation occurring at the stratigraphic contact between a felsic dome complex in the footwall and andesite flows and breccia in the hangingwall. The sulphide lenses are typically polymetallic, dominated by massive pyrite with sphalerite-chalcopyrite and galena. In addition to Arroyo Rojo the district contains many VMS prospects that have received limited exploration efforts (Ametrano et al., 2000; Broili et al., 2000).

The Jurassic volcanic sequences extend north into Chile where it hosts several massive sulphide deposits. Production from Punta del Cobre between 1800 and 1982 was 5 million tonnes at 4.8 % copper (Camus, 1985; Vivallo, 2000; Table 1). The deposits are hosted in the Upper Jurassic to Lower Cretaceous andesitic-dacitic volcanic rocks with local ferruginous cherts. The sulphide deposits are associated with dacitic volcanic rocks and consist of pyrite-chalcopyrite with lesser magnetite, pyrrhotite and sphalerite (Vivallo, 2000).

EARLY CRETACEOUS

Dominican Republic

Maimón Formation

The Early Cretaceous volcanism in the Dominican Republic (Fig. 5) defines a fore-arc and arc volcanic complex with the Cerro Maimón and correlated

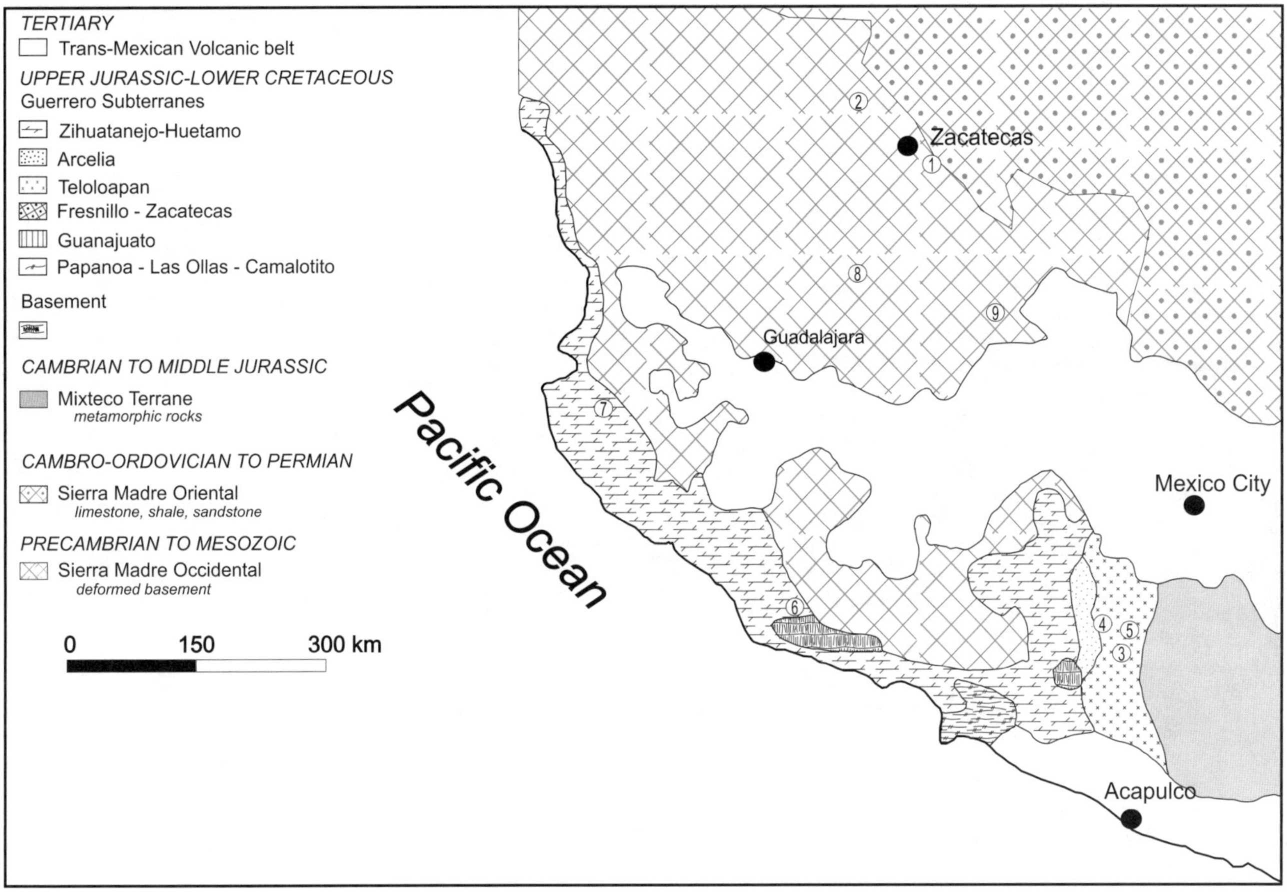

Figure 3. Geologic map of Mexico emphasising the Guerrero subterranes and VMS districts. After Campa and Coney (1983), Giles and García (2000), Hall and Gomez-Torres (2000,a,b,c), Johnson et al. (2000), Lewis and Rhys (2000), Miranda-Gasca (1995), Oliver et al. (2000), Rhys et al. (2000). 1. San Nicolás, 2. Francisco I Madero, 3. Campo Morado, 4. Rey de Plata, 5. Tizapa, 6. La Minta, 7. Cuale, 8. Los Gavilanes, 9. El Gordo

Amina Formation comprising the fore-arc and the Los Ranchos Formation the axial arc. There are several VMS-related occurrences in the Cerro Maimón and equivalent strata in the Greater Antilles but mineralization is largely restricted to epithermal subtypes in the Los Ranchos Formation such as the Pueblo Viejo deposit (Childe, 2000; Lewis et al., 2000).

The Maimón formation, in the Dominican Republic, is a lower Cretaceous bi-modal volcanic sequence that extends the full length of the Greater Antilles (Lewis and Draper, 1990). The Maimón formation is characterized by mafic rocks that range from tholeiities with bonnitic affinities to normal oceanic arc tholeiites (Lewis et al., 2000). The felsic volcanic rocks are generally quartz-plagioclase feldspar tuffs with flat REE patterns and enrichments in LILE and depletions in Nb, REE and HFSE with respect to N-type MORB (Lewis et al., 2000).

Cerro Maimón deposit (Fig. 5, Table 1), hosted by the Maimón Formation, is a polymetallic deposit hosted within a felsic assemblage which is generally enclosed within a dominantly mafic volcanic package (Lewis et al., 2000). It does contain a small secondary precious metal-rich oxide cap.

The San Antonio deposit is also hosted by the Maimón Formation where mineralization occurs in at least two stratigraphic intervals in a sequence dominated by felsic volcanic rocks (Holbek and Daubeny, 2000). Compared to Cerro Maimón the San Antonio deposit has higher Zn and Au and lower Cu.

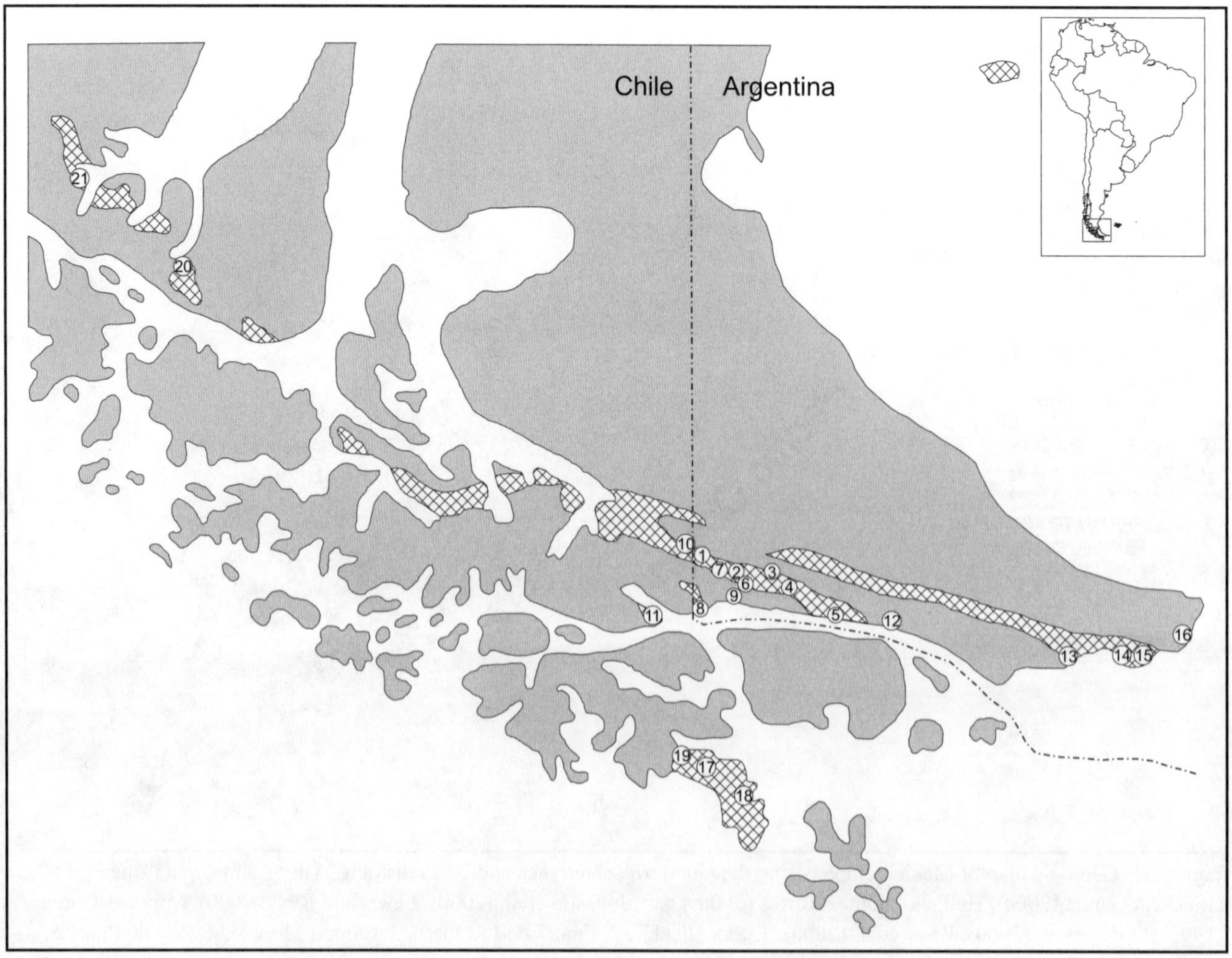

Figure 4. Geologic map of the Tierra del Fuego district with VMS deposits. Hatched area indicates the distribution of Jurassic volcanic rocks. After Broili et al. (2000), Ametrano et al. (2000), Vivallo (2000). 1. Rio Amarillo, Rio Café, 2. Lago Guanaco, 3. Rancho Hambre, 4. Pink Hill, 5. Puerto Almanza, 6. Arroyo Rojo, 7. Sargent, 8. Beatriz, 9. Estancia Túnel, 10. Hope, 11. Yendegaia, 12. Pampa Indios, 13. Pel Español, 14. Bania Aguírre, Río Bolsa, 15. B. Valentin, 16. B. Ben Suciso, 17. Gardiner, 18. Centinela, 19. Jackson, 20. Cutter Cove, 21 Cúpula

The Amina and Ile de la Tortue schists are correlated with the Maimón Formation based on similarities in lithologies, geochemistry and structural style (Draper and Lewis, 1982; Lewis and Draper, 1990; Kesler et al., 1991). Minor VMS prospects are seen in these formations.

Deposits similar to Cerro Maimón, but possibly younger, are seen at Rivière Mapou and Camp Coq in Haiti and the Santa Isabel and La Providencia areas of Villa de Cura Group in Venezuela (Kesler et al., 1990).

Cuba

Los Pasos Formation

Los Pasos Formation (Fig. 5), in Cuba, is inferred to be Early Cretaceous and is a bi-modal assemblage of basalt-rhyolite and clastic sediments. The formation has been described as a primitive Island Arc assemblage (Donnelly and Rogers, 1967; Russell et al., 2000) similar to others, such as the Maimón Formation, seen in the Greater Antilles. Significant volcanic associated mineralization is found at San

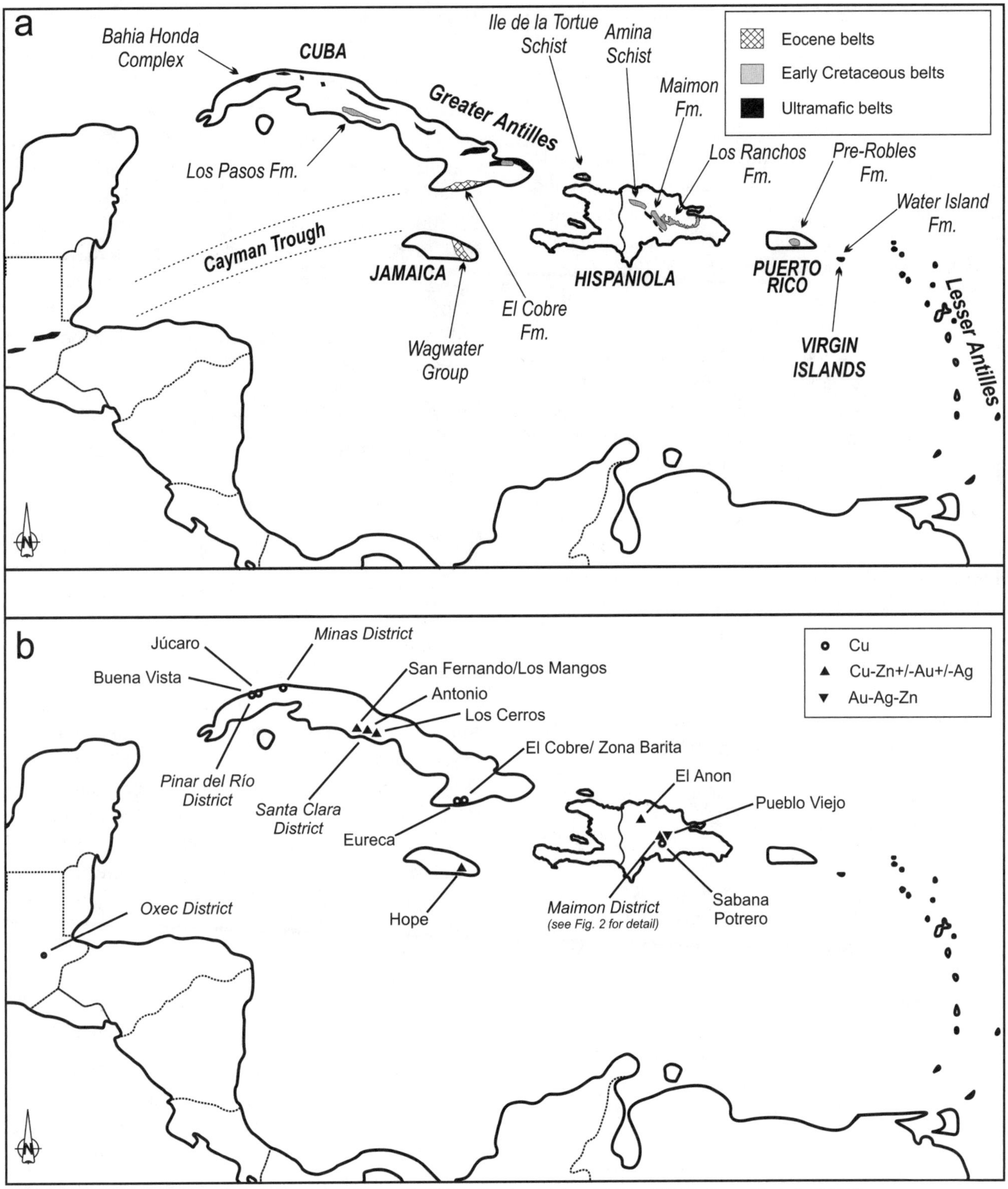

Figure 5. Geologic map of the Greater Antilles with VMS districts. After Childe (2000), Russell et al. (2000).

Fernando and Los Mangos (Bottrill et al., 2000). The Los Pasos Formation's extent in Cuba is limited dominated by mafic volcanic rocks and lesser felsic volcanic rocks. Its age is considered to be Neocomian and it is overlain by Aptian limestone that separates the formation from the overlying Upper Cretaceous calc-alkaline arc rocks (Russell et al., 2000). This period of limestone deposition may correlate with the Hatillo Limestone Formation in the Dominican Republic, which unconformably overlies the Los Ranchos Formation and represents a hiatus in volcanic activity (Russell and Kesler, 1991). Within the Los Pasos Formation are the massive sulphide deposits of Los Mangos-San Fernando, Antonio and Los Cerros deposits (Fig. 5, Table 1). The deposits appear to be at a similar stratigraphic level and are associated with felsic pyroclastic rocks (Russell et al., 2000).

The Los Mangos-San Fernando deposit (Fig. 1; Table 1) occurs as massive to semi-massive sulphide deposits in the Lower Cretaceous Los Pasos Formation. The deposit is at the stratigraphic contact between a footwall felsic lapilli-ash tuff and a hangingwall basaltic tuff (Bottrill et al., 2000). The Antonio deposit (Table 1), has a dacitic tuff as its footwall and a hangingwall of dacite lavas and flow breccias (Russell et al., 2000). The Los Cerros deposit is hosted within felsic rocks (Russell et al., 2000).

Esperanza Formation

The Guaniguanico block of western Cuba hosts several large Sedex deposits and also a number of Besshi-type deposits. The most northerly belt of deposits is the Esperanza Formation of Upper Jurassic to Lower Cretaceous age, and includes the Hierro Mantua orebody and the Juan Manuel - Unión deposits (Fig. 5; Table 1). Copper is the dominant base metal in this belt and lead-zinc are minor. Mineralization is hosted in limestones and calcareous schists with intercalations of siliciclastic sediments and concordant lenses of basalt to andesite (Russell et al., 2000). Although these deposits might also be included in the Sedex category, they appear to be associated with volcanic horizons and may be considered Besshi-type deposits (Kesler et al., 1996).

Margot Formation

The Margot Formation hosts small, mafic volcanic associated, VMS occurrences, the Margot and the América deposits (Russell et al., 2000). The formation has paleontologic ages of Upper Albian-Cenomanian or Aptian-Albian and has island arc tholeiitic to MORB geochemical affinities (Russell et al., 2000). The formation of these deposits is considered to be fore-arc or back-arc basins rather than Protocaribbean crust. The Margot and América deposits are hosted in fault bounded slices of basalt with sediment interbeds and brecciated serpentinite respectively (Russell et al., 2000).

Encrucijada (Bahia Honda) Formation

The Bahia Honda district, in Cuba, is an Early to Late Cretaceous ophiolite complex. Mafic volcanic-hosted copper-rich VMS deposits occur in the Bahia Honda ophiolite complex, Encrucijada Formation, in the eastern part of western Cuba (Fig. 5). These deposits include the Buena Vista, Júcaro, Cacarajícaro, Mendieta and Yagruma (Fig. 5; Table 1), which are described as lenses and stock-work veins of pyrite, marcasite and chalcopyrite with lesser sphalerite, pyrrhotite, enargite and bornite, hosted within mafic to ultramafic flows, sills and sediments (Bogdanov et al. 1966; Russell et al., 2000). The geochemistry of these host lithologies is consistent with MORB (Russell et al., 2000) and is believed to represent obducted oceanic crust. Case et al., (1984) have correlated the Bahia Honda complex with the Sierra de Santa Cruz ophiolite in Guatemala, which is the host to the Oxec VMS deposit.

Guatemala

Sierra de Santa Cruz ophiolite

The Oxec deposit in Guatemala (Petersen and Zantop, 1980; Petersen, 2000) is hosted by pillow lavas, part of the mid-Cretaceous Sierra de Santa Cruz ophiolite. The deposit is structurally disrupted with the mafic host lithologies structurally juxtaposed against the ultramafic lithologies of the ophiolite. The sulphide body itself is structurally disrupted and cross-cut by post-mineral mafic dykes. Sulphides consist of massive pyrite pyrrhotite and chalcopyrite

(Petersen and Zantop, 1980; Petersen, 2000).

Mexico: Guerrero Terrane

The Guerrero Terrane of western Mexico (Fig. 3), originally defined by Campa and Coney (1983) is the largest tectonostratigraphic terrane of Mexico and is the primary host of the VMS districts. The Guerrero terrane was initially subdivided into three subterranes (Campa and Coney, 1983) the Teloloapan, Zihuatanejo and Huetamo. However, recently (Centeno-García et al., 1993) Zihuatanejo and Huetamo have been considered a single subterrane. Other subterranes are Fresnillo-Zacatecas, Arcelia, Guanajuato and Papanoa-las Ollas-Camalotito (Fig. 3). Most significant in terms of VMS deposits are the Teloloapan, Fresnillo-Zacatecas, Guanajuato, and the Zihuatanejo-Huetamo subterranes.

Teloloapan Subterrane

The Teloloapan subterrane is dominated by calc-alkaline mafic volcanics, with lesser felsic volcanic rocks intercalated with greywacke-shales and limestones (Talavera et al., 1993). Fossils yield Late Jurassic – Early Cretaceous ages; no older basement rocks are recognized (Campa and Coney, 1983). This assemblage is metamorphosed up to greenschist facies and is often strongly deformed. Age relationships are grossly constrained by biostratigraphy of interlayered reefal limestones giving a general age of Hauterivian-Aptian, Aptian- Albian (Campa and Coney, 1983). The Teloloapan subterrane is interpreted as a calc-alkaline volcanic arc complex, composed of at least three lithotectonic elements (Monod et al., 1993).

- Paleozoic or Triassic metavolcanic and metasedimentary rocks of the Tierra Caliente complex and the Taxco Schist that forms the structural or stratigraphic basement
- Upper Jurassic to Lower Cretaceous andesitic to rhyolitic volcanic and sedimentary rocks that unconformably overly the basement assemblages.
- Mid-Upper Cretaceous limestones and clastic sediments.

Lower Tertiary felsic-intermediate volcanic and clastic rocks and Neogene to Quaternary volcanic rocks of the Trans-Mexican volcanic belt unconformably overlie the Teloloapan subterrane (Sedlock et al., 1993).

VMS deposits in the Teloloapan subterrane occur in the Upper Jurassic-Lower Cretaceous arc volcanic rocks in four districts (Miranda-Gasca, 1995),

- Tizapa-Esmeralda-Santa Rosa
- Azulaquez-Tlanilpa
- Rey de Plata
- Campo Morado-Suriana

Tizapa

The Tizapa mine (Fig. 3; Table 1) is a producing VMS deposit, operated by Servicios Industriales Peñoles S.A. de C.V. (Giles and García, 2000). The ore bodies are stratabound at or near the contact of footwall plagioclase-porhyritic sericitic and or chlorite schists interpreted as a bi-modal andesitic-rhyolitic sequence. The immediate footwall is interpreted to be a felsic tuff of variable thickness. The deposit is strongly deformed with west verging folding and imbricate thrust faults (Lewis and Rhys, 2000). The hangingwall sequence consists of locally carbonaceous phyllite and limestone (Lewis and Rhys, 2000). The mineralogy of the deposit is massive pyrite with sphalerite, chalcopyrite, galena, sulfosalts and rare stannite (Miranda-Gasca, 1995). The Esmeralda lens is located about 1 km Northeast of the Tizapa mine and may occupy a higher stratigraphic interval than the Tizapa deposit.

Azulaquez-Tlanilpa area

The Azulaquez-Tlanipa area consists of at least 15 sulphide occurrences (Miranda-Gasca, 1995). The deposit area is underlain by a bi-modal sequence of calc-alkaline volcanic rocks and intercalated sediments (Rhys et al., 2000). The lower portions of the stratigraphy are mafic volcanic rocks overlain by siliclastic sediments that form the immediate footwall to the massive sulphides. The hangingwall to the massive sulphides are felsic tuffs.

Rey de Plata

The Rey de Plata deposit (Fig. 3; Table 1) is operated by Servicios Industriales Peñoles S.A. de C.V. (Giles and García, 2000). The Rey de Plata area has several sulphide lenses and ore bodies the largest of which is the Tehuixtla followed by the Rey de Plata and Antares lenses, all of which are inferred to be hosted at the same stratigraphic interval. Two small lenses, Virgo and Libra, are at a higher stratigraphic interval (Miranda-Gasca, 1995). The immediate footwall is andesitic volcanic rocks which are conformably overlain by felsic volcanic rocks interbedded with black shales. Fine grained siliclastic sediments are overthrust on the volcanic sequence. Felsic volcaniclastic rocks generally immediately underlie the sulphides and fine grained sediments form the immediate hangingwall. The mafic and felsic rocks from the immediate mine stratigraphy are enriched in LREE and depleted in HREE indicating an evolved island-arc origin (Miranda-Gasca, 1995). The Tehuixtla lens is hosted in felsic volcanic rocks altered to a quartz-sericite pyrite assemblage and is zoned with a pyrite, chalcopyrite lower lens and a sphalerite, sulfosalt, galena dominated upper zone, capped by a thin jasper layer (Miranda-Gasca, 1995).

Campo Morado

The Campo Morado (Fig. 3; Table 1) volcanogenic massive sulphide deposits occur in a lower Cretaceous, bimodal, calc-alkaline volcanic sequence in a northerly trending belt in the Guerrero Terrane in northeastern Guerrero, Mexico. More then 20 massive sulphide lenses are recognized in the sequence (Miranda-Gasca, 1995; Oliver et al., 2000). At Campo Morado, massive sulphide deposits occur in a sequence of felsic to intermediate flows and tuffs, and heterolithic fragmental rocks. Many deposits occur in the area and at least four of these have had sufficient work to develop a resource figure (Oliver et al., 2000). Most of the deposits are in the upper part of the felsic sequence or at the contact with stratigraphically overlying, fine-grained chemical and clastic sedimentary rocks. The age of the felsic section is constrained by preliminary U-Pb data to be approximately 145 Ma or Lowest Cretaceous. Limited paleontology data support a Lower Cretaceous age for the sedimentary rocks in the section (Oliver et al., 2000).

Suriana

The Suriana deposit is located 5 km south of the Campo Morado district (Fig. 3; Table 1). The deposit was operated sporadically by Servicios Industriales Peñoles S.A. de C.V. between 1925-1942 producing high grade gold, silver and lead ore from oxidized material (Giles and García, 2000). The deposit is hosted in a dominantly andesitic volcanic sequence with volumetrically minor dacite which is the immediate footwall to the sulphides. The hangingwall consists of variably calcareous sandstones and fine grained clastic sediments.

Zihuatanejo-Huetamo Subterrane

The Zihuatanejo subterrane is made up of a series of complexes. The oldest of which is the Arteaga Complex that represents the basement upon which the arc was built. The Arteaga complex is comprised of up to 60 % sedimentary rocks and the rest mafic flows/intrusions and diorite intrusions. The Arteaga complex has Triassic aged radiolarian chert. The arc sequence, developed on the Arteaga complex, consists of a sequence of sediments and volcanic rocks. Magmatism is dated between 137-71.3 Ma (Ruiz and Centeno Garcia, 2000).

Cuale

The Cuale District (Fig. 3; Table 1) is hosted by a north-south elongated window, or roof pendant, which consists of Mesozoic volcanic and sedimentary rocks, and is roughly 25 by 5 km in size (Hall and Gomez-Torres, 2000c). Within this window are two felsic complexes that host the massive sulphide deposits of the Cuale and El Bramador Districts. The Cuale District consists of nineteen deposits that are past producers, plus an additional six that received work in the past and may have recorded some minor production. The total aggregate production is just over 2 million tonnes of sulphide (Hall and Gomez-Torres, 2000c; Giles and García, 2000). The Cuale district is hosted by the Zihuatanejo subterrane which generally consists of calc-alkaline andesitic to rhyolitic volcanics and interbeds of sediments. The deposits are hosted in a lower Cretaceous felsic volcanic sequence with a dacitic footwall generally occurring as flows or intrusions. The immediate host to the massive sulphides is the "ore-zone pyroclastics" consisting of fine tuff, lapilli tuff and breccias that are intercalated with the shale beds. The lapilli tuff fragments are generally dacitic, however, fragments of andesite, schist, mudstone and pumice have been observed. The estimated thickness of this unit is thought to be a maximum of 300 m. The hangingwall consists of dacitic tuffs (Berrocal and Querol, 1991).

The El Bramador district is located about 10 km SW of the Cuale district and has seen minor production in the 1800's. Deposits in this district occupy a similar stratigraphic interval at the top of a felsic sequence and are hosted by, or interlayered with, fine grained sediments (Berrocal and Querol, 1991).

Several sulphide deposits occur in the Cuale-El Bramador area such as the La América mine, El Rubí, and El Desmoronado (Table 1). These sulphide lenses are hosted in an analogous stratigraphic position as the Cuale and El Bramador districts with a felsic footwall and sedimentary hangingwall (Miranda-Gasca, 1995).

La Minita

The La Minita deposit (Fig. 3; Table 1) was mined by Servicios Industriales Peñoles S.A. de C.V., during the 1970's through to the 1990's (Giles and García, 2000). The lower most stratigraphic unit in the immediate mine area is a lower andesite to basalt sequence which is overlain by felsic volcanic rocks that host the baritic lenses. The hangingwall sequence consists of sandstones, shales and reefal limestones (Ortigoza-Cruz, 1988; Giles and García, 2000). The main deposit at La Minita is Vulcano, which is domal in shape and reaches a maximum thickness of 70 m. Several smaller lenses are also recognized at the same stratigraphic interval. Magnetite replacement bodies are hosted at the same startigraphic interval as the baritic lenses and grade laterally into sedimentary units and tuffs (Ortigoza-Cruz, 1988).

The Fresnillo-Guanajuato Subterrane

The oldest unit recognized of the Fresnillo-Guanajuato subterrane is the Triassic Zacatecas Formation, which likely represents the basement assemblages, upon which the arc sequences were built (Ruiz and Centeno-Garcia, 2000). The sequence was deformed and metamorphosed prior to the development of the Cretaceous arc assemblage. The Zacateas Formation is tectonically overlain by the Cretaceous arc volcanics (Ruiz and Centeno-Garcia, 2000). The arc sequence in the Fresnillo-Guanajuato subterrane consists of mafic, with lesser felsic, volcanic rocks interbedded with sandstone, chert and limestone.

VMS deposits in the Fresnillo-Guanajuato subterrane occur in both the Triassic basement and the Cretaceous arc volcanics (Miranda-Gasca, 1995). Deposits inferred to be hosted by the Triassic basement assemblage have been described previously and consist of the Francisco I Madero and Los Gavilanes/Guanajuato areas. Deposits in the Cretaceous arc include the San Nicolás deposit described below.

San Nicolás

The San Nicolás deposit (Fig. 3; Table 1) is hosted in an assemblage of marine volcanic and sedimentary rocks of Upper Jurassic – Lower Cretaceous age known as the Chilitos Formation (Johnson et al, 2000; de Cserna 1976). Rocks of this assemblage include deformed and lower greenschist-facies felsic to mafic flows, volcaniclastic rocks, chert, limestone and clastic sedimentary strata that form isolated exposures in an area largely covered by Quaternary sediments. From the few faunal assemblages that have been studied, at least part of the Chilitos Formation falls in the Tithonian to Hauterivian age range (Johnson et al., 2000), or approximately 152-124 Ma.

The San Nicolás deposit is hosted within volcanic and fine grained sedimentary rocks of the Chilitos Formation (Johnson et al., 2000). Felsic flow dome complexes, hosted within a mafic volcanic and sediment complex, form intervals up to 300 m thick and are the immediate footwall to sulphide mineralization at San Nicolás. Stratigraphic interpretations indicate two levels of mineralization that merge at the southeastern part of the deposit. Hangingwall units consist of black mudstones and mafic flows and sills (Johnson et al., 2000).

Peru-Ecuador

Extension and associated volcanism and sedimentation began in the Late Jurassic and continued until the Late Cretaceous in marginal basins along the western margin of Peru and Ecuador. Three distinct but interconnected sub-basins are recognized; the Loncones, Huarmey and Cañete basins (Fig. 6). These basins extend north into Ecuador where volcanism, coeval with the Lacones basal sequence, are recognized in the Macuchi and Célica formations that host massive sulphide deposits (Macellari, 1988).

In general the depositional environment of the western part of the basins was influenced by volcanism where the eastern part of the basin generally lacks volcanic activity and is characterized by siliciclastic and carbonate platform sedimentation (Steinmüller et al., 2000). The tectonic environment of these basins is generally characterized as rifted continental marginal basins (Jaillard et al., 1990).

The Lancones basin, in northern Peru hosts deposits in the Tambo Grande district. The Lacones basin can be extended intermittently northwards through Ecuador where it is coeval with the Macuchi and Célica formations that host the La Plata and the Macuchi massive sulphide deposits (Macellari, 1988; O'Dowd, 1999). The Huarmey basin hosts the Maria Teresa deposit and the Cañete basin hosts, the majority of Peruvian VMS deposits including; the Aurora Augusta, Perubar, Palma, Balducho, Raul, and Cerro Lindo (Vidal, 1987; Steinmüller et al., 2000).

Lacones Basin

The Tambo Grande series of deposits (Fig. 6; Table 1) are located in the Lancones basin, hosted within the pre-mid Cretaceous Ereo Formation. Several deposits are known and are currently the subject of a feasibility study; these include the TG-1, TG-3 and B5 (Table 1). These deposits are proximal to dacitic domes and associated volcaniclastic rocks emplaced within tholeiitic to transitional subalkaline volcanic rocks (Tegart et al., 2000). Synvolcanic faults and subbasins localized the distribution of volcanic rocks and accumulations of the sulphides. The Tambo Grande deposits represent some of the largest accumulations of sulphides ever discovered, comparable with deposits in the Iberian Pyrite Belt. The oxide cap at TG1, is the host to significant gold and silver mineralization, and likely represents a primary seafloor oxide precipitate (Tegart et al., 2000).

The Macuchi Formation (Fig. 6) is an Upper Cretaceous-Eocene aged basin located along the western flank of the north-south trending Cordillera Occidental of central Ecuador. The Macuchi Formation forms a N-S trending belt about 50 km in width and is the main constituent of the Cordillera Occidental. The formation, with a minimum thickness of 8,000 m, is composed mainly of fine grained marine sediments interbedded with mafic volcanic intervals. The Macuchi Formation is conformably overlain by the Silante Formation (O'Dowd, 1999). Many sulphide occurrences occur within the Macuchi Formation, the most important of them are the La Plata and Macuchi deposit, which geologically are similar but are separated by about 60 km. The hangingwall to the La Plata deposit is massive to brecciated andesite locally with hematite and jasper intervals near the mineralization. The footwall to the sulphides appears to be brecciated dacites-andesites, strong hydrothermal alteration makes this identification uncertain. Sulphides are massive to semimassive pyrite, chalcopyrite, sphalerite and lesser galena bornite and chalcocite (O'Dowd, 1999; Chiaradia and Fontboté, 2000).

Huarmey and Cañete basins

The Huarmey and Cañete basins (Fig. 6; Table 1) hosts several baritic zinc deposits in the Casma Group. The Casma Group comprises a 6,000 to 9,000 m thick sequence of submarine volcanic rocks and interbedded sediments ranging from about Albian to Cenomanian in age (Vidal, 1987). The western facies of the Casma Group consists of basaltic to andesitic volcanics and derived sediments with lesser sedimentary interbeds (Vidal, 1987). The eastern facies is characterized by a sequence of andesitic to dacitic volcanics and derived sediments with lenses of shale and limestone.

The María Teresa deposit is located with the Huarmey basin and is hosted by felsic tuffs of the Lower Cretaceous Casma Group (Vidal, 1987; Steinmüller et al., 2000). The mineralization consists of pyrite, galena, sphalerite, chalcopyrite lenses along with stratabound baritic zones up to 12 m thick. María Teresa is the only VMS occurrence known in the Huarmey basin (Steinmüller et al., 2000).

The Aurora Augusta deposit is hosted in the western facies of the Casma Group. The deposit consists of fine grained monomineralic barite (Vidal, 1987; Steinmüller et al., 2000).

The Perubar area collectively comprises the

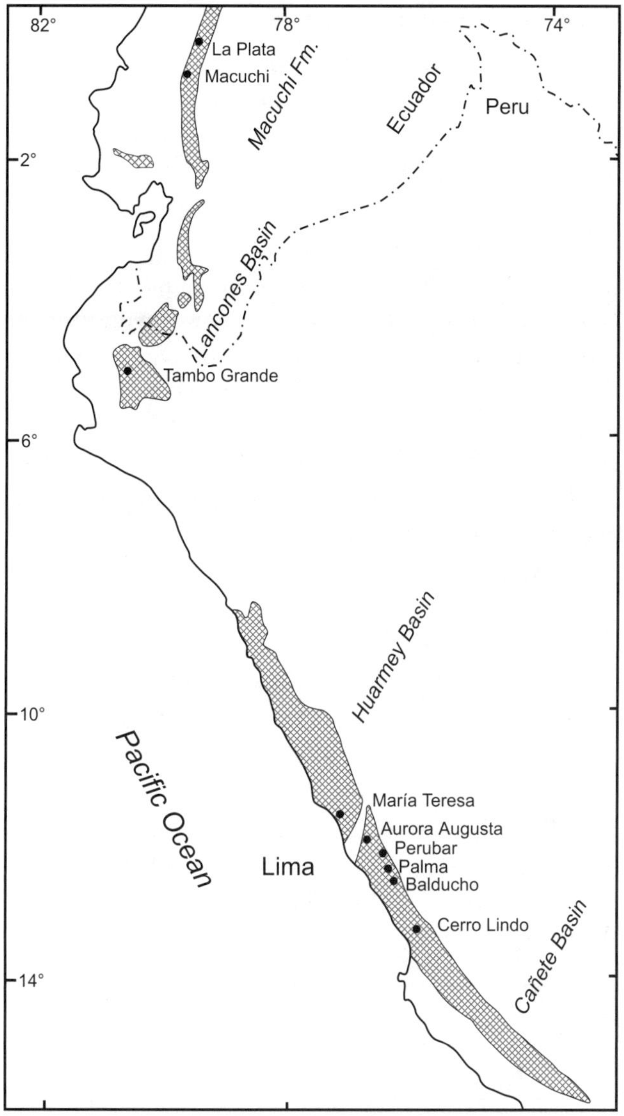

Figure 6. Geologic map of the Lower Cretaceous volcanic basins of western Peru and Ecuador, with VMS districts. After O'Dowd, (1999) Steinmüller et al. (2000), Tegart et al. (2000), Vidal (1987).

Leonila Graciela, Juanita, Santa Cecilia and Elenita deposits. This district is hosted by the eastern facies of the Casma Group that forms a roof pendant in the Late Cretaceous Coastal Batholith. The mineralized zones are hosted by mafic volcaniclastic rocks with interbeds of shales and limestones. The massive sulphide barite lenses consist of pyrite, pyrrhotite and sphalerite with increasing concentrations of barite towards the top of the lens. The sulphide-barite lenses are underlain by a stockwork zone that is strongly silicified and consists of pyrite and sphalerite veinlets and disseminations (Vidal, 1987; Polliand and Fontboté, 2000; Steinmüller et al., 2000).

The Palma deposit is hosted by rocks of the eastern facies of the Casma Group. The deposit is zoned, with pyrite and pyrrhotite at the base, pyrite, sphalerite and galena higher in the lense and barite dominated in the upper portions of the lense. The host rocks are mafic volcaniclastic rocks with lesser shales and limestones (Vidal, 1987; Steinmüller et al., 2000). The Cerro Lindo deposit is also hosted in the Casma Group forming a large baritic sulphide lense at the lithologic contact between mafic volcanic rocks and pelagic sediments (Ly, 2000).

LATE CRETACEOUS

Peralvillo Formation, Dominican Republic

Basaltic lavas of the Peralvillo Formation host the copper-rich VMS deposit at Sabana Potrero, where drilling has intersected pyrite and chalcopyrite-rich massive sulphides hosted by massive basaltic flows (Childe, 2000). Trace element geochemistry indicates that the basalts are similar to MORB (Donnelley and Rodgers, 1980; Espaillat et al., 1989) and are interpreted to have formed within a late Cretaceous back arc spreading centre, immediately following a reversal in subduction polarity and cessation of Lower Cretaceous primitive island arc volcanism (Draper and Lewis, 1991).

Calima Terrane, Colombia

The Calima Terrane in Colombia (Fig. 2; Table 1) is an ophiolitic sequence formed during the Late Cretaceous and hosts several VMS deposits. The volcanic sequences are generally mafic to intermediate volcanic rocks with pelagic sediments. The El Alacrán deposit is located in the western Cordillera and consists of sedimentary rocks interbedded with mafic and locally felsic volcanics (Jaramillo, 2000). A small gold resource has been identified in the oxidized cap. The Guadalupe deposit is located in the central Cordillera and hosted in the San Pablo formation which consists of sediments and mafic volcanic rocks. In addition, several other base metal sulphide occurrences have been identified in volcanic rocks of the Calima Terrane (Jaramillo, 2000).

TERTIARY

El Cobre Formation, Cuba

The Paleogene volcanic arc of eastern Cuba is thought to host felsic volcanic associated massive sulphides (Russell et al., 2000). Cobre Formation, is Lower Paleocene to Upper Eocene sequence of agglomerates, tuffs and andesitic flow breccias, along with local felsic pyroclastics, that host some Cu, Au and barite deposits, such as the El Cobre deposit. Much of the historic mineralization that was mined at the El Cobre deposit was in cross-cutting veins of possible epithermal origin although stratabound lenses of lead-zinc mineralization also occur. Between 1544 to 1998 El Cobre has produced an estimated 3 million tonnes of ore at grades ranging between 2 and 20 % copper.

Wagwater Group, Jamaica

The Wagwater Group, in eastern Jamaica, is a fault-bounded sequence of Paleocene to Early Eocene volcanic and volcaniclastic strata, conglomerate and minor limestone and evaporites that hosts several base and precious metal showings (Fenton, 1987). Water depths in the trough were variable, as evidenced by the presence of shallow water evaporates and deep water turbidite sequences.

The Hope Mine produced small scale copper and lead intermittently since the 1850's. The deposit is stratabound, moderately dipping pods or lenses of massive to semimassive pyrite, sphalerite, galena and chalcopyrite at the contact between Wagwater Formation volcaniclastic rocks and a plagioclase porphyritic andesite flow or sill, known as the Hope Mine Member (Carby, 1984; Russell et al., 2000). The genesis of massive sulphides at the Hope Mine is unclear. Carby and Jackson (1980) compare the deposit to Kuroko-type VMS deposits and Kesler et al. (1990) interpret the deposit to have formed as a replacement or vein.

QUATERNARY-HOLOCENE

Off the coast of Mexico, Central and South America are a series of spreading centres which define divergent plate margins. Associated with these are hydrothermal systems and seafloor sulphide mineralization (Rona, 1988). These are all characterized by mafic volcanic rocks and variable degrees of sedimentation. Often in the case of Guyamas Basin and the Galapogos spreading centre, these hydrothermal systems are in heavily sedimented rifts. Sulphide mineralization has been located at many sites along these spreading centres (Fig. 7), although much of these ridges remains to be explored. These sites represent modern day analogues to mafic volcanic and sediment associated massive sulphide deposits seen throughout Latin America.

SUMMARY

Given the geologic and geographic diversity of Latin America it is no surprise that volcanogenic massive sulphide deposits are found in rocks with a wide range of ages and geochemical affinities. Summarizing Table One provides a reasonable approximation of the distribution of deposits in Latin America. Figure 8A gives the average size of the deposits grouped into Precambrian, Paleozoic,

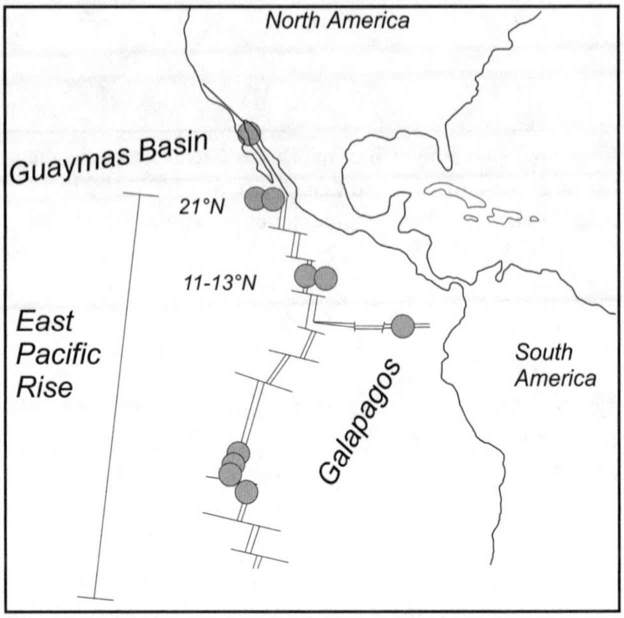

Figure 7. Active seafloor vent systems of the Eastern Pacific (Rona, 1988).

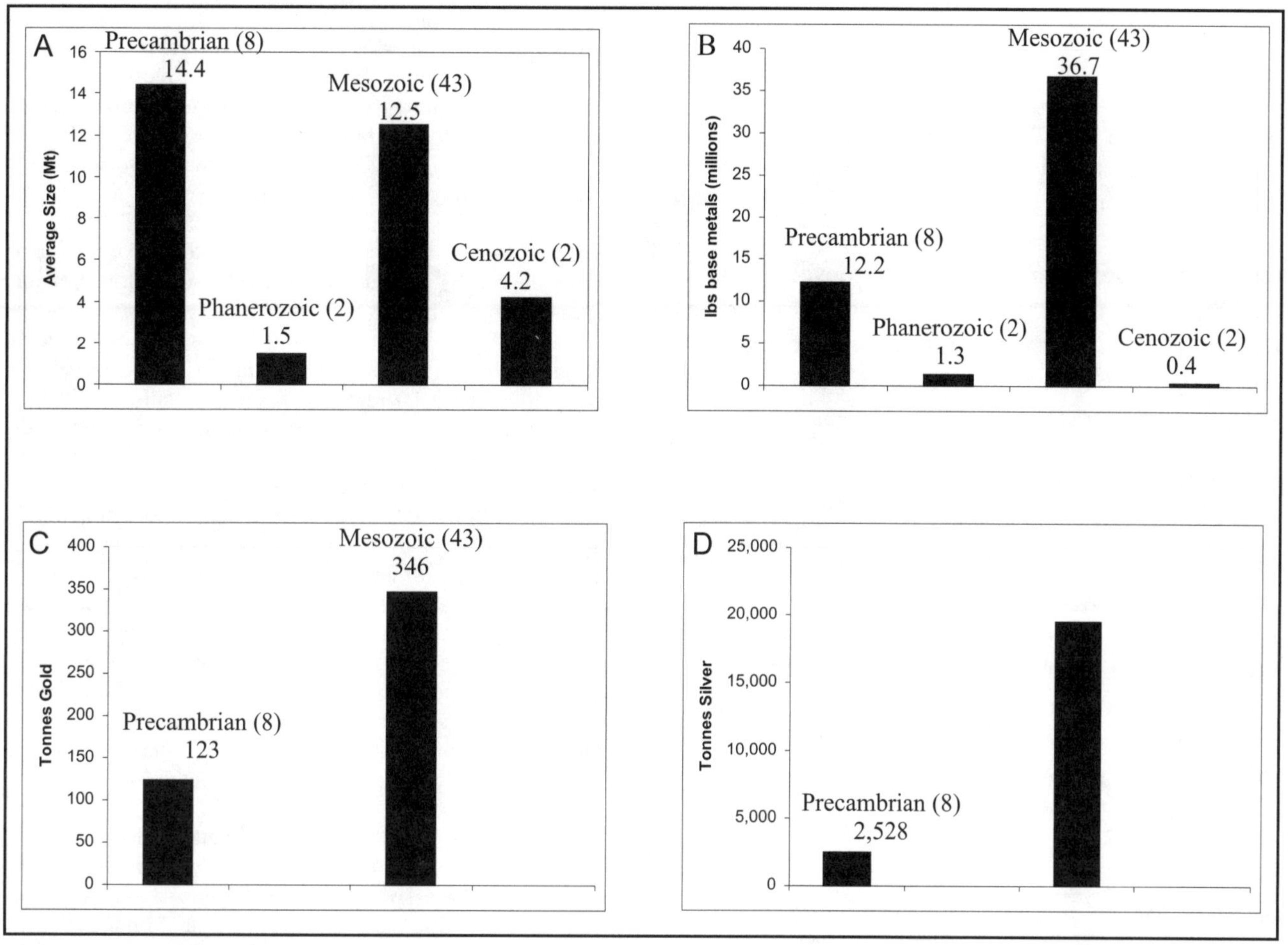

Figure 8. A. Average size of deposits by age group (Table 1). B. Pounds of contained base metal by age group (Table 1). C. Tonnes of contained gold by age group (Table 1). D. Tonnes of contained silver by age group (Table 1)

Mesozoic and Cenozoic. The average size of Precambrian deposits is 14.4 Mt based on an average of 8 deposits where the average size of the Mesozoic deposits is 12.5 Mt based on an average of 43 deposits. The sum of the contained metal (Fig. 8B,C,D) shows that the bulk of the resources are in the Mesozoic rocks however the Precambrian deposits have a total of 12.2 million pounds of base metals from 8 deposits, or an average of 1.5 million pounds of base metals per deposit. The Mesozoic deposits have a total of 36.7 million pounds of contained metal from a total of 43 deposits, or an average of 850,000 pounds per deposit.

The disparity in terms of numbers of deposits seen in Mesozoic versus Precambrian rocks as well as the apparent metal content and size is likely a reflection of the high prospectivity of the younger arc rocks as well as a general lack of exploration in the Precambrian terranes for base metal deposits. The Lower Cretaceous rocks are very prospective for VMS deposits, they tend to be associated with local accumulations of felsic volcanic rocks in submarine environments which are excellent localities to form polymetallic deposits. These deposits make excellent exploration targets and have a relatively long history of exploration and development particularly in the Caribbean and Mexico. As a result there are many VMS occurrences in these young rocks and the average size tends to be rather small despite the inclusion of some very large deposits such as Tambo Grande and San Nicolás.

The Precambrian Terranes of South America do not have a long history of base metal exploration, due to the relatively remote locations and poor infrastructure. These areas have generally been the focus of gold exploration. As a result few VMS deposits are known from these areas and the ones that are known tend to be larger as needed to justify development. It is likely with continued exploration and improved infrastructure in South America there will continue to be new discoveries of VMS deposits in the Precambrian Terranes of South America.

ACKNOWLEDGMENTS

This paper represents a compilation and summary of many of the deposits included within this volume. We would like to thank the many authors, who contributed papers, who's combined efforts will make the volume a significant contribution to VMS deposits in Latin America. Amelia Logan and an anonymous reviewer are thanked for their constructive reviews of this manuscript. Rachel Browne assisted in editing and drafting of figures.

REFERENCES

de Abreu, F.R. and Belo de Oliveira, O.A. 1998. Geologia e ocorrências de zinco e chumbo do Prospecto Salobro, Porteirinha, MG. In Anais do 40o Congresso Brasileira de Geologia, Sociedade Brasileira de Geologia, Núcleo de Minas Gerais, Boletim 15, pp. 140.

Ally, L. 1985. Volcanogenic massive sulfide potential in Northern Guayana. Memoria I, Simposium Amazonico, Boletin de Geología, Publicación Especial Nº 10, Ministerio de Energia y Minas. Dirección de Geología, 431-442.

de Almeida, F.F.M. and Hasui Y. (Editors) 1984. O Pré-Cambriano do Brasil. Edgard Blücher, São Paulo.

Ametrano, S., Etcheverry, R., Echeveste, H., Godeas, M. and Zubia, M. 2000. VMS district of Tierra del Fuego, Argentina. In Volcanogenic Massive Sulfide Deposits of Latin America. Edited by R.L. Sherlock and M.A.V. Logan, Mineral Deposit Division, Geological Association of Canada Publication.

Araújo, S.M. 1986. Petrologia e Mineralizações Sulfetadas da Seqüência Vulcano-Sedimentar de Palmeirópolis, GO. M.Sc. dissertation, Universidade de Brasília, Brasília, Brazil.

Araújo, S.M. 2000, The Palmeirópolis deposit, Tocantins State, Brazil: a typical metamorphosed volcanogenic massive sulfide deposit. In Volcanogenic Massive Sulfide Deposits of Latin America. Edited by R.L. Sherlock and M.A.V. Logan, Mineral Deposit Division, Geological Association of Canada Publication.

Araújo, S.M., Gorton, M.P. and Scott, S.D. 1996. Os anfibolitos enriquecidos em elementos traços da seqüência vulcano-sedimentar de Palmeirópolis, Tocantins: uma ferramenta na prospecção de metais básicos na região. In Anais do 39o Congresso Brasileira Geologia, Sociedade Brasileira de Geologia, Núcleo de Bahia - Sergipe, Volume 3, pp. 178-180.

Baars, F.J. 1997. The São Francisco Craton. In Greenstone Belts. Edited by M.J. de Wit and L.D. Ashwal. Clarendon Press, Oxford, Chapt. 5.5, 529-557.

Baltazar, O.F. and Pedreira, A.J. 1998. Associações litofaciológicas. In Projeto Rio das Velhas – Mapa Geológico Integrado, Escala 1:100.000, e Texto Explicativo. Edited by M. Zucchetti and O.F. Baltazar. Departamento Nacional de Produção Mineral / Companhia de Pesquisa de Recursos Minerais – Belo Horizonte, CD-ROM, pp. 43-48.

Barbosa, J.S.F. 1996. O embasamento arqueano e proterozóico inferior do Estado da Bahia. In Geologia da Bahia: texto explicativo para o mapa geológico ao milionésimo. Edited by J.S.F. Barbosa and J.M.L. Dominguez. Superintendência de Geologia e Recursos Minerais, Secretaria da Industria, Comércio e Mineração do Estado da Bahia, Salvador.

Berrocal, G.L. and Querol, F.S. 1991. Geological description of the Cuale District ore deposits, Jalisco, Mexico. The Geology of North America, vol. P-3 Economic Geology, Mexico, The Geological Society of America, 1991 p. 355-363.

Biste and Gourlay, 2000 Geology and Setting of the Miguela A-Zone, Guarayos Greenstone Belt, Eastern Bolivia. In Volcanogenic Massive Sulfide Deposits of Latin America. Edited by R.L. Sherlock and M.A.V. Logan, Mineral Deposit Division, Geological Association of Canada Publication.

Bogdanov, Y.V., Gur'yanova, V.N. and Mitayes, M. 1966. Outline of copper deposits of Cuba. International Geology Review, 8, 1218-1225.

Borba, R.P. 1998. O Magmatismo Ácido e sua Relação com a Mineralização Aurífera de Bico de Pedra, Greenstone Belt Rio das Velhas, Quadrilátero Ferrífero, Minas Gerais. M.Sc. dissertation, Universidade Estadual de Campinas, Campinas, Brazil.

Bottrill, T.J., Cortina, F.F. and Raman, K.S. 2000. Los Mangos-San Fernando deposit, Santa Clara, Cuba, geology and mineralization in a Cretaceous volcanic arc. In Volcanogenic Massive Sulfide Deposits of Latin America. Edited by R.L. Sherlock and M.A.V. Logan, Mineral Deposit Division, Geological Association of Canada Publication.

Broili, C., Klohn, M. and Hodder, R.W. 2000. Exploration, geology and mineral deposits of the Fin del Mundo VMS project, Tierra del Fuego, Argentina. In Volcanogenic Massive Sulfide Deposits of Latin America. Edited by R.L. Sherlock and M.A.V. Logan, Mineral Deposit Division, Geological Association of Canada Publication.

Campa, M.F. and Coney, P.L., 1983, Tectonostratigraphic terranes and mineral resource distribution in Mexico: Canadian Journal of Earth Sciences, v. 20, p. 1040-1051.

Camus, F., 1985. Los yacimientos estratoligados de Cu, Pb-Zn y Ag de Chile. In Geología y recursos minerales de Chile. Edited by J. Frutos, R. Oyarzún and M. Pincheira. Universidad de Concepción, Tome II, p. 538-635.

Carby, B.E. and Jackson, T.A. 1980. Kuroko-type mineralization in Jamaica. Abstract presented at the 9th Caribbean Geological Conference, Santo Domingo, Dominican Republic.

Carlson, G.,G. 1977. Geology of the Bailadores, Venezuela, massive sulfide deposit. Economic Geology , vol. 72, p.1131-1141.

de Carvalho, S.G. 1990. Geologia, petrologia e metalogenia da seqüência vulcano-sedimentar de Alpinópolis, Minas Gerais. Ph.D. thesis, Universidade de São Paulo, São Paulo, Brazil.

de Carvalho, S.G., Soares, P.C. and Barbour, A.P. 1992. Mineralizações nos terrenos granito-greenstone de Alpinópolis e Fortaleza de Minas. Universidade Estadual Paulista, Geociências, 11: 19-47.

Case, J.E., Holcombe, T.L. and Martin, R.G. 1984. Map of geologic provinces in the Caribbean region. Geological Society of America Memoir 162, 1-30.

Cassedane, J.P. 1972. Catalogue déscriptif des gîtes de plomb du Brésil. Ph.D. thesis, Université de Clermont-Ferrand, Clermont-Ferrand, France.

Centeno-Garcia, E., Ruiz, J., Coney, P.J. and Patchett, P.J. 1993. Guerrero Terrane of Mexico: Its role in the southern Cordillera from new geochemical data. Geology, vol. 21, pp. 419-422, May 1993.

Channer, D.A. and Anderson, P.F.N. 2000. Volcanogenic massive sulphide occurrences and potential in Venezuela, with emphasis on the Guayana shield. In Volcanogenic Massive Sulfide Deposits of Latin America. Edited by R.L. Sherlock and M.A.V. Logan, Mineral Deposit Division, Geological Association of Canada Publication.

Chiaradia, M. and Fontboté, L. 2000. Gold-rich VHMS deposits of the Western Cordillera of Ecuador: mineralogy. lead isotope and metal geochemistry. In Volcanogenic Massive Sulfide Deposits of Latin America. Edited by R.L. Sherlock and M.A.V. Logan, Mineral Deposit Division, Geological Association of Canada Publication.

Childe, F.C. 2000. Geology and tectonic setting of volcanogenic massive sulfide mineralization in the Greater Antiles. In Volcanogenic Massive Sulfide Deposits of Latin America. Edited by R.L. Sherlock and M.A.V. Logan, Mineral Deposit Division, Geological Association of Canada Publication.

Collao, S. and Alfaro, G. 1982. Mineralización sulfurada de hierro, cobre y zinc de la Cordillera de la Costa del sur de Chile. Revista Geológica de Chile, N° 15, p. 41-47.

de Cserna, Z. 1976. Geology of the Fresnillo area, Zacatecas, Mexico. Geological Society of America Bulletin, 87: 1191-1199.

Cunha, J.C.C. and Fróes, R.J.B. 1994. Komatiitos com textura spinifex do Greenstone Belt de Umburanas, Bahia. Companhia Baiana de Pesquisa Mineral, Série Arquivos Abertos, No. 7.

Donnelly, T. W. and Rogers, J. J. W. 1967. Crust vs. Mantle derivation of eastern Antillean igneous rocks [abs.]. EOS (American Geophysical Union Transactions), v. 48, p. 253.

Donnelly, T.W. and Rogers, J.J.W. 1980. Igneous series in island arcs: the northeast Caribbean compared with worldwide island arc assemblages. Bulletin Volcanologique, 43, 347-382.

Draper, G. and Lewis, J.F. 1982. Petrology, deformation, and tectonic significance of the Amina Schist, northern Dominican Republic. In Transactions of the 9th Caribbean Geological Conference, Santo Domingo, Dominican Republic. pp. 53-64

Draper, G. and Lewis, J.F. 1991. Metamorphic belts in central Hispaniola. In Geologic and Tectonic Development of the North American – Caribbean plate boundary in Hispaniola. Edited by P. Mann, G. Draper, and J.F. Lewis. The Geological Society of America, Special Paper 262, 29-45.

Espaillat, J. 1995. Revisión Litogeoquímica de la Formación Maimón. In Premier Congreso Nacional de Geología y Ciencias Afines de la Hispaniola y Reuníon de Proyecto IGCP 364, Santo Domingo.

Espaillat, J. Bloise, G, MacVeigh, J.G. and Lewis, J.F. 1989. Petrography and geochemistry of mafic rocks of the Peralvillo Formation in the Sabana Potrero area, Central Dominican Republic. In Transactions of the 12th Caribbean Geological Conference, St. Croix, Virgin Islands, 190-199.

Fenton, A. 1987. The (non-bauxite) metallic mineral potential of Jamaica. In Proceedings of a workshop on the status of Jamaican geology. Edited by R. Ahmad. The Geological Society of Jamaica, Special Issue 1987, 269-281.

Feoktistov, V.P., Aniyatov, I.A. and Norman, A. 1983. Metallogeny of western Cuba, International Geology Review, 25, 309-318.

Fleischer, R. and Espourteille, F.E. 1998. The Boquira Lead-Zinc Mine in central Bahia, Brazil. In Base Metal Deposits of Brazil. Edited by M.daG. da Silva and A. Misi. Ministério de Minas e Energia / Companhia de Pesquisa de Recursos Minerais / Departamento Nacional de Produção Mineral, Belo Horizonte, 44-53.

Franklin, J., Bertoni, C., Boudrie, M., Bout, J-P., Costelloe, D., Lillié, F., Sauvage, J-F., 2000. The Paul Isnard gold-copper occurrence, French Guiana: the first volcanogenic massive sulfide occurrence in the Guiana Shield. In Volcanogenic Massive Sulfide Deposits of Latin America. Edited by R.L. Sherlock and M.A.V. Logan, Mineral Deposit Division, Geological Association of Canada Publication.

Gibbs, A. K. and Barron, C. N. 1983. The Guiana shield reviewed. Episodes, Vol. 1983, No. 2, 7-14.

Gibbs, A. K. and Barron, C. N. 1993. Geology of the Guiana shield, Oxford University Press, 246 pp.

Giles, D.A. and García, J.F. 2000. Volcanogenic deposits in Mexico: the producing mines. In Volcanogenic Massive Sulfide Deposits of Latin America. Edited by R.L. Sherlock and M.A.V. Logan, Mineral Deposit Division, Geological Association of Canada Publication.

Gordillo , C. and Lencinas, A. 1979. Sierras Pampeanas de Córdoba y San Luis. II Simp. De Geol. Reg. Arg., Actas I: 577-650, Córdoba.

Gustin M.S. 1990. Stratigraphy and alteration of the host rocks, United Verde massive sulfide deposit, Jerome, Arizona. Economic Geology, vol. 85, p. 29-49.

Hall, B.V. and Gomez-Torres, P.P. 2000a. Geology and exploration of the Los Gavilanes deposit, Leon, Mexico – a bimodal siliciclastic volcanogenic massive sulfide deposit. In Volcanogenic Massive Sulfide Deposits of Latin America. Edited by R.L. Sherlock and M.A.V. Logan, Mineral Deposit Division, Geological Association of Canada Publication.

Hall, B.V. and Gomez-Torres, P.P. 2000b. The El Gordo volcanogenic massive sulfide deposit, Leon-Guanajuato district, central Mexico. In Volcanogenic Massive Sulfide Deposits of Latin America. Edited by R.L. Sherlock and M.A.V. Logan, Mineral Deposit Division, Geological Association of Canada Publication.

Hall, B.V. and Gomez-Torres, P.P. 2000c. Geology of the kuroko-type massive sulfide deposits of the Cuale district, Jalisco State, Mexico. In Volcanogenic Massive Sulfide Deposits of Latin America. Edited by R.L. Sherlock and M.A.V. Logan, Mineral Deposit Division, Geological Association of Canada Publication.

Holbek, P.M. and Daubeny, P.H. 2000. Geology of the San Antonio concession, Domincan Republic. In Volcanogenic Massive Sulfide Deposits of Latin America. Edited by R.L. Sherlock and M.A.V. Logan, Mineral Deposit Division, Geological Association of Canada Publication.

Jaillard E., Soler P., Carier G., Mourier T., (1990) Geodynamic evolution of the northern and central Andes during early to middle Mesozoic times: a Tethyan model, Journal of the Geological Society, London, v. 147, p. 1009-1022

Jaramillo, C. L. 2000. Marco geologico y potencial de SMV en Colombia. In Volcanogenic Massive Sulfide Deposits of Latin America. Edited by R.L. Sherlock and M.A.V. Logan, Mineral Deposit Division, Geological Association of Canada Publication.

Johnson, B.J., Montante-Martínez, A., Canela-Barboza, M. and Danielson, T.J. 2000. Geology of the San Nicolás deposit, Zacatecas, México. In Volcanogenic Massive Sulfide Deposits of Latin America. Edited by R.L. Sherlock and M.A.V. Logan, Mineral Deposit Division, Geological Association of Canada Publication.

Jost, H., Kuyumjian, R.M., Freitas, A.L.S., Costa, A.L.L., Nascimento, C.T.C., Vasconcelos, F.M., Galotti, L., Martins, M.C.A., Carvalho, M.N. and Condé, V.C. 1996. Geologia da porção norte do Greenstone Belt de Guarinos, GO. Revista Brasileira Geociências, 25: 51-60.

Kay S.M. Ramos V.A. and Kay R.W. 1984. Elementos mayoritarios y trazas de las vulcanitas ordovícicas de la Precordillera occidental: basaltos de rift oceánico temprano?próximo al margen continental. 9°Congreso Geológico Argentino. Pp.48-65. San Carlos de Bariloche.

Kerr, D. and Staff of Anglo American Brasil 2000 Volcanogenic Massive Sulphide Mineralisation in the Aripuanã District of Mato Grosso, Brazil. In Volcanogenic Massive Sulfide Deposits of Latin America. Edited by R.L. Sherlock and M.A.V. Logan, Mineral Deposit Division, Geological Association of Canada Publication.

Kesler, S.E., Levy, E. and Martin, C.F. 1990. Metallogenic evolution of the Caribbean Region. In The Caribbean Region. Edited by G. Dengo and J.E. Case. The Geological Society of America, Geology of North America Vol. H., 459-482.

Kesler, S.E., Russell, N., Reyes, C., Santos, L., Rodriguez, and Fondeur, L. 1991a. Geology of the Maimón Formation, Dominican Republic. In Geologic and Tectonic Development of the North American – Caribbean plate boundary in Hispaniola. Edited by P. Mann, G. Draper, and J.F. Lewis. The Geological Society of America, Special Paper 262, 173-185.

Kesler, S. E., Russell, N. and Bell, D. 1996. Gold-silver mineralization in Cuba and its geologic setting in the Greater Antilles. In Geology and Ore Deposits of the American Cordillera. Edited by A. R. Coyner and P. L. Fahey. Geological Society of Nevada Symposium Proceedings, Reno/Sparks, Nevada, April 1995. Pp. 1433-1441.

Kishida, A. 1979. Caracterização geológica e geoquímica das seqüências vulcanossedimentares do médio Rio Itapicuru (Bahia). M.Sc. dissertation, Universidade Federal da Bahia, Salvador, Brazil.

Leão Neto, R. and Olivatti, O. 1983. Projeto Palmeirópolis – Realtório de Etapa Preliminar. Departamento Nacional de Produção Mineral / Companhia de Pesquisa de Recursos Minerais, Goiânia.

Lewis, J.F. and Draper, G. 1990. Geology and tectonic evolution of the northern Caribbean margin. In The Caribbean Region. Edited by G. Dengo and J.E. Case. The Geological Society of America, Geology of North America Vol. H., pp. 77-140.

Lewis, J.F., Astacio, V.A., Espaillat, J. and Jimenez, J. 2000. The occurrence of volcanogenic massive sulfide deposits in the Maimon Formation, Domincan Republic; The Cerro de Maimon, Loma Pesada and Barbuito deposits. In Volcanogenic Massive Sulfide Deposits of Latin America. Edited by R.L. Sherlock and M.A.V. Logan, Mineral Deposit Division, Geological Association of Canada Publication.

Lewis, P.D. and Rhys, D.A. 2000. Structural geology and stratigraphic setting of the Tizapa mine, México state, México. In Volcanogenic Massive Sulfide Deposits of Latin America. Edited by R.L. Sherlock and M.A.V. Logan, Mineral Deposit Division, Geological Association of Canada Publication.

Lindberg, P.A. 1989. Precambrian ore deposits of Arizona. In Geologic Evolution of Arizona. Edited by J.P. Jenney and S.J. Reyolds, Arizona Geological Society Digest 17, p. 187-210.

Lobato, L.M., Baars, F.J. Jost, H., da Silva, M.G., Cunha, J.C. and Carvalho, S.G., (2000) The Potential for Volcanogenic Massive Sulphide Deposits in the Magmatic-Arc-Related Volcano-Sedimentary Belts in and Around the São Francisco Craton, Brazil. In Volcanogenic Massive Sulfide Deposits of Latin America. Edited by R.L. Sherlock and M.A.V. Logan, Mineral Deposit Division, Geological Association of Canada Publication.

Logan, M.A.V., Brodtkorb, M.K. and Schalamuk, I.B. 2000.

Mineral deposits associated with submarine volcanism in Argentina. In Volcanogenic Massive Sulfide Deposits of Latin America. Edited by R.L. Sherlock and M.A.V. Logan, Mineral Deposit Division, Geological Association of Canada Publication.

Ly Zevallos, P. 2000. Proyecto Cerro Lindo. In Volcanogenic Massive Sulfide Deposits of Latin America. Edited by R.L. Sherlock and M.A.V. Logan, Mineral Deposit Division, Geological Association of Canada Publication.

Macellari, C.E. 1988. Cretaceous paleogeography and depositional cycles of western South America. Journal of South American Earth Sciences, vol. 1, pp. 373-418.

Mascarenhas, J.d.F. and Silva, E.F.A. 1994. Greenstone Belt de Mundo Novo: Caracterização e implicações metalogenéticas e geotectônicas no Cráton do São Francisco. Companhia Baiana de Pesquisa Mineral, Série Arquivos Abertos, Vol. 5, 32p.

Mascarenhas, J.d.F., Pedreira, A.J.d.C.L., Misi, A., Motta, A.C., Sá, J.H.d.S. 1984. Província São Francisco. In O Pré-Cambriano do Brasil Edited by F.F.M. de Almeida and Y. Hasui. Edgard Blücher, São Paulo, Chapt. 4, pp. 46-122.

Miranda-Gasca, M.A. 1995. The volcanogenic massive sulfide and sedimentary exhalative deposits of the Guerrero terrane, Mexico. Unpublished Ph.D. Thesis, The University of Arizona, 294 pp.

Monod, O., Faure, M., Salinas, J. C., and Sabanero, H. 1993. What is the Guerrero Terrane made of ? In Proceedings of the first Circum-Pacific and Circum-Atlantic Terrane Conference, Guanajuao, Mexico, Universidad Nacional Autonoma de Mexico, p. 92.

Mourão M.A.A., Grossi Sad, J.H. and da Fonseca, E. 1997. Geologia da Folha Janaúba, Minas Gerais. In Projeto Espinhaço em CD-ROM (textos e anexos). Co-ordinated by J.H. Grossi Sad, L.M. Lobato, A.C. Pedrosa-Soares, B.S. Soares Filho. Companhia Mineradora de Minas Gerais, Belo Horizonte, pp. 9-123.

O'Dowd, P., 1999, La Plata Polymetallic property synthesis report Ecuador. Private Report for Cambior Inc. 37 pp.

Oliver, J., Payne, J., Kilby, D., Rebagliati, M. and Cluff, R. 2000 Precious metal-rich volcanic-associated massive sulfide deposits, Campo Morado, Guerrereo, Mexico. In Volcanogenic Massive Sulfide Deposits of Latin America. Edited by R.L. Sherlock and M.A.V. Logan, Mineral Deposit Division, Geological Association of Canada Publication.

Ortigoza-Cruz, F., 1988, The volcano-sedimentary deposits of La Minta, Michoacán, Mexico. MSc thesis, University of Alberta, 136 p.

Paes, V.J.C., Lobato L.M., Silva, S.L. and Baars, F.J. 1998. Geologia da Quadrícula de Alvarenga, Minas Gerais: Caracterização litológica e estrutural. In Anais do 40o Congresso Brasileiro de Geologia. Sociedade Brasileira de Geologia, Núcleo de Minas Gerais, Boletim 15, pp. 30.

Pedrosa-Soares, A.C., Noce, C.M., Vidal, Ph., Monteiro, R.L.B.P. and Leonardos Jr., O.H. 1992. Toward a new tectonic model for the Late Proterozoic Araçuaí (SE Brazil) – West Congolian (SW Africa) Belt. Journal of South American Earth Sciences, 6: 33-47.

Petersen, E.U. and Zantop., H. 1980. The Oxec deposit, Guatemala; an ophiolite copper occurrence. Economic Geology, vol. 75, p. 1053-1065.

Petersen, E.U. 2000. Geology of the Oxec, cyprus-type VMS deposit, Guatemala. In Volcanogenic Massive Sulfide Deposits of Latin America. Edited by R.L. Sherlock and M.A.V. Logan, Mineral Deposit Division, Geological Association of Canada Publication.

Polliand, M. and Fontboté, L. 2000. The Perubar Ba-Pb-Zn VHMS deposit, central Peru. In Volcanogenic Massive Sulfide Deposits of Latin America. Edited by R.L. Sherlock and M.A.V. Logan, Mineral Deposit Division, Geological Association of Canada Publication.

Resende, M.G. 1998. Estudo da Evolução das Supracrustais Metassedimentares dos Greenstone Belts de Goiás e Faina, GO. Ph.D. thesis, Universidade de Brasília, Brasília.

Resende, M.G., Jost, H., Osborne, G.A. and Mol, A. 1998. The stratigraphy of the Goiás and Faina greenstone belts, Central Brazil: a new proposal. Revista Brasileira de Geociências, 28: 77-94.

Rhys, D.A., Enns, S.G. and Ross, K.V. 2000. Geological setting of deformed VMS-type mineralization in the Azulaquez-Tlanilpa area, northern Guerrero state, México. In Volcanogenic Massive Sulfide Deposits of Latin America. Edited by R.L. Sherlock and M.A.V. Logan, Mineral Deposit Division, Geological Association of Canada Publication.

Ribeiro Filho, W. and Teixeira, N.A. 1981. Seqüência vulcano-sedimentar da borda oeste dos complexos de Niquelândia e Cana Brava. Sociedade Brasileira de Geologia, Núcleo do Centro-Oeste, Boletim Informativo 10, 157-173.

Ribeiro, A.F. and da Silva, M.d.G. 1998. O Greenstone Belt do Rio Salitre (GBS), Dominio Sobradinho, porção norte-nordeste do Cráton do São Francico, Bahia, e mineralizações associadas. In Anais do 40o Congresso Brasileiro de Geologia. Sociedade Brasileira de Geologia, Núcleo de Minas Gerais, Boletim 15, pp. 65.

Rocha, G.M.F. 1985. Caracterização faciológica da formação ferrífera de Boquira, encaixante da mineralização de Pb/Zn. M.Sc. dissertation, Universidade Federal da Bahia, Salvador, Brazil.

da Rocha Neto, M.B. and Pedreira, A.J. 1994. Geologia e recursos minerais do Greenstone Belt do Rio Itapicuru, Bahia. Companhia Baiana de Pesquisa Mineral, Série Arquivos Abertos, No. 4.

Rona, P.A. 1988. Hydrothermal mineralization at oceanic ridges. Canadian Mineralogist, vol. 26, p. 431-466.

Ruiz., J. and Centeno-Garcia, E. 2000. The Guerrero terrane of Western Mexico: geology and massive sulfide deposits. In Volcanogenic Massive Sulfide Deposits of Latin America. Edited by R.L. Sherlock and M.A.V. Logan, Mineral Deposit Division, Geological Association of Canada Publication.

Russell, N. and Kesler, S. E. 1991. Geology of the maar-diatreme complex hosting precious metal mineralization at Pueblo Viejo, Dominican Republic. In Geologic and Tectonic Development of the North America-Caribbean Plate Boundary in Hispaniola. Edited by P. Mann, G. Draper and J. F. Lewis. The Geological Society of America, Special Paper 262, pp. 203-215.

Russell, N., Moreira, J. and Sánchez, R. 2000. VMS deposits of Cuba. In Volcanogenic Massive Sulfide Deposits of Latin America. Edited by R.L. Sherlock and M.A.V. Logan, Mineral Deposit Division, Geological Association of Canada Publication.

Schrank, A, and da Silva, M.d.G. 1993. Os greenstone-belts do Cráton do São Francisco. In O Cráton do São Francisco. Edited by J.M.L. Dominguez and A. Misi. Sociedade Brasileira de Geologia, Núcleo de Bahia - Segipe / Superintendência de Geologia e Recursos Minerais do Estado da Bahia / Conselho Nacional de Pesquisa, Salvador, pp. 85-118.

Sedlock, R.L., Ortega-Gutierrez, F., and Speed, R.C., 1993. Tectonostratigraphic terranes and tectonic evolution of Mexico. Geological Society of America, Special Paper 278, 142 pages.

Sidder, G.B. 1995. Mineral deposits of the Venezuelan Guayana shield. U.S. Geological Survey Bulletin 2124, O1-O20.

Sidder, G.B. and Mendoza, V. 1995. Geology of the Venezuelan Guayana shield and its relation to the geology of the entire Guayana shield. U.S. Geological Survey Bulletin 2124, B1-B41.

Sidder, G.B., Brooks, W.E., Estanga, Y., Nuñez, F. and Garcia, A. 1991. Early to middle Proterozoic supracrustal rocks and mineralization of the southern Guayana shield, Venezuela. U.S. Geological Survey Circular 1062, p.69.

da Silva, M.d.G. 1987. Geochemic, Petrologie und geotektonische Entwicklung eines proterozoischen Grönsteingijrtels: Rio Itapicuru, Bahia, Brasilien. Ph.D thesis, Universität Freiburg, Freiburg.

Staargaard, C.F. and Carlson, G.G. 2000. The Bailadores volcanogenic massive sulfide deposit Venezuela. In Volcanogenic Massive Sulfide Deposits of Latin America. Edited by R.L. Sherlock and M.A.V. Logan, Mineral Deposit Division, Geological Association of Canada Publication.

Steinmüller, K., Chacón Abad, N. and Grant, B. 2000. Volcanogenic massive sulfide deposits. In Volcanogenic Massive Sulfide Deposits of Latin America. Edited by R.L. Sherlock and M.A.V. Logan, Mineral Deposit Division, Geological Association of Canada Publication.

Sureda, R.J. and Martín, J.L., 1990. Mina El Aguilar, provincia de Jujuy, Rep. Argentina. Un depósito SEDEX ordovícico, con metamorfismo de contacto sobreimpuesto, en la provincia metalogénica quiaqueña. Contribuciones al conocimiento de la mineralogia y geologia economica de la Republica Argentina. Asociación Argentina de Geólogos Economistas, Publicación Especial. Homenaje al prof. Ing. Victorio Angelelli, Buenos Aires, p78-91.

Talavera, M.O., Ramirez, E.J., and Guerrero, S.M., 1993, Geochemical evolution of the Guerrero terrane-Examples of a late Mesozoic multi-arc system. In Proceedings of the first Circum-Pacific and Circum-Atlantic Terrane Conference, Guanajuao, Mexico, Universidad Nacional Autonoma de Mexico.

Tegart, P., Allen, G. and Carstensen, A. 2000. Regional setting, stratigraphy, alteration and mineralization of the Tambo Grande VMS district, Piura department, northern Peru. In Volcanogenic Massive Sulfide Deposits of Latin America. Edited by R.L. Sherlock and M.A.V. Logan, Mineral Deposit Division, Geological Association of Canada Publication.

Thomas, A. 1973. Geología y perspectivas económicas del yacimiento Cutter Cove, Provincia de Magallanes. Informe Inédito, ENAMI, Santiago, Chile.

Vidal, C.E. 1987, Kuroko-type deposits in the Middle Cretaceous maginal basin of central Peru, Economic Geology, vol. 82, p/ 1409-1430.

Vieira, M.B., Lobato, L.M., Assis, C.M., Gomes, F.C., Silva, R.A., Nascimento, H.S and Orlandi, P.H. 1998. Contribuição ao estudo da alteração hidrotermal da mina de ouro de Fazenda Brasileiro, Bahia. In Anais do 40o Congresso Brasileiro de Geologia. Sociedade Brasileira de Geologia, Núcleo de Minas Gerais, Boletim 15, pp. 130.

Vivallo, W. 2000. Volcanic-exhalative massive sulfide deposits in Chile. In Volcanogenic Massive Sulfide Deposits of Latin America. Edited by R.L. Sherlock and M.A.V. Logan, Mineral Deposit Division, Geological Association of Canada Publication.

Walrond, G.W. 1985. A metallogenic scheme for the Guiana shield. Memoria I, Simposium Amazonico, Boletin de Geología, Publicación Especial Nº 10, Ministerio de Energia y Minas. Dirección de Geología, 609-624.

Winge, M. 1984. A seqüência vulcano-sedimentar do Grupo Capim - Bahia. In Geologia e Recursos Minerais do Estado da Bahia. Edited by P.V.S. Viveiros de Sá and F.B. Duarte. Secretaria de Minas e Energia do Estado da Bahia, Coordenação da Produção Mineral, Salavador, Textos Básicos, Vol. 5, pp. 43-103.

Winge, M. and Danni, J.C.M. 1980. Compartimentos geotectônicos pré-brasilianos entre Caratacá e Bedengo, municipio de Uauá, Bahia. In Anais do 31o Congresso Brasileira Geologia. Sociedade Brasileira de Geologia, Núcleo de Santa Catarina, Vol., pp.

Zappettini, E.O. and Brodtkorb, M. K., 2000. The VMS Santa Elena Deposit, San Juan Province, Argentina. In Volcanogenic Massive Sulfide Deposits of Latin America. Edited by R.L. Sherlock and M.A.V. Logan, Mineral Deposit Division, Geological Association of Canada Publication.

Zucchetti, M., Baltazar, O.F. and Raposo, F.O. 1998. Estratigrafia. In Projeto Rio das Velhas – Mapa Geológico Integrado, Escala 1:100.000, e Texto Explicativo. Edited by M. Zucchetti and O.F. Baltazar. Departamento Nacional de Produção Mineral / Companhia de Pesquisa de Recursos Minerais – Belo Horizonte, CD-ROM, pp. 13-42.

THE GUERRERO TERRANE OF WESTERN MEXICO: GEOLOGY AND MASSIVE SULPHIDE DEPOSITS

JOAQUIN RUIZ
Department of Geosciences, The University of Arizona, Tucson, Arizona 85721

ELENA CENTENO GARCIA
Universidad Nacional Autonoma de Mexico, Instituto de Geologia, Mexico, D.F. Mexico

ABSTRACT

The Guerrero terrane in western Mexico is one of the largest accreted terranes of oceanic affinity in the north American Cordillera and thus is an important exploration target for massive sulphide deposits. Small but economic deposits have been exploited in the past which has led to recent discoveries of larger gold-rich deposits. The diversity of deposits in the Guerrero terrane is the result of the complex geology consisting of accreted composite arc and back-arcs.

The basement of the Guerrero terrane is the Artega Complex and consists of pillow lavas with mid-ocean ridge chemistry and juvenile isotopic compositions. Chert associated with the pillowed basalt contains poorly preserved radiolarians of Triassic age. The Arteaga Complex also contains large volumes of greenschist to lower amphibolite metasedimentary rocks that derived their sediments from a Grenville age source, which was likely nuclear Mexico. Overlying the Arteaga complex is a mostly Cretaceous sequence of marine limestone interbedded with intermediate volcaniclastic rocks. These rocks represent the bulk of the Guerrero terrane and delineate an arc that was off the coast of western Mexico in the Cretaceous. Recent tectonic models suggest that there was a significant basin between Mexico and the incipient Guerrero terrane. Accretion of the Guerrero terrane occurred post Jurassic and deformation occurred during the Laramide Orogeny. After the accretion, the Guerrero terrane was affected by Cretaceous and Tertiary magmatism that is part of the Sierra Madre Occidental and Trans Mexican Volcanic Arcs.

Because of the oceanic nature of the terrane, as well as extensive and varied magmatic history that affected the original arc rocks, the Guerrero terrane has been considered an important target for many kinds of ore deposits including skarns, polymetallic veins and volcanogenic massive sulphide deposits. More than 60 volcanogenic massive sulphide and sedimentary exhalative occurences have been recognized in the Guerrero terrane, most of which have been categorized as Kuroko-type Zn-Pb-Cu. The deposits range from less than 100,000 metric tonnes to 75 million tonnes at San Nicolás.

INTRODUCTION

The Guerrero terrane, one of the largest accreted terranes with oceanic affinity of the North American Cordillera (Fig. 1), is a composite terrane mostly characterized by submarine and rarely subaereal volcanic and sedimentary sequences, that range in age from Upper Jurassic to middle Upper Cretaceous (Campa and Coney, 1983; Centeno-Garcia et al., 1993; Talavera-Mendoza, 1993) resting unconformable on deformed and partially metamorphosed oceanic sequences of Early Mesozoic age (de Cserna, 1982; Coney and Campa, 1987; Centeno-García, et al., 1993). The lithologic assemblages of the Upper Jurassic to Middle-Upper Cretaceous are generally recognized as representing accreted arcs and back arcs. However there is cotroversy as to whether the Guerrero terrane represents a continental arc that was built not far from its present position or whether the Guerrero terrane represents an oceanic arc that could be far-travelled, Structural evidence indicates that the timing of amalgamation of the Guerrero terrane, regardless of its origin, to nuclear Mexico is Late Cretaceous (Campa and Ramirez, 1979). The final events that affected the Guerrero terrane are arcs that have developed since Cretaceous time but culminated in mid-Tertiary time with the production of the Sierra

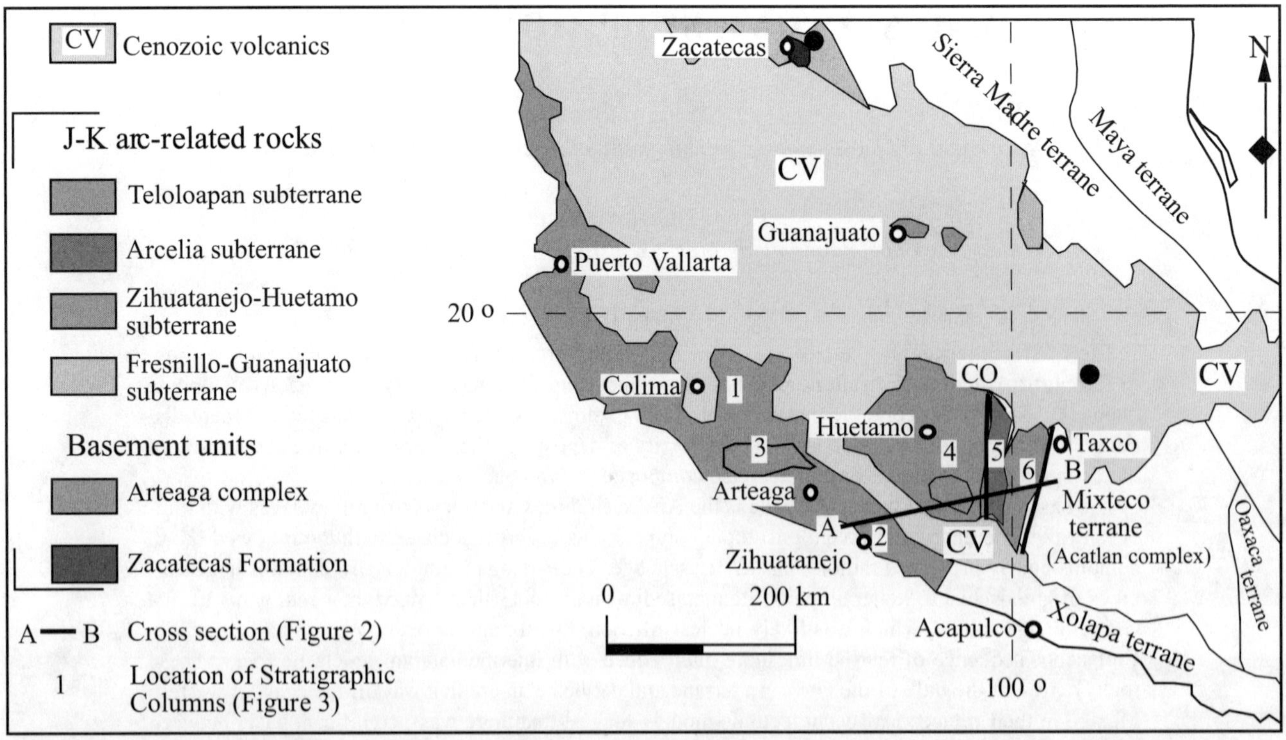

Figure 1. Location of the Guerrero subterranes, major assemblages and basement units (Arteaga complex and Zacatecas Formation) (modified from Campa and Coney, 1983, Centeno-Garcia, 1994).

Madre Occidental Volcanic Province and recently with the Trans Mexican Volcanic Arc. Volcanic and intrusive rocks of these arcs cover and affect large portions of the Guerrero terrane..

Because many parts of the Guerrero terrane are of oceanic affinity, massive sulphide deposits have been an obvious exploration target for the region. The complex history of the Guerrero terrane, which begins in the Triassic with a submarine origin near a mid-ocean ridge, followed by a long lived arc that lasted most of the Cretaceous, with intrusion of large magma bodies that range from diorite to granodiorite in composition and some minor highly peraluminous bodies, allows for a large range of targets that include volcanic massive sulphide deposits, sedimentary exhalative deposits, Fe and Au-rich skarns and Tertiary Au-Ag-polymetallic vein deposits.

REGIONAL SETTING OF THE GUERRERO TERRANE

Approximately the western half of Mexico, which includes the peninsula of Baja California is a complex but mostly volanogenic Mesozoic and younger arc assemblage that is known as the Guerrero terrane (Campa and Coney (1982) or the Guerrero Superterrane if Baja California is also considered (Dickinson and Lawton, in press). The Guerrero terrane was accreted to nuclear Mexico by arc-continent collision in early Cretaceous time (e.g. Ortiz et al., 1991; Freydier et al., 1996). Dickinson and Lawton (in review) argue that the collision occurred around 120 Ma in northern Mexico and around 110 Ma in the south.

The nomenclature of the Guerrero terrane is complex because although the Guerrero terrane consists of similar lithological units throughout, differences in the chemistry of the igneous rocks, as well as detailed variations in lithology and deformation styles indicate that the terrane is composite. Initially the Guerrero terrane was subdivided into three subterranes based on these differences. These subterranes are the Teloloapan, Huetamo and Zihuatanejo subterranes (Campa and Coney, 1983). However, recent work shows that the Huetamo and Zihuatanejo subterranes, have similar basement rocks and overlying lithologies (Centeno-Garcia et al., 1993a, 1993b; Centeno-

Garcia, 1994) and can probably be considered as a single subterrane.

The Teloloapan subterrane, however, has recently been subdivided into two different assemblages – Teloloapan and Arcelia - because of seemingly different histories (Talavera-Mendoza et al., 1995). A final subterrane, named the Arperos Bain by Lapierre et al (1992) and Fresnillo-Guanajuato by Centeno Garcia (1993) is exposed in the northeastern most parts of the Guerrero terrane near the cities of Guanajuato, Zacatecas, and Aguascalientes as described by Ortiz-Hernandez et al. (1991), Lapierre et al. (1992), Centeno and Silva-Romo (1993), and Martínez-Reyes (1994).

The Guerrero terrane was deformed and partially metamorphosed during the Laramide Orogeny, which affected southwestern North America in the Cretaceous (Campa and Coney, 1983). All the subterranes are presently limited by thrusts, and constitute nappes that verge toward the east over nuclear Mexico.

GEOLOGY OF THE GUERRERO TERRANE

Zihuatanejo Subterrane

The Zihuatanejo subterrane is exposed in the Huetamo region and along the Pacific Coast of Mexico (Fig. 1). The oldest unit of this subterrane, and of the whole Guerrero terrane, is the Arteaga Complex (Centeno-Garcia et al., 1993a), that represents the basement upon which the arc was built (Fig. 1, 2 and 3). The Arteaga complex is composed up to 60 % sedimentary rocks (Varales Formation and Jaltomate Member). The Varales Formation consists of siliciclastic turbidites, made up of interbedded black shale, quartz-rich sandstone and minor black chert. This formation locally shows intercalations of green shales interbedded with thin carbonate beds of the Jaltomate Member (Centeno-Garcia, 1994). Other lithologies, associated with the Varales Formation, are basaltic pillow lavas and lava flows, diabase dikes, and diorite intrusions. Large olistolithic blocks of previously deformed rocks are included in the Varales sediments. These blocks are made up of light-green thin to medium bedded chert, that is tightly folded and recrystalized. They contain radiolarians of Late Triassic (Ladinian-Carnian) age. There are also blocks of metamorphosed and recrystallized limestone that contains some light green chert bands and remains of recrystalized crinoids. The Arteaga complex was originaly deposited as an ocean-floor sequence that was deformed and locally metamorphosed during Middle Jurassic time (Centeno-Garcia et al., 1993a). The chert blocks containing radiolarians, and isotopic ages of deformation suggest a Late Triassic to Early Jurassic time of deposition for the Arteaga complex.

The arc sequence rests in angular unconformity on the Arteaga complex. Sedimentation began with a conglomerate formed by clasts derived from the complex. It is followed by interbedded basaltic-andesitic and some rhyolitic lava flows, pyroclastic and epiclastic deposits, limestone, and locally evaporites (Fig. 3; Pantoja, 1959; Ferrusquia et. al., 1978; Campa and Ramirez, 1979; Grajales-Nishimura and Lopez-Infanzón, 1984; Buitron, 1986; Pantoja and Estrada, 1986; Pantoja, 1990). Units of interbedded shale, sandstone, and conglomerate are found at different levels in the succession (Fig. 3). These are up to 2,000 m thick in the Huetamo region. Results from the analysis of composition and provenance of these sediments are discussed below. The arc was mostly submarine, although some units were deposited on transitional and subaereal environments (Pantoja, 1959; Ferrusquia et. al., 1978; Campa and Ramirez, 1979; Buitron, 1986; Pantoja and Estrada, 1986; Pantoja, 1990, Centeno-Garcia et al., 1993b). The arc magmatism along the coast of the Zihuatanejo subterrane is Valanginian to Campanian in age (Grajales-Nishimura and Lopez-Infanzón, 1984; Buitron, 1986), although fossils of Late Jurassic (Kimmeridgian) age have been reported from the Huetamo region (Pantoja, 1959). The total thickness of the arc sequence is unknown, at least 3,750 m have been measured from drilling (Grajales-Nishimura and Lopez-Infanzón, 1984).

A melange-like metamorphic complex (Las Ollas), with blueshist-facies, is exposed in Zihuatanejo (Fig. 1, 2, 3; Vidal-Serratos, 1991; Talavera-Mendoza, 1993). This unit is Albian in age, and it might represent a subduction complex related to the volcanic-arc (Delgado-Argote, 1982; Delgado-Argote et al., 1990; Vidal-Serratos, 1991; Talavera-Mendoza, 1993).

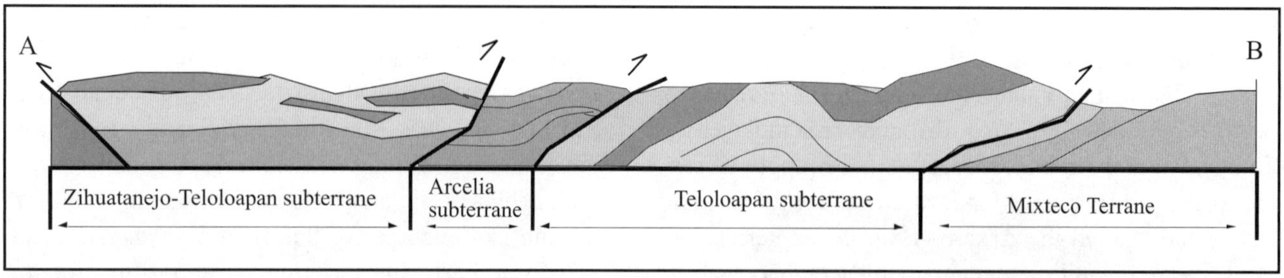

Figure 2. Cross-section A-B (Fig. 1) through the Guerrero terrane showing the structural juxtaposition of the various subterranes.

Arcelia Subterrane

The Arcelia subterrane (Fig. 1 and 3) shows deeper marine facies and less evolved magmatism than the rest of the arc sequences (Talavera-Mendoza et al., 1993; Talavera-Mendoza et al., 1995). It is made up of intensively deformed basaltic pillow lavas and ultramafic bodies, overlain by black shales, thin-bedded calcareous shales and chert, that thrusts over the Teloloapan subterrane (Fig. 1, 2, 3; Talavera-Mendoza et al., 1993; Ramirez-Espinosa et al., 1991). The chert layers contain radiolarians of Albian-Cenomanian age (Davila and Guerrero, 1990). The sequence grades upward into interbedded shales and sandstones (Fig. 3). The Arcelia subterrane is interpreted as an intra-arc or back arc basin that developed between the Huetamo and Teloloapan subterranes (Ramirez-Espinosa et al., 1991; Talavera-Mendoza et al., 1993). The nature of its basement is unknown.

Teloloapan Subterrane

The Teloloapan subterrane is deformed and partially metamorphosed to low-grade greenschist facies, and forms a thrust-fault system that verges eastward (Fig. 1, 2 and 3). It is characterized by lava flows, tuffs, epiclastics, and limestone, alternating with interbedded shale/sandstone at the top of the sequence, all deposited in shallow marine environments (Fig. 3; Campa and Ramirez, 1979, Guerrero-Suastegui et al., 1991). The magmatism is mostly Neocomian to Albian in age (Guerrero-Suastegui et al., 1991). At present, the nature of the basement of the Teloloapan subterrane is unclear. Metamorphosed volcanic-sedimentary sequence of the Tejupilco complex, that are interpreted as an older (Early Mesozoic) arc-assemblage, are suggested to be its basement (de Cserna, 1982; Elias-Herrera and Sanchez-Zavala, 1992; Sanchez-Zavala 1993). However, the same rocks have been interpreted as part of the Cretaceous arc assemblage by other authors (Campa and Ramirez, 1979; Ramirez-Espinosa et al., 1991; Talavera-Mendoza et al., 1995). The Teloloapan subterrane tectonically overrides either Cretaceous platform carbonates or clastic sediments of the Mexcala Formation of the Morelos subterrane (Fig. 2, 3; de Cserna, 1978; Campa and Ramirez, 1979).

Fresnillo-Guanajuato Subterrane

The older unit of the Fresnillo-Guanajuato subterrane is the Late Triassic (Norian) Zacatecas Formation (Burckhardt and Scalia, 1906; Monod and Calvet, 1991), that probably represents is its basement (Fig. 1, 2, 3). It is made up of black shale and quartz-rich sandstone, alternated with tuff, volcanic breccias, pillow lavas and thin bedded limestone (Fig. 3) (Ranson et al., 1982; and Monod and Calvet, 1991). The MORB geochemical and isotopic affinity of its basaltic lavas suggest that the Zacatecas Formation might have been an ocean-floor assemblage (Centeno-Garcia and Silva-Romo, 1993; Centeno-García, 1994). The sequence was deformed and low-grade metamorphosed prior to the development of the Cretaceous arc assemblage. The Zacateas Formation is tectonically overlain by the Cretaceous arc volcanics (Centeno-Garcia and Silva-Romo, 1993).

The arc sequence in the Fresnillo-Guanajuato subterrane is made up of basaltic pillow lavas and massive flows, interbedded with sandstone, radiolarian chert and limestone (de Cserna, 1976; Yta et al., 1990). This sequence is thrust over undated metamor-

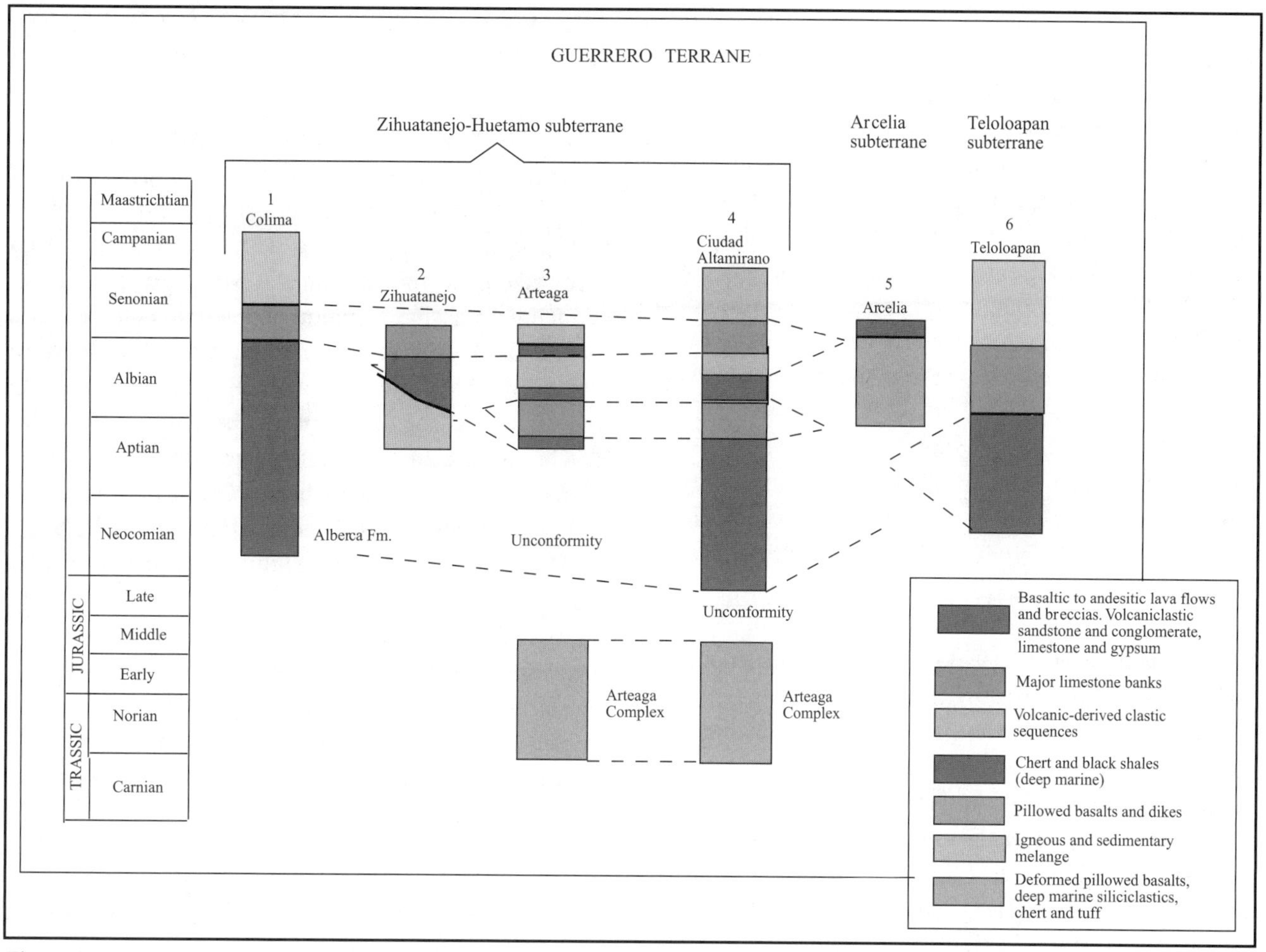

Figure 3. Stratigraphic columns of the Guerrero composite terrane (location on Figure 1).

phosed limestone in El Saucito area, east of Zacatecas city (Yta et al., 1990). Deep marine sedimentary facies are exposed near Guanajuato city (Fig. 1, 2 and 3), where the arc assemblage is made up of pillow basalts, interbedded with thin bedded siltstone, shale, sandstone and some limestone (Ortiz-Hernandez et al., 1991; Lapierre et al., 1992; Martínez-Reyes, 1994). This subterrane has been interpreted as relicts of an ocean basin (Arperos Basin) in the far-traveled arc models (Lapierre et al., 1992). However, the role of old rocks of the Zacatecas Formation in the Arperos basin is not discussed in such models. The boundary between the Sierra Madre and the Fresnillo-Guanajuato subterrane is covered by Cenozoic volcanic rocks (Fig. 1).

EVOLUTION OF THE GUERRERO TERRANE

The oldest rocks of the Guerrero terrane are in the Zihuatanejo subterrane and consist of pillow lavas of basaltic composition. The age of the basalt is thought to be Triassic based on poorly preserved radiolaria in chert coexisting with the basalt. Overlying and intermixed with the basalt is a sequence of metamorphic sedimentary rocks knows as the Arteaga Complex (Centeno-Garcia et al. (1993). The sediments that form the Arteaga Complex are recycled from a Grenville-age source that presumably was nuclear Mexico since all of nuclear Mexico's basement is of Grenville-age.

Because most of the lithologies of the Guerrero terrane are of magmatic origin, Geochemical analyses of the igneous rocks can constrain the tectonic regime in which the magmatism occurred. The pillow basalts, which form the base of the Zihuatanejo terrane, which has the oldest rocks of the Guerrero terrane, consists of basalt with mid-ocean ridge isotopic and trace element characteristics. The basalts are depleted in light-rare earth elements (LREE) and have initial ΣNd values of +10 to +6 (Centeno-Garcia et al., 1993a, 1993b; Centeno-Garcia, 1994). In contrast, REE and Nd isotopic signatures of the Jurassic-Cretaceous volcanic rocks suggests that they were formed in an evolved intra-oceanic island arc (Ruíz et al., 1991; Lapierre, et. al., 1992; Centeno-Garcia et al., 1993a, 1993b; Talavera-Mendoza, 1993; Talavera-Mendoza et al., 1993, 1995). Positive initial ΣNd values for the majority of the Jurassic-Cretaceous volcanic rocks, and most of the Tertiary granitoids are positive (ΣNd +2 to +8) (Schaaf, 1990; Ortiz-Hernandez et al, 1991; Lapierre et al., 1992; Centeno-Garcia et al, 1993a), indicating little or no assimilation of old crust by the magmas.

Dickinson and Lawton (in review) have evaluated the paleogeography of the Guerrero terrane and its relationship with North America. The Guerrero arc is thought to have been formed with a large basin between it and nuclear Mexico. The oceanic basin must have closed in Late Cretaceous time (Tardy et al, 1991a; 1991b, 1994; Lapierre, et. al., 1992; Dickinson and Lawton, in review). This model is in contrast to that of other authors that have suggested that the Guerrero terrane represents a marginal arc (Campa and Ramirez, 1979), which developed relatively close to the continent. Some authors (de Cserna, 1978; Elias-Herrera and Sanchez-Zavala, 1990) have also proposed that the presence of continental crust beneath the Guerrero terrane means that the terrane is of continental affinity and that it may represent a facies change from miogeoclyne to eugeoclyne from east to west in Mexico. The work by Centeno-Garcia et al. (1993) on the basement of the Guerrero terrane and the recent review of the geology of Mexico by Dickinson and Lawton (in review) strongly suggest that the evolved isotopic signatures in some places of the Guerrero terrane may represent assimilation of recycled sediments that were deposited in the ocean floor and not that the Guerrero terrane is an old terrane of continental affinity.

THE VOLCANOGENIC MASSIVE SULPHIDE AND SEDIMENTARY EXHALATIVE DEPOSITS OF THE GUERRERO TERRANE

Although we focus mostly with the geology of the Guerrero terrane, here we briefly summarize some of the salient features of volcanogenic massive sulphide and sedimentary exhalative deposits that have been recognized in this terrane. More than 60 volcanogenic massive sulphide and sedimentary exhalative occurences have been recognized in the Guerrero terrane by Miranda-Gasca (1995). Most of the deposits have been categorized as Kuroko-type Zn-Pb-Cu and are in the Zihuatanejo subterrane. These deposits range from less than 100,000 metric tonnes up to 75 million at San Nicolás (Johnson et al. 2000).

Miranda-Gasca (1995) shows that there are four groups of deposits in the States of Guerrero and Mexico. These are the Campo Morado-Suriana, Azulaquez, Tizapa and Rey de Plata. In western Jalisco there is another group of deposits around Cuale. Scattered occurrences of deposits deposits exist in Zacatecas, Guanajuanto and Michoacan. Very few volcanogenic massive sulphides have been economical in the Guerrero terrane. Among the most notable are Cuale, which was exploited mostly for silver, La Minita, which first produced barite but then was mined for polymetallic ore, Tizapa, and the small deposits El Rubi, Campo Morado, El Faisan, Suriana, Santa Rosa and Calmalli. These deposits were economic mainly because of silver production from oxidized ore.

The shale of the volcanogenic massive sulphide deposits is generally conformable with a stockwork at the base. However some important deposits that have been considered as volcanogenic massive sulphides, such as Tizapa, Aurora, San Ignacio and Arroyo Seco do not seem to have a stockwork zone at their base. Generally there seems to be mineralogical and chemical zoning of the deposits that are Pb-Ag at the top of the lenses and are Cu-rich at their bases.

REFERENCES

Anderson, T. H., and Silver, L. T., 1969, Mesozoic magmatic events of the northern Sonora coastal region, Mexico: Geological Society of America, Abstracts with Programs, v. 1, p. 3-4.

Anderson, T. H., and McKee, J. W., and Jones, N. W., 1990,

Jurassic (?) melange in north-central Mexico: Geological Society of America, Abstracts with Programs, v. 22, p. 3.

Aranda-Gomez, J., and Perez-Venzor, 1988, Estudio Geológico de Punta Coyotes, Baja California Sur: Universidad Nacional Autonoma de Mexico, Instituto de Geologia, Revista, v. 7, n. 1, p. 1-21.

Böhnel, H., Alva-Valdivia, L., Gonzalez-Huesca, S., Urrutia-Fucugauchi, J., Moran-Zenteno, D. J., and Schaaf, P., 1989, Paleomagnetic data and the accretion of the Guerrero terrane, Southwestern Mexico continental margin: in Deep structure and past kinematics of accreted terranes, American Geophysical Union, Geohpysical Monograph, n. 50, p. 73-92.

Buitrón, B. E., 1986, Gasterópodos del Cretácico (Aptiano Tardío-Albiano Temprano) del Cerro de Tuxpan, Jalisco: Sociedad Geológica Mexicana, Bulletin, v. XLVII, n. 1, p. 17-32.

Busby-Spera, C., 1988, Speculative tectonic model for the early Mesozoic arc of the southwest Cordilleran United States: Geology, v. 16, p. 1121-1125.

Burckhardt, C., and Scalia, S., 1906, Géologie des environs de Zacatecas: International Geological Congress, 10th Mexico, excursion guidebook 16, 26 p.

Campa, M.F. and Coney, P.J. (1983) Tectono-stratigraphic terranes and mineral resource distributions in Mexico: Canadian Journal of Earth Sciences, 20, 1040-1051.

Campa, M.F. and Ramirez, J., 1979, La Evolucion Geologica y la Metalogenesis de Guerrero: Universidad Autonoma de Guerrero, Serie Tecnico-Cientifica, n. 1, 84 p.

Campa, M.F.; Ramirez, J. and Bloome, C.,1982, La secuencia volcanico-sedimentaria metamorfizada del Triasico (Ladiniano-Carnico) de la region de Tumbiscatio, Michoacan. Soc. Geol. Mex., VI Conv. Nal., Resumenes, 48.

Cantu-Chapa, A., 1969, Una nueva localidad Triásico Superior en México, Revista Instituto Mexicano del Petroleo, v. 1, n. 2, p. 71-72.Centeno-García, Elena, 1994, Tectonic Evolution of the Guerrero Terrane, Western Mexico (Doctoral Dissertation): Department of Geosciences, University of Arizona, 200 p. (unpublished).

Centeno-Garcia E., 1994, Tectonic evolution of the Guerrero Terrane, Western México, Ph D. Dissertation, Department of Geosciences, University of Arizona, 220 p.

Centeno-García, E., and Silva-Romo, G., 1993, Geology of the San Luis Potosí-Zacatecas Region, Northeastern Limit of the Guerrero Terrane, in Ortega-Gutiérrez F., et al., eds., Terrane Geology of Southern México: UNAM, Instituto de Geología, First Circum-Pacific and Circum-Atlantic Terrane Conference, Gto. Mex., Guidebook of Field Trip A.

Centeno-García, E., Ruíz, J., Coney, P., Patchett, J. P., y Ortega-Gutiérrez, F., 1993a, Guerrero Terrane of Mexico: its role in the Southern Cordillera from new geochemical data: Geology, Geological Society of America, v.21, n. 5, p. 419-422.

Centeno-García, E., García, J.L., Guerrero-Suástegui, M., Ramírez-Espinosa, J., Salinas-Prieto, J. C., and Talavera-Mendoza, O., 1993b, Geology of the Southern Part of the Guerrero Terrane, Ciudad Altamirano-Teloloapan Area, in Ortega-Gutiérrez F., et al., eds., Terrane Geology of Southern México: UNAM, Instituto de Geología, First Circum-Pacific and Circum-Atlantic Terrane Conference, Gto. Mex., Guidebook of Field Trip B, p. 22-33.

Cole, G. L., 1990, Models of plate kinematics along the Western margin of the Americas: Cretaceous to Present, Ph. D. Dissertation (unpublished), University of Arizona, 115 p.

Coney, P.J., 1983, Un modelo tectónico de México y sus relaciones con América del Norte, América del Sur y el Caribe, Revista del Instituto Mexicano del Petróleo, v. 15, n. 1, p. 6-15.

Coney, P.J., and Campa, M.F., 1987, Lithotectonic Terrane Map of Mexico (west of the 91st meridian): Misc. Field Studies, Map MF 1874-D.

Davila, V. M., 1981, Radiolarios del Cretácico Inferior de la formación Plateros, Distrito Minero de Fresnillo, Zacatecas: Universidad Nacional Autonoma de Mexico, Instituto de Geologia, Revista, v. 5, p 119-120.

Davila, V. M., and Guerrero, M., 1990, Una edad basada en radiolarios para la secuencia volcánica-sedimentaria de Arcelia, Edo. de Guerrero: Sociedad Geológica Mexicana, X Convención Nacional, Abstracts, p. 83.

de Cserna, Z., 1976, Geology of the Fresnillo area, Zacatecas, México, Geological Society of America, Bulletin, v. 87, p. 1191-1199.

de Cserna, Z., 1978, Notas sobre la geología de la región comprendida entre Iguala, Ciudad Altamirano y Temascaltepec, Estados de Guerrero y México: Sociedad Geológica de México, Libro Guía de la excursión geológica a Tierra Caliente, p. 1-25.

de Cserna, Z., 1982, Hoja Tejupilco 14Q-g(9), and Resumen de la Geología de la Hoja Tejupilco, Estados de Guerrero, México y Michoacán, Insituto de Geología UNAM, Carta Geologica de Mexico, Series, map (1:100,00) and text, 28 p.

de Cserna, Z., Fries, C. Jr., 1981, Hoja Taxco 14Q-h(7), and Resumen de la Geología de la Hoja Taxco, Estados de Guerrero, México y Morelos, Insituto de Geología UNAM, Carta Geologica de Mexico, Series, map (1:100,00) and text, 47 p.

Delgado, L. A., 1982, Descripción preliminar de la geología y mecánica de emplazamiento del complejo ultrabásico de Loma Baya, Guerrero, México, Geofísica Internacional, v. 25, p. 537-558.

Delgado-Argote, L., López-M., M., York, D., and Hall, C. M., 1990, Geology and geochronology of ultramafic localities in the Cuicateco and Tierra Caliente complexes, southern Mexico: Geological Society of America, Abstr. with Progr., p. 326.

DePaolo, D.J., 1981, Neodymium isotopes in the Colorado Front Range and crust-mantle evolution in the Proterozoic: Nature, v. 291, p.193-196.

Dickinson, W.R., 1970, Interpreting detrital modes of graywacke and arkose: Journal of Sedimentary Petrology, v. 40, p. 695-707.

Dickinson, W.R., 1985, Interpreting provenance relations from detrital modes of sandstones: in Zuffa, G.G. (Editor), Provenance of Arenites. Dordrecht, Holl., Reidel, 333-361.

Dickinson W. R., 1992, Cordilleran sedimentary assemblages, in Burchfield, B. C., Lipman, P. W., and Zoback, M. L., eds., The Cordilleran Orogen: Conterminous U.S., G. S. A., The Geology of North America, v. G-3.

Dickinson W. R., Beard L. S., Brakenridge, G. R., Erjavec, J. L., Ferguson, R. C., Inman, K. F., Knepp, R. A., Lindberg, F. A., Ryberg, P. T., 1983, Provenance of North American Phanerozoic sandstones in relation to tectonic setting: Geological Society of America, Bulletin, v. 94, p. 222-235.

Dickinson W. R., and Suczek, C. A., 1979, Plate tectonics and sandstone compositions, Am. Ass. Petr. Geol., Bull., v. 63, p. 2164-2182.

Dickinson W.R., Lawton T. F., in review, Geotectonic Assembly and Fragmentation of Mexico, Geological Society of America Bulletin.

Elías-Herrera, M., Sánchez-Zavala, J. L., 1990 (1992), Tectonic implications of a mylonitic granite in the lower structural levels of the Tierra Caliente Complex (Guerrero Terrane), Southern México: Universidad Nacional Autonoma de Mexico, Instituto de Geologia, Revista, v. 9, n. 2, p. 113-125.

Evensen, M. N., 1978, Rare Earth abundances in chondritic meteorites, Geochemica et Chosmochemica Acta, v. 42, p. 1203.

Ferrusquía, I., Applegate, S. P., and Espinosa, L., 1978, Rocas volcanosedimentarias mesozoicas y huellas de dinosaurios en la región suroccidental pacifica de México: Universidad Nacional Autonoma de Mexico, Instituto de Geologia, Revista, v. 2, n. 2, p. 150-162.

Fries, C. Jr., 1960, Geología del Estado de Morelos y de partes adyacentes de México y Guerrero, región central meridional de México: Universidad Nacional Autonoma de Mexico, Instituto de Geologia, Bulletin, v. 60, 236 p.

Grajales-Nishimura, M. and Lopez-Infanzón, M.,1984, Estudio petrogenetico de las rocas igneas y metamorficas en el Prospecto Tomatlan-Guerrero-Jalisco: IMP Subdireccion de Tecnologia y Exploracion, Proyecto C-1160 (unpublished).

Grajales-Nishimura, M., Terrell, D. J., and Damon, P. E., 1992, Evidencias de la prolongación del Arco Magmático Cordillerano del Triásico Tardío-Jurásico en Chihuahua, Durango y Coahuila, Asoc. Mex. de Geol. Petr., Bull., v. XLII, n. 2, p. 1-18.

Guerrero-Suastegui, M., Ramirez-Espinosa, J., Talavera-Mendoza, O., Campa-Uranga, M. F., 1991, El desarrollo carbonatado del Cretácico Inferior asociado al arco de Teloloapan, Noroccidente del Estado de Guerrero, Convención sobre la evolución Geológica Mexicana, 1er Congreso Mexicano de Mineralogía, Pachuca, Memoir, p. 67-70.

Ingersoll, R. V.,1990, Actualistic sandstone petrofacies: discriminating modern and ancient source rocks, Geology, v. 18, p. 733-736.

Ingersoll, R. V., and Suczek, C. A., 1979, Petrology and provenance of Neogene sand from Nicobar and Bengal fans, DSDP sites 211 and 218, Journal of Sedimentary Petrology, v. 49, p. 1217-1228.

Johnson, B.J., Montante-Martínez, A., Canela-Barboza, M. and Danielson, T.J. 2000. Geology of the San Nicolás deposit, Zacatecas, México. In Volcanogenic Massive Sulfide Deposits of Latin America. Edited by R.L. Sherlock and M.A.V. Logan, Mineral Deposit Division, Geological Association of Canada Publication.

Jones, N.W., Mc Kee, J.W., Anderson, T.H., and Silver, L.T., 1995, Jurassic volcanic rocks in Northeastern Mexico: A possible remnant of a Cordilleran Magmatic Arc: in Jacques-Ayala C., Gonzalez-León, C., and Roldán Quintana, J., Studies of the Mesozoic of Sonora and Adjacent Areas, Geological Society of America, Special Paper 301, p. 179-190.

Kimbrough, D. L., 1985, Tectonostratigraphic terranes of the Vizcaino Peninsula and Cedros and San Benito Islands, Baja California, Mexico, in Howell, D. G., ed., Tectonostratigraphic terranes of the Circum-Pacific region, Circum-Pacific Council for Energy and Mineral Resources, Earth Science Series, n. 1, p. 285-298.

Köhler, H., Schaaf, P., Müller-Sohnius, R., Emmermann, R., Negendank, J.F.W., and Tobschall, H. J., 1988, Geochronological and geochemical investigations on plutonic rocks from the complex of Puerto Vallarta, Sierra Madre del Sur (México): Geofísica Internacional, v. 27, n. 4, p. 519-542.

Lapierre, H., Ortiz, L.E., Abouchami, W., Monod, O., Coulon, C., Zimmermann, J.L., 1992, A crustal section of an intra-oceanic island arc: The Late Jurassic-Early Cretaceous Guanajuato magmatic sequence, central Mexico: Earth Planetary Science Letters, v. 108, p. 1-77.

Lundberg, 1991, Detrital record of the early Central American magmatic arc: petrography of intraoceanic forearc sandstones, Nicoya Peninsula, Costa Rica, Geological Society of America Bulletin, v. 103, p. 905-915.

Marsaglia K.M., and Ingersoll, R. V., 1992, Compositional trends in arc-related, deep marine sand and sandstone: a reassessment of magmatic-arc provenance, Geological Society of America Bulletin, v. 104, p. 1637-1649.

Martínez-Reyes, J., 1994, Geologic map of Guanajuato area: Universidad Nacional Autonoma de Mexico, Instituto de Geologia, Map Series.

McLennan, S. M., McCulloch, M. T., Taylor, S. R., and Maynard, J. B., 1989, Effects of sedimentary sorting on neodymium isotopes in deep-sea turbidites: Nature, v. 337, p. 547-549.

McLennan, S. M., Taylor, S. R., McCulloch, M. T., and Maynard, J. B., 1990, Geochemical and Nd-Sr isotopic composition of deep-sea turbidites: Crustal evolution and plate tectonic associations: Geochemical et Cosmochemical Acta, v. 54, p. 2015-2050.

Monod, O., and Calvet, P., 1991, Structural and Stratigraphic reinterpretation of the Triassic units near Zacatecas, Zac., Central Mexico: evidence of a Laramide nappe pile, Zbl. Geol., Paläont., Teil I, 1991, p. 1533-1542.

Mullan, H. S., 1978, Evolution of part of the Nevadan Orogen in northwestern Mexico: Geological Society of America, Bulletin, v. 89, p. 1175-1188.

Nelson B., and DePaolo, D. J., 1985, Rapid production of continental crust 1.7 to 1.9 b. y. ago: Nd isotopic evidence from basement of the North American mid-continent: Geological Society of America, Bulletin, v. 96, p. 746-754.

Ortega-Gutiérrez, F., 1978, Estratigrafía del Complejo Acatlán en la Mixteca Baja, Estados de Puebla y Oaxaca: Universidad Nacional Autonoma de Mexico, Instituto de Geologia, Revista, v. 2, n. 2, p. 112-131.

Ortega-Gutiérrez, F., and Centeno-Garcia E., 1988, Caracterización tectonoestratigráfica de la "Cuenca Guerrero-Morelos": II Simposio sobre la Geología Regional de México, Universidad Nacional Autonoma de Mexico, Instituto de Geología, Memoir, p 59-60.

Ortiz-Hernandez, E., Yta, M., Talavera, O., Lapierre, H., Monod, O., Tardy, M., 1991, Origine intra-océanique des formations volcano-plutoniques d'arc du Jurassique-Crétacé inférieur du Mexique centro-méridional, C. R. Acad. Sci. Paris, t. 321, Série II, p. 399-406.

Pantoja, A.J. (1959) Estudio Geologico de Reconocimiento de la region de Huetamo, Estado de Michoacan, Consejo de Recursos Naturales no renovables, Bol 50, 1-33.

Pantoja, A.J., 1990, Redefinición de las unidades estratigráficas de la secuencia Mesozoica de la región de Huetamo-Altamirano, Estados de MIchoacán y Guerrero, Convención Geológica Nacional, Resúmenes, p. 66.

Pantoja, A.J. and Estrada, B.S.,1986, Estratigrafia de los alrededores de la mina de fierro de El Encino, Jalisco: Sociedad Geologica Mexicana, XLVII, v. 1, p. 1-15.

Patchett, P. J., and Ruiz, J., 1987, Nd isotopic ages of crust formation and metamorphism in the Precambrian of eastern and southern Mexico: Contributions to Mineralogy and Petrology, v. 96, p. 523-528.

Pearce, J. A., 1982, Trace Element characteristics of lavas from destructuve plate boundaries, in Thope, R. S., ed., Andesites: Orogenic andesites and related rocks, John Wiley and Sons, p. 227-239.

Pettijohn, F. J., Potter, P. E., Siever, R., 1987, Sand and Sandstone, Springer-Verlag, 553 p.

Quintero-Legorreta, O., 1992, Geología de la Región de Comanja, Estados de Guanajuato y Jalisco: Universidad Nacional Autonoma de Mexico, Instituto de Geologia, Revista, v. 10, n. 1, p. 6-25.

Ramírez-Espinosa, J., Campa, M. F., Talavera, O., Guerrero, M., 1991, Caracterización de los arcos insulares de la Sierra Madre del Sur y sus implicaciones tectónicas, Convención sobre la evolución Geológica Mexicana, 1er Congreso Mexicano de Mineralogía, Pachuca, Memoir, p. 163-166.

Ranson, W.A., Fernandez, L.A., Simmons, W.B. Jr, and de la Vega, E. S. 1982, Petrology of the Metamorphic rocks of Zacatecas, Mexico: Soc. Geol. Mex., v. XLIII (1), p. 37-59.

Roberts, S.J., and Ruiz, J., 1989, Geochemical zonation and evolution of the lower crust in Mexico: Journal of Geophysical Research, v. 94, p. 7961-7974.

Ruiz, J., Patchett, P.J., and Ortega-Gutierrez, F., 1988, Proterozoic and Phanerozoic basement terranes of Mexico from Nd isotopic studies: Geological Society of America, Bulletin, v. 100, p. 247-281.

Ruiz, J., Centeno-Garcia, E., Coney, P.J., Patchett, P.J., and Ortega-Gutierrez, F., 1991, Geology and Geochemistry of the Guerrero terrane, western Mexico and its possible correlation with rocks underlying the Greater Antilles and western Andes of Venezuela, Colombia and Ecuador: GSA, Abstracts with Programs, 1991 annual meeting, p. A218.

Sanchez-Zavala, J. L., 1993, Secuencia volcanosedimentaria Jurásico Superior-Cretácico Arcelia Otzoloapan (Terreno Guerrero), area Valle de Bravo-Zacazonapan, Estado de México: Petrografía, Geoquímica, Metamorfismo e Interpretación Tectónica, M. S. Thesis, Science Faculty, Univesidad Nacional Autónoma de México, Mexico, 91 p.

Schaaf, P., 1990, Isotopengeochemische Untersuchungen an Granitoiden Gesteinen eines aktiven Kontinentalrandes. Alter und Herkunft der Tiefengesteinskomplexe an der Pazifikküste Mexikos zwischen Puerto Vallarta und Acapulco: Dissertation, Ludwig-Maximilians Universität, München, 202 pp.

Sedlock, R. L., Ortega-Gutiérrez, F., Speed, R.C., 1992, Tectonostratigraphic Terranes and Tectonic Evolution of México, G.S.A., Special Paper, n. 278, 180 p.

Sholkovitz, E R., 1988, Rare earth elements in the sediments of the North Atlantic Ocean, Amazon Delta, and East China Sea: reinterpretation of terrigenous input patterns to the oceans, American Journal of Science, v. 288, p. 236-281.

Silva-Romo, G., 1993, Estudio de la Estratigrafía y Estructuras Tectónicas de la Sierra de Salinas, Edos. de San Luis Potosí y Zacatecas (M. S. Thesis): Science Faculty, Universidad Nacional Autónoma de México, Mexico, 111 p.

Stewart J, Blodgett R B, Boucot A J, y Carter J. L., 1993, Middle Paleozoic exotic terrane near Ciudad Victoria, NE Mexico, and the southern margin of Paleozoic North America: Proceedings of the First Circum-Pacific and Circum-Atlantic Terrane Conference, Gto Mex, p. 147-149.

Talavera-Mendoza, O., 1993, Les formations orogéniques mésozoïques du Guerrero (Mexique méridional). Contribution a la connaissance de l'évolution géodynamique des cordillères mexicaines, Ph. D. dissertation, Univ. Joseph Fourier-Grenoble I, France, 462 p.

Talavera-Mendoza, O., Ramírez-Espinosa, J., Guerrero-Suástegui, M., 1993, Geochemical evolution of the Guerrero terrane-example of a Late Mesozoic multi-arc system: Proceedings of the First Circum-Pacific and Circum-Atlantic Terrane Conference, p. 150-152.

Talavera-Mendoza, O., Ramírez-Espinosa, J., Guerrero-Suástegui, M., 1995, Petrology and Geochemistry of the Teloloapan subterrane: a Lower Cretaceous evolved intra-oceanic island-arc: Geofisica Internacional, v. 34, n. 1, p. 3-22.

Taylor, S. R., and McLennan, S. M., 1985, The Continental Crust: Its Composition and Evolution: Oxford, Blackwell ed., 311.

Tardy M., and Maury R., 1973, Sobre la presencia de elementos de origen volcanico en las areniscas de los flyschs de edad Cretásica superior de los Estados de Coahuila y de Zacatecas, Sociedad Geológica Mexicana, Bulletin, v. 34, n. 1 and 2, p. 5-12.

Tardy M., Lapierre, H., Bourdier, J. L., Yta, M., and Coulon, C., 1991a, The Late Jurassic-Early Cretaceous arc of western Mexico (Guerrero Terrane); origin and geodynamic evolution, Convención sobre la evolución Geológica Mexicana, 1er Congreso Mexicano de Mineralogía, Pachuca, Memoir, p. 213-215.

Tardy M., Lapierre, H., Bourdier, J. L., Coulon, C., 1991b,Ortiz-Hernandez, E., and Yta, M., 1992, Intraoceanic setting of western Mexico Guerrero terrane-implications for the Pacific-Tethys geodynamic relationships during the Cretaceous: Instituto de Geologia, Universidad Nacional Autonoma de Mexico, Revista, v. 10, n. 2, 118-128.

Tardy M., Lapierre H., Freydier C., Coulon C., Gill J.B., Mercier de Lepinay B., Beck C., Martinez J., Talavera M., Ortiz E., Stein G., Bourdier J. L., and Yta M., 1994, The Guerrero suspect terrane (western Mexico) and coeval arc terranes (the Greater Antilles and the Western Cordillera of Colombia): a late Mesozoic intra-oceanic arc accreted to cratonal America during the Creteaceous: Tectonophysics, v. 234, n. 4, p. 49-73.

Taylor, S. R., and McLennan, S. M., 1985, The Continental Crust: Its Composition and Evolution, Blackwell, Oxford.

Terrell, D. J., Surendra, P., Lopez, M., 1981, Geochemistry of some metamorphic and sedimentary rocks from the mineral district of Zacatecas, Zacatecas, Mexico: Geofísica Internacional, v. 17, n. 2, p. 151-166.

Torres-Vargas, R., Ruiz, J., Murillo-Muñetón, G., and Grajales-Nishimura, M., 1993, The Paleozoic magmatism in Mexico; evidences for the shift from circum Atlantic to circum-Pacific tectonism: Universidad Nacional Autonoma de Mexico, Instituto de Geología, First Circum-Pacific and Circum-Atlantic Terrane Conference, Guanajuato Mexico, p. 154-155.

Uribe, R. M., and Urrutia, J., 1992, Xenolitos de Corteza Inferior y Estratigrafía Volcánica en los maars de Valle de Santiago, Gto., GEOS, Unión Geofísica Mexicana, Abstracts, v. 12, n. 5, p. 263-GEOL-08.

Vidal-Serratos R., 1991, Estratigrafía y tectónica de la región de Zihuatanejo, Estado de Guerrero, Sierra Madre del Sur, Convención sobre la evolución Geológica Mexicana, 1er Congreso Mexicano de Mineralogía, Pachuca, Memoir, p. 231-233.

Yañez, P., Ruiz, J., Patchett, P.J., Ortega-Gutierrez, F., and Gehrels, G., 1991, Isotopic studies of the Acatlan Complex, southern Mexico: Implications for Paleozoic North American Tectonics: Geological Society of America, Bulletin, v. 103, n. 6, p. 817-828.

Yta, M., Lapierre, H., Monod, O., and Wever, P., 1990, Magmatic and structural characteristics of the Lower Cretaceous arc-volcano-sedimentary sequence of Saucito-Zacatecas-Fresnillo (central Mexico), geodynamic implications, Munich, Germany, Geowisenschaftliches Lateinamerika, kolloquium, Memoir, p. 21.11-23.11.

PRECIOUS-METAL-BEARING VOLCANOGENIC MASSIVE SULPHIDE DEPOSITS, CAMPO MORADO, GUERRERO, MEXICO

JIM OLIVER, JOHN PAYNE, MARK REBAGLIATI, ROBERT CLUFF
Farallon Resources Ltd., 1020 - 800 West Pender Street, Vancouver, B.C., Canada V6C 2V6

ABSTRACT

The Campo Morado precious-metal-bearing, volcanogenic massive sulphide deposits occur in a Lower Cretaceous, bimodal, calc-alkaline volcanic sequence in a northerly trending belt in the Guerrero Terrane, northeastern Mexico. During Upper Cretaceous to Lower Tertiary greenschist-facies regional metamorphism, the rocks were deformed strongly into a northeast-verging fold-and-thrust belt. Three later stages of weak deformation were dominated by kink-folds, broad warps, and extensional faults respectively. Most massive sulphide deposits occur in the upper part of a sequence of felsic flows and heterolithic volcanoclastic rocks or at its contact with overlying chert and argillite-sandstone. The Reforma and El Rey massive sulphide deposits are on the overturned limb of a major, thrusted anticline, and the Naranjo, El Largo, Estrella de Oro and El Profundo massive sulphide deposits are to the south on the upright limb of the same major fold. The La Lucha, San Rafael and G9 massive sulphide occurrences are in an upper plate to the southwest which was thrusted over the plate containing the Naranjo, El Largo, Estrella de Oro and El Profundo deposits. In most of the deposits, Au, Ag, Zn and Pb are concentrated near the stratigraphic top, and Cu is concentrated near the stratigraphic base. Major minerals are pyrite, quartz, ankerite, sphalerite, chalcopyrite and galena. Minor minerals are tennantite-freibergite, arsenopyrite and pyrrhotite. Gold and silver occur in argentian gold, and silver also occurs in tennantite-freibergite. The cumulative inferred resource of massive sulphide for the Reforma, Naranjo, El Rey and El Largo deposits exceeds 30 Mt, with the latter two deposits incompletely delineated. Underlying pyrite-quartz stockwork zones contain chalcopyrite, chlorite and sphalerite. Hydrothermal alteration minerals in the stratigraphic footwall are pyrite, quartz, chlorite, ferroan dolomite and ankerite. In the stratigraphic hangingwall, hydrothermal alteration minerals are sericite, calcite-dolomite and lesser clay minerals and quartz. The deposits belong to a volcanogenic massive sulphide system formed in a subaqueous environment, and are of the bimodal, siliciclastic type.

INTRODUCTION

The Campo Morado district is located in the Sierra Madre del Sur range in the north-central part of the state of Guerrero, Mexico, 160 km south-southwest of Mexico City. Exploration activities since November 1995 by Farallon Resources Ltd. have focused on a series of precious metal-bearing, volcanogenic massive sulphide deposits occurring at or near the contact of a sequence of felsic to intermediate flows, tuffs and heterolithic fragmental rocks with stratigraphically overlying fine-grained, chemical and clastic sedimentary rocks. Through diamond drilling, Farallon has outlined six massive sulphide deposits, five of which can be classified as new discoveries of which there is no surface expression. Current massive sulphide resources total in excess of 30 million tonnes.

EXPLORATION AND PRODUCTION HISTORY

The Reforma deposit was discovered in 1898. From 1903-1910, production totaled 3,387 kg gold, 125,229 kg silver and 4,157,150 kg lead. Minor production came from the Historic Naranjo deposit. In 1913, mining activity was interrupted by the Mexican Revolution, and since then production records are not available. The dates on gold, silver and copper coins minted at Campo Morado suggest that production continued during the revolution. From 1920-1927 and from 1937-1940 oxide ore and minor amounts of sulphide ore were mined. A calculation of resources in the Reforma and Historic Naranjo deposit prior to work by Farallon are shown in Table 1. From 1973-1977, a subsidiary of Union Oil rehabilitated 3.7 km of mine workings and cored 840 m in underground drilling. In 1986, Consejo completed 1:50,000 regional mapping and photo interpretation including mapping

Table 1 Inferred resources for the Reforma and historic Naranjo deposits*

Deposit	Tonnes	Au g/t	Ag g/t	Cu %	Pb %
Reforma	8,593,000	2.26	127	1.04	-
(includes)	2,700,000	4.87	247	1.14	-
Historic Naranjo					
low grade pyrite	198,000	0.96	60	1.03	-
silica sand ore	123,000	1.37	103	-	-
lead ore	24,000	23.66	627	-	8.8
iron oxide ore	81,000	2.68	278	-	0.2

*Unpublished report by O.R. Whitaker (1912) to the Canadian Agency Ltd., managers of the Reforma Syndicates.

of 16 massive sulphide occurrences in the Campo Morado area.

In late 1995, Farallon Resources Ltd. began an intensive geological and geochemical exploration program at Campo Morado. This program included regional and detailed geological mapping and multi-element soil-geochemical surveys. Emphasis was placed on assessment of the depositional environment, structural setting, alteration facies and vectors and the geochemical characteristics of prospective host units. From June 1996 to June 1998, a core-drilling program totaled 64,200 m in 320 holes. This included definition drilling of the Reforma deposit, the discovery and definition of the Naranjo deposit, and the discovery and partial definition of the El Largo and El Rey deposits and the discovery of the Estrella de Oro and G9 zones. Detailed geological, gravity, soil and geophysical surveys continue to define the resource potential of the district. Estimates of grade and tonnage of the Reforma, El Rey, Naranjo and El Largo deposits are shown in Table 2. Metallurgical, engineering, environmental and infrastructure studies are in progress to quantify the mineable resources.

Regional Geology

The Campo Morado district is in the Sierra Madre del Sur range in the north-central part of the state of Guerrero, Mexico, 160 km south-southwest of Mexico City at elevations ranging from 600 to 1600 m. The district occurs in the Guerrero Terrane; a large, fault-bounded composite terrane defined by Campa and Coney (1983), which contains three main sub-terranes defined as Teloloapan, Zihuantenejo, and Huetamo. The district is bounded to the east by the Mixteco Terrane, to the west by the Sierra Madre Occidental and to the north by the Trans-Mexican Neogene Volcanic belt (Fig. 1). The Teloloapan sub-terrane is a deformed Lower Cretaceous sequence which includes bimodal volcanic rocks, platform carbonate, quartz sandstone, shale and siltstone. The abundance of bimodal volcanic rocks is a main difference between the Teloloapan sub-terrane and the other two major sub-terranes, which have a higher percentage of volcanoclastic and clastic sedimentary rocks.

The evolution and origin of the Guerrero Terrane is in dispute. Campa and Coney (1983) described it as an allochthonous block of Upper Jurassic to Lower Cretaceous, volcano-sedimentary island-arc-derived rocks, which formed an accretionary prism onto the western margin of the Mexican craton in Campanian-Eocene time. Freydier et al. (1993) proposed a similar geodynamic model for the evolution of the Guerrero Terrane as a long-lived island arc, isolated from continental Mexico by an oceanic basin, the Arperos Basin. The allochthonous nature of the terrane, and even the existence of the terrane, was questioned by Lang et al. (1996), who found no evidence for the bounding faults which had been defined by other workers to separate the sub-terranes. A more-autochthonous origin was suggested by Centeno-Garcia et al. (1993) on the basis of the presence of cratonic-derived clastic sedimentary detritus in the Guerrero stratigraphic record.

During the Upper Cretaceous to Paleogene, Laramide age orogenesis, the region was deformed into a north-northeast verging fold and thrust belt and was metamorphosed to sub-greenschist to greenschist facies (Miranda-Gasca, 1995). The total amount of crustal shortening due to folding and thrust faults was 60 km (Lang et al. 1996).

PROPERTY GEOLOGY

At Campo Morado, precious-metal-bearing, volcanogenic massive sulphide deposits occur in a sequence of felsic to intermediate flows and tuffs, and heterolithic fragmental rocks. Precious metal-rich massive sulphide deposits are defined as containing gold greater than 2 g/t and/or silver greater than 100 g/t (Fig. 6.4-1 in Poulsen and Hannington, 1996). Preliminary geological descriptions of these deposits have been presented by Oliver et al. (1998). Most of the deposits are in the upper part of the felsic pile or at the contact with stratigraphically overlying, fine-

Table 2 Inferred resources for the Reforma, El Rey, Naranjo and El Largo deposits

Deposit	Tonnes (Millions)	Au (g/t)	Ag (g/t)	Cu %	Pb %	Zn %	Specific Gravity
Reforma	11.9	1.90	117	0.71	0.75	2.06	3.62
(including)	4.2	4.28	227	0.78	1.47	3.87	3.88
Naranjo	9.7	1.40	69	0.76	0.51	1.91	4.14
(including)	2.6	3.04	138	0.94	1.29	3.94	-
El Rey	3.7	1.35	74	0.48	0.53	2.38	4.18
(including)	1.4	2.73	138	0.47	1.10	4.29	-
El Largo	3.8	1.19	67	0.66	0.46	2.45	4.08
(including)	1.5	1.33	108	0.78	0.77	4.35	-
Total	29.0	1.57	89	0.69	0.60	2.10	
(including)	9.6	3.27	172	0.78	1.26	4.02	

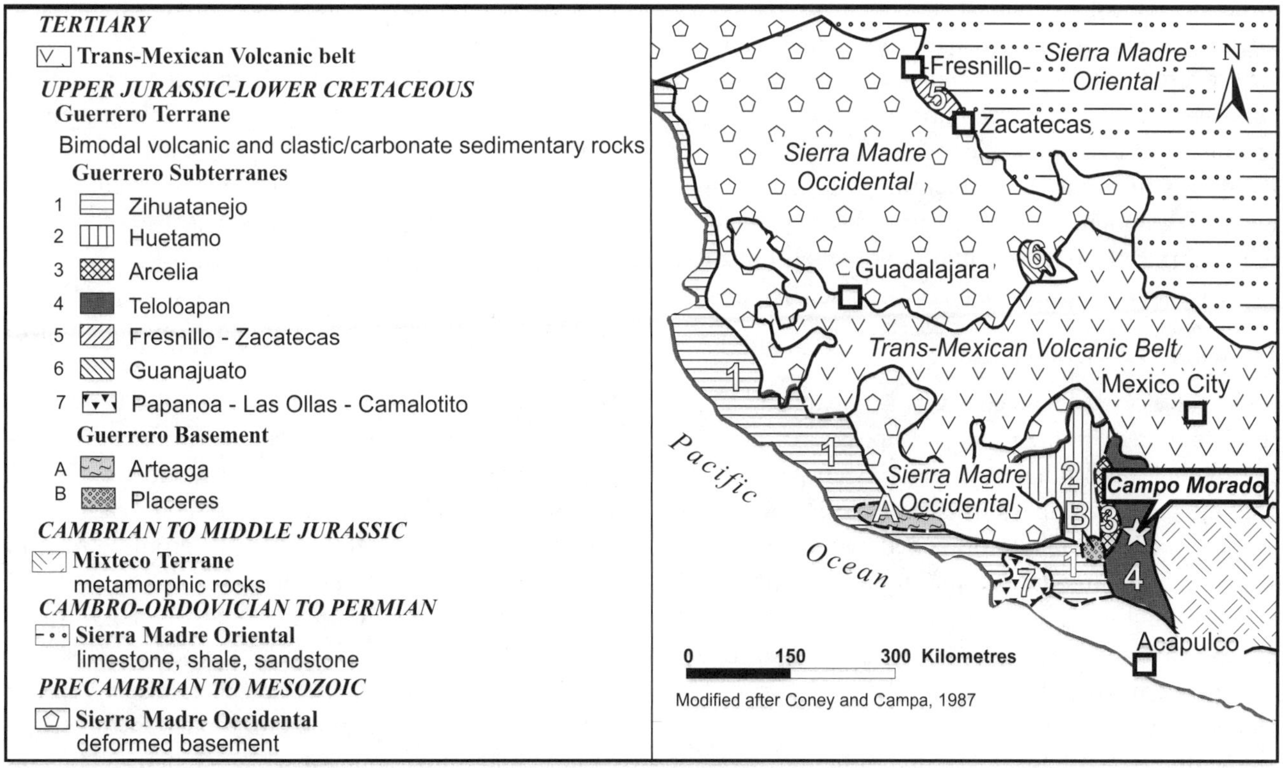

Figure 1. Regional geology and location of the Campo Morado VMS deposit

grained chemical and clastic sedimentary rocks. Surface geology (Fig. 2) based on mapping by Farallon geologists consists of five major lithostratigraphic units or formations. The age of the felsic section is constrained by preliminary U-Pb data to be approximately 145 Ma or Lowest Cretaceous. Limited paleontology data also suggests Lower Cretaceous ages of the sedimentary rocks in the section. Stratigraphic positions of some of these formations are uncertain, mainly because of incomplete knowledge of the early deformation.

La Cañita Volcanic Unit

This unit of felsic to intermediate volcanic and volcanoclastic rocks occurs southeast of the pueblo of Campo Morado. At the northwestern end, lenses of massive chert and siliceous rhyolitic flow occur. Along strike to the southeast, the flow contains 3-7 % plagioclase phenocrysts and locally up to 7 % quartz phenocrysts. Farther southeast is a zone of massive volcanic wacke. To the northeast is a porphyritic intermediate flow or subvolcanic intrusion, in part altered moderately to strongly to ankerite. At the structural top of the unit, to the southwest, a mixed zone of felsic and intermediate tuff and wacke are interlayered with argillite and one 10 m interval of fine to coarse, pebble conglomerate dominated by fragments of felsic volcanic rocks. This mixed zone is overlain structurally by a thick interval of limestone and lesser amounts of argillite, probably at the base of the Reforma Sedimentary unit. The overall thickness of the La Canita Volcanic unit is several hundred metres.

Reforma Sedimentary Unit

The Reforma Sedimentary unit is exposed above the Hinge fault in the Reforma deposit area and was intersected in drillholes in the lower part of the Naranjo and El Largo deposits. At Reforma, the stratigraphic section in the Reforma Sedimentary unit is as follows, from stratigraphic top to bottom: calcareous argillite, phyllitic limestone, rhythmically bedded siltstone-wacke-argillite marker unit and lapilli tuff/wacke interbedded with argillite and pyritic siltstone/argillite.

A single fossil (Distoloceras) from the western extremity of the Reforma area is indicative of the lower Cretaceous, upper Valanginian to lower Hauterivian (Haggart, 1997). The Hinge fault, a major thrust fault, separates this block from a lower overturned block containing rocks of the Campo Morado Felsic Volcanic unit and the Reforma massive sulphide deposit. At the Naranjo deposit, only the upright top of the Reforma Sedimentary unit was intersected in drill core. This top portion is dominated by calcareous argillite, cherty argillite and minor wacke. It overlies a thick interval of limestone exposed to the east, and conformably underlies rocks of the Campo Morado Felsic Volcanic unit.

Campo Morado Felsic Volcanic Unit

The lithology and internal stratigraphy of this unit are variable, and the thickness varies up to a few hundred metres, being thickest in the cores of felsic domes. In the Naranjo deposit area, a layer of chert and cherty argillite up to 10 m in thickness occurs along the lower contact. In general, the lower two-thirds of the section is dominated by massive felsic to intermediate flow and dome complexes, and by lesser amounts of lapilli tuff and lenses of heterolithic volcanic rock. The flows and domes range from massive to auto-brecciated to strongly brecciated; the last grades into volcanoclastic fragmental rocks with abundant juvenile fragments of felsite flow and minor to moderately abundant exotic fragments, commonly of argillite. In domes, the composition grades from intermediate near the base to felsic near the top.

At the Reforma and Naranjo deposits, the upper part of the unit consists of a clast-supported, heterolithic fragmental rock dominated by lapilli-size, angular to subrounded fragments of flow material, less abundant fragments of argillite, chert and siltstone and locally up to 3 % fragments of massive sulphide. These are set in a sparse to moderately abundant matrix of silt or fine tuff. Near the top of the section, this rock grades into a finer heterolithic rock in which fragments are supported in a matrix of silt sized fine tuff. Minor heterolithic rock also occurs in and directly above the massive sulphide bodies. Distal to the volcanic centre at Reforma, the felsic volcanic rocks comprise fine- to medium-grained tuff interlayered with argillite, some of which contains abundant fragments of felsite. At the north end of the Naranjo

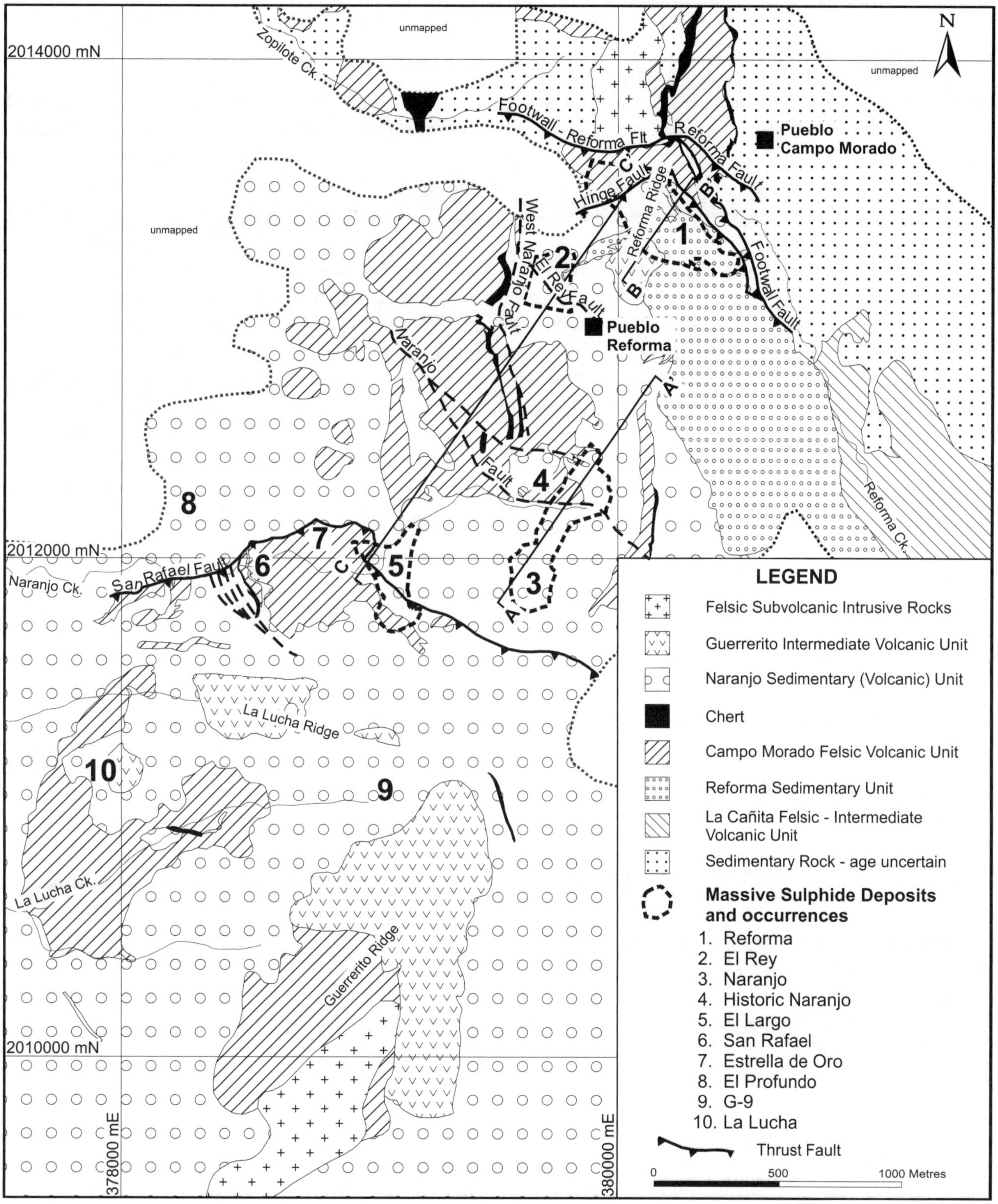

Figure 2. Propoerty Geology

deposit, outcrops of volcanic rocks consist of altered felsic to intermediate flows and lesser tuff, commonly with abundant hematite after pyrite.

At the El Largo deposit, a rapid, lateral transition is illustrated by the change from flows and domes to heterolithic fragmental rocks and massive sulphides, and then to distal sedimentary rocks.

Naranjo Sedimentary-(Intermediate Volcanic) Unit

This unit conformably overlies the Campo Morado Felsic unit and is at least several hundred metres thick. It contains intervals dominated by quartz sandstone and quartz siltstone interbedded with others dominated by siltstone and argillite. The argillite is calcareous in places and grades into argillaceous limestone and, locally limestone. Commonly present near quartz sandstone layers are irregular lenses of heterolithic fragmental rock up to 50 m thick. The heterolithic rocks contain angular to subrounded, pebble- to cobble-size fragments of quartz sandstone and quartz siltstone, with fewer fragments of siltstone and argillite, in a groundmass of finely comminuted material. The heterolithic rocks may have formed by slump into fault-bounded basins, some of which may represent reactivation of growth faults formed during the development of the Campo Morado Felsic Volcanic unit.

Guerrerito Ridge Intermediate Volcanic-Subvolcanic Unit

This unit contains two distinct sub-units of roughly similar composition, which may be related genetically. One, consisting of a massive porphyritic flow, occurs on Guerrerito and La Lucha ridges. In general, contacts are conformable with underlying rocks, but in detail they are irregular and along faults. Because the top of the unit was eroded, the overall thickness is unknown.

On Reforma ridge and north of Pueblo Reforma, a massive unit of andesitic wacke at least 30 m thick contains scattered angular fragments up to 30 cm across of porphyritic andesite flow. Locally, this rock overlies a 1 m thick basal zone of finely bedded green siltstone and wacke, which also contains scattered coarser blocks of porphyritic andesite flow. These rocks overlie thinly bedded siltstone and argillite of the Naranjo Sedimentary-(Volcanic) unit and many of the contacts are along moderately dipping faults.

Hypabyssal Intrusive Rocks

The Campo Morado Felsic Volcanic unit and Reforma and Naranjo Sedimentary units were intruded by high-level, massive felsic bodies. One large body north of and truncated by the Reforma fault contains two members: a plagioclase-phyric latite and a quartz- and plagioclase-phyric, leucocratic rhyodacite. At the south end of Guerrerito ridge occurs an intrusion of quartz- and plagioclase-phyric, leucocratic rhyodacite. The Reforma Sedimentary unit is intruded by irregular bodies of hypabyssal, aphanitic, commonly brecciated felsic bodies, which may have been intruded into wet sediments. The largest intrusion is structurally above the east side of the Reforma massive sulphide deposit. These intrusions probably represent subvolcanic equivalents of the Campo Morado Felsic Volcanic unit.

STRUCTURE

The deformation patterns are complex. In most outcrops only one major penetrative foliation is present. A second (later) foliation is present in a small percentage of outcrops and is generally weaker than the first. Faulting contributes an added complication to the structural complexity of the area. Large thrust faults follow the hinge line of large recumbent folds and allow for stratigraphy reversals. These thrust faults have been cut and stepped by a series of normal faults with movements in the order of 100 m. In all, at least four periods of deformation has been recognized.

A major, penetrative deformation event (D1) is characterized by north-northeast-verging, upright to slightly overturned F1 folds and thrust faults. The axial surface of the largest F1 anticline lies between the inverted Reforma and upright Naranjo stratigraphic sections (Fig. 3, section B-B[1]). D1 features are irregular and typical of zones containing blocks of highly varied strength. On limbs of folds in incompetent rocks, S0 was transposed parallel to S1. In competent rocks, transposition effects are limited and primary sedimentary features are preserved. D1 structural features were deformed slightly to moderately by later deformation events.

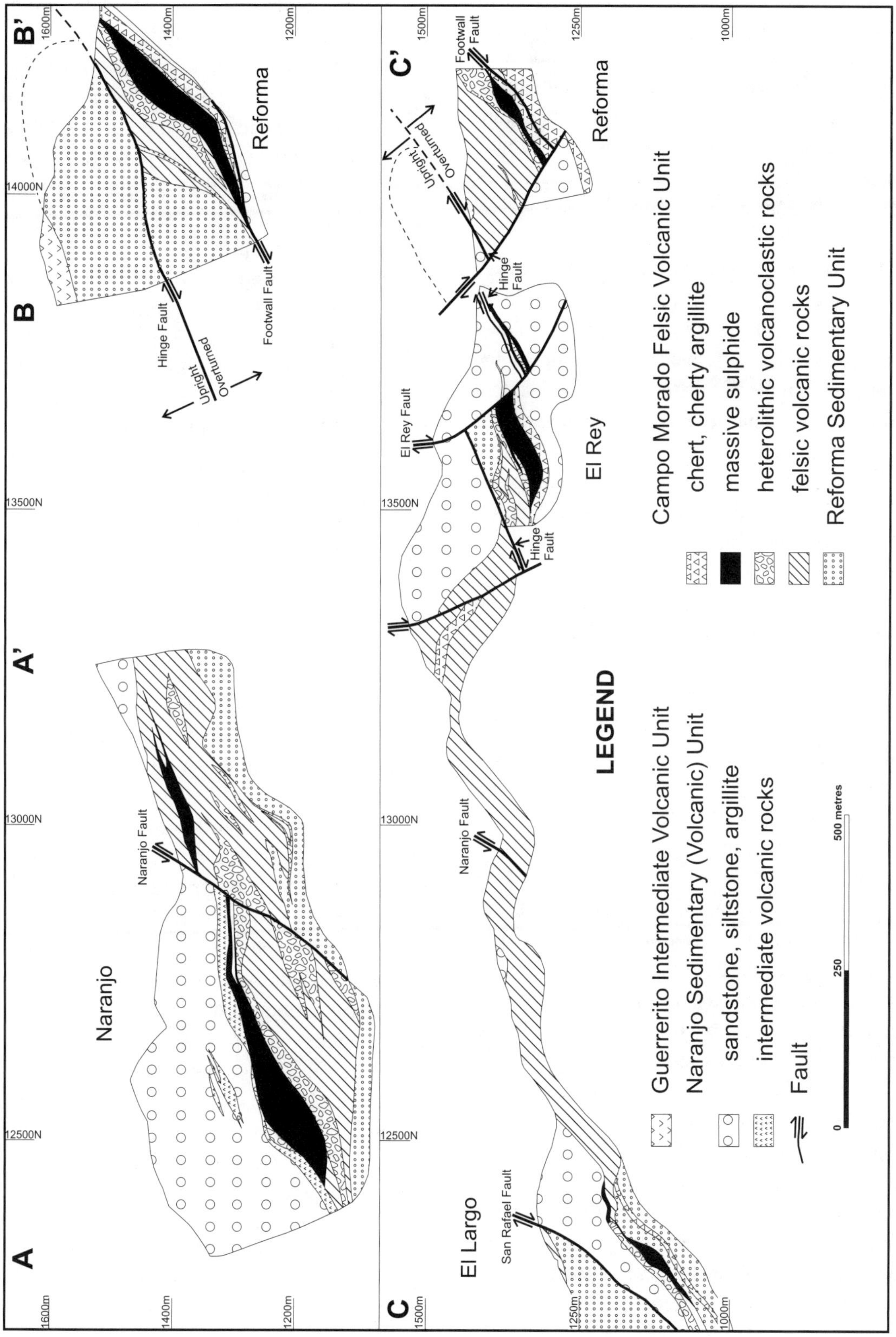

Figure 3. Geology cross section

At Reforma, D1 thrust faults include the Hinge, Footwall and Reforma faults. The Hinge fault separates overturned rocks of the Campo Morado Felsic Volcanic unit from upright rocks of the Reforma Sedimentary unit (Fig. 3). The Footwall fault and its northern splay, the Reforma fault, separate the Reforma zone from similar overturned felsic volcanic rocks and bedded chert to the north. The San Rafael thrust fault separates the Naranjo and El Largo zones from the San Rafael and Lucha zones to the west and southwest.

D1 features were formed during a major compressive deformation in the Upper Cretaceous - Lower Tertiary Laramide orogenic event. In the plate-accretion model, the deformation would be related to docking of the Guerrero Terrane with the North American continent.

D2 deformation is characterized by tight, angular kink folds, conjugate kink folds, and minor warps. These have a widespread distribution and variable orientations of fold axes and axial planes. Axial planes of kink folds commonly dip gently to the south, and cause a steepening of the southwesterly dipping S1 foliation. The variable orientation of D2 structural features indicates that D2 folds were deformed by later structural events.

D3 deformation produced open, upright folds with no macroscopic penetrative foliation. These include a broad syncline and tighter anticline pair between the Reforma and Naranjo deposits. This pair has an east-southeast-trending axis and shallow plunge to the southeast. This deformation produced a broad rotation of S1 foliation.

D4 deformation is dominated by extensional faults that offset stratigraphic and other structural elements. Slickensides indicate predominant dip-slip movement. Some early faults may have been reactivated and some faults are filled by massive mafic dykes, many of which were altered to clay. The Naranjo fault drops the stratigraphic section of the southern segment of the Naranjo deposit by 60 to 80 m (Fig. 3). The extensional north-dipping El Rey fault drops the north side of the El Rey massive sulphide deposit 30 to 60 m relative to the south side. The West Naranjo fault, which trends north and dips steeply east, drops the western edge of the El Rey area by at least 50 m. These faults may be part of regional Oligocene and younger crustal extension.

MASSIVE SULPHIDE DEPOSITS

Massive sulphide deposits occur in the Campo Morado Felsic Volcanic unit, mainly near its upper contact. A major thrust fault along the axial zone of a recumbent anticline separates the overturned Reforma and El Rey deposits from the upright Naranjo and El Largo deposits. In a thrust plate to the south of the Naranjo, El Largo and El Profundo deposits, the La Lucha and San Rafael massive sulphide occurrences contain lenses of auriferous massive sulphides up to a few metres thick and small stringer zones at the same stratigraphic level as the Naranjo deposit.

Figure 3 shows the spatial relationship between the Reforma and Naranjo massive sulphide bodies (composite section A-A^1 and B-B^1), and among the Reforma, El Rey, and El Largo deposits (section C-C^1).

Several other massive sulphide deposits, occurrences and stringer zones are associated with felsic to intermediate volcanic rocks in a 25 km long belt extending north-northwest and south-southeast of the Campo Morado district.

Reforma Deposit

The Reforma deposit occurs at the stratigraphic top (structural base) of the overturned Campo Morado Felsic Volcanic unit and is stratigraphically overlain (structurally underlain) by a prominent, well-bedded chert to cherty argillite. The massive sulphide body consists predominantly of pyrite with variable amounts of quartz and ankerite with minor to moderate sphalerite, chalcopyrite and galena. The deposit is zoned stratigraphically with a lower Cu-rich zone, a central pyrite-rich zone, which grades upwards to a pyrite-sphalerite zone and then to an upper sphalerite-galena-rich zone containing significant values in precious metals. Gold and silver occur in electrum (Au 65 Ag 35) and silver also occurs in tennantite-freibergite. Laterally, the central pyrite-rich zone diminishes in thickness and the lower copper zone merges with the upper Pb-Zn-Au-Ag zone (see assay intervals from holes 97260 and 97258 in Table 3).

The southeastern edge of the Reforma deposit is truncated along the Footwall fault. The southwestern edge is truncated by a north-dipping extensional fault parallel to the El Rey fault. Stratigraphically beneath the Reforma massive sulphides occurs a heterolithic fragmental rock. This fragmental unit thickest in the west-central part of the deposit and absent at either end. Below the heterolithic rock occurs massive felsic flow, flow-breccia and a minor volcanoclastic unit. This volcanoclastic unit is also most abundant in the centre of the zone and disappears off to the east and west. Figure 4 shows thicknesses of the Reforma massive sulphide body relative to the Campo Morado Felsic Volcanic unit. These spatial relations suggest the presence of a vent zone near 4750E with the massive sulphide body spilling onto the proximal flanks of the vent.

El Rey Deposit

The El Rey deposit, 200 m southwest of the Reforma deposit, appears overturned with the massive sulphides structurally beneath the Campo Morado Felsic Volcanic unit. The stratigraphic and structural setting is similar to that of the Reforma deposit. The Hinge fault occurs several metres above the structural top of the felsic pile, but is less prominent than at Reforma. The deposit is cut by extensional normal to oblique faults, of which the main one, the El Rey fault, dips northeasterly, with offset measured in tens of metres. The massive sulphide body is compositionally zoned and, like the Reforma deposit, has a zone rich in Au, Ag, Zn, and Pb at its structural base (stratigraphic top).

Naranjo Deposit

A train of coarse blocks and boulders of gossan, ferricrete and strongly hematitic felsic volcanic rocks represents the surface exposure of the historic Naranjo deposit. Drillholes in the historic Naranjo area intersected lenses of massive sulphides at three stratigraphic levels in the Campo Morado Felsic Volcanic unit. Also present are intervals of weak to strong stringer mineralization dominated by quartz and pyrite with less abundant chalcopyrite and sphalerite. The upper lens (which includes the historic Naranjo deposit) is oxidized and strongly leached. The lower two lenses and related stringer zones suggest the presence of a hydrothermal centre beneath the Naranjo deposit. At the base of the Campo Morado Felsic Volcanic unit, the Reforma Sedimentary unit is predominantly cherty to calcareous argillite with interbeds of chert. This interval overlies a thick section of limestone, which is well exposed on to the east.

The Naranjo deposit is at the upper contact of the upright Campo Morado Felsic Volcanic unit with the overlying Naranjo Sedimentary (Volcanic) unit. This is at the same stratigraphic level as the Historic Naranjo deposit. The former consists of felsic flows and heterolithic fragmental rocks with minor lapilli tuff and tuff. Above the massive sulphide deposit is a thin discontinuous zone of heterolithic fragmental rocks overlain by a zone of intermediate lapilli tuff and tuffaceous siltstone. Directly above this, the Naranjo Sedimentary (Volcanic) unit is predominantly siltstone and argillite. Stratigraphically higher the unit consists of interbedded sandstone and argillite, with two lenses of heterolithic fragmental sedimentary rocks.

The Naranjo deposit is an elongate massive sulphide lens that thickens to nearly 80 m in a steep-sided basin near its southern end. Many aspects of the deposit are similar to those of the Reforma deposit, although metal zonation is not as sharply defined. In the Naranjo deposit, an upper zone contains high values of Au, Ag, Zn and Pb, a central zone contains low to moderate values of Cu, and a lower zone of high

Table 3 Metal zoning Reforma deposit (structurally overturned)

DDH	From (m)	To (m)	Length (m)	Cu %	Pb %	Zn %	Ag g/t	Au g/t	Zone
97260	330.65	332.65	2.00	3.81	0.02	0.45	45.0	1.00	Lower Cu-rich
	332.65	338.65	6.00	0.84	0.01	0.28	19.0	0.54	Central Pyrite-rich
	338.65	358.65	20.00	0.43	0.68	3.04	124.0	4.76	Upper Pb, Zn, Ag, Au-rich
97258	83.06	91.74	8.68	0.81	0.44	3.67	57.0	0.92	Lower Cu-rich
	91.74	105.32	13.58	0.62	1.87	7.17	345.0	4.90	Upper Pb, Zn, Ag, Au-rich

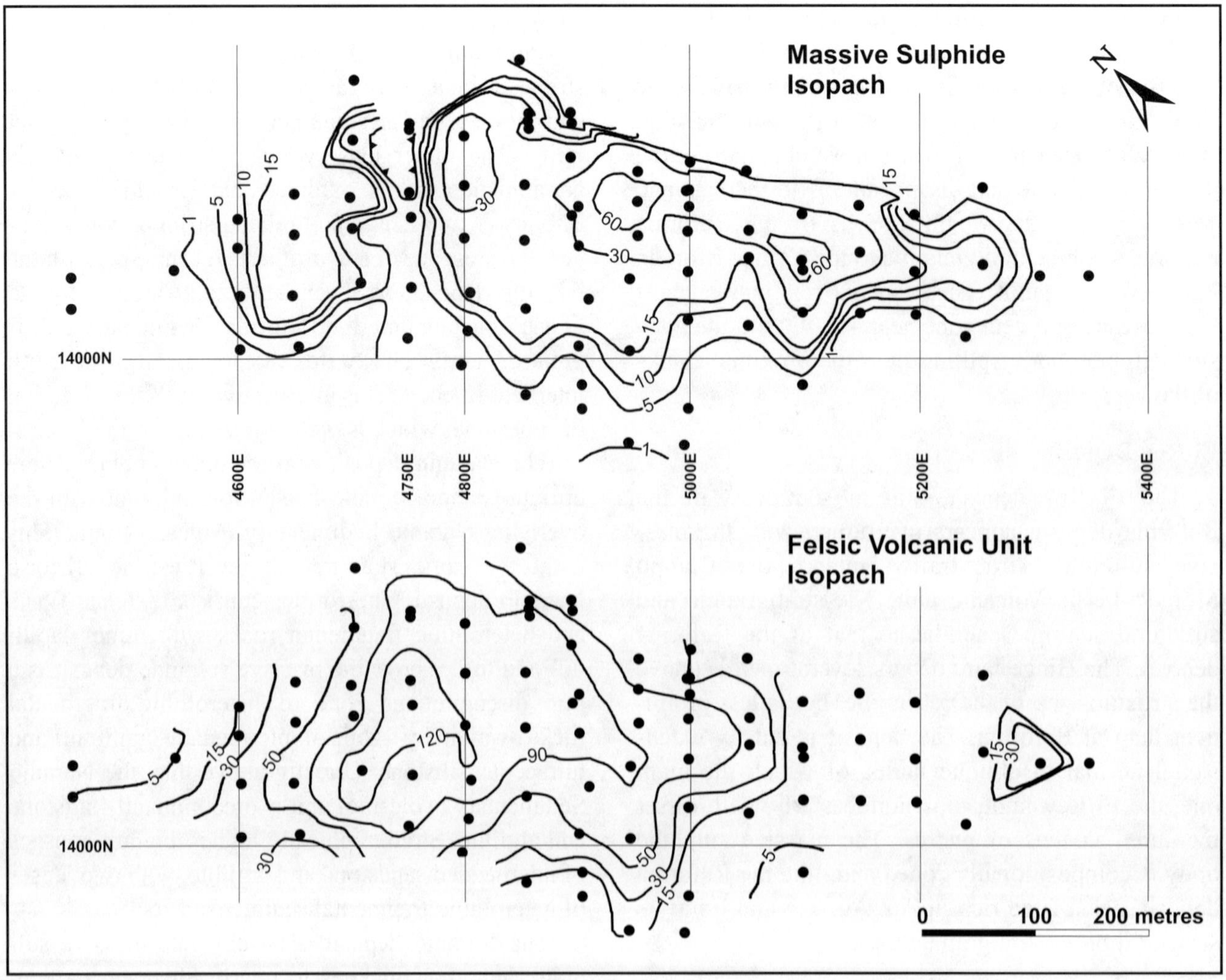

Figure 4. Reforma deposit massive sulphide and Campo Morado Felsic Volcanic unit Isopachs

values of Cu and rare high values of Zn and Au. Northeast of the main massive sulphide body, several drillholes intersected several metres of bedded to massive chert interpreted as a distal exhalite associated genetically with the massive sulphide body. In places the along strike transition is rapid from unmineralized chert to thick intercepts of massive sulphides. Unlike at Reforma, the chert zone does not extend over the top of the main part of the massive sulphide body. Beneath the massive sulphide body in heterolithic fragmental rocks and in an underlying felsic flow sequence is a replacement and stockwork alteration and vein system containing pyrite and quartz and locally abundant chalcopyrite and chlorite. This stockwork zone is thickest to the north of the main basin of massive sulphides suggesting that the former area is a vent zone for the hydrothermal solutions which produced both the stringer zone and the massive sulphide deposit.

El Largo Deposit

The El Largo deposit occurs in a felsic volcanic centre containing a massive steep-sided dome at the core surrounded by brecciated dome rocks and related coarse volcanoclastic debris on the flanks. To the south, these rocks grade rapidly outward into a sedimentary basin dominated by argillite. Near the top of the volcanic section is a 3 to 5 m thick continuous and stratabound copper mineralized zone in which chalcopyrite-pyrite veins, replacements and massive sulphides occur in felsic flows altered strongly to quartz-ankerite. Near or at the base of the section is an interval of Zn-rich massive sulphides up to 65 m thick. The thickest part is confined to a steep-sided basin, bounded by possible growth faults. Below the massive sulphide body, the upper part of the Reforma Sedimentary unit contains abundant bedded chert that grades downward into cherty, calcareous argillite and calcareous argillite. A second massive sulphide body occurs at the same stratigraphic level 200 m to the northwest again near the edge of the felsic dome. A third massive sulphide body occurs 400 metres to the north in the upper half of the felsic section on the north flank of the felsic dome.

Estrella de Oro Deposit

The Estrella de Oro deposit occurs 200 m west of the El Largo Deposit at the same stratigraphic level. It occurs near the middle of the interval of felsic volcanics and is in excess of 20 m thick. Only three drill holes have tested the Estrella de Oro deposit with the DDH 320 containing a massive sulphide intersection of 13.4 m with an average grade of 4.44 g/t Au, 357 g/t Ag, 0.55 % Cu, 2.57 % Pb and 2.76 % Zn.

San Rafael

The San Rafael zone occurs midway between the Estrella de Oro deposit and the El Profundo occurrence. Massive sulphide occurs within the Campo Morado felsic volcanic unit between rhyolitic flows and heterolithic debris flows. Channel sampling from underground workings returned 5.45 m of 2.65 g/t Au, 218 g/t Ag, 1.22 % Cu, 1.38 % Pb and 3.63 % Zn and 3.15 m of 3.41 g/t Au, 266 g/t Ag, 1.20 % Cu, 2.45 % Pb and 3.16 % Zn.

El Profundo

The El Profundo deposit was rediscovered on surface and is located 300 m west of the Estrella de Oro deposit at the same stratigraphic level in April of 1999. It occurs at the upper contact of the Campo Morado felsic volcanics with the overlying Naranjo sedimentary unit. A series of 7 adits expose a massive sulphide deposit up to 13 m in width and 120 m in length. Drilling has not commenced on this mineral occurrence.

G9 Deposit

The G9 deposit occurs 700 m to the south of the Naranjo deposit and its discovery was the result of an exploration drill test of a gravity anomaly. DDH 305 intersected 4.5 m of massive sulphides at the top of the felsic section beneath 300 m of sedimentary rocks of the Naranjo Formation. This intersection returned 3.30 g/t Au, 210 g/t Ag, 1.22 % Cu, 0.79 % Pb and 4.73 % Zn. The felsic section is 150 m thick and is characterized by abundant stockwork mineralization that contains up to 7 % Zn over widths of 3 m.

Volcanic environment

Many of the massive sulphide occurrences have similar paleographic and volcanological features. The steep sided felsic flow domes are stratigraphically overlain by blocky, mono-lithologic felsic carapace breccia which grades laterally into framework supported heterolithic fragmental rocks. The centres of the felsic flow sequences are massive, aphanitic and non-vesicular. Flow bands and lobe-hyaloclastite features are rare. Devitrified hyaloclastite fragments are widespread in the heterolithic fragmental rocks, but are volumetrically minor, generally less than 5 %. The rapid changes in thickness of the lenses of heterolithic fragmental rocks and of the overlying heterolithic sedimentary rocks suggest that both were confined in part by local, steep-sided depositional basins. Gibson et al. (1999) suggests these features are characteristic of small-volume, blocky flow domes, in contrast to larger volume, low relief, lobe hyaloclastite flows. Significant volumes of felsic synvolcanic dykes are present in the Reforma deposit but rare elsewhere. Many massive sulphide lenses have a close spatial relation to the flanks of the felsic pile, and at Reforma are elongate along the axis of the deposit. The axis of the felsic flow sequence likely is proximal to its central feeding fissure. The spatial relation of the massive sulphide sites to the central felsic flow axis also suggests a strong relationship between the feeding fissure and sulphide deposition.

Spatial Characteristics of Rock Alteration and Mineralization

Proximal, discordant patterns of rock alteration have strong similarities among most deposits of the

Campo Morado district. Alteration patterns have a striking asymmetry between stratigraphic hangingwall and footwall rocks. Stratigraphic footwall rocks were cut and replaced by extensive stockwork veinlets and patches of quartz and ferroan dolomite - ankerite. Locally they contain selvages of dark green chlorite and disseminated patches of pyrite, chalcopyrite and sphalerite. Near the footwall of the massive sulphide bodies, more intense replacement by chlorite is widespread. These alteration zones are best developed below the Naranjo deposit north of the main accumulation of massive sulphides, suggesting proximity to a vent zone.

At Reforma, ankeritic alteration of heterolithic fragmental rocks on the stratigraphic footwall is associated with intense veining and replacement by quartz and pyrite. Footwall ankerite alteration is less intense and less developed in the other deposits. In deeper footwall rocks, patchy replacements of sericite commonly replaced feldspar phenocrysts. In all deposits, kaolinite and quartz form the most distal alteration assemblages in footwall rocks.

In the footwall rocks of all deposits, alteration textures vary with rock type. In heterolithic fragmental rocks, alteration consists of patches of pervasive replacement along with disseminated sulphides. Many felsic flows contain moderate to strong quartz or sericite alteration, along with abundant stockworking and patches dominated by pyrite and quartz. Proximal to zones of hydrothermal venting, some rocks contain abundant chalcopyrite, and minor sphalerite. Near domes and in flows, alteration is strongest near their highly fractured upper margins.

Hydrothermal sericite occurs in hangingwall rocks directly above the massive sulphides. In places, the sericite-dominant alteration assemblage occurs in hangingwall heterolithic fragmental volcanic rocks that have macroscopic compositions similar to those of footwall rocks containing intense chloritic alteration. This demonstrates a major shift from Fe-Mg alteration in the stratigraphic footwall to K enrichment in the stratigraphic hangingwall. In the altered hangingwall rocks, calcite and dolomite are abundant, whereas ferroan dolomite, ankerite and siderite are sparse. Kaolinite, and quartz are abundant in both proximal and distal hangingwall rocks.

DEPOSIT CLASSIFICATION

The Campo Morado alteration assemblages, sulphide types and morphology of the alteration patterns are diagnostic of volcanogenic, massive sulphide systems as described by Hedenquist (1987). The predominance of felsic volcanic rocks over mafic ones, the abundance of clastic sedimentary rocks and the size of the deposits suggest that they belong to the bimodal siliciclastic type described by Barrie and Hannington (2000). Of all the deposit types they classified, this type of deposit has the highest average size, which is 23.7 Mt. The cumulative tonnage of massive sulphides at Campo Morado exceeds this number, and will increase as drilling continues.

CONCLUSIONS

The Campo Morado district contains precious-metal-rich, volcanic associated massive sulphide deposits in a Lower to Middle Cretaceous, volcano-sedimentary oceanic arc called the Guerrero Terrane. In Upper Cretaceous-Tertiary time, the region was deformed in a classic fold-and-thrust belt, which verges north-northeast.

The massive sulphide deposits occur in a sequence of felsic to intermediate flows and tuffs and heterolithic fragmental rocks, or at the contact of this unit with stratigraphically overlying fine-grained chemical and clastic sedimentary rocks. Most of the massive sulphide deposits were formed in steep-sided basins on the proximal flanks of felsic volcanic domes. The deposits belong to a class of bimodal, siliciclastic volcanogenic massive sulphide deposits.

The Reforma and El Rey deposits are on the overturned limb of a major north-northeast-verging, recumbent anticline whose axial plane was deformed further by a major thrust fault. The Naranjo, El Largo, Estrella de Oro and El Profundo deposits are to the south on the upright limb of the same recumbent anticline. The deposits exhibit a zoned sulphide stratigraphy. The Reforma deposit has an upper (stratigraphic) zone rich in Au, Ag, Zn and Pb, a central lower grade zone containing values mainly in Cu and Zn, and a lower zone rich in Cu, with occasional high values in Au, Zn and Ag. The El Rey deposit shows similar zonation but the Cu-rich zone is weaker. The Naranjo deposit shows similar, but less defined zonation as in the Reforma deposit, and has a prominent Cu-rich footwall stockwork zone. The El Largo deposit is Zn-rich and poorly zoned. In felsic flows well above the main El Largo massive sulphide deposit is a stratabound zone of high-grade Cu veins, replacement and massive sulphides associated with strong quartz-ankerite replacement.

The La Lucha, San Rafael and G9 massive sulphide and stringer occurrences to the southwest are separated from the underlying block containing the Naranjo, El Largo, Estrella de Oro and El Profundo deposits by a thrust fault. Late deformation includes numerous normal and sub-vertical faults, most with dip-slip or oblique movement. One of these drops the Naranjo deposit 60-80 m relative to its northern segment, and has an apparent right-lateral offset of up to 100 m.

Numerous other volcanogenic massive sulphide deposits and occurrences are present in and near felsic to intermediate volcanic rocks that form a north-northwest-trending belt at least 25 km long which extends through the Campo Morado district. Aggressive exploration of this prolific massive sulphide camp is ongoing.

ACKNOWLEDGEMENTS

A number of geologists not referenced in this text made important contributions to the development of the current level of understanding of the geology and to the success of the exploration program. These include Dan Kilby, Bernardine LeRoy, Martin Cons and Oscar Jiminez. The authors thank Farallon resources Ltd. for permission to publish this paper.

REFERENCES

Barrie, C.T. and Hannington, M.D., 2000. Classification of VMS deposits based on host rock composition. In Volcanic Associated Massive Sulphide Deposits: Processes and Examples in Modern and Ancient Settings. Edited by C.T. Barrie and M.D. Hannington. Reviews in Economic Geology, in press.

Campa, M.F. and Coney, P.J., 1983. Tectonostratigraphic terranes and mineral resources distribution in Mexico. Canadian Journal of Earth Sciences, 20, p.1040-1051.

Centeno-Garcia, E., Coney, P.j., Ruiz, J., Patchertt, J., and Orteg-Gutierrez, F., 1993. Tectonic significance of the sediments of the Guerrero Terrane from petrographic, trace-element, and Nd-isotope studies. In Proceedings of the First Circum-Pacific and Circum-Atlantic Terrane Conference. Edited by F. Ortega-Guitierrez, et al. UNAM, Instituto de Geologia, p. 30-33.

Freydier, C., Talavera-Mendoza, O., Tardy, M., Lapierre, H., Coulon, C., Ortiz-Hernandez, L.E., YTA, M., and Martinez-Reyes, J., 1993. Birth, growth, and accretion of Mesozoic intra-oceanic island arc (Guerrero Terrane) in the Mexican cordillera. In Proceedings of the First Circum-Pacific and Circum-Atlantic Terrane Conference. Edited by F. Ortega-Gutierrez, et al. UNAM, Instituto de Geologia, p. 50-51.

Haggart, J.W., 1997. Fossil Report No. JWH-1997-05; GSC loc. C-302912, Campo Morado, DDH 142 @ 29.36 m. Geological Survey of Canada.

Hedenquist, J.W. 1987: Mineralization associated with volcanic related hydrothermal systems in the Circum-Pacific basin. In Transactions of the Circum-Pacific Energy and Mineral Resources Conference, 4th, Singapore, August 17-22 , 1986, p. 513-524.

Lang, H.R., Barros, J.A., Cabral-Cano, E., Draper, G., Harrison, C.G.A., Jansma, P.E., and Johnson, C.A., 1996. Terrane deletion in northern Guerrero State. Geofisica Internacional, 35(4), p 349-359.

Lorinczi, I. and Miranda, J.C., 1978. Geology of the massive sulphide deposits of Campo Morado, Guerrero, Mexico. Economic Geology, 73, p.180-191.

Miranda-Gasca, M.A., 1995. The volcanogenic massive sulphide and sedimentary exhalative deposits of the Guerrero Terrane, Mexico. Ph.D. thesis, University of Arizona, Tucson, Arizona.

GEOLOGY OF THE SAN NICOLÁS DEPOSIT, ZACATECAS, MEXICO

BRADFORD J. JOHNSON, J. ANTONIO MONTANTE-MARTÍNEZ, MARIO CANELA-BARBOZA
Minera Teck, S.A. de C.V., Mariano Otero 2347, 3er Piso, Colonia Verde Valle, Guadalajara, Jalisco, Mexico 45050

THOMAS J. DANIELSON
Department of Earth and Ocean Sciences, University of British Columbia, 6339 Stores Road, Vancouver, British Columbia V6T 1Z4

ABSTRACT

The San Nicolás volcanogenic massive sulphide deposit in southeastern Zacatecas, Mexico, was discovered in 1997. Exploration in the area in 1996 led to the identification of a small (<1 Mt) massive sulphide lens on the El Salvador claim, 2 km east of San Nicolás, which was the first VMS discovery in the state of Zacatecas. The focus of exploration was shifted to the San Nicolás area because a copper showing and host rocks in nearby outcrops suggested that the geology was similar to that at El Salvador. Following results of a gradient-array induced polarization survey, the first hole drilled to test a 500 m x 500 m chargeability anomaly in the San Nicolás area intersected 175 m of massive sulphides. Subsequent drilling has outlined the largest VMS deposit yet discovered in Mexico, with an estimated mineral resource of more than 99 million tonnes.

The mineral resource consists of an upper Main Sulphide Zone with a high-grade polymetallic cap and a copper-rich Lower Sulphide Zone. The Main Sulphide Zone is a northwesterly trending elongate lens of massive sulphides 900 m long, over 200 m wide and up to 280 m thick. The Lower Sulphide Zone consists of massive to semi-massive sulphides and associated stringers inferred as being a feeder complex for the Main Sulphide Zone. The Main Sulphide Zone contains estimated mineable reserves of 75 million tonnes grading 1.40 % Cu, 2.11 % Zn, 0.53 g/t Au and 30 g/t Ag within a preliminary open pit model.

The deposit is hosted in a succession of volcanic and subordinate sedimentary rocks of the Upper Jurassic – Lower Cretaceous Chilitos Formation. The footwall of the deposit consists of rhyolite flows and breccias, mafic to intermediate flows and dikes, and siliceous sedimentary rocks. The hangingwall is a succession of mafic flows and flow breccias, siliceous to carbonaceous mudstones, volcaniclastic sediments and minor tuffs. Tertiary volcaniclastic breccias lie unconformably upon the Chilitos volcanic succession. Sulphide deposition was apparently structurally controlled by a syndepositional fault and by the steep flank of a rhyolite dome. Lithogeochemistry of the volcanic host rocks indicates a bimodal chemical distribution with tholeiitic affinities. The San Nicolás deposit is tentatively interpreted as having formed in an extensional back-arc setting.

INTRODUCTION

The San Nicolás volcanogenic massive sulphide (VMS) deposit was discovered in November 1997 during exploration of the El Salvador project, a joint venture between Teck Corporation (55 %) and Western Copper Holdings Ltd. (45 %) in which Teck is the operator. Industrias Luismin, S.A. de C.V., the original property owner, has the option to participate at up to a 25 % interest in the San Nicolás project development. The property covers an area of 22,500 ha and is located in central Mexico, approximately 60 km east-southeast of the city of Zacatecas (Fig. 1). The San Nicolás deposit is the largest VMS deposit yet discovered in Mexico. Its discovery sparked a renewed interest in the exploration of this area that traditionally was explored and developed for epithermal silver and gold. This paper summarizes the history of exploration leading to the discovery of the San Nicolás deposit and describes the geology of the deposit.

EXPLORATION HISTORY

The El Salvador project area hosts several small-scale workings of copper, manganese, phosphorous and kaolin that were exploited at various times during the past century. During the period between 1982 and 1995, the area was explored for epithermal Ag-Au

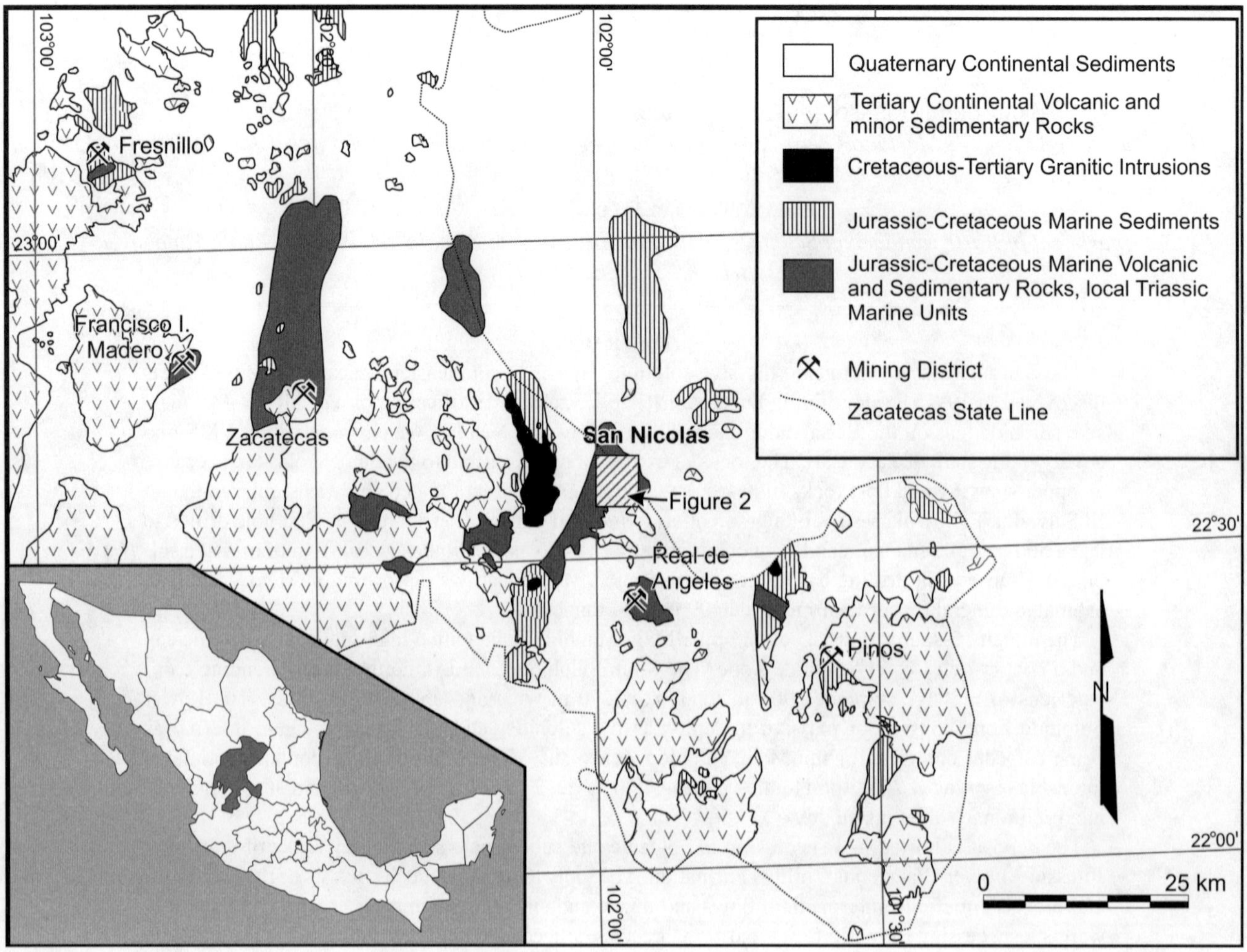

Figure 1. Geology of southeastern Zacatecas, modified from Consejo de Recursos Minerales (1992a). Inset shows location of Zacatecas state.

targets using geophysics, geochemistry and limited drilling. Companies involved during this period were Industrial Minera Mexico, S.A. de C.V., Industrias Luismin, S.A. de C.V., and Minera Santa Fe de Mexico, S.A. de C.V.

The Consejo de Recursos Minerales (1992b) completed a report on an oxide copper occurrence at El Salvador (Fig. 2) and concluded that the origin and nature of the mineralization was hydrothermal fracture filling. Minera Dolores, Angustias y Anexas, S.A. de C.V. explored the El Salvador claim by bulldozer trenching in 1994 and uncovered a new zone of copper oxide mineralization, from which they shipped several small lots of high-grade copper oxides to a local smelter. Minera Teck, S.A. de C.V. (the Mexican subsidiary of Teck Corporation) and Western Copper Holdings Ltd. conducted detailed mapping, geochemical sampling and air-track drilling in 1996, focusing on El Salvador and La Virgen copper oxide showings. The possibility that the copper mineralization was volcanogenic was recognized at this stage but efforts were focused more on delineating the oxide mineralization than on determining its origin. Diamond drilling at El Salvador commenced in October 1996 and a VMS target was identified when hole SAL-5 intersected 2.1 m of massive sulphides grading 2.07 % Cu, 1.53 % Pb, 16.57 % Zn, 3.68 g/t Au and 213 g/t Ag. Further drilling in 1996 and 1997 outlined a laterally persistent massive sulphide zone and laterally equivalent cherty sedimentary units at the contact

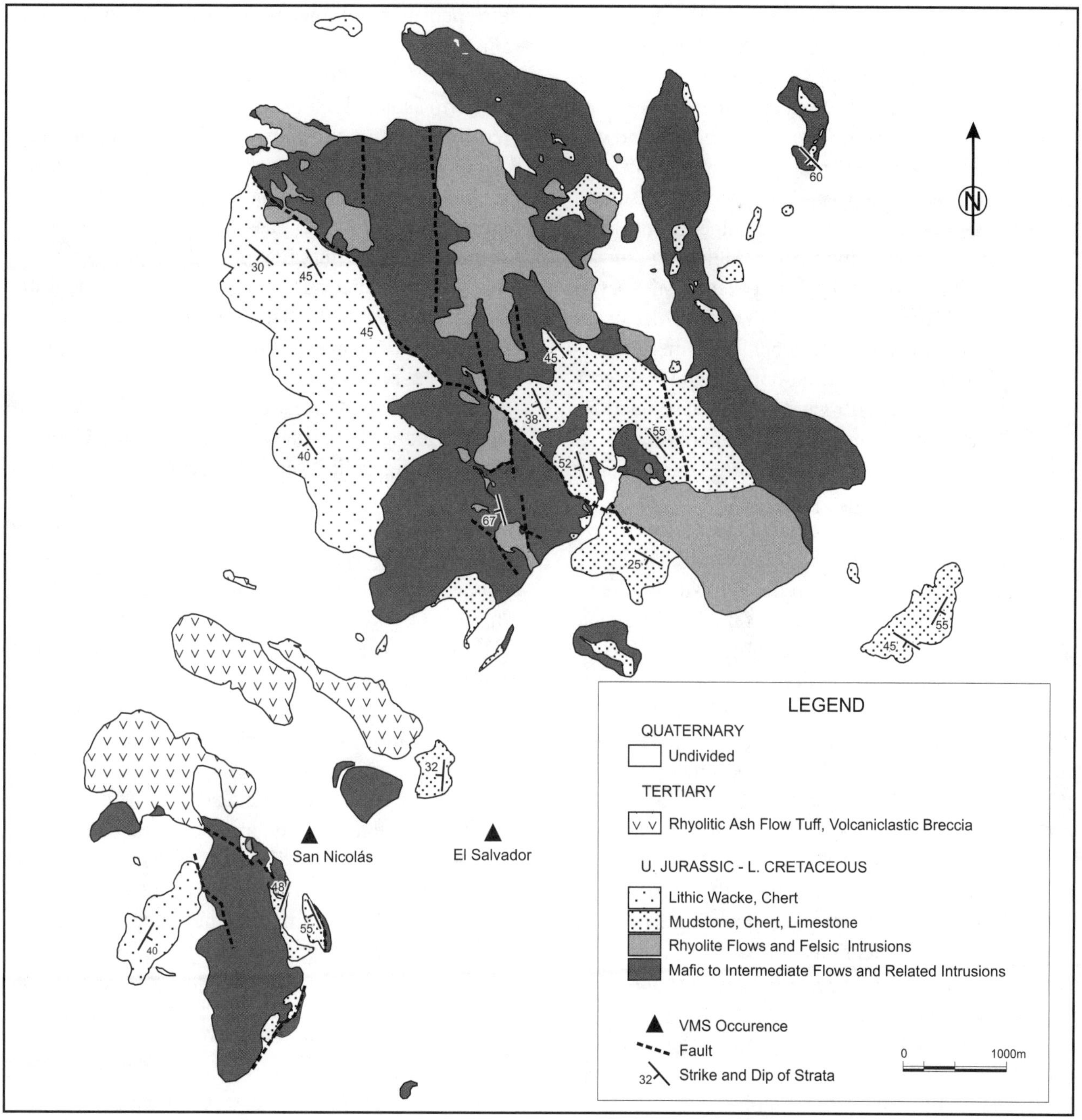

Figure 2. Geology of the El Salvador joint venture area. See Figure 1 for location.

between felsic volcaniclastic rocks and overlying andesite flows. A geological resource of approximately 1 Mt was estimated at El Salvador from the 26 holes that were drilled, with the most significant massive sulphide intersection (SAL-12) grading 1.04 % Cu, 1.06 % Pb, 5.99 % Zn, 1.98 g/t Au and 196 g/t Ag over 13.3 m.

Between October 1996 and March 1997, Teck completed reconnaissance prospecting and geochemical sampling of the joint venture area concurrently with regional mapping at 1:20,000 scale. Airborne geophysical surveys consisting of magnetics, electromagnetics, resistivity and radiometrics were also completed during this stage. The mapping program outlined the general geology of the property and identified geologically favorable targets for further exploration. Several copper anomalies, including one from old workings in the El Suavecito area located near San Nicolás, were identified by prospecting and confirmed through assays of rock chip samples. In association with the geology and prospecting, results of the airborne geophysical surveys helped to prioritize areas for further exploration, including the El Suavecito (San Nicolás) area. Orientation surveys were completed over the El Salvador VMS occurrence to test various ground geophysical methods and it was determined that time-domain gradient-array induced polarization (IP) gave the best response relative to cost. In the summer of 1997, approximately 22 km of gradient-array IP surveys were completed and a large anomaly (500 m by 500 m) characterized by high chargeability with associated low resistivity was detected at San Nicolás.

Diamond drilling began in the San Nicolás area in November, 1997. The discovery of the Main Sulphide Zone was made in hole SAL-25 at a vertical depth of 205.8 m, with the intersection of massive sulphides continuing for 179.7 m to a depth of 385.5 m (see Fig. 3 for hole locations; all are vertical holes). The structurally and stratigraphically deeper Lower Sulphide Zone was intersected in hole SAL-24 at a depth of 403.7 to 458.5 m, a 54.8 m interval. During the period from November 4, 1997, to July 25, 1998, more than 25,600 m of core were drilled in 58 vertical holes for definition and metallurgical sampling of the San Nicolás deposit. Attention shifted rapidly to delineation of open-pittable reserves and pre-feasibility work, including a geotechnical and hydrological study of the deposit and its hangingwall that was completed in September, 1998. As this paper goes to press (February 2000), the Main Sulphide Zone remains open to the north and the Lower Sulphide Zone is open to the west and south.

REGIONAL GEOLOGICAL SETTING

The San Nicolás deposit is hosted in an assemblage of marine volcanic and sedimentary rocks of Upper Jurassic – Lower Cretaceous age that in Zacatecas is known as the Chilitos Formation (de Cserna 1976). Rocks of this assemblage include deformed and non-metamorphosed to lower greenschist-facies felsic to mafic flows, volcaniclastic rocks, chert, limestone and clastic sedimentary strata that form isolated exposures in an area largely covered by Quaternary sediments (Fig. 1). Stratigraphic relationships among the various exposures are uncertain but in common practice the rocks of this assemblage are tentatively assigned to the Chilitos Formation. From the few faunal assemblages that have been studied, at least part of the Chilitos Formation falls in the Tithonian to Hauterivian age range (Cantú-Chapa 1974, Yta 1992), or approximately 152-124 Ma.

The Chilitos Formation and related rocks are exposed along the northeastern edge of the Guerrero tectonostratigraphic terrane (Campa and Coney 1983). This composite terrane of predominantly oceanic arc affinity is characterized by Upper Jurassic to Lower Cretaceous volcanic and sedimentary rocks and, according to most authors, was accreted to North America in mid-Cretaceous time by northeast-directed thrusting (Centeno-García et al. 1993, Tardy et al. 1994). An alternative interpretation is that Triassic assemblages that constitute the oldest known rocks in this part of the Guerrero terrane were accreted in the Middle or Late Jurassic and the Upper Jurassic – Lower Cretaceous volcanic and sedimentary rocks were deposited as an overlap assemblage (Sedlock et al. 1993). Northeast-directed thrusting in Late Cretaceous to Early Tertiary time resulted in imbrication of the Chilitos Formation and related rocks with Upper Jurassic to Upper Cretaceous carbonates and fine-grained siliciclastic sedimentary rocks of the Sierra Madre terrane. Mesozoic volcanic and sedimentary assemblages, throughout the region, are intruded by Late Cretaceous to Early Tertiary granite to granodiorite plutons and are overlain unconformably by extensive felsic volcanic flows and ashflow tuffs of Tertiary age (Consejo de Recursos Minerales 1992a).

On the El Salvador property, Upper Jurassic – Lower Cretaceous volcanic and sedimentary rocks are exposed over an area of approximately 30 km^2 (Fig. 2). The rocks include mafic to intermediate flows and related shallow intrusions, rhyolite flows and intrusions, felsic tuffs, and volcaniclastic lithic wackes.

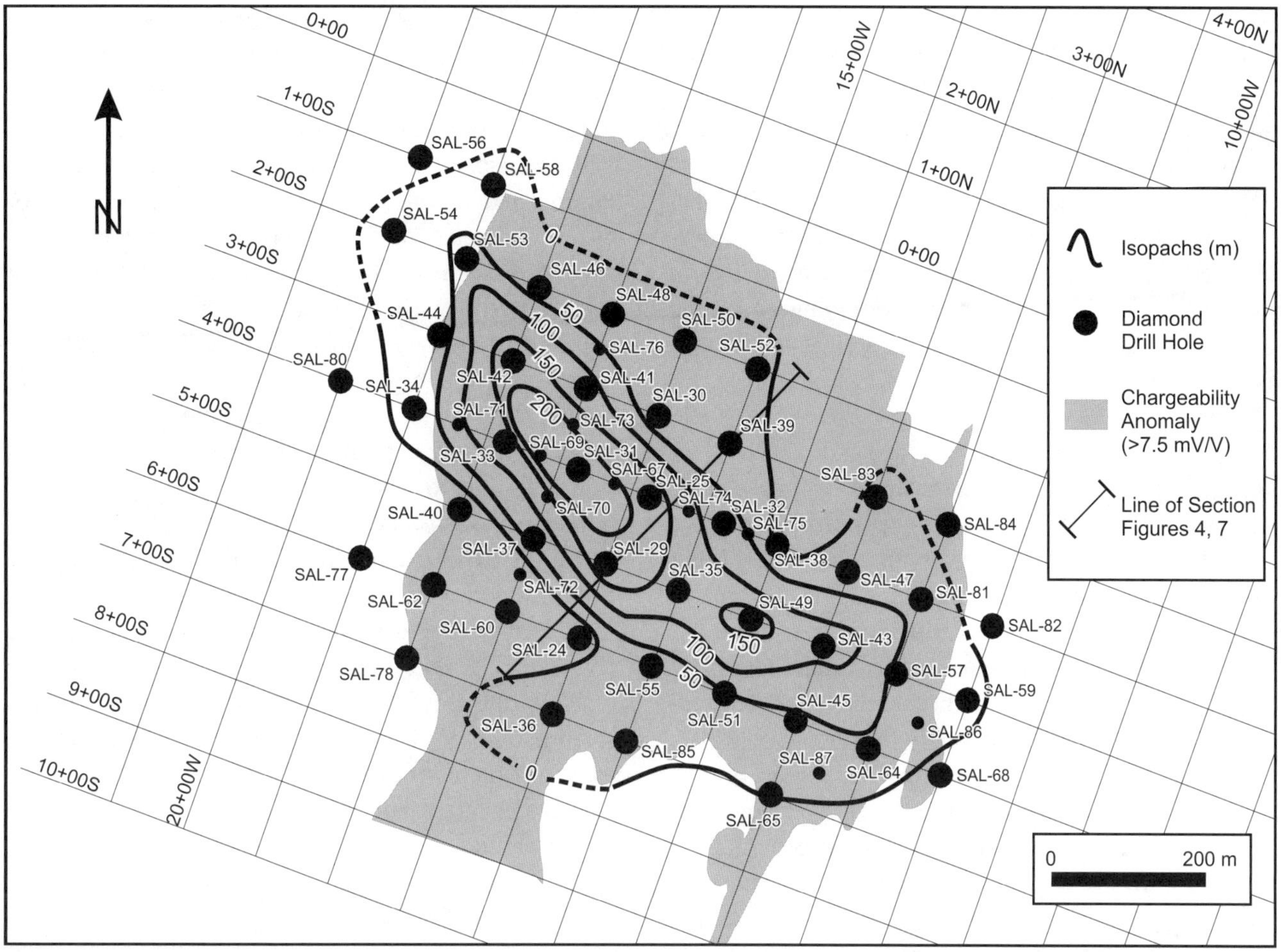

Figure 3. Drillhole locations and isopach map of the Main Sulphide Zone, San Nicolás deposit. Isopach contour interval 50 m.

Mudstone, chert and limestone are intercalated with the volcanic units. Tertiary volcaniclastic breccias and rhyolitic ash-flow tuffs lie in angular unconformity over the Mesozoic volcano-sedimentary succession south of the area shown in Figure 2. Most of the property is covered with Quaternary alluvium and caliche.

Stratification in the Mesozoic volcano-sedimentary assemblage over most of the property dips gently to moderately southwestward. Local northeasterly dips are due in part to northwest-trending folds and in part to tilting along faults. The assemblage is cut by northerly, northwesterly and westerly striking faults, most of which are of uncertain age and sense of displacement. Aeromagnetic data show a strong northwesterly structural grain across the property, and the San Nicolás deposit is itself controlled by northwest-striking structures that are probably, in part, synvolcanic extensional faults and in part postvolcanic (?) strike-slip faults. The geometry and relative ages of structures throughout the property are currently being studied through detailed mapping.

Geology of the San Nicolás deposit

The San Nicolás deposit is covered by gently northeast-dipping volcanic units and Tertiary breccias. Therefore, all interpretations of lithology and structural relations in the deposit are based entirely on drill core. Rock descriptions are supplemented by limited petrography.

Stratigraphy

The San Nicolás massive sulphides are hosted in volcanic rocks and associated fine-grained sedimentary rocks that are tentatively assigned to the Chilitos

Formation. Initial drilling indicated the presence of two massive sulphide zones at different positions in the stratigraphic section. Subsequent drilling has shown that these zones are separated by up to 200 m in the central part of the deposit, that they are apparently connected in the southeastern part, and that there are additional smaller tongues or lenses of massive sulphide. Rock units are described below in ascending stratigraphic order, beginning with the footwall of the deposit. A section through the deposit is shown in Figure 4.

Footwall Units

The lowermost unit intersected in drilling to date consists of black to medium grey graphitic mudstones with thin laminae and lenses up to 5 cm thick of light grey, fine-grained siltstone and limestone. The maximum thickness of this unit drilled to date is 70 m.

The graphitic mudstones are overlain by mafic flows, associated sills and dikes, and intercalated sediments and tuffs that collectively form units up to 120 m thick ("MVT" unit). The flows are olive green, massive, locally amygdaloidal, locally plagioclase phyric and commonly contain dark green chlorite pseudomorphs after pyroxene 1-2 mm across that give the rock a mottled appearance. Flow breccias are common and peperite textures occur at contacts between dikes/sills and sedimentary units. Medium to dark grey, massive or thickly bedded to laminated, cherty sediments form units up to 15 m thick. Medium to fine-grained volcaniclastic wackes up to 30 cm thick are interbedded with the cherty sediments. Light greenish-grey to dark green tuffs form units up to 4 m thick. The tuffs are composed of 10-20 % altered feldspar crystal fragments, 1-10 % quartz phenocrysts, 10-15 % volcanic lithic fragments and 5-15 % olive green, elongate to ribbonlike sericitic clasts (interpreted as formerly having been pumice) in a siliceous-sericitic matrix. The elongate clasts and sericite in the matrix define a moderate to strong foliation that dips shallowly based on high core-axis angles.

Rhyolite to rhyodacite flows and breccias (hereafter referred to as rhyolites) are intercalated with the MVT unit and form a complex up to 300 m thick, the top of which dips moderately to steeply northeast and forms the southwest footwall of the Main Sulphide Zone. The lower part of the rhyolite complex consists of massive flows that are light to medium grey to light green and contain ~5 % phenocrysts of sericitized white feldspar 1 to 2 mm long. These flows are overlain by, and complexly intercalated with, coarse autoclastic breccias and flow-laminated rhyolite. The flow-laminated rhyolite is commonly spherulitic and locally perlitic. The breccia clasts are composed of massive to flow-laminated rhyolite, are blocky and subangular to subrounded and commonly 5 to 15 cm across. Preliminary petrography indicates that the breccia clasts are silicified and the matrix is devitrified with altered glass being replaced by cryptocrystalline quartz, sericite and locally chlorite. Toward the top of the rhyolite complex, the breccias generally are finer-grained with angular to wispy clasts 1 to 5 cm long composed mostly of recrystallized hyaloclastite (Fig. 5a). The rhyolites are interpreted as representing a submarine flow-dome complex on the basis of the steep geometry of the upper contact and the complex intercalation of massive to banded flows and autoclastic to hyaloclastite breccias.

Distinctive porphyritic rhyolites 10 to 30 m thick occur within the MVT unit, locally directly overlying the lower graphitic mudstone unit. These rhyolites are pale yellowish green and contain 5-10 % quartz phenocrysts (anhedral, 2-3 mm), 1-10 % white feldspar phenocrysts (2-3 mm, replaced by sericite and minor carbonate) and 5-10 % disseminated pyrite. Tentative correlation of these rhyolites between drill holes suggests that they dip southwestward and crosscut other units (Fig. 4). Similar quartz-phyric rhyolite is rare but does occur locally within the flow-dome complex. Therefore, although contact relations in core are ambiguous due to strong alteration and local shearing, the quartz-phyric rhyolites are tentatively interpreted as dikes that may be subvolcanic equivalents to the flow-dome complex.

Massive Sulphides

The Lower Sulphide Zone consists of massive and semi-massive sulphides and sulphide stringers composed of fine-grained pyrite and chalcopyrite. Chalcopyrite is present throughout the zone, forming stringers up to several cm wide and locally forming

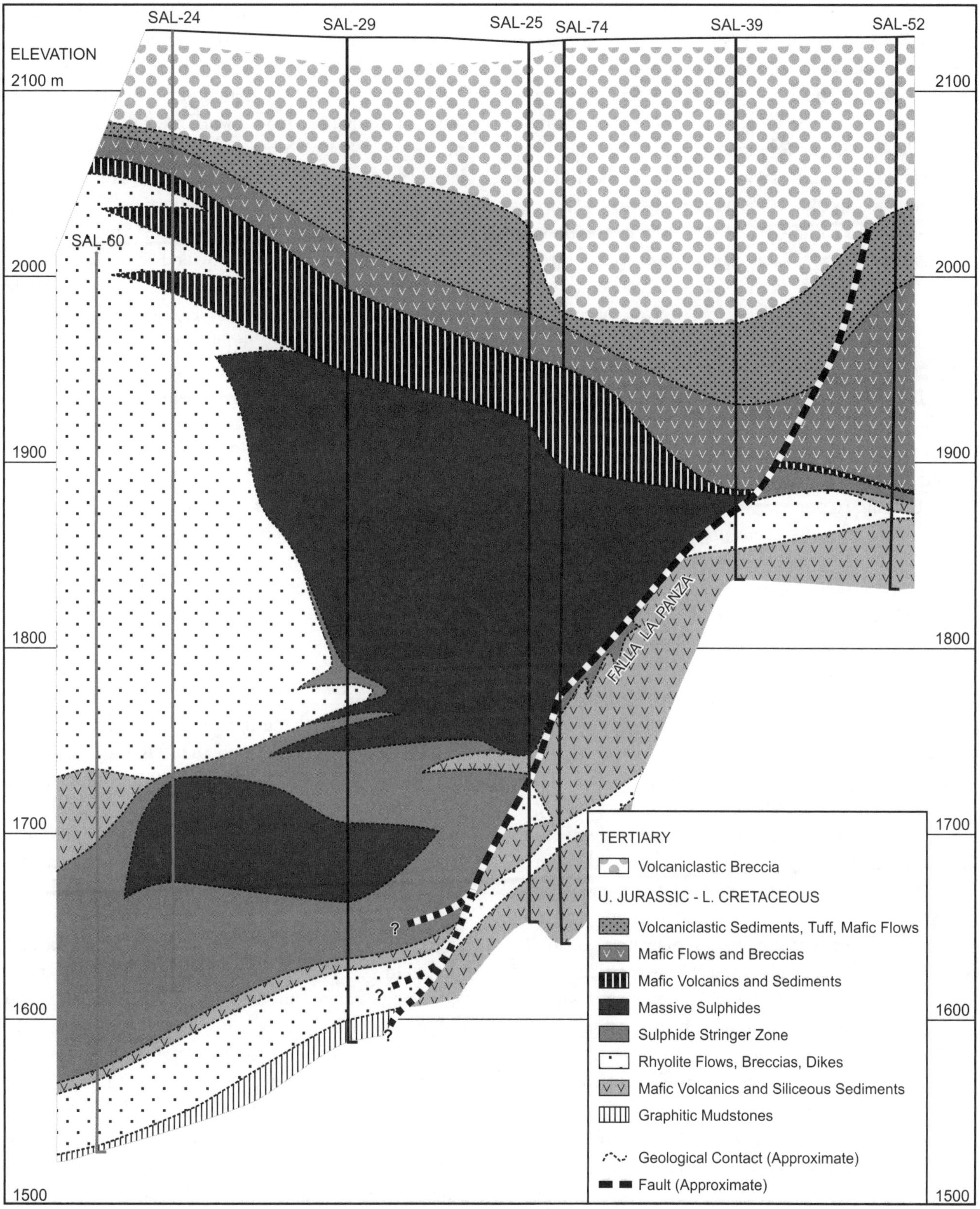

Figure 4. Geological cross section of the San Nicolás deposit. See Figure 3 for location.

massive intervals. Sphalerite is present locally. The Lower Sulphide Zone dips southwestward and has a generally tabular form, curved so that it is concave upward and to the southwest. The zone apparently merges with the southeastern part of the Main Sulphide Zone and terminates against a southwest-dipping fault beneath the axis of the Main Sulphide Zone to the northwest. Stringers within the Lower Sulphide Zone commonly follow flow laminations in the rhyolites that typically are the host rock, and textures within the massive sulphides suggest that they in part were formed by replacement of flow-laminated to brecciated volcanic rocks. The geometry of the Lower Sulphide Zone, its spatial relationship with respect to the Main Sulphide Zone and textural relationships within it suggest that it consists of multiple layers of massive sulphide connected and overprinted by coalesced stringers that represent a feeder system to the Main Sulphide Zone.

Sulphide stringers occur in volcanic rocks (mostly in the rhyolites) above, below and laterally from the massive core of the Lower Sulphide Zone, and to a lesser extent in the footwall of the Main Sulphide Zone. The rock is designated as a "stringer zone" in Figure 4 where it consists of >10 % stringers of pyrite with chalcopyrite or of >5 % stringers of chalcopyrite.

The Main Sulphide Zone is a northwesterly elongate lens of massive sulphide up to 280 m thick, more than 900 m long and from 200 m to more than 400 m wide (Fig. 3, 4). It is composed predominantly of fine-grained pyrite that ranges from massive and structureless to fragmental. Where fragmental, rounded pyrite clasts are cemented by fine-grained pyrite and/or fine-grained barite, locally with sphalerite. Some drill core exhibits textures that suggest a replacement or multi-stage origin for the sulphides. These include curved laminations that resemble flow laminations in the host rhyolite, textures that resemble hyaloclastite breccia replaced by sulphide, coarse-grained pyrite aggregates that form along crosscutting vein-like structures and between rounded breccia fragments of fine-grained pyrite (Fig. 5b), and domains several centimetres wide of alternating fine-grained and medium to coarse-grained pyrite. Whether pyrite has in part replaced host rocks, earlier-formed sulphides and/or gangue minerals is uncertain.

The upper 2 to 35 m of the Main Sulphide Zone contains high concentrations of sphalerite and chalcopyrite in addition to pyrite and generally displays laminated and brecciated intervals. Gold and silver concentrations are also elevated in the upper part of the sulphide body. Sphalerite occurs as thin black to dark brown laminae alternating with pyrite as well as in breccia matrix along with barite. Chalcopyrite forms wispy laminae and discordant stringers, irregular patches on massive pyrite and small crystalline aggregates along vuggy barite veins. In lower-grade intervals, chalcopyrite is only locally visible as very thin stringers, as patchy replacement of pyrite and as a yellowish sheen on the core, even though copper concentrations throughout the Main Sulphide Zone typically average >0.5 %.

The footwall contact of the Main Sulphide Zone is typically uneven and gradational over 5 to 20 cm into a stringer zone. In some drill intersections, the footwall contact is marked by brecciated clasts of massive pyrite in a grey matrix of cryptocrystalline quartz and barite. The hangingwall contact is typically sharp but is locally gradational over 5 to 10 cm into interlaminated sulphide and mudstone.

Hangingwall Units

The immediate hangingwall of the Main Sulphide Zone consists of black mudstones intercalated with light green mafic flows and sills ("MVS" unit). The mudstones are massive to laminated, commonly are internally brecciated, are siliceous to mildly carbonaceous and contain 1 to 5 % thin pyritic laminae. Where brecciated, they contain abundant barite and/or quartz stringers. The flows and sills are pale to olive green, aphyric, and range from glassy to aphanitic and amygdaloidal. The MVS unit generally contains intervals of intercalated mudstones and flows at the base and top of the unit and thicker intervals of flows and sills in the middle. Peperite is common along contacts between mudstones and flows or sills (Fig. 5c). Green crystal or crystal-lithic tuffs up to 2.5 m thick are locally intercalated with mudstones at, or near, the base of the unit. The MVS unit ranges from 3 to 80 m in thickness and is thickest over the central part of the Main Sulphide Zone.

The MVS unit is overlain by a succession of mafic

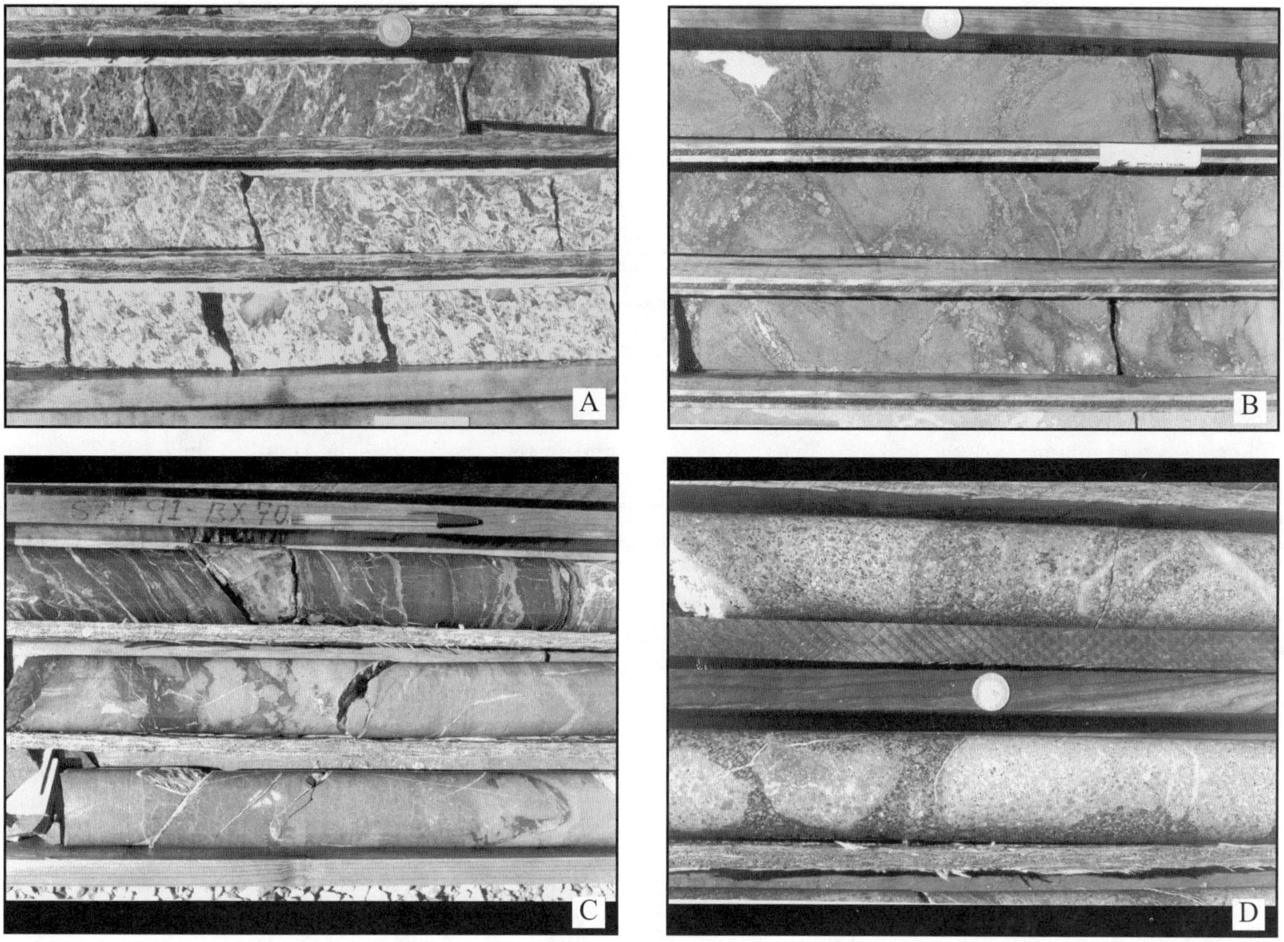

Figure 5. Photographs of San Nicolás core. In all photographs downhole is to the right and down. (A) Rhyolitic hyaloclastite breccia showing angular to wispy clasts and matrix variably altered by quartz-sericite-chlorite. SAL-40, 148-151 m depth. Coin is 20 mm in diametre. (B) Massive sulphides displaying rounded clasts of fine-grained pyrite cemented by medium to coarse-grained pyrite. Dark material between clasts is volcanic host rock intensely altered to quartz-sericite-chlorite. Light-coloured pod in upper left is a quartz vein. SAL-42, 338-342 m depth. (C) Mafic flows and sills (light grey) and carbonaceous mudstones of the hangingwall MVS unit. Peperite is developed in central and lower right portions of the photo. Lighter grey laminae in mudstones in upper part of photo contain pyrite. SAL-91, 209-212 m depth. (D) Mafic flow breccias of hangingwall. Light grey phenocrysts in clasts and matrix are pyroxene replaced by clay minerals and carbonate. SAL-88, 183-185 m depth.

flows and flow breccias that are 100 m thick in the north and pinch out near the southern edge of the area drilled to date. These rocks are light to olive green and are distinguished by the presence of 1-10 % pyroxene phenocrysts (euhedral, 2 to 5 mm, typically replaced by clay minerals, calcite, or epidote) and abundant amygdules variably filled by chlorite, clay minerals, calcite and quartz (Fig. 5d). In addition, they locally contain up to 15 % plagioclase (white to light green, 1 to 3 mm, typically destroyed by alteration), amphibole (1 to 3 mm, dark green to black, in part replacing pyroxene and in part euhedral prismatic phenocrysts) and chloritic fragments (1 to 3 mm, dark green to black) probably after glass. The groundmass appears glassy and the matrix of breccias within the unit is relatively dark in colour and probably consists of altered hyaloclastite.

The uppermost unit of the Chilitos Formation at San Nicolás comprises mafic flows, volcaniclastic rocks and minor siliceous sediments. This unit is up to at least 100 m thick and its upper contact is an angular unconformity. The mafic flows are amygdaloidal and aphyric to finely plagioclase-phyric. The volcaniclastic rocks include tuffaceous sandstone, feldspathic-lithic wacke, crystal-lithic tuff and hyaloclastite. Most of these rocks are light green where they are not oxidized. Very fine-grained, green, massive to laminated tuffaceous sandstones with intercalated purple-grey to black mudstones are characteristic of the unit. Laminations are commonly steeply dipping (based on low core-axis angles) and more gently dipping reactivation surfaces commonly separate steeply dipping domains, indicating that the steep dips are related to intraformational slump folds. The wackes are fine to very coarse-grained, are composed mainly of volcanic lithic clasts and angular feldspar, and form massive units up to several m thick. The composition and predominantly massive character of the volcaniclastic units, the presence of slump folds, and the association with intercalated flows and tuffs suggests that the volcaniclastic sediments were deposited rapidly by syneruptive mass-flow processes in relatively deep water.

A wedge of Tertiary volcaniclastic breccia overlies the Mesozoic rocks of the Chilitos Formation with angular unconformity. The breccia is medium to dark reddish brown, massive and polymictic, containing a wide variety of felsic to mafic volcanic and minor sedimentary clasts supported in a clay matrix. The clasts are angular to subrounded and range from sand to cobble size. The unit averages 40 to 50 m thick over the western part of the San Nicolás deposit, thickens to 185 m in the eastern part of the zone, and thins to zero along the southern limit of the area drilled. The range of clast types and massive character of this unit suggest that it was deposited rapidly by sedimentary mass-flow processes.

Alteration

The footwall rocks display strong to intense chlorite and quartz-sericite alteration along the southwestern margin of the Main Sulphide Zone, particularly near holes SAL-24, SAL-29 and SAL-36. The restricted distribution of strong chlorite alteration suggests proximity to a former fluid vent. Stringers of calcite, iron carbonate and barite are common throughout the footwall of the deposit, and barite veinlets locally cut the sulphides.

Almost all of the mafic volcanic rocks have at least weak clay or sericitic alteration. Mafic flows in the hangingwall of the Main Sulphide Zone have mild to intense alteration characterized by replacement of feldspars and amygdules by clay or sericite + epidote + calcite, replacement of groundmass by clay or sericite, and the presence of chlorite and calcite stringers. This alteration is most intense in the lower part of the mafic flows and breccias unit.

Structure

The northwesterly elongate geometry of the San Nicolás sulphide body is controlled in part by the steep margin of the rhyolite flow and breccia complex and in part by faults. The rhyolite dips 40-65° to the northeast and forms the southwest footwall of the Main Sulphide Zone. On the northeast flank of the Main Sulphide Zone, a fault zone characterized by up to 12 m of clay gouge and brecciated footwall rock is observed in the immediate footwall. This fault zone dips moderately southwest and probably has a more complex geometry than that depicted in Figure 4. Separation of footwall units across the fault suggests that it has a normal-sense component of displacement and the gentle northeasterly dip of hangingwall strata is consistent with antithetic tilting above a listric normal fault. The fault has not been traced downdip beyond the "keel" of the Main Sulphide Zone, possibly because it has been filled with sulphide stringers of the Lower Sulphide Zone or by quartz-porphyritic rhyolite dikes. Alternatively, the fault zone may sole into the graphitic mudstone unit. Breccias in the keel area are strongly silicified. Massive and stringer sulphides are relatively thin in the footwall (northeast) of the fault and strata of the immediate hangingwall are apparently not displaced more than a few tens of metres. These observations lead to the interpretation that displacement on this fault zone was coeval with sulphide deposition and that the fault controlled the northeast flank of the deposit, with relatively minor motion occurring after mineralization.

Fault zones along the southwest edge of the area explored by drilling apparently strike northwesterly, are steeply dipping and have an uncertain sense of displacement. These faults have only been documented in footwall rocks so far, and therefore their age relations with respect to mineralization are not yet known.

Lithogeochemistry

Lithogeochemical samples were collected from all stratigraphic levels of the volcanic succession at San Nicolás in order to characterize the geochemistry of the host rocks. Twenty major and trace elements were analyzed for each sample through X-ray fluorescence and inductively coupled plasma mass spectrometry (Table 1). The host rocks at San Nicolás have been subjected to extensive hydrothermal alteration, and therefore the reported element concentrations are not regarded as representing the original bulk composition of the rocks. For example, felsic volcanic rocks of the footwall exhibit dramatic sodium depletion and barium enrichment. In order to minimize the effect of alteration, only the immobile elements (determined through the use of bivariant discrimination diagrams) were considered in efforts to characterize the chemical nature of the rocks.

Based on the Zr-Y diagram of MacLean and Barrett (1993), volcanic rocks in both the footwall and the hangingwall of the San Nicolás deposit are tholeiitic (Fig. 6a). Geochemistry displays a bimodal distribution, as shown by the Nb/Y vs. Zr/TiO_2 diagram of Winchester and Floyd (1977) in which the analyses cluster in basaltic andesite and rhyolite to rhyodacite fields (Fig. 6b). This diagram also shows that all of the volcanic rocks are subalkaline. Immobile-element tectonic discrimination diagrams indicate an oceanic setting for the volcanic rocks. For example, in the Zr-Ti-Y diagram of Pearce and Cann (1973), volcanic rocks of the footwall and hangingwall plot in the ocean floor basalt field (Fig. 6c). Rare earth element patterns, measured on limited samples, are consistent with genesis at both normal (N-MORB) and enriched (E-MORB) mid-ocean ridge environments. The bimodal chemical distribution and the presence of both N-MORB and E-MORB affinities are consistent with deposition in an extensional setting such as a back-arc basin. Ongoing work will further characterize the chemical signature of the volcanic

Table 1. Geochemistry of Representative Volcanic Rocks [a]

Sample	9878	9879	9373	9543	B19281	9962
Unit [b]	MVS	MVS	HYA	FV	MVT	QRY
Al_2O_3	15.81	17.17	8.70	11.16	14.01	10.21
CaO	11.88	9.94	0.35	0.87	4.91	1.86
Cr_2O_3	0.05	0.06	0.03	0.01	0.03	<.01
Fe_2O_3	9.43	9.69	8.51	3.30	9.33	3.48
K_2O	0.12	0.10	1.10	4.25	4.14	3.75
MgO	8.21	9.28	4.73	1.56	6.68	1.37
MnO	0.16	0.15	0.04	0.03	0.28	0.06
Na_2O	2.29	2.32	0.11	0.21	0.13	0.11
P_2O_5	0.05	0.07	<.01	<.01	0.14	0.02
SiO_2	44.88	45.63	69.21	72.00	47.46	72.30
TiO_2	1.08	1.21	0.13	0.13	1.39	0.23
LOI	4.65	4.80	5.02	4.37	7.23	4.74
Ba	207.00	151.00	4230.00	1220.00	518.00	1660.00
Cs	10.00	10.00	7.00	13.00	20.00	16.00
Hf	1.00	2.00	6.00	9.00	2.00	9.00
La	4.00	3.00	15.00	29.00	6.00	22.00
Nb	1.00	1.00	6.00	10.00	1.00	8.00
Rb	5.00	6.00	28.00	94.00	42.00	72.00
Sr	256.00	266.00	52.00	46.00	60.00	48.00
Y	19.00	22.00	39.00	78.00	35.00	79.00
Zr	68.00	67.00	156.00	274.00	89.00	257.00

a Major element oxides given as weight percent, trace elements as ppm.

b Unit codes: MVS = hangingwall mafic flows, HYA = footwall rhyolite breccia, FV = footwall massive rhyolite, MVT = footwall mafic flow, QRY = footwall quartz-phyric rhyolite.

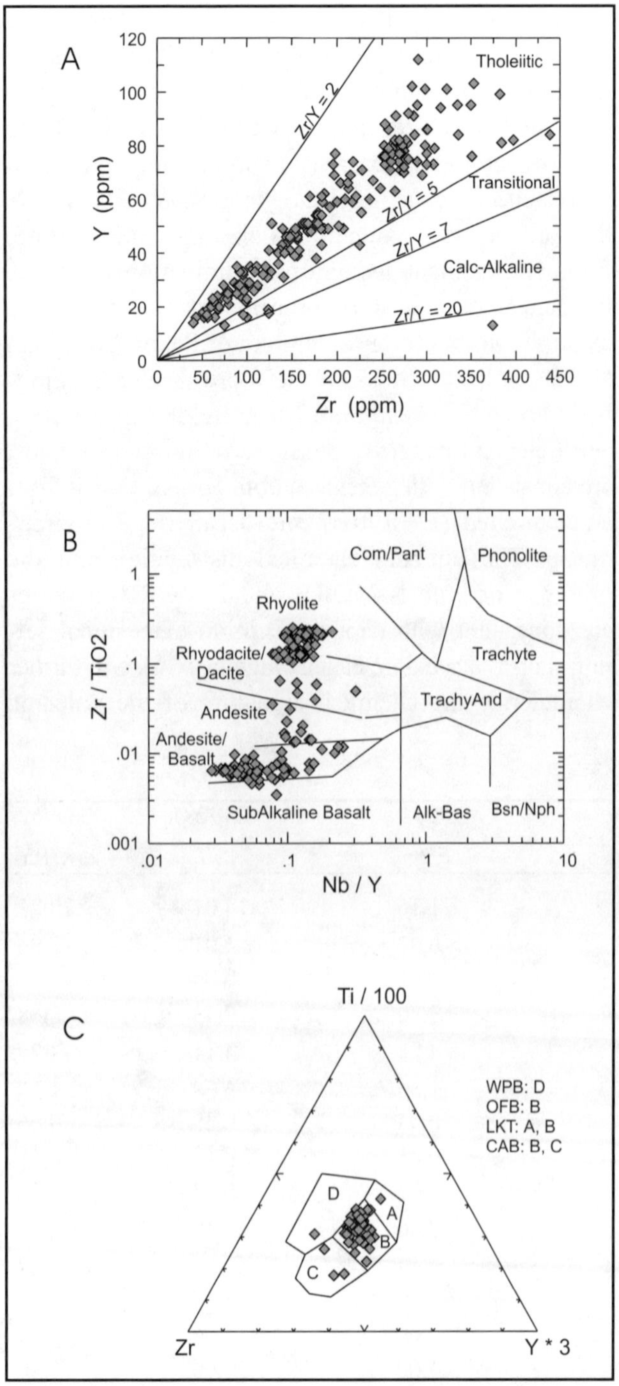

Figure 6. Lithogeochemistry of San Nicolás volcanic rocks. (A) Zr-Y diagram (MacLean and Barrett 1993) shows tholeiitic affinity. (B) Immobile-element classification diagram (Winchester and Floyd 1997) of all volcanic rocks in the deposit area shows strong bimodality. (C) Zr-Ti-Y diagram (Pearce and Cann 1973) of mafic rocks. A+B = low-potassium tholeiites, B = ocean floor basalts, B+C = continental arc basalts, D = within-plate basalts.

rocks that host the San Nicolás deposit.

Resource/reserve estimates and metal zonation

Teck Corporation made preliminary mineable reserve and resource estimates in mid-1998 based on assay results from 49 diamond drill holes (SAL-24 through SAL-78 excluding exploration holes outside the deposit area). A mineral resource of more than 99 million tonnes (Table 2) includes preliminary estimated open-pit reserves in the Main Sulphide Zone of 75 million tonnes grading 1.40 % Cu, 2.11 % Zn, 0.53 g/t Au and 30 g/t Ag. Resource estimates for massive and stringer mineralization of the Lower Sulphide Zone are 21.8 million tonnes grading 1.29 % Cu. The estimates do not include a portion of the Main Sulphide Zone that has low-grade copper-zinc mineralization.

A distinct metal zonation is noted in Table 2 and is illustrated by Figure 7. A stratiform polymetallic zone corresponding to the upper 2 to 30 m of the Main Sulphide Zone is characterized by high-grade zinc (>6 % on average) and 0.5 % to 1 % copper with elevated silver and gold. The high-grade zinc zone grades downward into a lower-grade zinc-copper zone that also has a lower content of precious metals. A massive pyrite zone up to 80 m thick, characterized by <1 % zinc and <1 % copper with only traces of silver and gold, gradationally underlies the mixed zinc-copper zone. This zone in turn grades into a copper-rich zone up to 70 m thick that grades 1.92 % copper on average. Finally, the Lower Sulphide Zone is enriched in copper (>1 %) with local intervals enriched in the other metals.

Discussion

The San Nicolás VMS deposit consists of (i) an elongate, lenticular Main Sulphide Zone, composed principally of fine-grained massive pyrite with a polymetallic cap, and (ii) a copper-rich Lower Sulphide Zone, characterized by massive and stringer sulphides. The Lower Sulphide Zone is tentatively interpreted as older massive sulphide lenses connected and overprinted by a feeder system. The deposit is hosted in a bimodal, tholeiitic volcanic succession with minor sediments. Textures in the volcanic rocks, particularly the abundant hyaloclastic breccias, indicate

Table 2. Preliminary Resource Estimation. Based on Holes SAL-24 through SAL-78

Unit	Tonnes	Au (g/t)	Ag (g/t)	Cu (%)	Zn (%)	Pb (%)
Main Sulphide Zone						
High-grade Zn	17,316,000	1.32	75.0	0.75	6.08	0.62
Mixed Cu/Zn	17,496,000	0.62	23.0	0.68	1.73	0.10
High-grade Cu	42,867,000	0.12	12.0	1.92	0.45	0.03
Subtotal	77,679,000	0.50	29.0	1.38	1.99	0.18
Lower Sulphide Zone						
High-grade Cu	9,745,000	0.16	12.0	1.57	0.78	0.07
Stringer Cu	12,099,000	0.01	2.0	1.07	0.05	0.00
Subtotal	21,844,000	0.08	6.0	1.29	0.38	0.03
Total	99,523,000	0.41	24.0	1.36	1.64	0.15

submarine deposition. The results of preliminary lithogeochemical studies also indicate that the volcanic units have an oceanic signature and may have formed in an extensional back-arc setting.

In terms of metal content, the San Nicolás deposit is similar to the Cu-Zn deposits described by Franklin et al. (1981), although the nearby El Salvador VMS occurrence has a slightly higher lead content. On the basis of host-rock composition, San Nicolás would best be classified as a bimodal-mafic type deposit as defined by Barrie and Hannington (1999) because, on both the property and regional scales, mafic volcanic rocks are more abundant than felsic rocks and are tholeiitic in composition. A comparison with Canadian deposits shows that San Nicolás has some characteristics of Archean Mattabi-type deposits such as Kidd Creek, for example an association with felsic flows and hyaloclastic breccias, the presence of stringer sulphides in the footwall, and the presence of abundant carbonate in the alteration assemblage (Morton and Franklin 1987). However, the apparently discrete zone of intense chlorite alteration in the footwall stringer zone, presumably related to a former conduit of hydrothermal fluids, is perhaps more akin to deposits of the Noranda type.

Other Mexican VMS deposits, such as Campo Morado (Oliver et al. 1998) and several small deposits in the Cuale district (Berrocal and Querol 1991), are also hosted in Upper Jurassic (?) – Lower Cretaceous volcanic and sedimentary rocks of the Guerrero terrane. These deposits are associated with felsic volcanic flows and tuffs in successions that generally have sediments in greater abundance than mafic or intermediate flows. The San Nicolás deposit, the largest VMS deposit yet discovered in Mexico, is hosted in a succession that, on the scale of the deposit, has mafic flows in far greater abundance than sediments.

ACKNOWLEDGMENTS

Our present knowledge of the San Nicolás deposit geology comes from several years of fieldwork on the El Salvador project by Minera Teck geologists, including Juan Benítez, Ricardo Contreras, Jorge Guerrero, Jim Janzen, Gillian Kearvell and Roberto Pulido. Other staff of Minera Teck and Teck Corporation that have contributed on a technical level include Paul Donkersloot, Jorge Ferrétiz, Juan García, Jim Gray, Joseph Kapler, Tom Lane, Alfonso Ochoa, Gabriel Ruvalcaba, Scott Smith and Craig Thorsen. Britton Hermanos Perforaciones de Mexico, Chemex Labs, Dighem, Quantec Geofísica de Mexico and Eva Schandl provided professional services that are

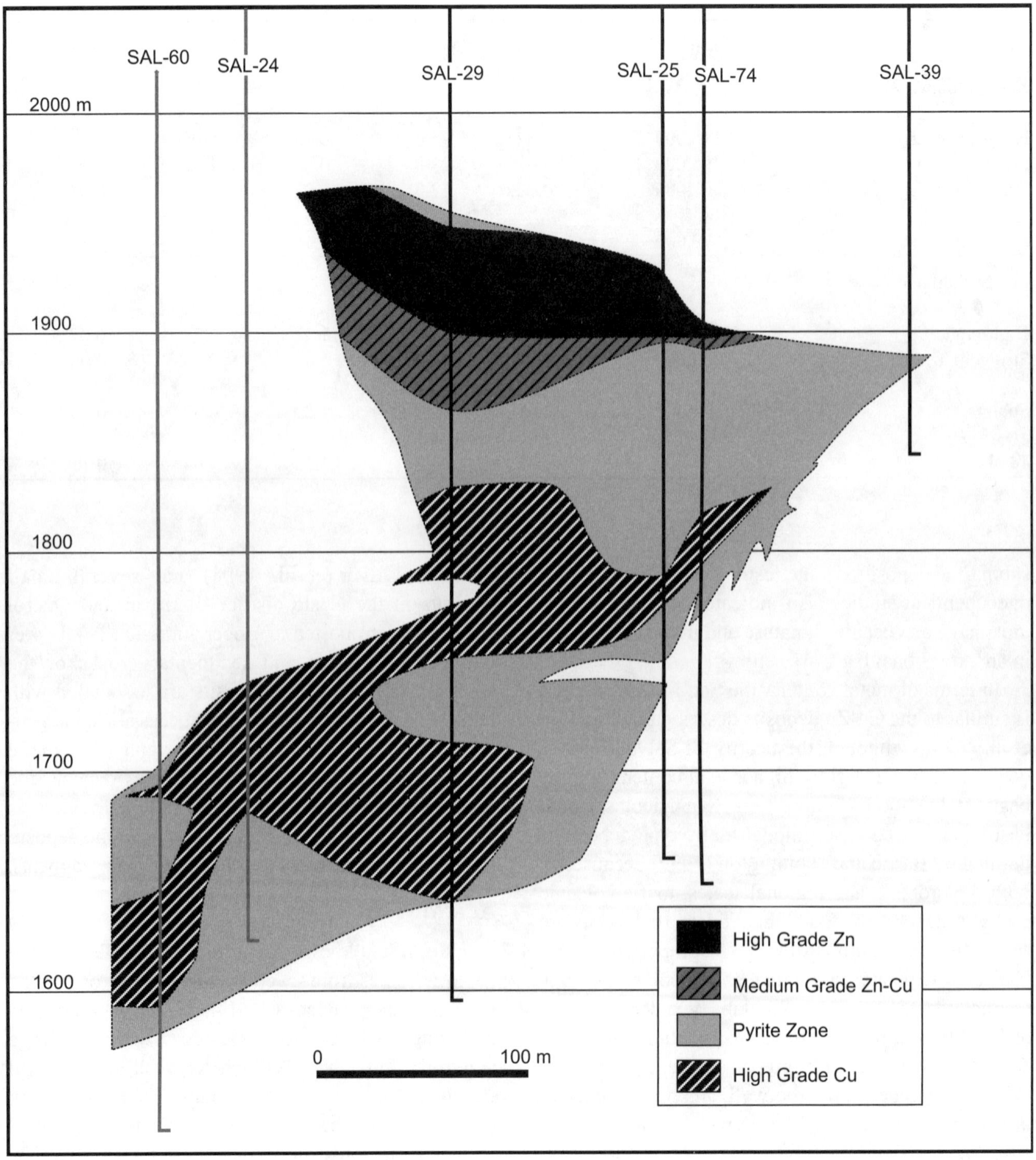

Figure 7. Cross section showing metal zonation of the San Nicolás deposit. See Figure 3 for location and Figure 4 for geology in same plane of section. Note that the pyrite envelope in the Lower Sulphide Zone corresponds to stringer zones and the high-grade Cu zone correlates well with massive sulphides.

reflected in our data and interpretations. Earlier drafts of this paper were reviewed internally by Joe Ruetz, Roger Scammell, John Thompson, George Thornton and Ken Thorsen. Reviews by Dave Adamson, Michael Gray and Ross Sherlock led to further improvements and clarifications. Finally, we thank Teck Corporation, Western Copper Holdings Ltd. and Industrias Luismin, S.A. de C.V., for permission to publish this paper.

REFERENCES

Barrie, C.T., and Hannington, M.D. 1999. Classification of volcanic-associated massive sulfide deposits based on host-rock composition. Reviews in Economic Geology, 8: 1-11.

Berrocal-L., G., and Querol-S., F. 1991. Geological description of the Cuale District ore deposits, Jalisco, Mexico. In Economic geology, Mexico. Edited by G.P. Salas. Geological Society of America, The Geology of North America, vol. P-3, Chapt. 45, pp. 355-363.

Campa, M.F., and Coney, P.J. 1983. Tectonostratigraphic terranes and mineral resource distributions in Mexico. Canadian Journal of Earth Sciences, 20: 1040-1051.

Cantú-Chapa, C.M. 1974. Una nueva localidad del Cretácico Inferior en México. Revista del Instituto Mexicano del Petroleo, VI: 515.

Centeno-García, E., Ruíz, J., Coney, P.J., Patchett, P.J., and Ortega-Gutiérrez, F. 1993. Guerrero terrane of Mexico: Its role in the Southern Cordillera from new geochemical data. Geology, 21: 419-422.

Consejo de Recursos Minerales 1992a. Geological-mining monograph of the state of Zacatecas. Secretaría de Energía, Minas e Industria Paraestatal, Subsecretaría de Minas e Industria Básica, Publicación No. M-2e.

Consejo de Recursos Minerales 1992b. Informe de visita de reconocimiento realizada al fundo minero "El Salvador" ubicado en el Mpio. de Villa González Ortega, Estado de Zacatecas.

de Cserna, Z. 1976. Geology of the Fresnillo area, Zacatecas, Mexico. Geological Society of America Bulletin, 87: 1191-1199.

Franklin, J.M., Lydon, J.W., and Sangster, D.F. 1981. Volcanic-associated massive sulfide deposits. Economic Geology, 75th Anniversary Volume, 485-627.

MacLean, W.H., and Barrett, T.J. 1993. Lithogeochemical techniques using immobile elements. Journal of Geochemical Exploration, 48: 109-133.

Morton, R.L., and Franklin, J.M. 1987. Two-fold classification of Archean volcanic-associated massive sulfide deposits. Economic Geology, 82: 1057-1063.

Oliver, J., Payne, J., and Rebagliati, M. 1998. Precious-metal-bearing volcanogenic massive sulfide deposits, Campo Morado, Guerrero, Mexico. Exploration and Mining Geology, 6: 119-128.

Pearce, J.A., and Cann, J.R. 1973. Tectonic setting of basic volcanic rocks determined using trace element analyses. Earth and Planetary Science Letters, 19: 290-300.

Sedlock, R.L., Ortega-Gutiérrez, F., and Speed, R.C. 1993. Tectonostratigraphic terranes and tectonic evolution of Mexico. Geological Society of America, Special Paper 278.

Tardy, M., Lapierre, H., Freydier, C., Coulon, C., Gill, J.B., Mercier de Lepinay, B., Beck, C., Martínez-R., J., Talavera-M., O., Ortiz-H., E., Stein, G., Bourdier, J.-L., and Yta, M. 1994. The Guerrero suspect terrane (western Mexico) and coeval arc terranes (the Greater Antilles and the Western Cordillera of Colombia): a late Mesozoic intra-oceanic arc accreted to cratonal America during the Cretaceous. Tectonophysics, 230: 49-73.

Winchester, J.A., and Floyd, P.A. 1977. Geochemical discrimination of different magma series and their differentiation products using immobile elements. Chemical Geology, 20: 325-343.

Yta, M. 1992. Etude géodinamique et métallogénique d'un secteur de la "Faja de Plata," Mexique: La zone de Zacatecas - Francisco I. Madero - Saucito. Ph.D. thesis, Université d'Orléans, Orléans, France.

GEOLOGICAL SETTING OF THE TIZAPA VOLCANOGENIC MASSIVE SULPHIDE DEPOSIT, MEXICO STATE, MEXICO

PETER D. LEWIS
Lewis Geoscience Services Inc., 15715 Mountainview Drive, Surrey, B.C. Canada V4P 2W9

DAVID A. RHYS
Panterra Geoservices Inc., 14180 Greencrest Drive, Surrey, B.C. Canada V4P 1L9

ABSTRACT

The Tizapa Zn-Pb-Cu-Au-Ag deposit in southwestern Mexico consists of stacked ore lenses within a Kuroko-style volcanogenic massive sulphide system. The deposit occurs within the Guerrero terrane, a Late Paleozoic to Cretaceous assemblage of calc-alkaline volcanic arc rocks and clastic sedimentary rocks, and overlying platform carbonates. Strata exposed in the deposit area are 1) grey phyllites of the Triassic (?) to Jurassic Tejupilco Schist, stratigraphically overlain by 2) Late Jurassic to Early Cretaceous intermediate to felsic metavolcanic rocks of the Teloloapan volcanic assemblage, and 3) calcareous carbonaceous phyllite and limestone of the Middle Cretaceous Amatapec Formation.

Massive sulphide lenses occur at the stratigraphic contact between the Teloloapan volcanic assemblage and the Amatapec Formation. The footwall metavolcanic rocks are bimodal and include a lower, andesitic plagioclase porphyritic sequence and an upper probable felsic tuff unit of highly variable thickness. Potassium feldspar megacrystic augen gneiss intrudes the Tejupilco schist south of the mine, and several compositional varieties and ages of dykes are present in both footwall and hangingwall of the deposit. Tertiary and Quaternary volcanic rocks unconformably overlie the deformed Mesozoic and Paleozoic sequence. All pre-Tertiary rocks are affected by mid- to upper greenschist facies metamorphism associated with the Laramide Orogeny.

Penetrative fabrics, contractional faults, and folds in the Tizapa area formed during two major ductile strain events (D1, D2). A D1 penetrative foliation (S1), is presently parallel to compositional layering, formed during regional metamorphism, and lacks correlative megascopic structures. It is overprinted by and transposed into a D2 spaced to penetrative foliation (S2) that is parallel to axial surfaces of major west-vergent mesoscopic and megascopic recumbent folds of S1 and compositional layering. A component of west-southwest directed shear strain, parallel to a west-southwest trending elongation lineation, is indicated by shear bands, oblique fabrics and asymmetric pressure shadows on porphyroclasts. West-directed D2 thrusts and nappes imbricate parts of the volcanic sequence and sulphide bodies at Tizapa.

The main ore bodies at Tizapa were a single continuous sulphide horizon that was deformed into a thrust-disrupted, west-verging and north-plunging recumbent syncline/anticline pair during D2. North-northwest plunging thickened ore shoots result from this deformation, and overturned fold limbs are substantially thickened relative to upright limbs.

Several phases of post-D2 crenulations affect the sequence, and a broad, west-trending anticline divides the area into south and north dipping S1/S2 domains. Dominant late brittle faults include the Falla Riolita, a west-striking structure separating the Tizapa mine area rocks from stratigraphically lower rocks to the south, and numerous northwest-striking faults with up to several tens of metres displacement.

Alteration beneath orebodies at Tizapa is characterized by banded and disseminated pyrite in (i) intensely sericitized phyllitic felsic metavolcanic rocks immediately below the sulphide horizon, and (ii) underlying intense chlorite alteration of andesitic metavolcanic rocks that extends for up to 50 m below the ore. Plots of metal distribution in the orebodies at Tizapa indicate several Cu-rich zones that correspond with areas of thick footwall alteration and abundant pyrite bands with variable Cu-content. These areas may be deformed stockwork feeders to the ore.

INTRODUCTION

The Tizapa base and precious metal mine is located in the state of Mexico approximately 70 km west-southwest of the city of Toluca, and 4 km southeast of the town of Zacazonapan (Fig. 1). The mine is operated by Servicios Industriales Peñoles S.A. de C.V. (referred to hereafter as "Peñoles") under the operating company Minera Tizapa S.A. de C.V. The Tizapa deposit comprises several highly deformed volcanogenic sulphide bodies, similar to occurrences distributed along the length of the Guerrero Terrane (e.g., Heredia-Barragán and Garcia-Fons, 1989; Parga, 1981). Mined and remaining proven and probable reserves at present total 4.5 Mt at 1.9 g/t Au, 325 g/t Ag, 1.8 % Pb, 7.9 % Zn, and 0.7 % Cu (Giles and Garcia, 2000).

Apart from drilling of the Esmeralda prospect, 0.7 km north of the mine (Fig. 2), little detailed exploration has been completed at Tizapa, outside of the immediate mine area, and significant potential exists to expand resources. This paper presents a structural and stratigraphic framework for the Tizapa mine area and region that is based on a recent (1997) field and analytical program by the authors. The work included detailed structural mapping of both underground workings and surface outcrops, regional mapping of the deposit area, geochemical sampling, structural analysis of drill hole data through interpretation of mine sections and mapped plans, evaluation of existing mine assay results, and petrographic analysis of selected samples.

Previous geologic studies in the Tizapa area, in addition to those completed by Peñoles for the purposes of mine exploration and development, include detailed and regional mapping-based studies by the Metal Mining Agency of Japan (MMAJ; 1989, 1991, 1993, 1994), reports on exploration progress and

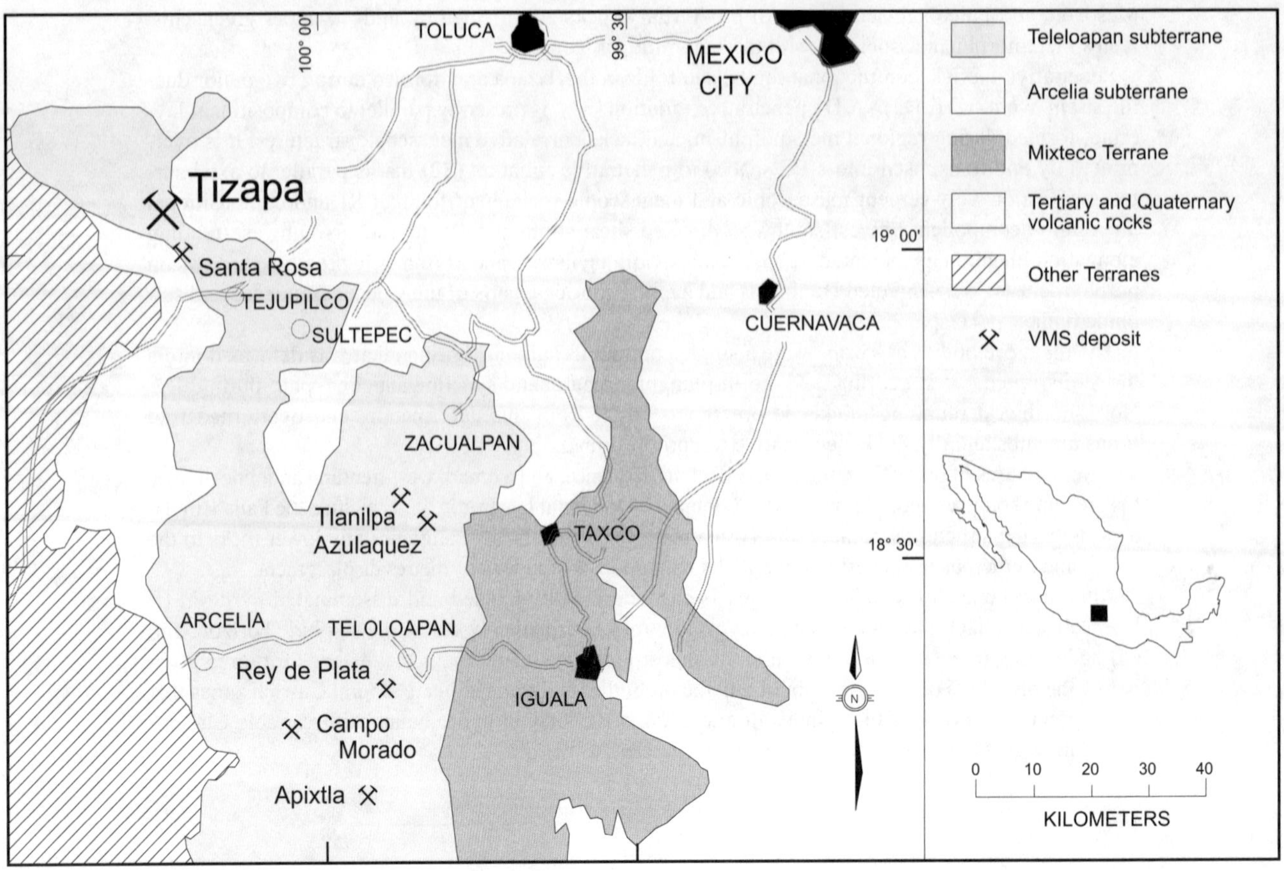

Figure 1. Location of the Tizapa mine, Mexico State.

mapping of the Tizapa and Esmeralda areas by Consejo de Resources Minerales (Parga-Perez at al., 1984), and several theses which addressed various aspects of the geology in the region (e.g. Parga-Perez, 1981). The history and development of the mine are outlined by Giles and Garcia (2000).

REGIONAL GEOLOGICAL SETTING

The Tizapa deposit is within the Teloloapan subterrane, a tectono-stratigraphic division of the Guerrero Terrane (Campa and Coney, 1983). This subterrane is a calc-alkaline volcanic arc sequence composed of at least three lithostructural elements (Monod et al., 1993): (i) Paleozoic or Triassic metavolcanic and metasedimentary rocks of the Tierra Caliente Complex and the Taxco Schist that form the structural or stratigraphic basement in the region, (ii) Upper Jurassic to Lower Cretaceous andesitic to felsic volcanic and clastic rocks of the Teloloapan volcanic arc that unconformably or tectonically overlie the basement units, and (iii) mid- to Upper Cretaceous limestone (Morelos and Amatapec formations) and clastic rocks. The Teloloapan Subterrane is bordered on the west by Cretaceous basalt and marine sedimentary rocks of the Arcelia Subterrane. Late Cretaceous to Early Tertiary polyphase shortening and greenschist facies metamorphism during the Laramide orogeny affected all

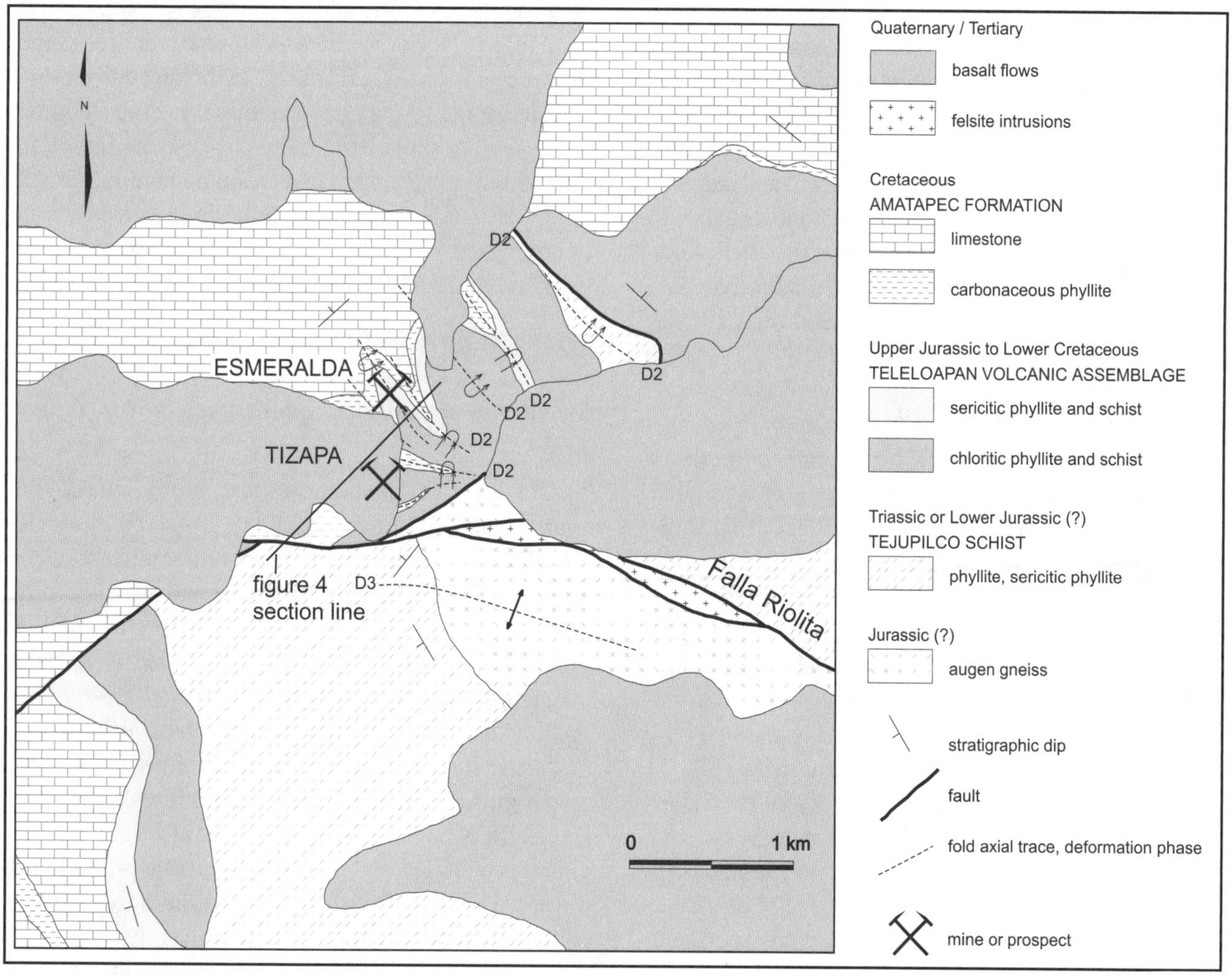

Figure 2. Simplified geology of the Tizapa mine area.

Mesozoic rocks in the region (Tolson, 1990), resulting in east- and west-vergent thrust faults and recumbent folds, and two generations of moderate to shallow-dipping foliation (Salinas-Prieto et al., 1993; Monod et al., 1993).

Lower Tertiary, felsic to intermediate volcanic and clastic rocks, and Neogene to Quaternary volcanic rocks of the Trans-Mexican volcanic belt unconformably overlie the deformed Mesozoic sequence (Sedlock et al., 1993), and cap many of the ridges in the Tizapa deposit area (Fig. 2). Tertiary, north and northwest-striking normal faults affect rocks as young as Oligocene in the region, and locally form grabens filled with Neogene volcanic rocks (Jansma and Lang, 1997).

Two dominant styles of mineral deposits occur in the Teloloapan Subterrane. The first consists of Early Cretaceous, Kuroko-type volcanogenic Zn-Pb-Ag-Au massive sulphide deposits in four districts (Fig. 1; Miranda Gasca, 1995): (i) Tizapa-Esmeralda-Santa Rosa, (ii) Azulaquez-Tlanilpa, (iii) Rey de Plata, and (iv) Campo Morado-Suriana. The second consists of northwest-striking Tertiary polymetallic sulphide-quartz veins associated with normal faults that have been exploited at Taxco and at several mines in the Zacualpan district (Noguez et al., 1991).

TIZAPA DEPOSIT AREA GEOLOGY

Rocks in the Tizapa deposit region comprise a sequence of northwest to north-striking, foliated, metasedimentary and metavolcanic rocks (Fig. 2, 3). The sequence is metamorphosed to lower to middle greenschist facies defined by assemblages of muscovite, chlorite, and at lower topographic elevations in the mine area, biotite and amphibole. Near Tizapa, the stratigraphic sequence is composed of two dominantly metasedimentary units that are separated by a band of intermediate to felsic volcanic rocks (Fig. 2). The lower sedimentary unit, the Tejupilco Schist, comprises phyllite with minor interbeds of sericitic phyllite of probable Triassic or Lower Jurassic age (Monod et al., 1993). It is overlain successively by an interval of volcanic rocks and by the upper metasedimentary sequence, which consists of metamorphosed limestone, carbonaceous mudstone, and siltstone. The volcanic sequence and the overlying limestone unit have been assigned to the Upper Jurassic to Lower Cretaceous Teloloapan volcanic sequence and the Amatapec Formation, respectively, by Monod et al. (1993) based on regional stratigraphic relationships and the presence of Albian fossils in the limestone.

A west-striking, subvertical to steeply north dipping brittle fault, the Falla Riolita, cuts the deposit area just south of the Tizapa mine. For much of its length, the fault coincides with a flow-banded to brecciated rhyolite dyke (Fig. 3). Stratigraphic separation is over 600 metres, with lower strata exposed south of the fault in a series of thrust panels.

The Tizapa ore bodies and other deposits in the region (e.g., Santa Rosa, Esmeralda) are stratabound and occur at or near a contact between lower, plagioclase-phyric, sericitic and/or chloritic schist and phyllite (Teloloapan volcanic assemblage), and an upper sequence of locally calcareous carbonaceous phyllite and limestone (Amatapec Formation). Five main ore lenses are presently being mined. These ore lenses are interpreted to have formed as a single continuous sulphide layer, that was subsequently imbricated through faulting and folding into the present complexely stacked configuration (Fig. 4).

Tizapa Mine Area Lithologic Units

K-feldspar megacrystic quartz metadiorite (augen gneiss)

Outcrops of medium-grained biotite-muscovite-quartz-plagioclase schist with 0.2 - 4 cm long K-feldspar porphyroclasts are exposed southeast of the Tizapa mine in the core of a regional west-trending anticline (Fig. 2). The homogenous nature and texture of this unit suggest that it is a deformed K-feldspar megacrystic diorite intrusion. A mineralogically similar but texturally distinct border phase of this unit lacks the megacrystic K-feldspar, and separates the augen gneiss from the overlying phyllites. This border phase is commonly up to 50 m thick, and formed either as a chilled margin or as a separate phase of the diorite. The ubiquitous presence of the border phase, combined with the lack of an unconformity breccia at the contact with the phyllitic sequence and the presence of ductilely deformed aplitic dykes emanating from the unit into the overlying section, indicate that

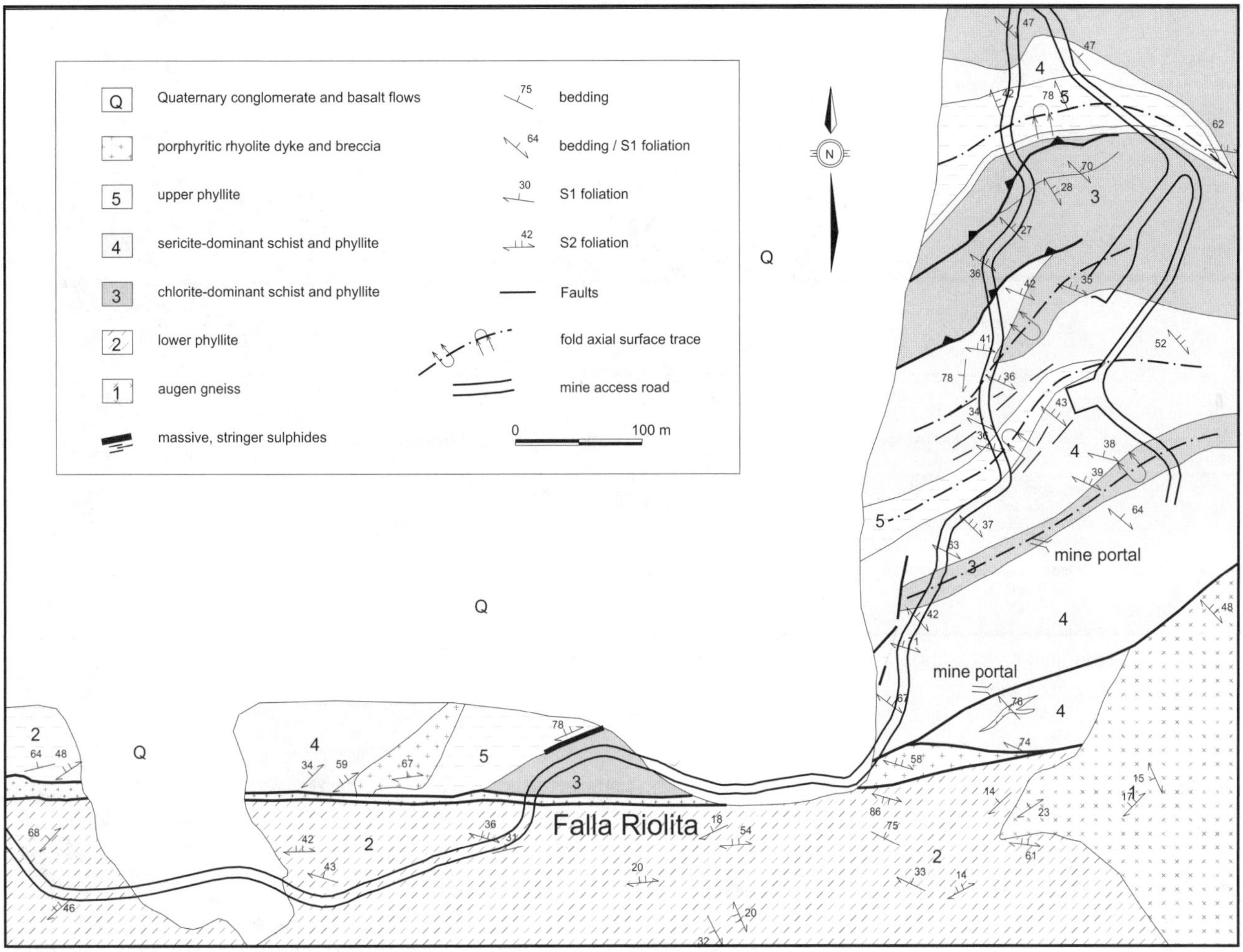

Figure 3. Detailed surface geology of the Tizapa mine area.

the augen gneiss is intrusive into the Tejupilco schist.

Lower phyllite unit (Tejupilco Schist)

Silver-grey to black phyllite of the Tejupilco Schist overlies the augen gneiss south of Falla Riolita (Fig. 2, 3). This phyllite is composed primarily of non-calcareous, silvery-grey metamudstone, and attains a thickness of approximately 800 m. Subordinate metasiltstone, and local 0.3 m to 10 m thick interbeds of pale grey to tan sericitic phyllite and schist representing possible tuffaceous or volcaniclastic beds, occur throughout the lower phyllite (Fig. 5). In lower parts of the sequence, the phyllites are commonly carbonaceous, and locally contain limestone and chert beds. Rocks equivalent to this unit have not been identified north of the Falla Riolita at the mine.

Metavolcanic sequence (Teloloapan volcanic assemblage)

Metavolcanic rocks of the Teloloapan volcanic assemblage are exposed extensively in eastern and northeastern portions of the Tizapa deposit area, as well as south of the Falla Riolita, 1.4 km southwest of the mine (Fig. 2). Near the Tizapa mine area, the volcanic rocks are structurally interleaved with calcareous carbonaceous phyllite of the overlying sequence (Fig. 3). The thickness of the volcanic sequence at the mine is uncertain due to this structural thickening, but it is probably greater than 200 m (Fig. 3). The volcanic section on the south side of Falla Riolita, 1.6 km southwest of the mine, is a structurally intact section that is approximately 220 m thick (Fig. 2).

The Teloloapan volcanic sequence in the Tizapa

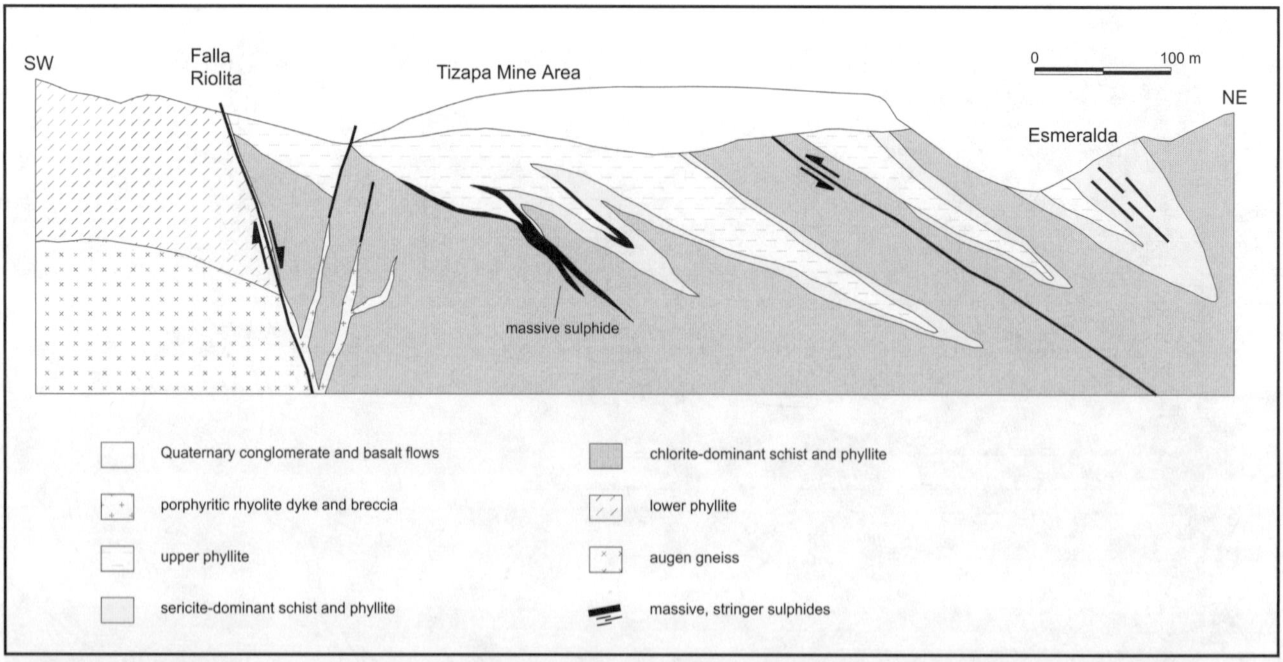

Figure 4. Geological cross section through the Tizapa mine and the Esmeralda prospect. View to the northwest. See Figure 2 for legend and section location.

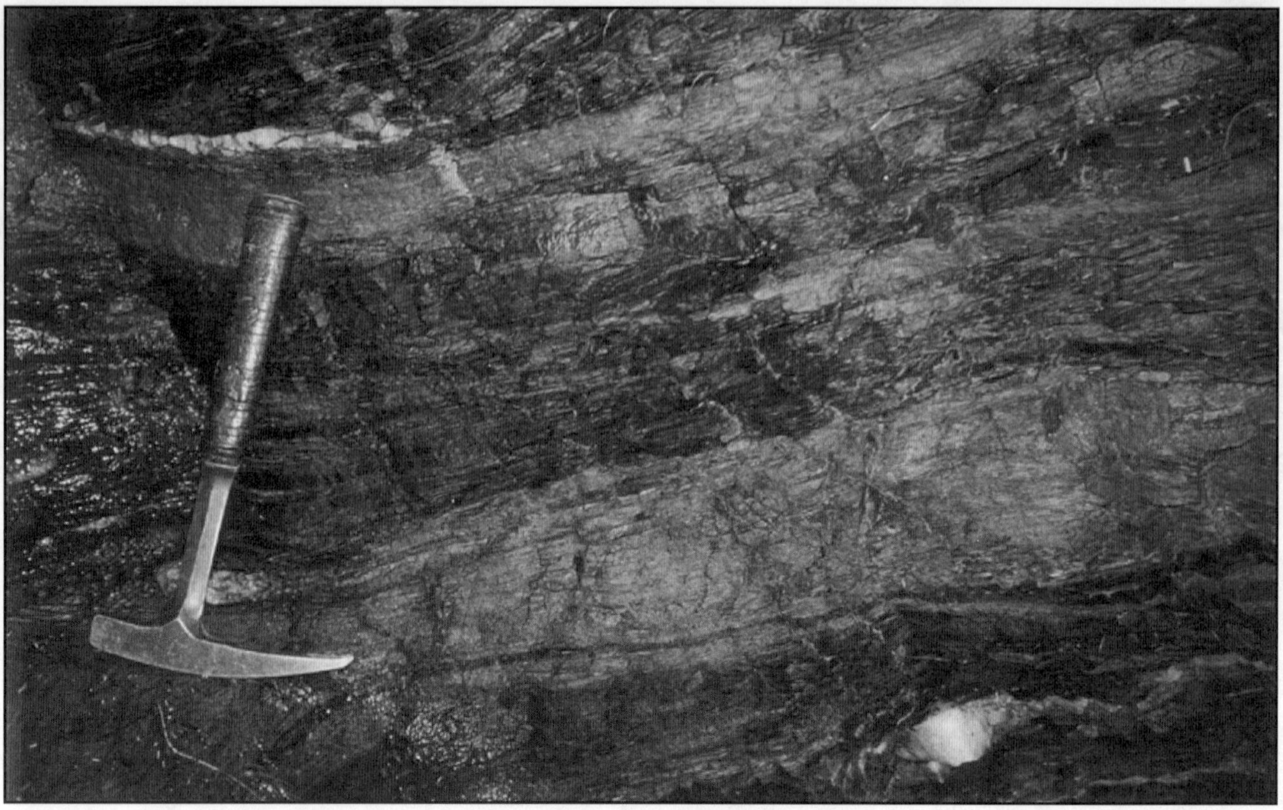

Figure 5. Lower phyllite sequence (Tejupilco Schist) south of the Falla Riolita, showing interbedded carbonaceous phyllite (dark grey) and sericite phyllite.

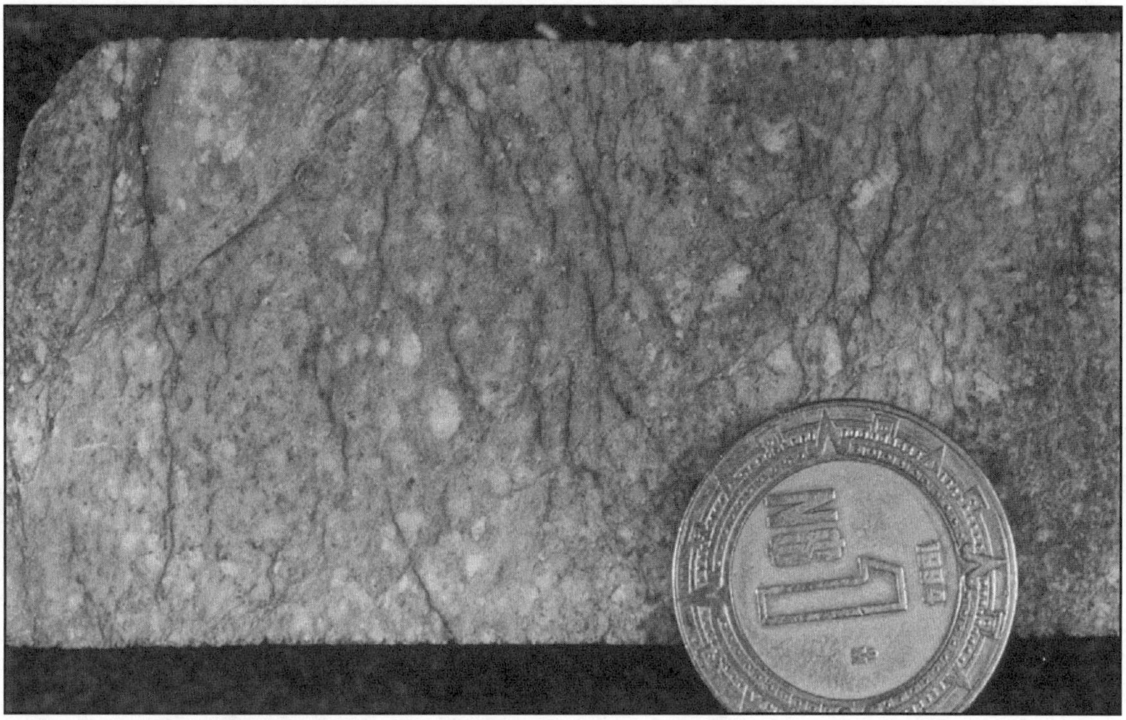

Figure 6. Typical example of porphyritic andesitic metavolcanic unit in the footwall of the Tizapa deposit. From drill hole MJM-5, 160.2 m.

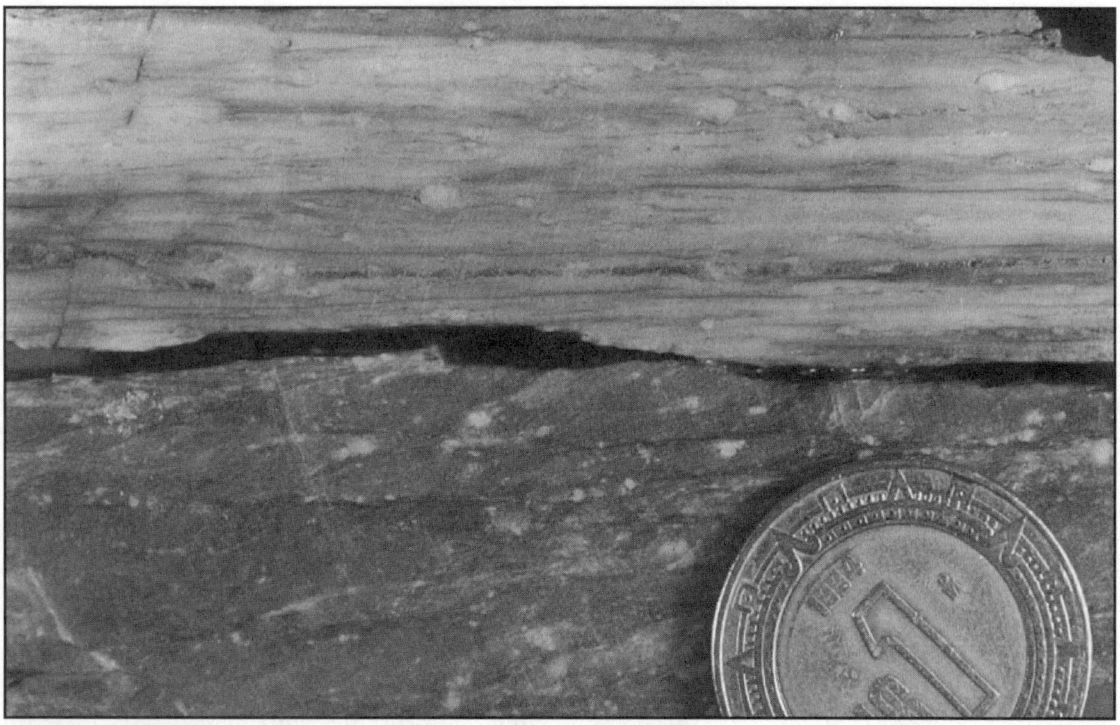

Figure 7. Examples of rhyolitic metavolcanic rocks, Esmeralda prospect. Note the laminated texture of the matrix of the top sample, which is typical of felsic volcanic units in the area, and the presence of quartz and plagioclase porphyroclasts in both samples. Coin is 2.1 cm in diametre.

area consists of chlorite, chlorite-sericite, and sericite schists. Their mineralogy and geochemical character (Fig. 7) support a bimodal sequence consisting of a thick, structurally lower andesitic unit and a thinner, less continuous structurally higher felsic volcanic unit. The felsic part of the sequence can be traced south of the Falla Riolita, but is absent 2 km to the northeast of the deposit (Fig. 2).

Chlorite and chlorite-sericite schist andesitic metavolcanic rocks

Green to tan plagioclase-porphyritic chlorite and chlorite-sericite schist form the dominant exposures near and to the northeast of the Tizapa mine (Fig. 2, 3). These schists contain 2-10 % plagioclase phenocrysts in a fine-grained, green to pale grey or tan, muscovite ± chlorite + plagioclase + quartz ± calcite matrix (Fig. 5). Biotite, tremolite, and actinolite occur locally on surface and in deep drill holes beneath the Tizapa deposit. Two subunits are distinguished based on dominant phyllosilicate phase: 1) schists composed primarily of chlorite with minor sericite, which are overlain by 2) mixed sericite-chlorite schist. Interbeds of grey phyllite occur locally near the top of the sequence in the Tizapa mine area, and several limestone beds occur within 50 m of its top to the northeast of the deposit area. Primary textures, other than the porphyritic character of the unit, are obscured in most areas by deformation and metamorphism. Most outcrops have a non-layered, homogeneous texture and an even distribution of feldspar porphyroclasts, suggesting a flow or intrusive origin. However, some areas contain interlayered mudstone and preserve fragmental textures (lapilli), indicative of interstratified tuffaceous or volcaniclastic intervals.

Sericite schist felsic metavolcanic rocks

Pale grey to white, plagioclase ± quartz porphyritic sericite-quartz phyllite and schist occur above the chlorite and chlorite-sericite schist in much of the Tizapa deposit area (Fig. 2). These rocks are distinguished from the underlying schists by (i) the lack of chlorite as a matrix phase, (ii) generally fewer or no plagioclase phenocrysts (0-3 %), (iii) the local presence of quartz as a phenocryst phase, and, (iv) a pale grey, yellow or white fine-grained quartz-rich matrix that commonly has 0.5-3 mm wide grey and white laminae (Fig. 7). Beds of grey sericite phyllite and carbonaceous phyllite occur locally within this unit at the Esmeralda prospect, 0.7 km north of the Tizapa mine (Fig. 2), where it is interlayered with carbonaceous mudstone. The texture and common presence of clastic interbeds suggest that this unit is a felsic meta-tuff. The thickness of the felsic metavolcanic unit varies from 1 to 40 m at Tizapa and up to 140 m at the Esmeralda prospect.

Upper metasedimentary rocks (Amatapec Formation)

The Teloloapan metavolcanic rocks are overlain throughout the Tizapa deposit area by calcareous carbonaceous phyllite and meta-limestone that together form the upper metasedimentary sequence (Fig. 2, 3). A stratigraphic contact between the volcanic sequence and the overlying calcareous sedimentary sequence is implied by: (i) the parallelism of bedding in the two sequences, (ii) the presence of sulphide beds (Tizapa orebody) at the contact in the Tizapa mine, and (iii) beds of felsic tuff that occur locally in the basal portions of the carbonaceous phyllite. Based on regional stratigraphic relationships and fossil assemblages, Monod et al. (1993) assign limestone of the upper metasedimentary sequence to the Albian Amatapec Formation.

Carbonaceous phyllite

Calcareous grey to black carbonaceous phyllite (Fig. 8) up to 100 m thick commonly forms the lower parts of the upper metasedimentary sequence (Fig. 2, 3). These phyllites can be distinguished from the phyllites of the Tejupilco Schist by their generally calcareous nature and the lack, except locally, of sericite phyllite interbeds. Thinly-bedded grey limestone is commonly interstratified with the carbonaceous phyllite, and increases in abundance higher in the section. No metavolcanic units occur in the carbonaceous phyllite at Tizapa, but at the Esmeralda prospect, beds of sericite phyllite that resemble the underlying felsic unit interfinger within the lower 50 m of the carbonaceous phyllites. Two kilometres to the northeast of the mine, the carbonaceous mudstone at the base of the upper sequence is only approximately 40 m thick and is highly gossanous due to the presence of abundant

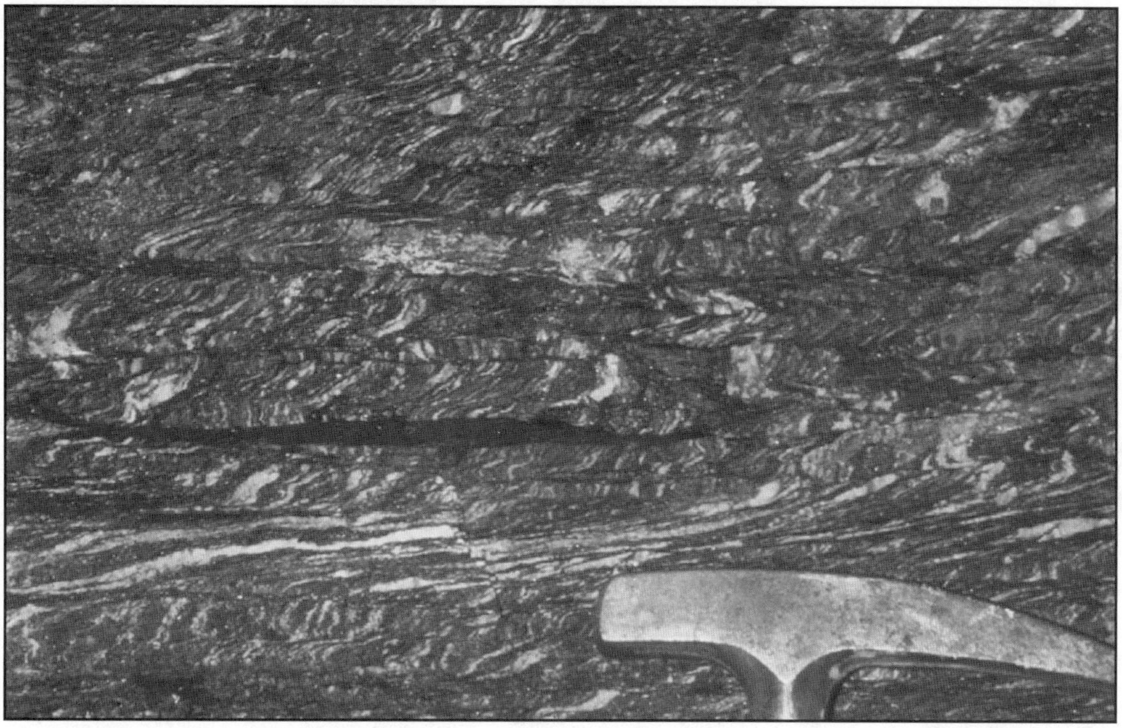

Figure 8. Carbonaceous phyllite in the stratigraphic hangingwall of the M0 orebody, 1180 level, Tizapa mine. Penetrative S1 foliation is folded and preserved in lithons between continuous, spaced S2 foliation surfaces.

Fe-oxide lamina. To the southwest, at Cerro de la Pila, the carbonaceous phyllite is absent and limestone directly overlies the volcanic sequence (Fig. 2).

Limestone

The calcareous carbonaceous mudstone at the base of the upper sequence grades upward into a thinly to thickly bedded pale grey, recrystallized and foliated limestone unit that is over 300 m thick (Fig. 2). The limestone contains pale to dark grey bands that probably reflect transposed bedding, and is commonly interlayered with thin beds and laminae of carbonaceous phyllite, sericite phyllite, and locally, greywacke.

Minor Intrusive Rocks

Dykes and small intrusions of several compositions are ubiquitous but volumetrically minor in the Tizapa mine area. The largest are white to pale grey rhyolite dykes up to 25 m wide that intrude the east-west striking Falla Riolita and related structures (Fig. 3). They are composed of 3-15 % quartz, plagioclase and locally, biotite phenocrysts in an aphanitic, pale grey matrix. Quartz phenocrysts are rounded and embayed. Planar to contorted flow banding defined by dark grey to black glassy bands is common. The dykes are often brecciated, with angular flow-banded fragments in grey, sandy matrix. They are probably Neogene in age.

Other minor intrusions include: 1) a sill of foliated, fine to medium-grained hornblende porphyritic metadiorite several tens of metres thick that occurs within phyllite on the ridge south of Falla Riolita; 2) pale grey, boudinaged, fine-grained plagioclase-phyric dykes and sills generally less than one metre thick that intrude all rock units in the mine area; 3) undeformed, fresh, fine-grained, grey to dark green dykes with pyroxene phenocrysts that may be cogenetic with nearby Quaternary basalt, and 4) aplitic dykes and stocks up to 10 m thick that occur south of the Falla Riolita within the augen gneiss.

Whole Rock Geochemistry

Geochemical analyses of samples of metavolcanic rocks collected from surface and undergound at the Tizapa mine area show distinctions between the mapped lithologic units (Table 1; Fig. 9). On a

Table 1. Whole rock geochemical data for altered volcanic rocks in the footwall to the Tizapa ore lenses, and their less altered stratigraphic equivalents from outside of the mine area. Abbreviations: U/G = underground sample; DDH = drill core sample; FW = footwall. Rock types are as follows: 1a = plagioclase porphyritic chlorite schist (least altered andesite); 1b = plagioclase porphyry with pale grey, quartz-bearing matrix; 2 = pale grey to white felsic schist (least altered felsite); 3 = sericite-pyrite-quartz schist (footwall alteration); 4 = chlorite-pyrite schist (footwall alteration); 5 = quartz-sericite-pyrite schist (M1/M2 hangingwall); 6 = K-feldspar megacrystic quartz diorite (augen gneiss). Analyses performed by Chemex Labs of Vancouver, British Columbia by XRF pressed pellet. Detection limit for major elements is 0.01%; for other elements detection limit is 2 ppm, except Zr (3 ppm).

(Table 1 continued on next page)

Sample Number	Location/description	Rock type	UTM easting	UTM northing
99910	Mine area	1a	9980.9	10394.8
99914	South ridge, west	1a	8383.2	8561.3
99916	U/G; Rampa Sur, above 1st bend	1a	9705.5	9909.0
99923	U/G; 1154L, M0 FW on Rampa Sur	1a	9572.5	9943.5
99928	DDH; Hole MJM-5, 240 m, >50m below ore	1b		
99933	U/G; 1157L, 15 m in FW of M0 orebody	1b	9416.5	10121.0
99937	Esmeralda showing; laminated tuff	1b	10015.9	10622.5
99951	DDH; Hole TIZS11, 451 m, 1.5 m below ore	1a		
99909	Mine area, north of mill; qz-plag porphyritic	2	9998.7	10358.6
99913	South ridge, west	2	8270.2	8366.6
99944	East of Esmeralda	2	10356.0	10925.5
99919	U/G; 1259B drift, 0.5m in FW of M1 lens	3	9691.0	9994.5
99920	U/G; 1154L, 2m in FW of M0 orebody, near L1	3	9581.0	10111.0
99931	U/G; 1157L, 3m in FW of M0 orebody	3	9422.5	10152.5
99949	U/G; 1100L, FW M0 near L1	3	9666.0	10063.5
99918	U/G; 1259A drift, 7m in FW of M2 lens	4	9704.0	10007.5
99921	U/G; 1154L, approx. 20m in M0 orebody FW	4	9613.0	9962.5
99926	U/G; 1100L, 7m in FW of M0 orebody near L1	4	9505.5	10229.0
99947	U/G; 1100L, FW M0 near L1	4	9664.0	10083.0
99945	Esmeralda east	5	10574.6	10912.3
99940	South ridge, foliated hornblende diorite	6	9709.5	9294.7
99939	Creek south of mine, augen gneiss unit	6	10158.2	9722.4

Table 1 (Continued from previous page)

Sample Number	Al2O3 %	CaO %	Cr2O3 %	Fe2O3 %	K2O %	MgO %	MnO %	Na2O %	P2O5 %	SiO2 %	TiO2 %	LOI %	TOTAL %	Ba ppm	Cs ppm	Hf ppm	La ppm	Nb ppm	Rb ppm	Sr ppm	Ta ppm	Y ppm	Zr ppm
99910	15.91	4.52	<.01	7.73	0.10	7.54	0.05	4.30	0.11	54.07	0.67	3.50	98.50	26	<1	4	13	4	2	225	<1	23	129
99914	14.76	4.71	<.01	5.98	0.72	4.61	0.07	3.30	0.10	60.63	0.63	2.77	98.28	145	<1	4	14	4	15	250	<1	26	112
99916	17.65	3.45	<.01	7.05	0.37	5.74	0.05	5.25	0.12	54.45	0.69	3.57	98.39	421	2	4	14	4	8	263	<1	24	115
99923	18.79	2.04	<.01	7.99	4.88	4.40	0.21	0.17	0.13	49.98	0.84	8.63	98.06	548	4	5	12	4	142	74	<1	21	132
99928	12.86	0.81	<.01	3.86	2.51	4.75	0.03	0.43	0.01	69.64	0.18	3.33	98.41	783	4	6	26	5	68	133	<1	34	167
99933	13.86	0.71	<.01	4.45	1.34	4.13	0.03	0.64	0.03	68.25	0.19	4.84	98.47	422	3	7	72	6	53	240	<1	53	211
99937	9.67	1.59	<.01	2.81	2.07	1.17	0.03	0.53	0.04	78.90	0.13	1.80	98.74	716	5	5	20	5	78	524	<1	21	149
99951	16.25	1.85	<.01	4.62	3.39	1.96	0.09	2.76	0.11	61.00	0.70	6.03	98.76	604	5	5	21	5	57	77	<1	28	165
99909	9.71	0.23	<.01	0.39	0.80	0.21	0.01	3.93	0.06	82.78	0.12	0.61	98.85	297	1	4	17	4	24	91	<1	24	110
99913	12.22	0.13	<.01	0.91	4.29	0.17	0.01	1.96	0.02	78.11	0.16	1.03	99.01	810	<1	5	13	4	76	62	<1	21	150
99944	10.36	0.38	<.01	0.40	0.37	0.03	0.01	5.54	0.03	81.19	0.12	0.45	98.88	104	<1	5	14	4	10	65	<1	35	150
99919	13.65	0.10	<.01	5.56	3.17	2.93	0.10	0.06	0.02	67.38	0.12	5.65	98.74	469	5	6	21	5	117	21	<1	35	149
99920	5.86	0.10	<.01	16.87	0.43	0.10	0.01	<.01	0.01	65.00	0.06	10.69	99.13	98	1	2	13	3	16	6	<1	17	62
99931	11.27	0.51	<.01	2.93	2.52	3.93	0.15	0.08	0.01	72.80	0.10	4.12	98.42	398	3	4	18	4	88	26	<1	27	118
99949	13.81	0.23	<.01	2.29	3.53	2.87	0.13	0.17	0.03	72.25	0.12	3.03	98.46	535	3	6	23	5	118	26	<1	35	132
99918	12.72	0.17	<.01	12.55	2.39	3.55	0.10	0.07	0.09	60.13	0.47	6.12	98.36	394	3	4	15	4	79	18	<1	19	122
99921	12.09	0.18	<.01	12.82	2.46	3.00	0.10	0.23	0.09	61.09	0.49	6.28	98.83	397	3	3	12	4	73	33	<1	18	106
99926	14.10	0.20	<.01	18.92	1.86	5.68	0.22	0.13	0.09	48.87	0.55	7.95	98.57	320	2	5	22	5	61	15	<1	23	159
99947	16.37	0.30	<.01	11.03	3.83	4.44	0.19	0.15	0.11	54.37	0.70	7.09	98.58	687	5	4	14	4	116	27	<1	23	126
99945	13.23	0.22	<.01	2.73	1.27	2.93	0.03	1.18	0.03	73.76	0.12	3.34	98.84	310	4	5	23	5	47	344	<1	32	140
99940	15.10	1.01	<.01	3.77	2.44	1.86	0.03	4.92	0.16	66.82	0.63	1.59	98.33	584	4	5	14	5	43	127	<1	30	159
99939	12.44	12.31	<.01	8.22	0.13	5.38	0.16	3.94	0.14	45.78	1.31	9.24	99.05	19	<1	2	4	2	4	198	<1	27	85

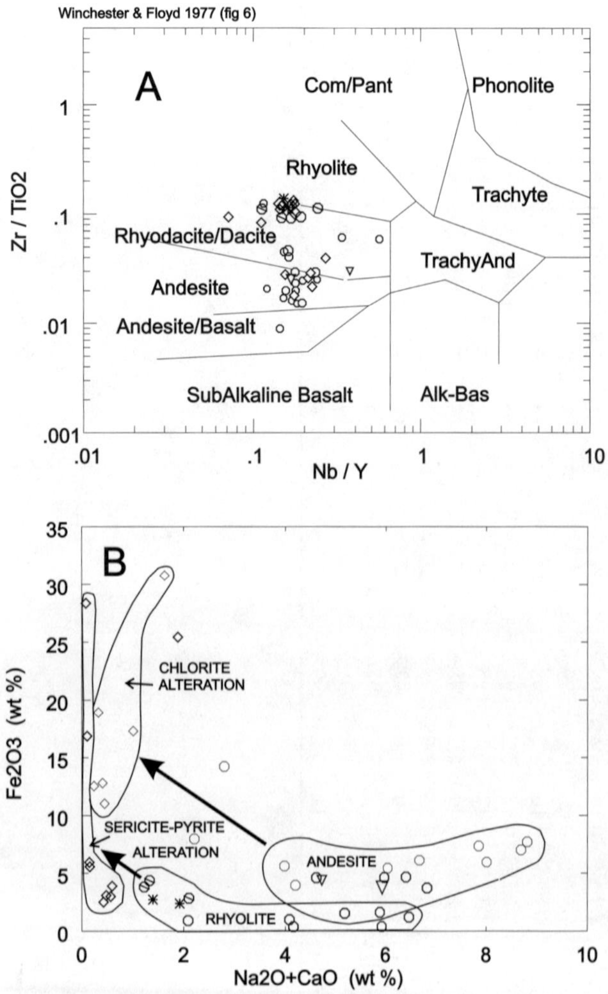

Figure 9. Chemistry of volcanic and igneous rocks in the Tizapa area, based on XRF pressed pellet analyses of representative samples. Note that sericite-pyrite-quartz altered units and chlorite altered units in the footwall of the Tizapa orebody have felsic volcanic and andesitic compositions, respectively, when plotted on a Winchester and Floyd (1977) diagram (A). Alteration is accompanied by decreases in relative $Na_2O + K_2O$, SiO_2, and $Na_2O + CaO$ content, and with increase in Fe_2O_3 (B). Complete geochemical analyses listed in Table 1.

Winchester and Floyd (1977) discrimination plot of immobile elements Zr/Ti versus Nb/Y, two distinct clusters are evident: samples of plagioclase porphyritic chloritic schist plot in the andesite field, while samples of the pale grey, felsic schist are chemically equivalent to rhyolite or dacite (Fig. 9a). Zr/Y ratios of least altered metavolcanic rocks in the Tizapa area typically range between 4.2 and 7.5, indicating compositions that are transitional between calc-alkaline and tholeiitic (Barrett and MaClean, 1999). The K-feldspar megacrystic metadiorite ("augen gneiss") plots in the same field as the andesitic volcanic rocks on Figure 9a, although field relationships dictate a younger age.

Samples collected from altered rocks beneath the orebodies in the Tizapa mine, where identification of protolith rock type is obscured by alteration, also cluster within rhyolite to dacite and andesite compositional fields. Samples of footwall pyritic sericite-quartz schist (sericite-pyrite alteration) collected from between 0.3 and 10 m beneath the Tizapa orebodies consistently plot with rhyolitic to dacitic rocks, while samples of chlorite + pyrite schist (chlorite-pyrite alteration) beneath the pyrite-sericite schist, and 5-50 m beneath the ore, consistently plot in the andesite field (Fig. 9a). These results indicate that a narrow band (5-10 m) of rhyolitic to dacitic volcanic rocks occurs at the top of the andesitic sequence beneath the Tizapa orebodies. The change from sericite-dominant to chlorite-dominant schist beneath the orebodies is a combined effect of both alteration and original lithology. Alternating layers of chloritic and sericitic units 5-15 m stratigraphically below ore at Tizapa may represent interstratification of andesitic and felsic tuff.

MINERALIZATION AND ALTERATION

The Tizapa orebodies have been traced by drilling and underground mining over an approximately 700 m by 500 m area. They comprise five major sulphide lenses denoted by their structural position in the mine: M0, L1, M1, M1.5 and M2 (Fig. 10, 11). Total mined and remaining proven and probable reserves at Tizapa as of December, 1998 were 4.5 Mt at 1.9 g/t Au, 325 g/t Ag, 1.8 % Pb, 7.9 % Zn, and 0.7 % Cu (Giles and Garcia, 2000). The style of mineralization, base metal signature (Zn + Pb >> Cu), associated felsic to intermediate volcanic rocks, and style of footwall alteration at Tizapa is typical of many Kuroko-type volcanogenic massive sulphide deposits.

Sulphide mineralization in the Tizapa area comprises stratabound sulphide bodies located primarily at the contact between metavolcanic rocks and overlying carbonaceous metasedimentary rocks (Fig. 12).

Widespread disseminated, banded, and stringer pyrite and chalcopyrite occurs in footwall metavolcanic rocks. Sulphide bodies consist of fine-grained pyrite with bands and disseminations of sphalerite, galena, arsenopyrite and chalcopyrite (Fig. 13). Contacts of sulphide bodies are sharp (Fig. 12). Tetrahedrite, friebergite, boulangerite and argentite are reported as accessory minerals that contain most of the precious metals (Monroy-Fernandez and Aragon-Pina, 1994). Sulphide bodies range from a few centimetres thick up to more than 20 m in parts of L1 and M2 (Fig. 10).

The M0 orebody can be traced underground through a disrupted fold closure into the L1 orebody, which in turn is traceable into the M1 and M2 orebodies, indicating that together they define a single sulphide horizon which is folded into a tight, west-verging recumbent fold (Fig. 10, 11). M0 and L1 both occur at the contact between calcareous carbonaceous phyllite in the stratigraphic hangingwall and underlying sericite phyllite at the top of the metavolcanic sequence. No metavolcanic rocks occur above these orebodies (Fig. 10). However, sericite phyllite geochemically similar to the footwall sericitic phyllite occurs in lowermost hangingwall of the M1 and M2 orebodies (Fig. 10). This sericitic phyllite may reflect (a) the presence of a felsic unit that was deposited locally over ore lenses M1 and M2 but not L1 and M0, after formation of the sulphide bodies, (b) that the sericite phyllite has been structurally inserted above the orebodies, or (c) that the M1 and M2 orebodies sit at a slightly different stratigraphic position than L1 and M0.

The Esmeralda prospect, 0.7 km north of the Tizapa mine (Fig. 2), consists of several discontinuous sulphide bodies that are up to 5 metres thick within a 400 metre (north-south) by 100 metres (east-west) area. Drilling here has defined a resource of approximately 350,000 tonnes grading 4 % combined Zn + Pb (Parga-Perez et al., 1984). The Esmeralda mineralization occurs in a similar stratigraphic position to the Tizapa orebodies, at the top of the volcanic sequence associated with felsic volcanic rocks. However, unlike the Tizapa ore, the Esmeralda sulphide bodies are entirely enclosed within felsic rocks. This felsic unit is up to 100 m thick, substantially thicker than at Tizapa, and may include units stratigraphically higher than at Tizapa. Abrupt interfingering of chlorite-sericite schist and carbonaceous phyllite in the prospect area may indicate thrust imbrication and/or recumbent folding.

Footwall alteration to the Tizapa orebodies

Recognition of hydrothermal alteration associated with the Tizapa orebodies is complicated by the metamorphic overprint, which has produced regional mineral assemblages similar to those found in the alteration zones. Criteria that distinguish rocks that have undergone hydrothermal alteration prior to metamorphism include (1) the presence of disseminated and banded pyrite, (2) more complete recrystallization and destruction of primary volcanic textures, and (3) a greater relative abundance of chlorite and/or sericite and lesser preservation of feldspars in the altered rocks than in their unaltered, metamorphic counterparts.

Footwall alteration zones display a consistent textural and mineralogical zoning with increasing distance (depth) from massive sulphide bodies:

Sericite-pyrite alteration occurs 3-10 m beneath the sulphide orebodies, and overprints felsic rocks. It usually comprises an upper zone (0.3-4 m) of abundant 0.5-25 cm wide bands of coarse-grained pyrite ± quartz ± chalcopyrite that are spaced at 2-30 cm apart, in a matrix of sericite + disseminated pyrite + quartz (Fig. 14). The bands commonly join obliquely and bifurcate, suggesting that they formed as footwall veins rather than sedimentary layers. Pyrite bands abruptly decrease in abundance with depth (Fig. 15), and grade into assemblages of intense sericite-disseminated pyrite-quartz in lower portions of this alteration zone. Elliptical, green chlorite-sericite blebs, possibly representing retrograde metamorphism of cordierite, occur locally in sericite-pyrite in the altered footwall rocks in peripheral portions of the Tizapa deposit.

Chlorite-pyrite alteration is present for up to 45 m beneath the sericite-pyrite alteration, primarily in the andesitic metavolcanic rocks. Assemblages of intense chlorite + disseminated pyrite ± Fe-carbonate define this zone (Fig. 16). Chlorite commonly forms >75 % of the rock in this zone. Coarse bands of pyrite, similar in texture and abundance to those in the sericite-pyrite zone, commonly occur in the upper 10 m of the

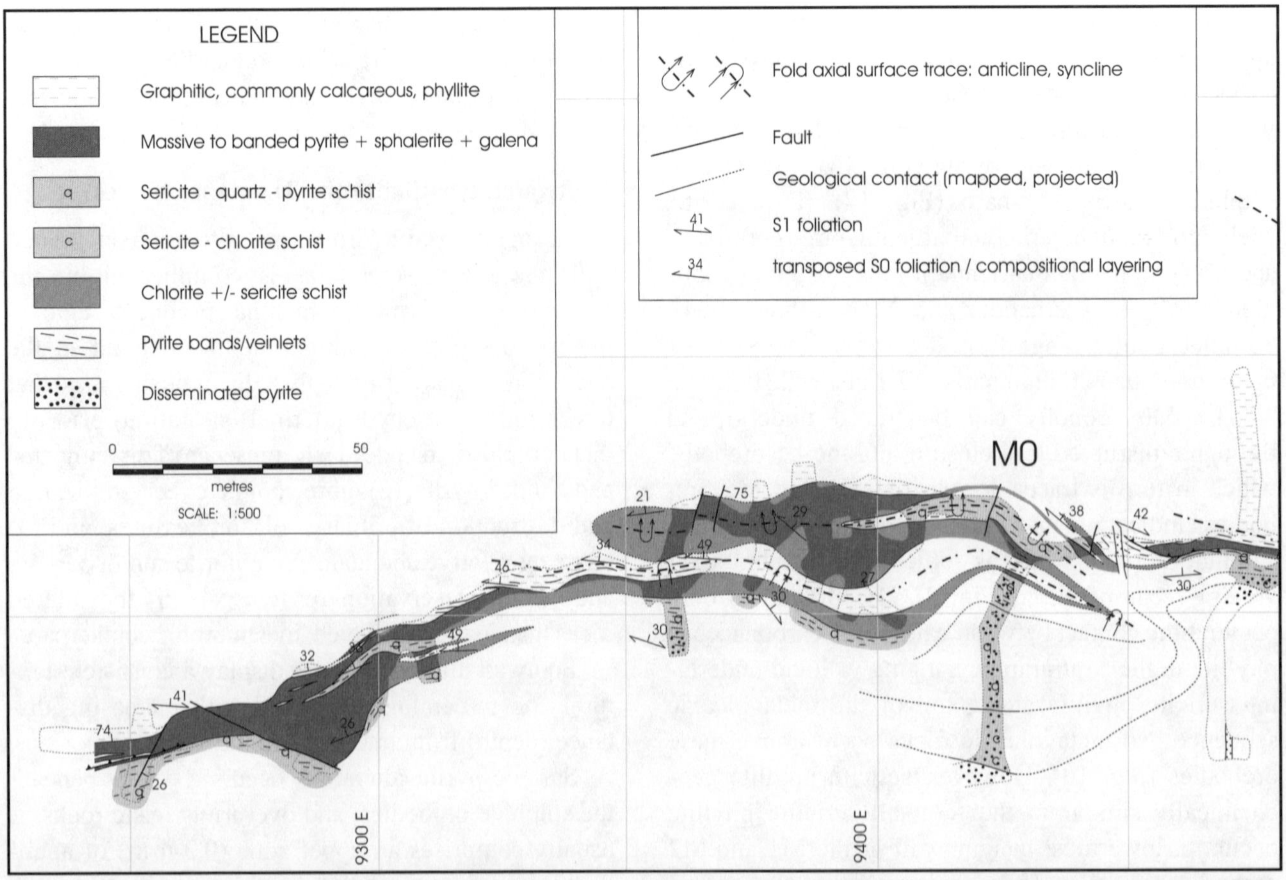

Figure 10. Composite geological plan of 1154 and 1163 m levels, Tizapa mine. The M0, L1, M1 and M2 orebodies form a single, folded horizon that occurs primarily at the contact between the metavolcanic and carbonaceous phyllite units. Note the tight, west verging morphology of D2 folds affecting the orebody. The thickened hinge of the minor fold on the M0 orebody between 9340E and 9450E forms an ore shoot that has been traced by drilling for several hundred metres to the north.

chlorite zone. Relict porphyritic textures are sometimes visible, but plagioclase phenocrysts are altered to sericite.

Beneath the chlorite alteration zone, primary plagioclase is preserved, and alteration is non-pervasive. Stringers of pyrite + quartz ± sphalerite are common, and calcite is abundant.

Carbonaceous phyllite within the hangingwall sequence contains no pyrite or any other visible indications of alteration, except for local slivers of pyrite-sphalerite within 5 m above ore that can usually be traced laterally back into the ore and may be tectonically imbricated.

Alteration Geochemistry

Geochemical characteristics of whole rock samples collected from footwall rocks at Tizapa and their stratigraphic equivalents outside of the mine area document changes in chemistry related to alteration. As described above, immobile element ratios (Fig. 9a) are similar for samples collected from footwall sericite-pyrite-quartz and chlorite-pyrite alteration zones at Tizapa and their least-altered stratigraphic equivalents. However, footwall rocks at Tizapa (both chlorite-pyrite and sericite-pyrite zones) contain significantly lower Na_2O and CaO concentrations and higher MgO, K_2O, and Fe_2O_3 concentrations than least altered samples (Table 1; Fig. 9b). These patterns are typical of alteration zones in volcanic rocks beneath Kuroko-type massive sulphide deposits in Japan (Date et al., 1983).

STRUCTURAL GEOLOGY

Four main periods of deformation can be docu-

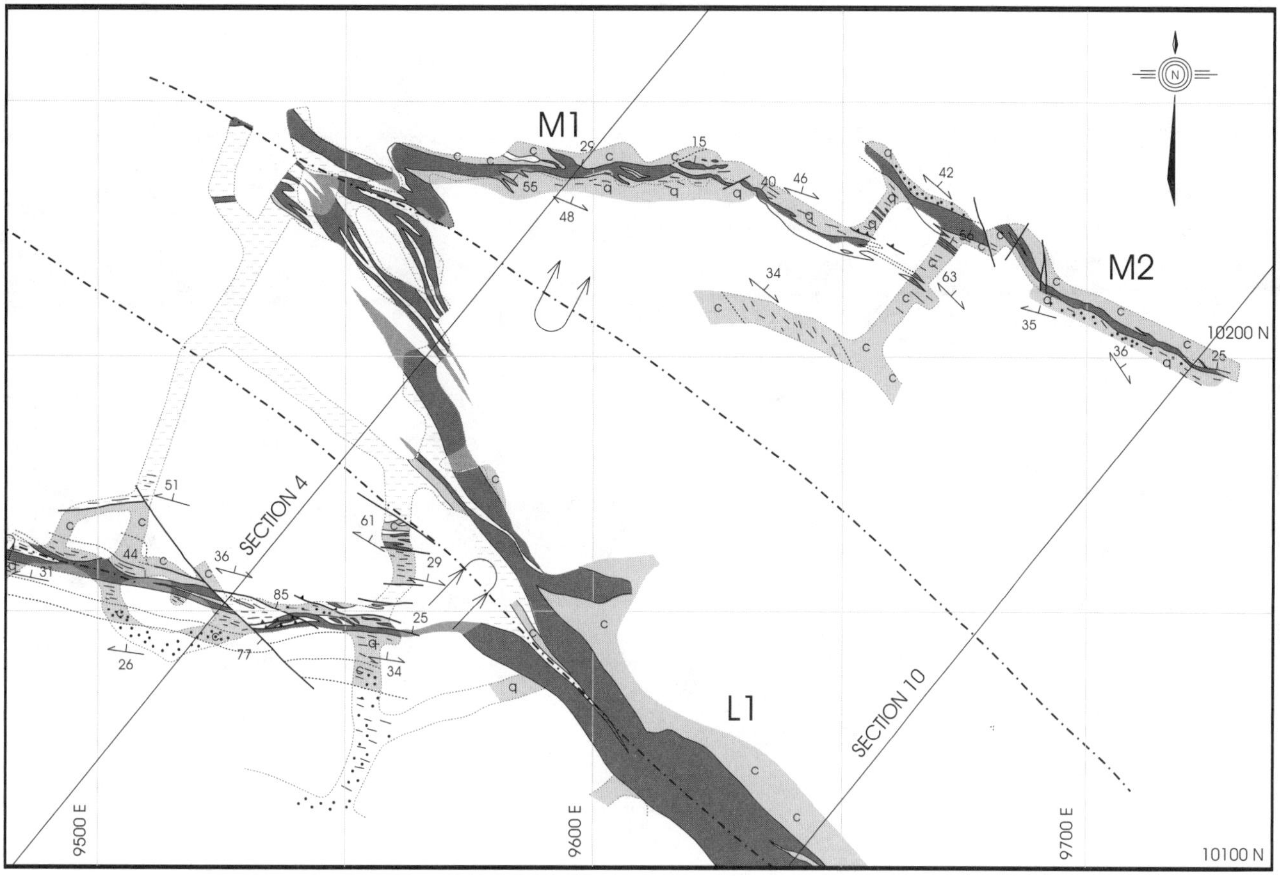

mented at the Tizapa deposit:

i) D1 development of penetrative foliation (S1), which is preserved only locally due to overprinting by later deformation events;
ii) D2 west-vergent folding, thrusting, and penetrative strain, which formed the dominant structures controlling the distribution of stratigraphic units and ore lenses at Tizapa;
iii) D3 folding about a regional west-trending anticline, accompanied by formation of west-trending crenulations; and
iv) D4 brittle faulting.

Possible faults of (pre-D1) synvolcanic origin, which may have localized mineralization and thus could serve as a guide to exploration, are suggested by patterns in metal zoning patterns within the Tizapa ore body (see below). If these structures existed, they are obscured by penetrative deformation.

D1 deformation

The earliest recognizable deformation at Tizapa is recorded as a locally preserved planar penetrative foliation (S1). No megascopic D1 structures are recognized in the Tizapa area; if such structures existed, they have been structurally overprinted to the extent that they are not distinguishable from D2 structures. S1 foliation is defined by penetrative micaceous folia, preserved in lithons between spaced S2 foliation surfaces (Fig. 8), and is syn-metamorphic. It is only detectable in about half of the Tizapa area, and elsewhere is transposed into S2 foliation. S1 surfaces dip moderately to steeply to the northeast; where both S1

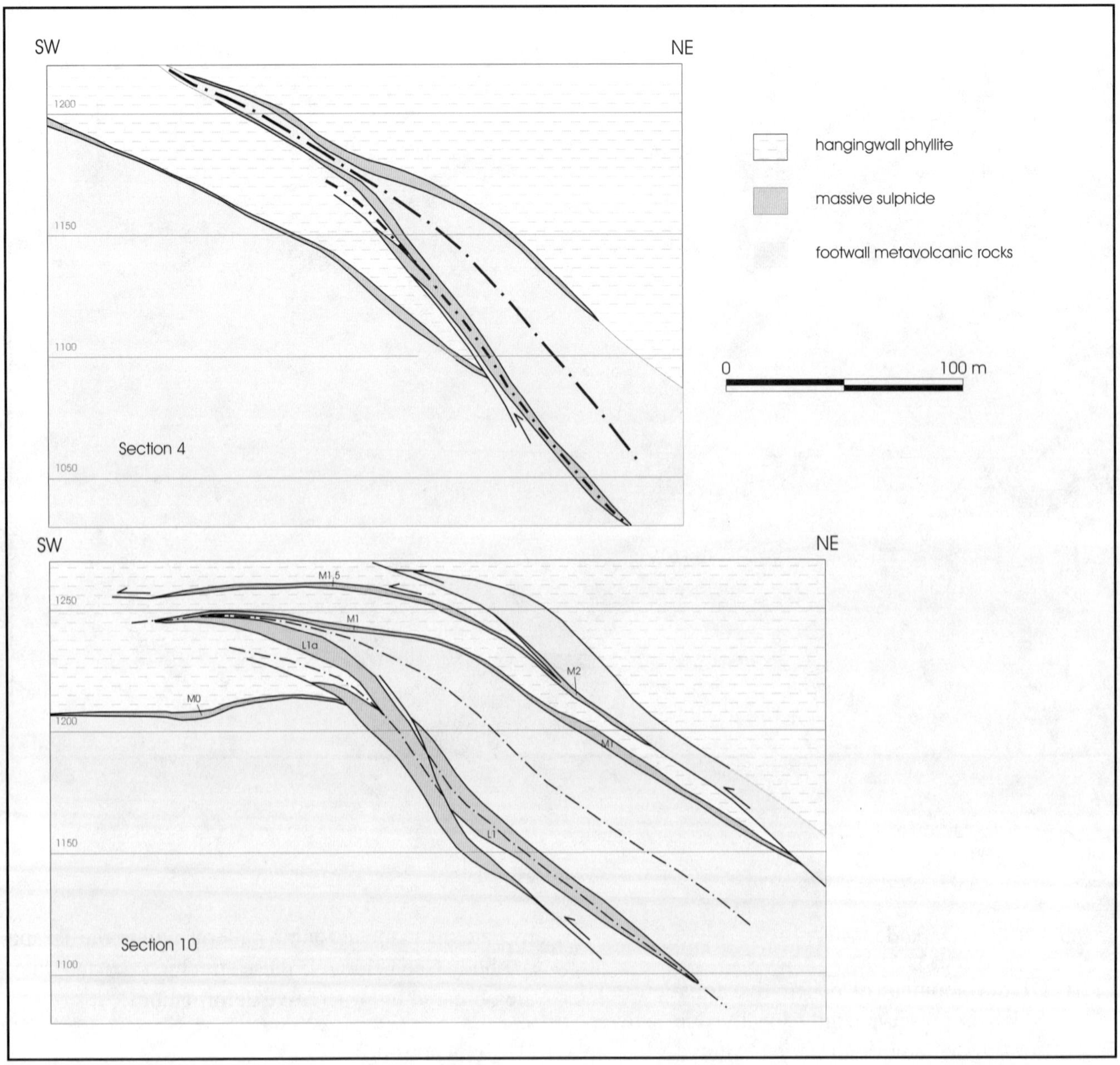

Figure 11. Simplified cross sections through the Tizapa mine oriented N40E, illustrating the distribution of orebodies and the effects of west verging folding and imbricate thrust faulting. Section lines on figure 10.

and S2 fabrics are visible S1 always has steeper dips than S2.

D2 deformation

D2 structures provide the dominant control on the geometry and distribution of lithologic units and ore lenses at Tizapa. Structures formed during D2 range from grain-scale cleavage fabrics, to map-scale, westerly-vergent tight to isoclinal recumbent folds and thrust faults (Fig. 17).

S2, L2 fabrics

D2 fabric elements include a penetrative to spaced S2 cleavage, which locally contains an L2 mineral elongation lineation. S2 is the dominant foliation in most outcrops, and provides the primary surface

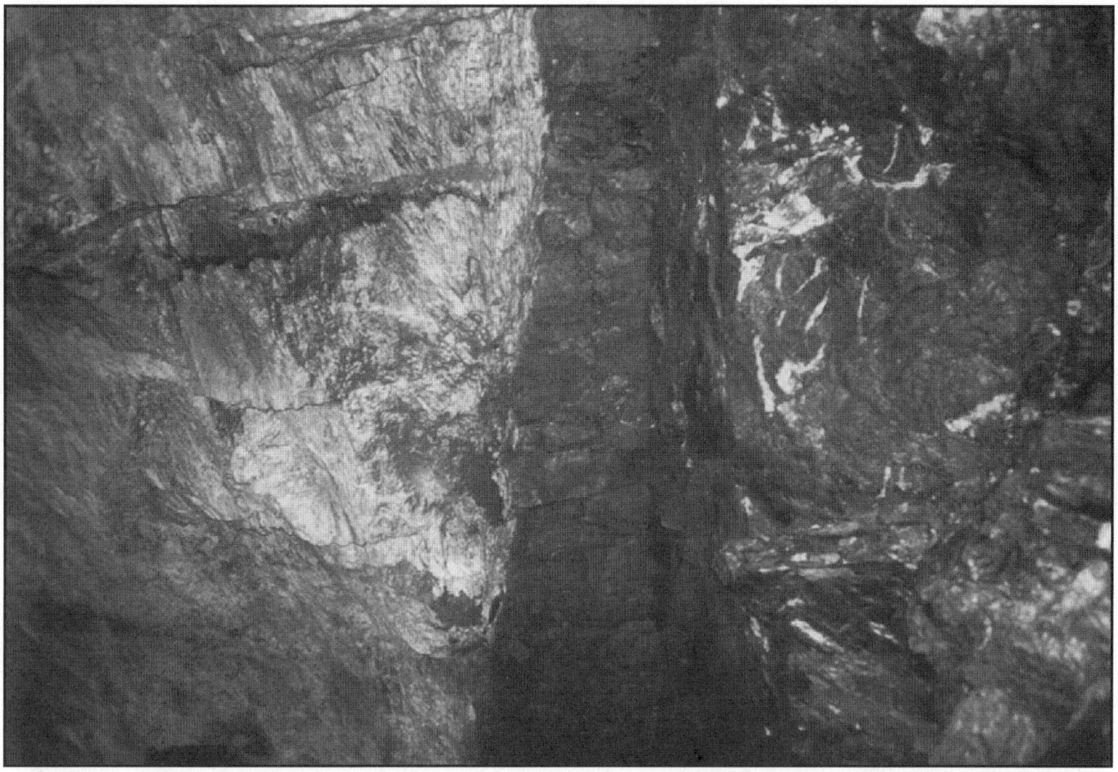

Figure 12. Sulphide ore (centre) at the contact between pale grey, sericite phyllite containing pyrite stringers (left) and carbonaceous, dark grey phyllite (right, with quartz veinlets); M0 orebody, 1154 level, Tizapa mine.

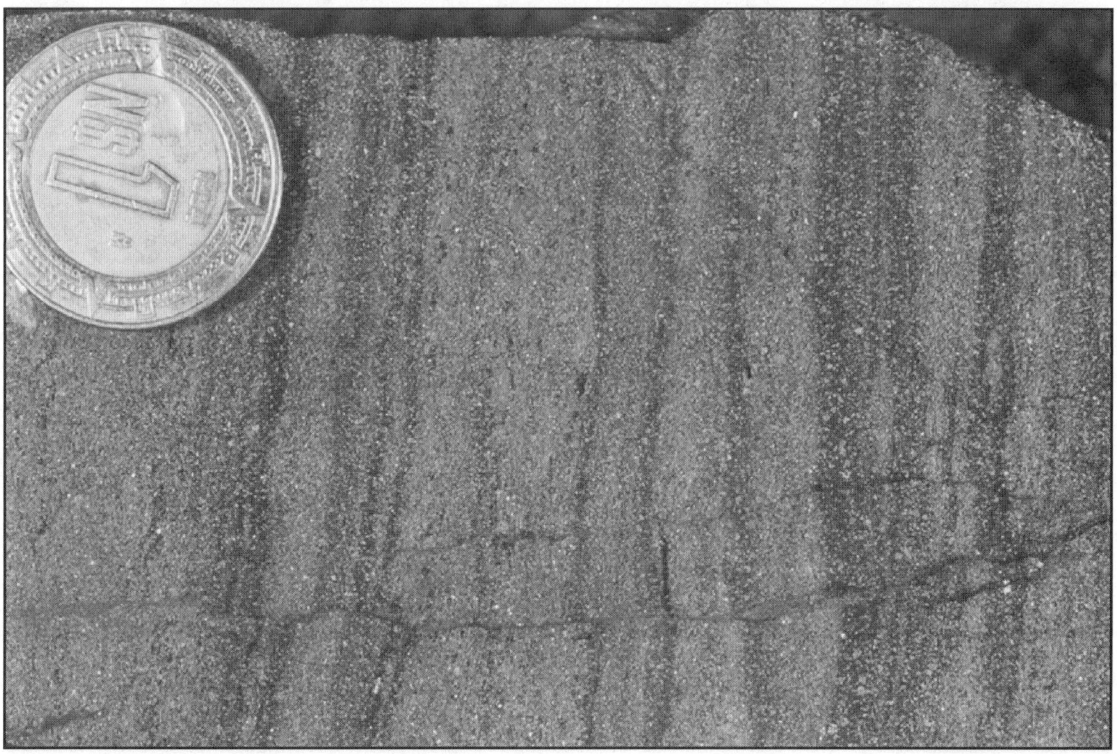

Figure 13. Typical ore, M2 orebody, 1259 level, Tizapa. The ore is composed of pyrite with bands of sphalerite + galena (dark grey). The coin is 2.1 cm in diameter.

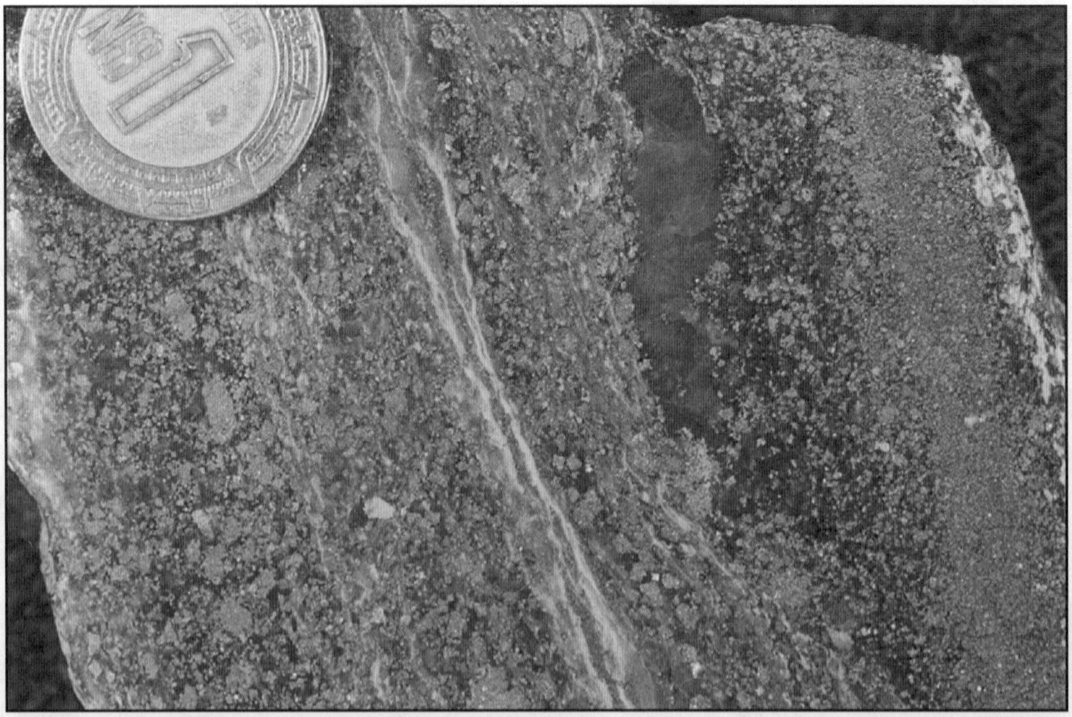

Figure 14. Banded pyrite-sericite from the base of the M0 orebody, 1100 level, Tizapa Mine. Pervasively disseminated pyrite occurs in a sericite-quartz matrix. The fine-grained sulphide band at right is the base of the M0 orebody. The coin is 2.1 cm in diametre.

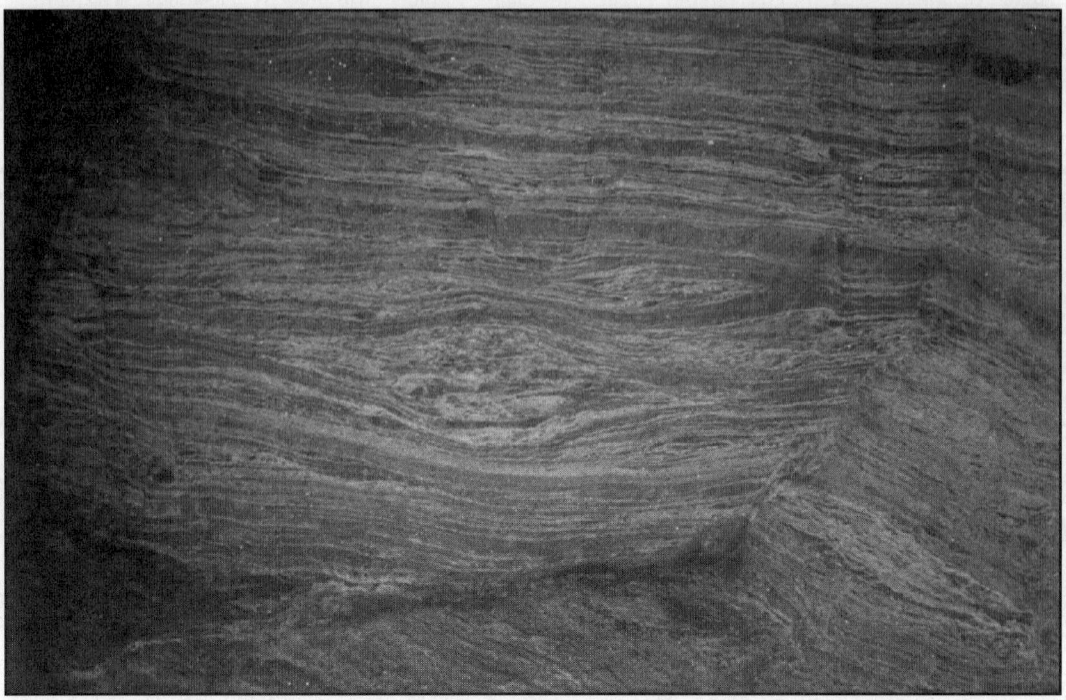

Figure 15. Pyrite bands in the footwall of the M0 orebody, 1154 level east, Tizapa. Bands of pyrite occur in sericite-quartz-pyrite schist approximately 1 m below ore. The pyrite bands are locally folded and may connect along strike; they may represent pyrite veinlets that are transposed into S2. Note the back-rotated foliation segments defined by oblique pyrite bends in the centre of the photograph. These suggest that a component of top to the west non-coaxial strain was accommodated on the S2 foliation. View to the south; width of view approximately 2 m.

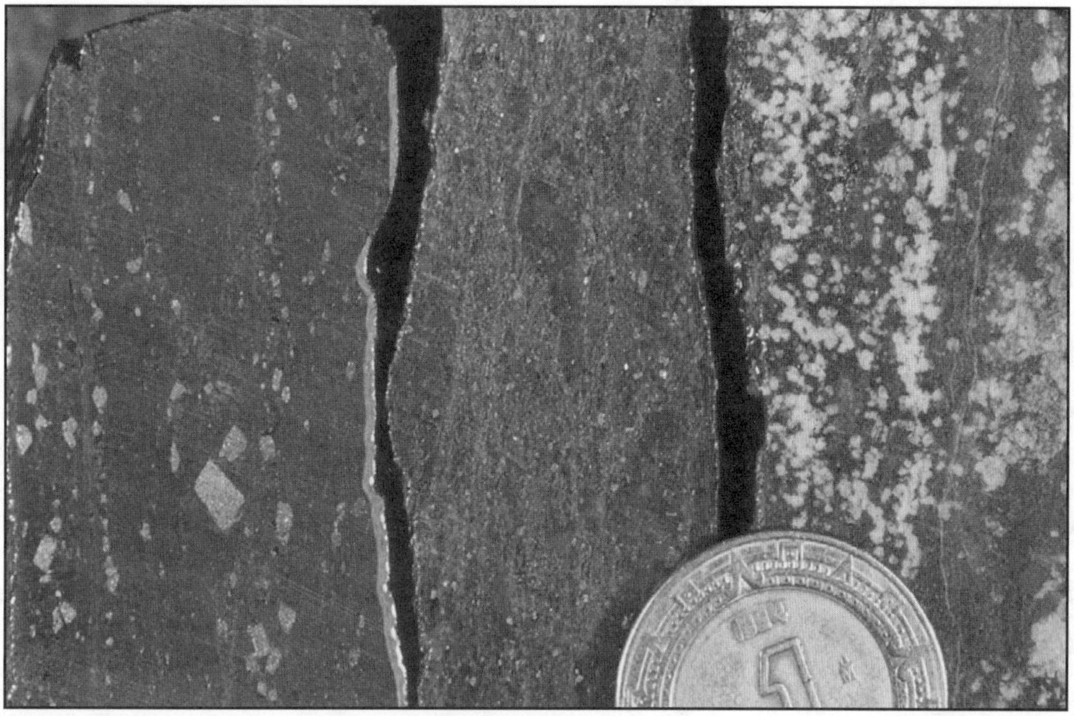

Figure 16. Representative samples of chlorite-pyrite phyllite in the altered footwall to the M0 (left and right) and M2 orebodies (centre). The samples were collected 5 to 20 m stratigraphically below the ore. Disseminated pyrite (left and centre samples) and Fe-carbonate + pyrite (right sample) occur in a chlorite matrix.

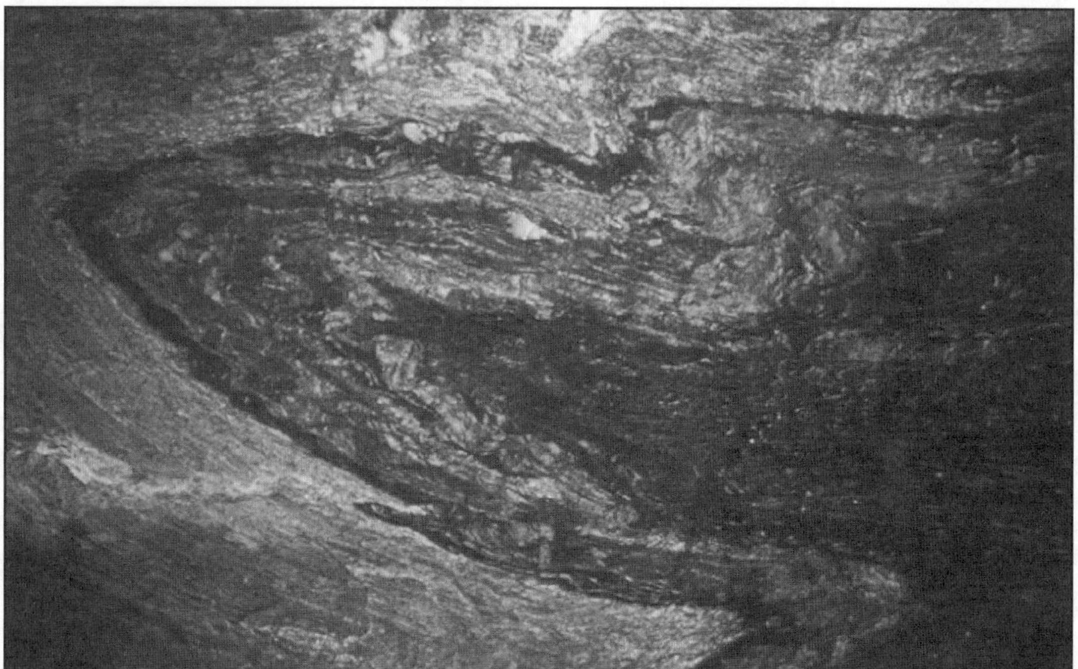

Figure 17. Recumbent D2 syncline in folded carbonaceous phyllite and sericite schist at the junction between the M0 and L1 orebodies. S2 is axial planar to the fold. Sulphide lenses up to 0.2 m thick occur locally along the contact here. View to the south; field of view is approximately 2.5 m.

along which rocks weather and exfoliate. It varies from a penetrative grain-orientation fabric defined by feldspar, quartz, and micas, to a spaced cleavage defined by planar concentrations of sericite or chlorite. S2 dips moderately to the northeast in most of the mine area, and to the southwest on the south side of the Falla Riolita due to D3 folding (Fig. 3).

Many areas show weak, top to the west S2 fabric asymmetry defined by numerous microscopic and mesoscopic indicators: 1) quartz pressure shadows mantling plagioclase porphyroclasts commonly have asymmetric forms and curved fibre growth. 2) Long axes of dynamically recrystallized quartz grains are inclined slightly to the S2 fabric. 3) Asymmetric shear bands cut shallowly across S2. 4) Long axes of feldspar megacrysts within the augen gneiss are inclined slightly to the surrounding S2 foliation. 5) Within highly strained parts of the footwall alteration zones, small asymmetric lenses containing back-rotated S2 are common (Fig. 15, 18). 6) Narrow, brittle-ductile shear zones that commonly deform layering contain internal fabric geometry indicating westerly-directed asymmetry.

An L2 mineral elongation lineation is variably developed in the Tizapa area, with its strongest expression in the augen gneiss unit. L2 plunges shallowly to moderately to the east or west, and is most intense in those areas with the strongest S2 foliation.

Massive sulphide lenses in the Tizapa mine are stacked vertically and in some instances overturned by D2 tight to isoclinal, west-vergent recumbent folds, faulted recumbent folds, and thrust sheets (Fig. 11). Structural and stratigraphic criteria used to define these map-scale structures in the mine include: 1) secondary structural indicators, such as parasitic fold geometry, fault cut-offs of stratigraphic layering, and cleavage/bedding angular relationships; 2) stratigraphic repetition, in particular the relative positions of the metavolcanic footwall and the carbonaceous phyllite hangingwall sequences; and 3) footwall alteration zoning patterns.

Megascopic D2 structures display a continuum of styles ranging from recumbent folds with relatively intact hinges, to thrust-faulted folds, to stacked thrust sheets. Intact folds include a major anticlinal closure between ore bodies L1 and M1 (Fig. 11), and smaller scale folds of the M0 ore body in the western part of the mine (Fig. 10). A megascopic fold closure bisects the L1 ore body, and the overturned L1 fold limb is structurally thickened, a pattern common in mesoscopic asymmetric folds both in the mine and on surface (Fig. 10). Second order folds of the major fold limbs produce local thickened north-plunging ore shoots. The M0 ore lens contains one such ore shoot, which can be traced through the vertical extent of the mine and has been intersected in exploration drill holes at deeper levels several hundred metres to the north. Megascopic fold axes and fault cut-off lines plunge shallowly (10 - 20°) towards the north-northwest, parallel to the measured axes of early mesoscopic folds.

Thrust sheets and faulted folds are most common at higher levels within the mine. For example, the M2 ore body occurs on an overturned synclinal fold limb, thrust westerly over the corresponding upright limb represented by ore bodies M1.5 and M1 (Fig. 11). Thrust faults also displace the upper limb of ore lens L1 from its inferred M0 continuation, and stack M1.5 over the hangingwall of M1 (Fig. 11). Thrust faults in the mine commonly follow flats along ore lenses, and ramp across hangingwall and footwall units. Structural imbrication and thickening of ore lenses by the thrust faults can have several geometric forms, depending on the magnitude of fault displacement and whether flat portions follow the hangingwall or footwall contacts of ore lenses. These include slivers of phyllite and/or schist completely enclosed within ore lenses; splays off of the primary ore lenses into either hangingwall or footwall rocks; and small isolated sulphide pods in either hangingwall or footwall. In addition, boudinage of massive sulphide layers commonly results in large variations in ore lens thickness over short distances (Fig. 19).

Post-D2 deformation

D3 folds

Broad, west-trending D3 folds deform D1 and D2 fabrics in the Tizapa mine area. The orientation of S2 bends gradually from northeast dipping north of the Falla Riolita, to southwest-dipping to the south of the fault, defining a major shallowly west-northwest

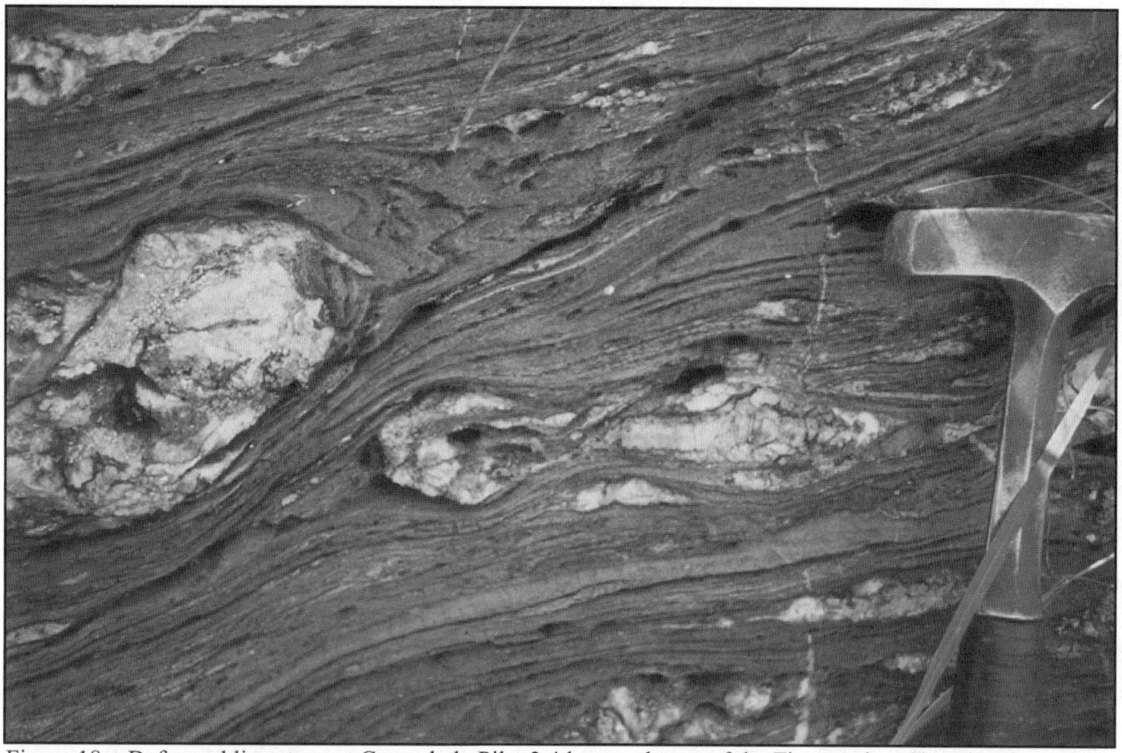

Figure 18. Deformed limestone at Cerro de la Pila, 2.4 km southwest of the Tizapa mine. Shear bands and back-rotation of intervening segments occur around a deformed quartz vein, and suggest a component of non-coaxial, westerly-directed strain on the dominant S2 foliation. View to the north.

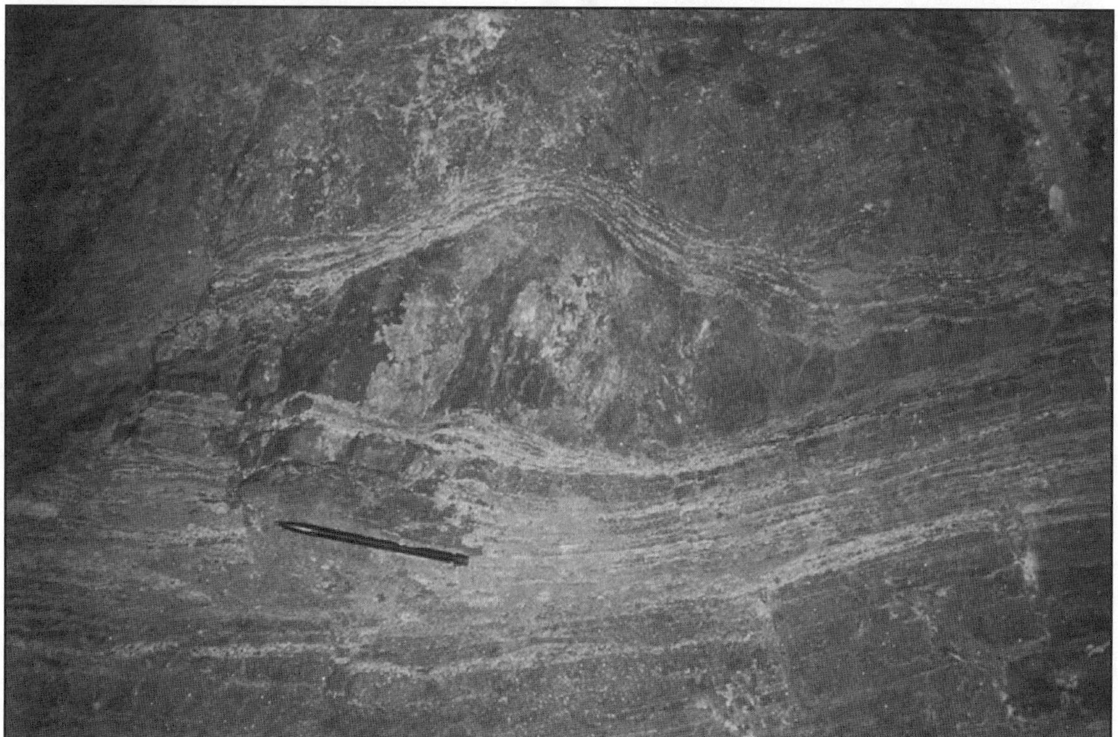

Figure 19. Boudinage of sulphide lenses, M0 orebody, 1154 level, Tizapa. Boudinage here affects a minor sulphide lens in the footwall of the main M0 orebody (above). Banded pyrite-sericite alteration occurs below. Field of view is approximately 1 m.

plunging D3 anticline subparallel to and just south of the fault.

Crenulations of S2 foliation planes are common. Crenulations plunge shallowly to the northeast or southeast, and both orientations may be present in a single outcrop. Associated crenulation cleavage is rare due to the low strain associated with the crenulation event. The parallelism between many crenulation lineations and D3 fold hinges suggest formation during D3 deformation.

D4 Faults

D4 faults in the Tizapa mine area include the west-striking Falla Riolita, numerous smaller southwest-dipping faults, and minor sub-horizontal faults.

Falla Riolita

The Falla Riolita strikes east-west across the entire Tizapa mine area, and forms the southern limit to known mineralization. It has been traced for over 5 km east of the mine area. Near the mine, the fault separates the mine sequence on the north from stratigraphically lower granitic schist/gneiss and overlying phyllites and schists on the south. It is intruded by a flow banded, commonly brecciated, rhyolite dyke for most of its known length. Rhyolite-cemented breccias along the dyke margins suggests synchronous fault movement and dyke emplacement. The Falla Riolita strikes westerly and dips 60°-75° northward in the western part of the Tizapa area. To the east, within an anomalously wide zone of rhyolite breccia, the fault splays into an east-west segment and a subvertical segment striking 070°.

Fault surfaces lack definite kinematic indicators. Stratigraphic distribution patterns can be accommodated by dip-slip displacement of 800 m (normal, north-side-up), strike-slip displacement of 1500 m (dextral), or oblique displacement.

Southwest-dipping faults: Falla Salas fault system

A system of northwest-striking, southwest-dipping faults, including the Falla Salas in the mine, offsets massive sulphide bodies with apparent normal displacement. Displacement magnitude increases to the southeast. Numerous minor parallel faults with centimetres to several metres of apparent normal displacement define this fault system underground (Fig. 10), and equivalent faults are present in surface outcrops. Narrow rhyolite dykes intrude these structures. These faults may be conjugate to, and branch from, the Falla Riolita (Fig. 4).

Flat Faults

Faults with subhorizontal to shallow westward dips occur in surface outcrops in several areas, and in the mine cut and displace lower portions of the L1 ore lens for up to several tens of metres. Most flat faults on the surface have upper plate displacements of several centimetres to the south. Foliation drag adjacent to the faults and oblique internal fault gouge fabrics are compatible with southerly-southwesterly displacements of upper plate rocks.

Metal zoning

Exploration and definition drilling at the Tizapa deposit provide several hundred assayed drill hole intersections that can be used to evaluate metal zoning within the orebodies. The structural imbrication of the sulphide lenses during D2 complicates metal distribution, and requires that major faults and folds in the mine be palinspastically restored to establish zoning. To remove the influence of D2 faulting and folding from the zoning patterns, sections through the mine area oriented N40E, or nearly perpendicular to fold axes and fault cut-off lines, were structurally interpreted and fault/fold displacements were balanced within sections and correlated between successive sections using line length perpendicular to transport direction. Deformation phases other than D2 are not expressed as mine-scale structures deforming the ore lenses. Because quantitative strain markers are unavailable, bulk strain is not restored in the sections. Drill hole ore intersections were assigned to specific ore bodies using the interpreted cross sections as a guide. Assay values were averaged for each ore body intersection. Because most ore intersections comprise only a few assay intervals, it is not possible to evaluate vertical zoning. Values for Au, Ag, Pb, Zn, and Cu, and several metal ratios were plotted at the midpoint of each ore lens intersection. These intersection midpoints and their assigned metal values were then restored in three dimensions by removing the fault displacements and restoring the folds shown in the

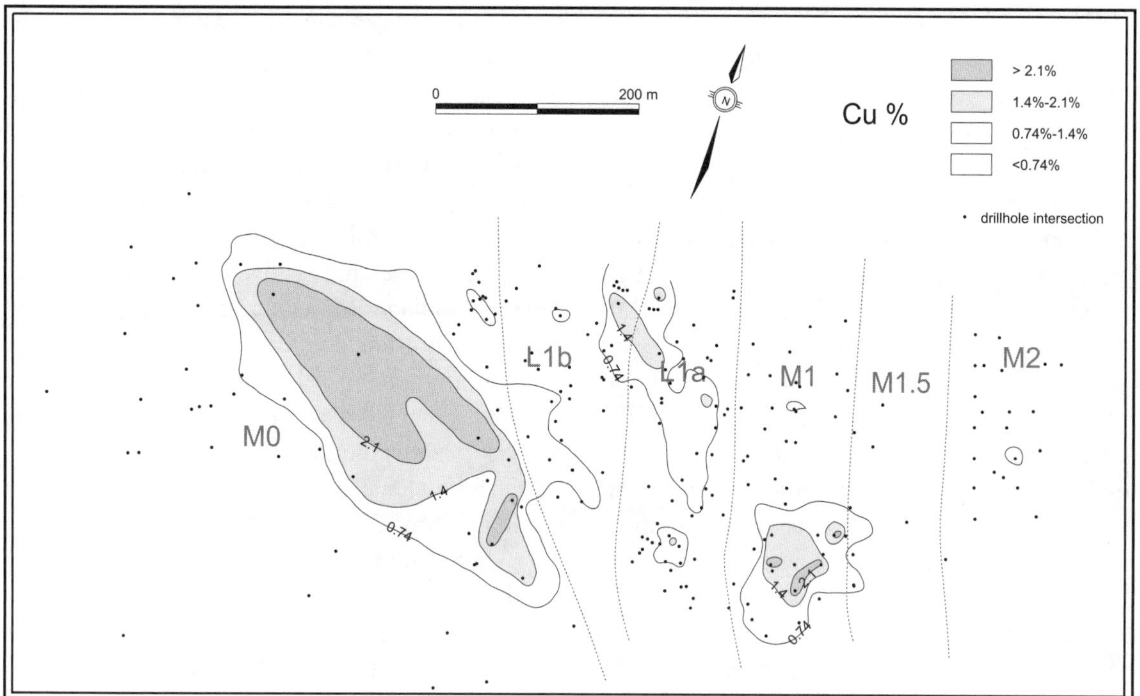

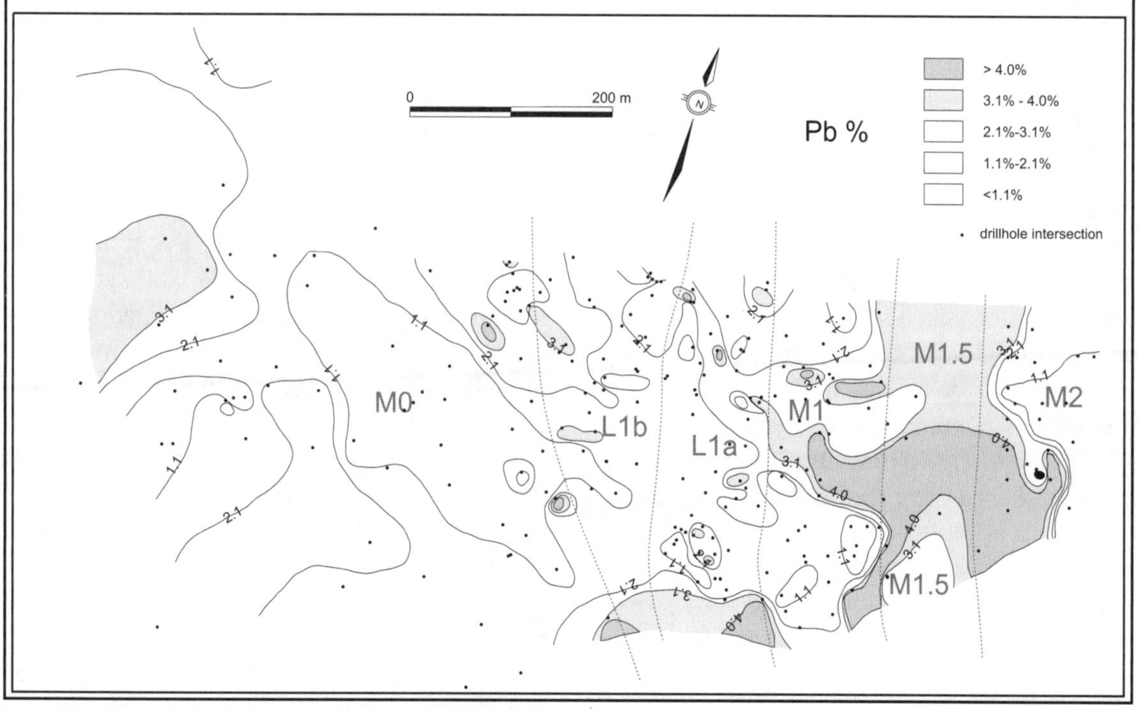

Figure 20. Plan view of contoured Cu and Pb diamond drill hole grades in the Tizapa orebodies in pre-deformational relative position, based on palinspastic restoration of the mineralized horizon. Note the zones of enriched Cu content in the M0, L1 and M1 orebodies (top). These correspond with the thickest areas of sericite-pyrite footwall alteration, and may represent feeder zones. Pb enrichment exhibits the opposite pattern (bottom), and is similar to the distribution patterns of Zn and Ag. The limits of contouring to the east, north, and west represent the limits of data, and not the limits of the orebody.

interpreted cross sections.

Most patterns of metal distribution show good continuity between ore bodies in their restored positions. Plots of Cu and Pb (Fig. 20) show the clearest zoning patterns, with several high Cu areas defined. The largest is a northwesterly-elongate zone of high values crossing ore body M0, with its eastern end extending onto the southern parts of ore bodies L1a and L1b. Smaller areas of high Cu on ore body M0 and the northern parts of ore bodies L1a and L1b are aligned in a northwesterly direction, possibly defining a second linear high (Fig. 20). Areas of highest Cu correspond with areas of thickest footwall alteration and abundant pyrite bands with variable Cu-content that locally range up to 5 % Cu over several metres, but are oblique to sulphide thickness trends. This footwall alteration may be deformed stockwork feeders to the ore bodies.

Plots of both Pb and Zn show an inverse correlation with Cu values. The northwesterly high-Cu trend in ore body M0, and the high-Cu areas on the southern part of ore body M1 and eastern part of ore body M2 all are low in Pb and Zn (Fig. 20). However, the smaller high-Cu anomalies on northern parts of ore bodies L1a and L1b contain erratic Pb and Zn values, and there is no northwesterly pattern of zoning here as suggested by the Cu plots. Au and Ag show patterns of distribution similar to Pb. The northwesterly high-Cu area of ore body M0 is low in Pb, Au and Ag, but is surrounded by a fringe of high values of these elements.

The metal zoning patterns likely represent primary zonation rather than deformation-induced mass redistribution because 1) the linear Cu+Pb high is oblique to mesoscopic structural fabric elements, 2) the Cu+Pb high trends approximately 30° west of the structurally thickened ore zones related to D2 folds, and 3) there is a strong spatial relationship between areas with high Cu+Pb values and thick footwall alteration zones. However, the shape and geometry of the primary zoning patterns were modified by subsequent penetrative strain events.

Discussion and conclusions

The Tizapa massive sulphide deposits occur at the contact between Late Jurassic to Early Cretaceous intermediate to felsic volcanic rocks of the Teloloapan volcanic assemblage and calcareous carbonaceous mudstones at the base of the Middle Cretaceous Amatapec Formation limestone. The volcanic rocks are bimodal and consist of a lower, andesitic plagioclase porphyritic sequence that is locally overlain by a felsic tuff unit of highly variable thickness (Fig. 21). Sulphide mineralization at Tizapa and Esmeralda is spatially associated with the felsic tuff at the top of the assemblage. Mineralization at Esmeralda is interlayered with felsic volcanic units that occur at a similar stratigraphic level as the Tizapa deposit, although the thicker felsic volcanic rocks here suggest that the felsic volcanism may have continued longer (Fig. 21). The Esmeralda deposit may have been closer to a felsic volcanic centre.

The stratigraphic position and setting of the Tizapa and Esmeralda deposits is similar to other deposits in the region, such as Campo Morado, Rey de Plata and the Tizapa-Azulaquez district, all of which occur within or above a felsic volcanic unit that overlies an andesitic volcanic sequence (Oliver et al., 2000; Rhys et al., 2000, Miranda-Gasca, 1995). The mid-Cretaceous age of fossils in the overlying Amatapec Formation at Tizapa is consistent with Albian fossils obtained from carbonate units stratigraphically above these other deposits, and with the Early Cretaceous age obtained from volcanic units and intrusions associated with deposits at Campo Morado and Azulaquez-Tlanilpa (Oliver et al., 2000; Rhys et al., 2000).

The style and zoning of alteration at Tizapa (inner sericite and outer chlorite), combined with the presence of Cu-rich pyrite stockwork zones, associated bimodal andesitic-rhyolitic volcanic sequence, and metal content of the sulphide bodies (Zn +Pb >> Cu) are typical of Kuroko-type volcanogenic massive sulphide deposits. Alteration beneath orebodies at Tizapa is characterized by banded and disseminated pyrite in (i) intensely sericitized phyllitic felsite immediately beneath the sulphide horizon, and (ii) underlying intense chlorite alteration of andesitic metavolcanic rocks that extends up to 50 m beneath the ore. Na_2O and CaO are depleted and Fe_2O_3 is enriched in these altered zones when compared with stratigraphically equivalent least-altered samples from the region. Pyrite bands probably represent transposed pyrite veins that originally formed stockworks beneath the

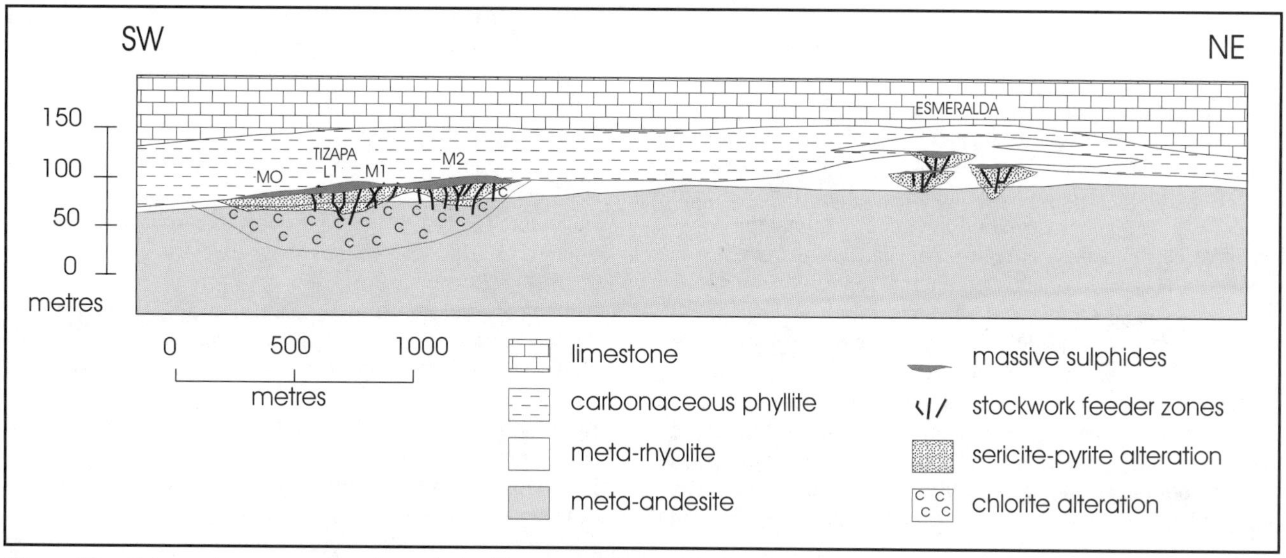

Figure 21. Schematic cross section through the Tizapa and Esmeralda deposits prior to penetrative deformation. Note the position of the orebodies at the top of the volcanic pile, associated footwall alteration, and the variation in the thickness of the felsic volcanic unit along strike.

ore. Alteration is thickest and pyrite banding best developed under Cu-rich areas of the orebodies in M0 and M2. The banded pyrite is Cu-rich in these areas and can contain several percent Cu. Footwall alteration associated with sulphide mineralization in the area can be distinguished from regional metamorphic affects by: (i) the presence of disseminated pyrite ± chalcopyrite, (ii) extremely sericite-rich or chlorite-rich schists lacking primary textures, (iii) sericite schists containing possible cordierite, and (iv) elevated Fe_2O_3 and low NaO + CaO contents in volcanic rocks.

Underground and surface mapping and interpretation of drill sections at Tizapa indicate that the main massive sulphide lenses were an originally continuous horizon that was subsequently deformed into a thrust-disrupted, west-verging, north-plunging tight recumbent D2 syncline/anticline pair. North-northwest plunging thickened ore shoots results from this structural thickening, either coinciding with overturned limbs or parasitic second order folds, rather than primary distribution patterns.

Patterns of metal zoning within the Tizapa ore bodies, when effects of D2 faults and folds are removed, show continuity across ore bodies, supporting their formation as a single continuous sulphide layer. Three areas enriched in Cu that overlie anomalously thick zones of footwall alteration may represent parts of the ore body closest to the feeder system. Northwest trends of these Cu-enriched zones are oblique to the more northerly-trending zones of D2 structural thickening, and may reflect the original geometry of the underlying structurally controlled feeder systems.

ACKNOWLEDGEMENTS

The authors are grateful to Servicios Industriales Peñoles for permission to publish this manuscript, and to the geology staff at the Tizapa mine for their help and geological discussions during the fieldwork.

REFERENCES

Barrett, T.J. and MacLean, W.H., 1999. Volcanic sequences, lithogeochemistry and hydrothermal alteration in some bimodal volcanic-associated massive sulphide systems. Reviews in Economic Geology, Volume 8, pp. 101-132.

Campa, M.F. and Coney, P.J. 1983. Tectono-stratigraphic terranes and mineral resource distribution in Mexico. Canadian Journal of Earth Sciences, Volume 20, pp. 1040-1051.

Date, J., Watanabe, Y. and Saeli, Y., 1983. Zonal alteration around the Fukazawa Kuroko deposits, Akita Prefecture, Japan. Economic Geology Monograph 5, pp. 365-386.

Giles, D.A. and Garcia, J.F. 2000. VMS orebodies in Mexico: the producing mines. This volume.

Heredia-Barragán, M.A. and Garcia-Fons, R.J. 1989. Distribución de yacimientos vulcanogénicos en la provincia norte de Guerrero - suroccidente del Estado de México. XVIII Convención Nacional AAIMMGM, Memorias técnicas, pp. 81-99.

Jansma, P.E. and Lang, H.R. 1997. The Arcelia graben: New evidence for Oligocene Basin and Range extension in southern Mexico. Geology, 25, pp. 455-458.

Metal Mining Agency of Japan, Japan International Cooperation Agency, 1989. Informe de la exploracion cooperativa de mineral en la region Arcelia, Estados Unidos de Mexico, (fase II). unpublished internal report.

Metal Mining Agency of Japan, Japan International Cooperation Agency, 1991. Informe de la exploracion cooperativa de mineral en la region Arcelia, Estados Unidos de Mexico, (fase IV). 74 pages, unpublished internal report.

Metal Mining Agency of Japan, Japan International Cooperation Agency, 1992. Informe del estudio fundamental en colaboration para la explotacion de los recursos, region de Tejupilco, Los Estados Unidos de Mexico, unpublished internal report.

Metal Mining Agency of Japan, Japan International Cooperation Agency, 1993. Informe de la exploracion cooperativa de mineral en la region Tejupilco, Estados Unidos Mexicanos (fase II). 260 pages, unpublished internal report.

Metal Mining Agency of Japan, Japan International Cooperation Agency, 1994A. Informe de la exploracion cooperativa de mineral en la region Tejupilco, Estados Unidos Mexicanos (fase III). 78 pages, unpublished internal report.

Metal Mining Agency of Japan, Japan International Cooperation Agency, 1994B. Informe de la exploracion cooperativa de mineral en la region Tejupilco, Estados Unidos Mexicanos (Sumario). 91 pages, unpublished internal report.

Metal Mining Agency of Japan, Japan International Cooperation Agency, 1994C. Reporte sobre la geologia y depositos minerales en la region Tejupilco, Estados Unidos Mexicanos. 44 pages, unpublished internal report.

Miranda-Gasca, M.A. 1995. The volcanogenic massive sulfide and sedimentary exhalative deposits of the Guerrero Terrane, Mexico. Ph.D. thesis, The University of Arizona, Tucson, Arizona.

Monod, O. and Busnardo, R., 1993. A late Albanian ammonite fauna in the carbonate cover of the Teloloapan arc volcanics, Guerrero, Mexico. in Proceedings of the first Circum-Pacific and Circum-Atlantic Terrane Conference, Guanajuao, Mexico, Universidad Nacional Autonoma de Mexico, pp. 90-91.

Monod, O., Faure, M., Salinas, J. C., and Sabanero, H. 1993. What is the Guerrero Terrane made of? In Proceedings of the first Circum-Pacific and Circum-Atlantic Terrane Conference, Guanajuao, Mexico, Universidad Nacional Autonoma de Mexico, p. 92.

Monroy-Fernandez, M.G. and Aragon-Pina, A., 1994. Estudio de caracterization del estado mineralogico del oro en colas de flotacion del mineral piritoso de Tizapa, Estados Unidos de Mexico. Servicios Industriales Penoles, S.A. de C.V., unpublished internal report.

Noguez, A., Flores, M., and Toscano, E., 1991. Zacualpan Mining District, State of Mexico. In Salas, G.P., editor, Economic Geology, Mexico. Boulder, Colorado, Geological Society of America, The Geology of North America, P-3, pp. 369-372.

Oliver, J., Payne, J., Kilby, D., Rebagliati, M., and Cluff, R., 2000. Precious metal-rich volcanic-associated massive sulphide deposits of Campo Morado, Guerrero, Mexico. This volume.

Parga-Perez. J. J., 1981. Geologia del area de Tizapa, Municipio de Zacazonapan, Mexico (M.Sc. thesis). Mexico D.F., Universidad Nacional Autonoma de Mexico, Facultad des Ciencas (Geologia), 135 p.

Parga-Perez. J. J. and Rodriguez-Salinas. J. J., 1991. Geology of the Tizapa Ag, Zn, Pb, Cu, Cd, and Au massive polymetallic sulphides, Zacazonapan, Mexico. In Salas, G.P., editor, Economic Geology, Mexico. Boulder, Colorado, Geological Society of America, The Geology of North America, Volume P-3, pp. 373-378.

Parga-Perez. J. J., Rodriguez-Salinas. J. J., Obregon-Ramos, E., and Romo-Vargas, E., 1984. Estudio Geologico-evaluativo del prospecto "La Esmeralda", Municipio de Temascaltepec, Estado de Mexico, Consejo de Recursos Minerales, 55 pages, unpublished internal report.

Rhys, D.A., Enns, S.G. and Ross, K.V. 2000. Geological setting of deformed VMS-type mineralisation in the Azulaquez-Tlanilpa area, northern Guerrero State, México. This volume.

Salinas-Prieto, J. C., Monod, O., and Faure, M., 1993. Deformacion ductil progresiva en el limite Oriental del Terreno Guerrero, soroeste de Mexico. in Proceedings of the first Circum-Pacific and Circum-Atlantic Terrane Conference, Guanajuao, Mexico, Universidad Nacional Autonoma de Mexico, pp. 130-132.

Sedlock, R.L., Ortega-Gutierrez, F., and Speed, R.C., 1993. Tectonostratigraphic terranes and tectonic evolution of Mexico. Geological Society of America, Special Paper 278, 142 pages.

Tolson, G., 1990. Structural development and tectonic evolution of the Santa Rosa area, SW state of Mexico, Mexico. Geological Society of America, Abstacts with programs, Volume 22, p. A328.

Winchester, J.A. and Floyd P.A. 1977. Geochemical discrimination of different magma series and their differentiation products using immobile elements. Chemical Geology, 20, pp. 1609-1622.

GEOLOGICAL SETTING OF DEFORMED VMS-TYPE MINERALIZATION IN THE AZULAQUEZ-TLANILPA AREA, NORTHERN GUERRERO STATE, MEXICO

DAVID A. RHYS[1], STEVE G. ENNS[2], KATHERINA V. ROSS[1]
1. Panterra Geoservices Inc., 14180 Greencrest Drive, Surrey, B.C., Canada V4P 1L9
2. 1696 Davenport Place, North Vancouver, B.C., Canada V7J 1N5

ABSTRACT

The Azulaquez-Tlanilpa area is one of four VMS districts in the Teloloapan subterrane, an Upper Jurassic to Lower Cretaceous calc-alkaline volcanic arc within the Guerrero Terrane in southern Mexico. Lithologies in the area comprise a bimodal volcanic sequence that is interbedded with marine sedimentary rocks. From the base upward, the stratigraphy consists of: a lower andesite flow and volcaniclastic sequence more than 400 m thick, a 20 to 130 m thick sequence of carbonaceous mudstone and limestone, a sequence of plagioclase-bearing felsic tuff with minor flows, more than 250 m thick, and an upper andesitic sequence of tuff and minor flows of unknown thickness. A synvolcanic diorite which cuts the lower andesitic and felsic sequences gave a U-Pb zircon age of 137 +/-1 Ma, providing a minimum Early Cretaceous age.

Upper Cretaceous-Lower Tertiary Laramide deformation produced recumbent folds and shallow dipping slaty cleavage in two events: (i) D1, associated with bedding parallel cleavage and east-verging folds, and (ii) D2, defined by recumbent, west-verging folds and foliation. Bedding parallel to discordant, late D2 shear zones, are localized in sedimentary rocks below the felsic tuff unit. Tertiary normal faults with a northwest-strike are widespread in the region.

Stratabound base metal sulphide mineralization comprises concordant lenses and disseminations that occur in carbonaceous mudstone and tuff at and near the base of the felsic tuff unit. The lenses are composed of tectonically laminated sphalerite - galena - pyrite - chalcopyrite – sulfosalts. Barite and chert may accompany the sulphides. Mineralization occurs in a series of four groups of showings that are exposed intermittently over a distance of 7 km. It is often transposed and entrained in shear zones, and may be tectonically displaced from its source. The mineralised bodies are elongate, parallel to the west-northwest trending D2 stretching lineation. Local zones of pyrite-chlorite-sericite alteration and silicification at a lower or similar stratigraphic position to the sulphide lenses may be footwall alteration. Quartz-sulphide breccia veins also occur within the region, but they post-date penetrative deformation and probably are genetically related to Tertiary normal faults.

The Azulaquez-Tlanilpa area shares several characteristics with other Early Cretaceous VMS districts in the Teloloapan subterrane. These include: (i) the occurrence of sulphide mineralization in carbonaceous sedimentary rocks which define a volcanic hiatus, (ii) an association with a felsic volcanic centre stratigraphically above andesitic volcanic rocks, and (iii) the intensity and style of overprinting deformation.

INTRODUCTION

The Azulaquez-Tlanilpa area, in north central Guerrero state, contains numerous stratabound base metal sulphide occurrences. The region is located 30 km west of the historic silver mining city of Taxco and 100 km southwest of Mexico City (Fig.1)

Silver mining activity in the study area may date back to Spanish occupation in the early 16th century (Holcapec, 1996). In the early 20th century, preceding the Mexican Revolution, and during the 1940's, limited production was obtained from small adits, shafts and pits at several showings. Consejo de Resources Minerales conducted reconnaissance exploration in the area between the early 1980's and 1994, during which time geological studies of some of the better-known showings were also made by Espinosa-Perea (1982) and Montes-Napoles (1984). Cominco Ltd. carried out geophysical surveys and drilled two holes on the Manto Rico prospect between 1976 and 1982 (Cominco Ltd., internal files).

Between 1995 and 1998 Valerie Gold Resources Ltd. and TVX Gold Inc. conducted base and precious metal exploration on their 208 square kilometre Mamatla Mineral Concession. More than 75 mineral occurrences were identified on the concession (Holcapek, 1996), the most significant being located between Azulaquez and Tlanilpa (Fig. 2). The exploration program consisted of soil sampling, prospecting, induced polarization and magnetometer surveys, airborne magnetometer-radiometric-electromagnetic surveys, geological mapping and diamond drilling of more than 140 holes. This paper is based largely on the geological mapping conducted by the authors during 1996 for Valerie Gold Resources Ltd. (Rhys and Ross, 1997; Enns and Findlay, 1997).

REGIONAL GEOLOGY

The study area (Fig. 1) is within the Teloloapan subterrane, a tectono-stratigraphic division of the Guerrero terrane (Campa and Coney, 1983). This subterrane is a calc-alkaline volcanic arc sequence that is composed of at least three lithostructural elements (Monod et al., 1993), which consist of: (i) Paleozoic or Triassic metavolcanic and metasedimentary rocks of the Tierra Caliente Complex and the Taxco schist that form the structural or stratigraphic basement in the region, (ii) Upper Jurassic to Lower Cretaceous andesitic to felsic volcanic and clastic rocks of the Teloloapan volcanic arc that unconformably or tectonically overlie the basement units, and (iii) Middle to Upper Cretaceous clastic rocks and limestone. The Teloloapan subterrane is bordered on the west by Cretaceous basalt and marine sedimentary rocks of the Arcelia subterrane. Lower to Middle Cretaceous carbonate rocks of the Morelos Formation to the east may interfinger with the Teloloapan arc rocks (Altamirano et al., 1979; Heredia-Barragán and Garcia-Fons, 1989). Lower Tertiary, felsic to intermediate volcanic and clastic rocks, as well as Neogene to Quaternary volcanic rocks of the Trans-Mexican volcanic belt unconformably overlie the deformed Mesozoic sequence (Sedlock et al., 1993).

Late Cretaceous to Early Tertiary shortening and greenschist facies metamorphism during the Laramide orogeny affected all Mesozoic rocks in the region. It occurred in at least two pulses, resulting in early east- and later west-vergent thrust faults and recumbent folds, and two generations of moderate to shallow dipping cleavage (Salinas-Prieto et al., 1993; Monod et al., 1993). Tertiary, north and northwest-striking normal faults affect rocks as young as Oligocene in the region, and locally form grabens that are filled with Neogene volcanic rocks (Jansma and Lang, 1997).

Two dominant styles of base metal mineralization occur in the Teloloapan subterrane. The first consists of Early Cretaceous, Kuroko-type volcanogenic Zn-Pb-Ag-Au massive sulphide deposits in four districts (Fig.1): (i) Tizapa-Santa Rosa, (ii) Azulaquez-Tlanilpa, (iii) Rey de Plata, and (iv) Campo Morado-Suriana (Miranda Gasca, 1995; Heredia-Barragán and Garcia-Fons, 1989). The second consists of northwest-striking Tertiary polymetallic sulphide-quartz veins, associated with normal faults, that have been exploited at Taxco and at several mines in the Zacualpan district (Noguez et al., 1991).

GEOLOGY OF THE AZULAQUEZ-TLANILPA AREA

The Azulaquez-Tlanilpa area is underlain by a polydeformed, bimodal sequence of volcanic rocks, and marine sedimentary rocks of the Teloloapan arc assemblage (Fig. 2). Extensive exposures of the Morelos Formation limestone occur to the east and southeast of the study area. The base of a felsic volcanic unit, recognizable throughout most of the map area, provides a useful datum to correlate lithologies in the area (Fig. 3). Zr/Y ratios of greater than 5 indicate a transitional to calc-alkaline affinity for andesitic volcanic rocks, felsic volcanic rocks and a diorite intrusion exposed in the map area (Table 1). Local exposures of mafic volcanic rocks have Zr/Y ratios of between 3 and 3.5, indicating tholeiitic compositions (Table 1; Barrett and MacLean, 1999).

Three geologically distinctive areas have been defined (Fig. 2):

1. In the northwestern portion of the study area between Otates and Tlanilpa, stratigraphy is upright and homoclinal. It is divisible into three conformable sequences, consisting of (i) a lower sequence of andesitic volcanic rocks, (ii)

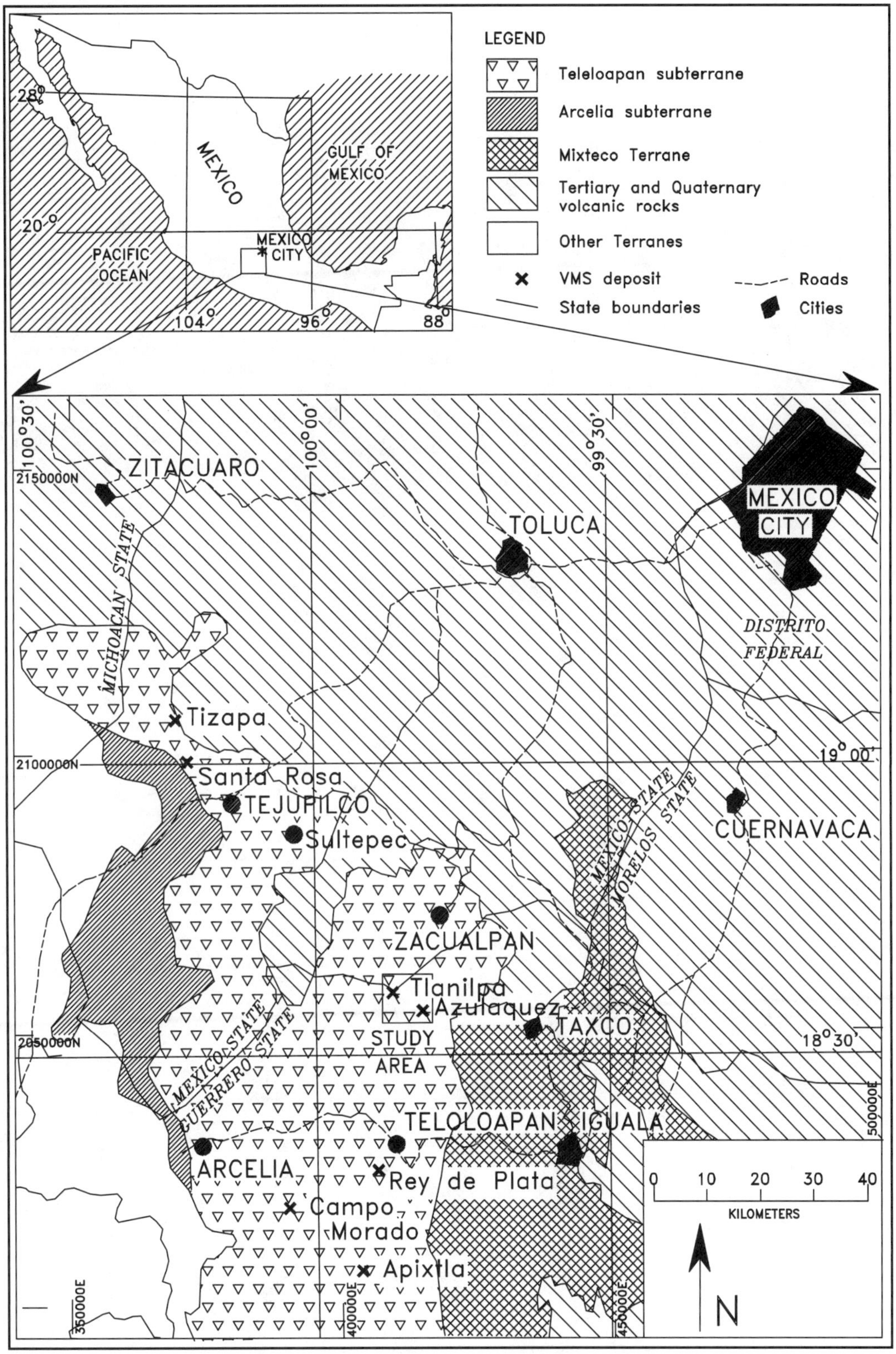

Figure 1. Location and geological setting of the Azulaquez-Tlanilpa area within the Teleloapan subterrane, southwestern Mexico.

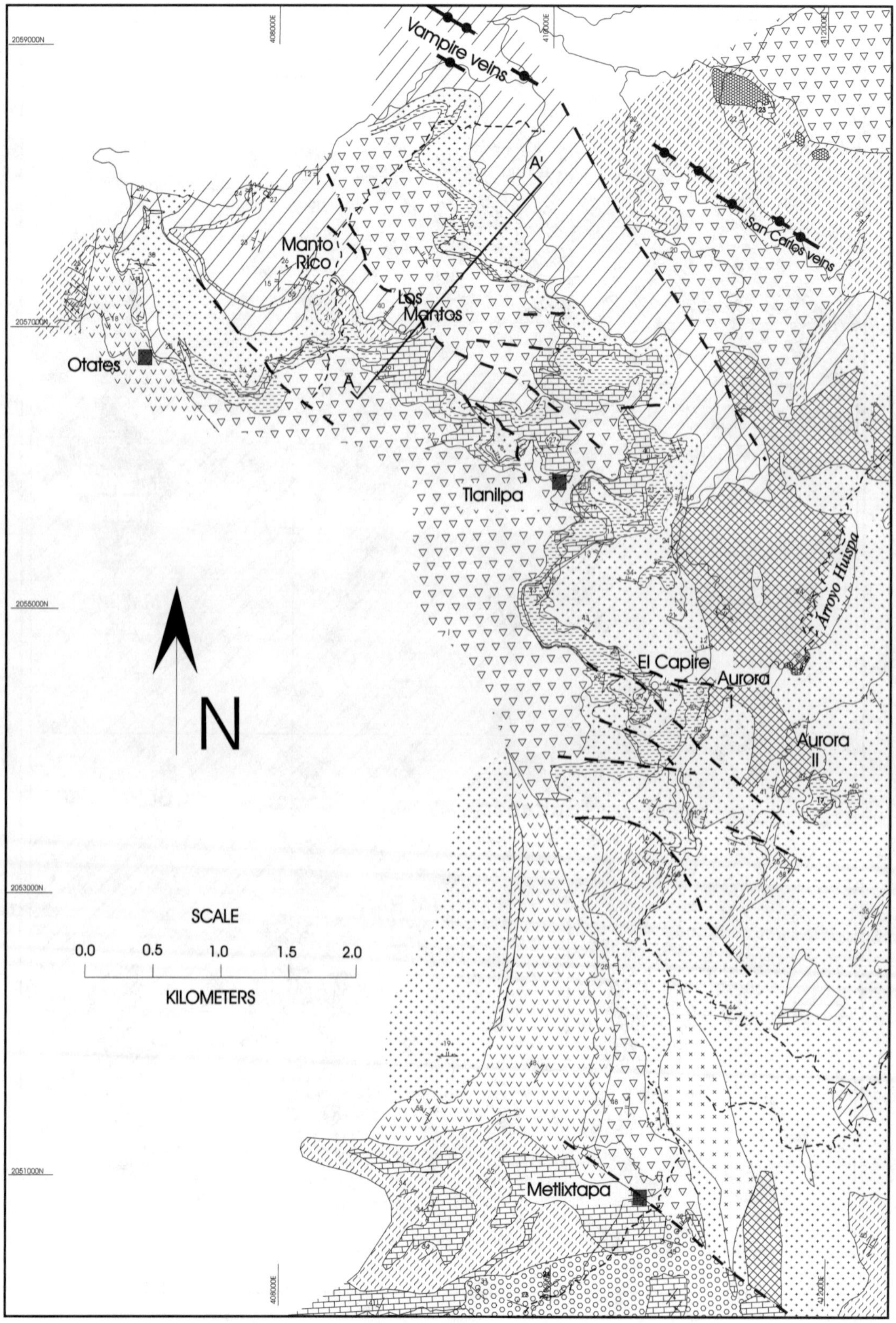

Figure 2. Geology of the Azulaquez-Tlanilpa area, Guerrero State, Mexico.

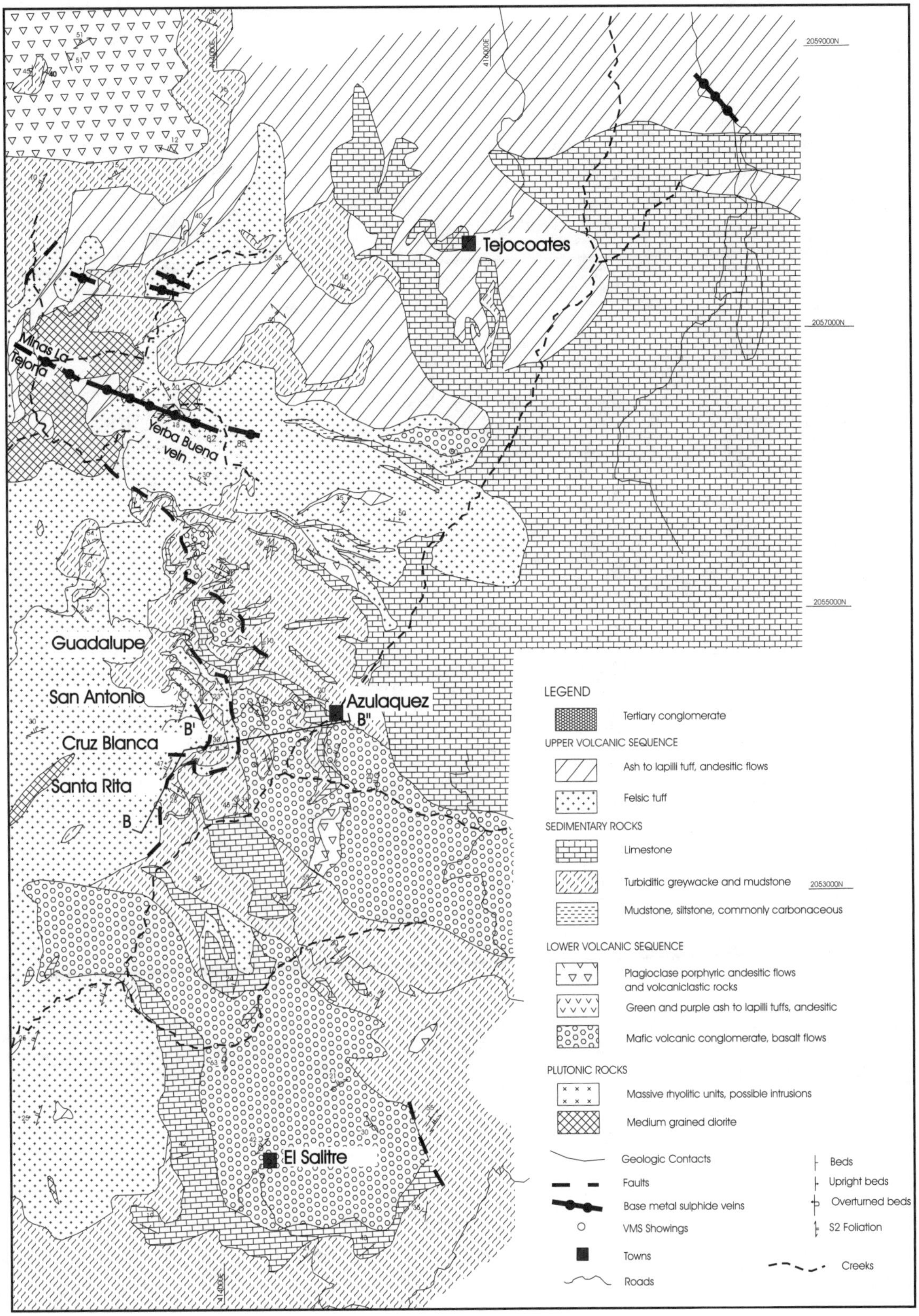

Tejocoates
Minas La Tejona
Yerba Buena vein
Guadalupe
San Antonio
Azulaquez
B'
B"
Cruz Blanca
Santa Rita
B
El Salitre
2059000N
2057000N
2055000N
2053000N
LEGEND
Tertiary conglomerate
UPPER VOLCANIC SEQUENCE
Ash to lapilli tuff, andesitic flows
Felsic tuff
SEDIMENTARY ROCKS
Limestone
Turbiditic greywacke and mudstone
Mudstone, siltstone, commonly carbonaceous
LOWER VOLCANIC SEQUENCE
Plagioclase porphyric andesitic flows and volcaniclastic rocks
Green and purple ash to lapilli tuffs, andesitic
Mafic volcanic conglomerate, basalt flows
PLUTONIC ROCKS
Massive rhyolitic units, possible intrusions
Medium grained diorite
Geologic Contacts
Faults
Base metal sulphide veins
VMS Showings
Towns
Roads
Beds
Upright beds
Overturned beds
S2 Foliation
Creeks

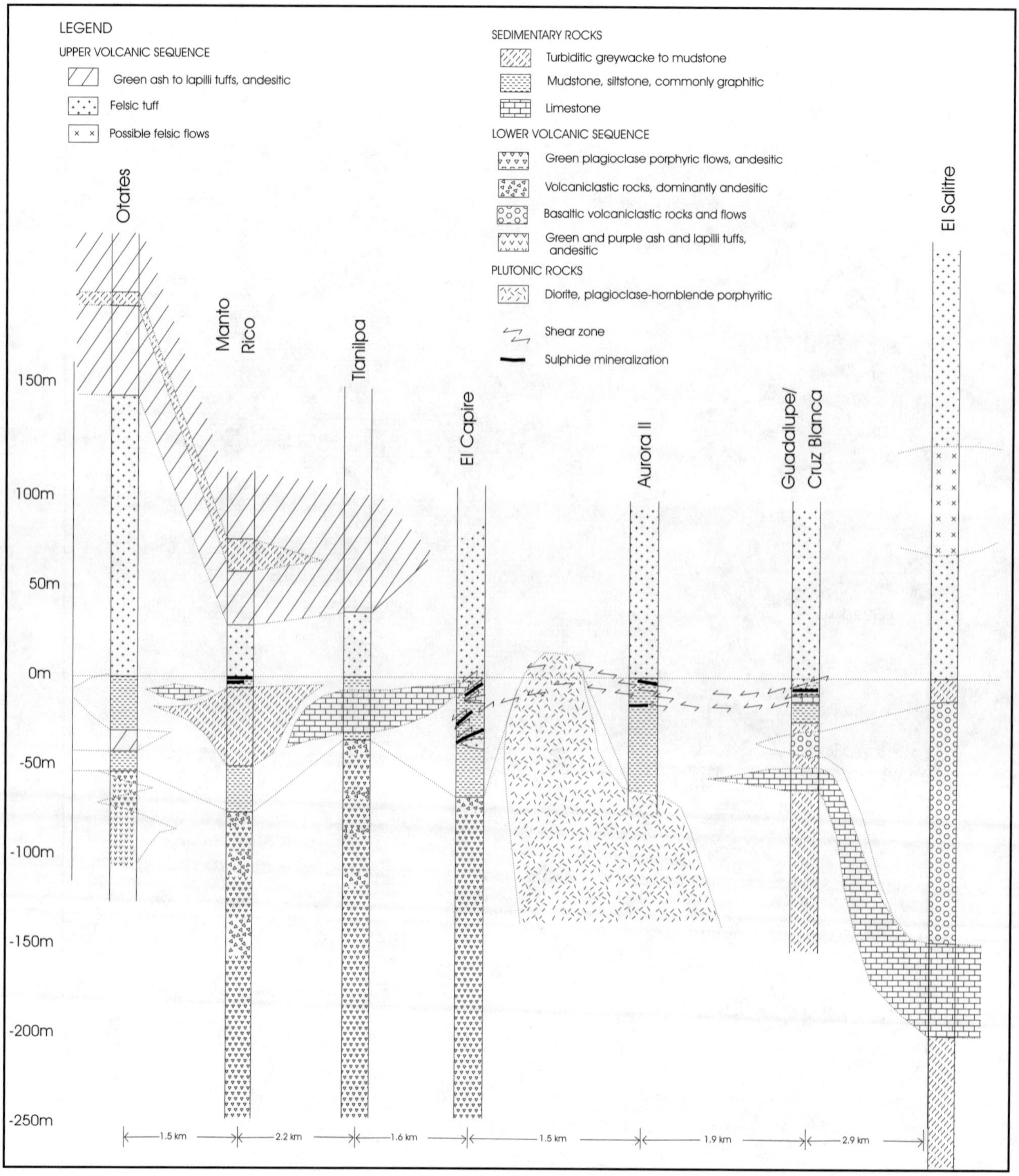

Figure 3. Stratigraphic columns through the Azulaquez-Tlanilpa area. See Figure 2 for locations. The base of the felsic tuff unit is used as a stratigraphic datum.

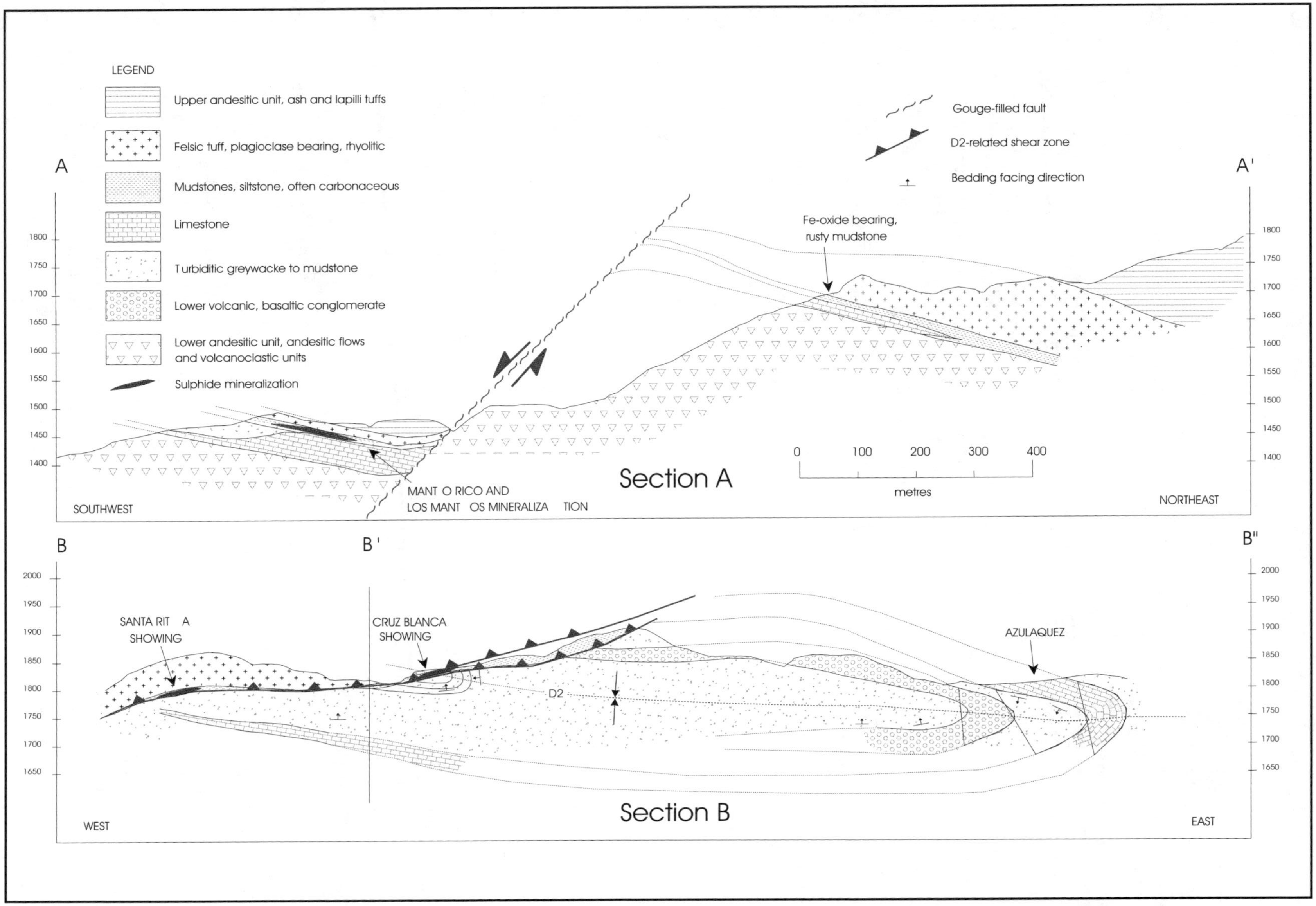

Figure 4. Cross sections illustrating stratigraphic and structural features. Both views are to the north-northwest. See Figure 2 for locations. Top: Cross section through the Manto Rico area. Bottom: Cross section in the Azulaquez area showing the effects of recumbent folding and the discordant nature of the shear zone beneath the felsic tuff unit.

a unit comprising clastic sedimentary rocks and limestone, that host stratabound sulphide mineralization, and (iii) an upper sequence composed of basal felsic (marker unit) and upper andesitic tuffs (Fig. 4A). Between Manto Rico and Otates, the lower andesitic rocks interdigitate with fine-grained clastic sedimentary rocks which become increasingly abundant to the north.

2. The central portion of the map area is underlain dominantly by felsic tuff and a diorite intrusion. Windows of clastic sedimentary rocks that are correlated with the clastic/limestone unit in the Otates-Tlanilpa area are locally exposed in topographic lows beneath the felsic tuff in this area.
3. In the south and east region of the map area, (between Azulaquez, El Salitre and Metlixtapa; Fig. 4B), a folded sequence of turbiditic greywacke, mudstone and siltstone, with lenses of limestone, basalt and basaltic volcaniclastic rocks, occurs beneath the felsic tuff unit. This sequence is in the same stratigraphic position as the mineralised clastic rocks and limestone at Otates and Tlanilpa, but a direct correlation was not established.

Lithologic Descriptions

Andesitic volcanic rocks

Extensive exposures of andesitic volcanic rocks that occur in the western and northern portions of the map area can be subdivided in two sequences based on their stratigraphic position relative to the felsic tuff unit (Fig. 3). Flow rocks in both sequences have compositions that range from basaltic andesite to andesite (Fig. 5).

Lower andesite sequence

Andesitic rocks stratigraphically beneath the felsic tuff unit are composed mainly of massive plagioclase +/- hornblende porphyritic flows, and subvolcanic dykes and sills with subordinate volcaniclastic rocks and tuff. The base of the lower andesitic volcanic sequence in the western map area was not encountered, and its overall thickness is greater than 400 m. The flows are generally composed of 3 to 15 % blocky plagioclase phenocrysts, and up to 10 % hornblende phenocrysts in a fine-grained or aphanitic, green to red groundmass (Fig. 6).

Discontinuous lenses and beds of volcanic conglomerate, tuff breccia, hyaloclastic breccia, and bedded tuff comprise approximately 20 % of the outcrops in the lower andesite sequence (Fig. 7). Clasts range from pebble to boulder size and may be angular or rounded. Matrix is green or maroon, and feldspar-rich, typically with numerous ash to lapilli sized fragments. The most common clast types are porphyritic andesite or dacite, although clasts of andesitic tuff, diorite, and clastic sedimentary rocks are locally present. Bedded block, lapilli and ash tuff is abundant in the Otates area and west of Metlixtapa (Fig. 2) where it is interlayered, or interfingers, with fine-grained clastic sedimentary rocks.

Upper andesitic sequence

In the north and northwestern parts of the map area, the felsic tuff unit is overlain by at least 250 m of grey, green and purple andesitic ash and lapilli tuff with local feldspathic greywacke and mudstone lenses and interbeds. Isolated exposures of andesitic volcanic rocks occur as erosional remnants above the felsic tuff unit in the southern portions of the map area. Flows are locally present, but are less abundant than in the lower volcanic sequence. They comprise massive, green, plagioclase-phyric andesite and occur above the andesitic tuffs along ridge tops north of Aurora I and east of Tlanilpa. Samples of ash tuff collected in the Otates-Tlanilpa area are andesitic, and have a similar chemistry to the lower andesite sequence (Fig. 5).

Mafic volcanic rocks

Mafic volcanic conglomerate and breccia, and intimately associated basalt flows are interbedded with turbiditic clastic sedimentary rocks and limestone in southeastern portions of the map area, between Azulaquez and Metlixtapa. These occur in at least one unit that is 30 to 200 m thick, and which lies stratigraphically above a 20 to 50 m thick limestone band, below the felsic tuff. Volcanic conglomerate is most abundant, and is composed of round to subround, cobble to boulder-size clasts of pale green, amygdaloidal pyroxene-porphyritic basalt in a green

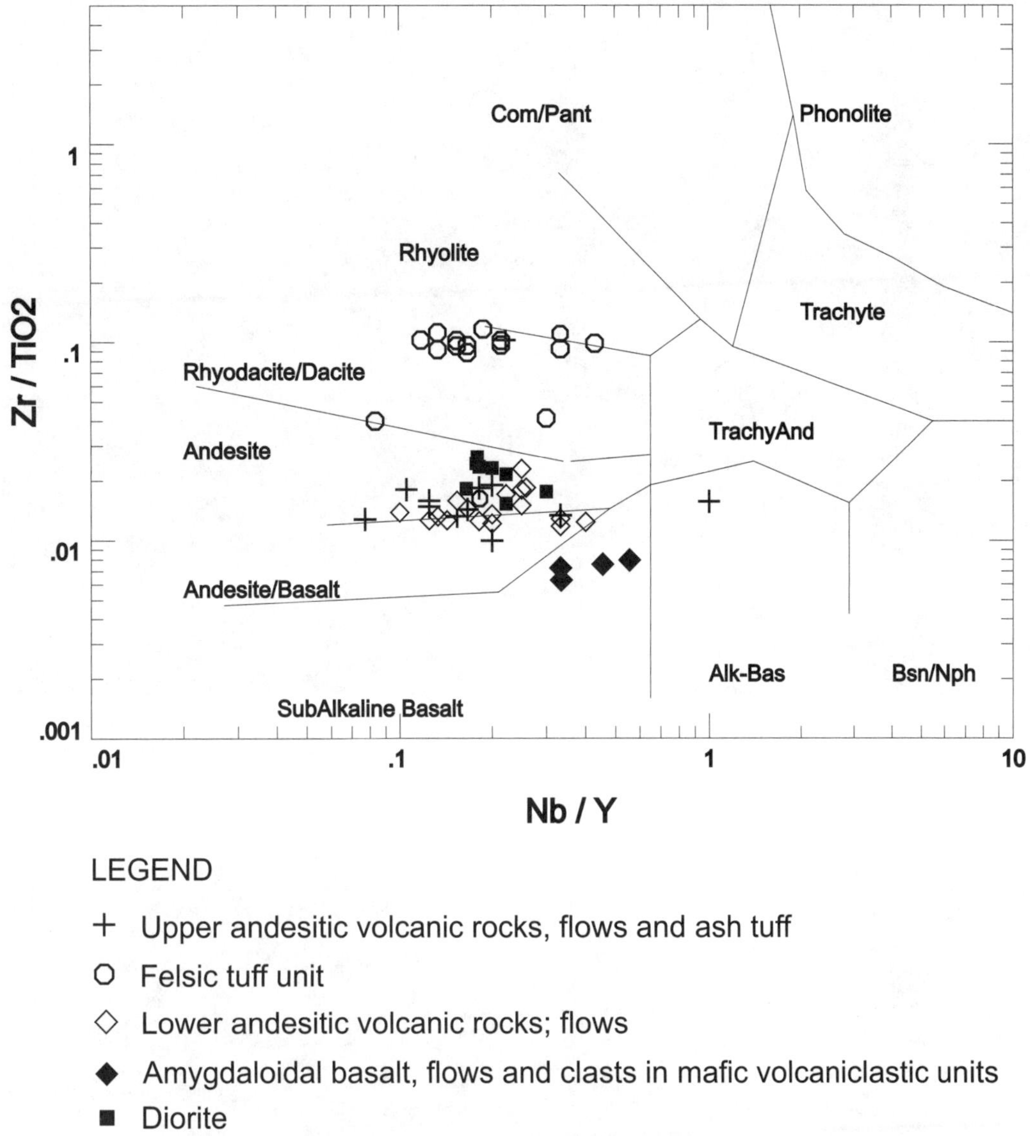

Figure 5. Winchester and Floyd (1977) plot of XRF whole rock geochemical data from samples of volcanic and plutonic units in the Azulaquez Tlanilpa area. See text for details.

to purple, plagioclase-rich sandy matrix. Clasts of limestone and mudstone occur locally. Discontinuous, pale green, pyroxene porphyritic and amydaloidal basalt flows and tuff are interlayered with the volcaniclastic rocks. These flows have distinctly higher P_2O_5 and TiO_2 content, and lower Zr than the andesitic volcanic rocks (Table 1).

In the northwestern parts of the map area, basalt is generally absent. A single flow approximately 10 m thick, occurs within basal portions of the felsic tuff unit in the western part of the map area, south of Tlanilpa. The flow is stratigraphically higher than basalts from the southeast, and indicates mafic volcanism continued at least to the early stages of felsic volcanism.

Sedimentary Rocks

Sedimentary rocks in the map area are dominated

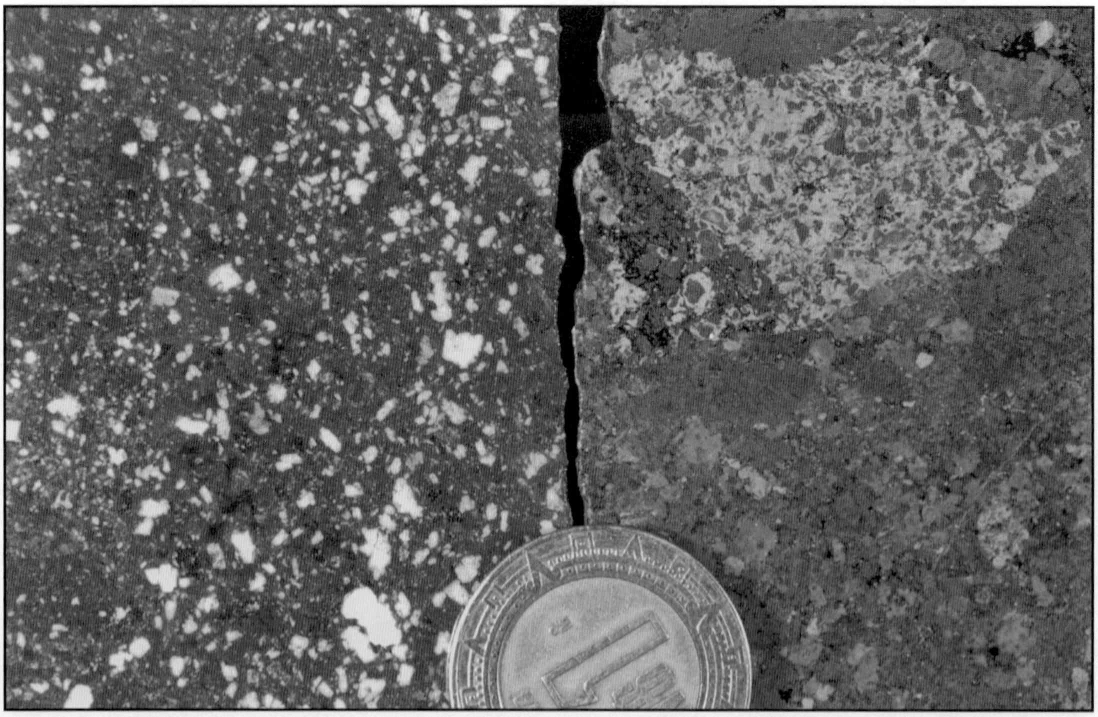

Figure 6. Photograph illustrating a typical plagioclase porphyritic andesitic flow (left) and volcaniclastic lithic breccia (right) from the lower andesitic sequence west of Tlanilpa. The coin is 2.1 cm in diameter.

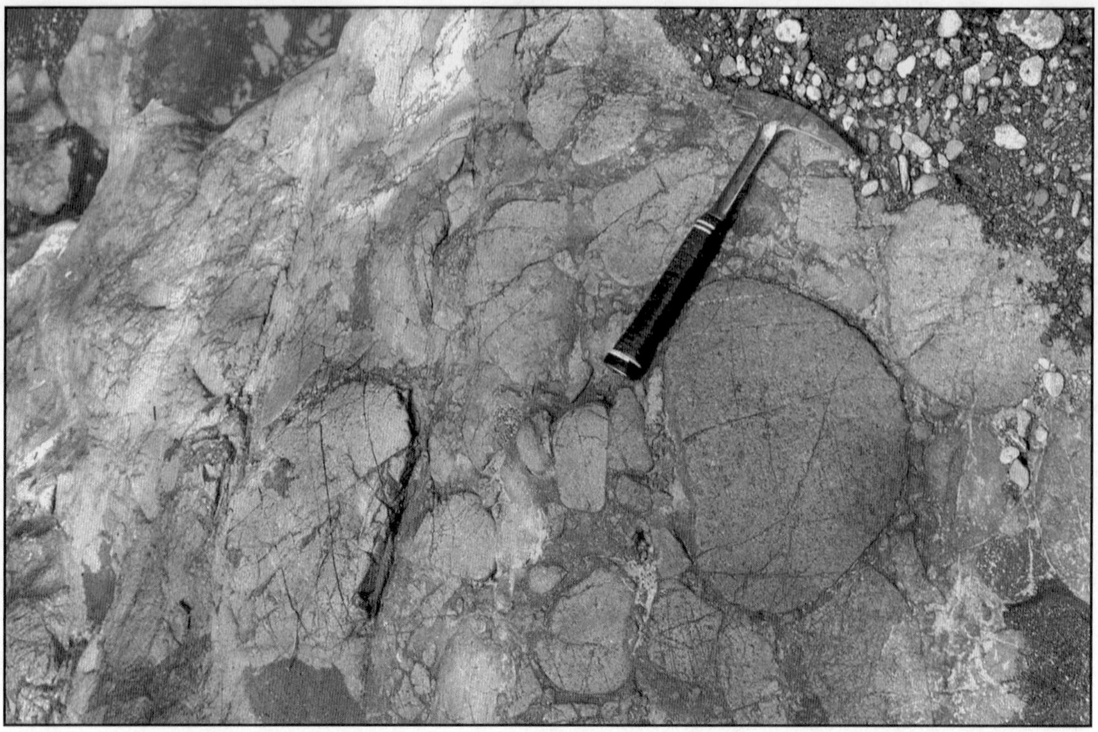

Figure 7. Volcanic conglomerate from the lower andesitic volcanic sequence west of the Capire showing. Clasts are mainly porphyritic andesite.

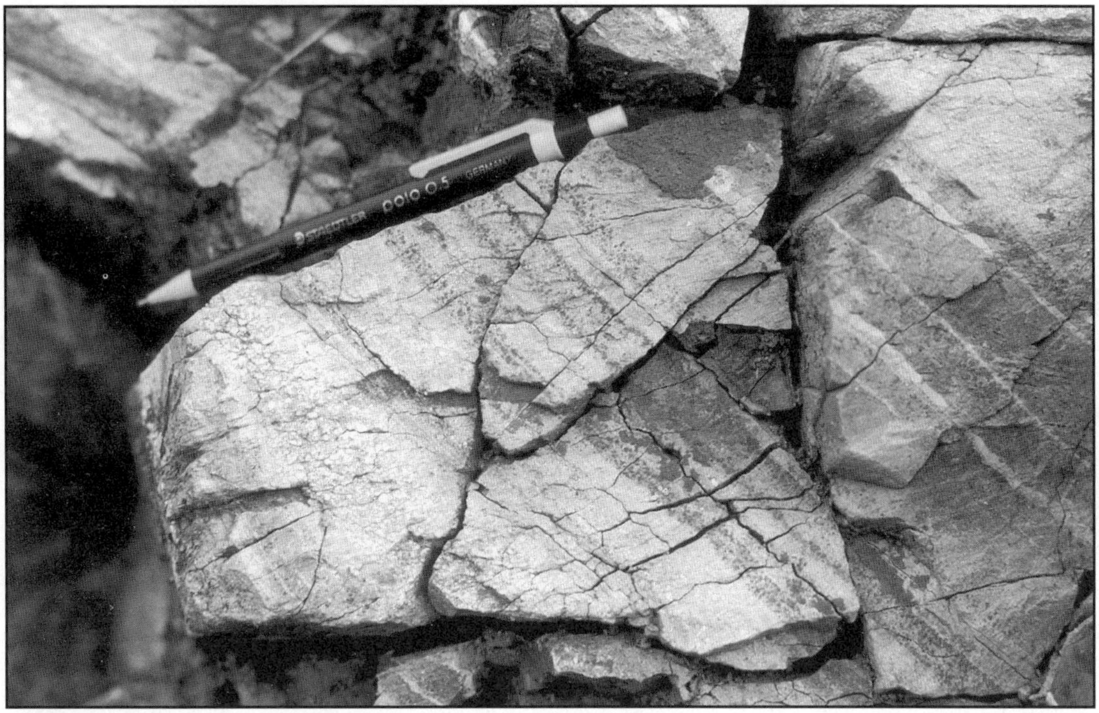

Figure 8. Plagioclase-rich volcaniclastic sandstone and interlaminated grey siltstone and mudstone from near the base of the felsic tuff unit at Tlanilpa. Porphyritic rhyolite clasts occur at the base of some sandstone beds.

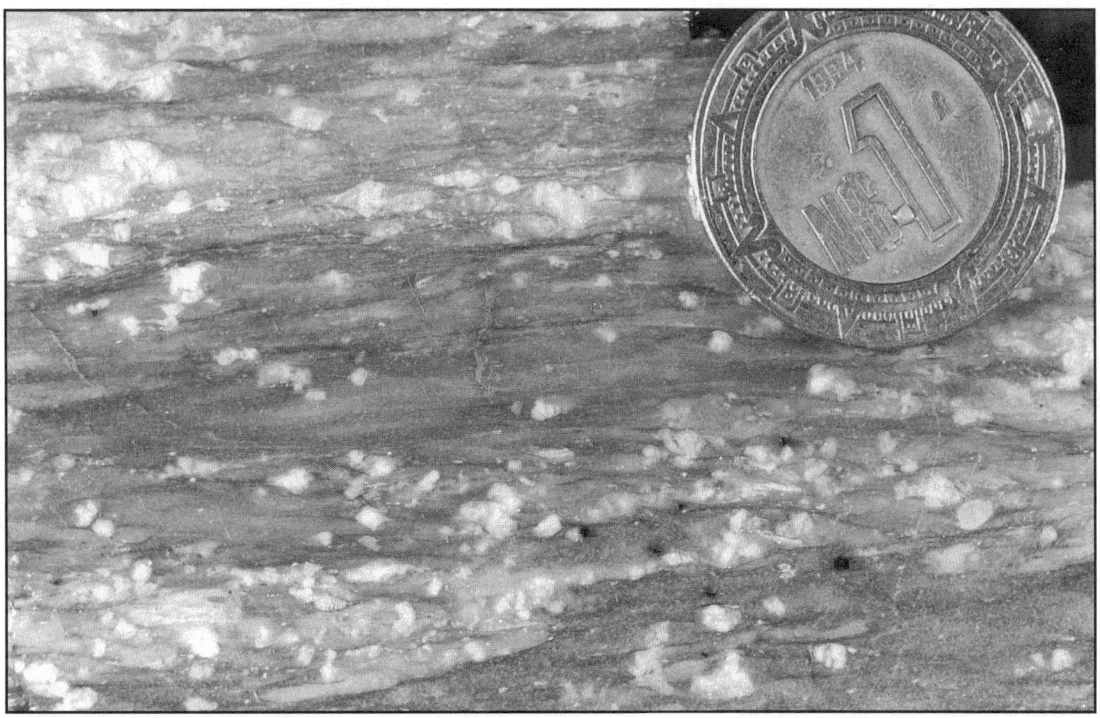

Figure 9. Typical example of the felsic tuff unit, comprising plagioclase +/- quartz crystals in a fine-grained, sericite-quartz matrix. The coin is 2.1 cm in diametre. The sample is from near Otates.

by turbiditic siltstone, mudstone and feldspathic greywacke, with interbeds and lenses of limestone. In lower portions of the stratigraphy, the belt of lower andesitic volcanic rocks is bounded to the north and northwest of the map area, and to the southeast between Azulaquez and Metlixtapa, by sequences of clastic sedimentary rocks that may represent a facies transition to basinal conditions. Most sedimentary rocks occur beneath the felsic tuff unit, but thin lenses of greywacke and siltstone occur higher in the sequence. Interbeds of felsic tuff, or plagioclase rich turbidites are common in the clastic sedimentary sequence 5 to 20 m stratigraphically below the felsic tuff unit (Fig. 8).

In the Tlanilpa area, between Otates and the El Capire showing, a 10 to 120 m thick unit of mudstone, siltstone and limestone overlies the lower andesitic volcanic rocks over a strike length of five kilometres (Fig. 2). This unit hosts several stratabound base metal showings. It is composed primarily of dark grey to black laminated siltstone, carbonaceous mudstone, minor greywacke and interbedded lenses of limestone. A 50 m thick lens of turbiditic, feldspathic greywacke and mud chip conglomerate occurs within the mudstone-limestone unit between Otates and Tlanilpa (Fig. 3), over a strike length of two kilometres. It may represent a submarine turbiditic fan. Between the El Capire showing and Metlixtapa, only discontinuous lenses of fine-grained clastic rocks and limestone occur between the felsic tuff unit and the underlying andesitic volcanic rocks. Several windows of clastic sediments that are exposed in topographic lows beneath the felsic tuff unit (e.g. at the Aurora II showing) in central portions of the map area may represent a continuation of the sedimentary unit to the east.

A folded sequence composed of feldspathic greywacke, siltstone and mudstone with interbedded limestone and lenses of basaltic volcaniclastic rocks occurs beneath the felsic tuff unit in the southern and southeastern portions of the map area between Azulaquez, El Salitre and Metlixtapa. It is at least 400 m thick. Limestone units range from 10 to more than 100 m in thickness and increase both in thickness and abundance to the east and south, where they join thick carbonate units of the Lower to Middle Cretaceous Morelos Formation. The limestone often contains bivalve fragments and chert nodules. The mafic volcaniclastic rocks are generally developed stratigraphically above the thickest and most continuous limestone band.

Felsic Tuff

The clastic sedimentary rocks are overlain in much of the map area by white weathering plagioclase-bearing ash, lapilli and crystal tuff that is accompanied by minor rhyolite flows. Felsic volcanic rocks are most abundant west and southwest of Azulaquez, where they attain a combined maximum thickness of more than 250 m. In the northern part of the map area, the felsic tuff is only 5 to 25 m thick at Manto Rico, and is absent north of the San Carlos veins (Fig. 2). Where it is thinnest, as in its basal section, the felsic tuff is frequently interbedded with the marine clastic sedimentary rocks.

Felsic tuff is composed of 2 to 30 %, 0.5 to 3 mm long subhedral plagioclase crystals in a pale green, waxy, and sericitic aphanitic matrix (Fig. 9). Quartz crystals occur locally. Coarser tuff units may contain 5 to 20 %, 1 to 5 cm long, subrounded felsic clasts that may be pumice. On a Winchester and Floyd (1977) compositional discrimination plot, samples of felsic tuff unit straddle the rhyolite-rhyodacite boundary (Fig. 5), and are distinguished from other volcanic rocks in the area by their high SiO_2, and low Fe_2O_3 (as total Fe) and TiO_2 contents (Table 1).

Several massive, siliceous, and locally brecciated rhyolite bodies up to 2 km in length are intercalated with felsic tuff in the southern parts of the map area northeast of Metlixtapa. These may represent felsic flows or flow domes.

Intrusive rocks

A diorite intrusion is exposed over more than 4 km along Arroyo Huispa, east of Tlanilpa. It is variably porphyritic, and contains 15 to 45 % fine- to medium-grained plagioclase, and 8 to 15 % hornblende phenocrysts that are set in an aphanitic, green groundmass. Dykes of this unit intrude felsic volcanic rocks north of the Yerba Buena vein and east of Metlixtapa. The presence of mineralogically and texturally identical diorite clasts in the andesitic volcanic sequence, and the geochemical similarity of this intrusion to the

Table 1. Representative whole rock lithogeochemical analyses of lithologies in the Azulaquez-Tlanilpa area. Chemex Labs of Vancouver, British Columbia performed the analyses by XRF pressed pellet. Detection limit for major elements is 0.01%; for other elements, detection limit is 2 ppm, except Zr (3ppm). Lithologic codes are as follows: 1a = lower andesitic sequence, flow; 1b = lower andesitic sequence, ash tuff; 2a = upper andesitic sequence, flow; 2b = upper andesitic sequence, ash tuff; 3a = mafic volcanic unit, amygdaloidal flow; 3b = mafic volcanic unit, amygdaloidal flow clast in volcaniclastic; 4 = diorite; 5 = felsic tuff.

Sample number	Easting	Northing	Lithologic code	Al_2O_3 %	CaO %	Cr_2O_3 %	Fe_2O_3 %	K_2O %	MgO %	MnO %	Na_2O %	P_2O_5 %	SiO_2 %	TiO_2 %	LOI %	TOTAL %	Ba ppm	Rb ppm	Sr ppm	Nb ppm	Zr ppm	Y ppm
9,031	410,007	2,055,797	1a	17.56	3.25	0.01	6.50	0.26	2.41	0.03	6.21	0.10	56.50	0.80	4.46	98.08	130	4	224	4	108	20
9,036	409,975	2,054,090	1a	15.97	4.92	0.01	7.62	0.99	3.11	0.15	4.25	0.12	56.55	0.91	4.72	99.31	245	22	198	4	114	22
9,010	410,026	2,054,519	1a	16.74	6.84	0.01	7.63	1.03	4.07	0.04	2.52	0.10	55.66	0.72	3.86	99.21	270	18	380	4	132	16
9,034	409,920	2,055,370	1a	17.85	5.80	0.01	7.64	1.12	4.51	0.03	2.47	0.08	53.20	0.88	4.86	98.44	330	20	266	4	132	16
9,045	408,510	2,057,750	1a	16.98	8.23	0.01	7.30	0.89	2.31	0.10	2.31	0.11	56.84	0.89	2.67	98.63	215	24	786	4	108	20
9,087	409,875	2,054,235	1a	16.29	7.62	0.01	6.29	1.03	2.48	0.11	2.73	0.12	57.88	0.85	4.04	99.44	305	20	352	4	123	24
9,080	409,775	2,055,940	1b	17.70	6.28	0.01	5.41	1.80	1.43	0.08	3.49	0.11	58.15	0.80	2.81	98.06	350	42	234	2	111	20
9,014	408,782	2,058,509	2a	17.38	0.09	0.01	7.34	6.76	2.02	0.18	1.60	0.06	59.46	0.70	3.60	99.19	575	180	26	4	126	38
9,049	408,415	2,057,460	2a	18.01	4.07	0.01	5.48	1.95	1.48	0.07	4.95	0.10	60.50	0.74	2.16	99.51	260	50	428	2	117	16
9,040	408,160	2,058,090	2b	19.42	4.57	0.01	7.04	1.78	1.86	0.08	4.07	0.17	53.75	0.85	5.92	99.51	285	42	314	4	126	32
9,038	409,904	2,058,366	2b	16.24	6.14	0.01	8.04	0.15	5.54	0.09	2.98	0.12	54.58	0.91	4.56	99.35	65	4	272	4	147	22
9,084	408,820	2,057,050	2b	18.90	2.33	0.01	5.34	2.40	1.84	0.06	4.63	0.08	58.99	0.75	3.95	99.27	650	72	288	4	138	22
9,081	408,452	2,057,548	2b	17.56	5.37	0.01	8.44	1.49	2.24	0.15	3.84	0.13	55.44	1.02	4.16	99.84	335	36	210	4	102	20
9,020	414,234	2,053,872	3	14.26	13.28	0.01	3.77	1.03	2.77	0.12	3.11	0.35	50.82	0.79	8.82	99.13	575	16	302	10	63	18
9,030	410,275	2,055,350	3	15.13	13.97	0.01	7.05	1.33	3.89	0.18	2.92	0.26	43.45	0.99	10.30	99.48	750	28	346	10	75	22
9,089	414,530	2,054,325	3	15.60	15.27	0.01	6.40	1.47	3.15	0.11	2.66	0.47	42.57	0.99	9.60	98.29	255	28	348	8	72	24
9,015	414,070	2,054,225	3	18.54	6.15	0.01	5.77	1.66	2.60	0.16	5.96	0.43	51.38	1.39	5.31	99.35	865	36	604	10	90	30
9,003	411,131	2,054,322	4	15.22	2.43	0.01	6.26	2.27	4.74	0.13	2.41	0.11	59.38	0.69	5.00	98.64	685	46	170	4	162	22
9,006	413,157	2,056,164	4	14.47	2.58	0.01	5.53	4.16	3.16	0.12	2.29	0.09	61.00	0.62	4.36	98.38	380	116	144	4	153	22
9,004	411,579	2,054,557	4	14.85	0.17	0.01	8.70	1.88	9.70	0.17	0.85	0.09	54.44	0.64	7.23	98.72	670	44	22	4	138	18
9,088	411,135	2,054,400	4	15.12	5.43	0.01	7.42	0.52	3.29	0.08	3.05	0.12	59.08	0.84	3.50	98.45	220	18	406	4	129	18
9,005	413,145	2,056,088	4	15.27	2.21	0.01	5.62	5.02	3.10	0.10	2.43	0.09	61.62	0.66	3.58	99.70	505	86	108	4	174	22
9,021	411,670	2,054,580	4	15.51	0.33	0.01	6.02	2.49	5.17	0.16	1.96	0.10	62.53	0.70	4.47	99.44	530	48	62	4	162	20
9,028	413,155	2,054,925	5	13.52	0.10	0.01	2.12	4.01	2.67	0.04	0.60	0.03	71.16	0.19	3.47	97.91	765	80	44	4	174	30
9,023	411,800	2,053,310	5	11.57	0.98	0.01	2.58	0.73	2.55	0.01	1.62	0.03	76.28	0.16	2.96	99.47	465	28	146	4	153	26
9,050	408,328	2,057,318	5	13.81	0.84	0.01	2.08	2.33	0.88	0.03	3.86	0.03	71.03	0.19	1.83	96.91	385	68	142	4	183	24
9,024	412,180	2,053,080	5	13.97	0.57	0.01	3.86	1.92	2.44	0.03	2.71	0.04	70.56	0.18	3.30	99.58	450	52	108	6	174	28
9,016	413,490	2,053,870	5	13.40	0.49	0.01	1.93	0.96	2.03	0.01	2.23	0.04	74.11	0.18	3.45	98.84	495	32	188	6	183	28
9,007	413,352	2,056,303	5	10.07	0.54	0.01	1.64	0.74	0.73	0.01	3.91	0.04	78.66	0.15	1.60	98.09	295	18	210	4	153	26
9,041	407,313	2,057,917	5	13.44	0.73	0.01	2.42	0.84	2.30	0.02	2.34	0.03	73.76	0.17	2.95	99.00	655	30	204	4	174	34
9,017	413,225	2,053,740	5	11.47	0.36	0.01	1.91	0.65	2.68	0.01	2.37	0.02	73.60	0.15	2.86	96.08	540	18	128	4	165	12

andesite units (Fig. 5), suggest that it may be a subvolcanic intrusion.

A sample of diorite collected from diamond drill hole A1-6, north of the Aurora I showing (Fig. 2), was submitted to the University of British Columbia Geochronology Laboratory for U-Pb zircon geochronometry. An Early Cretaceous age of 138.7 +/- 1 Ma was obtained (R. Friedman, personal communication, 1996).

Easterly-trending, green plagioclase porphyritic dykes that are up to 40 m wide intrude diorite and the surrounding felsic tuff south of Aurora I. These are unfoliated, and probably Tertiary in age. Rare, aphanitic to plagioclase porphyritic green and grey dykes also occur throughout the map area.

Conglomerate

Local erosional remnants of probable Tertiary conglomerate unconformably overlie the clastic sedimentary and andesitic rocks in the San Carlos area, and along Arroyo Huispa (Fig. 2). This unit is more than 70 m thick and contains round clasts up to 25 cm in diameter of quartz sandstone, siltstone and mudstone.

Structural geology

The rocks in the Azulaquez-Tlanilpa area are affected by two dominant, syn-metamorphic cleavage forming events (D1 and D2) that are associated with recumbent folding, and shallow dipping shear zones. These events define the main pulse of Upper Cretaceous-Early Tertiary, Laramide orogeny, which produced ubiquitous slaty cleavage, easterly-directed thrusts and recumbent folds throughout southwestern Mexico (Sedlock et al., 1993). Later fabrics accommodate only minor shortening and have little affect on the overall distribution of lithologies. Dips of bedding and cleavage in the area are generally shallow. Stratigraphy in the western parts of the map area defines an upright, shallow northwest to northeast dipping monoclinal sequence. In contrast, in the southeast part of the map area, rocks are affected by tight, recumbent folds which cause repetitions and inversions of stratigraphy.

D1 deformation

The earliest schistosity S1, is a shallow dipping, penetrative grain orientation fabric that is preserved mainly in western portions of the map area and is generally parallel to bedding. It is often transposed into the S2 foliation, or is preserved in lithons between S2 surfaces. Minor, east-verging probable F1 folds were identified at several locations. East-verging, megascopic F1 folds and thrust nappes are reportedly common elsewhere in the region (Monod et al., 1993), but no major D1 folds associated with S1 were recognized in the map area.

D2 deformation

D2 is the most widespread and intense deformation event recognized in the map area. S2 foliation, the dominant fabric element in the area, is a slaty to phyllitic cleavage that is defined by the planar alignment of phyllosilicate mineral grains, either as a penetrative or as a spaced foliation. The cleavage generally has shallow to moderate dips to the northwest. It is axial planar to megascopic, tight, and southwest-verging recumbent folds (F2) in the eastern parts of the map area (Fig. 4), and to minor folds with variable vergence in the west. An elongation lineation, L2, trends west-northwest in the plane of S2. It is defined by the elongation of phyllosilicate mineral grains, clasts and chert nodules in limestone, pressure shadows on feldspar grains in the felsic tuff unit, and elongation of clasts and lapilli in tuff and volcaniclastic units.

Shear zones are locally developed in carbonaceous clastic sedimentary rocks and in the basal part of the overlying felsic tuff unit. They are defined by intense S2 cleavage development and contain the L2 elongation lineation, suggesting a syn-D2 timing. However, these structures must have formed late during D2 since they locally truncate recumbent F2 folds (Fig. 4). Shear zones typically have shallow to moderate west dips and are 5 to 30 m wide. Intense shear zones affect carbonaceous sedimentary rocks and limestone between the Santa Rita, Cruz Blanca and Guadalupe showings (Fig. 2), at Aurora II, and between Aurora I, Capire and Tlanilpa. Extensive disruption and transposition of bedding, as well as intercalation of clastic sedimentary rocks, felsic tuff, and sulphide mineralization occurs in the shear zones. Where developed, kinematic indicators, including shear bands, oblique foliation, and asymmetrical boudinage provide conflicting shear sense on these structures, and their interpretation is complicated by widespread transposition of D1 fabrics. The superposition of felsic tuff on to older, folded clastic sedimentary and mafic volcanic rocks by the shear zone in the Cruz Blanca area is consistent with a component of top to the west shear on that structure (Fig. 4), and is compatible with top to the west imbrication of sulphide lenses at Aurora II.

Other structural elements

D3 is manifested by broad, open, north-northeast trending upright folds of bedding and S2. A spaced crenulation cleavage (S3) that strikes north-northeast and dips steeply, is axial planar to the folds, and crenulates S2 cleavage. Other structural elements include east-trending, steeply dipping kink bands in the Otates area (D4), and sets of subvertical, north-northeast striking quartz-calcite extension veins. The veins are oriented at a high angle to the L2 stretching lineation and may have formed late during D2.

Faults

The youngest structural features recognized in the area are gouge-filled normal faults. The most continuous faults with greatest displacement generally strike west-northwest and have moderate southwest dips (Fig. 2). Subvertical east-striking faults are also common. Displaced lithologies, and shallow-dipping gouge fabrics in exposed faults suggest that displacement is predominantly dip slip on the southwest-dipping faults with vertical displacements of up to several hundred metres (Fig. 4). Black carbonaceous sedimentary rocks are incorporated into many faults. Faults that cut andesitic volcanic rocks have bleached, rusty K-feldspar-bearing alteration with disseminated pyrite, and, or quartz-calcite-sphalerite veinlets.

MINERALIZATION

Both stratabound base-metal sulphide mineralization and younger, post-D2 quartz-sulphide breccia veins are represented in the Tlanilpa-Azulaquez area. Table II lists assays for selected mineralised drill intersections, which indicate the silver-rich nature of stratabound lead-zinc mineralization in this region.

Concordant mineralization (VMS)

Lenses of laminated base-metal sulphide mineralization occur as a series of prospects in four areas (Fig. 2): (i) the El Capire - Aurora I prospects, (ii) the Aurora II prospect, (iii) the Azulaquez area, containing the Guadalupe, Cruz Blanca, San Antonio and Santa Rita prospects, and (iv) the Manto Rico and Los Mantos prospects. All of these showings are hosted by dark grey calcareous, carbonaceous siltstone and mudstone and interlayered felsic tuff near the base of the felsic tuff unit. Locally, coarser clastic units occur in the stratigraphic footwall to mineralization. For example, the Manto Rico prospect occurs in interlayered carbonaceous mudstone and felsic tuff (Casselman, 1976) at the top of a turbiditic greywacke-conglomerate wedge. Lenses of felsic volcanic and mudstone clast breccia up to 1 m thick occur in the immediate stratigraphic footwall of sulphide mineralization at the Cruz Blanca prospect.

Although generally confined to the clastic sedimentary rocks, mineralization locally extends a few metres stratigraphically upward into the felsic tuff at the Aurora, Cruz Blanca and Guadalupe showings. Stratabound sulphide mineralization only occurs rarely in other parts of the stratigraphy. One exception is Mina Capulines, two kilometres east-northeast of San Carlos, where an east-dipping stratabound pyrite layer, 0.7 m thick, is hosted by lower andesitic tuff, about 15 to 20 m stratigraphically below the sedimentary rock contact.

Sulphide mineralization occurs in foliation-parallel, tectonically laminated lenses (Fig. 10), laminae (Fig. 11), and fine-grained disseminations. Pyrite, sphalerite, and galena, with subordinate chalcopyrite, tennantite and tetrahedrite are the dominant metallic minerals, and are accompanied by a variable amount of barite (Holcapec, 1996; Casselman, 1976). Typically, the sulphides occur as multiple bands comprising 40 to 75 % sulphide minerals that are 0.5 to 15 cm thick (Fig. 10), but locally, individual massive sulphide lenses are up to two metres thick. Multiple sulphide bands and disseminations define mineralised zones that typically range between 0.5 and 15 m in thickness, and which have a total sulphide content of 5 to 50 %.

The best defined zone of mineralization in the

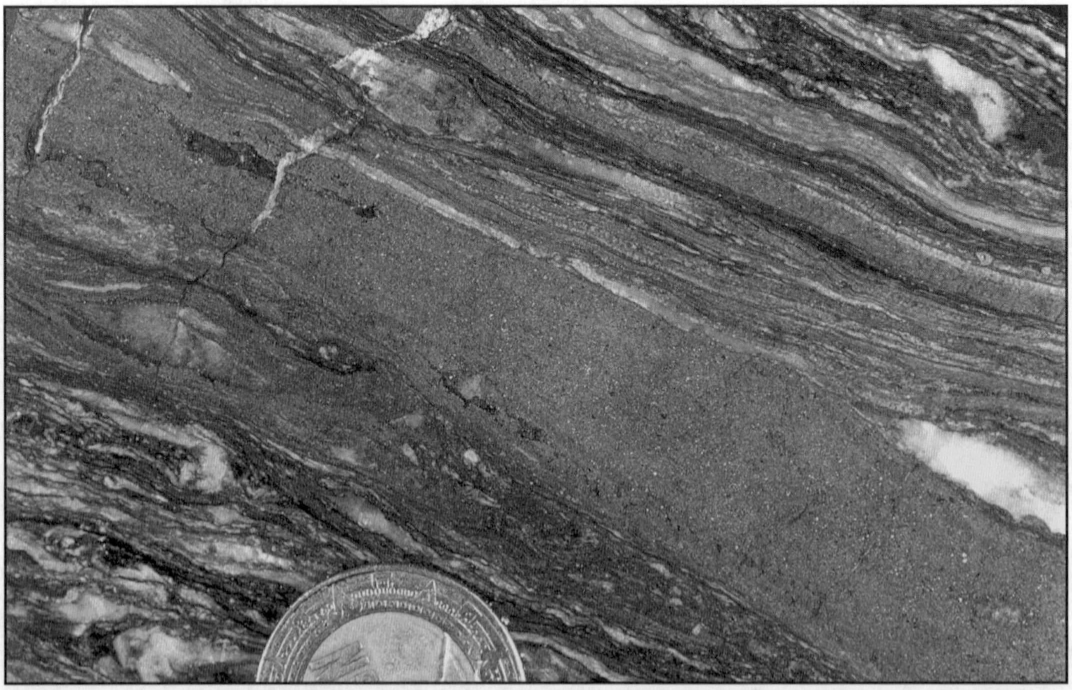

Figure 10. Deformed sulphide mineralization, El Capire deposit. Bands of sphalerite + galena + pyrite (homogenous grey band at centre and above) are interlaminated with deformed sericite phyllite, dark grey, carbonaceous phyllite (bottom left), and dismembered quartz and calcite veinlets (white). The sample is from a shear zone localized beneath the felsic tuff unit. Domains of oblique cleavage between S2 surfaces beside the coin suggest a top to the west shear sense was accommodated on the shear zone at this location.

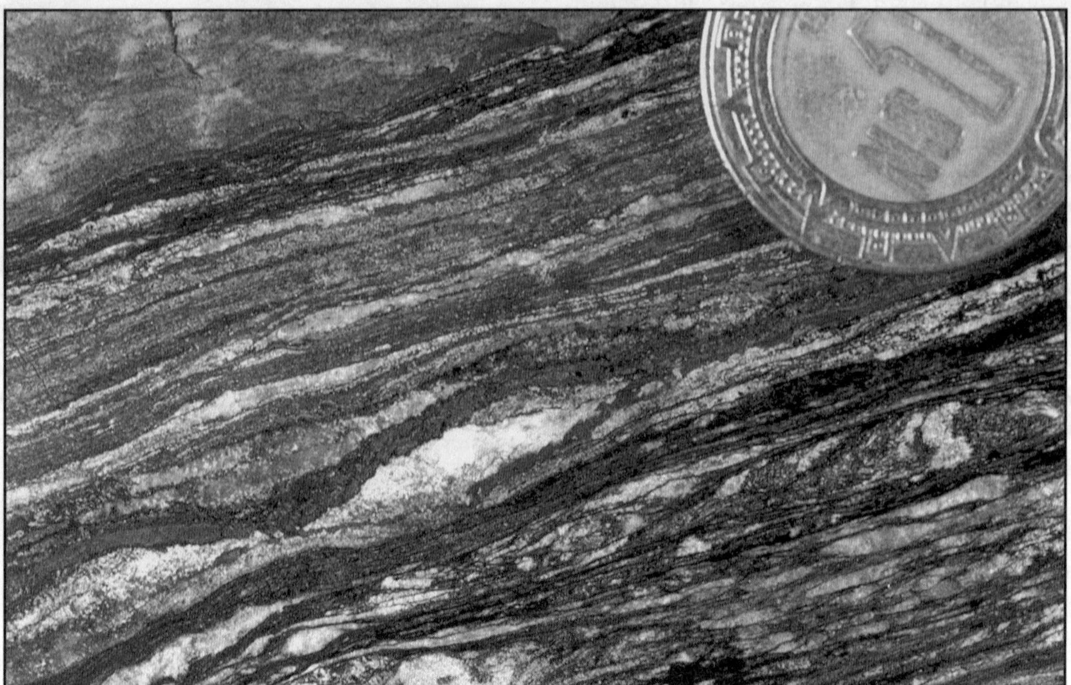

Figure 11. Transposed pyrite-sphalerite laminae occur in calcareous, carbonaceous phyllite with barite-rich layers (grey, top left corner) from the Aurora II prospect. Total sulphide content of the sample is approximately 5 % in laminae (medium grey bands to lower left of coin) and as pervasive disseminations. S1 foliation defined by deformed calcite laminae is preserved in lithons between S2 surfaces below the coin. The coin is 2.1 cm in diametre.

study area is at El Capire-Aurora I (Fig. 2). Here, a 600 m long and up to 300 m wide, flat-lying deposit has been defined by drilling. It is hosted by a 80 to 130 m thick unit of calcareous, carbonaceous mudstone and siltstone with minor felsic tuff interbeds that is overlain by felsic tuff and underlain by porphyritic andesite. Although generally 1 to 8 m thick, mineralization within a 200 m long and 50 m wide, northwest-trending elongate core area at El Capire occurs over a vertical thickness of between 30 and 60 m. Eleven drill holes in this thick core area averaged 0.24 g/t Au, 91.4 g/t Ag, 0.09 % Cu, 0.50 % Pb and 1.22 % Zn over an average width of 37.4 m. Higher grades were encountered over narrower intervals throughout the Capire-Aurora I deposit (Table 2).

Banded, pale grey barite occurs with the sulphides at many showings, in foliation-parallel bands or as laminae (Fig. 11). It is particularly abundant at the San Antonio and Manto Rico showings, where it occurs in lenses with disseminated pyrite at the same stratigraphic position, but along strike from, stratabound sulphide mineralization. Black chert is locally present at San Antonio, Cruz Blanca, Guadalupe, Capiri and Manto Rico, where it is spatially associated with mineralization. The barite and chert may represent chemical sediments that are laterally equivalent to mineralization.

The mineralised zones are highly strained and are frequently transposed into late D2 shear zones that are localized in the carbonaceous clastic rocks near the base of the felsic tuff unit. Shear zones may affect much of the width of the hosting sedimentary rocks. They locally obscure the stratigraphic position of sulphide mineralization in the Azulaquez area, where sulphide lenses are entrained in a shear zone that truncates the upper limb of a megascopic, recumbent F2 fold (Fig. 4). Individual sulphide lenses often are elongate and parallel to the west-northwest trending L2 elongation lineation. Structural intercalation of mudstone, siltstone, limestone and felsic tuff is common in deformed mineralised zones, resulting in lenticular lithons, lenses and wispy bands of felsic tuff and sulphides in black or calcareous sediments. The sulphide laminae have often localized significant shear strain, as evident from displacement and imbrication of lithons across them, and the fine-grained, mylonitic texture of many bands. Recumbent folds combined with S2 parallel slip surfaces cause local structural thickening and imbrication of sulphide lenses.

Apart from sericite-pyrite alteration of tuff beds directly associated with sulphide lenses, no alteration zones were identified stratigraphically below sulphide lenses. At showings that are affected by D2 shear zones, this may be due to tectonic transportation from their original hydrothermal source. Zones of pervasive and veinlet quartz, sericite, pyrite and chlorite alteration in diorite northeast of the Aurora I showing, in lower portions of the felsic tuff unit 600 m southeast of Aurora II and at a locality one kilometre north of the Yerba Buena showing may represent alteration associated with nearby mineralization. An extensive zone of pervasive, intense, quartz-sericite-pyrite alteration occurs in andesite near the town of Mamatla, north of the map area and 8 km north of Azulaquez.

Quartz-sulphide veins

Northwest-trending, steep southwest-dipping quartz-sulphide veins occur within a six kilometre corridor in the northern part of the map area. This area contains multiple, drusy quartz-sulphide breccia veins that are 0.2 to 4 m wide and are typically enveloped by K-feldspar-sericite-carbonate bearing and quartz veinlet stockworks. Purple amethyst is locally abundant in some veins. The Yerba Buena vein is the most continuous, with a strike length of at least 1.4 km. Other showings include Vampire, San Carlos, Esperanza, and Minas La Tejona (Fig. 2). The Yerba Buena and Vampire vein systems display a vertical mineralogical zoning, from coarse pyrite-quartz-sphalerite-galena breccia veins at deeper levels, to drusy, auriferous arsenopyrite-chalcopyrite-bearing quartz breccia veins on ridge tops. Sulphide-rich portions of veins intersected by drilling typically grade between 0.5 and 6 % Zn, 0.1 and 3 % Pb, 0.01 and 0.06 % Cu, 10 to 70 g/t Ag and 0.05 to 0.7 g/t Au.

Vein type mineralization in the Tlanilpa-Azulaquez region is younger than the deformed, stratabound base metal sulphide mineralization. The veins are undeformed; they truncate and brecciate all penetrative fabrics. Within hydrothermal alteration envelopes, pyrite and K-feldspar replace phyllosilicate minerals that define S2 cleavage. The vein-type

Table 2. Selected drilling and underground sampling results from stratabound sulphide deposits in the Azulaquez-Tlanilpa area. See Figure 2 for showing locations. Sample widths are apparent thickness. Information sources are as follows: 1 = Valerie Gold Resources Ltd., press release, July 15, 1996; 2 = Holcapec, 1996; 3 = Valerie Gold, press release, April 4, 1997; 4 = Valerie Gold, press release, Feb. 12, 1997; 5 = Cominco Ltd., internal files. NA = not analysed.

Showing	Sample type	Description	Sample width	UTM East	UTM North	Au ppm	Ag ppm	Cu %	Pb %	Zn %	Source
Manto Rico	channel	15 m long channel sample in drift	0.5 m	408,520	2,057,075	<1	625.0	1.65	14.20	22.60	5
Los Mantos	drill core	Hole LM-01, 95.51-96.51 m	1.0 m	408,927	2,056,971	1.03	1101.0	0.48	1.51	2.63	3
Los Mantos	drill core	Hole LM-03, 91.89-92.27 m	0.38 m	408,926	2,056,971	0.69	1200.0	2.31	5.78	9.77	3
Tlanilpa	drill core	Hole T-7, 86.6-89.7 m	3.1 m	409,280	2,057,619	0.03	51.9	0.22	1.88	7.55	3
El Capire	drill core	Hole C-1, 4.5-39.12 m	34.62 m	410,696	2,054,376	0.18	62.6	0.08	0.40	1.01	1
El Capire	drill core	Hole C-2, 33.0-39.0 m	6.0 m	410,660	2,054,391	3.65	2218.0	0.66	2.38	5.67	1
El Capire	drill core	Hole C-3, 40.0-45.0 m	5.0 m	410,641	2,054,385	0.47	189.4	0.37	2.59	5.58	1
El Capire	drill core	Hole C-4, 48.0-54.9 m	6.9 m	410,642	2,054,385	0.74	476.3	0.64	3.26	7.08	1
El Capire	drill core	Hole C-21, 87-89.2 m	2.2 m	410,783	2,054,348	0.33	200.5	0.34	1.50	3.62	3
El Capire	drill core	Hole C-38, 90.9-94.9 m	4.0 m	410,387	2,054,216	2.66	430.0	0.35	2.88	7.18	3
El Capire	drill core	Hole C-34, 87.4-93.1 m	5.7 m	410,840	2,054,260	0.14	57.2	0.39	2.18	4.14	4
El Capire	drill core	Hole C-40, 90-94.0 m	4.0 m	410,840	2,054,172	0.33	121.0	0.11	1.51	3.13	3
El Capire	drill core	Hole C-43, 45.1-51.1 m	6.0 m	410,747	2,054,195	0.22	55.7	0.16	1.22	3.57	3
Aurora I	drill core	Hole AUI-2, 26.45-36 m	9.55 m	411,040	2,054,363	3.04	267.7	0.52	3.17	5.59	1
Aurora I	drill core	Hole AUI-19, 40-47.5 m	7.5 m	411,056	2,054,426	0.54	230.0	0.44	3.67	6.71	3
Aurora II	drill core	Hole AU2-1, 6.5-15.1 m	8.6 m	411,910	2,053,761	1.16	480.7	0.18	0.93	2.11	1
Aurora II	drill core	Hole AU2-2, 20.5-23.7 m	3.2 m	411,946	2,053,828	1.27	346.0	0.35	1.85	4.34	1
Aurora II	drill core	Hole AU2-5, 93.2-95.2 m	2.0 m	411,720	2,053,788	1.82	247.0	0.26	1.68	3.40	3
Aurora II	channel	West incline, average of 6 samples	2.18 m average	411,715	2,053,635	2.66	576.1	NA*	2.19	6.40	2
Aurora II	channel	West drift, average of 7 samples	1.98 m average	411,705	2,053,625	0.90	130.5	NA*	0.78	2.52	2
Aurora II	channel	Sublevel 1, 15 samples	2.5 m average	411,700	2,053,620	5.46	297.1	0.30	2.06	5.11	2
Cruz Blanca	drill core	Hole CB-1, 23.0-27.5 m	4.5 m	413,740	2,053,970	0.82	282.8	0.26	0.90	2.10	1
Cruz Blanca	drill core	Hole CB-2, 5.0-10.5 m	5.5 m	413,776	2,053,962	0.26	113.2	0.16	0.62	1.65	1
Cruz Blanca	drill core	Hole CB-11, 25.8-27.3 m	1.5 m	413,758	2,053,985	0.43	350.0	0.30	1.40	3.70	4
Guadalupe	channel	Average of 10 drift samples	1.53 m average	413,225	2,054,880	0.88	471.2	0.69	2.43	8.40	2

mineralization probably formed along steep extensional fractures during Tertiary normal faulting in the region, since both veins and faults (i) have similar orientations, structural style and timing, (ii) are frequently enveloped by bleached K-feldspar alteration, and (iii) faults frequently contain disseminations and veinlets of base metal sulphides. The quartz-sulphide veins may be the same age as the historic Ag-bearing veins at Taxco and Zacualpan.

DISCUSSION AND CONCLUSIONS

Calc-alkaline volcanic rocks in the Azulaquez-Tlanilpa area form a bimodal volcanic arc that interfingers with a succession of clastic sedimentary rocks and limestone of unknown thickness in the east and southeast parts of the map area (Fig. 12). The upper part of the volcanic sequence interfingers with limestone of the Morelos Formation for which Albian fossils indicate an Early Cretaceous age (Altamirano et al., 1979). The distribution of lithologies suggests that in Early Cretaceous time, the volcanic rocks formed an arc that was developed 5 to 15 km offshore to the west-northwest of the Morelos carbonate platform (Fig. 12). Basaltic volcanism occurred locally in the sedimentary basin between the volcanic arc and the carbonate platform.

Sulphide deposits in the Azulaquez-Tlanilpa area occur on the northern margin of a felsic volcanic complex that was probably centred to the east of Metlixtapa, where the felsic succession is thickest and where possible felsic subvolcanic intrusions or flow domes are developed. The sulphide deposits occur near the stratigraphic base of the felsic volcanic unit in carbonaceous sedimentary rocks that define a volcanic hiatus between andesitic and overlying felsic volcanism (Fig. 12). Resurgence of andesitic volcanic activity followed deposition of the felsic volcanic unit, possibly fed by the diorite intrusion that occurs east of Tlanilpa. The 138.7 +/- 1 Ma U-Pb zircon age of this intrusion provides a minimum age for the volcanic sequence, which is consistent with the Albian age of fossils in the limestone of the Morelos Formation.

Mineralization in the Azulaquez-Tlanilpa area is Zn-Pb rich and Cu-poor, consistent with classification within the Zn-Pb-Cu group of VMS type systems (Franklin, 1995). The common occurrence of barite with sulphide mineralogy, and their association with calc-alkaline felsic volcanic rocks, and the paucity of mafic volcanic rocks in the footwall stratigraphy to the deposits, are all comparable with deposits of the Hokuroku district of Japan. The Azulaquez-Tlanilpa deposits occur in a stratigraphic position similar to other Zn-Pb-rich VMS-type deposits in the Teloloapan subterrane, including Rey de Plata, Campo Morado and Tizapa. All of these deposits are associated with felsic volcanic rocks that overlie intermediate volcaniclastic rocks and flows. The Rey de Plata deposits, 35 km south of the study area (Fig. 1), also occur with lenses of carbonaceous mudstone in basal portions of a 400 m thick metamorphosed rhyolite tuff unit (Herdia-Barragan and Garcia-Fons, 1989). This rhyolite tuff is developed above more than one kilometre of andesitic volcanic rocks, and may interfinger with early Cretaceous carbonate rocks to the east (Miranda-Gasca, 1995). At Campo Morado and Tizapa, felsic volcanism may have terminated before or during sulphide deposition, since the mineralization in these districts is directly overlain by clastic sedimentary rocks and limestone (Oliver et al., 2000; Lewis and Rhys, 2000). A U-Pb zircon age of 145 Ma from felsic volcanic rocks in the footwall of the Campo Morado orebodies (Oliver et al., 2000), and Early to Middle Cretaceous fossils obtained from overlying limestone in the Tizapa and Campo Morado areas (Monod and Busnardo, 1993) suggest that mineralization throughout the region is broadly coeval with the Azulaquez-Tlanilpa showings.

Like other deposits in the Teleloapan subterrane, the sulphide deposits in the Azulaquez-Tlanilpa area, have been affected by significant non-coaxial strain localized in clastic sedimentary rocks near volcanic contacts during the Late Cretaceous-Early Tertiary Laramide orogeny. Sulphide bodies are dismembered and elongated parallel to the west-northwest trending D2 stretching lineation. Consequently, future exploration in the Azulaquez-Tlanilpa area will require detailed stratigraphic mapping, and the tracing of tectonically transposed and dismembered sulphide bodies along D2 shear zones and across recumbent folds.

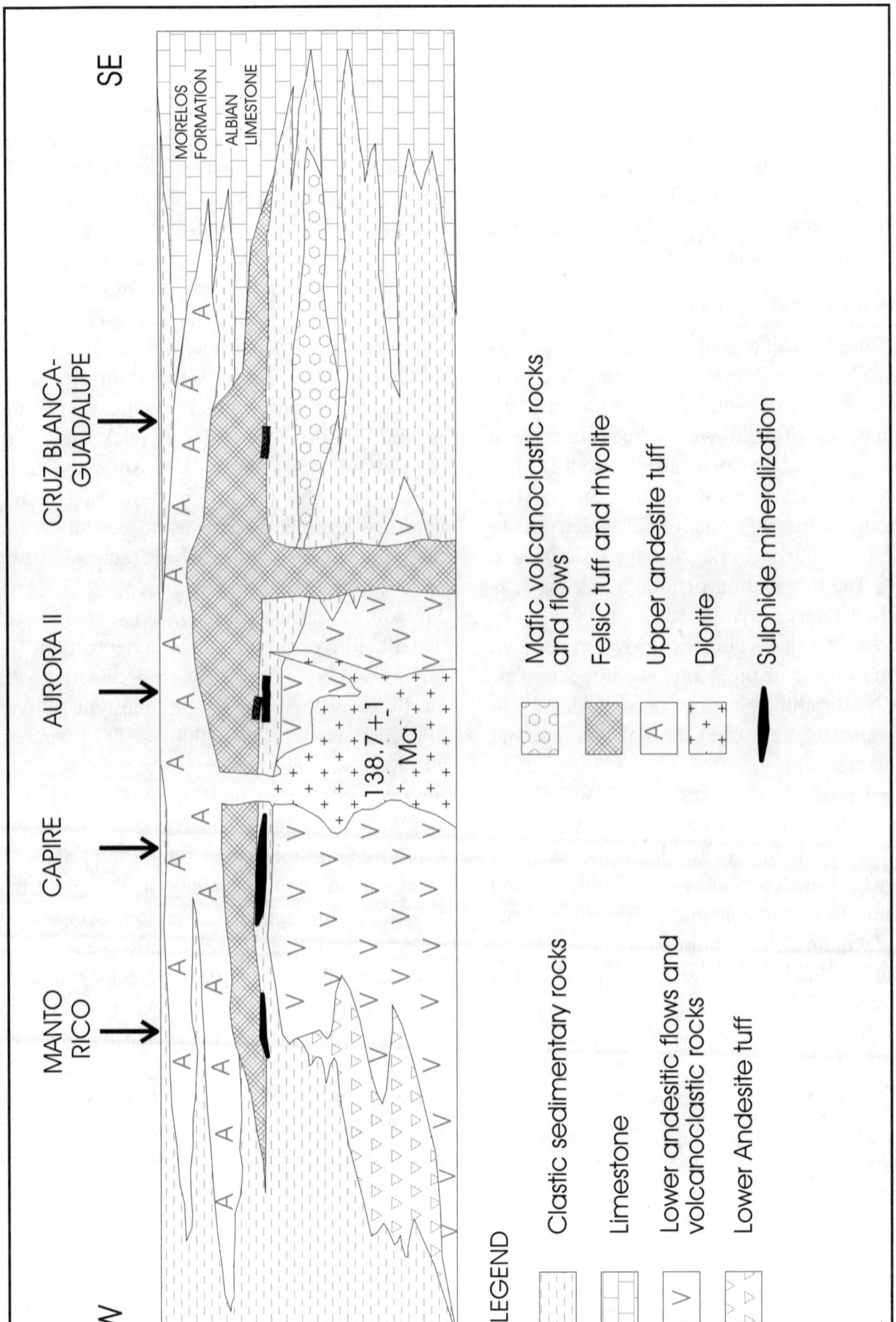

Figure 12. Schematic stratigraphic section of the Azulaquez-Tlanilpa area. View to the northeast.

Acknowledgments

The authors thank Valerie Gold Resources Ltd. for permission to publish this paper and acknowledge beneficial field discussions with Fred Holcapek. Alastair Findlay mapped parts of the area and assisted in the geological interpretation. Peter Walcott and Associates of Vancouver, Canada are gratefully acknowledged for providing logistical support and data processing services in the field, as well as retrieval and processing of archived data for preparing this paper. Art Troup kindly supplied drilling results obtained by Valerie Gold Resources Ltd., and Ian Paterson of Cominco Ltd. provided access to exploration results from the Manto Rico prospect. Reviews by Ross Sherlock and Christopher Lee helped to improve the manuscript.

References

Altamirano, F.J., de los Santos, J. de J., and Estevez, C.M. 1979. Geologia, tectonica y yacimientos minerales de la region norte central del Estado de Guerrero. A.I.M.M.G.M., Mem. Tec. XIII Convention, pp. 396-420.

Barrett, T.J., and MacLean, W.H., 1999. Volcanic sequences, lithogeochemistry and hydrothermal alteration in some bimodal volcanic-associated massive sulphide systems. Reviews in Economic Geology, Volume 8, pp. 101-132.

Campa, M.F., and Coney, P.J. 1983. Tectono-stratigraphic terranes and mineral resource distribution in Mexico. Canadian Journal of Earth Sciences, 20, pp. 1040-1051.

Casselman, M., 1976. Property examination report: Kerry property (Manto Rico). Cominco Ltd., internal report.

Enns, S., and Findlay, A. 1997. Report on geological mapping of the Mamatla property, Mexico. Unpublished report for Valerie Gold Resources Ltd.

Espinosa-Perea, V.J. 1982. Características geológicas de los yacimientos estratiformes de Tlanilpa, Guerrero. Thesis, Universidad Nacional Autónoma de México.

Franco-Serrano, A. 1983. Informe final de avance de los estudios realizados en el área de Azulaquez, Guerrero, durante 1983. Consejo de Recursos Minerales, internal report 120182.

Franklin, J.M. 1995. Volcanic-associated massive sulphide deposits. in Geology of Canadian Mineral Deposit Types, O.R. Eckstrand, W.D. Sinclair and R.I. Thorpe, editors, Geological Survey of Canada, Geology of Canada, no. 8, pp. 158-183.

Heredia-Barragán, M.A., and Garcia-Fons, R.J. 1989. Distribución de yacimientos vulcanogénicos en la provincia norte de Guerrero - suroccidente del Estado de México. XVIII Convención Nacional AAIMMGM, Memorias técnicas, pp. 81-99.

Holcapec, F. 1996. Summary report for the period September 1, 1994 to December 31, 1995, Mamatla mineral reserve. Valerie Gold Resources Ltd., internal report.

Jansma, P.E., and Lang, H.R. 1997. The Arcelia graben: New evidence for Oligocene Basin and Range extension in southern Mexico. Geology, 25, pp. 455-458.

Lewis, P.D., and Rhys, D.A. 2000. Structural geology and stratigraphic setting of the Tizapa mine and region, México State, México. This volume.

Miranda-Gasca, M.A. 1995. The volcanogenic massive sulfide and sedimentary exhalative deposits of the Guerrero Terrane, Mexico. Ph.D. thesis, The University of Arizona, Tucson, Arizona.

Monod, O. and Busnardo, R. 1993. A late Albian ammonite fauna in the carbonate cover of the Teloloapan arc volcanics, Guerrero, Mexico. in Proceedings of the first Circum-Pacific and Circum-Atlantic Terrane Conference, Guanajuao, México, Universidad Nacional Autónoma de México, pp. 90-91.

Monod, O., Faure, M., Salinas, J. C. and Sabanero, H. 1993. What is the Guerrero Terrane made of? in Proceedings of the first Circum-Pacific and Circum-Atlantic Terrane Conference, Guanajuao, México, Universidad Nacional Autónoma de México, pp. 92.

Montes-Napoles, J.V.B. 1984. Estudio geológico-minero del área Mamantla-Tlanilpa, Estados Guerrero y México. Thesis, Universidad Nacional Autónoma de México.

Noguez, A., Flores, M., and Toscano, E., 1991. Zacualpan Mining District, State of Mexico. In Salas, G.P., editor, Economic Geology, Mexico. Boulder, Colorado, Geological Society of America, The Geology of North America, P-3, pp. 369-372.

Oliver, J., Payne, J., Kilby, D., Rebagliati, M., and Cluff, R., 2000. Precious metal-rich volcanic-associated massive sulphide deposits of Campo Morado, Guerrero, Mexico. This volume.

Rhys, D.A., and Ross, K.V. 1997. Report on 1:2500 scale mapping of the central portion of the Mamatla property, Southeastern Mexico. Unpublished report for Valerie Gold Resources Ltd.

Salinas-Prieto, J.C., Monod, O., and Faure, M. 1993. Deformación dúctil progresiva en el limite oriental del terreno Guerrero, suroeste de México. in Proceedings of the first Circum-Pacific and Circum-Atlantic Terrane Conference, Guanajuao, México, Universidad Nacional Autónoma de México, pp. 90-91.

Sedlock, R.L., Ortega-Gutierrez, F., and Speed, R.C. 1993. Tectonostratigraphic terranes and tectonic evolution of Mexico. Geological Society of America, Special Paper 278.

Winchester, J.A., and Floyd P.A. 1977. Geochemical discrimination of different magma series and their differentiation products using immobile elements. Chemical Geology, 20, pp. 1609-1622.

VOLCANOGENIC DEPOSITS IN MEXICO: THE PRODUCING MINES

David A. Giles and Javier García F.
Industrias Peñoles S.A. de C.V., Av. de las Industrias 4335, Chihuahua, Mexico 31156

Abstract

Throughout its one hundred years of active participation in the Mexican mining industry, Industrias Peñoles has explored and operated numerous polymetallic deposits. The massive sulphide Ag-Pb-Zn deposits which are found in the volcanic sedimentary sequence of the Lower Cretaceous Guerrero terrane, at the western and central regions of the country, are considered to be of volcanogenic origin.

The Suriana Mine which consists of lenses hosted in a rhyolitic tuff unit near the andesitic tuff and lava, produced 0.7 Mt of ore with 7.7 g/t Au, 603 g/t Ag, 4.5 % Pb and 0.4 % Zn between 1927 and 1942. The production of the LaMinita Mine between 1981 and 1986 was 6 Mt with 60 g/t Ag, 0.3 % Pb, 3.0 % Zn and 34 % $BaSO_4$ hosted in a lens on the contact of andesitic tuff and a sequence of lutites and limestone. The Cuale Mine (1981-1986) exploited 6 lenses hosted in shales in contact with rhyolitic tuffs, with a total production of 1.3 Mt with grades of 0.8 g/t Au, 204 g/t Ag, 1.4 % Pb, 5.4 % Zn and 0.4 % Cu. The Tizapa Mine, in production since 1994, has reserves of 4.5 Mt with 1.9 g/t Au, 325 g/t Ag, 1.8 % Pb, 7.9 % Zn and 0.7 % Cu in four lenses emplaced in carbonaceous shale and phyllites. The Rey de Plata Mine is presently under development with resources of 3 Mt with 1.4 g/t Au, 240 g/t Ag, 2.1 % Pb, 8.7 % Zn and 0.5 % Cu hosted in a pyroclastic sequence with interfingering of carbonaceous lutite horizons. The Francisco I Madero project, also under development, has resources of 40 Mt grading 40 g/t Ag, 0.8 % Pb and 5.2 % Zn in a pyrite horizon hosted in the contact of argillaceous limestone and argillites.

The above described deposits form two groups distinguished by their volcanic association and relative proximity to the discharge vent and define massive sulphide belts suitable for exploration. Modern geochemistry and geophysics methods together with the identification of favourable geological environments, have proven useful in detecting drilling targets in deposits hidden by alluvial and post-mineral rocks.

Introduction

Throughout its one hundred years history of active participation in the Mexican mining industry, Industrias Peñoles has explored and operated a large number of polymetallic deposits, including Suriana, La Minita, Cuale, Tizapa, Rey de Plata and Francisco I Madero. These are massive sulphide silver-lead-zinc deposits hosted in volcanic sedimentary rocks of the Lower Cretaceous Guerrero terrane, located in the western and central region of Mexico (Fig. 1).

During the early years, between 1927-49, prospecting focused on the surface oxidation areas and some Au, Ag and Pb values were recovered from the Suriana and Rey de Plata Mines. From 1975 to 1985, with new technologies and a better understanding of the volcanogenic deposits around the world, Peñoles developed the La Minita and Cuale Mines, in addition to identifying sufficient reserves in Rey de Plata to develop a new mine, which is currently under construction. In 1992, the Peñoles-Dowa joint venture acquired the Tizapa project from the CRM (a government agency), carried out some mining activities and new geological interpretation that led to increased reserves. The Tizapa Mine entered into production in 1994. Since 1995, the exploration work based on a Sedex type geological model resulted in the Francisco I Madero project, which will start production in 2001 and will be the largest zinc producer in the country.

The producing mines

Suriana

The Suriana Mine is located in the State of

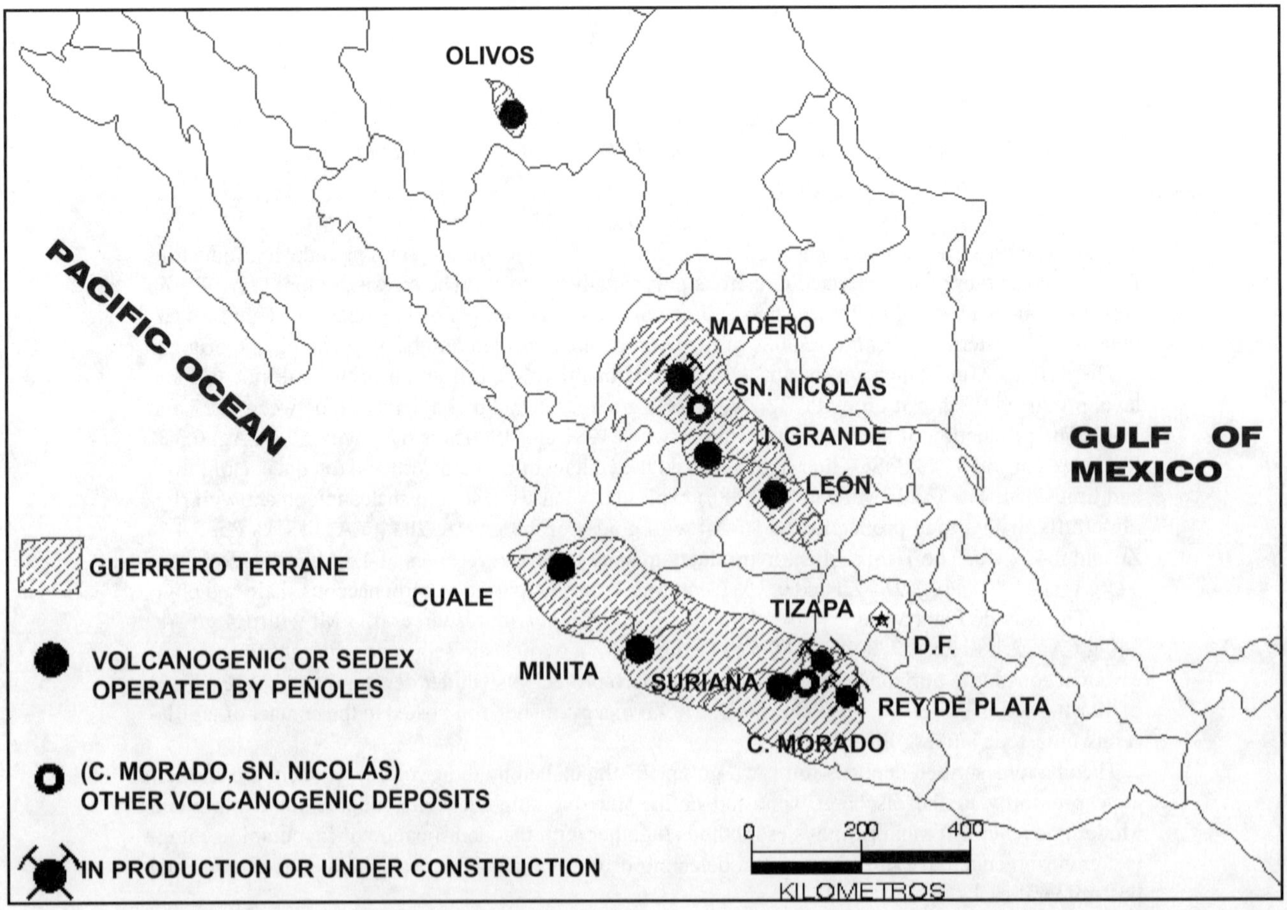

Figure 1. Mines and projects of volcanogenic deposits in Mexico

Guerrero, 160 km southwest of Mexico City, 5 km south of the Campo Morado district, and consists of a 25 km mineralized belt of volcanogenic showings.

In 1925 Peñoles leased the rights to exploit the Suriana Mines. These mines were worked on a fairly regular basis from 1903 to 1912 mining, in total 125 t of Ag, 3.9 t of Au and 4 t of Pb were produced from the supergene zone. The mines became inactive in 1912. Peñoles established an experimental plant in Temixco obtaining positive metallurgical results; therefore, in 1927 Peñoles built a 300 t/d plant. This plant was considered to be the only one of its kind, because the processing consisted of chloritizing roasting, followed by cyanidation, obtaining recoveries of 87 % Au and 90 % Ag from oxidized and mixed ore. The ore was delivered to the plant by a 10 km long aerial tramway, with a grade of 7 g/t Au and 565 g/t Ag. The company closed the mine in 1942. In 1989-90 Peñoles undertook an exploration campaign through geology, geochemistry, and 3,000 m of diamond drilling, but was unable to develop sufficient reserves to justify the reopening of the mine.

The deposit is located within the Lower Cretaceous volcano-sedimentary sequence of the Guerrero terrane, in the Teloloapan subterrane. The lithological sequence consists of andesitic marine volcanic rocks and dacitic-rhyolitic lenses underlying a sequence of lutites, sandstone and calcareous units. The Cretaceous sequence is covered by rhyolites and conglomerates of the Eocene-Oligocene. The mineralization is hosted in the upper part of a rhyolitic-tuff unit, close to the contact with tuffs and andesitic lava. It includes massive sulphide lenses, stringer and disseminated mineralization. The general strike of the mineralized horizons is NW with dips in the order of 40 to 75 degrees SW. The mineralized horizons reach a length of up to 1,200 m and thickness ranging from 2 to 80 m. The mineralization is associated to the felsic volcanism and consists of fine-grained pyrite, sphalerite, galena, chalcopyrite and tetrahedrite. In the oxidation areas, the mineralogy is dominated by hematite, goethite, limonite, argentojarosite and free gold. The most extensive hydrothermal alteration is a network of stringers and quartz replacements, sericite and disseminated pyrite which is associated with felsic rocks. It is closely related to the upper portion of the massive sulphide bodies. The region is affected by two fault systems with a N70E and N10E strike, which strongly displaced the mineralized horizons. The rocks are affected by regional foliation product of cataclastic stress and metamorphism.

There is no detailed information available on past production; however, there is evidence that a production of 600,000 tonnes of oxides and mixed ore were processed at the Peñoles Plant between 1927 and 1942. The grades of the ore mined during the 1927-30 period averaged 7.7 g/t Au, 603 g/t Ag, 4.5 % Pb and 0.4 % Cu.

La Minita

This deposit is located in the SW region of the State of Michoacan, 80 km SE of the city of Colima (Fig. 1). The first mining operations in this property go back to 1961 and were dedicated to mining barite for the company Minerales de Puebla. At the end of the sixties, Minera Autlán carried out a drilling program for manganese ore with negative results; however, they found anomalous values of Zn and Ag, but at that particular time, these minerals were not of interest. In 1974, Minerales de Colima continued to work the area looking for barite. In 1976 Peñoles initiated a volcanogenic lead-zinc exploration campaign The exploration of La Minita started in April 1979, when the mineral rights were acquired from Minerales de Colima, The mine was designed for open pit mining and beneficiation by selective flotation of 2,240 t/d of ore with silver, lead, zinc and barite. The mine was in operation from 1981 to 1995. This property was closed down because the mineral reserves were depleted.

The deposit is located in the rocks of the Guerrero terrane of the Lower Cretaceous. There are three main lithological units, the oldest consists of spherulitic tuffs and andesitic lithics overlain by a felsic tuff unit associated with the deposit. This sequence is covered by the rhythmic unit of lutites and sandstones and reef limestones. The deposit is hosted at the contact of the tuff and sediment units, with a double dipping regional dome, at the nose of a SE structure coinciding with the axial plane forming a dome shape. The lens has a maximum length of 600 m and thickness ranging from 6 to 70 m. This is a stratiform deposit of volcanogenic origin and may represent a secondary mobilization process which modified the original textures and caused replacement of limestones in the upper part of the body. It contains three types of orebodies: massive barite with sulphides; barite stringers with sulphides and massive magnetite with sulphides. The first of these orebodies is the economically attractive zone. It consists essentially of barite with Ag, Pb and Zn. More specifically, it is divided in a lower barite subzone, sulphides (Zn-Pb-Cu) and sulphosalts (Ag), an intermediate barite zone with sulphosalts (Ag) and sulphides (Zn-Pb) and a higher disseminated barite and jasper zone with sulphides (Pb-Zn) The main minerals are: barite, sphalerite, galena, stromeyerite, tetrahedrite, chalcopyrite, magnetite, native silver, cerussite and anglesite.

During the productive years of the mine, 1981-1995, 6 million tonnes of ore were mined with 60 g/t Ag, 0.3 % Pb, 3.0 % Zn and 34 % $BaS0_4$. There are no records available on the previous production of the mine.

Cuale

The Cuale mining district is located at the western tip of the Talpa de Allende municipality, some 200 km west of Guadalajara, Jalisco. The district has been known since 1804. It was mined intermittently during the last century, obtaining an estimated production of 250,000 t of selected ore, with grades of 900 to 1,000 g/t silver. The mines were closed down in 1900 and since then several companies, including Esperanza Co. (1918-22), Peñoles (1936-42) and Eagle Picher (1954-59) tried to reopen the mines. Compañía Fresnillo claimed the area in 1965 and in 1972 initiated intensive exploration work, including 7,400 m of diamond drilling. The exploration stage was completed in 1976 with encouraging results, prompting the construction of a new mine. Operations commenced in 1980 with a production of 500 t/d. In 1987 the mine closed because reserves were depleted.

The basement consists of a granite and granodiorite pluton underlying the volcanic sedimentary sequence of the Lower Cretaceous, part of the Guerrero terrane. The lower portion consists of tuffs and lava of rhyolitic composition. The upper portion is made up of lutites, limonites, sandstone and tuff. The sequence is partially covered by Tertiary rhyolitic breccia. The mineralized bodies known and exploited are Coloradita, Chivos de Arriba, Chivos de Abajo, Socorredora, Naricero and Grandeza. They are located in a favourable horizon in the upper portion of the lutites and limonites unit, close to the contact with the rhyolitic tuff unit. The orebody consists of fine grained banded lenticular massive sulphides with colloform textures and transported ores. In the Grandeza area of the deposit, it is associated with a stockwork structure. The mineralogy consists of pyrite, sphalerite, galena, chalcopyrite, argentite, tetrahedrite, covellite and bornite. Gold is associated with pyrite-sphalerite. Barite, carbonates and gypsum comprise the gangue. The bodies are located in a 2 x 2 km area forming lenses with a maximum width of 30 m.

Between 1981 and 1986 the production of the Cuale Mine totaled 1.3 Mt with 0.80 g/t Au, 204 g/t Ag, 1.4 % Pb, 5.4 % Zn and 0.4 % Cu. It is estimated that the Cuale District produced a total of 2.0 Mt with similar grades as those described above.

Tizapa

This deposit is located in the State of Mexico, 67 km south of Toluca (Fig. 1). Some small mining operations have been known in the area, which showed pyrite-rich thin lenses, but there is no information on the old mining production. The CRM started exploration in 1978 carrying out 10,000 m of diamond drilling between 1979 and 1985. The positive results obtained encouraged the Peñoles-Dowa joint venture which, from 1987 to 1990, drilled 63 additional holes (7,500 m) and a 750 m heading that cut across the main lenses. In 1992 the joint venture resumed exploration work and reinterpreted the geology allowing the construction of a new mine that started operations in August 1994, and currently has a capacity of 1,200 t/d.

The deposit is located in the Lower Cretaceous volcano-sedimentary sequence of the Guerrero terrane. Carbonaceous shales and phyllites make up the stratigraphic unit which hosts the massive sulphide deposits. This sequence is covered by conglomerates and plio-quaternary basalts. The massive sulphide lenses consist of pyrite, sphalerite, galena, chalcopyrite, bornite, argentite, tetrahedrite and pyrargyrite, with subordinate pyrrohotite, arsenopyrite, covellite and marcasite. Four main orebodies are hosted in a horizon, 10 to 50 m apart with thickness ranging 3 to 12 m, occupying an area of approximately 500 x 400 m. The bodies have been affected by compressional, extensive faulting, generating some interruptions and overthrusts of the mineralized horizons.

There was no production prior to 1995. The estimated reserves are in the order of 4.5 Mt with 1.9 g/t Au, 325 g/t Ag, 1.8 % Pb, 7.9 % Zn and 0.7 % Cu.

Rey de Plata

This deposit, located in the State of Guerrero 135 km directly SW of Mexico City, has been known since the last century. It was partially explored and mined by Peñoles between 1946 and 1949. From 1976 to 1980 an intensive exploration program was undertaken, including 11,000 m of drilling, which allowed to define the reserves in the Rey de Plata, Tehuixtla and the Zn-Cu lens in the order of 3 Mt with 1.4 g/t Au, 240 g/t Ag, 2.1 % Pb, 8.7 % Zn and 0.5 % Cu. Additional prospecting work with drilling and mining, including a 300 m shaft, generated sufficient mineral resources so that in 1998 Peñoles, in association with Dowa, approved the development of a mine, scheduled to start production at 1,100 t/d by the year 2000.

Rey de Plata is a volcanogenic massive sulphide deposit located in a pyroclastic sequence of rhyolitic-dacitic and andesitic composition with interfingered sedimentary horizons. Regionally, the pyroclastic sequence forms the lower portion of a volcanic unit covered by limestone and argillaceous rocks. The lenses and bands of massive sulphides are hosted in clay-pyrite altered rocks. The mineralogy consists of sphalerite and pyrite, with subordinated galena, chalcopyrite, tetrahedrite and sulphosalts.

The Tehuixtla body is the largest, its thickness ranges from 2 to 18 m and has a lenticular shape dipping 25 degrees to the SW. Lenses of barite are common, but not in economically significant concentrations. The quartz-sericite-pyrite alteration is the most common, forming a halo of up to 150 m over the mineralized layer. It consists of lenses of silica and pyrite with bandings of sericite and other clays. The mineralized layer outcrops in the Rey de Plata area and it dips to the SW where the Tehuixtla body is hosted, at a depth of over 250 m.

Francisco I Madero

The Francisco I Madero project is located 20 km west of Zacatecas, (Fig. 1). This property was part of the National Mining Reserve and from 1976 to 1983 the CRM carried out drilling, geophysical studies and other activities. The results of this work led to the suspension of the project. In 1994, Industrias Peñoles acquired the property and, on basis of geological, geochemical and geophysical interpretations, carried out 135,000 m of diamond drilling and, within a period of less than 2 years, was able to calculate proven (measured) and probable (indicated) reserves of 40 Mt with 40 g/t Ag, 0.8 % Pb, and 5.2 % Zn and 3 Mt with 89 g/t Ag and 1.33 % Cu.

The deposit lies in the middle portion of a limestone-clay sequence that overlies marine andesitic volcanics of the Guerrero terrane. In the region, the Guerrero terrane is covered to the west by a thick layer of rhyolites of the Tertiary, forming a contact with a SE-NW orientation. These rocks form the first steps of the Sierra Madre Occidental mountain range. At the east of the Guerrero terrane is the contact with the calcareous rock of the Sierra Madre terrane. In the deposit, the oldest rocks are argillites in laminar strata formed by carbonaceous clay with stringers and quartz lenses, characterized by a total absence of carbonates. Overlying this unit there is a layer consisting of pyrite-pyrrhotite with clay, chlorite, epidote and some magnetite. Its maximum thickness is 120 m and it has a characteristic banding, structures of synsedimentary collapse and a concentrical zoning of pyrrhotite-pyrite. This unit contains a major part of the economically mineable sulphides of the deposit. The overlying layer consists mainly of chlorite-epidote bands, tremolite-altinolite, silica and pyrite, with an irregular thickness (maximum 70 m). Covering the above units are thinly stratified recrystallized clayey limestones consisting mostly of calcite and carbonaceous matter. A maximum thickness of 400 m has been identified so far. Narrow dykes of dacitic composition dated (by Peñoles) at 61 Ma. intersect the above described sequence and are generally hosted in the N-S faults.

There are two types of orebodies: 1) Zn-Pb sulphide lenses included in the chlorite-epidote units and, 2) Lenses with Ag-Cu content within the pyrite-pyrrhotite unit. The Ag-Cu orebody consists of irregular lenses in a belt with an almost N-S direction in the middle portion of the pyrite-pyrrhotite unit. It forms laminations and bands of chalcopyrite-pyrite, cubanite and enargite with associated silver values. The Zn-Pb sulphides are contained within a series of interfingered lenses with thickness ranging from 6 to 65 m hosted in a 2.5 x 3.0 km area, forming a thicker axis with a N-S orientation. It consists of sphalerite bands and laminations with minor galena interbedded in silica with clay-pyrite or chlorite-epidote.

Conclusions

The deposits discussed above define a series of belts suitable for the exploration of massive sulphides within the volcano-sedimentary sequence of the Guerrero Terrane. The Suriana, Cuale and Rey de Plata deposits are closely related to the explosive felsic volcanism and show the characteristics of a proximal deposit with respect to the discharge source. The Tizapa and Francisco I Madero deposits, on the other hand, are associated with sedimentary rocks and their volcanic affinity is not evident, suggesting distal type mineralization. In neither case there is any evidence that correlates the size and content of the deposit with its deposition environment; however, the extension of the alteration zones may be indicative of the dimension of the mineralization process, which has an impact on the volume of the deposit.

Numerous mineralization showings have been studied by mapping the lithology and associated alterations, using geochemical methods, geophysical surveys, drilling and, above all, considering the regional location of the favourable environments which form the boundaries of the volcanogenic deposits. In recent years indirect prospecting methods have been used to investigate potential deposits, hidden by alluvial and postmineral rocks. Aeromagnetometry, induced polarization and gravimetry are valuable tools to detect the drilling targets. (A translation, original submitted in Spanish).

REFERENCES

García F. J., Juan M. Pérez I., Luis F. Novelo. Geología del Yacimiento Rey de Plata, Teloloapan, Meico. Technical Proceedings, AIMMGM Convention, 1981.

Giles, D. A., Exploration for Skarn and Stratabound Zinc-Lead-Silver Orebodies in Mexico, International Conference on Carbonate-Hosted Lead-Zinc Deposits, Society of Economic Geologists, 1995.

Giles, D. A., Garcia F. J., Gomez Torres S., Gonzalez Leopoldo. Geología y mineralización del Yacimiento FI Madero, Zac. Internal Report, Industrias Peñoles, 1997.

Gomez Torres S., Góngora Demetrio. Geología y distribución de Yacimientos del Terreno Guerrero. Internal Report, Industrias Peñoles, 1998.

Heredia M. A., and García F. J., Distribución de Yacimientos Vulcanogénicos en la provincia norte de Guerrero y suroccidente del Edo.de México. Technical Proceedings, AIM-MGM XVIII Convention, 1989.

Industrias Peñoles. El Primer Siglo de Peñoles. Special Edition, 1986.

Industrias Peñoles. Technical Reports on the Mining Units, 1995.

Franklin J. M., Lydon J. W., and Sangster D. F., Volcanic Associated Masive Sulfide Deposits. Economic Geology, 75th Anniversary Volume, 1981.

Scott S. D., Modern and ancient volcanogenic masive sulfide (VMS) deposits. Short Course presented to Industrias Peñoles, 1998.

GEOLOGY OF THE KUROKO-TYPE MASSIVE SULPHIDE DEPOSITS OF THE CUALE DISTRICT, JALISCO STATE, MEXICO

BRIAN V. HALL
International Croesus Ventures Corp., 1592 Eaglecliff Road, Bowen Island, British Columbia, V0N 1G0, Canada.

PEDRO PABLO GOMEZ-TORRES
Minera Croesus, S.A. de C.V., Loma Verde 623, Col. Loma Verde, San Luis Potosi, San Luis Potosi, Mexico

ABSTRACT

The Cuale District represents Kuroko-type volcanogenic massive sulphide mineralization that occurs in a relatively undeformed Cretaceous volcano-sedimentary package of the Guerrero terrane of Mexico. The deposits are polymetallic and, in comparison to massive sulphide deposits worldwide are relatively high-grade for silver, lead, zinc and copper. Supergene enrichment in the oxide portion of the orebodies has resulted in significantly enhanced precious metal grades. Pyrite, followed by sphalerite, galena and chalcopyrite are the dominant sulphides. Barite, tennantite, tetrahedrite, enargite, geocronite, proustite-pyrargyrite and stannite are also present.

To date twenty-five massive sulphide deposits have been recognized. These occur in a variety of depositional settings. The proximal deposits are associated with dacitic domes, and are underlain by exhalative centres represented by chloritization, sericitization and silicification, with veined and disseminated sulphides. Sulphide zoning is an important aspect of these deposits as they have sphalerite-galena on the top and the flanks, with pyrite-chalcopyrite underlying the central portions. The transported deposits are the result of slumping down the paleotopographic slopes, which has then caused the sulphides to be brecciated and fragmented. The distal deposits are located in basinal settings, with the sulphides exhibiting sedimentary bedding. A siliceous exhalite that is high in precious metal values occurs at the same stratigraphic horizons as the massive sulphides, and appears to connect a number of the deposits.

Spatially the deposits are most abundant in basinal settings composed of argillaceous sediments, which are adjacent to explosive rhyolitic or dacitic domes. The timing of the mineralization appears to be restricted to a relatively short period that is represented by less than one hundred metres of sedimentary stratigraphy.

INTRODUCTION

The Cuale District is located in the Sierra Madre del Sur range, approximately 30 kilometres southeast of Puerto Vallarta, in Jalisco State. It contains twenty-five of the roughly 150 massive sulphide occurrences that occur in the Guerrero terrane of western Mexico.

The district was discovered relatively late in the exploration history of Mexico (1804) and, by 1919, most of the known deposits had been discovered. The Kuroko-type massive sulphide deposits that characterize this district are very rich in silver, lead, zinc and copper in comparison with other massive sulphide deposits. Due to its higher than normal silver content (averaging over 500 g/t for the early producers), Cuale was one of the first places in Mexico where volcanogenic massive sulphide deposits attained commercial production.

Our understanding of the district has benefited from a number of individuals, whose work has formed the basis for this manuscript. Macomber (1962) was the first to provide a comprehensive study of the regional geology, and detailed descriptions of the mineral deposits. At the time of his work, volcanogenic massive sulphide deposits in North America were largely thought to be the result of replacement along fractures or favorable horizons. A number of experts in Kuroko-type deposits, including T. Sato, T. Urabe and D.J. Kirwin began studying the district in 1982. In conjunction with Mexican geologists working with Zimapan, S.A. de C.V. (a subsidiary of Penoles) a comprehensive understanding of the deposits and the district began to evolve. By the early 1990's this work had largely come to fruition in the excellent overview and deposit descriptions of Berrocal and Querol (1991).

REGIONAL SETTING

The Guerrero terrane underlies an area of over 350,000 square kilometres. It is the largest terrane in Mexico, and is best exposed and studied in the Sierra Madre del Sur, along the western coast of Mexico. Due to the intrusive activity in the Sierra Madre Occidental, and later Tertiary volcanic activity that occurred throughout much of central Mexico the distribution of the Guerrero terrane is, for the most part, restricted to isolated windows and roof pendants.

In general the Guerrero terrane is characterized by two major tectonic assemblages: the Triassic-Middle Jurassic "basement assemblage" that consists of ocean-floor sediments derived from continental sources, and the Late Jurassic-Cretaceous arc assemblage that formed in an oceanic island arc setting. During the Laramide orogeny this arc was accreted against the Mexican Craton. At this time the polarity of the sedimentation changed from westward to eastward, and the sediments from the arc-assemblage flooded onto the Mexican Craton. This process marks the "continentalization" of the Guerrero terrane, and represents a large addition of juvenile crust to the western North American Cordillera (Centeno-Garcia, 1994). The direction of subduction that produced the arc(s) is a matter of controversy; Coney (1983), and Tardy et al. (1991) have proposed westward subduction, and Ramirez et al. (1991) propose two subduction zones, one to the east and one to the west. Other associated tectonic environments such as marginal basins have been recognized (Tardy et al., 1991).

The Guerrero terrane is host to the only two volcanogenic massive sulphide deposits that are currently in production in Mexico (Tizapa and Rey de Plata), plus two others which are currently undergoing feasibility studies (Francisco I Madero and San Nicolas). Clustered in a number of areas of similar lithologic and tectonic settings are over 150 other occurrences (Fig. 1).

Several subdivisions of the Guerrero terrane have been proposed. The massive sulphide deposits of western Jalisco, Colima and Michoacan States are located within the Zituatanejo subterrane of the Guerrero terrane as defined by Ramirez et al. (1991) and Talavera et al. (1993), or the Nahuatl terrane as set out by Sedlock et al. (1993). The oldest rocks that outcrop are a series of zeolite to lower amphibolite facies metasedimentary and metavolcanic rocks that have been interpreted to be a magmatic arc/marginal basin assemblage which is likely Triassic to Middle Jurassic in age. This assemblage outcrops in the eastern portion of Guerrero and Mexico States and has informally been named the Tierra Caliente Complex by Ortega-Gutierrez (1981). Similar rocks are known near Arteaga in Michoacan State, where the name Arteaga Complex has been proposed (Centeno-Garcia, 1994).

The most recent regional mapping in the general vicinity of Cuale is in the Colima region, 200 km to the southeast (Centeno-Garcia, 1994). The oldest rocks are the Lower Cretaceous Tecalitlan, Alberca and Encino Formations, which are composed mostly of andesitic-basaltic lava flows with some rhyolite, interbedded with pyroclastic (intermediate tuffs and ignimbrites) and epiclastic deposits. This volcaniclastic sequence was deposited mostly in a submarine environment and records a major period of arc magmatism that hosts the volcanogenic massive sulphide deposits of western Mexico. The total thickness is unknown, but up to 2,400 metres has been measured from boreholes, without reaching the base. This volcanic activity decreased during the Early Albian, and almost ceased by the Mid-Late Albian. During Late Albian-Cenomanian time, thick calcareous sequences were deposited. One of the main formations during this period is the Tepalcatepec Formation. It is made up of relatively small limestone patches that are surrounded by lava flows, interbedded with horizons of volcaniclastic and rhythmically bedded clastic deposits, tuff, rhyolites, and minor evaporites. These units were deposited mostly in submarine and transi-

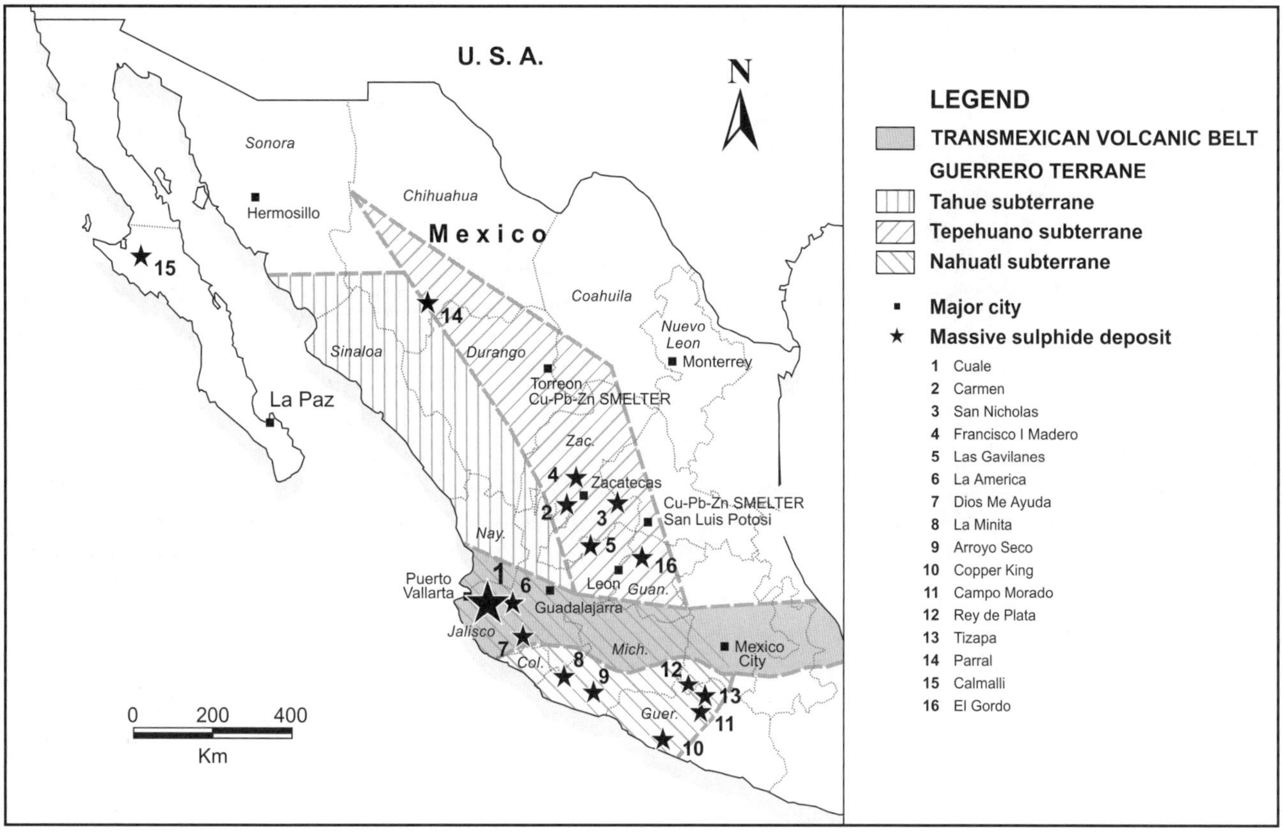

Figure 1. Volcanogenic massive sulphide deposits of the Guerrero terrane, Mexico

tional environments, with some subaerial layers recorded. The maximum observed thickness is 2,250 metres (Centeno-Garcia, 1994). The Albian-Cenomanian Madrid Formation consists of limestone, calcareous shale, gypsum and occasional andesitic flows and tuffs at the base. A borehole in central Colima State measured a 3,600 m section comprised mostly of limestone (Grajales and Lopez, 1984).

This stratigraphic package has been intruded by numerous mid-Cretaceous and Tertiary plutons, and is overlain unconformably by Tertiary volcanic rocks.

CUALE MINING DISTRICT

The Cuale District is hosted by a north-south elongated window, or roof pendant, which consists of Mesozoic volcanic and sedimentary rocks, and is roughly 25 by 5 km in size. Within this window are two felsic complexes that host the volcanogenic massive sulphide deposits of the Cuale and Bramador Districts. The Cuale District represents nineteen deposits that were in production, plus an additional six that received work in the past and may have recorded some minor production. They have been divided into three "camps" consisting of El Canton Mountain to the west, Mesa del Corozon in the centre and Descumbridora Mountain to the east.

The Bramador District is located 20 km to the south and hosts nine volcanogenic massive sulphide deposits (La Concha, La Trozada, Los Alpes, La Castellana, San Jose, Delicias, El Rosario, La Colaradas and San Pedro). Fifteen kilometres to the east in a smaller, separate window is the "Quatro Minas" (San Pedro, San Rafael, San Antonio and San Geronimo) of the Amaltea District.

Exploration and Mining History

Discovery of the Cuale District is credited to two local Indians searching for flint in the area of the Descumbridora Mountain in 1804. During the night one of them stole out with the samples, and took them to the Spaniards at Talpa de Allende. In 1810 the Spanish who had been operating the mines since 1805 were killed near Guadalajara when Mexican Independence was declared (Hoyle, 1919).

The earliest known claim on El Canton Mountain was registered on the Prieta orebody in 1823 (Table 1). The Prietita manto was discovered soon afterward, and both were worked intermittently by the Hernandez family (Beatty, 1899; Macomber, 1962; Chase, 1937).

In 1854 Jesus Camarena, a lawyer in Guadalajarra, who was engaged with the task of settling the estate of Luis Hernandez acquired the property and formed the "Union en Cuale Company". Norberto Vallarta was one of the initial shareholders (Hoyle, 1919). At the time Las Penas was a part-time fishing station located on Banderas Bay that supplied fresh fish to mining operations at Cuale. Through his friendship of Benito Juarez, then the President of Mexico, Jesus Camarena was able to secure a large harbor frontage on Banderas Bay, which in now Puerto Vallarta (Beatty, 1899).

The "Union en Cuale Company" operated the mines for 41 years until a drop in the price of silver forced their closing. Approximately 25 million ounces of silver were produced, mostly from the Preita orebody at a rate of 10 to 20 tonnes per day with a smaller tonnage coming from the lower grade La Prietita manto (Chase, 1937). Early in the history of the Prieta orebody the oxide ore (metal colorado) was exploited. Later production came from the primary sulphide minerals (Macomber, 1962).

Two tunnels were generally driven at a time, the upper tunnel was used for transportation and production, with the lower one for drainage, these were connected by raises to provide ventilation (Beatty, 1899). Shortly after the death of Jesus Camanera, in 1896 the lower workings were flooded due to one of the miners inadvertently breaking into La Prieta Fault. A disastrous mine fire later caused a large portion of the mine workings to cave in (Chase, 1937). Although a considerable amount of high-grade ore remained, the assets of the "Union en Cuale Company" were sold to Messers. Geist and Menzies for the relatively small sum of 60,000 pesos in 1898 (Chase, 1937).

Beginning at the time of Luis Hernandez the ores were treated at a several small reduction plants at San Francisco, which lay on the River Cuale. This site was chosen because it had a water supply steady enough to drive the water wheels that provided the milling power. From 1880 to 1882 there were twelve arrastras working in the district and in 1888 the process of lixiviation was introduced (Hoyle, 1919). During the time of "Union en Cuale Company" about 75 % of the silver was recovered and about eight tons of metal containing 80 % silver was transported to Guadalajara each month (Beatty, 1899).

Messers. Geist and Menzies had every intention of continuing the operation, however in 1900 when they learned that Felix Arrayze had registered the Estrella claim (which occupied the downdip extension to the Prieta orebody) they were so infuriated that drainage tunnel was dynamited to prevent Arrayze from entering the mine. The mine soon filled with water and, the lack of ventilation caused the timbers to rot. A later earthquake completed the damage (Chase, 1937).

Prior to 1919 a total of 35 mines had operated in the district, most of which were outside the lands controlled by the "Union en Cuale Company", but in total, their output did not equal that of the La Prieta (Hoyle, 1919).

The Esperanza Company took out an option in 1920, and in the early 1930's a syndicate comprised of Kennecott, Phelps-Dodge, and Real del Monte mapped and sampled the dumps (Chase, 1937). Minas de Penoles of Monterrey reopened two of the tunnels during the Second World War, and in 1954 Eagle Pitcher de Mexico carried out geological mapping and diamond drilling which lead to a much greater understanding of the district (Macomber, 1962).

Zimapan, S.A. de C.V. (a subsidiary of Industrias Peñoles S.A. de C.V.) acquired the Cuale District in 1965 and commenced exploration in 1971. Geological mapping was carried out 1972 along with a TURAM geophysical survey. Access roads were completed in 1975. From 1972 to 1978 a total of 215 drill holes, totaling 11,038 metres were completed mainly on the Chivos de Arriba, Chivos de Abajo, Socorredora, Naricero, Coloradita, Prieta and Minas del Oro (Grandeza) orebodies. This work indicated 1,471,000 tons of ore grading 1.15 g/t gold, 169 g/t silver, 1.27 % lead, 4.89 % zinc and 0.34 % copper, and on this basis a 20,000 tonne per month mill was commissioned in 1981 that operated until 1988

Table 1. Chronology of the mines and discoveries of the Cuale District

Mine	Deposit	Location	Date	Mine	Deposit	Location	Date
Carmen Tunnels	Carmen	Descumbridora	pre 1919	Las Tolvas Tunnel	La Prieta	El Canton	pre 1919
Cuepro Chivos Abajo	Chivos de Abajo	El Canton	1972	Upper Chivos Tunnel	La Prieta	El Canton	pre 1899
Los Chibos	Chivos de Arriba	El Canton	pre 1899	Lower Chivos Tunnel	La Prieta	El Canton	pre 1919
El Caldera Tunnels	El Caldera	Descumbridora	pre 1919	Coloradita Tunnel	La Prieta	El Canton	pre 1855
El Corazon Tunnel	El Corazon	El Canton	pre 1919	Obra de la Prieta	La Prieta	El Canton	pre 1899
	El Criste	El Canton	pre 1919	Prietita Obra	La Prieta	El Canton	pre 1899
	El Favor Copper	El Canton	pre 1899	Upper Prietita Tunnel	La Prieta	El Canton	pre 1899
Bolas Tunnel	El Oje de Agua	El Canton	pre 1919	Ancora Tunnel	La Prieta	El Canton	pre 1919
El Patrocinio Tunnels	El Patrocinio	El Canton	pre 1919	La Providencia Tunnel	La Providencia	Descumbridora	pre 1919
El Refugio Tunnel	El Refugio	El Canton	pre 1919	Bolas Drainage Tunnel	La Socorredora	El Canton	pre 1919
Esperanza Tunnel	Esperanza	El Canton	pre 1919		La Truenera	El Canton	pre 1919
Jesus Maria Tunnels	Jesus Maria	Descumbridora	pre 1899		La Zacaralampie	El Canton	pre 1919
	La Batalla	El Canton	pre 1919	Lower Paz Tunnel	Las Bolas	El Canton	pre 1919
	La Belle Aur 6	El Canton	pre 1919	Talpas Tunnels	Las Talpas	Descumbridora	pre 1919
Coloradita Tunnel	La Coloradita	El Canton	pre 1855	El Naricero Tunnel	Naricero	El Canton	pre 1919
Esperanza Tunnel	La Esperanza	El Canton	pre 1919	La Trinidad Tunnel	Naricero	El Canton	pre 1919
La Grandeza	La Grandeza	Descumbridora	pre 1919	Paz de Ceilo Tunnel	Paz de Ceilo	El Canton	pre 1962
La Guadalupe Tunnel	La Guadalupe	El Canton	pre 1919	Upper Paz Tunnel	Paz de Ceilo	El Canton	pre 1962
La Jesus Maria Tunnel	La Jesus Maria	El Canton	pre 1919	San Antonio Tunnels	San Antonio	Descumbridora	pre 1919
	La Lucema	El Canton	pre 1919	Lumbrera Tunnel	San Juan (?)	Descumbridora	pre 1899
Cristo Tunnel	La Paz / Cristo	El Canton	pre 1962	Lumbrerita Tunnel	San Juan (?)	Descumbridora	pre 1899
La Peregrina Tunnel	La Peregrina	Descumbridora	pre 1919	San Nicolas Tunnel	San Nicolas	El Canton	pre 1919
Jesus Tunnel	La Prieta	El Canton	1855	San Rafael Tunnel	San Rafael	El Canton	pre 1919
Esperanza Tunnel	La Prieta	El Canton	pre 1899		Vetarron	El Canton	pre 1962
Luz Tunnel	La Prieta	El Canton	pre 1899	Zapopan Tunnel	Zapopan	El Canton	pre 1919
Refugio Tunnel	La Prieta	El Canton	pre 1855		Zona de Pirita	El Canton	1972
Chorrillo Tunnel	La Prieta	El Canton	pre 1919				

Information from Beatty, 1899; Hoyle, 1919; Macomber, 1962

(Berrocal and Querol, 1991). Penoles continued its exploration efforts until 1990, and in total drilled 506 holes representing 28,500 metres, and mined almost 2.5 million tons of ore (Table 2).

In 1998 International Croesus Ventures Corp. was able to obtain a significant land position in the district through staking, and is currently studying the structure and stratigraphic setting of known deposits in order to commence a program of deep drilling.

Stratigraphy and Lithology

The most comprehensive mapping of the Cuale District was by a joint venture between the Japanese International Cooperation Agency and Metal Mining Agency of Japan (1986). Unless otherwise noted the nomenclature, most of the descriptions in this section are based on this work.

The oldest rocks are a series of Jurassic sediments that consist of pelitic schist, with intercalations of psammitic schist, sericite schist and chlorite schist. The base of this sequence is not exposed, but is estimated to be at least 800 metres thick (Berrocal and Querol, 1991).

An unconformity separates the Jurassic rocks from a shale-sandstone sequence that occurs within the Lower to Upper Cretaceous stratigraphy. These Cretaceous sediments host the dacite flows and pyroclastics, which are present throughout the sequence and form the volcanic edifaces. The thickness of this unit is estimated to be about 700 metres, with the

Table 2. Cuale District production figures (1980 to 1990)

Mine	Operation	Tonnes	Gold g/t	Silver g/t	Lead %	Zinc %	Copper %
Naricero	open pit	782,544	0.34	157	1.05	2.85	0.06
Grandeza	open pit	756,661	1.89	22	1.41	2.35	0.20
La Prieta-Rubi	underground	113,335	0.73	226	3.80	9.24	0.32
Socorredora	open pit	195,721	0.10	187	1.85	7.02	0.16
	underground	4,771	1.21	199	3.41	3.32	0.12
	total	200,492	0.13	187	1.89	6.93	0.16
Coloradita	open pit	170,055	0.66	85	1.99	6.51	0.37
Chivas de Abajo	open pit	85,771	1.08	179	1.48	4.71	1.54
Chivas de Arriba	open pit	23,588	2.79	70	0.85	2.18	0.74
Jesus Maria	open pit	46,751	0.06	109	1.85	3.31	0.09
Patrocinio	open pit	2,453	0.08	129	1.30	2.80	0.08
Caldera	open pit	13,004	0.90	140	0.09	0.20	0.01
Prietitas	open pit	13,662	0.16	139	2.25	5.30	0.22
Prietita	underground	2,401	0.15	34	1.72	3.43	0.11
	total	16,063	0.16	123	2.17	5.02	0.20
El Refugio	underground	34,569	0.14	156	0.89	1.95	0.10
San Nicolas	underground	79,965	0.19	121	1.57	3.18	0.13
San Rafael	underground	608	0.29	255	1.10	1.32	0.16
Las Talpas	underground	141,425	0.34	24	0.65	1.91	0.24
El Rosario	underground	473	1.25	84	0.19	0.15	0.06
San Pedro	underground	90	0.31	83	3.56	9.44	0.36
District Total		2,474,355	0.83	103	1.03	3.22	0.23

Data from Berrocal, Torres, and Franco 1990

dominant rock type an argillaceous shale.

The footwall dacite is the stratigraphically lowest volcanic unit. It is light gray to pale green, aphyric and locally weakly brecciated. Phenocrysts of quartz and plagioclase are locally abundant, with the matrix normally vitreous and devitrified. Phyllitic and/or argillic alteration in locally present in association with the massive sulphide deposits. Based on the geological cross sections the maximum thickness of this unit is estimated to be 500 metres.

The ore-zone pyroclastic unit is the most important stratigraphic interval in the district due to its proximity to the volcanogenic massive sulphide deposits. It is thought to represent a sequence of submarine pyroclastic flows that are very closely associated with the underlying footwall dacite lavas. In appearance they are pale green to gray, and mainly consisting of fine tuff, lapilli tuff and breccias that are intercalated with the shale beds. The lapilli tuff fragments are generally dacitic, however fragments of andesite, schist, mudstone and pumice have been observed. The estimated thickness of this unit is thought to be a maximum of 300 metres.

Overlying the ore-zone pyroclastic is the hanging-wall dacite pyroclastic. This unit consists of volcanic flows with overlying pyroclastic rocks consisting of fine tuff and tuff breccia. In appearance this unit is pale gray to gray in colour, and characterized by phenocrysts of quartz. The groundmass is glassy, cryptocrystalline, felsic and strongly silicified. The tuffs and tuff breccias exhibit grading on the scale of metres to tens of metres, and the maximum thickness of this unit is estimated to be 500 metres.

Tertiary rocks unconformably overlie the Cretaceous section with the base of this unit represented by a sandstone-conglomerate unit. Upwards, this package consists of a sequence of lavas and pyroclastics that alternate between andesite and dacite. Four distinct stages of andesitic volcanics are recognized, which are separated by three stages of dacitic lavas.

Granodiorite plutons have intruded the stratigraphy in the central portion of the Cuale window, and on the western and southern margins. They generally exhibit a phaneritic texture with euhedral quartz and feldspar along with variable amounts of biotite and hornblende. Isotopic dating indicates a range of 83 to 90 Ma (Gastil et al., 1979). Tertiary plugs of dacitic and andesitic composition have also intruded the central portions of the window.

Structure

Regionally the bedding trends north to northwest, with the dip undulating from 10 and 30°. A synclinal axis passes through the central portion of the Cuale District and any folds that are observed are generally broad open structures with wavelengths greater than 100 metres. Other small-scale folds are observed in the vicinity of faults. The steep paleotopography caused by the volcanic edifices results in steeper than normal attitudes for the contacts of some of the volcanic units.

A series of north-northwesterly trending normal faults cut the stratigraphy. The dip of these faults appears to be steep to the southwest, with displacements in the order of tens of metres. Another major structure, the La Preita Fault trends NE 52° and dips 50 – 65° to the northwest (Macomber, 1962). This structure can be traced for 2½ km and forms the northwesterly boundary of the Coloradita, La Prieta and Prietita orebodies (Fig. 2).

CUALE DISTRICT MINERAL PROPERTIES

El Canton Area

The most prolific portion of the Cuale District is the east slope of El Canton Mountain (elevation 2,380 metres). Within a southwesterly trending zone of the favorable stratigraphy measuring 2,500 by 800 metres there are ten massive sulphide deposits that were recently in production (Prieta, Preitita, Preititas, Chivos de Arriba, Chivos de Arriba, Coloradita, Socorredora, Naricero, El Refugio and San Nicolas). In addition, five other deposits have seen limited production in the past (Paz de Ceilo, Cristo, Vetarron, Polvorin and Las Bolas), or were deemed to be too low grade to mine (Zona de Pirita).

La Prieta

According to production figures in Table 2 and descriptions of the past production the La Prieta orebody has the highest grades in the district. Eight adits access a strike length of over 900 metres with the

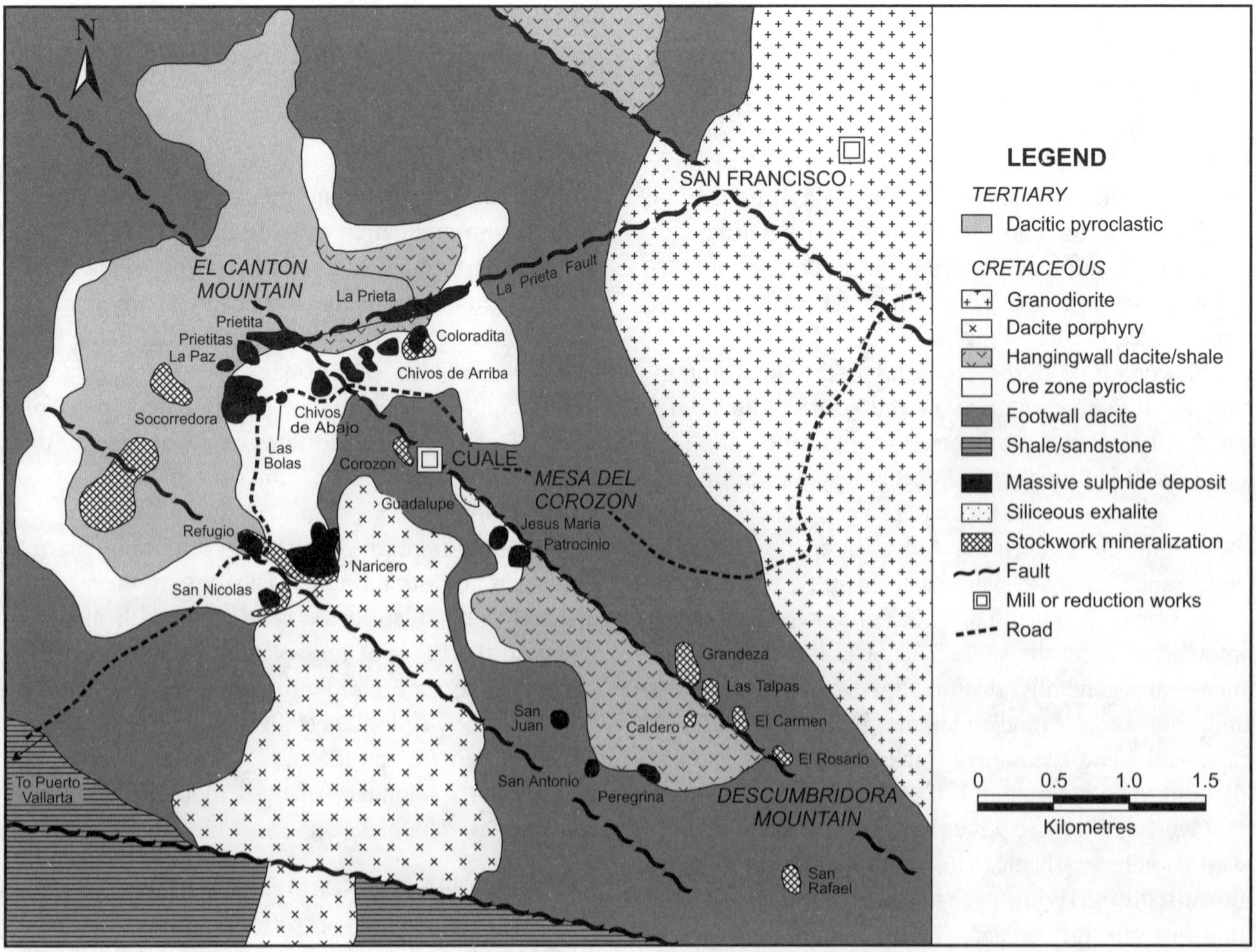

Figure. 2. Cuale District geology (modified from Japanese International Cooperation Agency and Metal Mining Agency of Japan, 1986)

early mining progressing from northeast to southwest.

The hangingwall stratigraphy is a massive to thick-bedded porphyritic rhyolite, with minor rhyolite tuff beds. The footwall consists mostly tuffs, felsic flows and argillaceous sediments (Macomber, 1962).

The orebody has been described as lying in the footwall of the La Prieta Fault (Macomber, 1962; Berrocal and Querol, 1991). The strike of the La Prieta Fault and the mineralization is N 50ºE, with the La Prieta Fault having a northerly dip of 65º. The work of Macomber (1962) suggests the dip of the mineralization steepens from 40º N on surface to 77º N over a vertical distance of roughly 200 metres. The plunge of the mineralization has been described as 40º to the west (Macomber, 1962). The shoots of massive sulphide mineralization range from a few centimetres to over 10 metres thick, 30 to 70 metres long, by 70 to 80 metres high (Berrocal and Querol, 1991).

The mineralization is zoned consisting of a silver-rich zone of massive sphalerite and galena that is between 0.5 and 4.0 metres in thickness at the hangingwall. Below this is a lower grade zone of massive pyrite that is 5 to 6 metres thick, which then grades into altered volcanic and sedimentary rocks over a 10 to 30 m interval (Macomber, 1962). Assay samples of the higher grade material range up to 1.8 g/t gold, 894 g/t silver, 15.1 % lead, 22.0 % zinc, with trace amounts of copper (Chase, 1937). Within the massive sulphides barite, tetrahedrite, stannite and chalcopyrite have been observed. Sedimentary banding is also

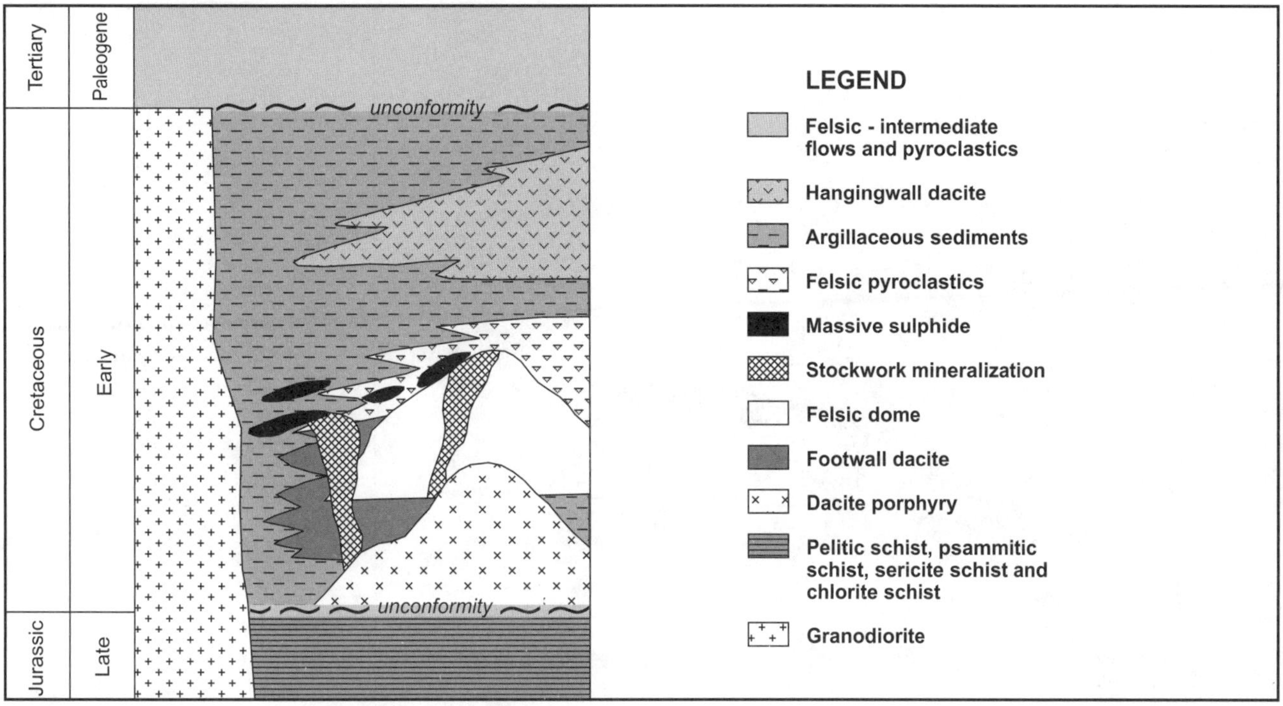

Figure 3. Stratigraphic column for the Cuale District (modified from Japanese International Cooperation Agency and Metal Mining Agency of Japan, 1986)

present (Lowther, 1949; Kirwin, 1982; Berrocal and Querol, 1991). Abundant disseminated sphalerite and galena has been observed in the argillaceous sediments to the footwall of the mineralization. Immediately above the mineralization is a zone of choritized clays with occasional elongated siliceous nodules, and a distinctly brecciated zone that appears to represent the La Prieta Fault (Berrocal and Querol, 1991).

There is some confusion as to the origin of the mineralization. The early references, when the mine workings were open, refer to the orebody as a vein hosted by the La Prieta Fault (Macomber, 1962). Figure 4 indicates the La Prieta orebody is the downdip extension to the Chivas de Arriba orebody (Berrocal and Querol, 1991). Portrayed in this cross section is a scenario whereby the Chivas de Arriba orebody was deposited at the edge of a submarine plateau and portions of it slide down accumulating along a slope to form an oreshoot of the La Prieta. The same scenario exists for the Coloradita orebody and another oreshoot of the La Prieta located to the east. It is suggested by Berrocal and Querol (1991) that these oreshoots accumulated independently along the slopes of a presumed submarine plateau.

Prietita and Prietitas

Access to the Prietita orebody was provided by approximately 1,500 metres of underground workings. Peñoles recommenced underground mining of the Prietita orebody in the early 1980's, along with the open pit mining of the Prietitas, which appears to be the surface manifestation of the Prieta orebody (Berrocal, 1985).

The geology of the Prietita orebody is very similar to the La Prieta orebody. The thickness averages about three metres, with the thickest portion being 15 metres. The maximum strike length as defined by the underground workings is 150 metres, and based upon these figures an orebody of about 300,000 tonnes can be inferred for the top 50 metres (Macomber, 1962). Assays for the massive sulphide mineralization vary from 1.0 – 2.0 g/t gold, 171 – 714 g/t silver, 1.3 – 19.7 % lead, 5 – 27.6 % zinc and 0.2 – 6.6 % copper. It was also noted that the lead and zinc content increase to the east, where the thickness of the mineralization is greatest (Macomber, 1962). The sulphide

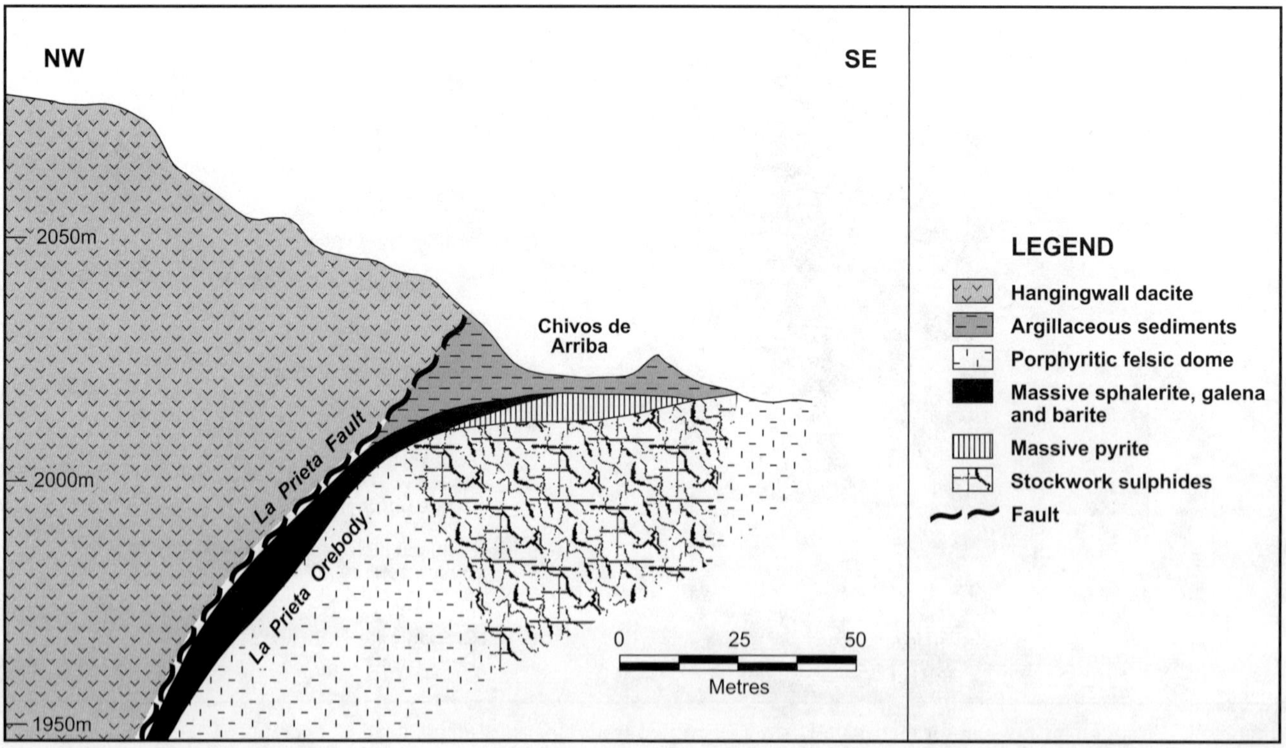

Figure 4. La Prieta and Chivos De Arriba Mines – Cross Section (modified from Berrocal and Querol, 1991)

mineralogy consists of pyrite, galena, sphalerite and chalcopyrite. The high-grade ore occurs as balls, small pipes and irregular streaks in an envelope of lower grade pyritic material (Macomber, 1962).

The Prietitas orebody has a northerly dip of 10º on surface, which steepens to 45º at a depth of 50 metres. The mineralization in the Preititas orebody is hosted by a porphyritic rhyolite tuff/breccia that appears to represent the upper volcanic sequence that lies above a disconformity. A massive porphyritic rhyolite lies approximately 20 metres above the mineralization; whereas to the footwall several thin bands of black shales are present.

In the Prietita orebody, the footwall rocks consist of thin-bedded to massive black shales and beds of metarhyolite, with the hangingwall consisting of a massive to thick-bedded quartz porphyritic felsic volcanic (Macomber, 1962). In the underground workings the mineralization appears to coincide with a zone of faults (La Prieta Fault) which are in part subparallel (dipping at 60ºN) with the stratigraphy and mineralization (Macomber, 1962).

Chivos de Arriba

The Chivas de Arriba orebody was discovered during the 1800's (Beatty, 1899), while driving the Lower Chivas Tunnel to provide ventilation and drainage to the La Preita orebody. At the time, the sulphide mineralization was considered to be too low grade to mine, but was later mined by Peñoles through open pit and underground operations during the early 1980's.

The stratigraphy is similar to the Coloradita consisting of the same basal rhyolite porphyry. This rhyolite dome is overlain by rhyolite porphyry tuff/breccia that is up to 25 metres thick and is the host to the massive sulphide mineralization. Overlying this sequence is a tuffaceous arenite that has been truncated by the La Prieta Fault (Fig. 4). On the hangingwall side of this fault is a rhyolite lapilli tuff. On surface the stratigraphy is generally flat lying, whereas in the underground workings to the north, the dip steepens to 45ºNW.

Sphalerite, galena, pyrite, chalcopyrite and barite are the main constituents of the massive sulphide mineralization. On surface the oxidized ore attains grades of 11.71 g/t gold over a 6.25 m thickness (Ontiveros, 1980). At depth one of the better drill intersections contained 0.78 g/t gold, 354 g/t silver, 5.29 % lead, 20.88 % zinc and 0.69 % copper over a 9.35 metre interval. In appearance the massive sulphide ore is brecciated and reworked, suggesting transport down a slope. Large blocks, up to 1.5 metres across consisting of sphalerite-galena-barite and massive pyrite are scattered in a fine-grained matrix of pyrite-chalcopyrite. The upper surface of the fragmental ore is ragged and is overlain by a clayey tuff that is less than one metre thick (Urabe, 1982). Adjacent to the massive sulphide mineralization in the footwall rhyolite porphyry is a well-developed pyrite-quartz stockwork zone (Kirwin, 1982).

Coloradita

Historically the Coloradita orebody has been interpreted as a massive sulphide vein that is situated at the junction of the La Prieta Fault and a crosscutting structure. The older workings consist of four tunnels that were relatively short and likely date from the time of the "Union en Cuale Company" (Macomber, 1962). During the late 1970's Peñoles drilled 22 surface and underground holes, and open pit mining was carried out between 1982 to 1984. Based upon this work the Colaradita is now considered to be a classic example of a proximal volcanogenic massive sulphide deposit (Berrocal and Querol, 1991).

The stratigraphy consists of a basal rhyolite porphyry that is characterized by phenocrysts of quartz and feldspar that are set in an aphanitic matrix. Overall this unit has the configuration of a domal structure. It is overlain by a porphyritic rhyolite breccia, which is composed of the same material as the underlying dome, and grades upward into a rhyolite tuff. Uppermost in the sequence is a tuffaceous sandstone, which represents a mixing of tuffaceous and sedimentary material.

The mineralization consists of two main lenses of massive sulphides that are draped over the top, and flank of the rhyolite dome. A vertical distance of roughly 20 metres separates these massive sulphide horizons. Several smaller discontinuous horizons (less than 1.0 metre thick) are also present. The lowermost horizon appears to be hosted by the porphyritic rhyolite breccia, and the upper horizon is hosted by the rhyolite tuff. The lower horizon is the largest, having the lateral dimensions of 120 by 80 metres, with an average thickness of 11.0 metres (Luna-Barcelo, 1979). Over the top portions of this dome the massive sulphide bodies dip at 15 to 35° to the southwest, steepening to 45 to 50° along the flank (Berrocal and Querol, 1991). Figure 5 shows the position of the La Prieta Fault, which in this case is completely unrelated to the mineralization, but does occur at roughly the same orientation as the massive sulphides.

A well-defined stockwork zone consisting of veins of pyrite, chalcopyite, sphalerite, galena and quartz underlie the massive sulphide horizons. Silicification and chloritization are the dominant forms of alteration, and the sulphide content is semi-massive, approaching massive over small intervals. Overlying the massive sulphide horizons is an altered zone that is not as intensely developed as the footwall zone. It consists of silicification and possibly kaolinite, with disseminated and veined sulphides.

The uppermost massive sulphide horizon appears to be lead-zinc rich, with some barite; whereas the lower horizon exhibits classic zoning patterns consisting of a lead-zinc rich top that is underlain by pyritic massive sulphides that are enriched in copper. Illustrating this point is Hole 40E from the central portion of the deposit, which contains 0.5 g/t gold, 129 g/t silver, 6.96 % lead, 18.43 % zinc and 0.37 % copper over the top 4.56 metres; and 0.54 g/t gold, 41 g/t silver, 0.32 % lead, 0.53 % zinc and 3.82 % copper over the bottom 6.15 metres (Ontiveros, 1980). The precious metal values appear to be hosted by tetrahedrite, along with native silver and gold. Silver and gold rich oxide zones occur where sulphide zones come to surface.

Chivos de Abajo

A TURAM electromagnetic survey conducted in 1971 initially located the Chivos de Abajo orebody. Drilling conducted by Penoles from 1972 through 1977, plus underground exploration resulted in the delineation of a small orebody that was mined by an open pit in 1982.

Two porphyritic rhyolite units are present which

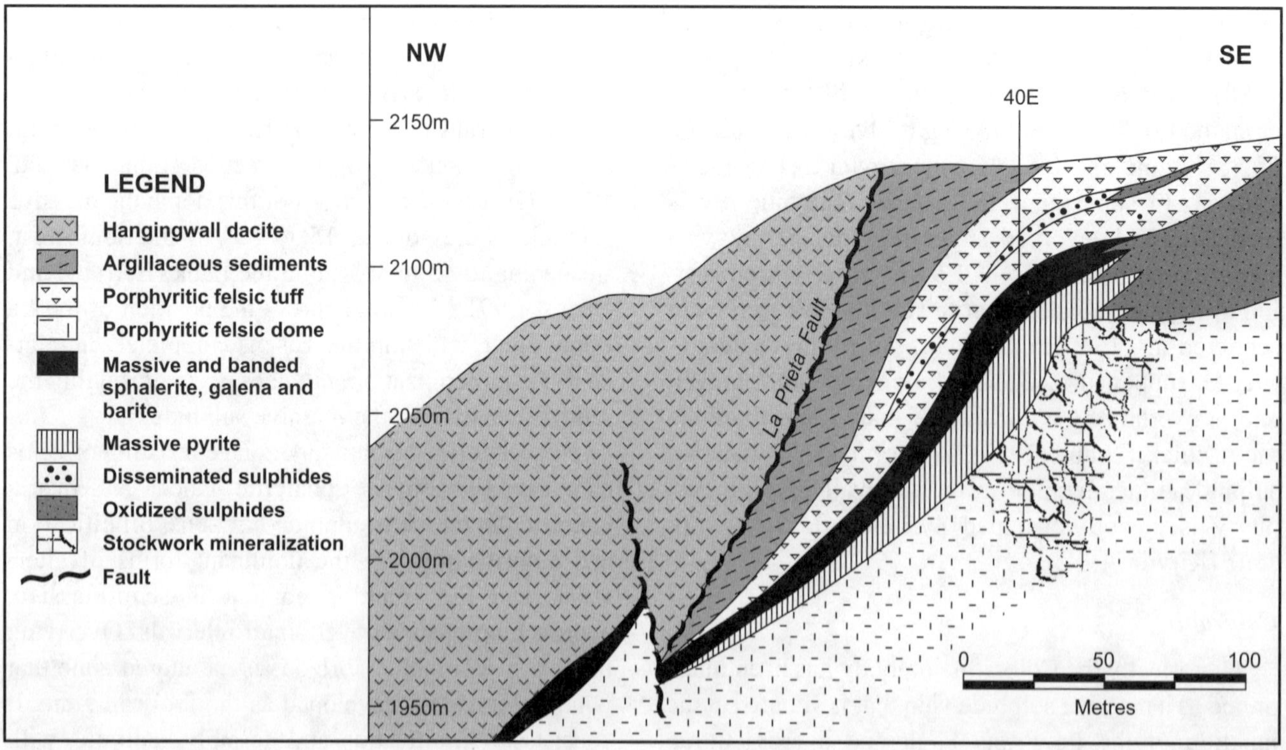

Figure 5. Coloradita Mine – Cross Section (modified from Kirwin, 1978)

are separated by approximately 20 metres of argillaceous sediments. Uppermost in the sequence is a felsic unit, which likely represents a tuff. Overall the stratigraphy is essentially flat-lying, with the northwestern extremity exhibiting a 10 to 20º degree dip to the north.

The argillaceous sediments are the host to several massive sulphide lenses. The internal structure of these lenses is quite complicated, as they appear to represent transported sulphide bodies. Typically the sulphides exhibit a fragmental texture. All the ore breccias are pyritic and show northeasterly imbrications that are hosted within a powdery pyrite-chalcopyrite matrix. The clast size is distinctly smaller than in the Chivas de Arriba orebody, averaging about 20 cm in diametre. Cross bedding at a 30º angle to bedding is consistent throughout the orebody (Urabe, 1982). A quartz-pyrite stockwork that is hosted by the basal porphyritic rhyolite and the lowermost portion of the argillaceous sediments represents the exhalative centre. Immediately to the west, within the argillaceous sediments is an oblate pod of massive fine-grained pyrite (Fig. 6). Further to the west is an overlapping pod of massive and banded fine-grained sphalerite, galena and barite. The horizon immediately above the massive sulphides contains "balls" and lenses of sphalerite, galena and barite along with siliceous carbonate nodules. Below the massive sulphide horizon the argillaceous sediments contain small concordant pyrite laminae (Urabe, 1982). In the centre of the deposit the massive pyritic mineralization is enriched in copper having grades of 71 g/t silver, 0.16 % lead, 0.83 % zinc and 1.90 % copper over 14.1 metres. The lead-zinc rich portions can grade up to 1,484 g/t silver, 3.56 % lead, 13.84 % zinc and 1.15 % copper over a thickness of 9.9 metres. It is suggested that this lateral zoning is also the result of the sulphides sliding down the slope of a rhyolitic dome, with the lead-zinc rich portions that likely formed on top of massive pyrite sliding the furthest (Kirwin, 1982; Urabe, 1982).

Zona de Pirita

The Zona de Pirita is a small pyritic orebody that was located by drilling in 1972, by the first hole of what became an eighteen-year drilling campaign by

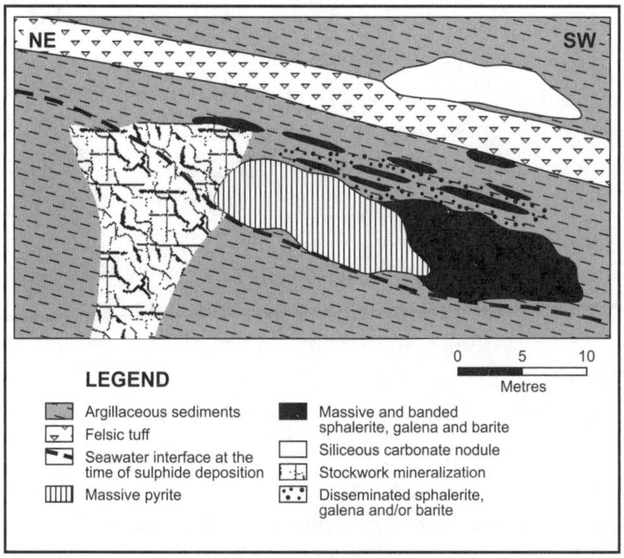

Figure 6. Chivos De Abajo Mine – Diagramatic cross section of the southeast face of the open pit (from Kirwin, 1982)

Peñoles. This hole encountered a 9.3 metre intersection of massive pyritic sulphides, but the grades and tonnage for this massive sulphide body were too low to justify mining.

The Zona de Pirita area represents the first appearance of basinal sediments outward from the rhyolite dome that underlies the Coloradita and Chivos de Arriba orebodies. The stratigraphic package consists of a 20 to 80 metre thick unit of argillaceous sediments that is enclosed by a porphyritic rhyolite. This argillaceous unit is host to the mineralization, which consists of massive pyrite, with lesser amounts of sphalerite, galena and chalcopyrite.

Las Bolas

The mine workings of the Las Bolas area consist of several short adits. These exploited a number of "concretionary balls" of massive sulphides which are similar to mineralization found in the Zona de Pirita and Chivas de Abajo orebodies, only smaller in size (the largest being only several hundred tons). They are found within the argillaceous sediments over a stratigraphic interval of 30 to 40 metres, and are sometimes stacked. According to the detailed mapping of Macomber (1962) this stratigraphic interval lies about 70 metres below the horizon that hosts the Socorredora deposit.

The mineralogy consists of massive pyrite, with lesser amounts of fine-grained sphalerite, galena and barite, with minor tetrahedrite and enargite (Macomber, 1962). Some pods are banded, and likely represent small lenses of stratiform sulphides, whereas others are zoned in a concentric fashion (Kirwin, 1982). A weighted average for the mineralization in Upper Bolas Tunnel which intersects one of these lenses indicates a grade of 0.26 g/t gold, 84 g/t silver, 0.39 % lead, 1.09 % zinc, with trace amounts of copper. Indicative of the higher grade material from the district, which was the target of early high-grading operations, are samples from the dump at the Bolas mine that assayed 752 g/t silver, 10.5 % lead, 35.8 % zinc and 1.11 % copper (Macomber, 1962).

La Paz

The workings consist of the two main tunnels (Upper and Lower Paz), plus three smaller adits, and a number of open cuts. The stratigraphy consists of an upper porphyritic rhyolite, which is underlain by 90 metres of argillaceous sediments, and finally a rhyolite tuff that is porphyritic. Sulphide bearing intervals occur over the entire stratigraphic interval represented by the argillaceous sediments, with a 2.5 m interval of massive sulphides grading 0.23 g/t gold, 47 g/t silver, 0.78 % lead, 25.8 % zinc and 0.13 % copper occurring near the top. Within the footwall rhyolite tuff are quartz veinlets containing pyrite and chalcopyrite within a zone of chloritic alteration.

Socorredora

The Socorredora Deposit is typical of a distal-type massive sulphide deposit (Fig. 7). It consists of a series of massive sulphide lenses in which the sulphides are well bedded, and occur in argillaceous sediments that are well removed from an alteration zone. Around the turn of the century a number of independent operators high-graded this deposit through a series of irregular tunnels. Following drilling campaigns by Peñoles between 1973 – 1982, the deposit was mined by a large open pit from 1982 to 1984.

The stratigraphic package consists of a porphyritic rhyolite tuff that is overlain by a series of intercalated argillaceous sediments, tuffaceous argillites and rhyolite tuffs. Above this is a small unit of rhyolite lapilli tuff that appears to have a disconformable contact with the overlying porphyritic quartz latite. The thicker intervals of the argillaceous sediments are up to forty metres, with the rhyolite tuffs seldom exceeding ten metres. The thickest unit is the porphyritic quartz latite that is more than 120 metres. Overall the shape resembles an inverted bowl with the bedding in the central portion of the deposit flat-lying, but at the edges dipping at 10 - 30°.

The massive sulphide mineralization occurs in three horizons that are roughly elliptical in shape, tapering gradually in all directions. The lower horizon is hosted entirely by the upper sequence of argillaceous sediments. The middle horizon is the largest and occurs at the top of the upper sequence of argillaceous sediments in the northern portion of the deposit, but appears to upwardly transgress the stratigraphy into the overlying porphyritic rhyolite tuffs in the central and southern portions. This horizon is the largest measuring roughly 150 by 200 metres, with a maximum thickness of 11 metres. The upper horizon is only present in the southern extremity of the deposit, and is less than two metres thick.

Within these horizons the sulphides generally occur as disseminated aggregates, lenticular aggregates, and discrete crystals (Urabe, 1982; Kirwin, 1982). The mineralogy consists of pyrite, sphalerite, galena, chalcopyrite, barite, quartz and gypsum, plus minor amounts of boulangerite, tennantite and stromeyerite that are generally associated with the galena. Within some of the bands of massive sphalerite, colloform nodules of chalcopyrite are present, and in the argillaceous sediments discrete grains of sphalerite that are rimmed by barite have been observed (Kirwin, 1982). The copper and gold grades are distinctly lower than the other deposits in the district (Ontiveros, 1980), and there does not appear to be a zoning pattern for the base metals within the sulphide horizons (Berrocal and Querol, 1991). The silver and gold grades are distinctly higher in the southern portion of the deposit. One of the better intersections from the central portion of the deposit contains

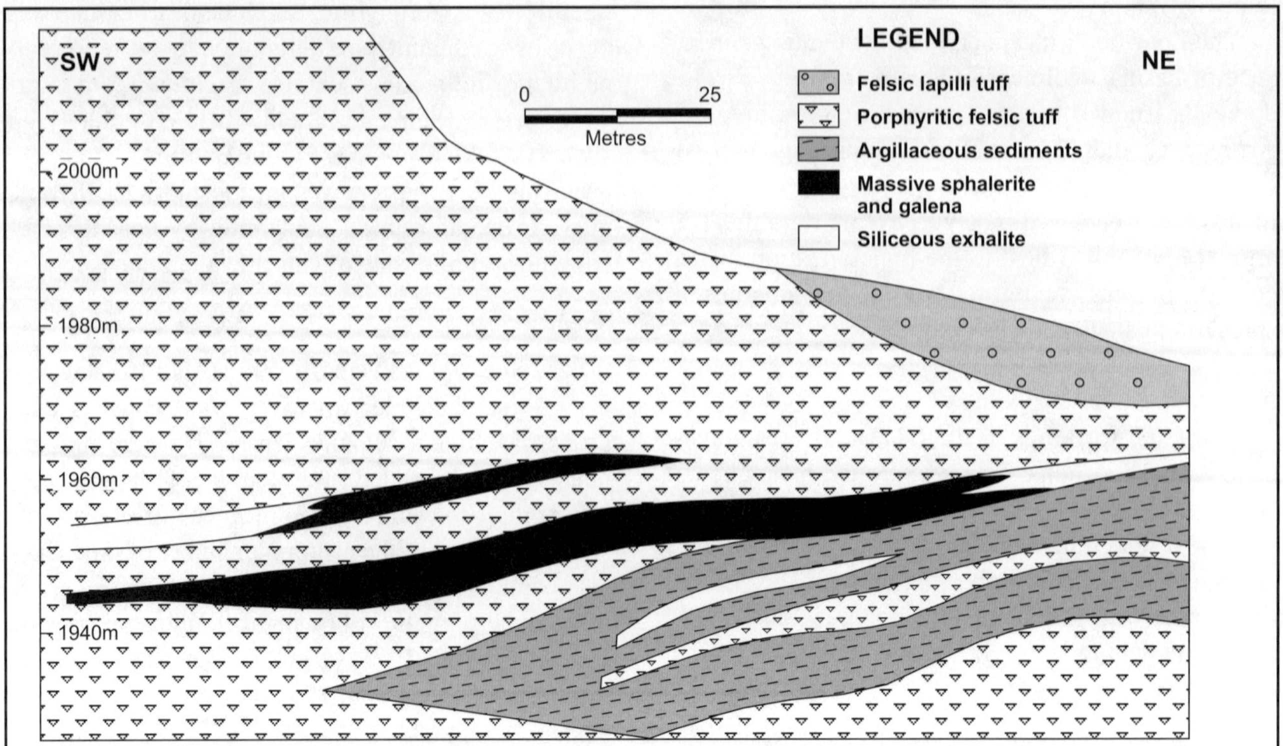

Figure 7. Socorredora Mine – Cross Section (modified from Ontiveros, 1978)

1.1 g/t gold, 835 g/t silver, 9.42 % lead, 24.44 % zinc and 0.33 % copper over a 4.22 metre interval (Ontiveros, 1980).

Naricero

The Naricero deposit was the largest producer for the district (Fig. 8). During the early to mid 1900's it was high-graded by small underground operations that were run by a number of independent operators. Penoles conducted a number of drilling campaigns between 1974 and 1989, and commenced mining on a larger scale through underground and open pit methods between 1982 and 1987.

The stratigraphic succession for the Naricero deposit is similar to the Socorredora in that the mineralization is hosted by an intercalated sequence of argillaceous sediments and porphyritic rhyolite tuffs. Above this is a thick interval of porphyritic quartz latite that appears to have a disconformable contact with the underlying stratigraphy. The argillaceous sediments are up to 30 metres thick, whereas the porphyritic rhyolite tuffs tend to be thinner. A rhyolite dome is located approximately 150 metres to the north, and may have a bearing on the origin of this deposit. The bedding is undulating, but in general dips to the northeast between 10 and 25°. A number of northeasterly dipping normal faults have dissected the stratigraphy, producing offsets up to 30 metres (Berrocal and Querol, 1991). These faults do not appear to be present in the overlying porphyritic quartz latite, and might be contemporaneous with the formation of the ore (Urabe, 1982). A large alteration zone consisting of veins, veinlets and disseminations of pyrite, along with chloritization, sericitization and intense silification is lies immediately under the Naricero deposit.

The massive sulphides are contained within two horizons that are separated by a stratigraphic interval of 30 metres. The argillaceous sediments are the preferred host, although some portions transgress into the rhyolite tuffs. The lower horizon is the thickest, and more laterally extensive having the dimensions of 390 by 195 metres, with an average thickness of 2.7 metres (Luna-Barcelo, 1979). The mineralization is composed of subangular fragments of massive and disseminated sulphides with reworked volcanic mate-

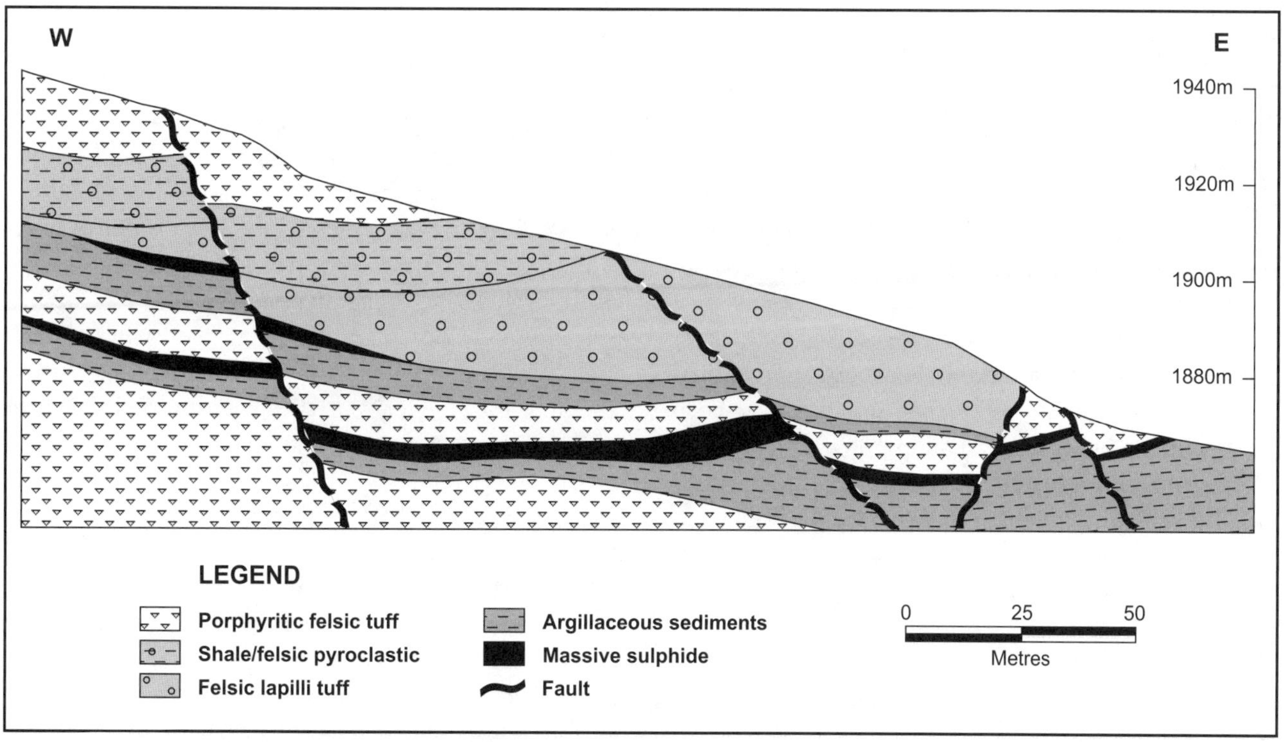

Figure. 8. Naricero Mine – Cross Section (modified from Ontiveros, 1980)

rial (Kirwin, 1982). According to Berrocal and Querol (1991) the mineralogy exhibits a "fragmental transported" texture in which the principal ore minerals are disseminated or evenly sized large sphalerite grains with chalcopyrite exsolutions and veinlets, as well as mixed pyrite-galena grains. Sphalerite is more abundant than pyrite, with the galena content very low. Lesser amounts of tetrahedrite-tennantite, geocronite and proustite-pyrargyrite are also present. The overall grade is relatively low; however one of the better grade intersections did contain 0.94 g/t gold, 500 g/t silver, 3.08 % lead, 18.76 % zinc and 0.37 % copper over a 3.25 metre interval. This material was likely indicative of the higher-grade ore that was exploited by the early independent operators.

San Nicolas

The workings of the San Nicolas deposit consist of two short adits, plus several open cuts. They are located to the west of a northerly trending arroyo that hosts a major fault. The stratigraphy and structure consists of a westerly dipping rhyolite porphyry at the base that is overlain by an intensely altered chloritic tuff, and a thick interval of rhyolite tuff on top. Adjacent to the adit, to the west of the arroyo is a five metre thick stratabound sequence of rocks that are intensely silicified and, altered to chlorite and sericite. This also contains disseminated and veined pyrite, sphalerite and galena. Samples of this material carry up to 2.4 g/t gold, 356 g/t silver, 2.9 % lead, 0.54 % zinc and 0.21 % copper (Mendoza-Hdez, 1985). Samples from one of the waste dumps consist of massive coarse-grained sphalerite and galena, with trace amounts of pyrite and chalcopyrite. The recrystallized, or coarse-grained appearance of these rocks suggests a thermal metamorphic overprinting that could have been caused by the underlying dacite porphyry.

In the general vicinity of the San Nicolas deposit are the underground workings of the Refugio and Esperanza, both of which are thought intersect small massive sulphide deposits.

Mesa del Corozon Area

The Mesa del Corazon area occupies a series of small plateaus that are roughly in the centre of the Cuale District. Three small massive sulphide occurrences (Jesus Maria, Patrocinio and Mesa del Corazon) are present. These occur in the ore-zone pyroclastic unit that is a continuation of the stratigraphy hosting the San Juan deposit to the south.

Jesus Maria

As with most of the early mining efforts, the oxidized ore of the Jesus Maria had been initially worked from surface, or by short adits. During the late 1950's there were four tunnels in the area (Macomber, 1958). Penoles conducted drilling over an area measuring 175 by 150 metres in 1977 and 1984, and between 1982 - 1983 most of the ore had been removed by open pit mining.

The stratigraphy consists of a porphyritic rhyolite that is overlain by a thin (10 – 40 metre thick) unit of felsic breccia (Fig. 9). This in turn is overlain by a porphyritic quartz latite. Two stratiform lenses of massive sulphide mineralization are present consisting of pyrite, sphalerite and galena that range from 2 to 10 metres in thickness. Both the stratigraphy and mineralization strike north-south and dip at about 30° to the west, steeping to 50° in the westernmost portion. The upper horizon is situated at the contact between the felsic breccia and porphyritic rhyolite. A small tonnage of 43,000 tonnes grading 0.34 g/t gold, 182 g/t silver, 1.47 % lead, 3.35 % zinc and 0.15 % copper was outlined in the upper horizon by the 1977 drilling (Ontiveros, 1980). Grades in the thicker portions of this lens attained 0.37 g/t gold, 134 g/t silver, 3.54 % lead, 9.44 % zinc and 0.33 % copper over an 8.55 metre thickness. However to the east, in the up-dip direction the mineralization becomes considerably thinner (approximately 1.0 metre) with the base metal grades dropping off to 0.10 % lead, 0.24 % zinc and 0.03 % copper, but the precious metal values increasing to 0.5 g/t gold and 428 g/t silver.

To the south, the 1984 drilling outlined two stacked orezones that were hosted by the porphyritic rhyolite, plus some additional mineralization in the overlying felsic breccia. This mineralization has been described (Berrocal-Gonzalo, 1984) as consisting of veinlets and disseminations of pyrite, sphalerite and galena that are hosted by a zone of silicification and argillic alteration. Significant intersections include a 2.7 metre thick section grading 0.06 g/t gold, 12 g/t

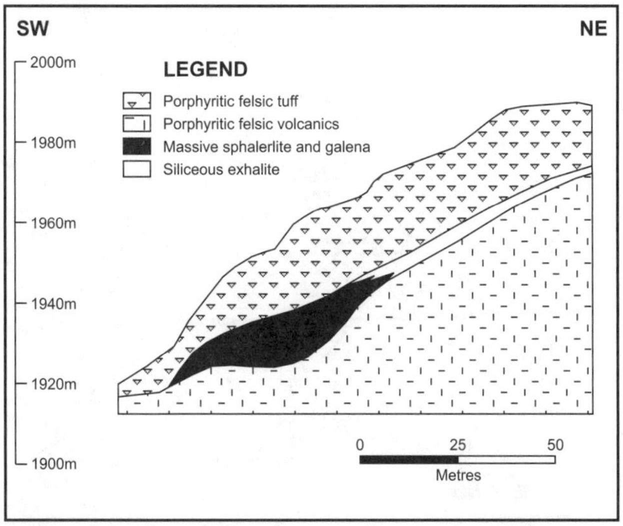

Figure 9. Jesus Maria – Cross Section (modified from Ontiveros, 1980)

silver, 3.39 % lead, 4.69 % zinc and 0.06 % copper (Berrocal-Gonzalo, 1984). It is likely this mineralization represents a feeder zone to the overlying massive sulphide mineralization.

Patrocinio

The Patrocinio is located approximately 250 metres to the southeast of the Jesus Maria, and likely represents a continuation of this mineralization. Four short adits (less than 50 metres long) are present. These adits along with a minor amount of drilling that was completed by Peñoles in 1977 and 1983 outlined a small resource of 3,444 tonnes grading 4.07 g/t gold, 791 g/t silver, 1.59 % lead, 4.75 % zinc and 0.13 % copper (Luna-Barcelo, 1978a).

The stratigraphy consists of a porphyritic rhyolite that is overlain by porphyritic quartz latite that grades into a rhyolite breccia to the east. The mineralization is confined to a westerly dipping stratiform zone that is up to four metres thick. Samples from the waste dump contain veinlets of sphalerite, galena and pyrite that are hosted by a pervasively silicified rhyolite (Kirwin, 1982). Significant intersections include a 4.40 metre section grading 0.35 g/t gold, 93 g/t silver, 3.40 % lead, 8.10 % zinc and 0.20 % copper (Luna-Barcelo, 1978a). As with the lower zones of the Jesus Maria this mineralization appears to be hosted by the porphyritic rhyolite and likely represents the same stratigraphic interval.

Guadalupe

The workings for the Guadalupe consist of an adit that is over 150 metres in length, plus several inclined winzes. According to Macomber (1962) these workings developed a manto that was located within a thin-bedded metachert (argillite) which lies beneath a massive metarhyolite. A small tonnage of hand picked material that was reported to contain 2 kilograms per tonne silver was taken out prior to 1936, and a sample from a small pile of siliceous material from the dump averaged 273 g/t silver and 0.5 g/t gold (Chase, 1937).

Corozon

Underlying the general office at the Cuale millsite is a northerly trending zone of stockwork mineralization measuring 60 by 150 metres. The workings are located to the northwest of this zone and, consist of a shaft, plus a number of short adits and open cuts (Macomber, 1962). Drilling conducted by Peñoles in 1978 intersected three narrow zones containing native copper, cuprite and malachite (Kirwin, 1982) that assayed up to 7.10 % copper over 1.85 metre interval (Luna-Barcelo, 1978b). Channel sampling conducted in 1985 by Penoles on an oxide zone northwest of the general office produced intervals longer than seven metres grading better than 1.0 g/t gold. The stratigraphy hosting this mineralization consists of a felsic tuff/breccia that appears to be overlain by a rhyolite.

Descumbridora Area

Situated on the east slope of Descumbridora Mountain in the eastern portion of the Cuale District are a large number of stockwork zones. Further down the hill to west are several massive sulphide deposits that occur in the overlying stratigraphy. A total of 41 old workings are known in this area, most of which consist of shallow openings and shafts. During the mid-1930's there were five small mills and approximately 150 men produced about 1½ kilograms of gold a week.

The stockwork zones are represented by the Grandeza (Minas del Oro), Las Talpas, El Caldero, El Rosario, El Carmen and San Rafael deposits, and are hosted by a porphyritic rhyolite unit that represents the footwall stratigraphy to the massive sulphide deposits. The strike extent of these deposits between the Grandeza, and San Rafael is approximately 1,300 metres. Generally these stockwork deposits consist of a crosscutting array of sulphide veins and veinlets consisting of pyrite, sphalerite, galena and chalcopyrite that in general have a steep southwesterly dip. In some cases chlorite, sericite and silicification envelope the sulphide veins. The smaller deposits such as the El Caldera, El Roserio, El Carmen and San Rafael vary from small irregular stringers, to pipes five to six metres in diametre that can be stoped for more than 30 metres (Macomber, 1962). Supergene enrichment has enhanced the precious metal grades significantly. In the case of the No. 1 adit of the San Rafael a weighted average over 17.2 metres graded 0.36 g/t gold, 236 g/t silver, 0.40 % lead, 0.29 % zinc and 0.16 % copper. Gold grades in the range of 12 - 14 g/t have been obtained from hand picked samples (Macomber, 1962).

The massive sulphide deposits of the Descumbridora camp include the Peregrina, Lumbrera, San Juan and San Antonio.

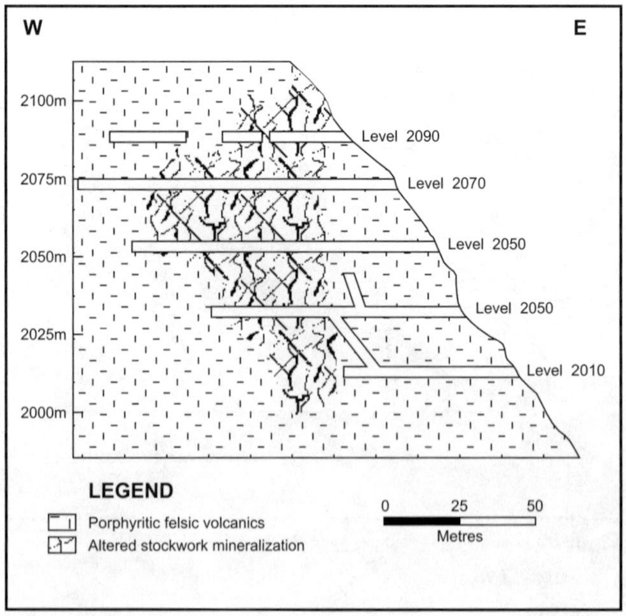

Figure 10. Grandeza (Minas Del Oro) Mine – Cross Section (modified from Berrocal and Querol, 1991)

Grandeza (Minas del Oro)

It was largest producer in the Descumbridora camp, and ranks second overall for the Cuale District. The orebody is roughly elliptical in outline, 20 to 50 metres wide, by more than 125 metres long in a north-south direction, and 70 metres high. Five tunnels access the Grandeza orebody at various elevations (Fig. 10). Peñoles conducted drilling between 1976 and 1982, and mined the deposit as a large open pit during the mid-1980s.

The ore occurs in seams, pockets and pipes within a shattered quartz porphyry in which the groundmass has been altered to a mixture of sericite and quartz (Kirwin, 1982). The gold and zinc values tend to be erratic occurring in narrow (1-2 mm to 10 cm thick) irregular, multidirectional veinlets and veins. The most abundant sulphide minerals are pyrite and sphalerite. The pyrite generally appears as idiomorphic crystals that are generally fractured. The sphalerite commonly has inclusions of galena, chalcopyrite and pyrite (Berrocal and Querol, 1991). The oxidized ore consists of a mixture of limonite, vuggy quartz, kaolin and barite (Macomber, 1962). Also present are bornite, covellite and native gold (Berrocal and Querol, 1991).

Las Talpas

The Las Talpas is located approximately 150 metres to the southeast of the Grandeza orebody. The mineralization is confined to two steeply dipping pipe-like bodies consisting of veined and disseminated sulphides that appear to be elongated in a northwesterly direction. They have a vertical extent in excess of 100 metres and are 10 to 25 metres wide. The host rock is a porphyritic rhyolite that is crosscut by a series of felsic dykes. The workings consist of five adits, from which a number of underground holes were drilled. In the Talpa No.4 tunnel one of the better intersections contained 0.15 g/t gold, 29 g/t silver, 1.04 % lead, 1.58 % zinc and 0.54 % copper over a 16.5 metre interval. Reserve calculations carried out in 1988 indicated roughly 200,000 tonnes of material grading 1.82 g/t gold, 67 g/t silver, 1.15 % lead, 1.34 % zinc and 0.10 % copper (Bravo-Medina, 1988).

Lumbrera

The Lumbrera claim was one of the first claims to be located in the District and was in production by the

"Union en Cuale Company". From 1891 to 1897 it produced 693 tons of ore (Beatty, 1899). A Company Report dated 1891 states the following "*the strike of the Lumbrera vein is given as N 70° E, and the dip 46° to 58° to the NW*" and "*The ores occur in shales. The minerals which predominate are galena, silver sulphides, black blende (sphalerite), and copper pyrites (chalcopyrite). The width of the vein is reported to be 26 metres*" (Hoyle, 1919). Although the present location of this mine is not known, based upon the description, it would appear to be in the general vicinity of the San Juan deposit.

San Juan

The workings of the San Juan mine consist of eleven short adits, plus a number of open cuts that can be traced for approximately 250 metres along the contact between a rhyolite breccia and the underlying rhyolite porphyry. An old millsite dating back to the early 1800's is also present, suggesting that the San Juan may in fact be the Lumbrera deposit.

The stratigraphy consists of a basal unit of massive gray rhyolite porphyry, which varies from porphyritic to aphanitic. In places this unit is strongly silicified, and contains finely disseminated pyrite. It is reported that a possible unconformity separates this unit from a cream coloured rhyolite that contains minor phenocrysts of quartz. A moderate amount of silicification is present in this unit, along with veinlets of quartz. The uppermost unit representing the hanging-wall to the massive sulphides is a yellow coloured rhyolite tuff/breccia that contains phenocrysts of quartz and fine grains of feldspar. In general the stratigraphy strikes to the north-northwest, and dips to the west at 34° (Mendoza-Hdez, 1985).

The thickness of the mineralization varies from 70 cm to 2.0 m, and is generally comprised of finely disseminated pyrite, sphalerite and galena that is hosted by quartz. In places the sulphides become massive to semi-massive, and exhibit a variety of replacement textures such as crosscutting veins and large clots of pyrite, which are up to 2 centimetres in diametre. In the southernmost adits, barite and quartz are present. Silver is the main commodity of interest. Sampling of the waste dumps in 1985 by Penoles indicated an average grade of 0.21 g/t gold, 142 g/t silver, 0.28 % lead, 0.04 % zinc and 0.02 % copper (Mendoza-Hdez, 1985), which is consistent with grades obtained through drilling.

Peregrina and San Antonio

The Peregrina and San Antonio prospects are located within the ore-zone pyroclastic unit, and occur along the contact between a rhyolite breccia and the underlying rhyolite porphyry. Two short adits, plus a number of shallow open cuts are present at the Peregrina and San Antonio. On surface the mineralization at the San Antonio is very oxidized and has been described as disseminated pyrite that is associated with a series of quartz veinlets. These quartz veinlets occur over an 80 centimetre thickness. Silver is main economic commodity, with the average grade of 948 tonnes at the San Antonio waste dumps of 0.6 g/t gold, 374 g/t silver, 0.09 % lead, 0.11 % zinc and 0.01 % copper.

SUMMARY

The Cuale District exhibits similar characteristics to the Kuroko volcanogenic massive sulphide deposits of Japan. The abundance of the deposits in the Cuale district that display a variety of different diagnostic features, plus the paucity of deformational and metamorphic complications has created an ideal setting for the study of this class of deposit.

The Cuale massive sulphide deposits are Lower Cretaceous in age, and bear a spatial and likely a genetic relationship to the felsic volcanism of the ore-zone pyroclastic unit. They appear to be related to the explosive rhyolitic domes, but are most abundant in adjacent basinal settings composed of argillaceous sediments. The mineralization appears to be restricted to a relatively short period of time that is represented by less than one hundred metres of sedimentary stratigraphy.

The deposits occur in a number of different settings. The stockwork mineralization is generally restricted to the porphyritic rhyolite of the footwall statigraphy (Grandeza, Los Talpas, El Caldera, El Roserio, El Carmen, San Rafael, Coloradita, Chivas de Arriba and Naricero deposits). This form of mineralization consists of disseminations, and crosscutting veinlets and veins of sulphides (pyrite, chalcopyrite, sphalerite and galena) that are enclosed in sericitic, chloritic and silicified zones. Immediately beneath the massive sulphide mineralization this form of mineralization coalesces to create a dense stockwork sulphide veins and silicification (Jesus Maria, San Juan, Patrocinio, Chivas de Arriba and Coloradita deposits). In the proximal deposits (Coloradita, Chivas de Arriba, Jesus Maria and La Prieta) the overlying massive sulphide mineralization is zoned with "yellow ore" (pyrite-chalcopyrite) lying beneath the "black ore" (sphalerite-galena). Transported sulphides that are inferred to have slid down the paleotopographic slopes occur along the flanks of the rhyolite domes, and in the adjacent sedimentary basins (Chivos de Abajo, Naricero and Las Bolas). Distal massive sulphide deposits such as the Socorredora and possibly the Las Bolas exhibit fine sedimentary features, and are well removed from the exhalative centres. A siliceous exhalite consisting of quartz, with elevated values precious metal values occurs distal to the massive sulphide deposits (Corazon, Guadalupe, San Nicolas, Peregrina, San Juan and San Antonio). Supergene enrichment of gold and silver in the oxidized portions has resulted in bonanza type grades for the early producers that are especially evident in the siliceous exhalite deposits.

ACKNOWLEDGEMENTS

A number of individuals have helped in the preparation of this manuscript such as my colleges at International Croesus Ventures Corp. Bob Cathro and Greg Crowe whose insights seemed to take less time to formulate than the authors. David Jennings of Farallon Resources Ltd. is thanked for his editorial comments, as are the two reviewers of this manuscript Tina Roth and Ross Sherlock. The exploration team headed by Matt Wunder of Noranda Exploracion, Mexico, S.A. de C.V. provided important insights into the district, as did Enrique Ontiveros and Martin Garcia, the caretaker at Cuale. Industrias Peñoles S.A. de C.V. is thanked for providing access to the property and the information.

REFERENCES

Beatty, E.C. 1899. Report on the property of the "Union in Cuale Company" State of Jalisco, Mex. Compania Minera Penoles Report.

Berrocal G. L. and Querol, F.S. 1991. Geological description of the Cuale District ore deposits, Jalisco, Mexico. The Geology of North America, Vol. P-3 Economic Geology, Mexico, The Geological Society of America, 1991 pp. 355-363.

Berrocal-Gonzalo, L. 1984. Zimapan S.A. de C.V., Company Report, March 29, 1984.

Berrocal L.G., Torres, G.D. and Franco, S.M. 1990. Zimapan, S.A. de C.V. Company Report.

Bravo-Medina, N. 1988. Zimapan S.A. de C.V., Company Report.

Centeno-Garcia, E. 1994. Tectonic evolution of the Guerrero Terrane, Western Mexico. University of Arizona, Ph.D. thesis, 220 p.

Chase, P.W. 1937. Prieta, Prietita, Socorredora & other mines, Cuale District, Jalisco. Compania Minera de Penoles S.A. Company Report, 24 p.

Coney, P.J 1983. Un modelo tectonico de Mexico y sus relaciones con America del Norte, America del Sur y el Caribe. Revista del Instituto Mexicano del Petrolio, vol. 15(1), pp. 6-15.

Gastil, G.D., Krummenbacher, M.A. and Jensky, H. 1979. Reconnaissance geology of West-Central Nayarit, Mexico. Summary: Geological Society of America Bulletin, vol. 90, pp. 15-18.

Grajales, M. and Lopez, M. 1984. Estudio petrogenetico de las rocas igneas y metamorficas en el Prospecto Tomatlan-Guerrero-Jalisco en Chihuahua, Durango y Coahuila. Association Mex. De Geol. Petr., Bulletin vol. XLII, no. 2, pp.1-18.

Hoyle, C. 1919. Report on properties of "LA UNION EN CUALE". Company Report, 55 p.

Japan International Cooperation Agency / Metal Mining Agency of Japan 1986. Report on the Cooperative Mineral Exploration in the Jalisco Area, The United Mexican States.

Kirwin, D.J. 1982. Investigation Report Concerning "Kuroko Type" Massive Sulphide Mineralization at Cuale, Jalsico. Compania Fresnillo S.A. de C.V. Company Report.

Lowther, G.K. 1949. Notes on the Cuale Area, Jalisco, May 4, 1949. Company Report, 9 p.

Luna-Barcelo, R. 1978a. Zimapan S.A. de C.V., Company Report, April 26, 1978.

Luna-Barcelo, R. 1978b. Zimapan S.A. de C.V., Company Report, May 6, 1978.

Luna-Barcelo, R. 1979. Yacimientos Minerales y Exploracion del Cuepro "Naricero" en el Distrito Cuale, Mpio. De Talpa de Allende, Jalisco. I.P.N. Tesis Profesional.

Macomber, B.E. 1958. Summary of Exploration at Cuale, Jalisco. Eagle Pitcher de Mexico, S.A. de C.V., Company Report, May 26, 1958.

Macomber, B.E. 1962. Geology of the Cuale Mining District, Jalisco, Mexico. Rutgers * The State University, Ph.D. Thesis, New Brunswick, New Jersey, U.S.A. 386 p.

Mendoza-Hdez, H. 1985. Compania Fresnillo S.A. de C.V., Company Report.

Ontiveros, E. 1978. Seccion Geologica, Barrenos 4-P, 4-O, 4-H, 4-D Area Socorredora. Zimapan, S.A., Company Report.

Ontiveros, E. 1980. Estudio geologico de exporacion del distrito minero de Cuale. Etado de Jalisco, Mexico. Tesis Profesional, University Autonoma de San Luis Potosi, Mexico.

Ortega-Guiterrez, F. 1981. Metamorphic belts of southern Mexico and their tectonic significance. Geofisica Internacional, vol. 20, pp. 177-202.

Ramirez-Espinosa, J., Campa-Uranga, M.F., Talavera-Mendoza, O. and Guerrero-Suastegui, M. 1991. Caracterizacion de los arcos insulares de la Sierra Madre del Sur y sus implicaciones teconicas. Convencion sobre la evolucion geologica de Mexico. Primer congreso Mexicano de mineralogia. Pachuca, Hgo. Memoria, p. 163-166. Abstract.

Sedlock, R.L., Ortega-Gutierrez, F. and Speed, R.C. 1993. Tectonostrotigraphic Terranes and Tectonic Evolution of Mexico. Geological Society of America, Special Paper, no. 278, 180 p.

Talavera-Mendoza, O., Ramirez-Espinoza, J. and Guerrero-Suastegui, M. 1993. Geochemical evolution of the Guerrero Terrane-Example of a late Mesozoic multi-arc system, in Proceedings of the first circum-Pacific and circum Atlantic terrane conference. Univ. Nal Auton. De Mex., Instituto de Geologia, Ortega-Gutierrez, F., et al. Editors, 5-22 Noviembre, 1993.

Tardy, M., Lapierre, H., Boudier, J.L., Yta, M. and Coulon, C. 1991. The late Jurassic-early Cretaceous arc of Western Mexico (Guerrero terrane): Origin and geodynamic evolution. Abstract. In Conv. Sobre las evolucion geologica de Mexico, Primer congr. Mexicano de Mineralogia, memoria, Pachuca, Hgo., Jun. 23-28, 1991, p. 213-214.

Urabe, T. 1982. Geological Overview and Mineral Deposits of the Talpa Area, Jalsico. Japanese International Cooperation Agency-Consejo de Recursos Minerales, Report of Activity, No. 3.

THE EL GORDO VOLCANOGENIC MASSIVE SULPHIDE DEPOSIT, LEON-GUANAJUATO DISTRICT, CENTRAL MEXICO

Brian V. Hall,

Golden Temple Mining Corp., 1592 Eaglecliff Road, Bowen Island, British Columbia, V0N 1G0, Canada.

Pedro Pablo Gomez-Torres

Templo Dorado, S.A. de C.V., Loma Verde 623, Col. Loma Verde, San Luis Potosi, San Luis Potosi, Mexico

Abstract

The El Gordo is a volcanogenic massive sulphide deposit hosted by volcano-sedimentary rocks of the Guerrero terrane located near the city of Guanajuato, in central Mexico. These oceanic rocks belong to the Esperanza Formation, which is exposed in a northwesterly trending window that is surrounded by Tertiary volcanic and sedimentary rocks.

The massive sulphide potential of the property was first recognized by Golden Temple Mining Corp. in February of 1997 through a program of regional prospecting that focussed on massive sulphide deposits of the Esperanza Formation. Shortly after the sale of the Leon-Guanajuato Mineral Reserve in summer of 1998 to Grupo Mexico (IMMSA) and Industrias Penoles S.A de C.V., the property was optioned to Noranda Exploracion, Mexico S.A. de C.V. whose work forms the basis of this manuscript.

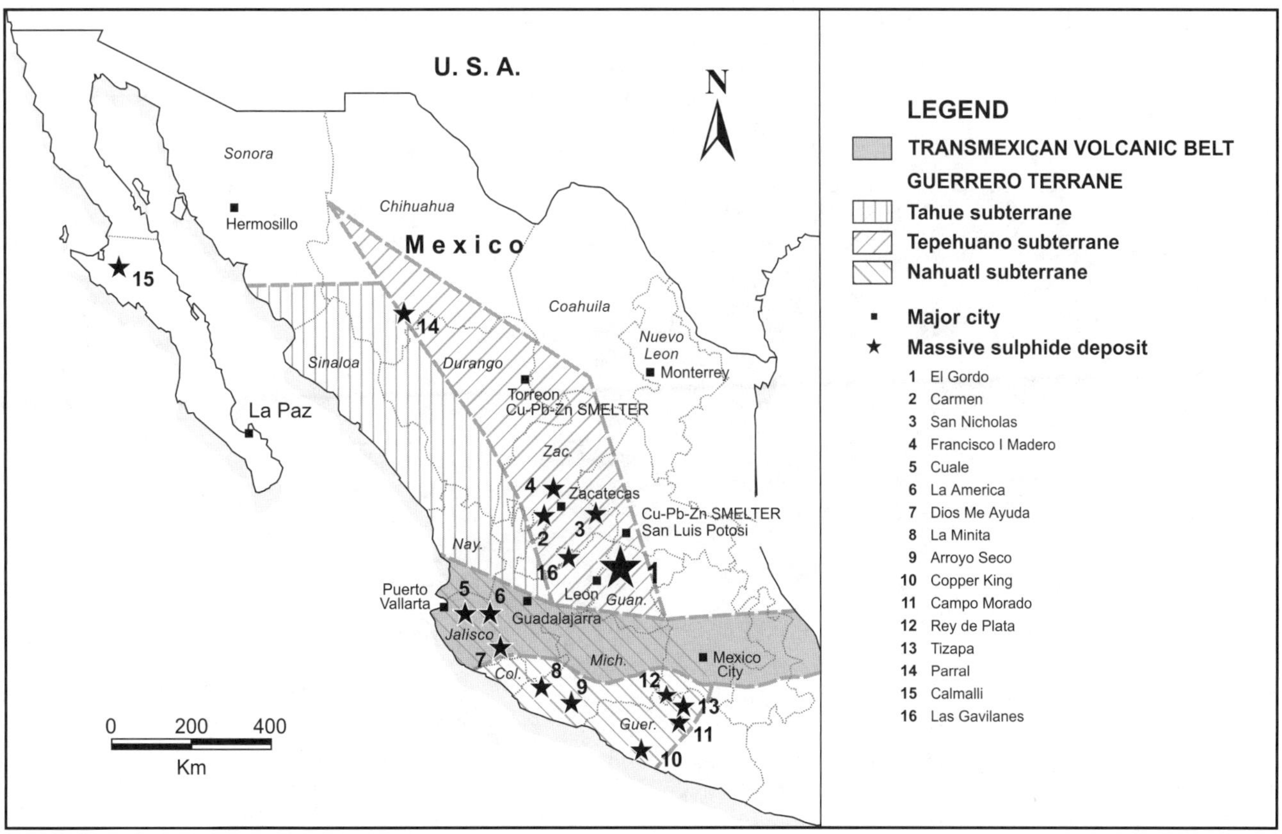

Figure 1. Volcanogenic massive sulphide deposits of the Guerrero Terrane, Mexico

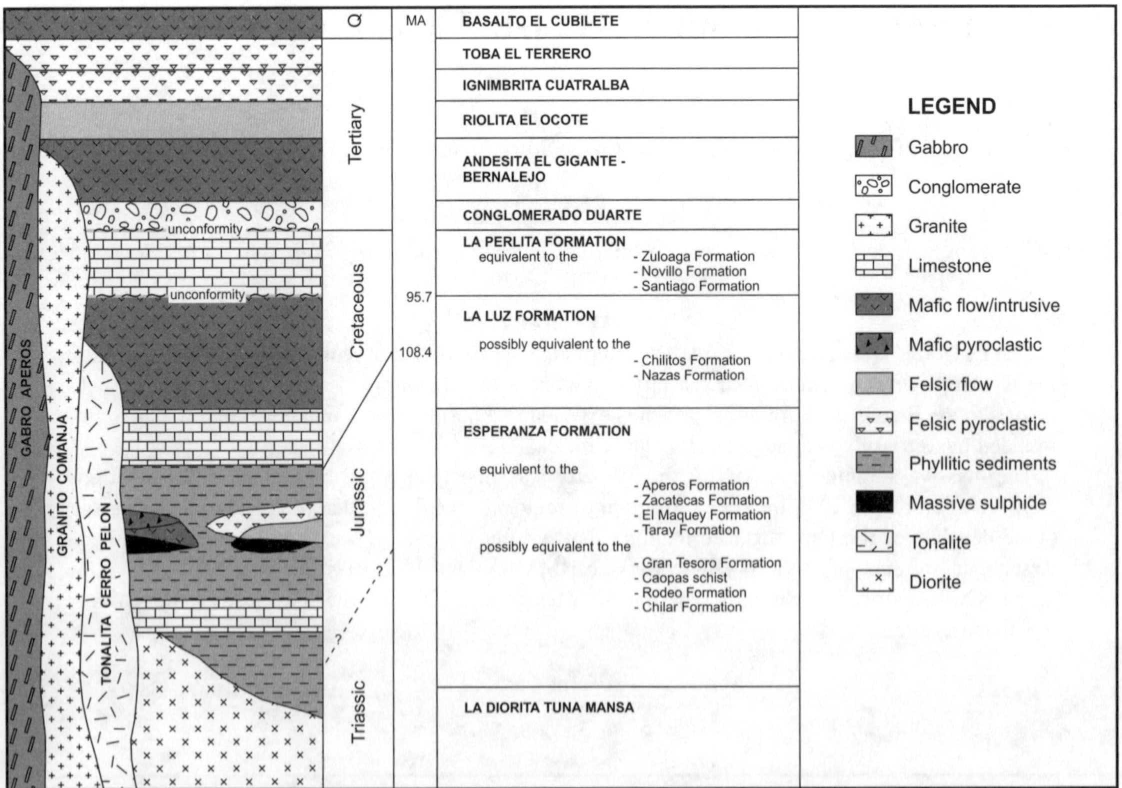

Figure 2. Stratigraphic Column for the Leon-Guanajuato District (modified from Consejo de Recuros Minerales, Carta Geologico – Minera, Guanajuato F14-C43; Sedlock, et al., 1993; Martinez-Reyes, et al. 1995)

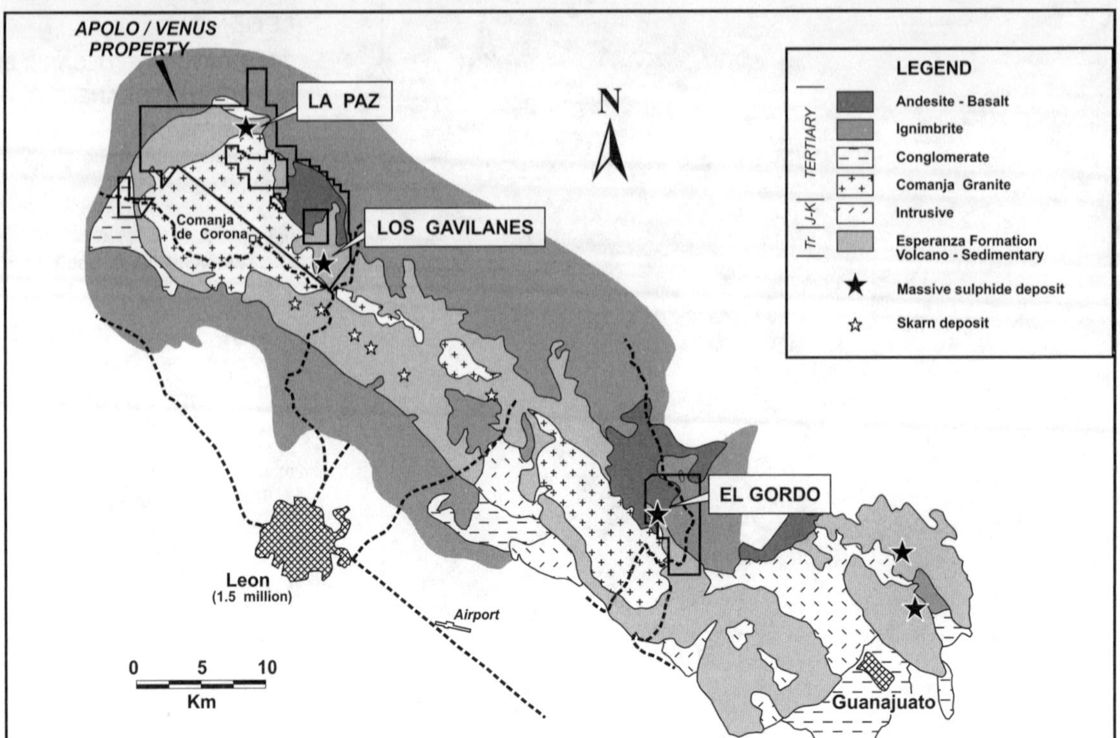

Figure 3. Geology of the Leon-Guanajuato District (modified from Martinez-Reyes, Vassallo and Franco-Ibarra, 1995)

The age of the Esperanza Formation is poorly constrained and a subject of much controversy. Based upon regional correlations with the Aperos, Zacatecas, El Maguey and Taray Formations an Upper Triassic appears to be most appropriate (Sedlock, et al., 1993), while others feel it is Jurassic in age (Ortiz-Hernadez, et al., 1990).

The stratigraphy consists of micritic limestones and argillaceous sediments that are overlain by a 100 metre thick sequence of felsic flows and pyroclastics, which host the El Gordo massive sulphide mineralization. Regionally, the Esperanza Formation can be correlated with the Zacatecas Formation, which in turn hosts the Francisco I Madero deposit in Zacatecas State. Recent estimates for the Francisco I Madero deposit indicate 40 million tonnes grading 36 g/t silver, 0.8 % lead and 4.7 % zinc, with a 3 million tonne copper zone grading 80 g/t silver and 1.1 % copper (Giles and Garcia, this volume). The stratigraphy of El Gordo prospect can also be correlated with the Los Gavilanes volcanogenic massive sulphide deposit located 30 km to the northwest and other occurrences within the Leon-Guanajuato Mineral Reserve (Hall and Gomez-Torres, this volume)

Exposures of massive to disseminated pyrite up to 50 metres in thickness can be traced along strike for approximately 1,200 metres in a small arroyo. Surrounding this arroyo is a 200 metre thick section of Quaternary basalt (Basalto El Cubilete) that has covered much of the massive sulphide mineralization, and stratigraphy of the Esperanza Formation.

Two phases of deformation have affected the Esperanza Formation. The F1 folds are rootless, isoclinal structures, with the F2 folds being open, symmetrical structures that have a vertical, close-spaced cleavage. Bedding of the Esperanza Formation and F1 folds strike northwesterly (N40°W), and dip steeply to the northeast. The axial planes for the F2 folds are strike at N50°W.

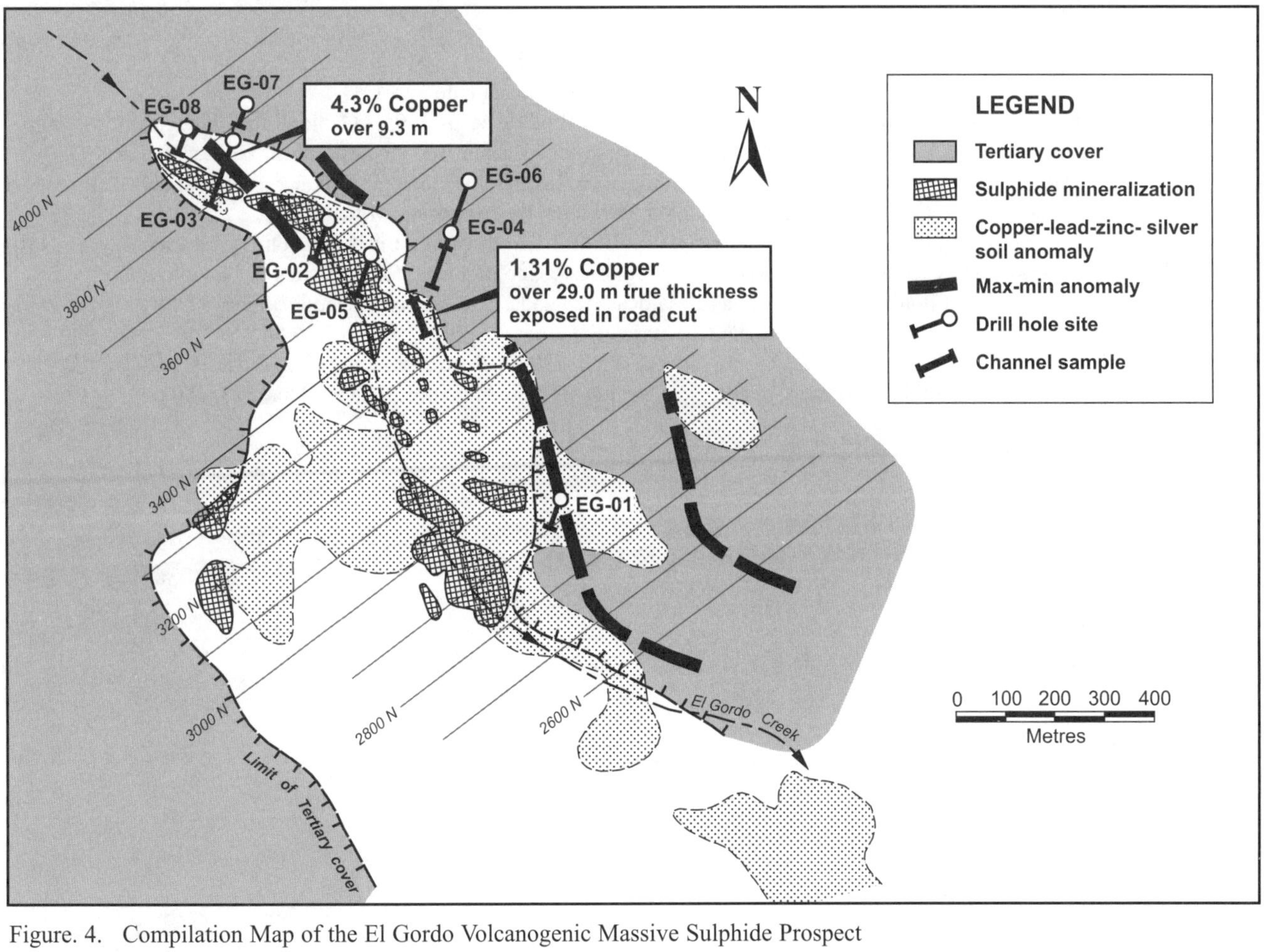

Figure. 4. Compilation Map of the El Gordo Volcanogenic Massive Sulphide Prospect

The sulphides are stratiform and well bedded, with the mineralogy consisting of pyrite, with lesser amounts of sphalerite, chalcopyrite, pyrrhotite, chalcocite, digenite, bornite, galena, magnetite and barite. Drilling has encountered three to five distinct sulphide horizons in one limb of the folded stratigraphy. Within these horizons, the sulphide bands vary from 0.5 cm to 12.9 metres in thickness, with the thickest and highest-grade intersection occurring in hole EG 99-03. Within a 46.6 metre intersection of massive to semi-massive sulphide a 9.3 metre interval assayed 4.37 % copper, 0.38 g/t gold, 33.5 g/t silver, 0.01 % lead, and 0.02 % zinc. Wallrock alteration consisting of sericite, chlorite and quartz underlies the massive sulphide horizons. A siliceous exhalite consisting of fine-grained quartz with fine laminations of pyrite and sphalerite occurs to the southeast, in holes EG 99-04 and 06.

Soil sampling has indicated an anomaly for copper-lead-zinc-silver-gold that is 1,700 metres long by 800 metres wide. A Max-Min electomagnetic survey has indicated four discrete anomalies. The mineralization of hole EG 99-03 is associated with one of the weaker anomalies.

Analogous deposits in terms of tectonic setting and stratigraphic relations to the Leon-Guanajuato District and Francisco I Madero deposit belong to a class known as "Bimodal-Siliciclastic". These occur in the Iberian Pyrite Belt, Ural Mountains of Europe and the Bathurst District of eastern Canada. This class of deposit hosts most of the world's largest volcanogenic massive sulphide deposits and is characterized by mafic to felsic volcanism that is hosted by a dominantly sedimentary package.

ACKNOWLEDGEMENTS

A number of geologists in addition to those referenced in this manuscript have made significant contributions to the development and understanding of this deposit. These include Curt Hogge, Hipolito Monje, Chris Moreton and Carlos Cham. Noranda Exploracion, Mexico, S.A. de C.V. is thanked for providing access information and for the excellent fieldwork that was carried out on the behalf of this project.

REFERENCES

Consejo de Recuros Minerales, Carta Geologico – Minera, Guanajuato F14-C43.

Martinez-Reyes, J., Vassallo, L.F. and Franco-Ibarra, Felipe de Jesus 1995. Geologfia y Potencial Minero de la Procion Central-Poniente de Estado de Guanajuato, La Zona de la Ex-Reserva Minera "Leon-Guanajuato". Folleto de divulgacion, Instituto de Geologia Estacion Regional del Centro, Secretaria de Desarrollo Economico, Direccion de Promocion Minera.

Ortiz-Hernadez, E., Lapierre, H. and Monod, O. 1990. El Arco Introceanico Aloctono (Cretacico inferior) de Guanajuato-Caracteristicas Petrograficas, Geoquimicas, Estructurales el Isotopicas del Comlejo Filoniano y de las Lavas Basalticas Asociada; Implicaciones Geodinamicas. Univ. Nal. Auton. de Mex., Inst. Geologia, Revista, vol. 9, num. 2, 1990 (1992) p. 126-145.

Sedlock, R.L., Ortega-Gutierrez, F. and Speed, R.C. 1992. Tectonostratigraphic Terranes and Tectonic Evolution of Mexico. Geological Society of America, Special Paper, No. 278, 180 p.

GEOLOGY AND EXPLORATION OF THE LOS GAVILANES DEPOSIT, LEON, MEXICO – A BIMODAL-SILICICLASTIC VOLCANOGENIC MASSIVE SULPHIDE DEPOSIT

BRIAN V. HALL

Golden Temple Mining Corp, 1592 Eaglecliff Road, Bowen Island, British Columbia, V0N 1G0, Canada.

PEDRO PABLO GOMEZ-TORRES

Templo Dorado, S.A. de C.V., Loma Verde 623, Col. Loma Verde, San Luis Potosi, San Luis Potosi, Mexico

ABSTRACT

The Los Gavilanes volcanogenic massive sulphide deposit is hosted by volcano-sedimentary rocks the Guerrero terrane of central Mexico. These oceanic rocks belong to the Esperanza Formation, which is exposed in a northwesterly trending window of the Sierra de Leon-Guanajuato. Tertiary volcanic and sedimentary rocks enclose this window. The age of the Esperanza Formation is loosely constrained and can be interpreted to be either Upper Triassic, or Jurassic.

At the Los Gavilanes deposit the stratigraphic succession consists of limestone, followed by argillaceous sediments, which are overlain by a thin sequence of felsic to intermediate flows and pyroclastics. This stratigraphic interval appears to be same as the Francisco I Madero deposit located near Fresnillo in Zacatecas State (40 million tonnes grading 36 g/t silver, 0.8 % lead and 4.7 % zinc), and other massive sulphide occurrences of the Leon-Guanajuato District.

The stratigraphy strikes northwesterly, and dips to the southwest between 20 and 40°. The F1 folds strike at N80°W, and are southwesterly dipping, recumbent folds, which are rootless, isoclinal structures. The F2 folds are symmetrical open structures that have vertical close-spaced axial plane cleavage that strike at N50°W.

Preliminary drilling has outlined massive to semi-massive sulphide mineralization over a lateral extent of 500 by 600 metres. The sulphides are stratiform, and appear to represent an undulating body that is flat-lying to moderately dipping to the southwest. Intermediate to felsic volcanics host this mineralization, with the sulphide mineralogy consisting of pyrite, pyrrhotite and marcasite, with lesser amounts of sphalerite, chalcopyrite and galena. The massive sulphides occur as bands that vary from 0.5 cm to 5.4 metres in thickness with the overall thickness of the massive sulphide-bearing horizon 0.6 to 49.4 metres. The thickest sulphide intersections occur to the south and west. Pyrite is in general more abundant than pyrrhotite, except in the southern portion where pyrrhotite becomes the dominant sulphide. Chalcopyrite is more abundant than sphalerite and galena in the proximal northeastern portion of the deposit where the wallrock alteration is most intense. The gold content is highest to the northeast, as is the gold:silver ratio. The distal portion of the deposit is located to the southwest, and has higher zinc values.

Analogous deposits in terms of tectonic setting and stratigraphic relations to the Los Gavilanes and Francisco I Madero deposits occur in the Iberian Pyrite Belt of Europe, the Ural Mountains, and the Bathurst District of eastern Canada. Based upon their tectonic and stratigraphic setting these deposits belong to a class known as "Bimodal-Siliciclastic", which host the majority of the world's largest massive sulphide deposits.

INTRODUCTION

The Los Gavilanes deposit is located within the westernmost portion of Jalisco State, in roughly the centre of Mexico. The industrial city of Leon is located 15 km to the south in Guanajuato State. Several other volcanogenic massive sulphide occurrences (Paz de Mexico, La Pena Rica, Centenario and Tres Estrellas) in addition to the Los Gavilanes are situated on the 10,000 hectare Apolo/Venus property. The farming village of Comanja de Corona is located near the centre of the property. The surrounding terrain is somewhat mountainous with elevations ranging from 2,000 to 2,600 metres.

In the fall of 1996 Golden Temple Mining Corp. recognized that the Apolo/Venus Property hosted volcanogenic massive sulphide mineralization in an area of Mexico where this type of deposit was previously unrecognized. In 1998 Noranda Exploracion de Mexico S.A. de C.V. acquired an option from Golden Temple and commenced exploration. Preliminary surveys in the form of geological mapping, ground and airborne geophysics, geochemical surveys, trenching and diamond drilling have been carried out over the past year. To date this work has outlined a small, flat-lying volcanogenic massive sulphide body measuring roughly 600 by 500 metres that is currently open to the east, south, and west. Intersections of massive to semi-massive sulphides up to 50 metres in thickness have been encountered in wide spaced drilling. Currently there is no estimate of the tonnage and grade as many of the intersections are not economic at current metal prices.

The Los Gavilanes deposit is a new discovery in an emerging district in Mexico. It is the intention of this manuscript to review the geological setting, and exploration methodologies that were used for the Los Gavilanes deposit.

REGIONAL SETTING

The Guerrero terrane is the largest tectonic unit in Mexico. It underlies most of western Mexico, comprising an area of over 350,000 square kilometres. Due to the intrusive activity of the Sierra Madre Occidental, and later Tertiary volcanic activity that occurred throughout much of central Mexico, the Guerrero terrane is only exposed in small isolated windows.

A number of subdivisions of the Guerrero terrane have been proposed; 1) three subterranes: Teloloapan-Ixtapan, Zihutanejo and Huetamo (Campa and Coney, 1983), 2) three terranes: Tahue, Tepehuano and Nahuatl (Sedlock et al., 1993), with the southern and central portions subdivided further into, 3) five subterranes: Las Ollas, Zihuatanejo, Huetamo, Arcelia and Teloloapan (Ramirez et al., 1991; Talavera et al., 1993).

The Guerrero terrane is interpreted to be an island arc that is floored by oceanic and continental crust. It is characterized by two major tectonic assemblages: a Triassic-Middle Jurassic "basement assemblage" that corresponds to ocean-floor sediments derived from continental sources, and a Late Jurassic-Cretaceous assemblage that formed in an oceanic island-arc setting. During the Laramide orogeny, this arc was accreted to the Mexican Craton. At this time the polarity of the sedimentation changed from westward to eastward, and the sediments that were derived from the arc-assemblage flooded onto the Mexican Craton. This process marks the "continentalization" of the Guerrero terrane, and represents a large addition of juvenile crust to the western North American Cordillera (Centeno-Garcia, 1994). The direction of subduction that produced the arc(s) is a matter of controversy; Coney (1983) and Tardy et al. (1991) have proposed westward subduction, while Ramirez et al. (1991) has proposed two subduction zones, one to the east and one to the west. Other associated tectonic environments such as marginal basins have also been recognized (Tardy et al., 1991).

The Guerrero terrane hosts two volcanogenic massive sulphide deposits that are currently in production (Tizapa and Rey de Plata), plus two others that are currently undergoing feasibility studies (Francisco I Madero and San Nicolas). There are also over 150 other occurrences of volcanogenic massive sulphides that are clustered in a number of areas of similar lithologic and tectonic settings (Fig. 1).

The Apolo/Venus Property is located in the Mesozoic stratigraphy of the southern portion of the Tepehuano terrane. The oldest rocks are metamorphosed greenschists of the Aperos Formation. These greenschists consist of volcaniclastic flysch, tuff, chert, limestone and shale that have been assigned a Triassic to Jurassic age. In the northern portion of the Tepehuano terrane, the Aperos Formation tentatively can be correlated with the Zacatecas Formation of Norian age (Servais et al., 1982). Based upon stratigraphic similarities, the Zacatecas Formation may be correlated with the same stratigraphic sequence that hosts the Francisco I Madero massive sulphide deposit (Miranda-Gasca, 1995). Elsewhere in the Tepehuano terrane, the Aperos Formation is known as the

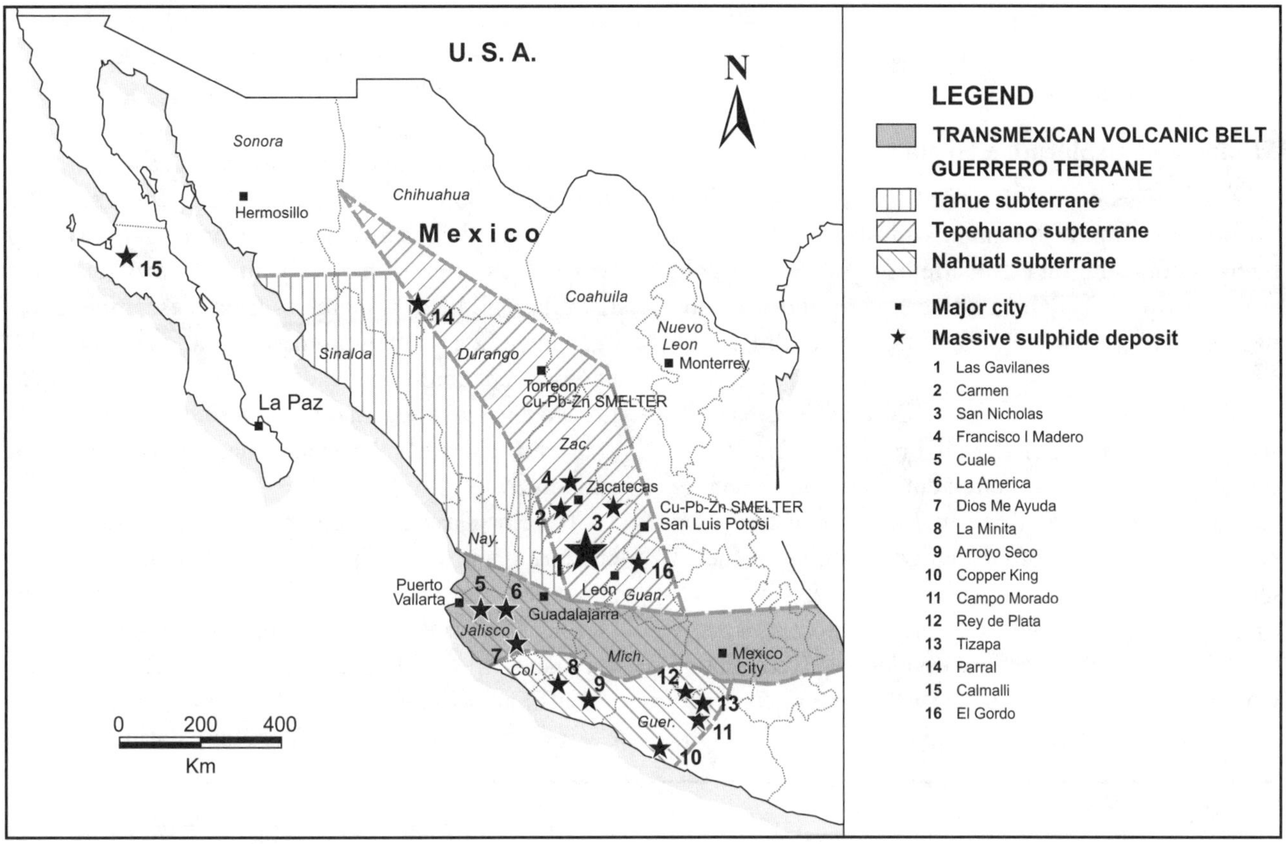

Figure 1. Volcanogenic massive sulphide deposits of the Guerrero terrane, Mexico

Esperanza and/or the El Maguey Formations (Sedlock et al., 1993). The age of the Esperanza Formation is a subject of much controversy. In the northern part of the Tepehuano terrane, the Esperanza Formation has been assigned a probable Triassic or Jurassic age, and is tentatively correlated with the Upper Triassic Zacatecas Formation. Radiolarians of probable Early Cretaceous age (Davila-Alcocer and Matinez-Reyes, 1987) indicate the entire assemblage is probably post-Jurassic. Deformational features in the Zacatecas Formation include first phase folds which are evident by a well-developed foliation and tight folding; and a second phase which produces open to tight folding and local thrust faulting (Centeno-Garcia, 1994).

The relationship with older stratigraphy and the overlying Cretaceous stratigraphy is unknown, although a major angular unconformity exists between the metamorphic rocks of the Arteaga Complex and the arc-related rocks in western Mexico (Centeno-Garcia et al., 1993). The nearest exposure is the Cretaceous (possibly Jurassic) Chilitos Formation located in Zacatecas State, which hosts the San Nicolas massive sulphide deposit. The Chilitos Formation is composed of mafic to intermediate flows and related shallow intrusions, felsic flows, felsic tuffs, volcaniclastic lithic wackes and cherts (Johnson et al., 1999).

Lower Cretaceous (Albion) carbonates that are interpeted as the western continuation of the platformal carbonates of the Gulf of Mexico unconformably overlie the Aperos Formation in the Guanajuato area (Chiodi et al., 1988). To the south and east the Aperos Formation is structurally overlain by faulted slabs of mafic and ultramafic igneous rocks that have been interpreted as an ophiolite complex (Monod et al., 1990).

APOLO/VENUS PROPERTY

The Apolo/Venus Property occupies the northern portion of a northwesterly trending window of the Triassic Esperanza Formation (Fig. 2). This window is roughly 70 km long by 15 km wide. The city of Guanajuato lies to the southeast, and Lagos de Moreno to the north.

Mining and Exploration History

Mining has occurred in the Guanajuato area since the middle of the 16th century with some of the mines being among the oldest in Mexico. Silver and gold were the primary commodities, with most of the mining activity focussed on the Veta Madre ("the Mother Vein").

The village of Comanja de Corona, located near the centre of the Apolo/Venus Property is one of the oldest in Mexico. A monument in the town centre suggests it was established in 1534, about ten years earlier than the city of Guanajuato. Mining at the El Orcon mine began in the 16th century, and was continued in the late 19th and early 20th centuries. A smelter was established in the village of Comanja de Corona towards the end of the 18th century for treating the auriferous ore of this mine. Other mines in the area that exploited the precious metal-bearing quartz veins include the El Orita, San Ignacio de Loyola, La Esperanza y Villegas and El Roblecito (Consejo de Recursos Minerales, 1992).

A number of other small properties have seen limited production in the past (La Paz de Mexico, La Esperanza, Pichichahua and the Comanja-1). In 1990 two mines were operating in the district (Tres Estrellas and El Dore). Grades from these mines averaged about 2.1 - 2.9 g/t gold, 32 - 100 g/t silver and 3 to 6 per cent combined lead and zinc. The mineralization consists of veins and veinlets of quartz with lesser pyrite, galena, sphalerite, along with native gold and silver.

The Los Gavilanes adit appears to have been driven during the early Spanish Colonial period, likely about the same time as the early mining at the El Orcon. The only known previous work on Los Gavilanes was by Las Cuevas S.A. de C.V. (a previous affiliate of Noranda), and Minera Gamma SA de CV (a past subsidiary of Noranda) during the late

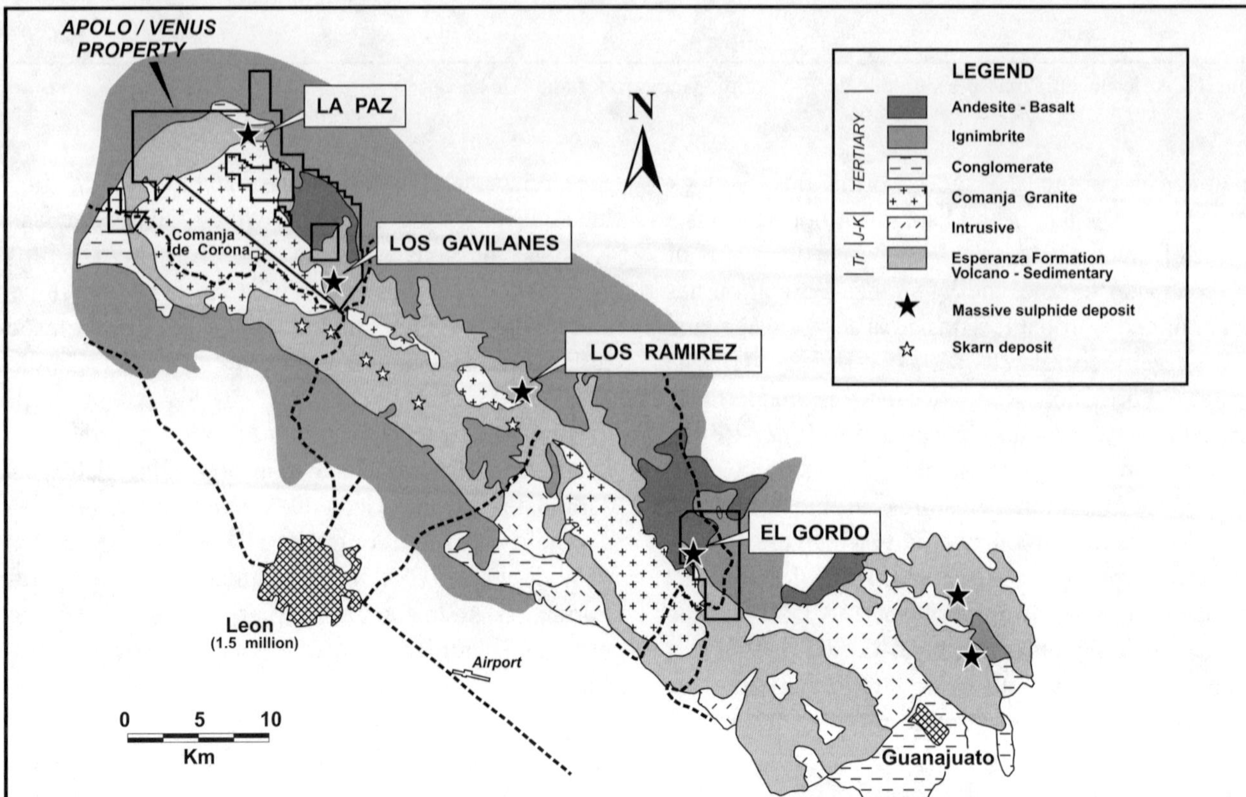

Figure 2. Geology of the Leon-Guanajuato District (modified from Martinez-Reyes, et al., 1995)

1960's. At the time, it was known as the Carmen property. The work consisted of underground sampling of the Los Gavilanes adit, geological mapping, an induced polarization (IP) survey and diamond drilling. The program was somewhat limited in nature, and focussed entirely on copper, as the price of gold at the time was pegged at $35 per ounce.

A total of eleven short drill holes were attempted, the deepest reaching 75 metres. Recoveries were poor, but the drilling did confirm the presence of a large alteration system containing elevated copper values. The induced polarization survey was conducted over four lines, spaced 100 metres apart. A strong anomaly was outlined immediately to the south of the Los Gavilanes adit, which is consistent with the southerly dip to the mineralization. The underground mapping indicated several extensions to the workings that are presently caved in. Sampling from these extensions indicated 62 metres of additional mineralization containing a weighted average of 1.38 % copper. For the entire 101 metre sampled interval, the weighted average was 1.18 % copper. Higher grade intervals included 2.23 % copper over 17 metres, 1.62 % copper over 16.5 metres and 1.92 % copper over 17 metres, which likely represent massive sulphide mineralization. Only three gold assays were reported from the underground sampling. These ranged from 1.0 to 2.4 g/t, which is consistent with the gold values from the most recent underground sampling.

In 1980, the Consejo de Rescursos de Minerales established the Leon-Guanajuato Mineral Reserve which covered what is now the Apolo/Venus Property. The purpose of this mineral reserve was to conduct exploration on behalf of the government. Soon after the government released this portion of the

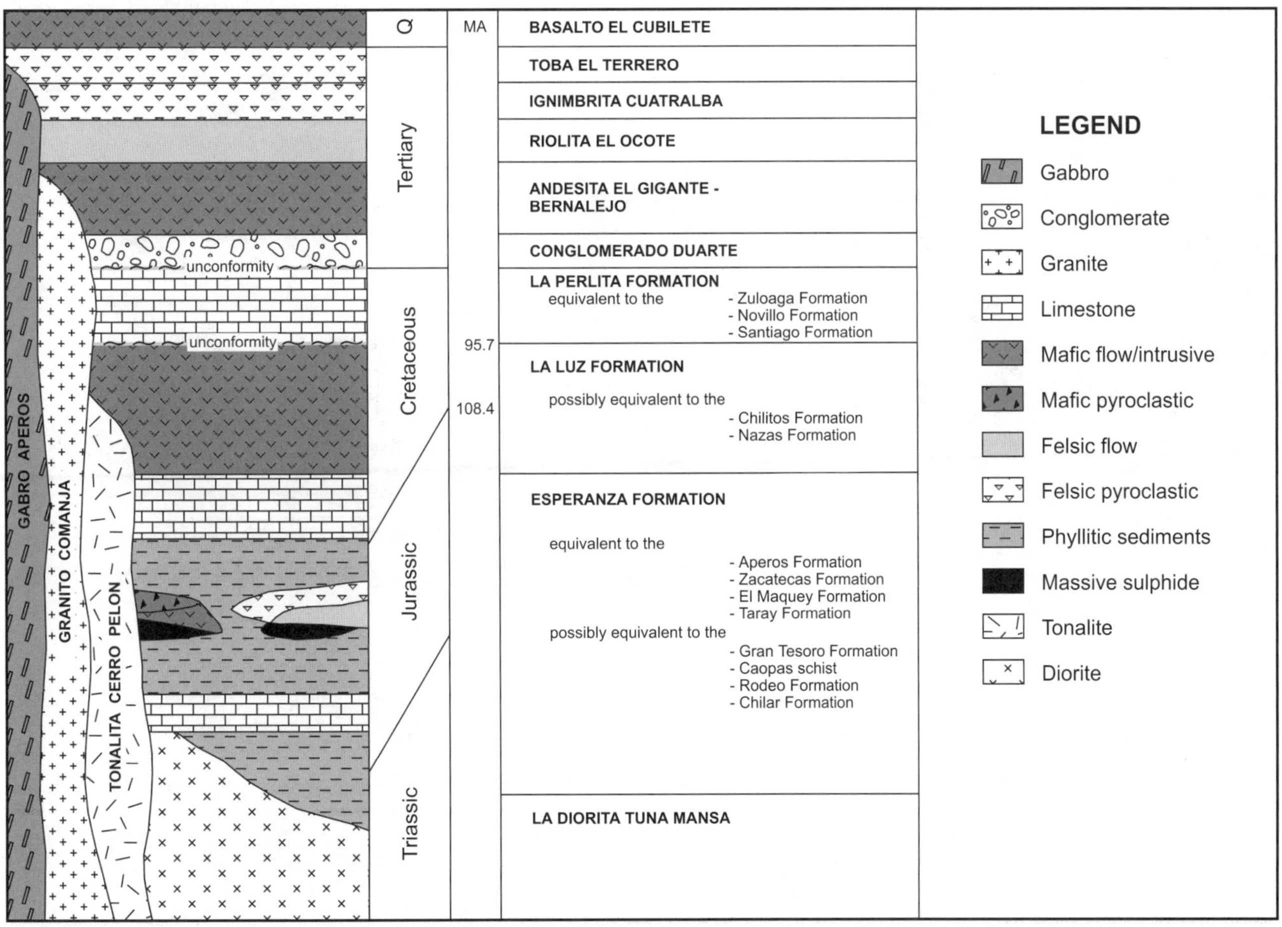

Figure 3. Stratigraphic Column for the Leon-Guanajuato District (modified from Consejo de Recuros Minerales, Carta Geologico – Minera, Guanajuato F14-C43; Sedlock, et al., 1993; Martinez-Reyes, et al. 1995).

reserve in 1996, two medical doctors from Zacactecas staked the Apolo/Venus Property.

In the summer of 1996 Minera Dolares S.A. de C.V. carried out a limited amount of rock sampling over the Apolo/Venus Property on behalf of Minera Teck S.A. de C.V. Also at this time, a portion of the Los Gavilanes adit was rehabilitated and sampled, and four shallow trenches were excavated immediately to the north of the adit.

In the fall of 1996 Golden Temple Mining Corp. recognized that the massive sulphide and alteration assemblages in the Los Gavilanes adit were indicative of volcanogenic massive sulphide mineralization, and immediately acquired the property through an option agreement. Shortly after the sale of the Leon-Guanajuato Mineral Reserve in summer of 1998 to Grupo Mexico (IMMSA) and Industrias Penoles S.A de C.V., the property was optioned to Noranda Exploracion, Mexico S.A. de C.V.

Stratigraphy and Lithology

The Esperanza Formation underlies the northern and eastern portion of the property. It has been exposed along a northwesterly axis due to uplift that is related to the intrusion of the Tertiary Comanja Granite. Surrounding and overlapping onto the Esperanza Formation and Comanja Granite are Tertiary volcanic and sedimentary rocks (Fig. 4).

The Esperanza Formation consists of carbonaceous shales, with the upper portions containing calcareous shales and clayey limestones that are interbedded with sporadic intermediate and felsic flows. The geochemistry of the volcanic flows indicates an alkalic affinity (Martinez-Reyes et al, 1995).

A limestone unit that is locally known as the La Perlita Limestone is found in the northern portion of the Apolo/Venus Property. It overlies the Esperanza Formation and is likely equivalent to Cretaceous limestones found elsewhere in the Leon-Guanajuato District.

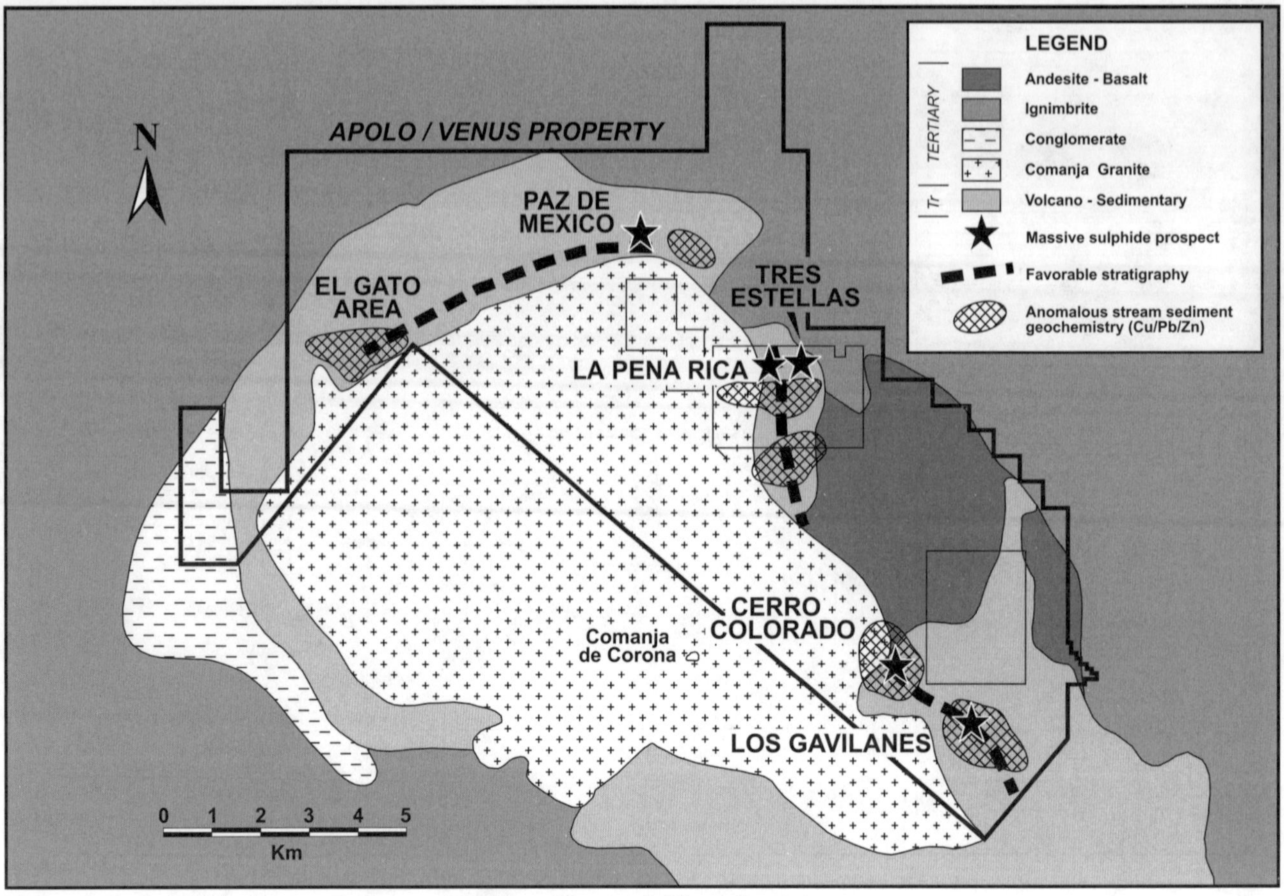

Figure 4. Geology and stream sediment geochemistry of the Apolo/Venus Property.

The Comanja Granite occupies the central portion of the Apolo/Venus Property. It is equigranular, medium to coarse grained, and consists mainly of quartz, plagioclase and potassium feldspar, with minor pyroxene. Recent mapping by the Univerisdad Nacinal, Autonoma de Mexico (Martinez-Reyes et al, 1995) suggest it is Tertiary in age.

Surrounding the Esperanza Formation and La Perlita limestone is the Durarte Conglomerate. This unit is thought to be Tertiary in age (Martinez-Reyes et al, 1995), and an unconformity represents the time interval between this unit and the La Perlita limestone.

Other members of the Tertiary stratigraphy include the El Gigante-Bernalejo andesites and an ignimbrite unit known as the Cuatralba. The El Gigante-Bernalejo andesites occur to the northeast of the Apolo claim, while the Cuatralba ignimbrites surround the entire uplifted sequence of the Leon-Guanajuato District.

Structure

Bedding of the Esperanza Formation strikes mainly in a west to northwesterly direction, with shallow to moderate dips to the southwest. Two main phases of folding are present. The first phase (F1) folds are recumbent, rootless, isoclinal structures that can result in structural repetitions of the stratigraphy. The second phase (F2) folds are northwesterly trending, open symmetrical structures that are characterized by a vertical axial planar fracture cleavage. Changes in bedding orientations can be used to recognize these folds. There is also evidence for the rotation of some of the F2 folds at the margins of the Comanja Granite (Moreton, 1999).

A north northwesterly striking series of fractures, which are most pronounced in the Tres Estrellas to Los Gavilanes area are readily discernable from the air. In some cases these structures represent faults and host mineralized quartz veins. They are thought to be Tertiary in age as this fracture pattern cuts through the Comanja Granite.

Los Gavilanes deposit

The Los Gavilanes Deposit has been the focal point for an ongoing program of fieldwork, with most of the work focussed on the Los Gavilanes – Cerro Colorado Grid (Fig. 5).

Stratigraphy and Lithology

Within the Los Gavilanes-Cerro Colorado Grid the stratigraphy consists of silicified black argillites, siltstones, variably altered limestone, quartz-sericite schists and iron-rich cherts that belong to the Esperanza Formation. These have been intruded by the Tertiary Comanja Granite (Moreton, 1999).

Based upon the current structural interpretation, the limestone situated to the north of the Los Gavilanes adit is the oldest stratigraphic unit, and appears to represent the core of a F1 recumbent fold (Fig. 5). Locally this limestone has been silicified due to later alteration. Metamorphism has developed calc-silicate assemblages consisting of actinolite-tremolite, wollastonite and garnet.

This limestone is overlain by silicified black argillites and siltstones, which are well stratified and thinly bedded. These are overlain by a 20 to 80 metre thick interval of felsic to intermediate volcanic flows and tuffs. It is these volcanic rocks that host, and in part overlie, the massive sulphide mineralization (Fig. 6). Also associated with the massive sulphide horizons are irregular intervals of siliceous exhalite. A second sequence of silicified black argillites and siltstones overlie the felsic to intermediate volcanic rocks.

Structure

In general the stratigraphy strikes northwest and dips 20 – 40º to the southwest. The F1 folds are rootless, isoclinal structures that strike N80ºW and have a moderate southwest dip. These folds have caused small structural repetitions of the stratigraphy. To the northwest of the Los Gavilanes adit, a silicified limestone unit cores one such fold. The fold axis for these folds are thought to be shallow and doubly plunging about a northeasterly trending axis that passes through the area of the Los Gavilanes adit.

The F2 folds are symmetrical open structures that have vertical close-spaced axial planer cleavage (Moreton, 1998). The axial planes for these structures strike N50ºW. In places these folds have refolded the F1 folds resulting in a complex interference pattern.

Faults which strike east west and at N10ºE have been recognized. The former are the more significant in terms of displacement (Moreton, 1998), such as the fault that appears to have truncated the Southern

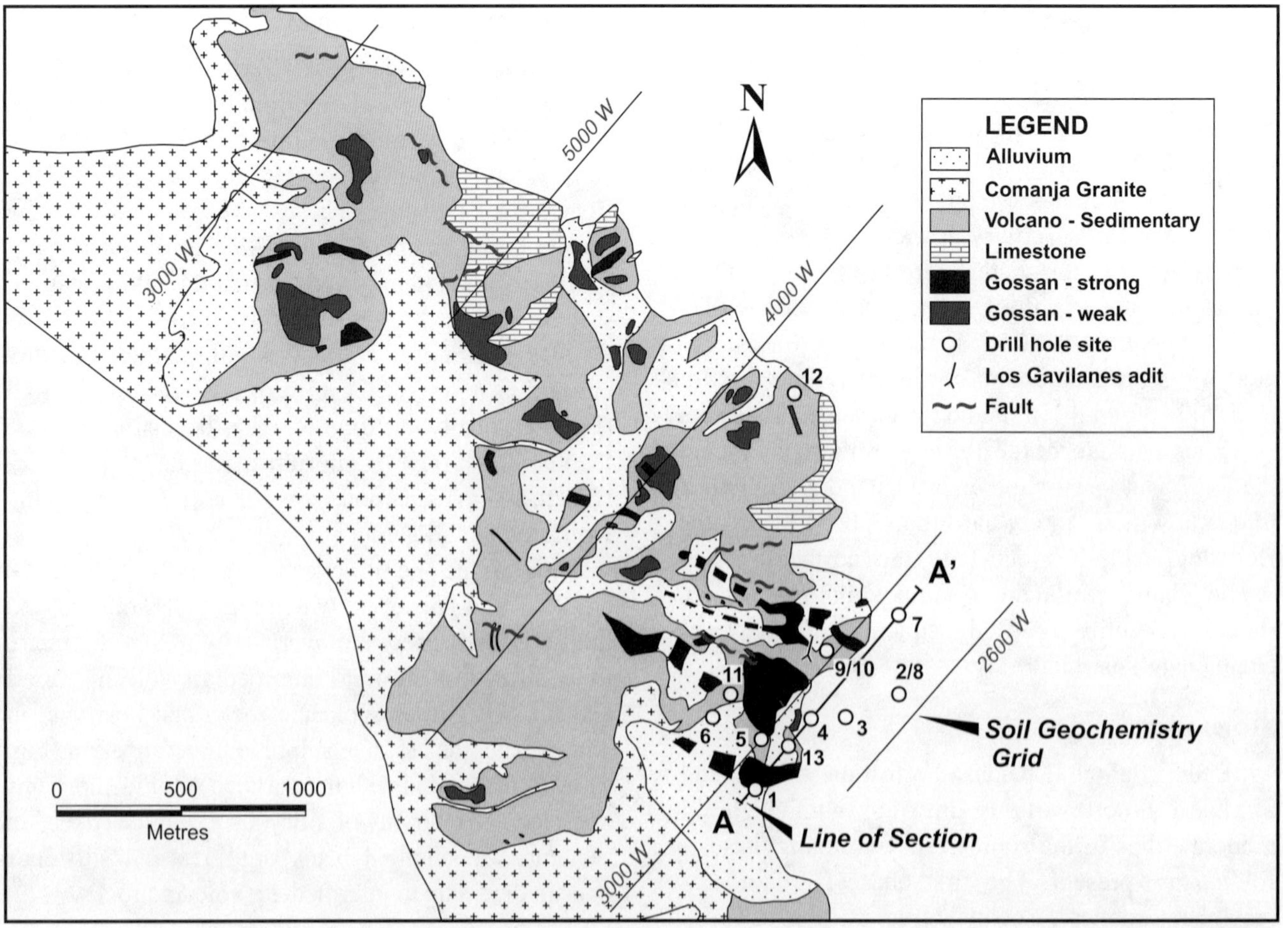

Figure 5. Geology of the Los Gavilanes – Cerro Colorado Grid

IP anomaly, or the fault that occurs in the Los Gavilanes adit.

Mineralization

Stratiform and relatively flat-lying massive to semi-massive sulphide mineralization has been outlined by drilling over an area of 600 by 500 metres. This mineralization was initially discovered in the Los Gavilanes adit, with most of our current understanding based upon a recently completed 13-hole drill program.

The intent of this drill program was to test a number of the geophysical, geological and geochemical targets that were generated as a result of the recent fieldwork. In general the drilling was too wide spaced to accurately define the structure or shape of the mineralization. The F1 folds shown on Figure 6 are isoclinal and southwesterly dipping, while the southernmost F2 fold is a broad open feature, that is also southwesterly dipping.

In the deposit area the base of the stratigraphic sequence consists of thinly bedded black argillites that have been intruded by a granodiorite (Comanja Granite). Overlying the argillites is a sequence of felsic to intermediate volcanic tuffs and flows, which attain a maximum thickness of 80 metres. To the southwest this volcanic sequence thins to 20 metres. The felsic volcanic flows and tuffs are most abundant along a northeasterly trending axis that passes through the central portion of the deposit. At the margins of this axis the intermediate volcanic flows and tuffs are more abundant. The felsic volcanic flows tend to occur to the footwall of the volcanic packages, and are generally overlain by felsic tuffs and breccias.

The massive to semi-massive sulphides consist of pyrite, pyrrhotite, marcasite and lesser amounts of

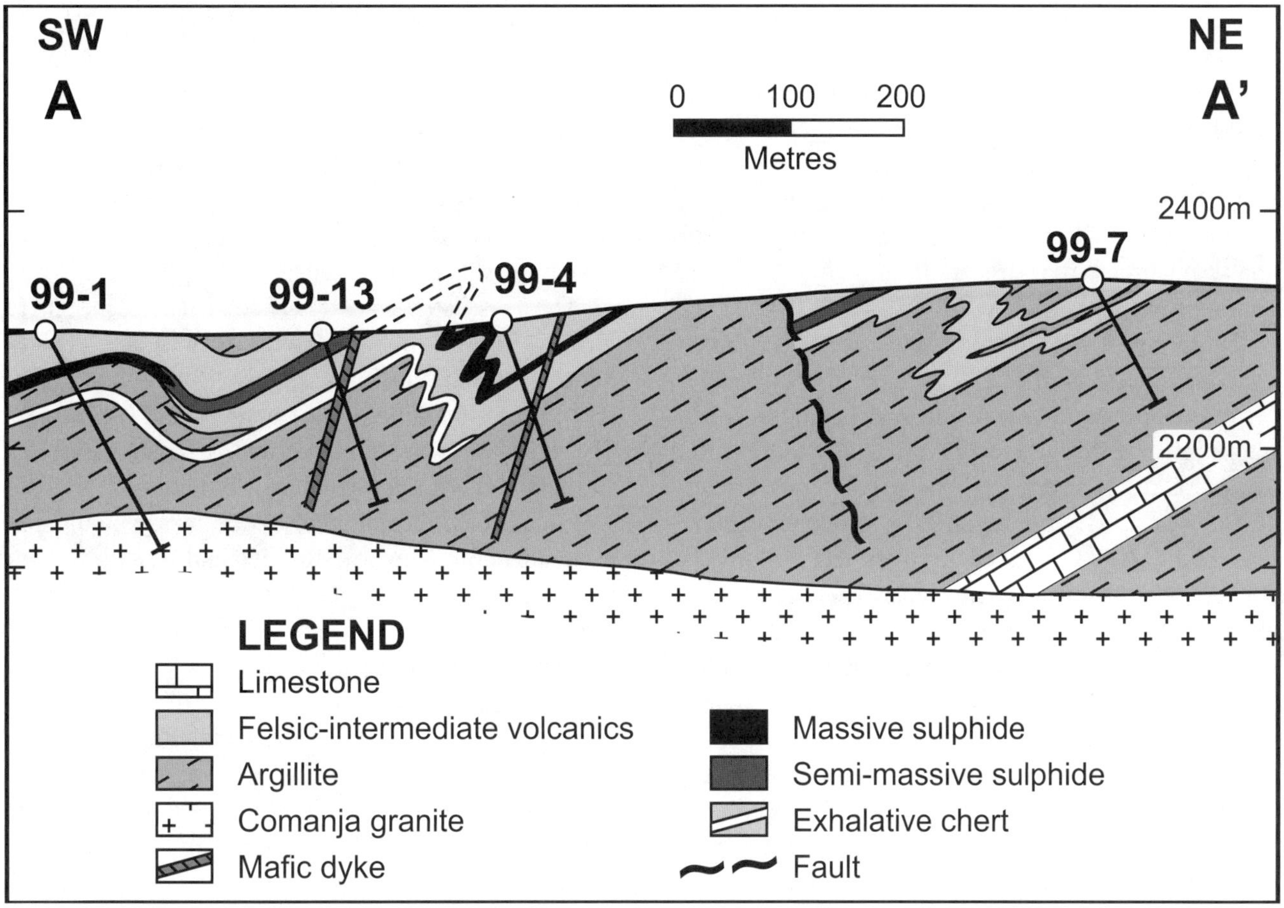

Figure 6. Los Gavilanes Cross Section at 2800 W.

sphalerite, chalcopyrite and galena. In general the massive sulphides occur as beds that vary from 0.5 centimetres to 5.4 metres in thickness. Separating these beds are layers of felsic tuff, or a siliceous exhalite. The overall thickness of the sulphide-bearing horizon varies from 0.6 to 49.4 metres, with the thicker intersections occurring to the south and west. Pyrite is generally more abundant than pyrrhotite, although in the southwestern portion of the deposit pyrrhotite becomes the dominant sulphide. Chalcopyrite is more abundant than sphalerite and galena in the northeastern portion of the deposit where the wallrock alteration is most intense. The gold content is highest in the northeast, as is the gold:silver ratio.

The sulphides are generally coarse-grained and display textures that are indicative of replacement and/or metamorphic recrystallization. Sedimentary banding within the massive sulphide bands is relatively rare, but can be displayed by all the sulphide minerals. The pyrite is generally fractured and locally displays a framboidal texture. Where pyrrhotite and pyrite are present together, the pyrite tends to occur as large idiomorphic grains (up to 3 cm in diametre) which are surrounded by pyrrhotite. Chalcopyrite generally occurs as blebs within pyrrhotite, or as infilling fractures in pyrite. The sphalerite is generally brown, and banded.

The best base metal grades occur in Hole 99-4 (0.02 g/t gold, 157 g/t silver, 2.24 % copper, 4.16 % lead and 10.35 % zinc), which was also the narrowest intersection (0.60 metres). Distal massive sulphides at the western margin of the deposit grade 0.07 g/t gold, 18.5 g/t silver, 0.81 % copper, 0.03 % lead and 3.02 % zinc over 5.45 metres in Hole 99-6. This is contrasted by the northeastern, proximal portion which contains

0.34 g/t gold, 11.9 g/t silver, 0.59 % copper, 0.22 % lead and 0.38 % zinc over 21.0 metres in Hole 99-9.

Wallrock alteration has affected local areas associated with the massive sulphide mineralization producing irregular zones of quartz-sericite schist, which are now heavily oxidized. Within the oxidized portions of the alteration zones relict sulphide veins and boxworks after disseminated sulphides are a common feature.

Sampling of the Los Gavilanes adit in 1996 produced an intersection of 1.78 g/t gold, 20.0 g/t silver, 1.14 % copper, 0.02 % lead and 0.03 % zinc over a 48 metre interval that was estimated to represent a true thickness of 31 metres. Massive sulphides grading 1.15 g/t gold, 31.4 g/t silver, 2.33 % copper, 0.02 % lead and 0.06 % zinc occur over the bottom 7.7 metres, with the base of the massive sulphides not exposed. The upper portion consists of hydrothermally altered and oxidized, volcanic and sedimentary rocks that contain 2.17 g/t gold, 26.0 g/t silver, 0.40 % copper, 0.02 % lead and 0.02 % zinc over a 23.3 metre thickness. Supergene enrichment has likely enhanced the gold, silver and copper grades. Oxidized and hydrated copper in the form of chalcanthite is present as stalactites in those portions of the underground workings that contain the massive sulphides. Malachite and azurite also occur within the massive sulphides. The hangingwall alteration consists of sericite, quartz and/or chlorite. Goethite and limonite, after sulphide veins and boxworks are also present.

OTHER OCCURRENCES

Regional geological mapping has outlined the favorable stratigraphic interval over a strike length of approximately 16 km. Several other occurrences of massive sulphides and gossanous outcrops after massive sulphides, have been located (Cerro Colorado, Tres Estrellas, La Pena Rica and Paz de Mexico). At present, none of these prospective areas have been evaluated in any detail, although they will likely be the subjects of future work.

The Cerro Colorado area is located on a small gossanous hill roughly four kilometres northwest of the Los Gavilanes adit. Local areas of gossanous float after semi-massive sulphides occur within a large area of quartz-sericite-pyrite and chlorite-pyrite-quartz alteration. Also present is an intensely altered, thinly laminated marble, with local strong development of calc-silicate mineral assemblages (tremolite, cummingtonite, epidote and garnet). This calc-silicate unit is exposed for a strike length of approximately 800 metres, and is estimated to be up to 50 metres thick. Along strike this calc-silicate unit grades into a siliceous exhalite.

The Tres Estrellas and La Pena Rica prospects are located 10 km to the northwest of the Los Gavlanes adit, in the centre of the property. Both contain massive to semi-massive pyrite bands up to 50 cm thick. The host rocks are metasediments, felsic volcanics and andesites of the Esperanza Formation. The felsic volcanics form the footwall of the massive sulphide mineralization. They are silicified and sericitized with disseminated pyrite. Within the metasediments a dark green chlorite is present as an alteration mineral.

The Paz de Mexico prospect is located in the north-central portion of the property. The mineralization consists of banded massive sphalerite and galena. Geological mapping has traced two stratiform sulphide horizons that average three metres in thickness for approximately 275 m along strike. Hosting this mineralization is a sequence of felsic volcanic rocks and sediments of the Esperanza Formation. Channel samples from one of these horizons graded 1 g/t silver, 0.01 % copper, 0.01 % lead and 2.94 % zinc over a 3.4 metre thickness. Assay values from a 15 kilogram float boulder found in an area of subcrop graded 90.9 g/t silver, 8.1 % lead and 12.7 % zinc.

GEOCHEMISTRY

Geochemical data was obtained for 124 stream sediment samples. With the exception of the southwestern portion of the property, which was not sampled because it was underlain by the Comanja Granite, the sampling density is approximately two samples per square kilometre.

Four areas of anomalous geochemistry were outlined by the stream sediment sampling (Los Gavilanes-Cerro Colorado, Tres Estrellas, Paz de Mexico and El Gato) (Fig. 4). All appear to be caused by massive sulphide mineralization. Anomalous levels of silver, copper, lead and zinc and to a lesser degree iron and barium occurs in these areas. The most anomalous samples were from the Los Gavilanes (74 ppm silver, 954 ppm copper, 670 ppm zinc and 278 ppm lead) and Cerro Colorado (1.6 ppm silver, 107 ppm copper, 1,710 ppm lead and 932 ppm zinc).

Soil sampling was carried out over the entire Los Gavilanes-Cerro Colorado Grid, with 914 samples of the B-horizon collected intervals of 50 metres. Gold, silver, copper, lead and zinc and to a lesser degree iron and barium were used to identify the anomalous areas (Figures 7c – 7f).

The Southern Soil Anomaly measures roughly 900 by 500 metres and is anomalous for zinc and copper, and to a lesser degree gold and lead. It is associated with a prominent gossan that occurs within the Comanja Granite.

The Los Gavilanes Soil Anomaly measures about 700 by 500 metres, and is anomalous in gold (up to 346 ppb), copper (up to 668 ppm) and lead (up to 2,863 ppm). The anomaly approximates the area of a prominent gossan, with the Los Gavilanes adit occurring to the north, or uphill side.

The Northern Soil Anomaly has the largest lateral extent. Anomalous values in lead (up to 3,321 ppm), followed by zinc (up to 2,163 ppm), then gold and copper outline an anomalous area that measures roughly 2,700 by 500 metres, with the northwestern end of this anomaly continuing off the grid. Geological mapping has encountered relatively few gossanous outcrops that are associated with this anomaly.

The Cerro Colorado Soil Anomaly is located on small hill. Lead and zinc values are anomalous over an area of 500 by 700 metres. Several gossanous outcrops are present which appear to be along strike from gossanous outcrops that are exposed in the southern portion of the Northern Soil Anomaly.

Geophysics

An airborne geophysical survey was conducted over the entire Apolo/Venus Property, with ground magnetometer and induced polarization surveys over portions of the Los Gavilanes-Cerro Colorado Grid.

The airborne geophysical survey covered 20 square kilometres on lines spaced 200 metres apart, for a total of 905 line kilometres. The survey included 1) five electromagnetic systems having vertical and horizontal coaxial coils using frequencies ranging from 490 Hz to 4,600 Hz; 2) a proton magnetometer system; and 3) a radiometrics system. Unfortunately the somewhat rugged terrain resulted in flight elevations that were higher than the survey specifications, which caused the depth of penetration for electromagnetic data to be very shallow (estimated to be less than 7 metres in places).

The airborne geophysical survey did prove useful in distinguishing the main rock types. The Comanja Granite showed up as a pronounced high for the potassium and total count radiometric surveys, with very high resistivities on the 490 Hz horizontal coil. The Esperanza Formation exhibited lower resistivities, a low count for the potassium radiometrics, and a mixed magnetometer response. The lowest resistivities and magnetic responses were associated with the phyllites in the area of the Los Gavilanes-Cerro Colorado Grid.

Several small magnetic anomalies were located within the Los Gavilanes-Cerro Colorado Grid. Hole GV 99-1 tested one such anomaly (Fig. 7a) that was associated with a moderately strong induced polarization anomaly. This hole intersected 7.8 metres of semi-massive to massive pyrrhotite and pyrite. The resisitivity response for the 490 Hz horizontal coaxial coil of the electromagnetic survey produced several anomalies that were coincident with low resistivities of the induced polarization survey. Holes GV 99-1, 3, 5 and 6 tested these features and in every case found massive to semi-massive pyrite and pyrrhotite intersections between 7.6 and 29.8 metres thick.

The proton ground magnetometer survey was carried out over the immediate vicinity of the Los Gavilanes adit. Several discontinuous highs were outlined. The most prominent is coincident with the airborne magnetometer anomaly located near Hole GV 99-1.

The induced polarization (IP) survey covered 30 line kilometres of grid. The electrode array was dipole-dipole with a fifty-metre separation that was used to measure six levels. Four main anomalies were located that parallel the stratigraphy, and a somewhat confusing pattern of disconnected anomalies that lie to the west and north of the Los Gavilanes adit (Fig. 7b).

The Southern IP Anomaly is the strongest. It can be traced for 1,100 metres and appears to dip moderately to the southwest. The chargebilities range from

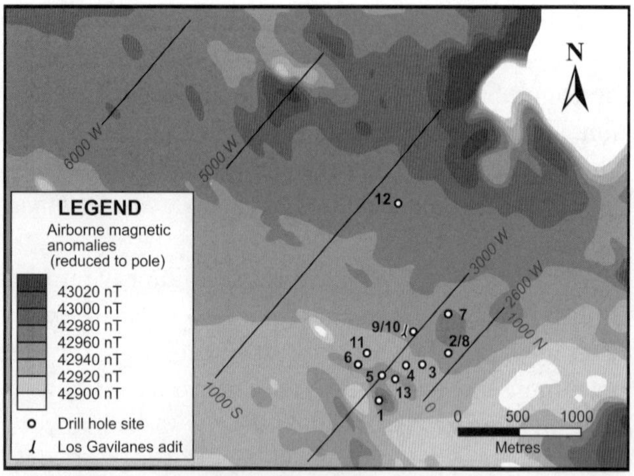

a) Airborne magnetometer survey

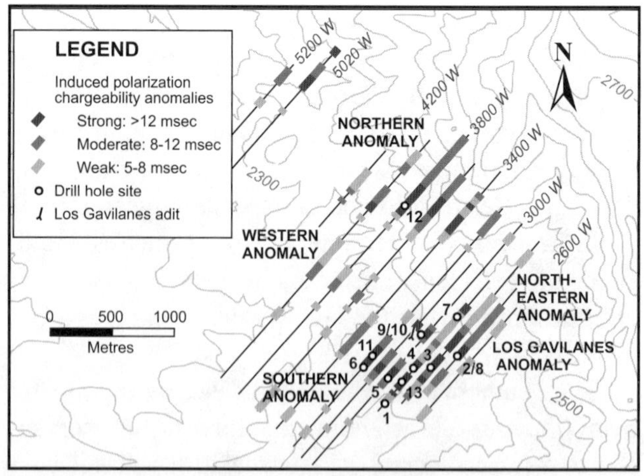

b) Induced polarization survey and topography

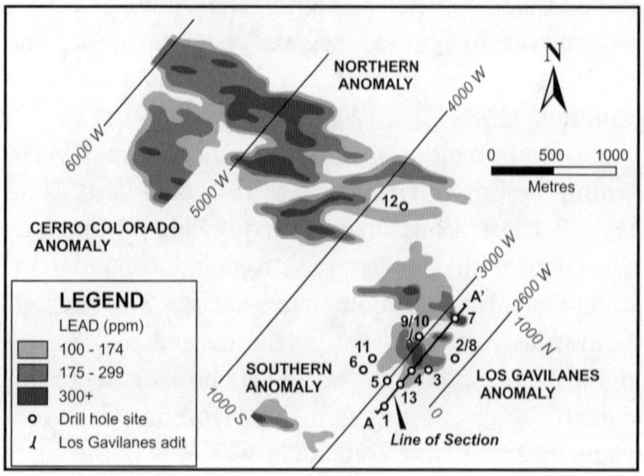

c) Lead distribution in soil samples

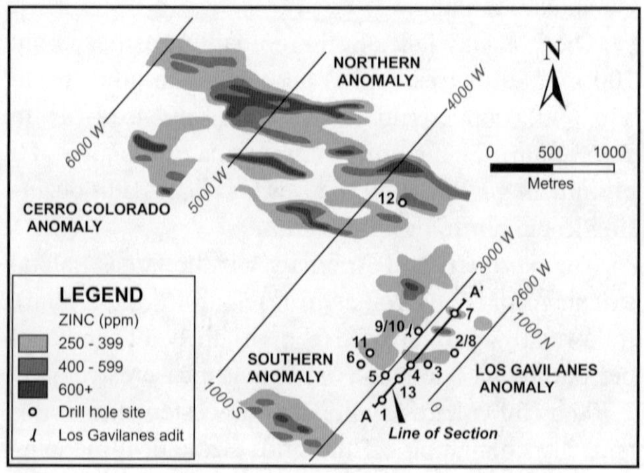

d) Zinc distribution in soil samples

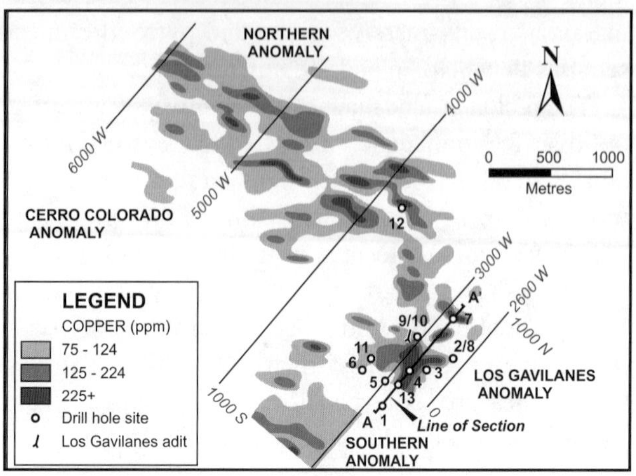

e) Copper distribution in soil samples

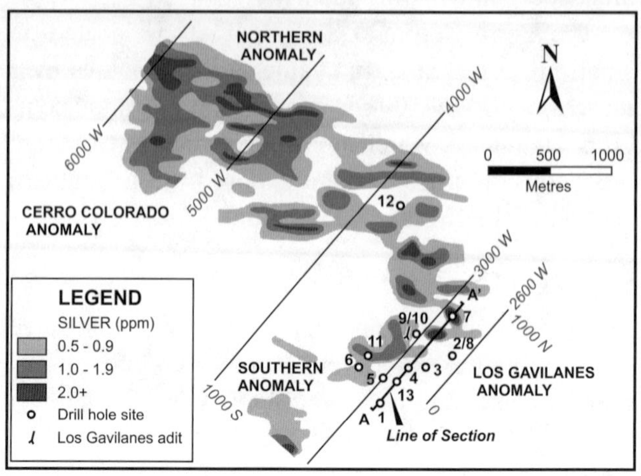

f) Silver distribution in soil samples

Figure 7. Geophysical and Soil Geochemical data for the Los Gavilanes – Cerro Colorado Grid

10-12 milliseconds (3 to 4 times background), attaining a high of 21 milliseconds in the area of Hole GV 99-5. The four drill holes (GV 99-5, 6, 11 and 13) that tested this anomaly encountered massive to semi-massive pyrite-pyrrhotite mineralization with lesser amounts of chalcopyrite and sphalerite over a strike length of 400 metres. The thickest intersection occurred in Hole GV 99-5. This IP anomaly weakens considerably to the northwest, where the massive sulphides become thinner and more sphalerite rich. It is quite likely that the Western IP Anomaly may represent the faulted extension of the Southern IP Anomaly.

The Los Gavilanes IP Anomaly is approximately 400 metres long and occurs in the immediate vicinity of the Los Gavilanes adit. This anomaly is up to 22 milliseconds in strength, relatively narrow, and appears to dip moderately to the southwest. Holes GV 99-9 and 10 tested this anomaly and encountered massive to semi-massive pyrite, with minor amounts of chalcopyite in a siliceous matrix.

The Northeastern IP Anomaly is about 400 metres long, with a north-south strike and a moderate dip to the west. It was tested by three holes (GV 99-2, 7 and 8), all of which failed to intersect significant volcanogenic massive sulphide mineralization.

The Northern IP Anomaly is situated roughly 800 metres northeast of the Los Gavilanes adit. It is the largest and can be traced for at least 1,200 metres where it continues off the surveyed portion of the grid to the northwest. This anomaly is interpreted to be caused by a flat lying to southwesterly dipping planar body, although the geological mapping suggests the presence of an antiform in this area. Gossanous outcrops have been mapped in this area. The one drill hole (GV 99-12) that tested this anomaly failed to encounter significant mineralization.

COMPARISON WITH OTHER DEPOSITS

In Mexico, deposits similar to the Los Gavilanes occur within and adjacent to the Leon-Guanajuato Mineral Reserve and in the case of the Francisco I Madero deposit, 170 km to the northwest (Fig. 1).

Along strike from the Los Gavilanes deposit to the southwest the following occurrences exhibit characteristics of volcanogenic massive mineralization: Barbosa, Buenas Aires, Madrono, Mina Honda, Ricon Ibarra, El Saltio, Los Rameriz and El Gordo. All appear to be hosted by sediments and/or volcaniclastic rocks of the Esperanza Formation and represent the same stratigraphic interval as the Los Gavilanes deposit. This package can be traced for at least 50 km stretching from the El Gato area of the Apolo/Venus property (Fig. 4), to the El Gordo deposit located immediately to southeast of the Leon-Guanajuato Mineral Reserve (Fig. 2).

At the El Gordo deposit, a 100 metre thick sequence of felsic flows and pyroclastics that is underlain by micritic limestones and argillaceous sediments host the massive sulphide mineralization. Exposures of massive to disseminated pyrite up to 50 metres thick can be traced along strike for approximately 1,200 metres in a small window of the Esperanza Formation. The sulphides are stratiform and well bedded, with the mineralogy consisting of pyrite and lesser amounts of sphalerite, chalcopyrite, pyrrhotite chalcocite, digenite, bornite, galena, magnetite and barite. Drilling has encountered three to five distinct sulphide horizons in one limb of the folded stratigraphy. Within these horizons, the sulphide bands vary from 0.5 cm to 12.9 metres in thickness. Within a 46.6 metre intersection of massive to semi-massive sulphide a 9.3 metre interval assayed 4.37 % copper, 0.38 g/t gold, 33.5 g/t silver, 0.01 % lead and 0.02 % zinc. Wallrock alteration consisting of sericite, chlorite and quartz underlies each of the massive sulphide horizons. A siliceous exhalite consisting of fine-grained quartz with fine laminations of pyrite and sphalerite is located along strike, 400 metres to the southeast of the massive sulphides (Hall and Gomez, this volume).

In the area of the El Gordo deposit two phases of deformation have affected the Esperanza Formation. The F1 folds are rootless, isoclinal structures, with the F2 folds open, symmetrical structures that have a vertical, close-spaced cleavage. Bedding of the Esperanza Formation and F1 folds strike northwesterly (N40°W), and dip steeply to the northeast. The axial planes for the F2 folds strike at N50°W (Hall and Gomez, this volume).

Within the Leon-Guanajuato Mineral Reserve, the Los Ramirez is the best example of volcanogenic massive sulphide mineralization. This prospect is exposed in a small arroyo, located midway between the Los Gavilanes and El Gordo deposits (Fig. 2). Hosting this prospect are argillaceous sediments and felsic pyroclastic rocks of the Esperanza Formation that display a pronounced schistosity. Sulphides consisting of pyrite, sphalerite and galena occur in stratiform bands ranging from 0.1 to 10 centimetres in thickness, which are exposed over an interval of 2.0 metres. A 60 centimetre wide channel sample taken perpendicular to bedding graded 0.49 g/t gold, 50 g/t silver, 0.36 % copper, 0.14 % lead and 5.82 % zinc.

Elsewhere in central Mexico are two world class volcanogenic massive sulphide deposits that have recently been the subject of extensive drill campaigns (Francisco I Madero and San Nicolas). The Francisco I Madero deposit is located near the town of Fresnillo in Zacatecas State. A recently completed ore reserve estimate indicates 40 million tonnes lead-zinc material grading 36 g/t silver, 0.8 % lead and 4.7 % zinc, with a copper zone containing 3 million tonnes grading 1.1 % copper (Giles and Garcia, this volume). The Francisco I Madero deposit is thought to be hosted by the Zacatecas Formation (Miranda-Gasca, 1995), which is considered to be Upper Triassic in age (Burckhardt, 1905 and 1930), and correlative with the Esperanza Formation (Sedlock, et al., 1993). At the Francisco I Madero deposit three main sedimentary units are present: a lower unit composed of sericite-chlorite schist; a middle one composed of calc-silicate horizons that are interbedded with argillaceous sediments; and an upper one that contains a higher proportion of calc-silicate horizons. The lower portion of the basal unit hosts approximately 90 % of the reserves in a mineralized zone that is up to 200 metres in thickness. Graphitic layers of this unit are interbedded within a groundmass of epidote, sphene, actinolite, diopside and hedenbergite (Miranda-Gasca, 1995).

The sulphides at the Fransciso I Madero consist of pyrrhotite in massive bands that contain sphalerite, galena, chalcopyrite, galena, bismuthinite and native bismuth. These appear to be stratiform, and are up to several metres thick (Miranda-Gasca, 1995). Sulphide textures in the upper and middle portions consist of pyrite bands that parallel beds of graphite, sericite, quartz, actinolite and chlorite. The pyrite is generally fractured, exhibits pull apart textures and is recrystallized. Colloform pyrite is a rare feature. The chalcopyrite, sphalerite and galena are generally found as fillings between the pyrite crystals, or as bands that parallel the graphite bands (Miranda-Gasca, 1995). It is generally interpreted that the Fransciso I Madero deposit is syngenetic in origin (Giles and Garcia, this volume; Miranda-Gasca, 1995), although the lower massive sulphide lens has been interpreted to be part of a skarn that is associated with Tertiary intrusive activity (Miranda-Gasca, 1995).

The Late Cretaceous to possibly Jurassic Chilitos Formation hosts the San Nicolas deposit, located near the city of Zacatecas, in Zacatecas State. This volcano-sedimentary package has an island arc affinity and based upon the relative lack of deformational features appears to be younger than the Los Gavilanes deposit. A resource of 83.4 million tonnes, consisting of 72 million tonnes in the main zone grading 0.53g/t gold, 30 g/t silver, 1.35 % copper and 2.27 % zinc; and 11.4 million tonnes in the lower zone grading 1.62 % copper has recently been estimated. The footwall stratigraphy consists of mafic to intermediate flows and dykes, siliceous sedimentary rocks, and felsic flows and breccias. The hangingwall stratigraphy is a succession of mafic flows and flow breccias, siliceous to carbonaceous mudstones, volcaniclastic sediments and minor tuffs (Johnson, et al., 1999).

A class of volcanogenic massive sulphide deposits known as "Bimodal-Siliciclastic" is likely analogous in terms of tectonic setting and volcanic association to the Leon-Guanajuato District, and possibly the Francisco I Madero deposit. Other deposits that belong to this class occur in the Iberian Pyrite Belt, Ural Mountains and the Bathurst District of eastern Canada. "Bimodal Siliclastic" massive sulphide deposits are defined as having roughly equal portions of volcanic and siliciclastic rocks, with felsic volcanics generally more abundant than mafic volcanics (Barrie and Hanington, 1997). The felsic host rocks are generally calc-alkalic, and in some cases it can be argued that they were derived by partial melting of sedimentary sources. The mafic volcanics are generally tholeiitic, but both the Bathurst district and the Iberian Pyrite belt have mildly alkaline basalts high in the stratigraphic section. As a class of deposit they are have an average size of 23.7 million tonnes and are the largest (Barrie and Hanington, 1997).

The Iberian Pyrite Belt is host to 90 volcanogenic massive sulphide deposits (Carvalho, et al. 1997) which includes 11 out of the 25 largest deposits in the world. In general terms the stratigraphy consists of the Upper Devonian Phyllite-Quartzite Group (consisting entirely of phyllites and quartzites, with minor limestone lenses) which is overlain by the Lower Carboniferous Volcanic-Siliceous Complex, and finally the Flysch Group. The Volcanic-Siliceous Complex varies between 100 and 1,000 metres in thickness, and consists of shales, greywackes, quartzwackes and quartzites, with felsic and mafic volcanics. In the western and southern portions of the Iberian Pyrite Belt, lavas and dolerites having a chemical signature comparable to within-plate alkaline basalts are also present (Thieblemont, et al., 1998). The massive sulphide deposits are generally found on top of the felsic volcanism in close association with black shales and siliceous shales (Carvalho, et al., 1997). Characteristic of the Iberian Pyrite Belt is the thick sequence of sediments that occurs below the Volcanic-Siliceous Complex.

The tectonic setting of the Iberian Pyrite Belt considered to be extensional. Melting of a mafic crustal protolith at low to medium pressures with a steep geothermal gradient is thought to be the cause for the felsic rocks that are associated with the massive sulphide deposits (Leistel, et al., 1998)

CONCLUDING REMARKS

The Los Gavilanes deposit exhibits the following features that are in common with volcanogenic massive sulphide deposits in general: 1) a sulphide mineralogy consisting of pyrite and pyrrhotite, with lesser amounts of sphalerite, galena and chalcopyrite; 2) massive sulphide mineralization that is stratiform; 3) wallrock alteration consisting of sericite, quartz and chlorite; 4) metal zoning with copper-gold enriched in the vent area, and lead-zinc enriched in the more distal portions; 5) a stratigraphic association with felsic volcanic rocks that were deposited in a submarine setting; 6) sedimentary banding of the sulphides; and 7) sulphide textures that indicate they predate the last major metamorphic and deformational event.

In central Mexico world class volcanogenic massive sulphide deposits occur in Mesozoic volcano-sedimentary stratigraphy. The Late Cretaceous to possibly Jurassic volcanic rocks of the Chilitos Formation have an island arc affinity. The Upper Triassic (possibly Jurassic) rocks which host the Los Gavilanes deposit are comprised of oceanic sediments and volcanics of the Esperanza Formation, which is correlative with the Zacatecas Formation that hosts the Franscisco I Madero deposit.

The Los Gavilanes resembles the Francisco I Madero deposit in that both appear to be massive sulphide deposits hosted by sericite-chlorite schists and black shales of a similar age. The calc-silicate assemblages in the silicified limestone that underlies the Los Gavilanes is similar to the Francisco I Madero deposit, as is the sulphide mineralogy consisting of pyrite, pyrrhotite, chalcopyrite, sphalerite and galena, along with similar silver and gold grades.

The volcanogenic massive deposits of the Esperanza Formation share a similar stratigraphic setting as a worldwide class of deposits known as "Bimodal-Siliciclastic". This class of deposits is characterized by a dominantly sedimentary stratigraphy in which the volcanic rocks associated with the massive sulphide mineralization are bimodal.

ACKNOWLEDGEMENTS

A number of geologists in addition to those referenced in this manuscript have made significant contributions to the development and understanding of this deposit. These include Curt Hogge, Luis Mayoral and Carlos Cham. Noranda Exploracion, Mexico, S.A. de C.V. is thanked for providing access information and for the excellent fieldwork that was carried out on the behalf of this project. Tim Barrett and Ross Sherlock are thanked for their constructive comments while reviewing this manuscript.

REFERENCES

Barrie, T. and Hannington, M. 1997. Classification of VMS deposits based on host rock compositions. In Volcanic-Associated Massive Sulphide Deposits: Processes and Examples in Modern and Ancient Settings, A volume to accompany a short course co-sponsored by: The Geological Association of Canada (GAC), Mineral Deposits

Subdivision (MDD) of the GAC, and the Society of Economic Geologists (SEG), May 17-18, 1997, pp. 1-12.

Burckhardt, C. 1905. La Faune Marine du Trias Superieur de Zacatecas, Mexico. Bol. Inst. Geol., Univ. Nal. Auton de Mexico, vol. 21, 44 p.

Burckhardt, C. 1930. Etude Sythetique sur le Mesozoque Mexicain. Soc. Paleontologique Suisse Mem., vol. 50, pp. 157-158.

Campa, M.F. and Coney, P.J. 1983. Tectonostratigraphic terranes and mineral resource distributions in Mexico. Canadian Journal of Earth Sciences, vol. 20, pp. 1040-1051.

Centeno-Garcia, E. 1994. Tectonic Evolution of the Guerrero Terrane, Western Mexico. University of Arizona, Ph.D. thesis, 220 p.

Centeno-Garcia, E., Ruiz, J., Coney, P.J. and Patchett, P.J. 1993. Guerrero Terrane of Mexico: Its role in the southern Cordillera from new geochemical data. Geology, vol. 21, pp. 419-422, May 1993.

Carvalho, D., Barriga, F.J.A.S. and Munha, J. 1997. Bimodal Siliciclastic Systems – The Case of the Iberian Pyrite Belt. In Volcanic-Associated Massive Sulphide Deposits: Processes and Examples in Modern and Ancient Settings, A volume to accompany a short course co-sponsored by: The Geological Association of Canada (GAC), Mineral Deposits Subdivision (MDD) of the GAC, and the Society of Economic Geologists (SEG), May 17-18, 1997, pp. 385-418.

Chiodi, M., Monod, O., Busnardo, R., Gaspard, D., Sanchez, A. and Yta, M. 1988. Une discordance ante albienne datee par une faune d'Ammonites et de Brachiopades de type Tethysien au Mexique central. Geobios, vol. 21, pp. 125-135.

Coney, P.J. 1983. Un modelo tectonico de Mexico y sus relacionees con America del Norte, America del Sur y el Caribe. Revista del Instituto Mexicano del Petroleo, vol. 15 (1), pp. 6-15.

Consejo de Recursos Minerales, 1992. Geological-Mining Monograph of the State of Jalisico. Consejo de Recursos Minerales, Secretaria de Energia, Minas e Industria Paraestatal, Subsecretaria de Minas E Instria Basica, p.122.

Consejo de Recuros Minerales, Carta Geologico – Minera, Guanajuato F14-C43.

Davila-Alcocer, V. and Martinez-Reyes, J. 1987. Una edad Cretacica para las rocas basales de la Sierra Guanajuato. Simposio sobre la geologia de la region de la Sierra de Guanajuato (Resumenes), April 1987, pp. 19-20.

Giles D.A. and Garcia, J. this volume. Yacimientos Vulcanogenicos en Mexico: Las Minas Productoras.

Johnson, B., Montante, A., Gearvell, G., Janzen, J. and Scammell, R. 1999. Geology and Exploration of San Nicolas Polymetallic (Zn-Cu-Au-Ag) Volcanogenic Massive Sulphide Deposit. In: VMS and Carbonate-Hosted Polymetallic Deposits of Central Mexico, British Columbia and Yukon Chamber of Mines, Cordilleran Roundup, January 1999, pp. 45-54.

Leistel, J.M., Marcoux, E., Thieblemont, D., Quesada, C., Sanchez, A., Almodovar, G.R., Pascual, E. and Saez, R 1998. The volcanic-hosted massive sulphide deposits of the Iberian Pyrite Belt. Mineralium Deposita, vol. 33, pp. 2-30.

Martinez-Reyes, J., Vassallo, L.F. and Franco-Ibarra, Felipe de Jesus 1995. Geologfia y Potencial Minero de la Procion Central-Poniente de Estado de Guanajuato, La Zona de la Ex-Reserva Minera "Leon-Guanajuato". Folleto de divulgacion, Instituto de Geologia Estacion Regional del Centro, Secretaria de Desarrollo Economico, Direccion de Promocion Minera.

Miranda-Gasca, M.A. 1995. The volcanogenic massive sulphide and sedimentary exhalative deposits of the Guerrero Terrane, Mexico. Univeristy of Arizona, Ph.D. thesis, 294 p.

Monod, O., Lapierre, H., Chiodi, M., Martinez, J., Calvet, P., Ortiz, E. and Zimmermann, J.L. 1990. Reconstitution d'un arc insulaire intra-oceanique au Mexique central. La sequence volcano-plutonique de Guanajuato (Cretace inferieur), Comptes Rendus l'Academie des Sciences, vol. 310, pp. 5-51.

Moreton, C. 1998. Notes on the detailed mapping in the Cerro Colorado area. Noranda Exploracion de Mexico, Report dated December 9, 1998, p.2.

Moreton, C. 1999. Mapping in the Cerro Colorado area. Noranda Exploracion de Mexico, Report dated July 24, 1999, p. 3.

Ramirez-Espinosa, J., Campa-Uranga, M.F., Talavera-Mendoza, O. and Guerrero-Suastegui, M. 1991. Caracterizacion de los arcos insulares de la Sierra Madre del Sur y sus implicaciones teconicas. Convencion sobre la evolucion geologica de Mexico. Primer congreso Mexicano de mineralogia. Pachuca, Hgo. Memoria, pp. 163-166. Abstract.

Sedlock, R.L., Ortega-Gutierrez, F. and Speed, R.C. 1992. Tectonostratigraphic Terranes and Tectonic Evolution of Mexico. Geological Society of America, Special Paper, No. 278, 180 p.

Servais, M., Rojo-Yaiz, R. and Colorado-Lievano, D., 1982. Estudio de las rocas basicas y ultrabasicas de Sinaloa y Guanajuato. Postulacion de un paliogulfo de Baja California y de una digitacion Tethysiana en Mexico central, Geomimet, vol. 115, pp. 53-71.

Talavera-Mendoza, O. Ramirez-Espinoza, J. and Guerrero-Suastegui, M. 1993. Geochemical evolution of the Guerrero terrane-Example of a late Mesozoic multi-arc system. In Proceedings of the First Circum-Pacific and Circum Atlantic Terrane Conference. Univ. Nal. Auton. de Mex., Instituto de Geologia, (Ortega-Gutierrez, F., et al. Editors), 5-22 Noviembre, 1993.

Tardy, M., Lapierre, H., Boudier, J.L., Yta, M. and Coulon, C. 1991. The late Jurassic-early Cretaceous arc of western Mexico (Guerrero terrane); Origin and geodynamic evolution. Abstract, In Conv. Sobre las Evolucion Geologica de Mexico, Primer congr. Mexicano de Mineralogia, Memoria, Pachuca, Hgo., Jun. 23-28, 1991, pp. 213-214.

Thieblemont, D., Pascual, E. and Stein, G. 1998. Magmatism in the Iberian Pyrite Belt: petrologiclal constraints on a metallogenic model. Mineralium Deposita, vol. 33, pp. 89-110.

VOLCANOGENIC MASSIVE SULPHIDE MINERALIZATION IN THE GREATER ANTILLES

FIONA CHILDE
iMAP Interactive Mapping Solutions, 2170-1050 West Pender Street, Vancouver, BC, Canada V6E 3S7

ABSTRACT

Volcanogenic massive sulphide (VMS) mineralization in the Greater Antilles occurs on the islands of Cuba and Hispaniola; stratabound deposits in the Wagwater Formation suggest that VMS mineralization may also be present on the island of Jamaica. Despite a long history of exploration and mining, recent discoveries suggest the potential for future VMS discovery in this region.

Volcanogenic massive sulphide mineralization in the Greater Antilles is hosted within specific belts that can be grouped on the basis of magmatic affinity, lithology, metal signature and known or inferred age of host strata. The oldest group of deposits, inferred to have formed during the early stages of development of the Greater Antilles island arc, are characterized by zinc-copper-silver ± gold mineralization and Lower Cretaceous (Aptian-Albian?) bimodal volcanic and volcaniclastic host rocks with a primitive island arc affinity. This group includes deposits in the Los Pasos Formation in central Cuba and the Maimón Formation and Amina Schist in the Dominican Republic. In western Cuba mafic- to ultramafic-hosted copper-rich VMS mineralization of Late to Early Cretaceous (Aptian-Turonian?) age occurs in the Bahia Honda Ophiolite Complex and Las Minas District. These copper-rich VMS deposits are hosted within slices of obducted oceanic crust and have been correlated with similar mineralization in the Oxec District of Central America. Copper-rich VMS mineralization hosted within massive to pillowed basaltic flows of MORB affinity and Late Cretaceous (Cenomanian-Turonian?) age has been documented at one locality in the Peralvillo Formation in the Dominican Republic. This style of mineralization is interpreted to have formed in a back-arc spreading centre formed in response to the obduction of peridotite belts and a reversal in the subduction polarity of the Greater Antilles arc in early Late Cretaceous time. This change in arc polarity has been correlated with an evolution from tholeiitic to calc-alkaline magmatism; it also correlates with a marked decrease in the abundance of VMS mineralization. Subsequent to this change in the tectonic regime in early Late Cretaceous time, VMS mineralization is restricted to calc-alkaline strata of Eocene age, deposited in localized back-arc rift basins, such as the Cobre Formation in eastern Cuba and possibly the Wagwater Formation in Jamaica.

INTRODUCTION

The Greater Antilles is a Mesozoic to Cenozoic island arc system extending from Cuba eastward to the Virgin Islands (Fig. 1a). It is host to a wide range of arc-related mineral deposits, including precious metal epithermal, copper ± gold porphyry, base and precious metal skarn and volcanogenic massive sulphide (VMS) deposits. This paper gives an overview of the geology, style, magmatic affinity and tectonic setting of VMS mineralization in the Greater Antilles.

With the exception of Cuba, economic concentrations of VMS hosted base and precious metal mineralization is relatively scarce in the Greater Antilles. Volcanogenic massive sulphide deposits have been exploited on a small scale since at least the sixteenth century, however historic production records are virtually non-existent. A map complied in 1975 of the principal copper and lead-zinc deposits of the Caribbean region shows no lead or zinc deposits of any type and only a handful of copper deposits (Guild and Cox, 1975). The copper deposits consist mainly of porphyry, skarn and sedimentary exhalative (Sedex) deposits, and include only one VMS occurrence, the San Fernando deposit in central Cuba. The scarcity of VMS deposits is incongruous, since regional work has clearly established that the Greater Antilles formed as island arc assemblages in a largely subaqueous environment. As such, the region represent an ideal tectonic setting for the formation of VMS mineralization. An increase in base metal exploration of volcanic belts beginning in the mid-1970's, combined with a reexamination of historic base metal districts has resulted in the discovery of a number of copper or copper-zinc rich VMS deposits.

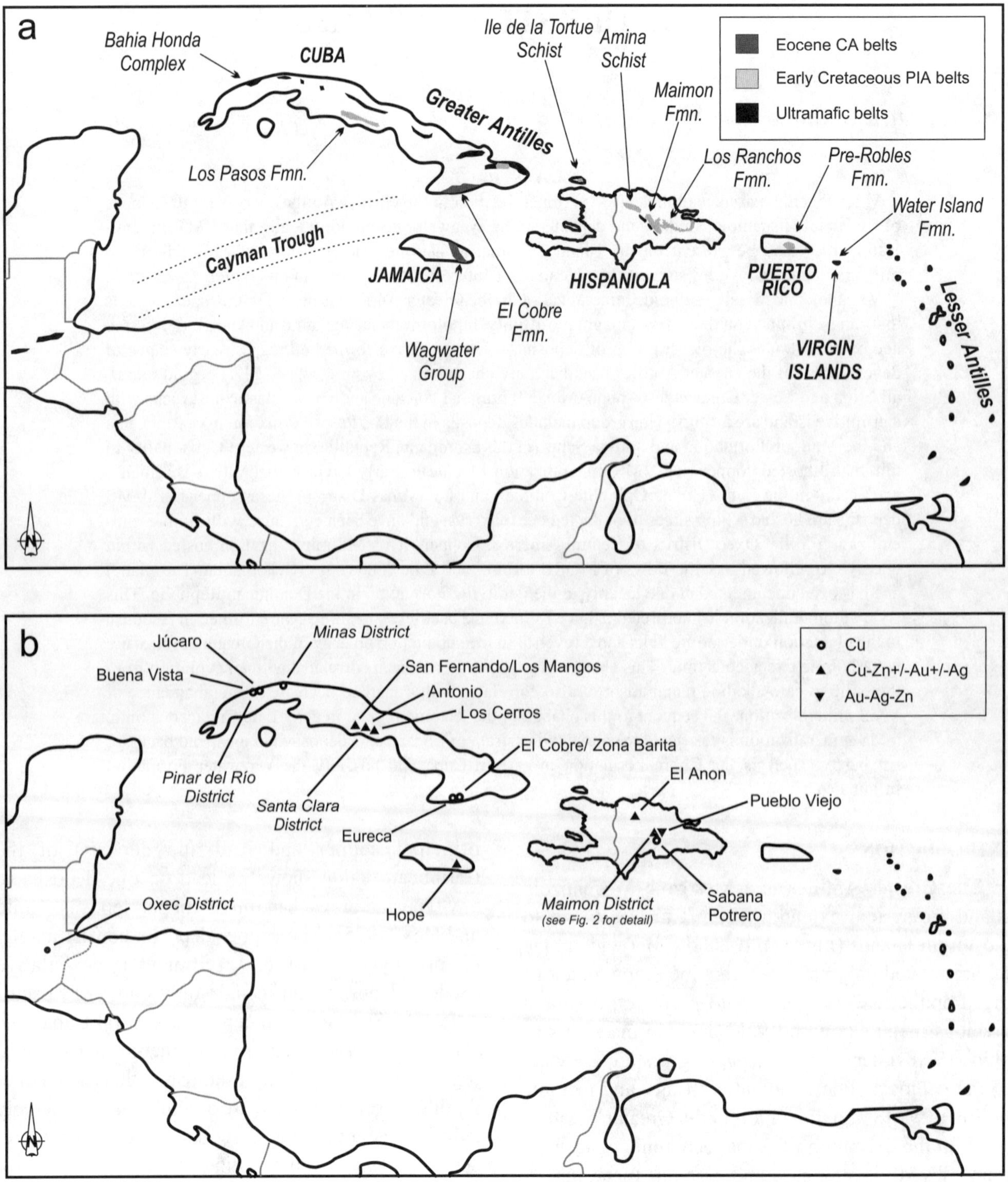

Figure 1. a) Distribution of Eocene calc-alkaline, Early Cretaceous primitive island arc and ultramafic assemblages in the Greater Antilles; b) location of VMS deposits and prospects in the Greater Antilles.

The distribution of these deposits is typical of other well established VMS districts, as the deposits tend to cluster within specific, favorable formations within the arc system (Figs. 1a and b). In general, VMS deposits in the Greater Antilles tend to be relatively small, but high grade, often with significant precious metal values. They are typically copper- or copper-zinc-rich, the scarcity of truly polymetallic (copper-lead-zinc) or lead-rich deposits is consistent with the tectonic setting, that is, arc formation predominantly on a juvenile oceanic substrate.

Several classification schemes have been proposed to categorize VMS deposits, the most widely accepted being the threefold classification of Sawkins (1976), which divides deposits into Kuroko-, Besshi- and Cyprus-type, based on tectonic setting, host lithologies and metal content. However, this system of classification has limitations in the Greater Antilles. Although some of the copper-rich, mafic volcanic and volcanic-sediment hosted deposits in this region have fundamental similarities to the Cyprus and Besshi deposits, the compositionally bimodal volcanic-hosted deposits are distinct from true Kuroko-type mineralization in terms of tectonic setting, magmatic affiliation of host lithologies and metal content. Therefore in this paper VMS mineralization is categorized simply by host rocks, known or inferred age, metal association and when known, magmatic affinity, without using commonly used VMS classification schemes (cf. Thompson et al., 1994; Sherlock et al., 1996) (Table 1).

Tectonic Evolution of the Greater Antilles

The Greater Antilles is a Cretaceous to Tertiary arc system which was deformed by Late Mesozoic to Cenozoic tectonic processes (Lewis and Draper, 1990). Rocks in western and central Cuba are thought to have formed, at least in part, on a continental substrate and contain continentally-derived detritus, suggesting formation proximal to an evolved emergent landmass. Strata in western Cuba have been correlated with similar assemblages in Guatemala and the Yucatan Peninsula (Khudoley and Meyerhoff, 1971). In contrast, assemblages from eastern Cuba eastward to the Virgin Islands, including the islands of Hispaniola, Puerto Rico and Jamaica, formed in a primitive island arc environment on an oceanic substrate.

Although lateral facies variations, limited exposure and post-depositional faulting have hampered precise stratigraphic correlations within and between the islands of the Greater Antilles, volcanic and intrusive rocks of similar age and magmatic affinity can be traced across this region. Donnelley and Rogers (1980) have defined three distinct igneous suites within this arc system, consisting of mid-ocean ridge basalt (MORB), primitive island arc (PIA) and calc-alkaline (CA) assemblages. In addition to the three magmatic suites, ophiolitic rocks of Early to Late Cretaceous age, representing obducted slices of oceanic crust, form discrete belts across the Greater Antilles (Pindell and Barrett, 1990).

Mid-ocean ridge basalt of Early Cretaceous (Aptian to Coniacian) age is interpreted to have erupted in the early stages of development of the Greater Antilles arc, perhaps as early oceanic plateaus or seamounts whose formation was roughly coincident with the onset of pre-Albian age PIA volcanism. Donnelley and Rogers (1980) and Donnelley et al. (1990) interpret compositionally bimodal, subaqueous to locally subaerial PIA assemblages to have formed in response to early subduction within the arc system. Widespread Late Cretaceous volcanic and intrusive rocks of intermediate composition in the Greater Antilles have a CA magmatic affinity (Donnelley et al., 1990). Throughout the Greater Antilles these more evolved CA assemblages are separated from older MORB and PIA assemblages by a regional unconformity. Draper and Lewis (1991) and Lebrón and Perfit (1994) have suggested that this abrupt change in magmatic affinity is coincident with a reversal of subduction polarity, from northeast to southwest directed subduction in Early Cretaceous (Albian) time. Lebrón and Perfit (1994) further speculate that the evolution of the magmatic rocks may be in direct response to a change in the composition of both the subducted slab and entrained sediments. Draper et al. (1996) correlate reversal of subduction polarity with obduction of ophiolite assemblages in Hispaniola and Puerto Rico, followed by extrusion of basalts of the Peralvillo Formation and other mafic volcanic sequences in this region in Late Cretaceous time.

Table 1. VMS mineralization in the Greater Antilles

Deposit	Country	Formation	Age	Metals	Host Lithologies	Status, Reserves & Past Production
El Cobre/ Zona Barita	Cuba	El Cobre	Eocene	Cu-Au	andesite porphyry & pyroclastics	Past Producer at El Cobre, drilling at Zona Barita in late 1990's (1)
Eureca	Cuba	El Cobre	Eocene	Cu-Au	andesite porphyry & pyroclastics	Past Production: 63,500 t of 7-9% Cu (2)
Hope	Jamaica	Wagwater	Eocene	Pb-Zn-Cu-Ag	andesite & volcanic-derived sediments	Past Cu-Pb Producer (3)
Sabana Potrero	D.R.	Peralvillo	Late Cretaceous (Cenomanian -Turonian?)	Cu>>Zn	pillowed to massive basalt flows	Drilled prospect (late 1980's), cut >10 m of low grade massive sulphides (4)
Buena Vista	Cuba	Encrucijada (Bahia Honda Complex)	Early-Late Cretaceous (Aptian-Turonian)	Cu	ophiolite (flow & pyroclastic rocks)	Past production: 0.363 Mt of medium quality sulphide & oxide ores (2); Proven & Probable Reserves: 0.106 Mt of 2.58% Cu (13)
Júcaro	Cuba	Encrucijada (Bahia Honda Complex)	Early-Late Cretaceous (Aptian -Turonian)	Cu	ophiolite (flow & pyroclastic rocks)	Past producer; Proven & Probable Reserves: 0.589 Mt of 1.38% Cu, 0.31% Zn+Pb (2, 13)
Minas	Cuba	Bahia Honda equivalent	Early-Late Cretaceous (?)	Cu	ophiolite (flow & pyroclastic rocks)	Several small past-producers and prospects (1,5)
Los Mangos-San Fernando	Cuba	Los Pasos	Early Cretaceous (Albian-Aptian?)	Zn-Cu -Ag	bimodal volcanic	Past Production: 1840-1942: 13,600 t @ 17-20% Cu; 1955-1961: 0.2 Mt @ 2.75% Cu, 7.0% Zn, 3.0g/t Au, 205g/t Ag. 1997 Indicated Resource: 1.0 Mt of 1.84% Cu, 3.35% Zn (2,6)
Antonio	Cuba	Los Pasos	Early Cretaceous (Albian-Aptian?)	Cu	bimodal volcanic	Past Production from oxide zones; Sulphide Resource: 1.67 Mt of 0.5-0.6% Cu (2, 13)
Los Cerros	Cuba	Los Pasos	Early Cretaceous (Albian-Aptian?)	Cu	bimodal volcanic	Past Production from oxide zones; low grade pyritic sulphides (up to 0.38% Cu, 0.49% Zn, 0.09% Pb, 0.45g/tAu, 0.8g/t Ag) (13)
Cerro de Maimon	D.R.	Maimon	Early Cretaceous (Albian-Aptian?)	Cu-Zn-Au-Ag	bimodal volcanic	Inferred Resource: 3.5 Mt of 3.77% Cu, 2.04% Zn, 0.62g/t Au, 46.36g/t Ag in sulphides; 0.30 Mt of 0.31% Cu, 0.02% Zn, 3.10g/t Au, 59.9 g/t Ag in oxides based on drilling in 1970's to 1980's (7)
San Antonio	D.R.	Maimon	Early Cretaceous (Albian-Aptian?)	Cu-Zn-Au-Ag	bimodal volcanic	Drilled prospect, exploration ongoing at time of publication, short (0.5-4m) high grade massive sulphides at 3 stratigraphic levels over a 2 km strike length (8)
Loma La Mina	D.R.	Maimon	Early Cretaceous (Albian-Aptian?)	Cu-Zn -Au-Ag	bimodal volcanic	Historic Cu production in oxide zones, Drilled Prospect (1960's to 1990's) (9,10,11)
Loma Pesada	D.R.	Maimon	Early Cretaceous (Albian-Aptian?)	Cu-Zn	bimodal volcanic	Drilled Prospect (1991) Indicated Resource: 1.105 Mt of 2.13% Cu, 0.77% Zn, 4.37g/t Ag, 0.16g/t Au (14)
Loma Barbuito	D.R.	Maimon	Early Cretaceous (Albian-Aptian?	Cu-Zn	bimodal volcanic	Drilled prospect (1990's) cut low grade massive sulphides up to 26m thick, including 6.16m of 4.4% Cu, 3% Zn, 108.3g/t Ag, 1.4g/t Au (12, 14)
El Altar	D.R.	Maimon	Early Cretaceous (Albian-Aptian?)	Cu-Zn	bimodal volcanic	Drilled prospect (12)
El Anon	D.R.	Amina	Early Cretaceous (Albian-Aptian?)	Cu-Zn	bimodal volcanic	Drilled prospect, Indictaed Resource of 0.3 Mt of 1.58g/t Au in oxides in the Cerro Verde Zone & 0.27Mt of 2% Cu, 1.67% Zn, 1.28g/t Au, 13.6g/t Ag at Anomaly B (4, 14)
Pueblo Viejo	D.R.	Los Ranchos	Early Cretaceous (Albian-Aptian?)	Au-Ag-Zn	bimodal volcanic	Past Production: 5.3 Moz. Au & 24.4 Moz. Ag from oxides, reserves of >20 Moz. Au, 200 Moz. Ag & 3 Mt

abbreviations: t=tonnes, Mt=million tonnes, Moz=million ounces, m=metres, km=kilometres, D.R. = Dominican Republic

footnotes:
(1) Feoktisov et al. (1983) (2) Bogdanov et al. (1966) (3) Carby (1985) (4) Espaillat et al. (1989)
(5) Kesler et al. (1990) (6) Bottrill et al. (this volume) (7) Lewis et al. (1989) (8) Energold Mining Ltd. & Atna Resources Inc. News Release, March 12, 1999
(9) Vaughan et al. (1921) (10) Koschmann and Gordon (1950) (11) Energold Mining Ltd. News Releases, August 12, 1998 and January 18, 1999
(12) Espaillat, 1995 (13) Russell et al. (this volume) (14) ACA Howe, 1998

By Paleocene to Eocene time arc magmatism in the Greater Antilles was confined to CA volcanism localized within in small basins such as those of the El Cobre Formation in the Sierra Maestra of eastern Cuba and the Wagwater Group in Jamaica. The present day tectonic regime of the Greater Antilles is dominated by post-Eocene left-lateral strike-slip movement, which has formed the Cayman Trough. Cuba is now part of the North American plate, whereas the other islands of the Greater Antilles lie on the Caribbean plate. The Caribbean plate is bounded to the east and west by subduction zones, with the oceanic Cocos and Nazca plates being subducted under Central America to the west and Atlantic ocean crust being subducted under the Lesser Antilles to the east (Mann et al., 1991).

Within the Greater Antilles copper and copper-zinc-gold-silver VMS mineralization is found within Lower to lowermost Upper Cretaceous volcanic rocks of PIA and MORB affinity, as well as Lower to Upper Cretaceous mafic-ultramafic ophiolitic assemblages. In addition, gold-enriched baritic to massive sulphide mineralization, of probable VMS origin, occurs within Eocene CA strata.

VMS mineralization in the Greater Antilles

Cuba

Cuba is host to a wide range of styles of massive sulphide mineralization, including VMS and Sedex deposits. This paper discusses the tectonic setting, magmatic affinity and VMS metallogeny of the principal belts which host VMS mineralization in Cuba. For a more comprehensive review of specific VMS deposits in Cuba the reader is referred to Russell et al. (this volume). Feokistov et al. (1983) and Kesler et al. (1990) present reviews of Sedex mineralization in the Pinar del Río district of western Cuba.

Predominantly copper–rich VMS mineralization is abundant in Cuba in comparison to other islands of the Greater Antilles and has been a significant source of base metals intermittently throughout the twentieth century, and possibly much earlier (Bogdanov et al., 1966). Historic VMS districts include Pinar del Río, Minas and Santa Clara (Fig. 1). Despite a long history of exploration in Cuba, recent VMS discoveries, such as the Los Mangos–San Fernando deposit, in the Santa Clara district, suggest potential for future discoveries.

Los Pasos Formation

The Los Pasos Formation consists of volcanic and volcaniclastic rocks of inferred Early Cretaceous (pre-Albian) age, which crop out in the Santa Clara district of central Cuba (Figs. 1a and 1b). The Los Pasos Formation is compositionally bimodal, with massive to amygdaloidal basalt and basaltic andesite and rhyolitic to dacitic flows, subvolcanic intrusives and tuffs; minor intercalated sandstone and shale occur within the sequence (Iturralde-Vinent, 1996). Massive sulphide mineralization hosted within highly altered felsic volcanic and volcaniclastic rocks of the Los Pasos Formation occurs at the Los Mangos-San Fernando, Antonio and Los Cerros deposits (Table 1 and Fig. 1b).

The copper-zinc-rich San Fernando Mine was discovered in 1827 and mined intermittently from 1840 to 1942, with an estimated 13,600 tonnes of ore grading 17-20 % copper recovered from near-surface oxide zones (Bottrill et al., this volume). The mine was reopened in 1955 and mining to 1961 produced a further 200,000 tonnes at an average grade of 2.75 % copper, 7.0 % zinc, 3.0 g/t gold and 205 g/t silver (Bogdanov et al., 1966; Bottrill et al., this volume). Exploration in the late 1990's in the vicinity of the old mine led to the discovery of the Los Mangos orebody; the discovery hole at Los Mangos intersected 3.25 m of 14.09 % zinc, 0.81 % copper, 0.32 % lead, 272 grams of silver per tonne and 1.71 grams of gold per tonne (Holmer Gold Mines Ltd. News Release, January 16, 1997). Further drilling has outlined an indicated resource of 1,000,000 tonnes of 3.35 % zinc and 1.84 % copper and an inferred resource of a further 1,000,000 tonnes of comparable grade; gold and silver were omitted from the calculations due to a lack of data for these elements in older drill holes (Bottrill et al., this volume). Mineralization consists of finely laminated zinc-rich (pyrite>sphalerite>chalcopyrite) sulphides overlying massive copper-rich (pyrite>chalcopyrite>>sphalerite) sulphides hosted within and locally at the top of a sequence of felsic lapilli to ash tuff, altered to a quartz-sericite-pyrite assemblage. The mineralized sequence is overlain by a thin rhyolite-dacite tuff unit, which is capped by a mafic sequence consisting of basalt to basaltic-andesite lapilli tuff with lesser flows (Bottrill et al., this volume).

The Antonio deposit is located approximately 27 km southeast of Los Mangos-San Fernando. Sulphide mineralization at Antonio consists of pyrite and chalcopyrite with lesser sphalerite and sulphosalts, hosted at the top of a sequence of altered felsic volcanic breccias overlain by basalt flows and breccias. Sulphide reserves of 1,666,300 tonnes grading 0.52 to 0.6 % copper have been calculated for the Antonio deposit; enriched oxide zones overlying the massive sulphides are mined out (Bogdanov et al., 1966; Russell et al., this volume).

Some 15 km southeast of Antonio, the Los Cerros deposit is also the site of past production from near-surface secondary oxide zones. Remaining primary sulphide mineralization consists of pyrite with lesser chalcopyrite and sphalerite hosted by dacite and rhyolite altered to a quartz-chlorite-epidote-sericite-albite assemblage (Russell et al., this volume).

Bahia Honda Complex

Mafic volcanic-hosted copper-rich VMS deposits occur in the Bahia Honda ophiolite complex in the eastern part of the Pinar del Río District of western Cuba (Fig. 1a). Deposits of this type include Buena Vista and Júcaro (Table 1 and Fig. 1b). Bogdanov et al. (1966) describe VMS mineralization at the past-producing Buena Vista deposit as lenticular to stock-like zones of pyrite and chalcopyrite hosted within mafic to ultramafic flows and pyroclastic rocks. Some 20 km away at Júcaro, copper-rich massive to semi-massive sulphide mineralization is hosted within similar strata.

Lewis and Draper (1990) suggest that the Bahia Honda Complex represents an overturned oceanic succession of allochthonous affinity. Strata associated with VMS mineralization form a 50 km long, 1-7 km wide belt of mafic lavas and tuffs, subvolcanic intrusions and marine sediments of Early to Late Cretaceous (Aptian-Turonian) age (Feokistov et al., 1983). Case et al. (1984) correlate the Bahia Honda complex with ophiolitic rocks which host similar mineralization in the Oxec District of Guatemala; Kesler et al. (1990) suggest a correlation with massive sulphide mineralization in the Minas District of Cuba, some 100 km to the east.

El Cobre Formation

The Paleocene to Upper Eocene El Cobre Formation in eastern Cuba consists primarily of water-lain pyroclastic strata, with minor basaltic and dacitic flows lower in the sequence and limestone higher in the sequence (Lewis and Draper, 1990) (Fig. 1a). Copper-gold-rich baritic VMS mineralization occurs in the Cobre Formation at the past-producing El Cobre deposit and the nearby Zona Barita (Guild and Cox, 1975; Joutel Resources News Release, March 7, 1999) (Fig. 1b). Based on textural evidence, mineralization at El Cobre and Zona Barita may have formed primarily as a subseafloor replacement (T. Bottrill, pers. comm., 1999). Also within the Cobre Formation, a similar style of mineralization has been described at the Eureca deposit by Bogdanov et al. (1966). Massive to semi-massive mineralization at Eureca consists of a barite-pyrite-chalcopyrite lens which, prior to mining contained 63,500 tons of ore with an average copper grade of 8 %, as well as pyrite-chalcopyrite "vein-incrustations" which cut pyroclastic rocks and andesite porphyry. Based on similarities in alteration and mineralogy, Bogdanov et al. (1966) suggest Eureca has similarities to VMS mineralization at Rio Tinto in Spain. However, Kesler et al. (1990) suggest that the mined-out deposit represents epithermal vein style mineralization. Based on the information available, barite-sulphide-gold mineralization at Eureca, El Cobre and the nearby Zona Barita is tentatively included as VMS mineralization of probable Eocene age.

Hispaniola (Dominicanf Republic and Haiti)

The island of Hispaniola is divided into the Dominican Republic to the east and Haiti to the west, with the roughly north-south political boundary obliquely cutting the northwest trend of the principal belts and tectonic features of Hispaniola (Fig. 1a). The most significant ore deposit on Hispaniola is the world class Pueblo Viejo gold-silver-zinc deposit, hosted by the Los Ranchos Formation in the central Dominican Republic (Fig. 2). Known VMS mineral-

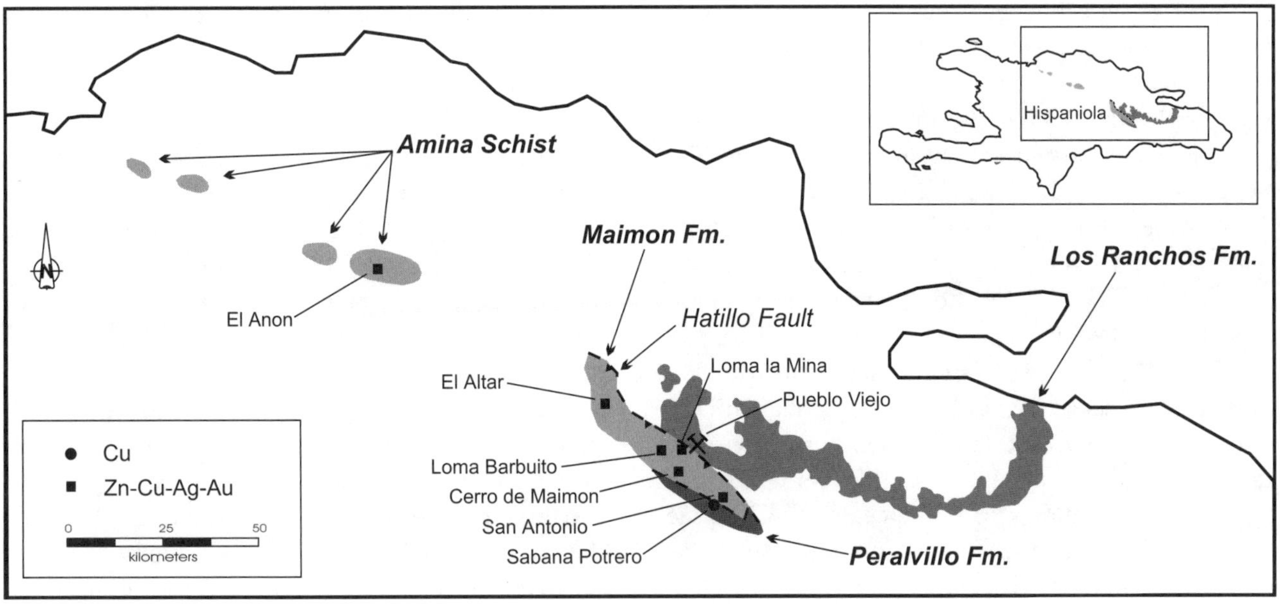

Figure 2. Location of VMS deposits and prospects in the Dominican Republic, island of Hispaniola.

ization on Hispaniola is hosted by bimodal volcanic rocks of the Maimón Formation and Amina Schist, as well as basalt of the Peralvillo Formation. Copper- and copper-zinc-rich VMS deposits in the Maimón Formation are known for their historic production, however, no development has occurred in the latter half of the twentieth century.

Maimón Formation

The Maimón Formation crops out as a 1-10 km wide by 65 km long, northwest trending, volcanic and sedimentary belt in the central Dominican Republic (Fig. 1a); palentological and isotopic age constraints are scarce. Geological relations suggest an Early Cretaceous (pre-Albian) age, which is consistent with unpublished lead isotopic model ages (S. Horan, unpublished data, 1995), fossil data (S.K. Donovan, unpublished data, 1994) and correlation with other PIA assemblages in the Greater Antilles.

Copper-rich base metal deposits in the Maimón Formation have been exploited on a small scale since at least the time of Spanish colonization (Vaughan et al., 1921; Koschmann and Gordon, 1950). Modern base metal exploration in the Maimón Formation beginning in the 1970's led to the discovery of a number of VMS deposits and prospects (Table 1 and Fig. 2). General features common to VMS mineralization in the Maimón Formation include a spatial association with bimodal volcanic and volcaniclastic rocks, zinc-copper mineralization with low lead concentrations and significant precious metal grades that are enhanced in near-surface, secondary oxide zones.

The two most advanced VMS deposits in the Maimón Formation are Cerro de Maimón and San Antonio (Fig. 2). The geology and mineralization of these two deposits, along with Loma la Mina, a small-scale historic producer, is summarized below. For greater detail on Cerro de Maimón and San Antonio the reader is referred to Astacio (1998), Lewis et al (this volume) and Holbek and Daubeny (this volume). Other VMS mineralization in the Maimón Formation is found at the drill-tested Loma Barbuito, Loma Pesada and El Altar prospects, as well as at several grassroots prospects (Table 1).

The Maimón Formation contains volcanic and volcaniclastic strata with minor intercalated marine sedimentary strata, all of which are metamorphosed to greenschist to sub-greenschist facies. Volcanic strata consist of massive to pillowed mafic flows and felsic flows, tuffs and fragmental rocks with coeval dykes and small intrusive bodies. Marine sedimentary strata include greywacke, shale, conglomerate, limestone and chert. The sedimentary assemblage and lack of terrestrial fossils indicated formation in a relatively deep water environment.

Strata of the Maimón Formation strike northwest and dip steeply to moderately to the southwest. The sequence is bound to the northeast by the Hatillo Fault, which thrust rocks of the Maimón Formation northeastward, over younger sedimentary rocks of the Hatillo, Las Lagunas and Los Ranchos Formations, probably in the Late Eocene. The Hatillo Thrust is locally imbricate, with small slices of Maimón Formation rocks lying northeast of the principal fault trace. To the southwest, the Maimón Formation is in fault contact with the Loma Caribe Peridotite and Peralvillo Formation; drill intercepts at Cerro de Maimón show the Peralvillo-Maimón contact to be strongly sheared (Lewis et al., 1998). Deformation in the Maimón Formation may be related to obduction of the Loma Caribe peridotite in mid-Cretaceous time, resulting in an increase in the intensity of deformation of the Maimón Formation southwest towards the peridotite belt (Draper et al., 1996). Strata on the southwest side of the Maimón Formation are highly deformed and locally mylonitic, whereas strata on the northeastern side is less deformed and can retain primary volcanic and sedimentary textures (Draper et al., 1996). The exception to this is immediately adjacent to the Hatillo Thrust, where strata are typically well foliated and locally sheared.

Major element lithogeochemical studies indicate that volcanic strata of the Maimón Formation are compositionally bimodal, with relatively low primary potassium and high sodium concentrations (Kesler et al., 1991a; Holbek and Daubeny, this volume). Trace element analyses of Maimón Formation rhyolite and basalt yield low concentrations of high field strength (HFSE) and rare earth (REE) elements, along with enrichment of large ion lithophile elements (LILE) (Espaillat, 1995; Lewis et al., 1998); Maimón Formation volcanic rocks have a tholeiitic affinity characteristic of PIA assemblages (Donnelley and Rogers, 1980).

Volcanogenic massive sulphide mineralization at Cerro de Maimón was discovered in the mid-1970's during the early stages of modern base metal exploration of the Maimón Formation. Drilling indicates a primary sulphide resource of 3.36 million tonnes of 3.93 % copper, 1.93 % zinc, 0.56 g/t gold and 47.3 g/t silver, overlain by a secondary oxide resource of 0.32 million tonnes of 3.10 g/t gold and 59.9 g/t silver (Lewis et al., 1998). The deposit is hosted by variably deformed and metamorphosed flows, volcaniclastic rocks and chert near the southwestern margin of the Maimón Formation. The hangingwall is metamorphosed, but not hydrothermally altered, and consists of tuffs of intermediate composition, mafic flows and thin lenses of chert. The footwall consists of metamorphosed quartz-sericite-pyrite altered felsic volcaniclastic and intermediate composition tuffaceous rocks (Astacio, 1998; Lewis et al., 1998).

Massive sulphide mineralization at Cerro de Maimón extends from surface, where it occurs as gossan, to depths of at least 200 m. At depth, primary sulphides form massive to semi-massive lenses of pyrite with lesser chalcopyrite and sphalerite and minor bornite, tetrahedrite-tenantite, galena and idalite (Astacio, 1998). Supergene processes have resulted in enhancement of precious metal grades and replacement of primary sulphides by chalcocite.

Volcanogenic massive sulphide mineralization was discovered at San Antonio in the late 1980's; a small drill program in 1990-91 at the La Parcela zone intersected massive sulphide mineralization in two of four holes drilled. The discovery hole cut 15.6 m of low grade, massive to semi-massive pyrite with minor amounts of sphalerite and chalcopyrite. Drilling of a further sixteen holes in 1999 intersected thinner (1.2-4.6 m) intervals of high grade massive sulphides, including 3.1 m of 3.39 % copper, 8.55 % zinc, 0.13 % lead, 185.2 g/t silver and 1.38 g/t gold (Energold Mining Ltd. and Atna Resources Ltd. News Releases, March 12, 1999). San Antonio occurs within a compositionally bimodal volcanic and volcaniclastic sequence. Mineralization occurs at three or more stratigraphic horizons, including at or near the contact between unaltered felsic hangingwall tuffs and fragmental rocks and footwall quartz-sericite±pyrite altered schists in the La Parcela zone, as well as within footwall quartz-sericite±pyrite altered schists in the Copper zone. At the time of writing (March, 2000) drilling is ongoing at San Antonio.

The Loma la Mina deposit, located approximately

10 km west of Cerro de Maimón, is the site of historic copper mining (Vaughan et al., 1921; Koschmann and Gordon, 1950); evidence of mining activity remains in the form of old pits, trenches and dumps, as well as small piles of slag. From the 1960's to present three small drill campaigns have been conducted on the property in the search for base and precious metals (Energold Mining Ltd. News Releases Aug. 12, 1998 and January 18, 1999).

Chlorite and quartz-sericite-pyrite schists of the Maimón Formation are exposed on top and down the west side of Loma la Mina, in the hangingwall of the northwest trending Hatillo thrust fault. Strata at Loma la Mina are considerably more deformed than at Cerro de Maimón and San Antonio, with primary textures rarely preserved. Late brittle (?) faults which cut and offset stratigraphy, along with intense deformation and paucity of outcrop have hampered recognition of the primary stratigraphic sequence at Loma La Mina and prevented direct correlation with stratigraphy which hosts massive sulphide mineralization at Cerro de Maimón and San Antonio. Schists at Loma la Mina are gossanous and commonly malachite and azurite stained, particularly in the vicinity of old workings. At surface, primary iron and copper sulphides are almost completely weathered to oxides. A strong gold in soil anomaly is roughly coincident with surface oxide mineralization. Drilling has intersected multiple lenses of deformed but broadly conformable, low grade volcanogenic massive to semi-massive sulphides, with thicknesses locally exceeding ten metres.

Amina and Ile de la Tortue Schists

The Amina Schist, in northwestern Dominican Republic and the Ile de la Tortue Schist, off the north coast of Haiti have been correlated with the Maimón Formation on the basis of similarities in lithology, magmatic affinity and structural style (Draper and Lewis, 1982; Lewis and Draper, 1990; Kesler et al., 1991a) (Fig. 1a). The Amina Schist is geochemically similar to the Maimón Formation, with a weakly compositionally bimodal assemblage of basaltic andesite and dacite to rhyolite with low primary potassium concentrations and high iron to magnesium ratios (Draper and Lewis, 1982; Kesler et al., 1991a).

In contrast to the Maimón Formation, which contains abundant flows and contemporaneous sub-volcanic intrusive rocks, the Amina and Ile de la Tortue Schists are comprised of volcanic-derived sedimentary material, with little or no lava. Draper and Lewis (1982) suggest that these facies variation may reflect a more distal setting for the Amina Schist; this analogy may be extended to the Ile de la Tortue Schist. A distal setting may in part be responsible for the scarcity of known VMS mineralization in the schists relative to the Maimón Formation. El Anon, in northwestern Dominican Republic, represents the only documented VMS prospect known in this belt. At El Anon copper- and zinc-rich sulphides hosted within quartz-sericite-pyrite and chlorite schists have been cut in drill holes in four zones, namely Cerro Verde, Elias Gossan, Anomaly A and Anomaly B (Brouwer et al., 1989, ACA Howe, 1998) (Fig. 2). An oxide-hosted indicated resource of 300,000 tonnes of 1.58 g/t gold, thought to be derived from the secondary concentration of underlying low grade pyritic ore, was calculated for Cerro Verde and a massive sulphide indicated resource of 272,667 tonnes of 2 % copper, 1.67 % zinc, 1.28 g/t gold and 13.6 g/t silver was calculated for Anomaly B (ACA Howe, 1998).

Los Ranchos Formation

The Los Ranchos Formation is a Lower Cretaceous (Aptian-Albian), compositionally bimodal volcanic and volcaniclastic assemblage of PIA affinity, which is thought to have formed contemporaneously with or slightly later than the Maimón Formation (Donnelley and Rodgers, 1980; Kesler et al., 1991b) (Fig. 1a). In contrast to the Maimón Formation, a fossil assemblage that includes terrestrial plant debris suggests formation in a subaerial to shallow subaqueous environment. Near its faulted western margin, the Los Ranchos Formation is host to the world class Pueblo Viejo gold-silver-zinc deposit, from which 5.3 million ounces of gold and 24.4 million ounces of silver has been mined from oxide ore bodies and sulphide-hosted reserves are estimated to be in excess of 20 million ounces of gold, 200 million ounces of silver and 3 million tones of zinc (Fig. 2). Russell and Kesler (1991) interpret Pueblo Viejo to have formed from acid sulphate (high sulphidation) fluids in a maar-diatreme setting, however, new insights into geologic relations at Pueblo Viejo and a general shift away from the maar-diatreme model has led to reevaluation of this model by Kesler (1998). Recent reexamination of well-known VMS deposits, such as the Boliden deposit in Sweden, as well as the discovery of the precious metal-rich VMS Eskay Creek deposit in Canada has led to the recognition of a group of deposits which formed in a subaqueous, transitional setting with characteristic of both epithermal and VMS mineralization (Sillitoe et al., 1996). Features of this style of mineralization include high precious metal concentrations relative to traditional VMS mineralization, an epithermal (As-Sb-Hg) trace element signature and the presence of low pH alteration assemblages (alunite, pyrophyllite, dickite).

At Pueblo Viejo the presence of alunite, pyrophyllite, and enargite attest to the high sulphidation nature of the mineralizing fluids. Characteristics such as the high zinc concentration and bedded pyritic-carbonaceous sediments of probable exhalative origin suggest that Pueblo Viejo is a transitional epithermal-VMS deposit.

Peralvillo Formation

Basaltic lavas of the Peralvillo Formation crop out around the southern end of the Maimón Formation in the central Dominican Republic; where observed, the contact is faulted (Espaillat et al., 1989; Lewis et al., 1998) (Fig. 2). Trace element geochemistry indicates that the basalts have a geochemical signature similar to MORB (Donnelley and Rodgers, 1980; Espaillat et al., 1989) and are interpreted to have formed within a back arc spreading centre in probable Late Cretaceous time, immediately following a reversal in subduction polarity and cessation of Early Cretaceous PIA volcanism (Draper and Lewis, 1991).

Copper-rich VMS mineralization within the Peralvillo Formation has been identified at Sabana Potrero, where drilling has intersected pyrite- and chalcopyrite-rich massive sulphides with lesser sphalerite, hosted by pillowed to massive basaltic flows cut by diabase (Brouwer et al., 1989; Espaillat et al., 1989) (Fig. 2). Massive sulphide mineralization is structurally overlain by altered basalt containing an anastamosing stockwork of quartz-sulphide±chlorite veins suggesting that drilled section at Sabana Potrero is overturned, imbricated or that multiple, stacked lenses may be present.

Puerto Rico

Much of Puerto Rico is underlain by three fault-bounded igneous sequences which record a similar tectonic evolution to the arc assemblages of Hispaniola (Schellekens, 1991; Schellekens, 1998). Base metal exploration beginning in the 1950's resulted in the discovery of several significant Late Cretaceous porphyry copper deposits, including Tánama and Río Viví (Guild and Cox, 1975). Volcanogenic massive sulphide mineralization is not recognized in Puerto Rico. However, limited exposures of a Lower Cretaceous bimodal, mainly volcaniclastic sequence of PIA affinity, the pre-Robles Formation, which was emplaced at least in part in a subaqueous setting, suggests limited potential for Early Cretaceous Zn-Cu-Ag-Au VMS mineralization (Fig. 2).

Virgin Islands

Volcanogenic massive sulphide mineralization is not documented in the Virgin Islands. However, similar to Puerto Rico, the Virgin Islands contains limited exposures of prospective bimodal stratigraphy of PIA affinity in the Water Island Formation (Donnelley, 1966) (Fig 1a). Bimodal volcanic rocks of the Water Island Formation consists mainly of subaqueous lavas with minor volcaniclastic rock and as such represent prospective stratigraphy for the discovery of VMS mineralization.

Jamaica

The surface area of Jamaica is dominated by Tertiary limestone, overlain by alumina-rich soil from which bauxite is mined. Exposures of volcanic and intrusive strata are limited to the Wagwater Trough and several small Cretaceous inliers. Non-bauxite mineral exploration in Jamaica has focused mainly on porphyry copper and epithermal gold potential, in large part due to discovery of these styles of mineralization on the nearby islands of Puerto Rico and Hispaniola (Fenton, 1987). Possible VMS mineralization occurs within the Wagwater Group at the Hope Mine, near Kingston (Figs. 1a and b).

Wagwater Group

The Wagwater Group, in eastern Jamaica, is a fault-bounded sequence of Paleocene to Early Eocene volcanic and volcaniclastic strata, conglomerate and minor limestone and evaporites that hosts several base and precious metal showings (Fenton, 1987). The interpreted tectonic setting of the Wagwater Group is equivocal. Draper (1979) suggests formation in a back arc basin, in response to southeast directed subduction, whereas Jackson and Smith (1979) favour formation within a pull-apart basin, in response to short-lived right-lateral shear. Lewis and Draper (1990) suggest that subsequent to major Cretaceous arc building, a northwest trending rift basin formed in what is now eastern Jamaica. Rifting was synchronous with dacitic to basaltic calc-alkaline volcanism and infilling of the resultant trough with conglomerate and marine sediments. Water depths in the trough were variable, as evidenced by the presence of shallow water evaporates and deep water turbidite sequences.

The Hope Mine represents the only non-bauxite deposit to produce significant amounts of ore in Jamaica; with small-scale sporadic copper and lead production since the 1850's (Fenton, 1987). The average grade of a subset of samples collected from the deposit yielded 4.7 % zinc, 1.8 % lead, 5 g/t silver and 3 g/t gold (Carby, 1985). Mineralization at the Hope Mine occurs as stratabound, moderately dipping pods or lenses of massive to semi-massive pyrite-sphalerite-galena-chalcopyrite at the contact between Wagwater Formation volcaniclastic rocks and a plagioclase porphyritic andesite flow or sill, known as the Hope Mine Member (Carby, 1984). Although the Hope Mine Member overlies mineralization, Carby (1984) suggests that this highly altered and pyritic unit originally formed the stratigraphic footwall and that the deposit is overturned. Geochemistry reveal an asymmetric alteration halo around the mineralization, with a decrease in sodium and a corresponding increase in potassium with increasing intensity of alteration in the Hope Mine Member (Carby, 1984).

The genesis of massive sulphide mineralization at the Hope Mine is equivocal. Carby and Jackson (1980) compare the deposit to Kuroko-type VMS deposits and although the metal signature is polymetallic, the lack of intimately associated felsic volcanism and interpreted tectonic setting is inconsistent with Kuroko deposits. In contrast, Kesler et al. (1990) interpret the deposit to have formed as a replacement or vein, rather than through exhalative processes. The concordant nature of mineralization and intense alteration of the interpreted footwall resulting in strong sodium depletion and potassium enrichment suggest that this deposit may have formed in Paleocene to Early Eocene time as rift-related polymetallic andesite-hosted VMS mineralization by either replacement or exhalative processes.

DISCUSSION

Volcanogenic massive sulphide mineralization occurs throughout the Greater Antilles and can be grouped by inferred age, metal signature, host lithology and magmatic affinity as follows:

Early Cretaceous (Aptian-Albian?) PIA-hosted Zn-Cu-Ag±Au mineralization

Deposits in this group include San Fernando/Los Mangos in the Los Pasos Formation of Cuba, Cerro de Maimón, San Antonio and Loma La Mina in the Maimón Formation of the Dominican Republic and El Anon in the Amina Schist of the Dominican Republic. These deposits consist of copper-zinc massive sulphide mineralization with appreciable precious metal contents that are hosted by PIA bimodal volcanic and volcaniclastic strata of Early Cretaceous age. The relative abundance of VMS mineralization in the Los Pasos and Maimón Formations relative to the other PIA assemblages in the Greater Antilles may in part be related to water depth and proximity to active volcanism. However, the presence of VMS mineralization in Lower Cretaceous PIA assemblages in Cuba and Hispaniola suggests the potential for discovery within similar strata throughout the Greater Antilles.

The precious metal-rich Pueblo Viejo deposit, hosted by Lower Cretaceous sedimentary strata and PIA volcanic rocks of Los Ranchos Formation in the Dominican Republic, is interpreted to be a transitional epithermal-VMS deposit. Pueblo Viejo represents a distinct outlier to an otherwise generally similar group of deposits in terms of size, metal content and depth of formation.

Early-Late Cretaceous (Aptian-Turonian) Ophiolite-hosted Cu mineralization

This style of mineralization is restricted to western Cuba and includes deposits such as Buena Vista and Júcaro in the Bahia Honda ophiolite complex and deposits in the Las Minas district. These cupriferous pyrite deposits are hosted within mafic volcanic strata interpreted to represent fragments of obducted oceanic crust. Correlation of the Bahia Honda deposits with ophiolite-hosted copper-rich massive sulphide mineralization in the Oxec district of Guatemala suggests that this style of VMS mineralization was relatively widespread in Aptian-Turonian time and as such, ophiolite sequences of comparable age in the northern Greater Antilles and Central America hold potential for future VMS exploration.

Late Cretaceous (Cenomanian-Turonian) MORB-hosted Cu-rich mineralization

Interpreted reversal of subduction polarity in Albian time corresponds with an end to PIA volcanism and a marked decrease in development and preservation of VMS mineralization in the Greater Antilles. Only one deposit, Sabana Potrero in the Peralvillo Formation of the Dominican Republic, falls into this classification.

Eocene andesite-hosted Cu-Au and Pb-Zn-Cu-Ag mineralization

This group consists the El Cobre, Zona Barita and Eureca deposits in the Cobre Formation, Cuba and possibly the Hope deposit in the Wagwater Group, Jamaica. These deposits are interpreted to have formed as andesite-hosted polymetallic subseafloor mineralization within Eocene rift basins.

Conclusions

Review and classification of Cretaceous to Tertiary VMS deposits and prospects in the Greater Antilles arc demonstrates a variety of styles and ages of mineralization. Tropical weathering, leading to the formation of secondary, oxide-hosted precious metal-rich ore has been a significant factor in terms of historic mining and delineation of reserves in this region. The presence of districts with abundant VMS deposits and prospects such as Santa Clara and Maimón, as well the world class Pueblo Viejo deposit suggests high potential for future VMS discoveries in the Greater Antilles.

Acknowledgements

Ian Thomson and Terrence Bottrill are gratefully acknowledged for sharing their insights on the Hope and Zona Barita deposits, respectively. Grenville Draper is thanked for his assistance in acquiring difficult to obtain papers on Caribbean geology and mineralization. The reviewers are thanked for their comments and suggestions, which greatly improved this manuscript.

References

ACA Howe, 1998. Unpublished Report Prepared for Sarmin Exploration Corp. September 24, 1998.

Astacio, T.V. 1998. Mineralogy, lithogeochemistry and oxygen isotope study of the Cerro de Maimón massive sulfide deposit, Dominican Republic. M.Sc. thesis, New Mexico Institute of Mining and Technology, Socorro, New Mexico.

Bogdanov, Y.V., Gur'yanova, V.N. and Mitayes, M. 1966. Outline of copper deposits of Cuba. International Geology Review, 8, 1218-1225.

Bottrill, T.J., Formell, F., Raman, K.S. 2000. Los Mangos - San Fernando deposit, Santa Clara, Cuba: Geology and mineralization in a Cretaceous volcanic arc. In VMS Deposits of Latin America, Geological Association of Canada Special Publication. Edited by R. Sherlock and A. Logan.

Brouwer, S.B., MacVeigh, J.G., Espaillat, J., Jimenez, J. and Pizano, O. 1989. Geological setting of some polymetallic massive sulphide occurrences in the Median Belt, Central Dominican Republic. In Transactions of the 12th Caribbean Geological Conference, St. Croix, Virgin Islands.

Carby, B.E. 1984. The alteration halo of the Hope lead-zinc deposit, Jamaica: Major element chemical changes. In Transactions of the 11th Caribbean Geological Conference, Barbados. pp. 22.1-22.9.

Carby, B.E. 1985. The geology, mineralogy and geochemistry of the Hope lead-zinc deposit. Ph.D. thesis, University of the West Indies, Kingston, Jamaica.

Carby, B.E. and Jackson, T.A. 1980. Kuroko-type mineralization in Jamaica. Abstract presented at the 9th Caribbean Geological Conference, Santo Domingo, Dominican Republic.

Case, J.E., Holcombe, T.L. and Martin, R.G. 1984. Map of geologic provinces in the Caribbean region. Geological Society of America Memoir 162, 1-30.

Donnelly, T.W., 1966. Geology of St. Thomas and St. John, U.S. Virgin Islands, In Caribbean Geological Investigations. Edited by H.H. Hess. Geological Society of America Memoir 98, 85-176.

Donnelly, T.W. and Rogers, J.J.W. 1980. Igneous series in

island arcs: the northeast Caribbean compared with worldwide island arc assemblages. Bulletin Volcanologique, 43, 347-382.

Donnelley, T., Beets, D., Carr, M., Jackson, T., Klaver, G., Lewis, J., Maury, R., Schellekens, H., Smith, A., Wadge, G., and Westercamp, D. 1990. History and tectonic setting of the Caribbean magmatism. In The Caribbean Region. Edited by G. Dengo and J.E. Case. The Geological Society of America, Geology of North America Vol. H., pp. 339-374.

Draper, G. 1979. Tectonics of the regionally metamorphosed rocks of eastern Jamaica. Ph.D. thesis, University of the West Indies, Kingston, Jamaica.

Draper, G. and Lewis, J.F. 1982. Petrology, deformation, and tectonic significance of the Amina Schist, northern Dominican Republic. In Transactions of the 9th Caribbean Geological Conference, Santo Domingo, Dominican Republic. pp. 53-64

Draper, G. and Lewis, J.F. 1991. Metamorphic belts in central Hispaniola. In Geologic and Tectonic Development of the North American – Caribbean plate boundary in Hispaniola. Edited by P. Mann, G. Draper, and J.F. Lewis. The Geological Society of America, Special Paper 262, 29-45.

Draper, G., Gutiérrez, G and Lewis, J.F. 1996. Thrust emplacement of the Hispaniola peridotite belt: Orogenic expression of the mid-Cretaceous Caribbean arc polarity reversal? Geology, 24, 12, 1143-1146.

Espaillat, J. 1995. Revisión Litogeoquímica de la Formación Maimón. In Premier Congreso Nacional de Geología y Ciencias Afines de la Hispaniola y Reuníon de Proyecto IGCP 364, Santo Domingo.

Espaillat, J. Bloise, G, MacVeigh, J.G. and Lewis, J.F 1989. Petrography and geochemistry of mafic rocks of the Peralvillo Formation in the Sabana Potrero area, Central Dominican Republic. In Transactions of the 12th Caribbean Geological Conference, St. Croix, Virgin Islands, 190-199.

Fenton, A. 1987. The (non-bauxite) metallic mineral potential of Jamaica. In Proceedings of a workshop on the status of Jamaican geology. Edited by R. Ahmad. The Geological Society of Jamaica, Special Issue 1987, 269-281.

Feoktistov, V.P., Aniyatov, I.A. and Norman, A. 1983. Metallogeny of western Cuba, International Geology Review, 25, 309-318.

Guild, P.W. and Cox., D.P. 1975. Mineral Resources of the Caribbean. Edited by J.W. Draper. Geology Geophysics and Resources of the Caribbean, 150p.

Holbek, P and Daubeny, P. 2000. Geology of the San Antonio concession, Dominican Republic. In VMS Deposits of Latin America, Geological Association of Canada Special Publication. Edited by R. Sherlock, and A. Logan.

Iturralde-Vinent, M.A. 1996. Ofiolitas y arcos volcánicos de Cuba: IUGS-UNESCO International Geological Correlation Programme, Project 364, Caribbean Ophiolites and Volcanic Arc Special Contribution 1, 254 p.

Jackson, T.A. and Smith, T.E. 1979. The tectonic significance of basalts and dacites in the Wagwater Belt, Jamaica. Geological Magazine, 116, 365-374.

Kesler, S.E., 1998. Geologic relations between Pueblo Viejo mineralization and the Los Ranchos Formation: the status in 1998. In Mineral Deposit of the Dominican Republic. Edited by P.G. Feiss. The Society of Economic Geologists, March 1998 Field Trip, Dominican Republic.

Kesler, S.E., Levy, E. and Martin, C.F. 1990. Metallogenic evolution of the Caribbean Region. In The Caribbean Region. Edited by G. Dengo and J.E. Case. The Geological Society of America, Geology of North America Vol. H., 459-482.

Kesler, S.E., Russell, N., Reyes, C., Santos, L., Rodriguez, and Fondeur, L. 1991a. Geology of the Maimón Formation, Dominican Republic. In Geologic and Tectonic Development of the North American – Caribbean plate boundary in Hispaniola. Edited by P. Mann, G. Draper, and J.F. Lewis. The Geological Society of America, Special Paper 262, 173-185.

Kesler, S.E., Russell, N., Polanco, J., McCurdy, K. and Cumming, G.L. 1991b. Geology and geochemistry of the early Cretaceous Los Ranchos Formation, central Dominican Republic. In Geologic and Tectonic Development of the North American – Caribbean plate boundary in Hispaniola. Edited by P. Mann, G. Draper, and J.F. Lewis. The Geological Society of America, Special Paper 262, 187-201.

Khudoley, K.M. and Meyerhoff, A.A. 1971. Paleogeography and geological history of Greater Antilles: Geological Society of America Memoir 129, 199p.

Koschmann, A.H. and Gordon, M. 1950. Geology and mineral resources of the Maimón-Hatillo district, Dominican Republic, United States Geological Survey Bulletin 964-D, 359 p.

Lebrón, M.C. and Perfit, M.R. 1994. Petrochemistry and tectonic significance of Cretaceous island-arc rocks, Cordillera Oriental, Dominican Republic. Tectonophysics, 229, 69-100.

Lewis, J.F., Astacio, V.A., Espaillat, J., Jimenez, J. 2000. The occurrence of volcanogenic massive sulfide deposits in the Maimon Formation, Dominican Republic: The Cerro de Maimon, Loma Pesada and Loma Barbuito Deposits. In VMS Deposits of Latin America, Geological Association of Canada Special Publication. Edited by R. Sherlock and A. Logan.

Lewis, J.F. and Draper, G. 1990. Geology and tectonic evolution of the northern Caribbean margin. In The Caribbean Region. Edited by G. Dengo and J.E. Case. The Geological Society of America, Geology of North America Vol. H., pp. 77-140.

Lewis, J.F., Astacio, T, and Espaillat, J. 1998. The Maimón Formation. In Mineral Deposit of the Dominican Republic. Edited by P.G. Feiss. The Society of Economic Geologists, March 1998 Field Trip, Dominican Republic.

Mann, P., Schubert, C. and Burke, K. 1991. Review of Caribbean neotectonics. In The Caribbean Region. Edited by G. Dengo and J.E. Case. The Geological Society of America, Geology of North America Vol. H., pp. 307-338.

Pindell, J.L. and Barrett, S.F. 1990. Geological evolution of the Caribbean region; a plate tectonic perspective. In The

Caribbean Region. Edited by G. Dengo and J.E. Case. The Geological Society of America, Geology of North America Vol. H., pp. 405-432.

Russell, N. and Kesler, S.E. 1991. Geology of the maar-diatreme complex hosting precious metal mineralization at Pueblo Viejo. In Geologic and Tectonic Development of the North American – Caribbean plate boundary in Hispaniola. Edited by P. Mann, G. Draper, and J.F. Lewis. The Geological Society of America, Special Paper 262, 203-215.

Russell, N., Moreira, J. and Sánchez, R. 2000. Volcanogenic Massive Sulphide deposits of Cuba. In VMS Deposits of Latin America, Geological Association of Canada Special Publication. Edited by R. Sherlock and A. Logan.

Schellekens, J.H. 1998. Geochemical evolution and tectonic history of Puerto Rico. Geological Society of America Special Paper 322, 35-66.

Schellekens, J.H. 1991. Late Jurassic to Eocene geochemical evolution of volcanic rocks of Puerto Rico: Geophysical Research Letters, 18, 553-556.

Sillitoe, R.H., Hannington, M.D. and Thompson, J.F.H. 1996. High sulphidation deposits in the volcanogenic massive sulphide environment. Economic geology, 91, 204-212.

Sawkins, F.J. 1976. Massive sulphide deposits in relation to geotectonics. Geological Association of Canada Special Paper, 14, 221-240.

Sherlock, R.L., Barrett, T.J., Thompson, J.F.H., Macdonald, R.W.J., McKinley, S.D., Roth, T., Sebert, C., and Childe, F., 1996. Geology of volcanogenic massive sulfide deposits in the Cordillera of British Columbia, Canada. In: Geology and Ore Deposits of the American Cordillera. A.R. Coyner and P.L. Fahey, editors. Symposium sponsored by: Geological Society of Nevada - U.S. Geological Survey - Sociedad Geológica de Chile. April 1995, Reno/Sparks, Nevada. Symposium Proceedings, v. 3, p. 1253-1280.

Thompson, J.F.H., Barrett, T.J., Childe, F. and Sherlock, R.L. 1994. Volcanogenic massive sulphide deposits of the Canadian Cordillera, Geological Society of America Annual Meeting, Seattle, Washington, Program with Abstracts, p. A-27.

Vaughan, T.W., Cooke, W., Condit, D.D., Ross C.P., Woodring, W.P. and Calkins, F.C. 1921. A geological reconnaissance of the Dominican Republic, Memoirs, v. 1, Gibson Brothers Inc., Washington, D.C.

GEOLOGY OF THE SAN ANTONIO CONCESSION, DOMINICAN REPUBLIC

PETER M. HOLBEK AND PETER H. DAUBENY
Atna Resources Ltd., 1550-409 Granville Streeet, Vancouver, B.C. V6C 1T2
atna@atna.com; www.atna.com

ABSTRACT

The San Antonio concession is situated within the Cordilleran Central of the Island of Hispaniola, approximately 30 km NNW of Santo Domingo, Dominican Republic. The Early Cretaceous volcanic and sedimentary rocks that underlie the San Antonio concession are part of the Maimon Formation that occurs within the central part of the Dominican Republic. The volcano-sedimentary sequence on the San Antonio concession is approximately 1,500 metres thick. Immediately north of the concession, the Maimon Formation is thrust over the slightly younger Los Ranchos Formation, while to the south, the Maimon Formation is in fault contact with the dominantly basaltic Upper Cretaceous Peralvillo formation. Volcanic stratigraphy of the Maimon Formation is characterized by mafic volcanic flows and associated fragmental rocks, felsic pyroclastic rocks, and a variety of reworked volcaniclastic rocks. The chemistry of the volcanic rocks and their stratigraphic setting suggests deposition within a primitive island arc setting. The rocks underlying the concession have been metamorphosed to lower greenschist facies and exhibit moderate to intense strain. Micro to minor scale, tight to isoclinal, folds are common but mapping has not delineated any large scale fold structures.

Volcanogenic sulphide mineralization and exhalative barite and jasper occur at three or more stratigraphic levels within the San Antonio concession, two of which have been drill tested. The Parcela deposit is a small sheet-like zone of massive sulphide mineralization at the upper stratigraphic level which has been defined by nine diamond drill holes over a 400 m strike length and a 275 m width (down dip). The zinc, copper, silver and gold bearing massive sulphide mineralization ranges in thickness from 0.3 to 15.9 m, and occurs at the contact of footwall felsic pyroclastic rocks and hangingwall epiclastic rocks. The Copper zone is located 1.5 km east of the Parcela deposit. This zone lies lower in the stratigraphy than the Parcela deposit, and is partially defined by five drill holes over a strike length of 400 m and up to 180 m down dip. The Copper zone mineralization occurs at or near the contact between footwall mafic rocks and hangingwall felsic pyroclastic rocks. The mafic rocks consist of pillow basalt and related fragmental rocks. Copper zone mineralization ranges from thin massive sulphide bands to extensive sections of intercalated sulphide bands and sericite-altered, felsic protolith, probably representing deformed stockwork mineralization. Both the Copper zone and Parcela deposits are accompanied by minor hangingwall alteration and moderate to intense footwall alteration consisting of quartz, sericite, and minor Fe-carbonate and chlorite.

Chemical zoning within the mineralization and peripheral alteration, and deposit morphology indicate that stratigraphy is facing upwards.

INTRODUCTION

Volcano-sedimentary rocks of the Early Cretaceous Maimon Formation are host to a number of volcanogenic massive sulphide prospects, showings and deposits. The geology, and to some extent the mineralization, of the Maimon Formation and adjacent rocks has been described by Kesler (et al., 1991) and Russell (et al., 1982). Both of these works are regional in scope and cover the western part of the Formation. This paper describes the detailed geology, geochemistry and mineralization of the San Antonio concession, a 58 square kilometre exploration concession and VMS prospect located at the southeastern end of the Maimon Formation.

The San Antonio concession is located approximately 30 km NNW of Santo Domingo, the capital city of the Dominican Republic (Fig. 1), in the Cordilleran Central, 1 km west of the town of Yamasa. Topography on the concession is characterized by moderately incised terrain that is covered by either dense, second growth, tropical jungle or small cultivated plots. Outcrop exposure is poor, except

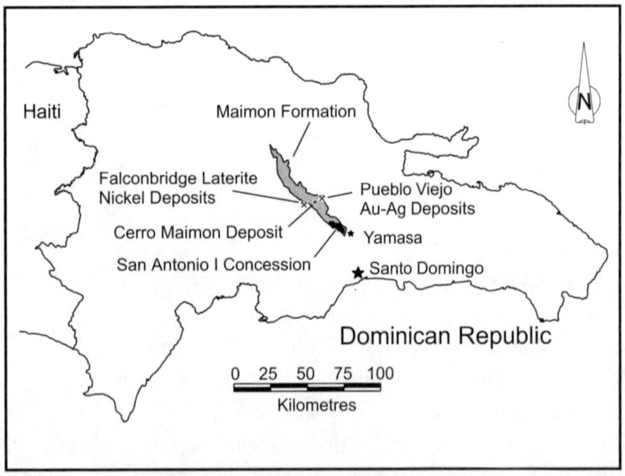

Figure 1. Location of the San Antonio 1 Concession and the Maimon Formation VMS Belt.

locally in creeks, on ridge tops and road cuts. Paved or gravel roads traverse the length of the concession and a network of trails provides access to the remainder of the property. Elevations on the concession range from 55 to 380 m.

Geologic mapping, geochemical sampling, geophysics and diamond drilling on the San Antonio concession has resulted in the discovery of two zones of volcanogenic massive sulphide (VMS) mineralization.

HISTORY

The area of the San Antonio concession has been explored intermittently for the last 25 years, due in part to its proximity to the large Pueblo Viejo gold deposit (Fig. 1). Falconbridge Mines Ltd. followed by Standard Quimica, a Venezuelan company, both undertook gold exploration in the area between 1973 and the early 1980's. Canyon Resources Ltd., in a joint venture with Battle Mountain Gold Ltd., further examined the gold potential of the Yamasa area and applied for the current concession in 1988. The joint venture drilled four holes on the concession, one of which intersected 15.9 m of semi-massive to massive sulphide grading 1.0 % Cu, 0.5 % Zn, 6.7 g/t Ag and 0.3 g/t Au, within what was later to be termed La Parcela zone. Energold Mining Ltd. acquired all of Canyon Resources-Battle Mountain exploration concessions in the Dominican Republic in 1996. Atna Resources Ltd. optioned the concession in late 1998 and carried out a program of pole-dipole IP, geological mapping and diamond drilling. A total of 2,727 metres in 16 drill holes has been completed at the time of writing (Jan, 2000). Highlights from the drilling include hole SA99-02, in the La Parcela zone that returned grades of 3.4 % Cu, 8.55 % Zn, 185 g/t Ag and 1.38 g/t Au over a 3.1 metre thickness. The discovery hole in the Copper Zone (SA99-07) assayed 1.2 % Cu, 15.9 % Zn, 24.0 g/t Ag and 1.3 g/t Au over 1.9 metres.

GEOLOGY

Regional setting

The VMS bearing stratigraphy of the San Antonio concession is part of the Maimon Formation (Bowin, 1960; Kesler et al, 1991), which together with the Peralvillo Formation, form a narrow, northwest trending, arcuate belt of volcano-sedimentary rocks that extends for 65 km, forming the northern flank of the Cordillera Central (Fig. 2). The rocks of the Maimon Formation were likely deposited in a submarine environment of an Early Cretaceous ocean island arc setting (Kesler et al. 1991) and are characterized by andesite to rhyolite flows, felsic pyroclastic rocks, marble, carbonaceous shale, iron formation, and a number of volcanogenic massive sulphide showings. The Peralvillo Formation, consisting of basalt flows, argillite, shale and chert, is in fault contact with the Maimon Formation along its northeastern edge. The Amina schist, which may be Maimon equivalent, is located to the west of the Maimon-Peralvillo belt and collectively these rocks represent Early Cretaceous fore-arc and island arc volcanism (Lewis and Draper, 1991).

The Maimon-Peralvillo belt is bounded by two major structures. The northeastern limit of the Maimon Formation is defined by the Hatillo Fault zone, a late Eocene, southwesterly dipping thrust fault (Kesler et al. 1991), that places Maimon Formation stratigraphy over volcanic rocks of the slightly younger and less deformed Los Ranchos Formation to the northwest of the San Antonio concession, and over limestone of the Late Cretaceous Don Juan Formation, northeast of the concession (Fig. 2). On the southeastern edge of the concession rocks of the Peralvillo Formation are separated from serpent-

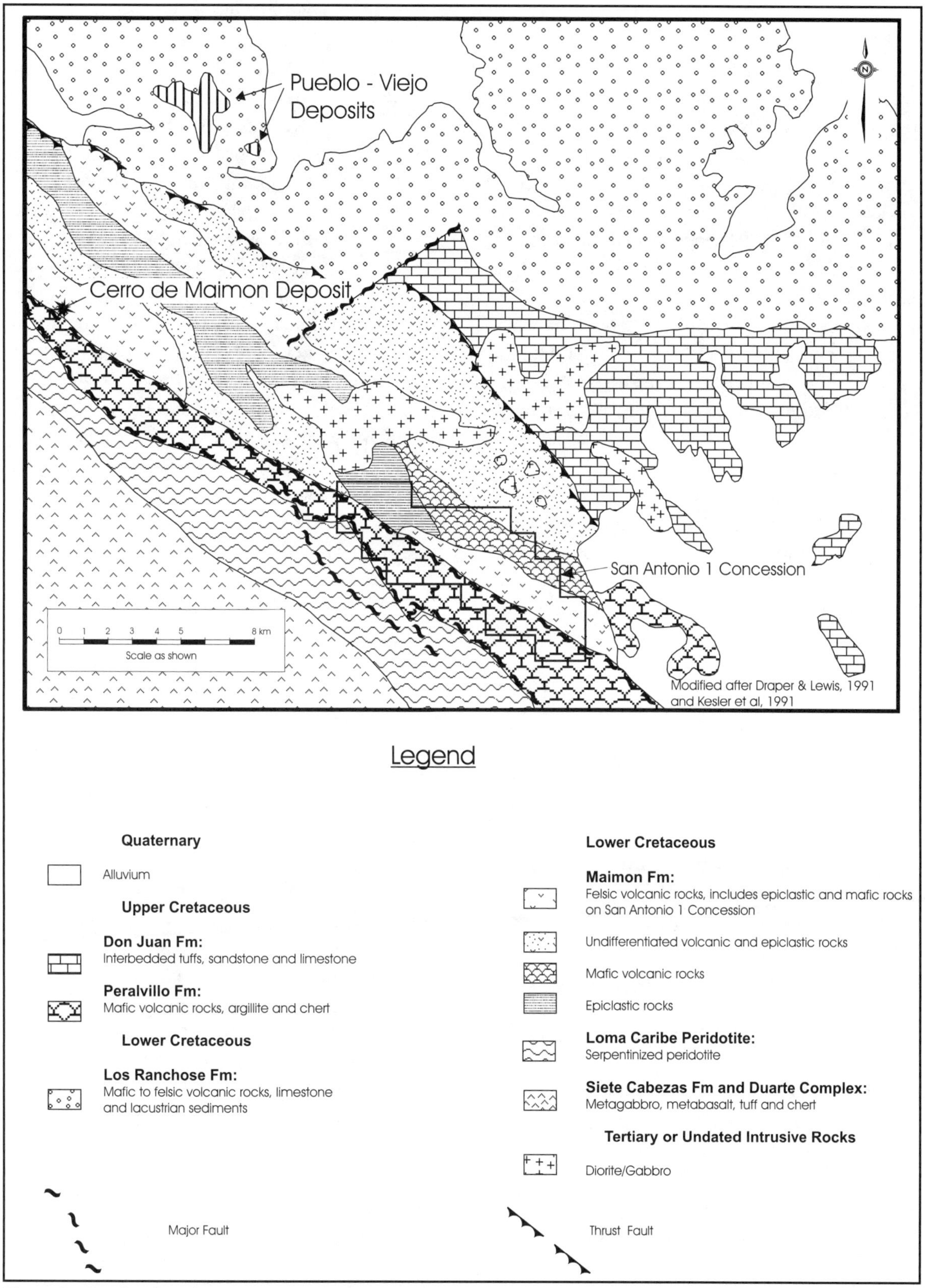

Figure 2. Regional geology.

enized peridotite of the Early Cretaceous Loma Caribe terrane by the left-lateral, strike-slip Hispaniola Fault Zone (Mann et al., 1991) (Fig. 2). A northwest striking, moderately southwest dipping foliation and essentially parallel, primary layering dominates the structural grain of the Maimon Formation. Metamorphism of the Maimon Formation rocks is variable, but typically of lower greenschist facies. Kesler (et al., 1991) reports that metamorphic grade and deformation of the belt increases from southeast to northwest.

The Maimon Formation and the bounding packages of rocks are highly metaliferous (see Childe, this vol.). The Maimon Formation is host to at least one VMS deposit and a number of prospects and showings. The best documented of these occurrences is the Cerro de Maimon deposit, which is located 14 km northwest of the San Antonio concession and hosts approximately 3.5 million tonnes grading 4 % Cu, 2 % Zn, 44 g/t Ag and 0.6 g/t Au, (Kesler et al. 1991). Northeast of the Maimon Formation, the Los Ranchos Formation is host to the +20 million ounce Pueblo Viejo gold deposits. South of the Maimon Formation, the Peralvillo Formation contains volcanogenic massive sulphide mineralization and a number of gold in quartz-vein showings (Russell et al. 1982).

Property geology

Mapping on the San Antonio concession is hampered by generally poor exposure and tropical weathering. Individual lithologies can be difficult to identify, as colour and texture are often obscured by weathering. However, excellent exposures occur in some of the larger creeks as well as the Rio Yamasa, which provides coverage over much of the property. Additionally, diamond drill core has provided exposure of a narrow band of stratigraphy in the central property area. With few exceptions, tracing individual volcanic or volcaniclastic units in surface exposures is difficult. However, grouping of rocks primarily on the basis of gross composition, has proven effective, particularly as these groups can commonly be distinguished by multi-element soil geochemistry.

Most of the San Antonio concession is underlain by the Maimon and Peralvillo Formations. Serpentinized peridotite of the Loma Caribe ultramafic complex occurs in the southwestern most edge of the property (Fig. 3). The lower contact of the Maimon Formation occurs north of the property boundary and has not been mapped. The contact between the Maimon Formation and the overlying Peralvillo Formation is rarely exposed, but is well constrained by mapping; the straightness of the this contact suggests a steeply dipping to vertical fault.

Volcanogenic massive sulphide mineralization on the San Antonio concession occurs at two or more stratigraphic positions within a sequence dominated by felsic volcanic rocks. These felsic rocks are in conformable contact with a thick section of underling mafic flows and fragmental rocks. To the southwest, the felsic volcanic unit is conformably overlain by a fineing upward sequence of volcaniclastic and epiclastic rocks and a second package of interlayered felsic and mafic volcanic rocks. All of these units strike west northwesterly and dip moderately to the southwest (Fig. 3).

Maimon Formation:

Rocks of the Maimon Formation have been subdivided into four units (Fig. 4) on the basis of composition, texture and assumed stratigraphic position, essentially following the sub-divisions of Kesler (et al. 1991). These four subdivisions have been given informal unit names reflecting local geographic features near the areas of best exposure. Collectively, these four units are greater than 1,500 metres thick. Contacts between the units appear to be conformable, and the sequence is believed to be upright, younging from north to south. Maimon Formation rocks extend north of the concession but this area has not been mapped in any detail; it is probable that an additional band of felsic rocks occurs north of our mapping on the basis of Kesler's map in Lewis and Draper (1991).

The Lambedera mafic unit (Mf1) is the lowest unit of the Maimon Formation which is exposed on the San Antonio concession. This unit is greater than 700 metres thick and consists of mafic volcanic flows to mafic volcaniclastic rocks and agglomerates or conglomerates with felsic fragments within a mafic matrix. In general, surface exposures of this unit consist of roughly equal proportions of massive, fine grained flows and matrix to clast supported fragmental

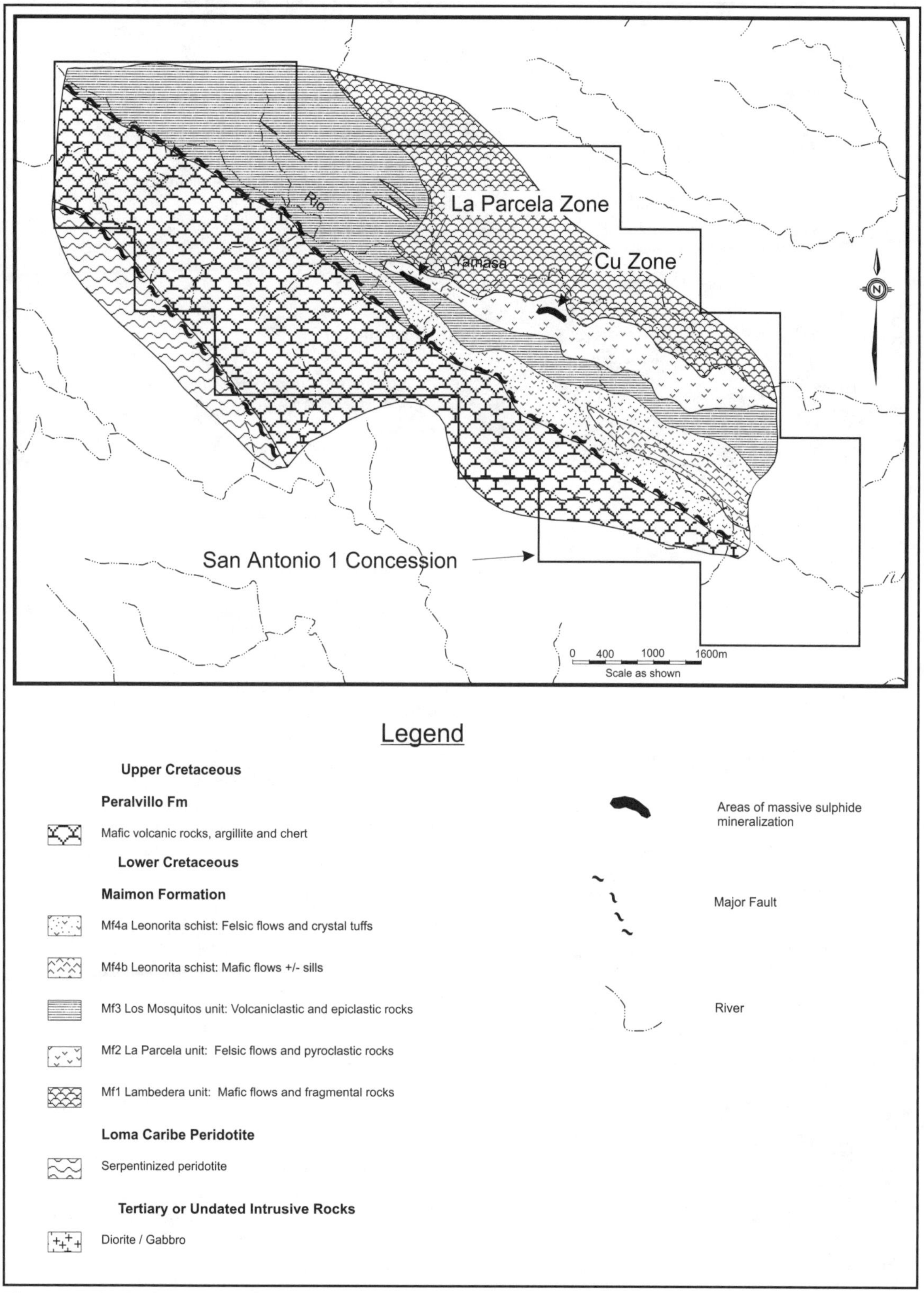

Figure 3. Geological map of the San Antonio 1 Concession.

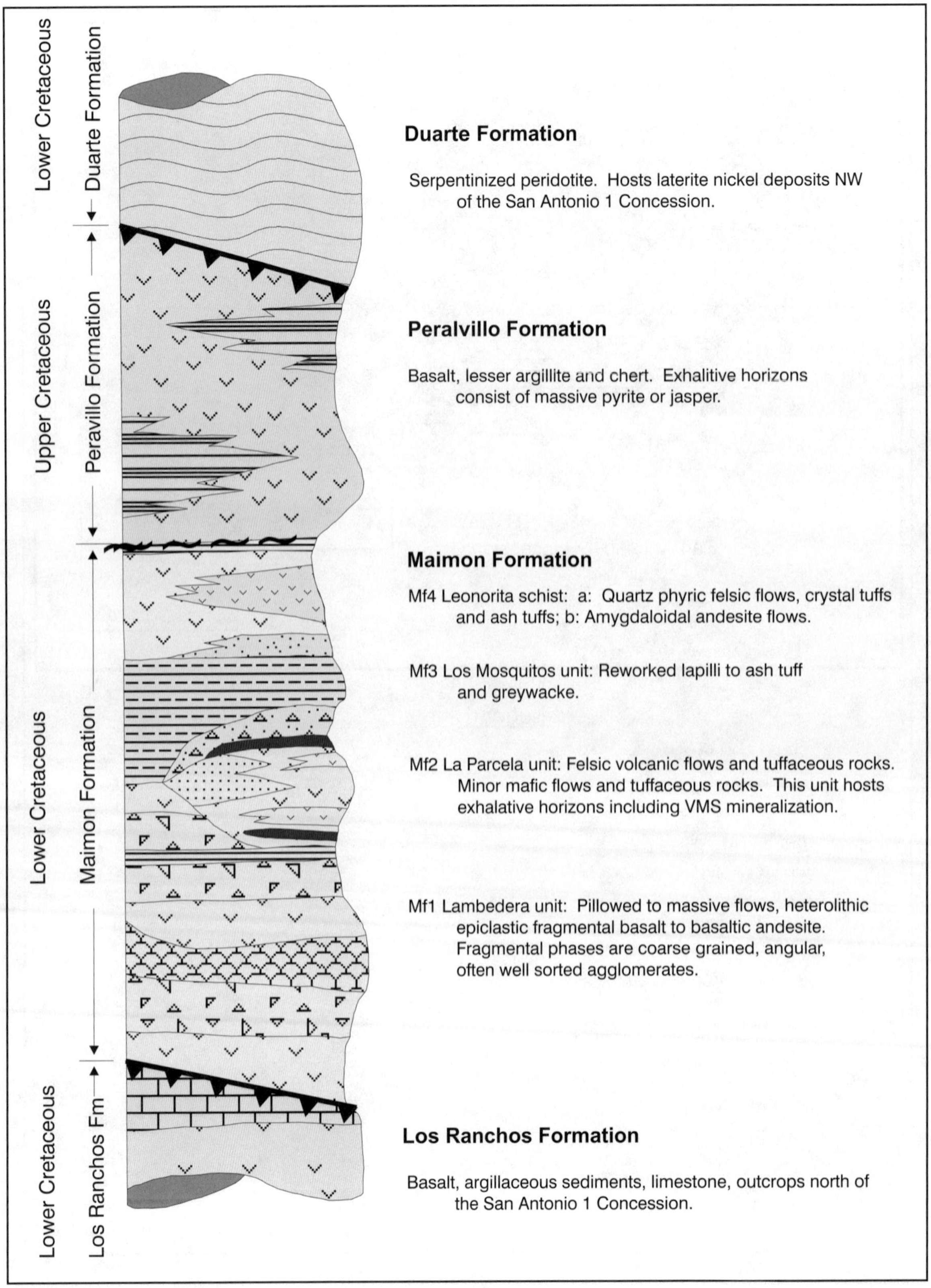

Figure 4. Schematic stratigraphy of San Antonio 1 Concession.

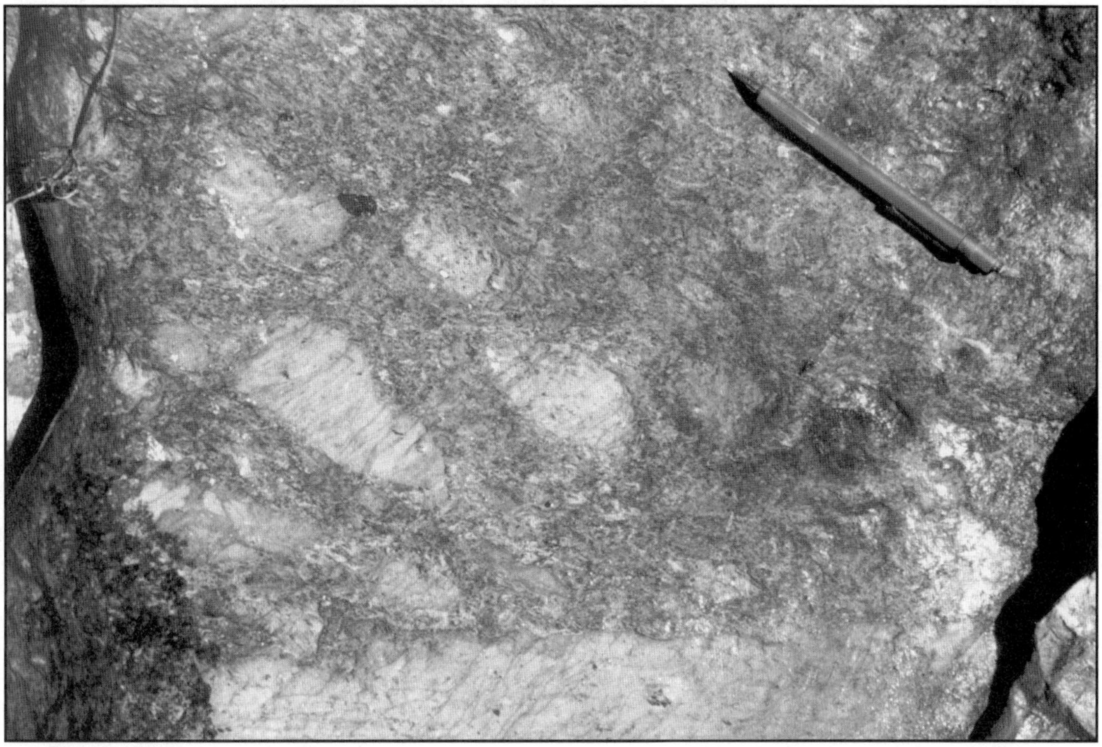

Figure 5A. Heterolithic, predominantly felsic clasts hosted in a chloritic matrix, an example from the Lambedera unit fragmental rocks near the contact with Los Mosquitos sediments on the northwestern part of the San Antonio concession

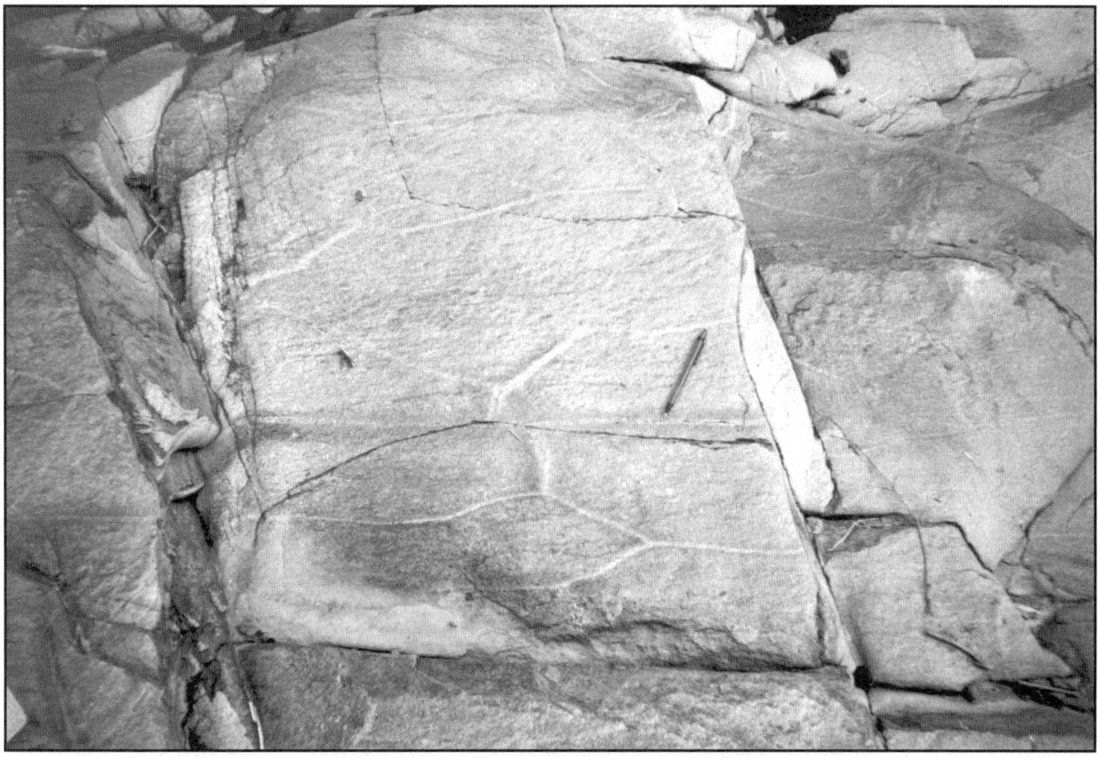

Figure 5B. Slightly deformed pillow textures in Lambedera flow rocks near Rio Yamasa.

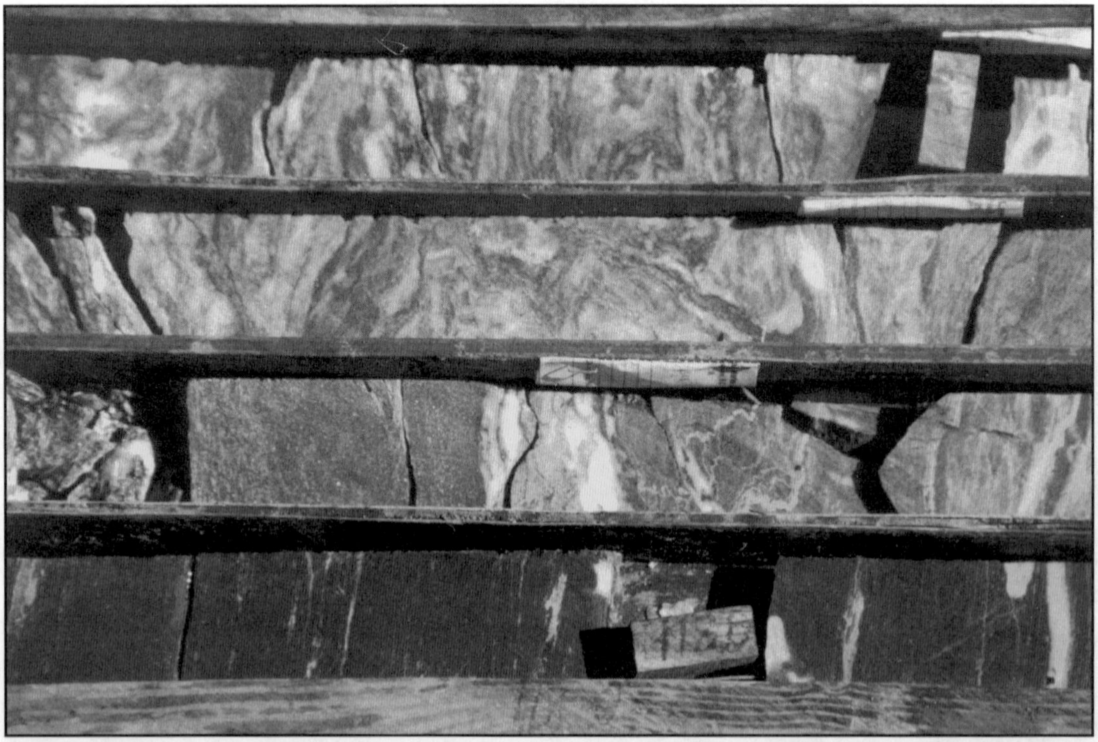

Figure 5C. Diamond drill core from drill hole SA99-12 showing a relatively sharp, silicified contact between stringer-type sulphide mineralization (+/- silica exhalite) in altered felsic ash tuff and underlying mafic tuffs of the Lambedera unit from the Copper zone. The contact is located at the base of the 5 cm band of siliceous exhalite located in the middle of the 3rd row from the top.

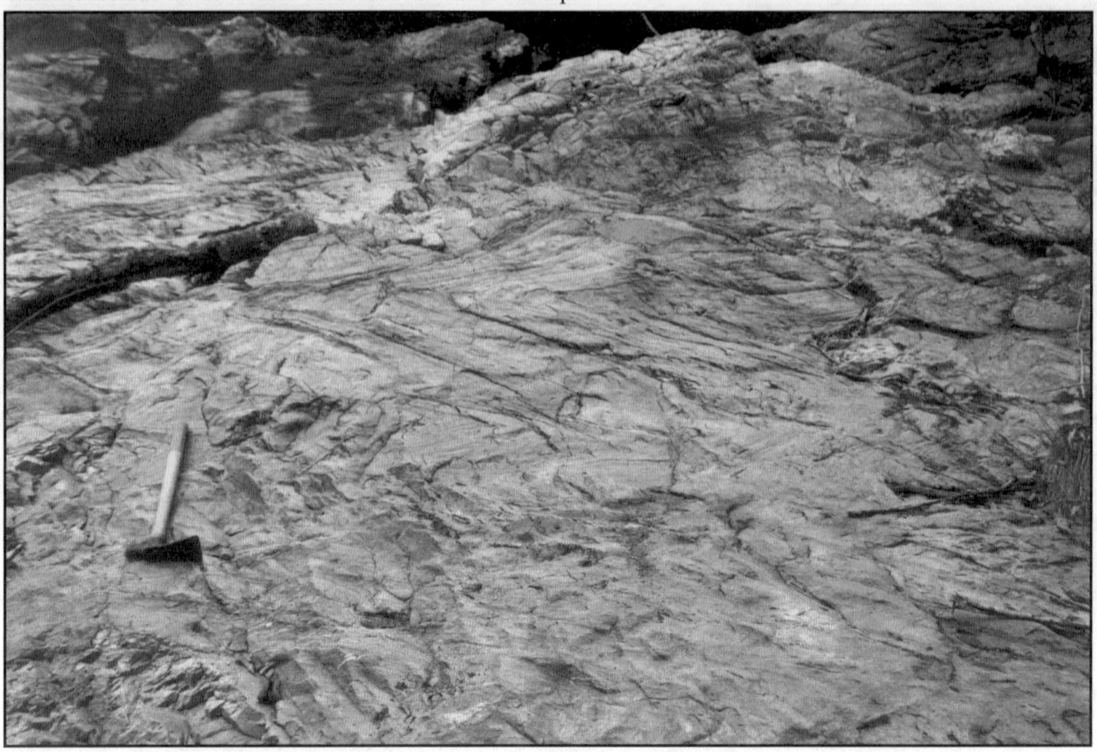

Figure 5D. Symmetrical, metre-scale, tight folds within fine grained epiclastic rocks of the Los Mosquitos unit in the Rio Yamasa high strain zone.

rocks. The fragments range from ash to lapilli size and are usually monolithic with rare exotic, sometimes felsic, clasts (Fig. 5a). Clasts are typically flattened and supported by a mafic matrix, giving outcrops a dark green colour. Well preserved pillow textures (Fig. 5b) are exposed in outcrops along the Rio Yamasa and intervals of epidote-quartz-chlorite breccia observed in drill core likely represent brecciated pillow material.

Character of the Lambedera unit changes both along strike and with depth. In the eastern part of the concession, fine-grained, weakly porphyritic flows with minor interbedded argillite are prevalent, whereas fragmental rocks predominate in the western part of the concession. The lower contact of the unit has not been investigated. At the upper contact the rocks typically become thin bedded and tuffaceous. Jasper horizons are common in the upper parts of this unit and, near areas of mineralization, the upper contact is silicified. In the central area of the concession the Parcela felsic unit (Mf2) overlying the Lambedera mafic rocks pinches out and the sediments of Los Mosquitos unit (Mf3) form the upper Lambedera contact. This mafic-sediment contact swings to the northeast for 500 metres before resuming the regional northwesterly trend (Fig. 3). Actual mafic-sediment contacts were not observed, but outcrop patterns suggest that the contact is at least in part depositional with the two units being interdigitated, perhaps indicating the formation of a small sedimentary basin to the northwest. However, the deflection of the volcanic-sedimentary contact could also be partly controlled by unrecognized structures.

The Parcela volcanic rocks, consist of a 500 metre thick section dominated by felsic volcanic flows and lapilli to ash tuffs. These felsic rocks are intercalated with lesser amounts of mafic flows, mafic tuffs, jasper horizons and massive sulphide mineralization (Fig. 5c). Rocks of the Parcela unit are typically well foliated and sericitic; consequently, apart from quartz phenocrysts, primary textures in outcrop are obscured. On surface, extensive areas of the felsic volcanic unit are altered to sericite-limonite-hematite ± quartz assemblages, commonly with gossans indicative of weathered sulphides. These gossans are interpreted to be the surface expression of stringer mineralization associated with volcanogenic massive sulphide mineralization. The more siliceous parts of the Parcela unit form localized topographic highs within the concession area. Although most outcrops of this unit are only recognizable as a quartz-sericite schist, in drill core, moderate to thick flows of quartz-phyric rhyolite, lapilli tuffs and crystal tuffs can be identified. Thickness of the various lithologies is variable from drill hole to drill hole.

Contacts between mafic and felsic lithologies are generally sharp, however, because these lithologies are commonly thinly interbedded along the upper and lower margins of the Parcela unit, contacts between the major units can be somewhat arbitrary. A strong gold, barium, and lead soil geochemical anomaly is associated with the central part of the Parcela unit and extends for 5 km along the eastern part of the San Antonio concession.

Los Mosquitos unit (Mf3) consists of volcaniclastic to epiclastic rocks that range in thickness from about 100 metres to greater than 900 metres. These rocks may have been deposited in a basin that now dominates the geology of the western half of the concession. On the eastern half of the concession, where unit Mf3 overlies the altered felsic volcanic rocks of the Parcela unit, it consists of reworked, fine to coarse-grained tuffs and thin bedded, variably siliceous (chemical?) sediments, and occasionally bedded or laminated jasper. These rocks are unaltered, except locally, where moderate to strong chlorite alteration occurs above massive sulphide mineralization in the Parcela deposit. Sections of this unit observed in drill core, consist of ash to heterolithic lapilli tuffs intercalated with lesser fine-grained, thinly laminated, grit or greywacke. Primary sedimentary structures are ubiquitous in these intervals and a number of features, such as graded bedding, load casts and flame structures, indicate that stratigraphy is upright, younging to the south. Primary sedimentary layering is also common in surface exposures of this unit. Mapping indicates the unit fines upwards from coarse-grained volcaniclastic rocks, possibly agglomerates, at its basal contact, to thin-bedded, fine-grained, greywacke at the upper contact. Some of the fine-grained epiclastic sections of this unit are sufficiently siliceous to form property-scale topographic highs.

The uppermost units of the Maimon Formation within the map area have been termed the Leonorita schists which consist of a felsic unit (Mf4a) and mafic unit (Mf4b) which are similar to units Mf2 and Mf1, respectively. The spatial distribution of the Leonorita schists is suggestive of a fold, but structural data does not support this, and the apparent closure may be an artifact of the scale of mapping and the lack of outcrop. Thus, the current interpretation is that the felsic and mafic lithologies are interbedded.

The Leonorita felsic unit consists of massive to thick bedded quartz-phyric, and locally also feldspar-phyric, flows and possibly crystal tuffs. Quartz phenocrysts range from 1 to 5 % of rock volume. Coarse fragmental rocks were not observed as they were in the Parcela unit. The Leonorita mafic rocks are dark green chlorite-epidote schists with rare chlorite and quartz filled amygdules and epidote spots. In outcrop these rocks are very similar in appearance to the more massive mafic rocks seen in the Lambedera unit. Bedded volcaniclastic and epiclastic rocks are a minor component within the mafic sequence and are similar to those observed in the underlying Los Mosquitos unit. All of the rocks in the Leonorita units display a strong penetrative foliation. Locally, the felsic rocks host alteration and mineralized similar to the stockwork alteration and mineralization observed in the Parcela unit. Gossans and soil geochemistry associated with this mineralization form a discontinuous, four kilometre long, primarily gold in soil geochemical anomaly.

Peralvillo Formation:

The Peralvillo Formation overlies the Maimon Formation along a regional scale fault contact. On the San Antonio concession, the Peralvillo Formation is in excess of 1,500 metres thick, and is composed of fine-grained massive to moderately foliated, monolithic, mafic volcanic rocks with lesser argillite, graphitic argillite, and chert. At its upper contact, the Peralvillo Formation is likely separated from the Duarte Complex serpentinized peridotite by the Hispanoila Fault (Mann et al, 1991).

Within the San Antonio concession, the Peralvillo Formation hosts intervals of jasper, a number of formational barite-copper geochemical anomalies, at least two gossanous zones and a small stratiform lens of massive pyrite; all of which indicate potential for massive sulphide mineralization. The Sabana-Poterro prospect, a predominantly copper with minor zinc bearing massive sulphide occurrence is located within the Peralvillo Formation immediately south of the San Antonio concession (Espaillate, et al. 1990).

Loma Caribe Peridotite

Serpentinized peridotite, interpreted to be part of the Loma Caribe ultramafic complex which separates rocks of the Peralvillo Formation from the similar aged rocks to the south underlies the southwest corner of the concession. The peridotites display a strong tectonic fabric and consist of slickenslided masses of serpentine surrounding less deformed blocks of fine-grained to medium-grained dunite. Soil geochemistry from areas underlain by these ultramafic rocks is highly anomalous in nickel (1,000 to 7,073 ppm).

Intrusive Rocks

A small number of undeformed, fine to medium grained, holocrystaline, gabbro dykes intrude the Maimon Formation. These intrusive rocks maybe related to Eocene diorite intrusives (Draper and Lewis, 1991) that outcrop north and northwest of the concession. Rare mafic dykes from 2 to 10 metres thick occur in the hangingwall to the Parcela zone mineralization and are fine grained, dark green and contain up to 20 % medium-grained amphibole phenocrysts. Chemically, these dykes are distinct from both the mafic volcanic rocks and the diorite-gabbro intrusions.

STRUCTURE

A weak to strong, WNW striking, foliation, typically parallel to bedding, is developed in most of the volcanic and sedimentary units underlying the San Antonio concession. Small scale minor folds are common in drill core and locally in outcrop. However, the largest folds observed in outcrop are tight, regular folds with amplitudes of 1 metre which occur near the Rio Yamasa in Los Mosquitos sediments (Fig. 5d). No direct evidence of regional scale folding has been observed although indirect evidence for megascopic folds occurs in drill hole SA99-11, where stringer type mineralization is structurally underlain by a succession of massive sulphide mineralization, massive barite and unmineralized felsic volcanic rocks suggesting a locally overturned sequence. Significant amplitude folds are probable, given the regional setting, and would be difficult to discern due to outcrop limitations and nature of stratigraphy, however, it is also possible that the minor folds are caused by localized ductile strain proximal to shear zones.

The San Antonio concession is roughly centreed on the Rio Yamasa valley which is localized by a high strain zone where rocks are strongly foliated, locally sheared and phyllonitic. Observations of minor folds, which range from locally abundant centimetre sized isoclinal folds to rare, metre-scale, tight asymmetrical folds, are generally confined to the high strain zone. This zone is, at least in part, coincident with hydrothermally altered quartz-sericite schists. The high strain zone is 500 to 800 metres wide and foliation becomes less pronounced peripheral to the zone. Within the strain zone, primary layering is nearly always parallel to foliation, coincident to the orientation of the strain zone. North of the strain zone, layering, and to a lesser degree, foliation measurements become much less consistent and may mimic the asymmetical minor folds at a much larger scale.

Rocks of the Peralvillo Formation lack a penetrative foliation except for within 50 metres of the contact with the underlying Maimon Formation. This observation supports the interpretation for a regional scale fault contact between the Peralvillo and the Maimon Formation (Draper and Lewis, 1991).

MINERALIZATION

Exploration drilling to date, has defined two zones of volcanogenic massive sulphide mineralization on the concession; the Parcela deposit and the Copper zone (Table 1). Both zones of mineralization occur within the Parcela felsic volcanic unit near the centre of the concession (Fig. 2). The discovery hole in the Parcela zone was drilled in 1990 and intersected two closely spaced zones of massive sulphide mineralization: an upper, narrow (30 cm) zinc and gold rich (15.2 % Zn and 5.8 g/t Au) zone; and a lower high pyrite but low-grade zone extending 15.9 metres. The two sulphide zones are separated by 4 metres of highly altered ash tuff. Sulphide mineralization consists of stratiform pyrite, sphalerite, chalcopyrite and bornite in a gangue of quartz and barite. An additional hole drilled in 1991 and a further six holes drilled in 1999 within the Parcela zone have defined a generally, thin (0.5 to 3 m), sheet-like body of mineralization over a 400 metre strike length and approximately 275 metres down-dip. One drill hole appears to close the zone off at depth and other drill holes indicate that the zone is thinning along strike in both directions from the discovery hole. Due to weathering, mineralization is not exposed at surface, although it is reflected by anomalous soil geochemistry and gold-rich float samples.

The Copper zone, named for the abundant malachite present within the discovery outcrop, is marked by a coincident soil geochemical and IP geophysical anomaly. The initial drill hole (SA99-07) intersected 1.2 % Cu, 15.8 % Zn, 24g/t Ag and 1.3g/t Au over 1.9 metres. A further four drill holes have defined a massive sulphide lens that measures over 400 metres strike length and approximately 180 metres in the down dip direction. The zone lacks sufficient thickness for exploitation but remains open to expansion.

The massive sulphide textures in both zones are variable, but generally consist of weakly laminated sulphide minerals. Zinc-rich bands are composed of cream to gray coloured, fine-grained, net-textured sphalerite with interstitial 'buckshot' pyrite, chalcopyrite and gangue. Copper-rich bands are generally narrow and consist of wispy to irregular aggregates of primary bornite, chalcocite and chalcopyrite. Chalcopyrite occurs as scattered blebs within pyrite layers or as copper-rich bands within massive pyrite. Generally, sulphide intersections are zoned from zinc-rich at the top to more pyrite-chalcopyrite dominated at the base. Siliceous sulphide zones, and more rarely, barite sulphide zones, commonly overlie the massive mineralization whereas the lower contacts are typically gradational, with pyrite- chalcopyrite laminae and disseminations fading in quartz, sericite schists. Precious metal grades, particularly gold can be significant with grades of up to 16 g/t Au within a 20 cm thick massive sphalerite band. Gold distribution is somewhat erratic, whereas the best silver grades correlate with high copper values. There is a moderate correlation of gold with barite. Galena is rarely

Table 1. San Antonio concession, significant 1999 drill results.

Hole number	From (m)	To (m)	Width (m)	Cu %	Zn %	Ag g/t	Au g/t
SA-99-01	88.2	91.6	3.4	5.88	3.52	85.7	2.27
	135.1	136.5	1.4	2.43	10.52	141.9	3.10
SA-99-02	152.4	155.5	3.1	3.39	8.55	185.2	1.38
SA-99-03	99.0	100.0	1.0	1.17	2.07	69.7	1.87
SA-99-04	148.2	151.5	3.3	2.24	3.60	19.7	3.40
SA-99-05	15.1	17.2	2.1	0.02	0.28	122.5	2.79
SA-99-07	56.1	58.0	1.9	1.20	15.84	24.0	1.31
SA-99-08	139.7	140.9	1.2	1.29	5.30	16.3	1.48
SA-99-11	54.4	57.4	3.0	0.43	2.20	26.1	2.37
	59.2	61.1	1.9	0.21	2.85	28.7	2.04
	101.4	101.5	0.1	2.27	8.24	68.2	3.67
SA-99-12	81.2	84.3	3.1	1.55	14.60	77.7	2.85
	85.4	85.8	0.4	1.05	3.40	14.7	1.17
	92.1	96.6	4.5	1.17	1.70	33.5	1.30
	103.1	106.1	3.0	1.29	5.32	5.5	0.55
SA-99-13	273.3	273.8	0.5	2.51	6.33	101.4	6.86

observed and the weighted average for lead in most of the massive sulphides is less than 1000 ppm. Banded semi-massive to massive barite up to 2 metres thick has been mapped on surface in a number of localities and massive barite has been intersected in one drill hole on the west side of the Copper zone.

Mineralization at the Parcela deposit is located at the upper contact of altered felsic pyroclastic rocks of the Parcela unit (Mf2) with overlying sediment-volcaniclastic rocks of Los Mosquitos unit (Mf3). The Copper zone mineralization is hosted within the Parcela unit approximately 300 metres stratigraphically below the mineralization in the Parcela zone and near the lower contact with the mafic rocks of the Lambadera unit.

Within both areas of mineralization, the thicker sulphide intersections are accompanied by thicker and more intense zones of alteration, and occur in areas where geological mapping has indicated a pronounced and localized thickening of the felsic host rocks. This observation, combined with the relatively rapid decrease in alteration and mineralization thickness along strike, suggests the possibility that the best mineralization may be related to graben-like structures which rake steeply down-dip. Additional work will be required to verify this hypothesis.

LITHOGEOCHEMISTRY

Table 2 lists the major and selected trace element compositions of representative rocks from the various units of the Maimon Formation. These rocks were selected from a much larger (102 sample) database as being the least altered on the basis of appearance and LOI values, and are plotted (Fig. 6) as closed symbols whereas the remainder of the database are plotted as open symbols. Samples were collected for the purpose of determining chemical variations between the units and degree of chemical alteration of various samples. Samples were analyzed by Acme Laboratories of Vancouver using ICP techniques following a LiBO2 fusion and HNO3 digestion; trace element values are not sufficiently accurate to determine tectonic settings or petrogenetic processes.

In general, the Maimon Formation rocks have relatively low primary potassium and high sodium contents, a feature also noted by Kesler (et al. 1991), suggesting the possibility that the rocks have been spillitized, although total alkali values are not high. Classification of the rocks by the silica versus Zr/TiO_2 plot (Winchester and Floyd, 1977) indicates that the Parcela unit rocks plot in the rhyolite and rhyodacite fields whereas the Lambedera unit plots in the

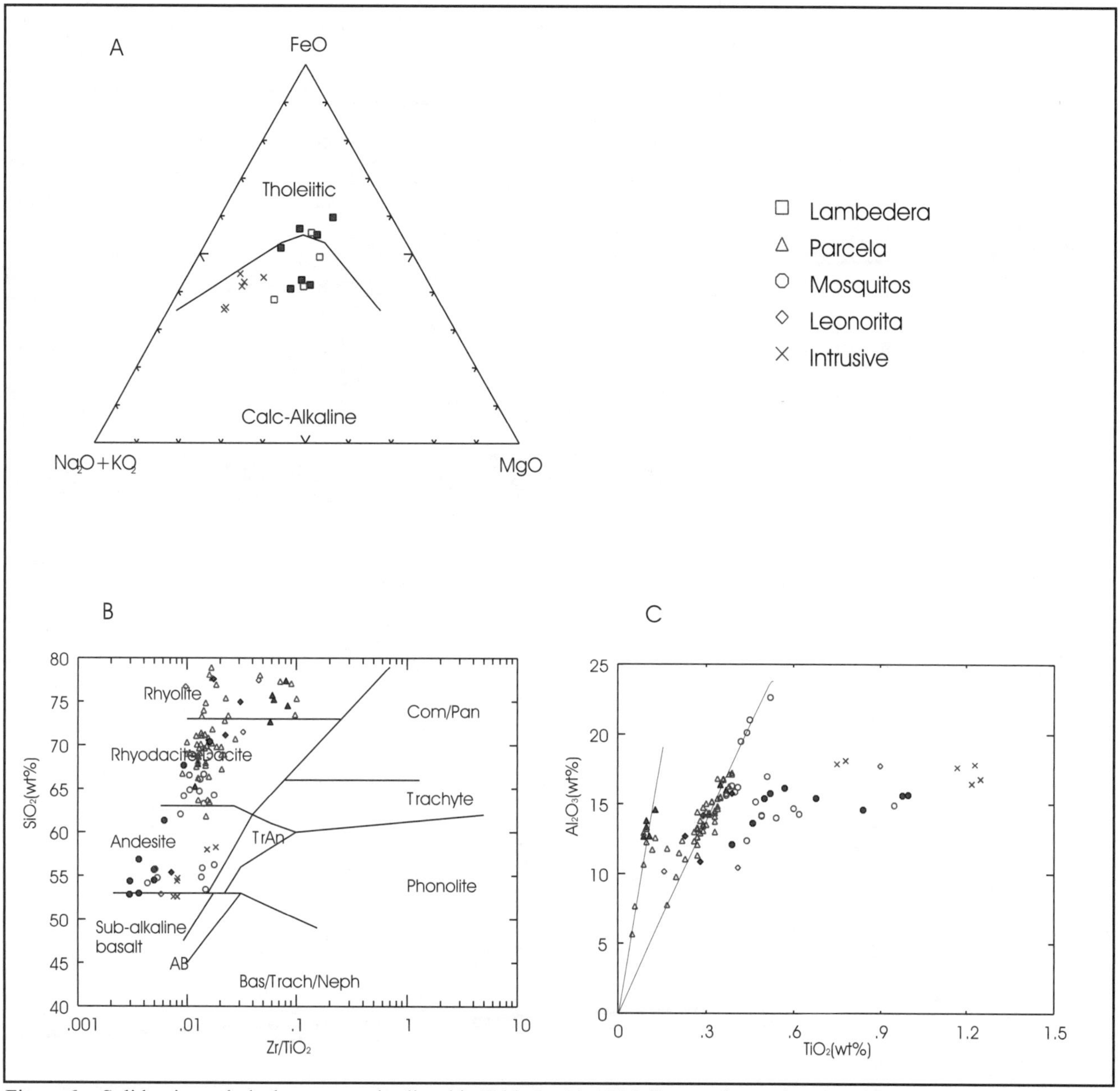

Figure 6. Solid unit symbols denote samples listed in Table 2. (a) AFM diagram for unaltered Maimon Formation mafic volcanic rocks and selected dyke rocks underlying the San Antonio concession from Irvine and Baragar (1971). (b) SiO_2 versus Zr/TiO_2 for Maimon Formation and dyke rocks on the San Antonio concession from Winchester and Floyd (1977). (c) Al_2O_3 versus TiO_2 diagram for Maimon Formation and dyke rocks on the San Antonio concession.

andesite to basalt fields (Fig. 6a). Without the epiclastic rocks, which tend to plot the dacite field, the Maimon Formation rocks display a bimodal character on the basis of silica content. The weakly unimodal distribution of silica noted by Kesler (et al., 1991) was likely caused by sampling of unidentified fragmental rocks. Unaltered (Na_2O > 3 wt. %, LOI< 3 wt. %) mafic volcanic units and dyke rocks on the San Antonio concession plot in both the calc-alkaline and tholeiite fields on the AFM diagram (Irvine and Baragar, 1971), a feature compatible with more primitive island-arc type basalts (Fig. 6b). More detailed

Table 2. Selected San Antonio whole rock data.

Sample number	Unit	Lithology	Sample type*	SiO2 %	Al2O3 %	Fe2O3 %	MgO %	CaO %	Na2O %	K2O %	TiO2 %	P2O5 %	MnO %	Cr2O3 %	Ba ppm	Ni ppm	Sr ppm	Zr ppm	Y ppm	LOI %	SUM %
72882	Lambedera	Mafic flow	C	52.8	15.6	13.33	5.34	4.87	2.67	0.11	0.98	0.1	0.22	0.015	74	<20	134	29	23	3.7	99.8
72906	Lambedera	Mafic flow	C	53.0	15.7	13.68	4.42	4.22	4.40	0.60	1.00	0.05	0.17	0.013	275	< 20	81	36	22	2.9	100.1
72908	Lambedera	Mafic tuff	C	54.5	15.8	10.34	5.94	3.65	5.72	0.59	0.52	0.07	0.37	0.027	273	35	63	26	14	2.6	100.1
72909	Lambedera	Mafic tuff	C	56.9	15.4	9.27	5.33	3.33	6.51	0.24	0.50	0.06	0.40	0.023	193	24	55	18	13	2.1	100.0
73001	Lambedera	Fragmental	S	55.7	15.4	11.73	4.83	3.60	1.38	2.40	0.68	0.06	0.13	0.010	133	50	132	34	12	4.0	100.0
73002	Lambedera	Pillowed flow	S	61.3	14.6	8.55	2.76	4.43	3.74	0.72	0.84	0.11	0.10	0.004	179	< 20	140	52	18	2.5	99.7
73188	Lambedera	Fragmental	S	54.4	16.1	9.88	6.40	3.19	4.13	1.81	0.57	0.01	0.15	0.020	88	25	348	17	14	3.4	100.1
72861	Parcela	Felsic flow	C	74.5	13.8	2.11	0.72	0.81	4.62	1.99	0.10	0.03	0.06	0.020	515	< 20	48	84	27	1.3	100.2
72895	Parcela	Felsic tuff	C	75.2	13.3	2.02	0.62	0.77	4.84	1.92	0.10	0.01	0.06	0.024	432	< 20	41	63	27	1.2	100.2
72897	Parcela	Felsic flow	C	77.4	12.7	2.10	0.20	0.38	6.74	0.14	0.09	0.02	0.03	0.024	42	< 20	27	73	24	0.3	100.1
72903	Parcela	Felsic flow	C	72.7	14.6	2.43	1.37	2.08	3.02	1.93	0.13	0.03	0.14	0.022	784	23	122	76	27	1.6	100.1
72916	Parcela	Pyroclastic	C	65.3	16.0	5.39	2.96	4.05	2.64	1.26	0.37	0.08	0.07	0.025	562	< 20	168	44	12	2.2	100.4
72983	Parcela	Felsic flow	C	67.9	16.4	3.91	0.93	2.14	5.89	1.24	0.35	0.07	0.03	0.021	463	< 20	58	44	16	1.4	100.3
73093	Parcela	Felsic flow	S	75.7	12.7	2.55	0.85	0.74	3.20	2.53	0.11	< .01	0.05	0.027	583	30	83	67	20	1.4	100.0
72704	Mosquito	Volcaniclastic	C	70.4	12.1	4.40	2.30	3.60	2.40	1.00	0.40	0.1	0.10	0.021	667	24	229	63	30	3.0	100.0
72631	Mosquito	Ash tuff	C	67.7	13.6	5.28	2.97	2.64	1.20	2.78	0.46	0.08	0.10	0.019	1163	< 20	280	43	24	2.6	99.6
73043	Leonorita	Felsic flow?	S	77.6	10.9	2.32	1.47	0.38	5.50	0.07	0.28	0.06	0.06	0.019	61	23	42	49	17	1.1	99.7
73086	Leonorita	Felsic flow	S	75.0	12.7	2.36	1.13	0.35	4.49	1.35	0.23	< .01	0.02	0.022	189	< 20	47	71	20	2.3	99.9
73111	Leonorita	Felsic tuff?	S	71.1	14.2	4.01	0.65	1.67	5.06	0.66	0.29	< .01	0.04	0.023	79	21	163	65	17	2.2	100.0
73082	Leonorita	Mafic flow	S	55.4	15.8	9.10	6.90	4.80	4.20	0.40	0.40	<.01	0.17	0.024	42	44	398	28	12	3.6	100.1
73177	Parcela area	Mafic dyke	S	58.3	18.1	5.92	1.98	4.06	4.94	2.60	0.78	0.38	0.19	0.017	1497	20	531	143	22	2.1	99.6
72814	Parcela area	Mafic dyke	C	58.0	17.9	6.01	2.01	4.97	4.67	3.20	0.75	0.34	0.17	0.017	1671	22	610	115	22	1.5	99.8
73190	Diorite associated?	Mafic dyke	S	54.4	17.6	7.40	2.32	5.14	4.24	2.84	1.17	0.64	0.19	0.012	1848	< 20	825	95	46	3.0	99.3
73972	Diorite associated?	Mafic dyke	S	54.7	16.4	8.67	2.15	4.83	4.83	2.64	1.22	0.82	0.21	0.002	1304	< 20	692	100	34	3.1	99.9

*C = core, S = surface

analysis of the Maimon geochemistry was carried out by Lewis (et al., 1998) who interpreted the low, but variable TiO_2 contents and low concentrations of the high field strength elements as well as REE as indicative of "primitive" oceanic island-arc tholeiites as in the PIA series of Donnelly and Rogers, (1978).

Degree of alteration may be inferred from the Al_2O_3 versus TiO_2 plot (Fig. 6c). The felsic rocks show two groupings where covariance of aluminum and titanium indicate the addition or subtraction of minerals without these elements (ie: silica or carbonate). The trend of Lambedera unit rocks, variable TiO_2 with constant Al_2O_3, suggests magmatic or depositional processes that result in variable titanium compositions. Mafic dykes and the diorite intrusive rocks have distinctly different geochemistry from the mafic flow rocks.

CONCLUSIONS

The Maimon Formation is an Early Cretaceous bimodal volcanic sequence that has been subdivided into four units: a lower mafic unit consisting of pillowed flows and related fragmental rocks; a felsic unit characterized by quartz-phyric flows, pyroclastic rocks and massive sulphide mineralization; a sedimentary to epivolcaniclastic unit derived from both mafic and felsic volcanic source rocks; and an upper unit of interbedded felsic and mafic flows with minor pyroclastic and epiclastic rocks. The Maimon Formation occurs in a fault-bounded northwest trending linear belt, which together with the adjacent Peralvillo Formation and arc volcanic rocks of the Los Ranchos Formation represent parts of an early or basal island-arc sequence. This setting, together with northeasterly directed transpression has resulted in thrust and strike-slip fault contacts between the associated formations and high strain zones within the Maimon Formation. The lithologies and geochemistry of the Maimon Formation are compatible with a primitive arc environment.

Volcanogenic massive sulphide mineralization of the San Antonio Concession occurs at two, or more, stratigraphic positions within felsic flows and pyroclastic rocks. Mineralization is copper-zinc or zinc-copper with significant gold and silver credits and is accompanied by moderately extensive haloes of quartz-sericite-pyrite-barite alteration. The mineralization is laterally very extensive giving rise to soil geochemical and geophysical anomalies with strike lengths of up to five kilometres. Potentially economic mineralization appears to be much more restricted, occurring as thin sheet-like bodies over a few hundreds of metres, however drill testing is still at an early stage. Locii of the more significant areas of mineralization may be controlled by narrow, near vertically dipping, basins or graben-like structures but further work is required to confirm this.

ACKNOWLEDGEMENTS

This work was undertaken as part of an exploration program carried out by Atna Resources Ltd. on a project optioned from Energold Mining Ltd. and the support of both companies is appreciated. Rob Wilson of Atna Resources assisted in editing the manuscript and in the creation of the graphics. The manuscript was greatly improved through the comments of the reviewers.

REFERENCES

Bowin, C.O., 1966. Geology of the central Dominican Republic; a case history of part of an island arc. In Caribbean geological investigations. Ed. by H.H. Hess. Geological Society of America Memoir 98, pp. 11-84.

Childe C., 2000. Geology and Tectonic Setting of the Volcanogenic Massive Sulphide Mineralization in the Greater Antilles. In VMS deposits of Latin America, Geological Association of Canada Special Publication. Ed. by R. Sherlock and A. Logan.

Donnelley, T.W. and Rogers, J.J.W., 1980. Igneous series in island arcs: the northeast Caribbean compared with worldwide arc assemblages. Bulletin Volcanologique #43, pp. 347-382.

Draper, G. and Lewis, J.F. 1991. Geologic Map of the Central Dominican Republic. In Geologic and Tectonic Development of the North America-Caribbean Plate Boundary in Hispaniola. Edited by Mann, P. Draper, G. and Lewis. J. F. Geological Society of America Special Paper 262, map 2b.

Espaillat, J. Bloise, G. MacVeigh, J.G. and Lewis, J.F. 1990. Petrography and geochemistry of the mafic rocks of the Peralvillo Formation in the Sabana Potrero area, central Dominican Republic. Transactions 12th Caribbean Geological Conference, St. Croix, 1989.

Irvine, T.N. and Barragar, W.R.A. 1971. A guide to chemical classification of the common volcanic rocks. Can. Journal of Earth Sci. vol. 8 pp. 523-548.

Kesler, S.E. Russell, N. Reyes, C. Santos, L. Rodriguez, A. and Fondeur, L. 1991. Geology of the Maimon Formation, Dominican Republic. In Geologic and Tectonic

Development of the North America-Caribbean Plate Boundary in Hispaniola. Edited by Mann, P. Draper, G. and Lewis. J. F. Geological Society of America Special Paper 262, pp. 173-186.

Lewis, J.F. and Jiminez, J.G. 1991. Duarte complex in the La Vega-Jarabocoa-Janico Area, Central Hispaniola: Geologic and geochemical features of the sea floor during the early stages of arc evolution. In Geologic and Tectonic Development of the North America-Caribbean Plate Boundary in Hispaniola. Edited by Mann, P. Draper, G. and Lewis. J. F. Geological Society of America Special Paper 262, pp. 115-142.

Lewis, J.F. and Draper, G. 1990. Geology and tectonic evolution of the northern Caribbean margin. In The Caribbean Region. Edited by G. Dengo and J.E. Case. The Geological Society of America, Geology of North America, Vol. H, pp. 77-140.

Lewis, J.F., Astacio, T., and Espaillat J. 1998. The Maimon Formation. In Mineral Deposits of the Dominican Republic. Ed. by P.G. Fiess. The Society of Economic Geologists, March 1998 Field Trip, Dominican Republic.

Mann, P., Draper, G., and Lewis, J.F., 1991. An overview of the geological and tectonic development of Hispaniola. In Geologic and Tectonic Development of the North America-Caribbean Plate Boundary in Hispaniola. Edited by Mann, P. Draper, G. and Lewis. J. F. Geological Society of America Special Paper 262, pp. 1-28.

Russell, N., Brouwer, S., and Kesler, S.E., 1982. Economic geology of the central Dominican Republic. In Society of Economic Geologists Fall Field Trip Guide Book, 1982. Edited by S.E. Kesler.

Winchester, J.A. and Floyd, P.A., 1977. Geochemical discrimination of different magma series and their differentiation products using immobile elements. Chemical Geology, vol. 20, pp. 325-343

THE OCCURRENCE OF VOLCANOGENIC MASSIVE SULPHIDE DEPOSITS IN THE MAIMON FORMATION, DOMINICAN REPUBLIC: THE CERRO DE MAIMON, LOMA PESADA AND LOMA BARBUITO DEPOSITS

JOHN F. LEWIS

Dept. of Earth and Environmental Sciences, The George Washington University, Washington D.C. 20052

VINCENTE A. ASTACIO[1]

Dept. of Earth and Environmental Sciences, New Mexico Institute of Mining and Technology, Socorro, New Mexico

JULIO ESPAILLAT[2] AND JORGE JIMENEZ[2]

Corporation Minera Dominicana, Avenida Maximo Gomez H 29 B, Santo Domingo, Dominican Republic

[1]*Present address: 949 S.Longmore, Apt. #255, Mesa, Arizona, 85282*

[2]*Formerly Dept. of Exploration, Falconbridge Dominicana*

ABSTRACT

Exploration over the past 25 years has led to the discovery of several volcanogenic massive sulphide (VMS) deposits within the Maimon Formation, central Dominican Republic. Rocks of the Maimon Formation of apparent Lower Cretaceous (pre Albian) age form a narrow 73 km long belt composed of mainly low grade metamorphosed volcanogenic rocks. The southwestern part of the Maimon belt, where the Cerro de Maimon and Loma Pesada VMS deposits are located is a high strain greenschist facies ductile shear zone consisting of interlayered mafic phyllonites and felsic mylonites. The rocks are much less deformed in the northern part of the belt, the location of the Barbuito deposit, and original textural features can be recognized. Much of the volcanic pile consists of bedded submarine volaniclastic units with lesser amounts of volcanic flows and shallow intrusions. Minor black shales, cherts, limestone and exhalite horizons are also present.

The Maimon protolith, as determined from analyzing least-altered rocks, is comprised of a bimodal spilite-keratophyre suite, best seen at Loma Pesada. Basaltic rocks range from low TiO_2 (0.2-0.4 %) high MgO (up to 15.4 %) tholeiites with boninitic affinities to typical oceanic arc tholeiites (TiO_2 = 0.5-0.8 %; MgO < 8.0 %). The boninitic basalts have depleted (<<N-type MORB) concentrations of HFSEs and REEs. A short interval of basalts in the Loma Pesada section shows elevated TiO_2 and high Fe/Mg ratios reflecting a more evolved series.

Felsic rocks are quartz-plagioclase tuffs and porphyries (keratophyres) with flat chondrite normalized REE patterns and negative Eu anomalies. Like the basalts the keratophyres have a clear subduction zone signature with enrichment in LILEs, and depletion in Nb, REE and HFSEs with respect to N-type MORB.

Characteristic features of the Maimon VMS deposits are their pyrite-rich nature, copper-zinc mineralization (Cu:Zn~2:1), low lead concentrations (<1000 ppm) and significant precious metal values (0.69 g/t Au and 44.7 g/t Ag at Cerro de Maimon). Of the four massive sulphide deposits that have been located only the Cerro de Maimon deposit is economically feasible at the present time.

The application of geochemical techniques has shown that the original rocks at Cerro de Maimon, formed prior to the deposition of the sulphides, were mafic to intermediate tholeiitic basalts. The hydrothermal alteration in footwall rocks involved the loss of calcium and sodium and the extensive introduction of silicon and potassium in the form of quartz and sericite. Oxygen isotope values of altered footwall rocks at Cerro de Maimon and Loma Barbuito range from 8.1 to 13.4 ‰ whereas hangingwall rocks and least altered rocks range from 3.4 to 4.7 ‰. The unusually high oxygen isotope values are considered to be due to the introduction of hydrothermal silica during mineralization.

The VMS deposits in the Maimon Formation were formed in a nascent primitive island arc, probably in the forearc area.

INTRODUCTION

Copper rich sulphides in the Maimon area in the central Dominican Republic have been known and exploited since the time of the Spanish colonization (Rodríguez, 1965). However, the discovery of several massive sulphide deposits of volcanogenic origin in the Maimon Formation did not occur until systematic exploration was begun in the late 1970s. A first general account of the Maimon Formation was given by Bowin (1966), as a result of his studies in the area between 1957 and 1960 but for some 18 years little work was done on the these rocks. The massive sulphide deposit at Cerro de Maimon was located by Falconbridge on their Quisqueya concession from the occurrence of gossanous outcrop. It was first drilled in 1978. In 1983 Rosario Dominicana obtained the concession rights to explore all the Maimon Formation. This work, which included geological surveys, defined several exploration targets and resulted in a geological map at 1:25,000 scale and report (Rosario Dominicana, 1985) summarized by Kesler et al., (1991). Falconbridge Dominicana (Falcondo) took over the Maimon concession in 1990 and in 1991 located and drilled the Loma Pesada deposit. Through mineral exploration by Rosario Dominicana, Falconbridge and other companies over the past 15 years, four volcanic-hosted massive sulphide deposits have been located within the Maimon Formation. The location of these deposits and other exploration targets that have been investigated are shown in Figure 2. As part of the Falcondo exploration program, more detailed studies of the structure, petrography, whole rock geochemistry and isotope geochemistry of the Maimon Formation have been undertaken, the results of which are described below. More detailed descriptions of the Cerro de Maimon deposit have been published (Astacio, 1997; Lewis et al., 1998; Astacio et al., 2000). In this report we summarize the main features of the Cerro de Maimon, Loma Pesada and Loma Barbuito deposits, as presently known. The San Antonio deposits are discussed by Holbek and Daubeny (2000, this volume).

THE MAIMON FORMATION

General Geology

The Maimon Formation, along with the Amina schists to the west, are part of a belt of early

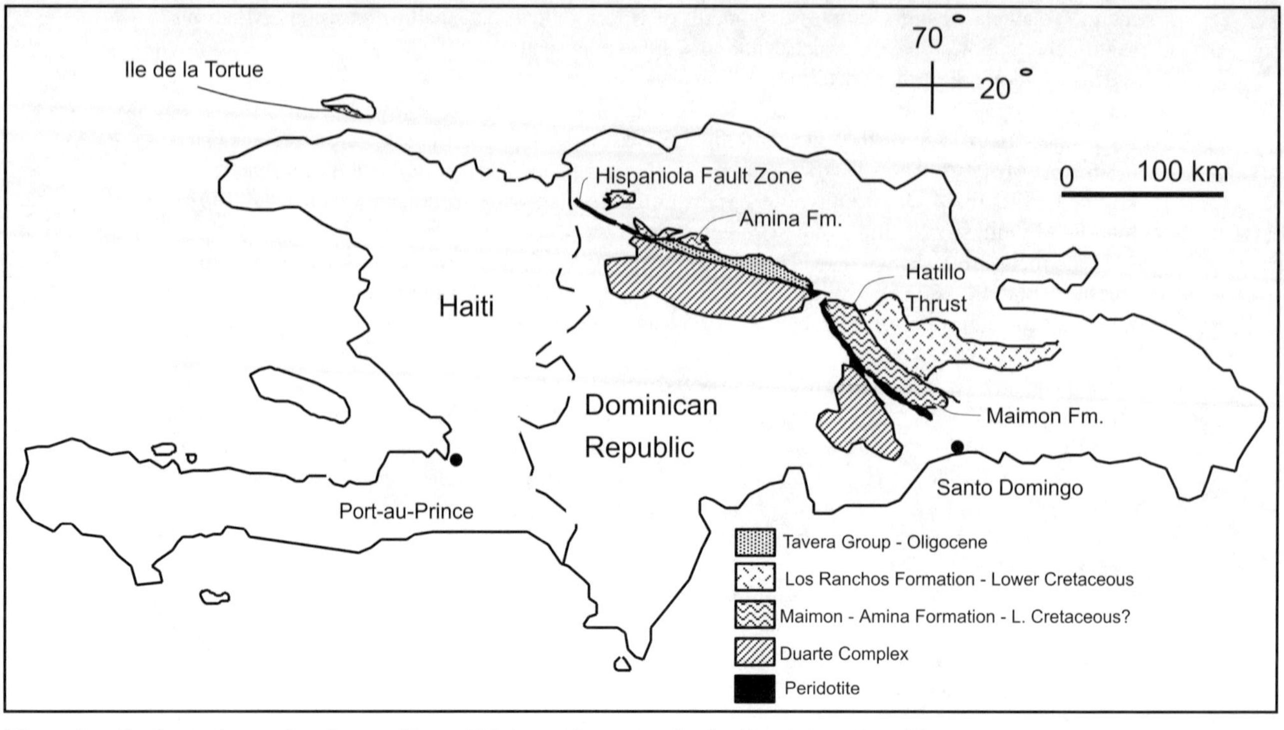

Figure 1. Geological map showing position of Maimon Formation in the Dominican Republic.

Cretaceous (pre-Albian) bimodal volcanism that extends the full length of the present day Greater Antilles arc (Lewis and Draper, 1991, Lewis et al., 1996; Childe, 2000). In the Dominican Republic, the fore-arc and island arc components of this early volcanism are preserved as the Maimon and Amina Formations (fore-arc) and the Los Ranchos Formation (axial island arc).

The Maimon volcaniclastic rocks of the fore-arc basin host several exhalitive massive sulphide deposits whereas the extensive mineralization throughout the Los Ranchos Formation is of the epithermal type. Many features of the structure and lithologies of the Maimon protolith are analogous with those found in the Eocene basement of the Izu-Bonin-Mariana fore-arc (Bloomer et al., 1995).

A regional unconformity, recognized on all the main islands of the Greater Antilles and marked by rudist-bearing limestones of Albian age, seperates the early Cretaceous arc tholeiite bimodal volcanism from the extensive calc-alkaline volcanism that took place through the Late Cretaceous.

The Maimon Formation is a northwest trending belt, about 9 km wide and 73 km long, of mainly metamorphosed volcaniclastic rocks, that lies between the Loma Caribe peridotite belt and the Los Ranchos Formation to the north (Figs 1, 2). At the southern contact a thin belt of mainly mafic volcanic rocks, the Peralvillo Formation of Late Cretaceous age, separates the Loma Caribe peridotite from the Maimon Formation. At the contact between the Peralvillo and Maimon Formation, the rocks are highly sheared as seen in drill cores. At the northern contact along the Hatillo Thrust the Maimon Formation

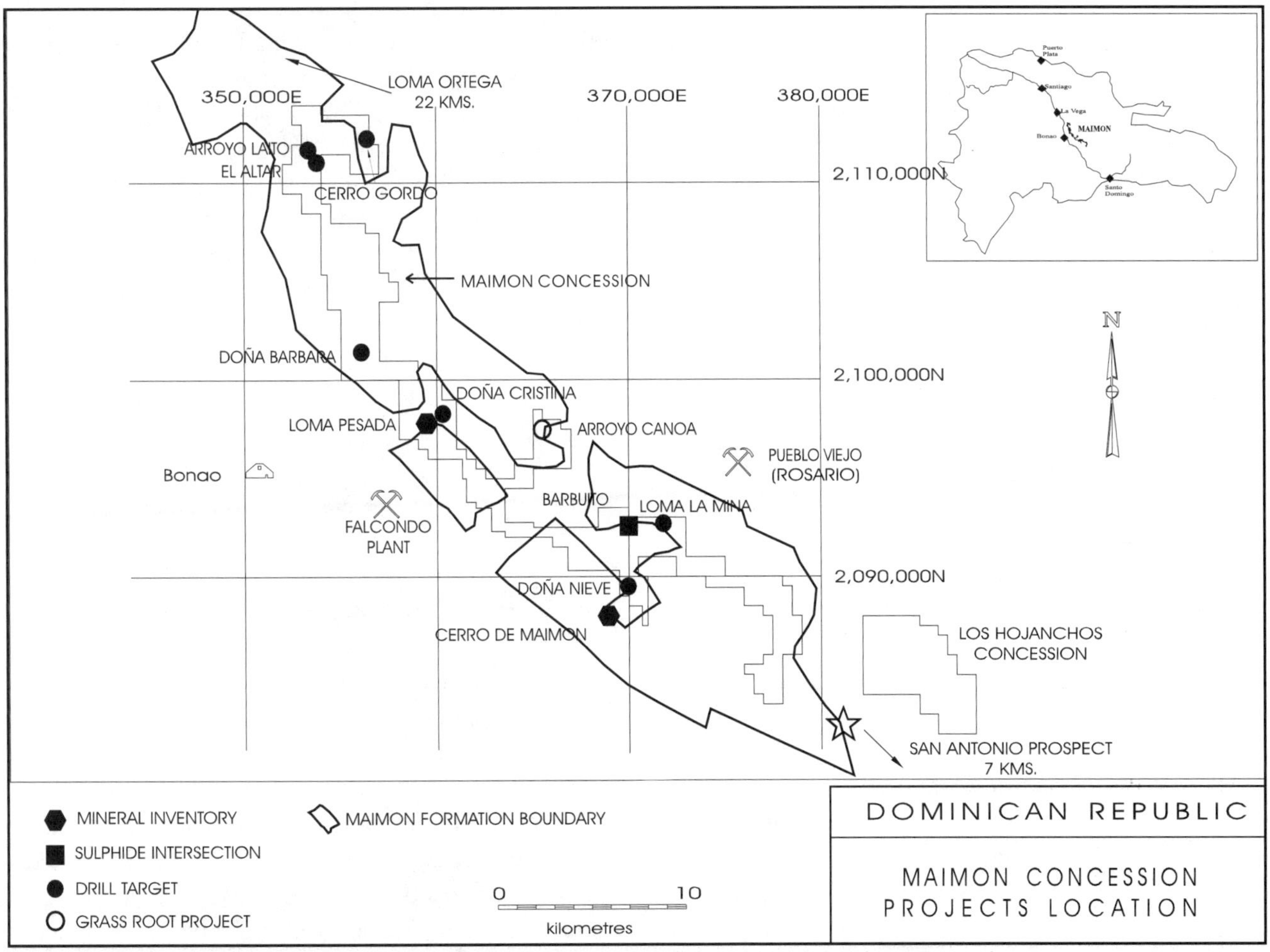

Figure 2. Map showing the Maimon concession and principal localities within the Maimon Formation.

overthrusts the Las Lagunas Formation of Late Cretaceous age and Hatillo limestone of Albian age. The Hatillo Limestone overlies the Los Ranchos Formation unconformably. The Maimon Formation extends to the west as the Amina Formation (Fig. 1). Amina rocks have similar lithologies to the Maimon, but the metamorphism is more uniform, the deformation is more complex, and the rocks are more highly recrystallized (Draper and Lewis, 1982; 1991).

Rocks of the Maimon (and Amina) Formation constitute a bimodal spilite-keratophyre suite. Much of the volcanic pile consists of bedded submarine volcaniclastic units with lesser amounts of intercalated volcanic flows and shallow intrusives. The volcaniclastic rocks are mainly tuffs but horizons of breccias and conglomerates can be recognized in less deformed rocks. A belt of well-laminated rocks of obvious sedimentary origin occurs through much of the central part of the Maimon Formation outcrop area. These are mainly fine-grained laminated metatuffs but cherts, dark shales and limestones are also present. These meta-sedimentary rocks appear to be totally conformable with the more typical Maimon Formation meta-volcaniclastic rocks. Layers of manganese oxide, hematite iron concentrations and cherty layers interbedded with the volcaniclastic units are considered to have resulted from exhalitive activity.

The age of the Maimon Formation is not well established. The general structural/tectonic relations suggest the Maimon Formation is Early Cretaceous in age. Model ages calculated from the lead isotope data (Horan, 1995) suggest an early Cretaceous age similar to model ages calculated from the lead isotope data for the Los Ranchos Formation (Cumming and Kesler, 1987). Fragments of echinoid spines found in a meta-limestone interbedded with tuffs in the central part of the Maimon Formation are similar to those of hemicidarids from the Early Cretaceous of Mexico and Jamaica (S.K. Donovan, unpublished data, 1994).

The regional strike of the foliation in the Maimon Formation rocks is northwest parallel to the regional strike of the Median Belt (Bowin, 1966; Draper and Lewis, 1991). The foliation and apparent bedding dips to the south over most of the area of Maimon. The stratigraphic relations of the sulphide deposit to the host rocks and the younger Peralvillo Formation at Cerro de Maimon are the main reason for the assumption that the youngest units of the Maimon are to the north. Kesler et al. (1990) reported that pillow lavas are clearly upright along the northeast side of the belt.

The Maimon Formation is divided into two structural metamorphic provinces parallel to the northwest-southeast structural trend of the belt (Draper et al., 1996). The Ozama shear zone in the southwest of the Maimon belt is a high-strain greenschist facies ductile shear zone consisting of interlayered mafic phyllonites and felsic mylonites. The extreme deformation in this zone has obliterated most of the original textures. The Altar Zone in the northeast part of the Maimon belt is composed of much less deformed rocks which can be recognized as interlayered mafic and felsic tuffs, breccias and flows. These show variable degrees of schistosity and exhibit both pure and simple shear fabrics. These structural data suggest that the deformation feature, and in particular the Ozama shear zone in the Maimon Formation, resulted from northward thrust emplacement obduction of the peridotites over the arc rocks of the Maimon Formation. Most of the deformation and metamorphism of the Maimon Formation rocks, particularly in the Ozama mylonite zone, resulted from the obduction of the Loma Caribe peridotite on to the early Antillean arc in the mid Cretaceous (Draper, et al., 1996). This obduction event was followed by the deposition of limestone over the early arc rocks and was accompanied by a polarity reversal so that subduction changed from northwest-dipping to southwest-dipping (Draper, et al., 1996). The new volcanism beginning in the early Cenomanian was of the calc-alkaline type and continued to Eocene time.

In the middle to late Eocene, Hispaniola underwent northeast-southwest contraction (Mann et al., 1991). Many of the mid-Cretaceous thrust structures were reactivated at this time, including the Hatillo thrust (Bowin, 1966), which juxtaposed the Maimon belt against the lower Eocene and upper Cretaceous rocks. Reactivated thrusts emplaced the peridotites in a northeast direction over the Peralvillo Formation of Late Cretraceous age. Horizontal axis rotation accompanying contraction steepened earlier faults and foliations. The Eocene reactivation probably faulted out high-grade metamorphic rocks, which are expected to have formed adjacent to the sole thrust of the ophiolite as well as tectonically thickening the Maimon belt.

Geochemistry

A total of more than six hundred major element whole rock analyses have been made of samples from the Maimon Formation. This includes samples taken from five transects across the Maimon belt. Samples were selected for analysis to determine the range in lithologies and whole rock chemistry from the entire area. Many of the samples used for geochemical studies come from the drill cores of the areas where the mineral exploration has been focused. This allows the selection of unweathered rocks for detailed geochemistry.

Samples were analyzed at several different laboratories allowing a cross-check to be made. Major element analyses on Cerro de Maimon rocks were made by XRAL and later by ACME Laboratories Canada. Many of the trace element determinations on drill core samples were determined by XRF by Shannon Horan at the University of Florida at Gainesville (Horan, 1995). A selected group of these samples was analyzed for Rare Earth Elements by ICP-MS at the Geological Survey of Canada. Other high precision trace element analyses were made by ICP-MS techniques at Activation Laboratories, Canada.

Several data sets of the geochemistry of Maimon rocks have been compiled. The first group to be examined here is a compilation of 134 whole rock major element analyses of least altered rocks from throughout the Maimon outcrop area and from drill cores.

The second data set is composed of 64 analyses of a selected group of least altered rocks for which satisfactory trace element analyses have been made. Only those rocks that have undergone the least hydrothermal alteration were selected for this study. This was determined from petrographic examination and the major element geochemistry. Samples with obvious quartz or carbonate veining or alteration were not included. Depending on the composition, samples with low values for CaO and Na_2O were also excluded from the data set. In order to examine the protolith of the Maimon rocks only the immobile high field strength (HFS) and rare earth elements (REEs) have been used. Other data sets are of the hydrothermally altered rocks associated with the massive sulphide deposits.

Table 1 lists the major and trace element compositions of representative examples of the least altered samples of Maimon rocks. These samples are chosen to illustrate the range in chemistry of the Maimon in comparison with rocks from Izu-Bonin-Mariana arc systems, which have similar composition for both major and trace elements.

Using the above data bases, plots have been selected to show variation in composition of Maimon rocks. These are TiO_2-SiO_2, TiO_2-Zr, and Ni-SiO_2 shown in Figures 3a, 3b and 3c respectively. It can be seen from these plots that TiO_2 is a useful geochemical discriminant and that the rocks plot in distinct groups according to locality and composition. The TiO_2/Zr plot (Fig. 3b) reflects two trends in the evolution of the Maimon magmas. The increase in TiO_2 with a slight increase in Zr is typical of the tholeiitic trend whereas the trend in increasing Zr at a low concentrations of TiO_2 is a feature shown by the Izu-Bonin-Mariana arc boninitic rocks (Bloomer et al, 1995).

Multi-element trace element and rare earth element plots are used to examine separately the compositions of the mafic and felsic rock groups (Figs. 4 and 5).

Maimon Formation rocks can be conveniently classified into three groups: mafic, intermediate and felsic according to their silica content. Least altered Maimon rocks range in composition from mafic (basaltic) types mainly between 50 to 60 % SiO_2, intermediate between 60 to 70 % SiO_2 and felsic (acidic) between 70 to 80 % SiO_2.

The mafic (basaltic) rocks are present as several metamorphic mineral assemblages. Samples with little deformation from the northern part of the Maimon belt include flows as well as various volcaniclastic lithologies and it is assumed that the protolith to the deformed lithologies in the Ozama zone to the south included similar rock types.

Basaltic members of the Maimon Formation have a low but variable TiO_2 content and low concentrations of HFSE and REE, characteristic of oceanic island-arc tholeiites, the primitive island-arc (PIA) series of Donnelly and Rogers (1978). The mafic rocks range from low TiO_2-high MgO basalts with depleted (<<N-type MORB) concentrations of HFSEs which have boninitic affinities (Pierce et al., 1992), to those with slightly higher TiO_2 and lower MgO, more

Table 1. Representative chemical analyses of Maimon Formation rocks with comparisons from the Izu Bonin area. EA-01/93.45 metabasalt El Altar drill core; LP-04/87.0 chlorite-epidote schist, Loma Pesada; LB -16/30.0 aphyric metabasalt Loma Barbuito; LP-04 quartz-sericite schist, Loma Pesada; 91-122A Keratophyre north of Rincon; LP-09/153.4 Dacite intrusive into the Maimon, Loma Pesada; 62R-3 Boninite ODP Leg 125; 66R-1 Rhyolite ODP Leg 125 (Pierce et al., 1992).

	EA-01/93.45	LP04/87	LP-139	LB-16/30	LP-04	91-122A	LP-09/153.4	62R-3	66R-1
SiO_2	48.76	49.25	52.1	48.28	76.5	74.5	69.9	53.47	68.95
TiO_2	0.36	0.27	0.59	0.73	0.15	0.2	0.26	0.2	0.26
Al_2O_3	11.47	12.05	17.05	17.25	12.5	12.18	15.6	12.05	13.41
Fe_2O_3t	9.09	8.85	8.21	10.9	1.4	2.1	2.1	8.47	4.07
MnO	0.37	0.16	0.17	0.12	0.01	0.03	0.03	0.13	0.08
MgO	15.41	14.4	7.45	6.51	0.66	0.49	1.13	13.04	0.82
CaO	6.35	9.05	6.95	8.92	0.33	0.66	2.94	5.27	2.26
Na_2O	2.03	1.14	5.23	1.15	5.6	5.33	4.9	3.19	3.70
K_2O	<0.04	0.14	0.06	0.08	0.76	1.02	0.82	0.67	3.12
P_2O_5	0.05	0.04	0.1	0.12	0.03	0.06	0.05	0.03	0.08
CO_2					0.5		0.3		
H_2O					1.3		1.3		
LOI	6.4	4.35	3			1.32		4.33	2.36
TOTAL	100.45	99.7	100.89	100.89	99.8	97.9	99.4	100.85	99.11
Sc	31	40	37	38	4.7	20	3	29	11.8
Cr	634	826	<10	37	28	2	25	1036	33
V	192	191	351	285	30	10	63		166 31
Ni	182	304	9	55	3	<5	**	306	9
Co	47.6	46.5	40.8		2	<5	10	45	5.6
Cu	5	55	53	40	1	<5	28	60	50
Zn	172	30	122	65	28	30	56	63	92
Zr	19.6	23.5	101	40	99	123.3	46	35	81
Y	10	6.6	38	18	24	43	11	7.2	10.7
Nb	0.4	0.1	1.7	0.8	1	1.4	<1	0.53	0.98
Rb	<0.1	1.6	0.4		<1	13.9	**	6.4	29
Sr	12.2	62.8	135.2	96.6	58	41.8	564	107	104
Ba	7.3	33.3	26.4	7	104	261	325	47	388
Hf	0.7	0.4	2.8	0.7		3.6	1.1	0.9	2.1
Th	0.36	0.09	0.27	0.5		0.5	0.3	0.27	0.67
La	1.6	0.5	3.6	0.9	2.1	2.5	1.5	1.81	3.6
Ce	3.9	1.3	11.7	3	6.1	12	3.7	3.86	8.1
Pr	0.51	0.2	1.8		0.99		0.52	0.59	1.41
Nd	2.9	1.1	9.8	<5	4.5	9	2.6	2.84	5.9
Sm	0.9	0.5	4	1.1	1.7	2.8	0.8	0.81	1.39
Eu	0.35	0.18	1.28	0.5	0.34	0.5	0.34	0.27	0.46
Gd	1.4	0.6	5		2.2		0.87	0.97	2.16
Tb	0.3	0.2	1	<.5	0.46	0.8	0.15	0.16	0.26
Dy	1.6	1.1	6.1		2.9		0.84	1.05	1.82
Ho	0.3	0.3	1.4		0.66		0.16	0.23	0.38
Er	1.1	0.9	4.4		1.9		0.39	0.69	1.21
Tm	0.15	0.13	0.67		0.35		0.07	0.11	0.18
Yb	1.1	0.9	4.2	1.3	2.4	4.7	0.4	0.8	1.17
Lu	0.21	0.14	0.65	0.21	0.37	0.81	0.06	0.14	0.19

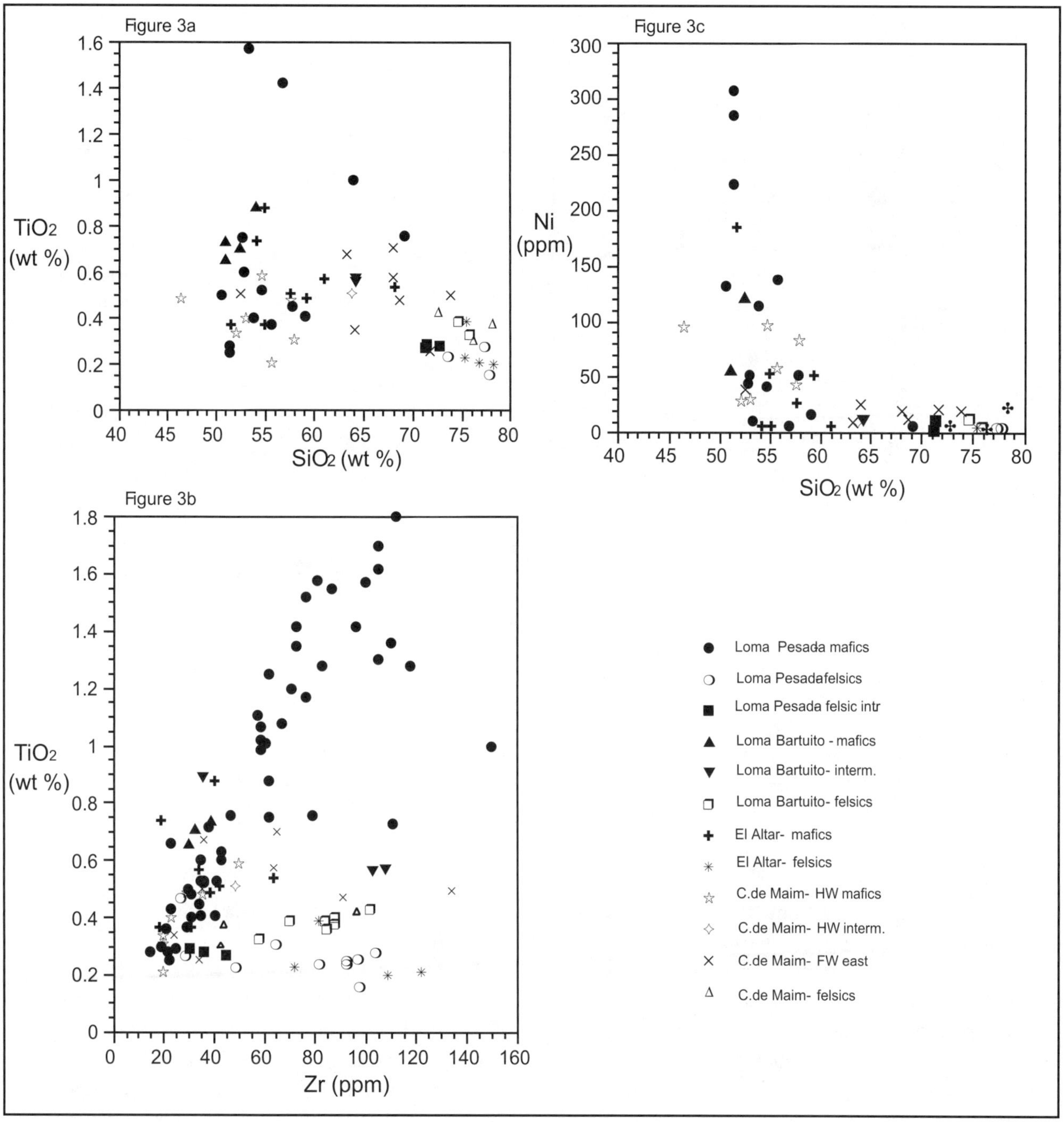

Figure 3. TiO_2 - SiO_2, TiO_2 - Zr, Ni-SiO_2 variation diagrams of least altered Maimon rocks. Samples are labeled according to locality.

typical of oceanic arc tholeiites (Fig. 3 and 4a). Rocks with the highest MgO and highest NiO are those from the hangingwall at Cerro de Maimon. TiO_2 ranges from 0.2 to 0.4 % in rocks with boninitic affinities, up to 0.9 % in most of the mafic rocks in the Maimon. However, in a small section over no more than 250 m in thickness in the Loma Pesada drill cores TiO_2 increases to 1.8 % reflecting a more evolved series.

Rocks of intermediate composition are mainly

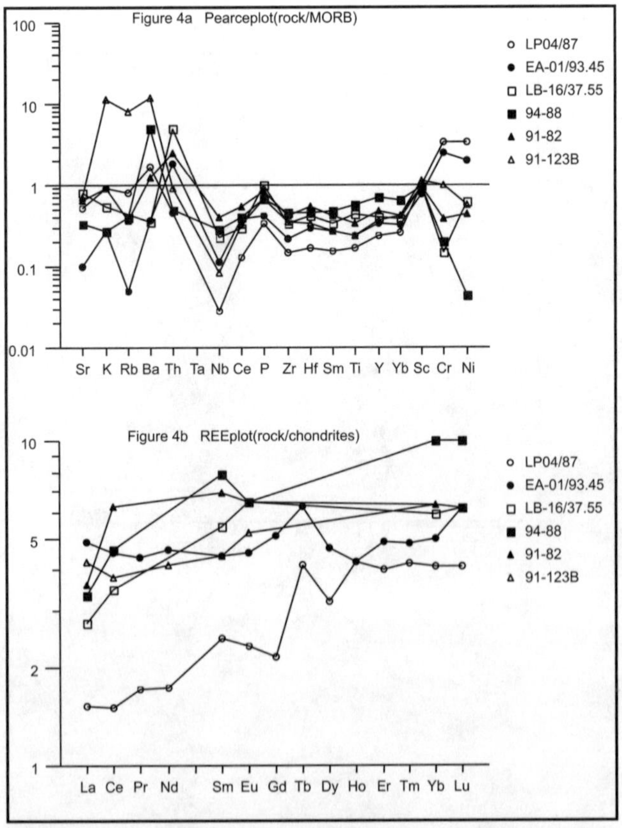

Figure 4(a). Multi-element plots (Pearce, 1983) normalized to N-type MORB of representative samples of least altered meta-mafic rocks from the Maimon Formation.

Figure 4(b). REE plots normalized to chondrite of representative samples least-altered meta-mafic rocks from the Maimon Formation.

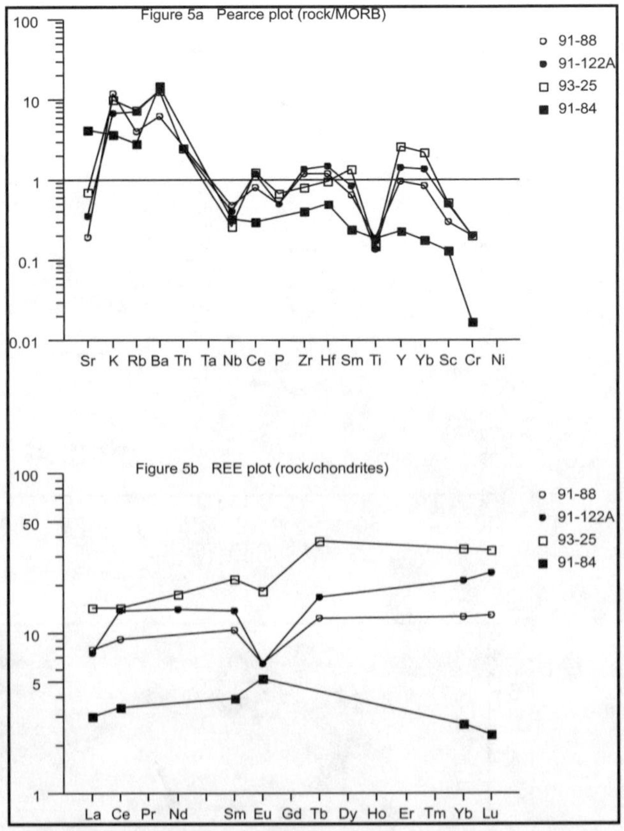

Figure 5(a). Multi-element plots (Pearce, 1983) normalized to N-type MORB of representative least altered felsic rocks from the Maimon. 91-84 is an intrusive feldspar porphyry (dacite).

Figure 5(b). REE plots normalized to chondrite of representative least altered felsic rocks from the Maimon.

chlorite and epidote-bearing quartz felspathic schists. In comparison with rocks of mafic composition, the intermediate rocks show more uniform composition. They have lower MgO (< 6.0 %) and Ni (< 50ppm) in contrast to the mafic rocks (Fig. 3). In most of the rocks of intermediate composition from the central area, Loma Barbuito and Cerro de Maimon TiO_2 ranges from 0.3 % to 0.7 %. On the other hand mafic rocks from Loma Barbuito and two samples from Los Hojanchos area in the northeast have relatively high TiO_2 between 0.6 % to 0.8 %.

It is considered that most of the rocks of intermediate composition are volcaniclastic in origin and have resulted from mechanical mixing between the basaltic and rhyolitic (keratophyric) end member lithologies. This mixing of volcaniclastic lithologies is seen clearly at Loma Pesada both in the field and in drill cores.

Rocks of felsic composition are metarhyolites or meta-quartz keratophyres that consist of phenocrysts of plagioclase and quartz in a quartzo-felspathic matrix. These occur as large plugs or flows along the northern margin of the Maimon Belt where the rocks are less deformed. In the Loma Pesada and Loma Barbuito areas, the felsic lithologies are interbedded with the mafic lithologies. Quartz and felspar are detrital in origin and the felsic rocks in these areas are clearly volcaniclastic in origin.

Sericite commonly occurs in the felsic rocks and a common assemblage in schistose rocks in the Ozama zone is sericite-quartz-plagioclase. The sericite in most of the rocks is probably related to the metamor-

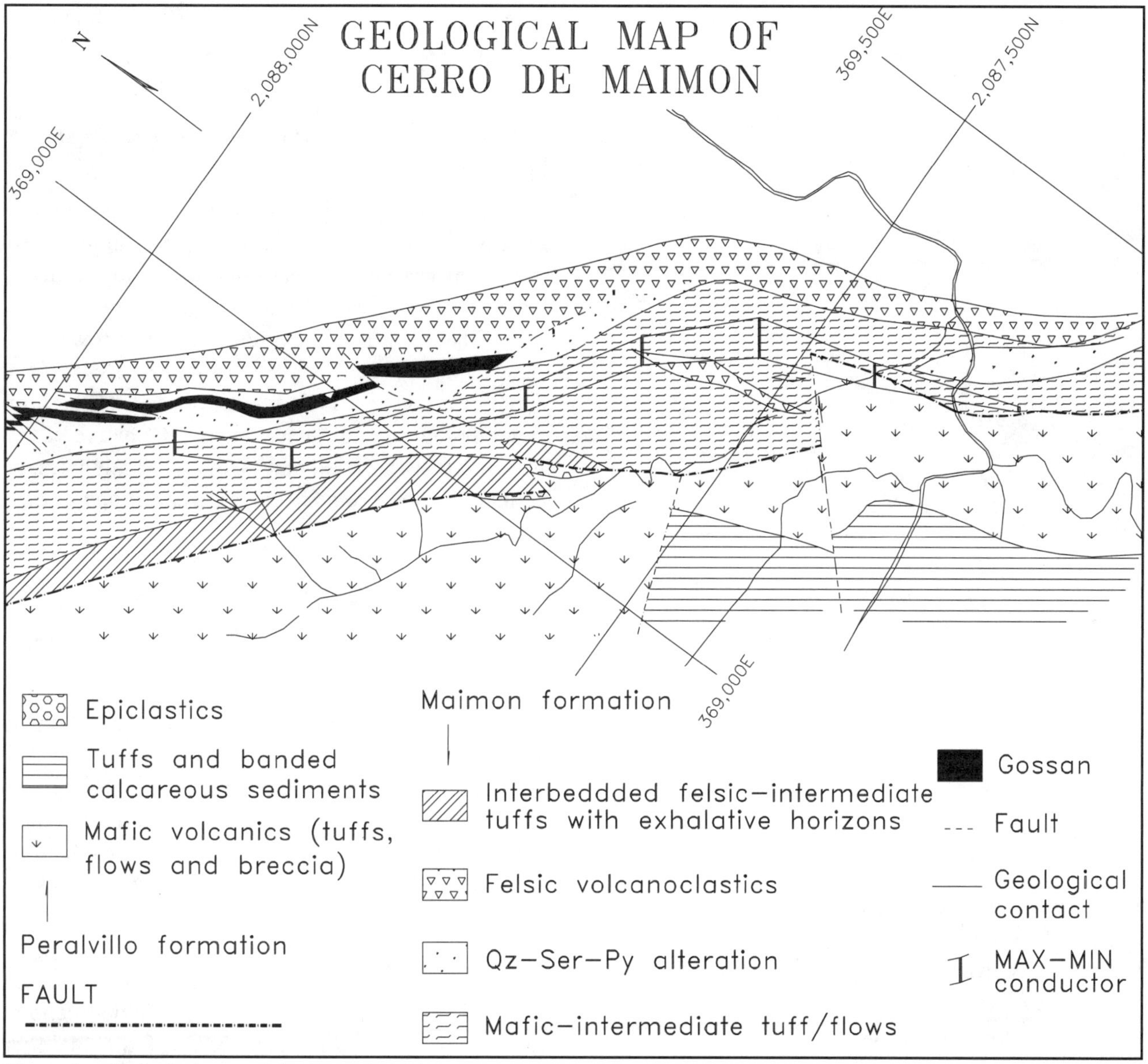

Figure 6. Geological map of the Cerro de Maimon area.

phism. However, the sericite in sericite-quartz-plagioclase "felsic" rocks associated with the massive sulphides is considered to have resulted from the mobilization and addition of potassium as a result of hydrothermal alteration.

The multi-element plot (Fig. 5a) shows that Maimon meta-quartz keratophyres are depleted in TiO_2, HFSEs, and REEs compared with other arc rhyolites. Like the basalts the rhyolites have a clear subduction signature with enrichment in LILE's, depletion in Nb, REEs and HFSEs with respect to N-type MORB. The REE patterns for three least altered felsic rocks of primary igneous origin are shown in Figure 5b. Note the flat pattern and negative Eu anomalies in these rhyolites (keratophyres), a feature typical of arc rhyolites from the Pacific (e.g., Bloomer et al. 1994). Sample 91-84 from Loma Pesada is an intrusive felspar porphyry probably of Eocene age.

Lead isotope ratios

Isotopic compositions for Sr, Nd and Pb have been determined for selected representative rocks from

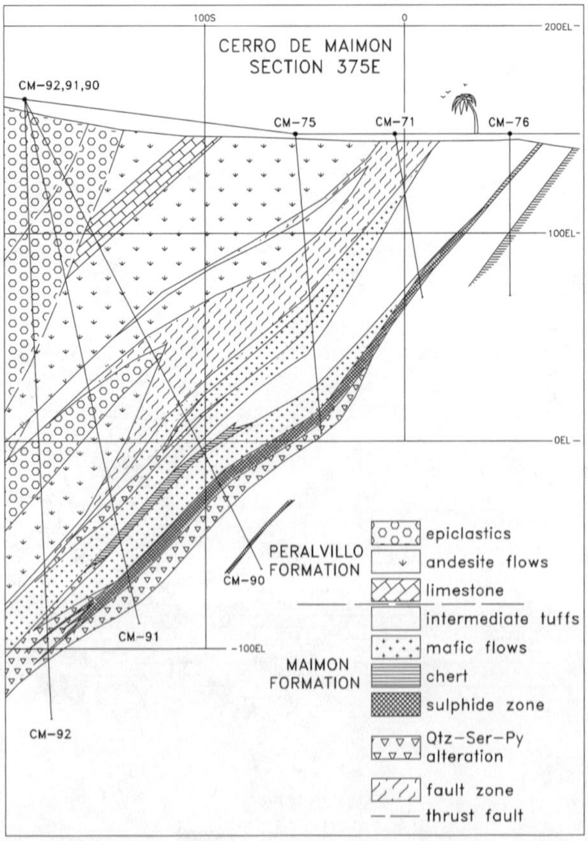

Figure 7. Geological cross section through the Cerro de Maimon deposit.

Maimon Formation (Horan, 1995). Plots of the $^{207}Pb/^{204}Pb$ ratios for samples of the sulphides and the whole rocks from the Maimon are compared with other Cretaceous arc rocks from the Caribbean. Both mafic and felsic rocks of the Maimon have low $^{207}Pb/^{204}Pb$ and $^{208}Pb/^{204}Pb$ ratios and fall in the Pacific MORB field. The chemically similar Water Island suite from the Virgin Islands has similar primitive Pb-isotope ratios whereas the other PIA suites (e.g., Los Ranchos) which are more evolved chemically, have slightly more enriched Pb-isotope arrays. The Pb data indicates a similar MORB source for all the initial bimodal volcanism in the Greater Antilles.

The isotopic and trace element data indicate the basalts and keratophyres have a common parent. It is difficult to derive the keratophyres by direct melting of a mantle source because of their large volume and the low compatible element concentrations in the keratophyres. Two possibilities are that the keratophyres were derived from a more mafic magma by fractional crystallization or that they are dehydration melts of arc crust (e.g., Beard and Lofgren, 1991).

Massive sulphide deposits in the Maimon Formation

Massive sulphide deposits have been found in four areas of the Maimon Formation. For each area, a geologic map has been prepared. The lithologies differ considerably from one area to another. It is for this reason that it is difficult to draw a generalized geological map of the Maimon Formation. Below is a summarized description for each deposit, of the host rock lithologies, their geochemistry, the nature of the hydrothermal alteration and the massive sulphides. A summary of the results of the oxygen isotope studies is also given.

Cerro de Maimon

The Cerro de Maimon deposit is located along the southern margin of the Maimon Formation immediately below the contact with Peralvillo Formation, about 7km east of the town of Maimon (Fig. 2). The following is a summary of the main features of the deposit. A more complete account is given in Astacio (1998), Lewis et al. (1998) and Astacio et al. (2000). Figure 6 is a geological map of the Cerro de Maimon area and Figure 7 is a cross section through the deposit.

Host rock lithologies

The Cerro de Maimon massive sulphide deposit lies within the Ozama shear zone of the Maimon Formation and hence the rocks are strongly deformed, and have the fabric of mylonites and phyllonites typical of shear zones. Few primary features can be recognized not only because of the deformation but because of the strong hydrothermal alteration particularly of the footwall rocks.

The host rocks to the ore body were mainly mafic to intermediate submarine volcaniclastic and volcanic rocks prior to alteration and metamorphism. Many of the pale quartzo-feldspathic lituologies at Cerro de Maimon that were mapped or logged as felsic rocks are the result of the extensive hydrothermal alteration and metamorphism. A cross section through the ore

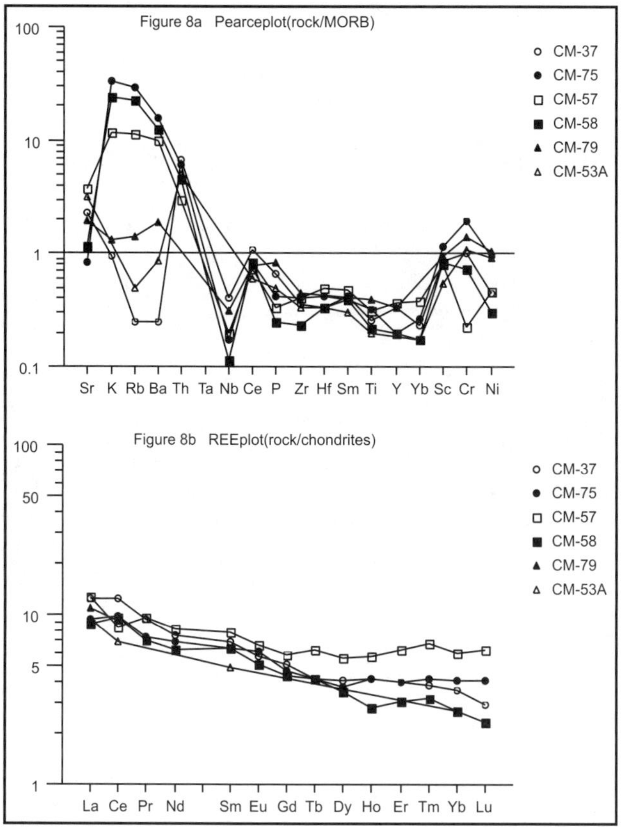

Figure 8(a). Multi-element plots (Pearce, 1983) normalized to N-type MORB of representative samples of hangingwall meta-mafic rocks from Cerro de Maimon.
Figure 8(b). REE plots normalized to chondrite of hangingwall meta-mafic rocks from Cerro de Maimon.

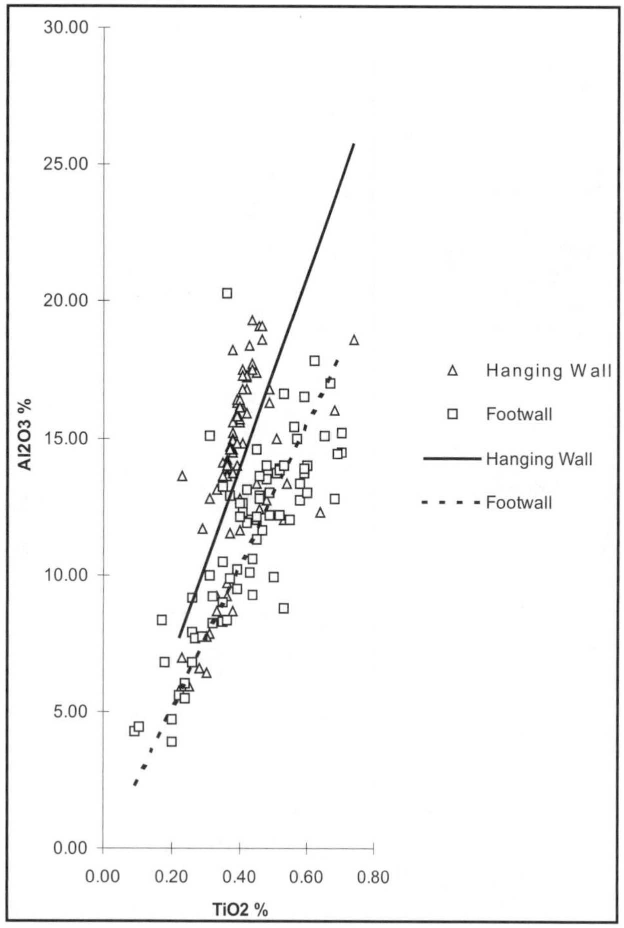

Figure 9. TiO_2 - Al_2O_3 % diagram to test element mobility in altered footwall and hanging rock samples from Cerro de Maimon. Well-defined alteration lines corresponding to homogeneous units are shown for footwall and hangingwall rocks.

body shows the distribution of lithologies (Fig. 7).

Two dominant lithologies are found in the hangingwall rocks:

(1) pale epidote-bearing mafic schists spotted with chlorite flakes;
(2) dark green chlorite schists with prominent calcite-quartz veins.

These two lithologies grade into one another. Cherty horizons are prominent in the western hangingwall whereas thin graphitic and hematitic beds are found in the eastern hangingwall rocks. Watkins (1989) identified several horizons of siliceous exhalites in the hangingwall.

Quartz-sericite-pyrite schists are the dominant footwall rocks below the western and central parts of the ore body. In places quartz-sericite-pyrite schists extend above the main massive sulphide orebody into the hangingwall. Footwall rocks in the east are mainly mafic to intermediate chlorite-rich rocks with minor quartz-sericite lenses. With depth these footwall rocks grade into chlorite-quartzo-feldspathic schists of mafic to intermediate composition.

The high concentration of quartz veins associated with the strong hydrothermal alteration in the western-most area suggests that the western footwall zone is a sulphide stockwork and possibly the alteration pipe so that the footwall rocks to the east are distal to the main centre of hydrothermal alteration.

Host Rock Geochemistry

Representative analyses of mafic rocks from the

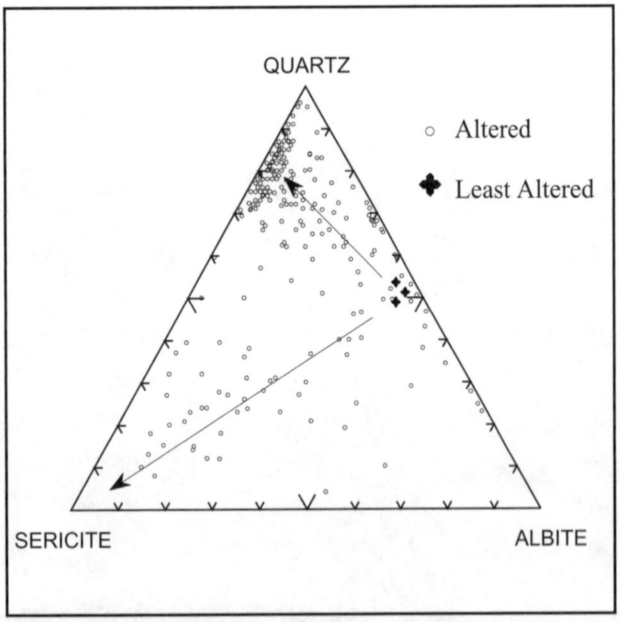

Figure 10. Quartz-Sericite-Albite ternary plots of altered rocks from the Cerro de Maimon.

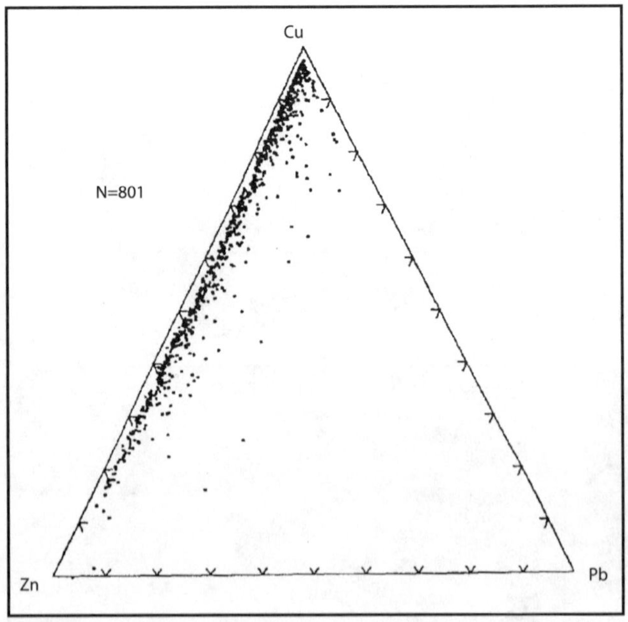

Figure 11. Cu - Zn - Pb diagram of 801 massive sulphide samples from the Cerro de Maimon deposit.

hangingwall and least altered rocks from the footwall for Cerro de Maimon are given in Table 2. Both types of mafic lithologies in the hangingwall have high MgO content (up to 15.4 %) and high Ni. The pale-coloured epidote-bearing group contains higher contents of CaO and appears to have compositions closer to typical tholeiitic basalts compared with the dark green chlorite-rich group. The latter are often sericitised and have relatively high K_2O content (up to 6 %). Figure 8a is a multi-element plot of examples of meta-basalts from Cerro de Maimon. Note the variable concentration in the large ion lithophile elements and the high Cr and Ni contents in three samples. The HFSE and HREEs are all uniformly depleted with respect to N-type MORB. These meta-basaltic rocks have distinct REE patterns (Fig. 8b) with enrichment in the light REEs, a feature not seen elsewhere in the Maimon Formation.

Hydrothermal Alteration

Examples of the compositions of the altered rocks from the footwall and hangingwall sections of the Cerro de Maimon are given in Table 2. Note that CaO and Na_2O have been depleted in the western footwall rocks by the hydrothermal alteration. On the other hand Na_2O has not been totally removed in the eastern footwall rocks but MgO has probably been added. It is considered that the lithologies and chemistry of the eastern footwall rocks resulted largely from seawater alteration followed by a relatively mild overprint of hydrothermal alteration.

Because the Cerro de Maimon rocks were volcaniclastic in origin, it is not possible to establish exact precursors before the rocks were altered and metamorphosed. However, using the composition of least altered rocks from Cerro de Maimon and rocks outside the area of hydrothermal alteration it is possible to obtain some idea of the extent of mass loss and mass gain during alteration and metamorphism.

Detailed studies of the lithogeochemistry of the hydrothermally altered rocks associated with massive sulphide deposits has shown that the elements Ti, Al, Zr and REE are immobile under typical conditions of hydrothermal alteration and greenschist grade metamorphism (eg., McLean and Barret, 1993).

Primary and alteration relationships between immobile elements have been examined on the Cerro de Maimon rocks using plots of Al_2O_3-TiO_2 and

Table 2. Representative chemical analyses of drill core from Cerro de Maimon.
CM-90/218.5 and CM-59/111 quartz-sericite schists, footwall zone; CM 71/54 intermediate footwall rock (west); CM 96/143.9 intermediate footwall rock (east); CM-97/252 mafic footwall rock -eastern section; CM-90/191.4 chlorite-epidote schist, hangingwall zone.

	CM-90/218.5	CM-59/111	CM-71/54	CM-96/143.9	CM-97/252	CM-90/191.4
SiO_2	70.5	83.65	61.9	64.9	49.75	55.35
TiO_2	0.3	0.26	0.5	0.7	0.5	0.47
Al_2O_3	8.62	6.57	14.5	11.26	17.55	16.24
Fe_2O_3t	9.13	3.35	8.80	5.81	10.03	7.72
MnO	0.01	0.02	0.08	0.11	0.20	0.16
MgO	0.91	1.35	3.64	2.72	12.93	6.97
CaO	0.15	0.03	5.21	6.34	0.20	5.93
Na_2O	0.33	0.21	0.60	3.10	2.51	1.02
K_2O	2.07	1.40	1.36	0.06	0.38	1.75
P_2O_5	0.08	0.05	0.05	0.11	0.02	0.04
CO_2	0.10		0.20			
H_2O			3.50			
S	7.19		< 0.02			
LOI	6.6	2.5		5.2	6.3	5.12
TOTAL	99.7	99.81	100	100.35	100.52	100.75
Cr	36		22	8.66	31.8	56
Ni	1	20	8	<10	37	42
Co	5		4		33	37
V	51		97	66.4	36.3	208
Cu	52		49		<50	40
Zn	128		95		196	96
Zr	43	35	50	66.4	36.3	37
Y	10	14	19	24.8	8.7	11
Nb	1		2	1.44	0.95	0.7
Ba	4217	2330	923	36.3	267	200
Rb	11		26	1.23	3.17	22.6
Sr	21	21	407	161	16	451
Sc	11	<10	22	19	30	32
Th				<0.5	<0.5	0.59
La	0.25		1.9	2.7	0.7	4.2
Ce	0.81		5.2	9	3	7.3
Sm	0.43		1.7	2	0.6	1.6
Yb	0.97		2.2	2.1	1.3	0.6

TiO_2-Zr. The Al_2O_3-TiO_2 plot (Fig. 9) shows clearly the distinct alteration lines for the footwall and hangingwall rocks at Cerro de Maimon. These data suggest a change in the magma system at the end of the deposition of the sulphides.

The Quartz-Sericite-Albite diagram (Fig. 10) and a SiO_2-Zr plot (not shown) highlights the high degree of silica and potassium mobility during the hydrothermal alteration. The diagram also demonstrates the breakdown of plagioclase and that considerable silica

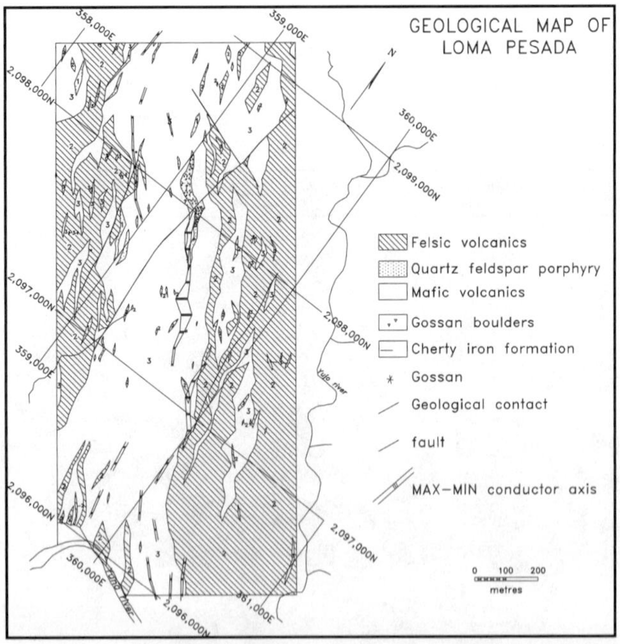

Figure 12. Geological map of the Loma Pesada area. Where there was no exposure, the dominant lithology was determined by taking auger samples every 20 metres to a depth of 0.6 metres along grid lines 50 metres apart.

was added to the western footwall zone.

Massive Sulphide

Cerro de Maimon is a volcanic hosted copper and zinc rich exhalitive massive sulphide deposit 200 m wide and 800 m long. It is 40 m thick near the surface, but narrows to a 5 m thick zone down plunge. The deposit plunges south at 25 degrees, dips 50 degrees, and flattens to 20 degrees. The estimated reserve is 2.9 metric tonnes of sulphide grading 4.05 % Cu, 1.93 % Zn, 44.7 ppm Ag and 0.47 ppm Au. Although the Cu/Cu+Zn ratio varies through the ore body, there is no clear trend evident. Supergene enrichment has significantly increased the copper grade of the deposit to a depth of 120 m below the surface.

Ore Petrography and sulphide chemistry

Pyrite, forming rounded to angular grains (~ 200 microns) is the dominant mineral in the massive sulphide ore body with lesser amounts of 5-50 micron chalcopyrite and sphalerite. Minor bornite and traces of tetrahedrite and galena fill the interstices and also occur as small inclusions within the pyrite. Quartz, sericite, chlorite, rare calcite and barite are the interstitial gangue minerals. Bornite is the dominant mineral in the supergene zone. Chalcocite and covellite are found in the supergene zone although chalcocite also occurs as minor veins in the primary ore.

Figure 11 is a Cu-Zn-Pb ternary diagram for 801 samples of massive sulphide from Cerro de Maimon (Watkins, 1989). Note that although the samples range from copper-rich to zinc-rich there are no samples with greater than 90 % in their Zn/Cu ratio. On the other hand a high concentration of samples have greater than 90 % in their Cu/Zn ratio. No samples have more than 21 % Pb on the Cu-Zn-Pb ternary diagram. There is decided enrichment in the Cu/Cu+Zn ratio in the supergene zone but in the hypogene assemblage there is no trend in zinc enrichment or copper depletion. There is however an increase in the Zn/Cu ratio toward the eastern section of the orebody. This suggests that the copper-rich part of the orebody in the west might be the area of discharge of the metal-bearing hydrothermal fluids whereas the Zn-rich eastern part might represent the outer fringes of the system.

Detailed fabric and microtextures of the massive sulphides at Cerro de Maimon and elsewhere in the Maimon Formation are principally controlled by the degree of metamorphism and deformation in a particular part. Along with the strongly folded sericite, pressure fringes, composed of mainly silica, are developed on the euhedral edges of pyrite.

Oxygen isotope geochemistry

Whole rock oxygen isotope compositions have been determined for 32 rocks from drill cores transecting all the rock type through the Cerro de Maimon deposit (Astacio, 1998; Astacio et al. 2000). Details of the analytical techniques used are given in these papers. The most highly altered rocks found in the eastern footwall area have $\delta^{18}O$ rocks ranging from 7.9‰ to 12.9‰ with the majority between 9-11‰. These unusually high values for footwall zone rocks are considered to have resulted from the intense silicification and seritization during hydrothermal alteration of the original mafic and intermediate volcanic rocks. No $\delta^{18}O$ zonation is evident within the altered

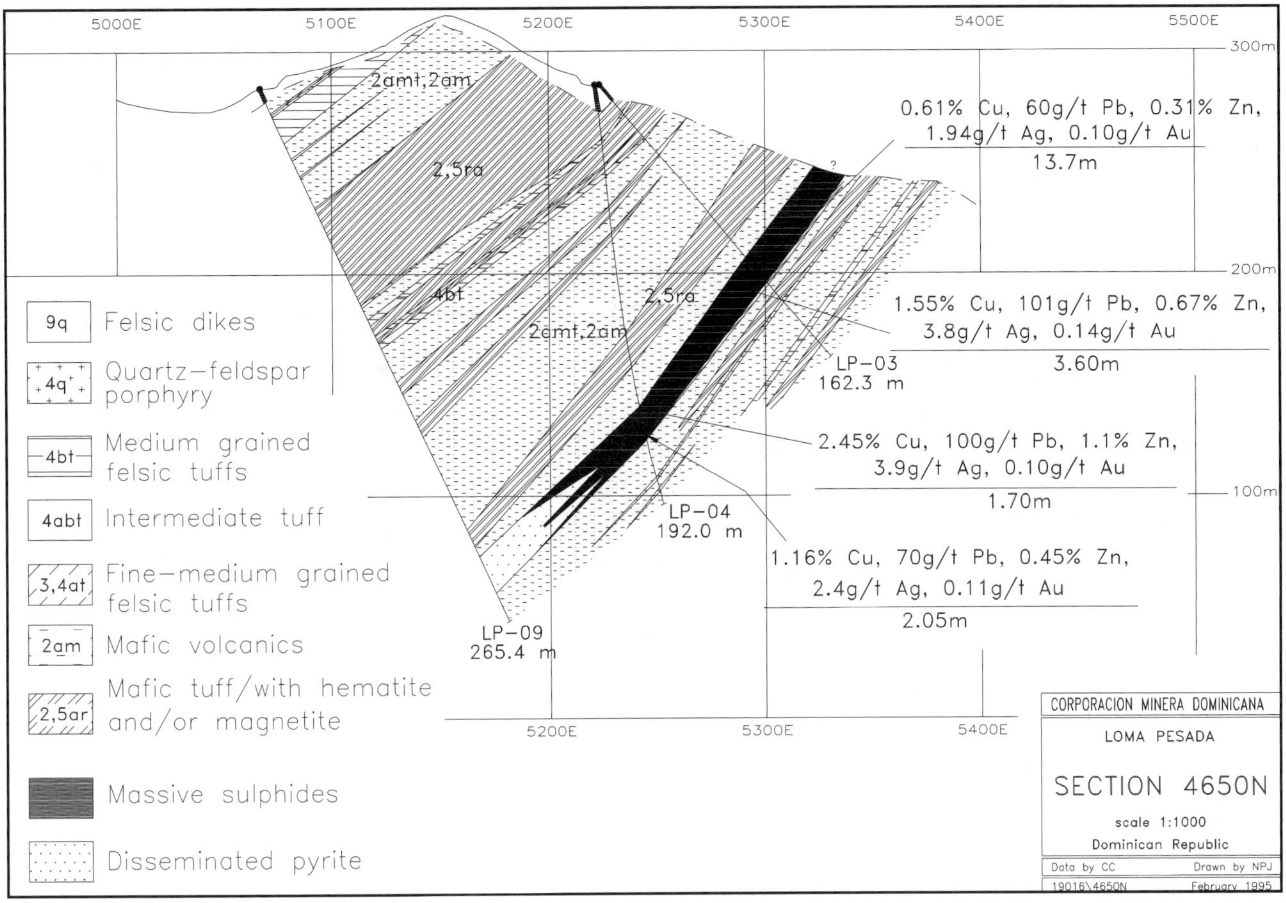

Figure 13(a). Cross section through drill cores LP-03, LP-04 and LP-09 at Loma Pesada.

footwall rocks. $\delta^{18}O$ in the hangingwall rocks ranges from 7.9‰ to 10.1‰ (average 8.9‰ in 8 samples). $\delta^{18}O$ values for rocks in the eastern footwall least altered rocks ranges from 4.9 to 7.6‰ (average 6.68‰; 8 samples). Calculated values for $\delta^{18}O$ for the parental hydrothermal fluids range from 3.4 to 4.7‰ and temperatures of ore deposition are from 309°C to 358°C.

Loma Pesada

The Loma Pesada deposit is located 4 km north of the site of the Falconbridge Dominicana nickel plant. Figure 12 is a geological map and Figures 13a and 13b are cross sections through the Loma Pesada area.

Host Rocks

Strongly foliated to laminated greenschists composed of the assemblage plagioclase + quartz + epidote + chlorite ± amphibole ± sericite ± magnetite are the most abundant rock type in the Loma Pesada area. These mafic schists are intercalated with minor thin horizons of pale coloured, sericitic quartz-feldspar schistose rock. Most of the Loma Pesada rocks are foliated and recrystallized. However, some rocks are massive or only weakly foliated and the original textural features and minerals are at least partly preserved.

LP-09/67.1 is an example of a porphyritic mafic lava with boninitic affinities containing relic phenocrysts of pyroxene and olivine? in a matrix of fibrous amphibole.

Detailed traverses showed a higher percentage of felsic lithologies intercalated with mafic lithologies northeast and southwest of the drill core area as reflected on the map (see Fig. 12 for details). In places there is a rapid change from dominantly mafic to dominantly felsic lithologies over a few metres. The thickness of the mafic or felsic layers (units) varies

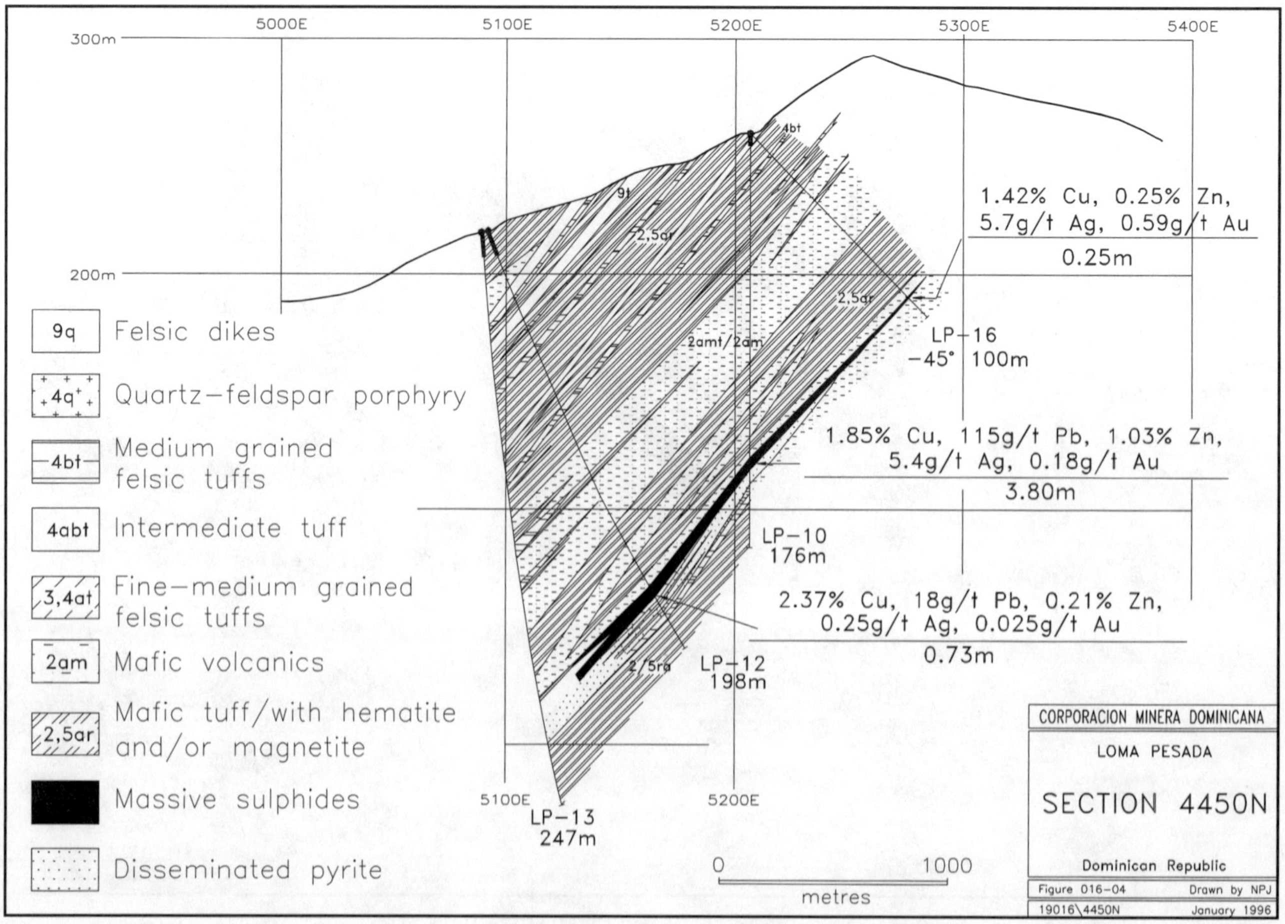

Figure 13(b). Cross section through drill cores LP-10, LP-12, LP-13 and LP-16 at Loma Pesada.

from a few centimetres to about 60 metres although felsic layers are rarely thicker than 4 metres. In other parts of the section mafic lithologies are dominant over tens of metres with only minor intercalations of felsic rock.

The fine laminations are considered to reflect compositional differences produced during the deposition of the original rock and mineral grains. The coarser-grained plagioclase found in the mafic lithologies, and the quartz (seen as quartz eyes in the field) and plagioclase in the felsic lithologies, are considered to be clastic in origin. This together with the laminations suggests the rocks are a sequence of fine to medium-grained tuffs. On the other hand horizons of weakly foliated rock are probably flows but could be more massive beds in the volcaniclastic sequence.

The rocks of the Loma Pesada area are therefore interpreted to be a sequence of mainly mafic volcaniclastic rocks (tuffs) interspersed with thin intervals of felsic quartz-bearing volcaniclastics. Mafic rocks that are probably flows are also present in minor quantity. The sequence of layered volcaniclastics is clearly bimodal in composition but in some horizons particularly outside the drilled area, the clastic layers are compositionally gradational and intermediate compositions are present.

Based on the chemical analyses, core logs and measured thicknesses in the field, it is estimated that 96 % of the Loma Pesada drill core section is composed of mafic volcaniclastic rocks with some mafic flows. The individual "beds" of intercalated felsic tuffs vary from a thickness of a few millimetres to about 35 m. This layered volcaniclastic sequence is intruded by small massive bodies of non-foliated feldspar porphyry.

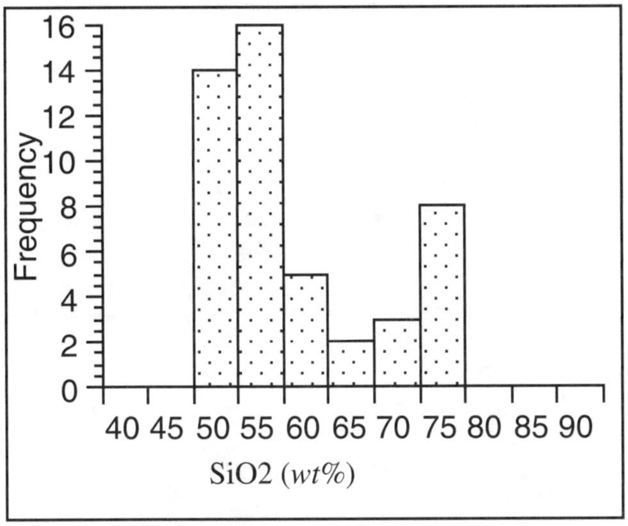

Figure 14. Distribution in terms of silica for Loma Pesada rocks.

Host Rock Geochemistry

Whole rock major element analyses have been made for this study of 75 selected rock samples from the Loma Pesada area. Sixty-two of these are from the drill cores; the remainder from the field area immediately around the drill sites. Since the rocks at Loma Pesada show little of the strong hydrothermal alteration seen at Cerro de Maimon a fairly detailed study has been made of the variation in chemical composition through the section. Representative analyses of some least altered rocks from Loma Pesada are listed in Table 1. Loma Pesada analyses show a clear bimodal distribution in terms of silica variation (Fig. 14). Most of the analyses of mafic rocks range from 50 to 55 % SiO_2. In this mafic group MgO varies from 4.59 % to 14.4 % and TiO_2 from 0.27 % to 1.8 %. CaO shows considerable variation and presumably has been mobilized during epidotization. Na_2O is consistent (up to) 5.83 % and K_2O ranges from 0.02 to 0.56 % with the exception of samples with clear evidence of sericitization.

Detailed trace element analyses have been determined for six samples considered to be representative of the mafic rocks from Loma Pesada. Figure 15a is a multi-element plot of these data. The two high MgO/low TiO_2 samples have very depleted patterns including Th and the LILs. In terms of their chemistry, these two samples have definite boninitic affinities. LP-12/121.9 and LP-09/211.9 are typical of the arc tholeiites and their composition falls in the same general field as identified for other arc tholeiites in the Maimon Formation (Fig. 4). Samples LP-09/157.04 and LP-03/79.8 containing 0.99 and 1.56 % TiO_2 respectively and low MgO and high FeO/MgO ratios are the more fractionated basaltic types in the Loma Pesada section. Although their HFSE concentrations are similar to N-type MORB suggesting a similarity in origin N-type, MORB basalts are less fractionated as measured by their FeO/MgO ratio at a particular TiO_2 content. Arc tholeiites with a similar range in chemistry are those from Hakone, Japan (Arculus et al., 1991).

The felsic tuffs show a small and consistent range in composition (8 samples analyzed for major elements) with silica varying from 68.4 to 76.5 % (Table 1, Fig.14). CaO is consistently low at less than 1 %. MgO is variable and is related to the amount of chlorite present. Na_2O ranges from 3.95 to 5.12 % and K_2O from 0.42 to 1.34 %. The percentage of K_2O is related to the degree of sericitization. The major element chemistry of the felsic tuffs and the intrusive porphyries is similar (Table1). All the intrusive porphyries are slightly lower in SiO_2 except one sample. The other main difference in composition is that the intrusive porphyries have slightly higher Al_2O_3 and CaO contents. Both have similar alkali contents.

Detailed trace element analyses have been made of three samples of the felsic tuffs from Loma Pesada - two from the drill cores and one from the field. Figure 16a is a multi-element plot of these data normalized with respect to N-type MORB. Figure 16b is a chondrite-normalized REE plot of the same samples. For comparison, the data for three felsic porphyries that intrude the Loma Pesada sequence are also plotted on the same diagrams (Fig. 16). Both the multi-element and REE patterns of all three tuffs are similar to those of the two keratophyre plugs from the northern part of the Maimon (Fig. 5). The more depleted composition of the felsic tuffs is more typical of rhyolite formed in the early stages of arc development (Bloomer et al., 1994). The intrusive porphyries (samples LP-09/153.4, LP-12/71.8 and 91-84) have relatively high concentrations of Sr and Ba but show marked depletion in the HFSE and HREEs and have sloping REE

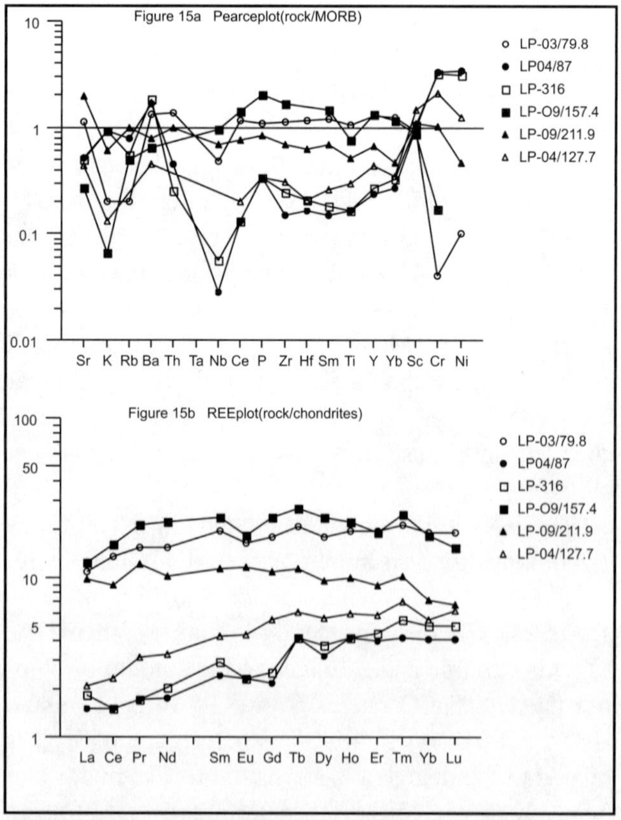

Figure 15(a). Multi-element plots (Pearce, 1983) normalized to N-type MORB of meta-mafic rocks from Loma Pesada. 15(b). REE plots normalized to chondrite of meta-mafic rocks from Loma Pesada.

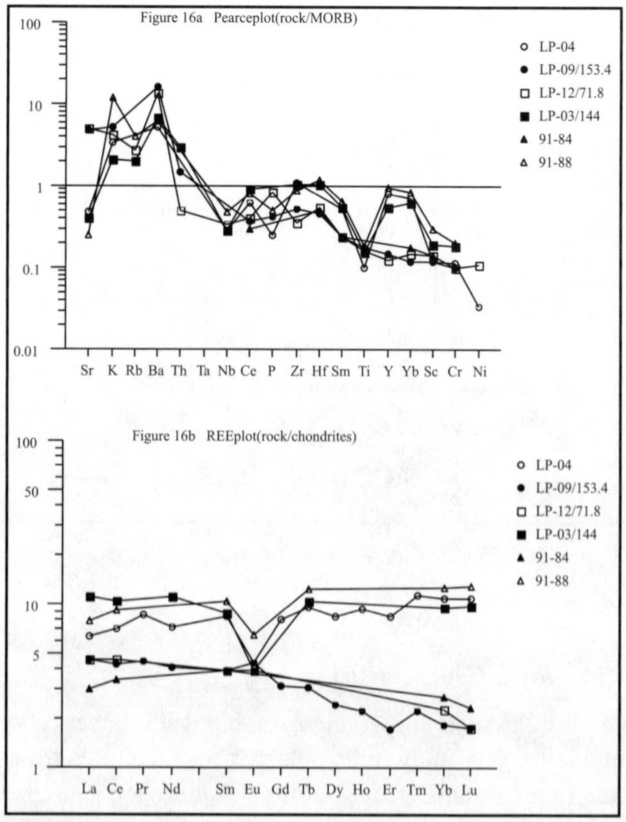

Figure 16(a). Multi-element plots (Pearce, 1983) normalized to N-type MORB of meta-felsic rocks from Loma Pesada. 16(b). REE plots normalized to chondrite of meta-felsic rocks from Loma Pesada. See text for explanation of samples.

patterns more typical of calc-alkaline series rocks. Their trace element patterns differ significantly from those of the felsic tuffs. These felsic porphyry intrusives found in the Loma Pesada area are probably related to the dioritic bodies that also intrude the eastern part of the Maimon Formation.

Hydrothermal Alteration

Chlorite and epidote are the most prominent alteration minerals at Loma Pesada. Epidote is a common mineral phase in both footwall and hangingwall rocks. This is in contrast to Cerro de Maimon where epidote is confined mainly to the hangingwall rocks. Epidote occurs in most rocks as small grains about 200 microns intergrown with the quartz-felspar matrix as an integral part of the rock. Granular epidote is often highly concentrated and gives the rock a greyish appearance in contrast to the dark greenish black of the chlorite-rich rocks. The epidote also concentrates in bands or layers parallel to the foliation.

Aggregates or clots of epidote vary from 1-2 mm to 3 cm across. Epidote, quartz, chlorite and/or calcite are commonly associated. Much of the deposition and distribution of epidote is probably the result of hydrothermal activity related to the initial magmatism. On the other hand, most of the granular epidote developed in the matrix of the rocks is probably the result of metamorphic recrystallization.

Sericite-quartz-pyrite alteration at Loma Pesado is clearly hydrothermal in origin and directly related to the massive and disseminated pyrite. Examples of this type of alteration are seen in LP-09 (231-248 m) and in the footwall to LP-10 (Figs. 13a and b). However, unlike Cerro de Maimon, sericitic and hydrothermal silica alteration is not pervasive through either footwall or hangingwall rocks at Loma Pesada. Traces of sericite can be found in most rocks, however, and stringers of sericite are ubiquitous in the felsic tuffs. Sericite appears to be more concentrated in the weathered mafic rocks as observed in the upper 30 m of the drill core. This is probably due to preferential leaching of the other mineral components during weathering.

Thin bands, 1-2 cm thick, of oxidized pyrite are found at the contact between layers of contrasting lithology.

Although the general nature of the alteration associated with the mineralization at Loma Pesada is understood, no quantitative study of the chemical trends has been made. The data indicate very little mobilization of silica, potassium or sodium although calcium has probably been depleted to some degree and redeposited during the epidotization process. Because all the rocks in the immediate area of Loma Pesada have been metamorphosed and/or hydrothermally altered, it is difficult to select any precursors.

Massive Sulphides

The discovery of the Loma Pesada massive sulphide deposit by Corporación Minera Dominicana in 1990 was based on EM37 geophysics, geochemistry and detailed field mapping. The massive sulphide body consists of a 4 to 15 m thick wedge shaped layer, dipping approximately 45° to the southwest and extending about 200 m along strike. The deposit is still open to the southeast.

The total massive sulphide as outlined to date amounts to about 3 million metric tons mainly of massive pyrite but with up to about 6 % chalcopyrite and less than 5 % sphalerite. It is estimated that within the deposit there are 1.1 million metric tons containing 2.13 % Cu, 0.77 % Zn, 41.6 ppm Pb, 4.37 g/t Ag and 0.16 g/t Au. No intersection was found in the four holes drilled in 1995 to test the extension of the body to the southeast. A geophysical anomaly located 250 m to the northeast, similar to the anomaly associated with the deposit, has yet to be tested.

Features of the zonation of mineralization are illustrated in the two examples of cross sections through six drill holes shown in Figures 13a and 13b. In several intersections Cu, Au and Ag tend to be concentrated with very fine-grained massive pyrite that encloses a coarser-grained barren pyrite zone (e.g., LP-04 in Fig. 13a). In this section, the contact of the massive sulphide with mafic rock is sharp at both the hangingwall and the footwall.

The second section (Fig. 13b) shows the massive sulphide with a thickness of 3.80 m as in LP-12 but thins to 0.25 m in LP-16. The thicker part of the massive sulphide grades down-dip into pyrite bands and disseminated pyrite in a quartz-sericite matrix (LP-13). The footwall to the thicker part of the massive sulphide as seen in LP-12 is a fine-grained chlorite-rich mafic rock (tuff) that grades rapidly into disseminated pyrite in a quartz-sericite matrix. This suggests that precipitation of base metal sulphides and precious metals is related to a certain level of quartz-sericite hydrothermal alteration.

Oxygen Isotopes

Oxygen isotope measurements were made on eight samples taken from four drill cores through the Loma Pesada deposit (Table 3). The mineralogy of the samples analyzed is given in Table 4. Histograms of these data are shown in Figure 17. The two samples of mafic hangingwall rocks from LP-05 gave values of 1.4 and 4.7‰, the lowest values recorded for all Maimon samples so far measured. The five samples taken from the immediate footwall to the massive sulphide, all of which showed some evidence of hydrothermal alteration, gave $\delta^{18}O$ values ranging from 5.5 to 8.3‰. These values are considerably lower than those from the footwall rocks at Cerro de Maimon and reflect the low amount of hydrothermal silica in the Loma Pesada footwall rocks. Sample LP-10/149.4 is a felsic rock with 8.3 ‰. This corresponds to the average value of 8.7‰ given by four quartz separates. Note that these values are considerably lower than those given by the Cerro de Maimon samples with dominant hydrothermal quartz.

Calculation for the quartz-sericite mineral pair at Loma Pesada gave a temperature of $\delta^{18}O$ of 118°C and $\delta^{18}O$ of -9.6‰ for the ore bearing fluid. These low numbers can be explained by assuming a subaerial environment and the long-lived presence of meteoric water later in the system that might have shifted original $\delta^{18}O$ values for the mineralizing hydrother-

Table 3. Oxygen Isotope Compositions of Footwall and hangingwall rocks for Loma Pesada and Loma Barbuito.

Sample #		$\delta^{18}O$(‰)	Locality
LP-04-163.9	WR	5.5	FW
LP-05-120.4	WR	1.4	HW
LP-05-123.5	WR	4.7	HW
LP-07-125.4	WR	7.1	FW
LP-10-141.5	WR	7.1	FW
LP-10-141.9	WR	6.1	FW
LP-10-144.5	WR	6.7	FW
LP-10-149.4	WR	8.3	FW
LB-16-54.4	WR	9.5	HW
LB-16-77.3	WR	13.4	FW
LB-16-82.9	WR	11.4	FW
LB-16-104.6	WR	9.9	FW
LB-18-72.4	WR	13.2	FW
LB-18-85.9	WR	9.8	FW

LP = Loma Pesada; LB = Loma Barbuito;
WR = whole rock; FW = footwall; HW = hangingwall

mal fluid.

Loma Barbuito

The Loma Barbuito deposit is located 2 km southeast of the town of Hatillo along the northern margin of the Maimon belt. Figure 18 is a geological map of the Loma Barbuito area and Figures 19a and 19b are cross sections based on drill cores.

Host Rocks

The dominant rock type at Loma Barbuito is a sequence of intermediate to felsic volcanics dipping at about 30º to the southwest. These rocks are dacitic to rhyolitic (keratophyres and quartz keratophyres) flows, crystal-lithic tuffs, lapilli tuffs and breccias. In the upper 140 m, intermediate and mafic flows and tuffs are intercalated with the felsic volcanics (Fig. 19). Below this is a section consisting of more than 120 m in which a pale greenish felsic lapilli tuff is the most dominant rock. The massive and disseminated sulphides are contained within this felsic volcaniclastic unit. The host rocks to the mineralization are strongly altered to quartz-sericite-pyrite and the original textures are destroyed. The hydrothermally altered rocks are exposed at the surface over an area of about 16,000 m and the area is covered by numerous blocks of gossans (Fig.18).

Host rock geochemistry

Major and trace element analyses of examples of least altered samples of the main lithologies at Loma Barbuito are given in Table 1. As mentioned previously the mafic rocks are characterized by relatively high TiO_2. Figures 20a and b are multi-element and REE plots of two basaltic rocks and one andesitic rock. Note that the basaltic rocks both show depletion in the LREEs and the patterns resemble those of the basalts from Loma Pesada (Fig 15). The andesitic rock has an enriched flat pattern.

Complete trace element data are available for two of the volcaniclastic felsic rocks. These data are plotted on Fig. 21a and 21b together with the andesitic rock (LP-237) and a quartz-plagioclase felsic tuff from Loma Pesada (LP-04) for comparison. The concentration levels of the REEs in the two felsic volcaniclastic rocks are similar but not identical. The concentrations of HREE are lower in the Barbuito samples compared with Loma Pesada. The strong negative Eu anomaly in the Loma Pesada sample is absent from the Loma Barbuito samples since the alteration has largely destroyed the plagioclase in the Loma Barbuito rocks, Chlorite is a minor component of the alteration.

Hydrothermal Alteration

The mafic, intermediate and felsic rocks in the hangingwall are little altered, although, in places they show evidence of shear. Relict pyroxene phenocrysts are present in some of the basaltic rocks. The plagioclase is albitized and chlorite, epidote and some hydrothermal silica are the main alteration minerals. Veins and stringers of quartz, calcite and sericite are common.

Rocks in the ore zone and footwall rocks are moderately to strongly altered to quartz-sericite-pyrite. Plagioclase phenocrysts are replaced by sericite and the matrix is filled with hydrothermal silica. The alteration style is similar to that at Cerro de Maimon, but at Loma Barbuito the original rocks were intermediate to felsic rather than mafic.

Table 4. Mineralogy of rock samples analyzed for $\delta^{18}O$.

LP-05/120.4 (HW)	Quartz 40-45%; Chlorite 25-30%; Epidote 23-25%; Sericite 2-3%; Plagioclase <1%
LP-05/123.5 (HW)	Epidote 55-66%; Quartz 20-24%; Plagioclase 8-10%; Chlorite 5%; Calcite 2-3%
LP-10/141.6 (ore zone/FW)	Quartz (fine-grained and fringes) 35-40%; Sericite 45 50%; Sulphides10-15%; Chlorite<1%
LP-10/141.9 (FW)	Epidote 55-60%; Quartz 20-24%; Plagioclase 8-10%; Chlorite 5%; Calcite 2-3%
LB-10/149.4 (FW)	Quartz 90%; Sericite 5%; Chlorite 1-2%; Epidote 1-2%; Albite 1%
LB-16/54.4 (HW)	Quartz 50%; Epidote 24%; Chlorite 24%; Calcite 2-3%
LB-16/77.3 (ore zone/FW)	Quartz+Feldspar (?Albite) 63-68%; Sericite15-20%; Sulphide 8-12%
LB-16/82.9 (ore zone/FW)	Quartz 80%; Sericite 14-16%; Sulphides 4-6%
LB-16/104.6(ore zone/FW)	Quartz-60%; Sericite 35%; Sulphides 5%
LB-18/72.4 (ore zone/FW)	Quartz 70-75%; Sericite 15-20%; Plagioclase 2-3%; Suphides 4-5%
LB-18/85.9 (altered FW)	Sericite 55-60%; Quartz Vein 35-40%; Quartz Phenocryst 2-3%; Epidote 1-2%

LP=Loma Pesada; LB=Loma Barbuito;
WR=whole rock; FW=footwall; HW=hangingwall

Massive and Disseminated Sulphides

The Barbuito prospect was identified as an important target by Rosario Domincana early in their exploration of the Maimon Concession. Drilling in the early 1980's resulted in nine intersections. The mineralization consists of massive to disseminated sulphide with a maximum thickness of about 20 m. The sulphide lens strikes at 160° and is at least 120m long. It dips approximately 30° to the SW with a gentle plunge to the south. The best intersection consisted of 6 m of massive sulphide containing 4.45 % Cu and 3 % Zn. The range in values were as follows: Cu: 0.24-4.45 %; Zn: 0.29 - 3.78 %; Ag: 3.2 - 108.5 g/t; Au: 0.3 - 2.7 g/t. Lead analyses were unsatisfactory but values determined on massive sulphides were consistently less than 1000 ppm. Falcondo drilled three holes in 1995 to test the extension of the mineralization to the east but obtained only one significant intersection with massive sulphide.

Oxygen Isotopes

Five samples of footwall rocks and one sample from the hangingwall from two drill cores LB-16 and LB-18 from Loma Barbuito were analyzed for oxygen isotopes (Table 3). The mineralogy of the samples analyzed is given in Table 4. Histograms of these data are shown in Figure 17. The high $\delta^{18}O$ values of 8.9 to 13.6‰ for the footwall rocks are comparable to those from the footwall at Cerro de Maimon. This is as expected because the type of alteration is similar.

A temperature of 152°C and of $\delta^{18}O$ of -32.4‰ for the mineralizing fluids was calculated for the mineral pair in sample LB-16/77.3, whereas 352°C and $\delta^{18}O$ of 5.5‰ was calculated for a mineral pair in sample LB-16/106.5. The difference in temperature and $\delta^{18}O$ of the fluids can be explained by the nature and position of the samples. The samples are from the same drill core but are separated by 29 m. Sample LB-16/106.5 lies immediately below the copper sulphide mineralization at 106 m whereas there is only semi-massive pyrite without copper values at 77 m the locality of LB-16-77.3. It can be implied therefore that a more isotopically enriched/evolved fluid at a temperature capable of carrying copper in solution (300 - 350°C) was responsible for copper mineralization around 106 m below surface. An isotopically depleted fluid at lower temperatures failed to do so higher up in the stratigraphic section due to the dominance of seawater fluid at a higher water/rock ratio.

San Antonio and other prospects

Massive sulphide lenses have been located in the San Antonio area south of Yamasa along the south-

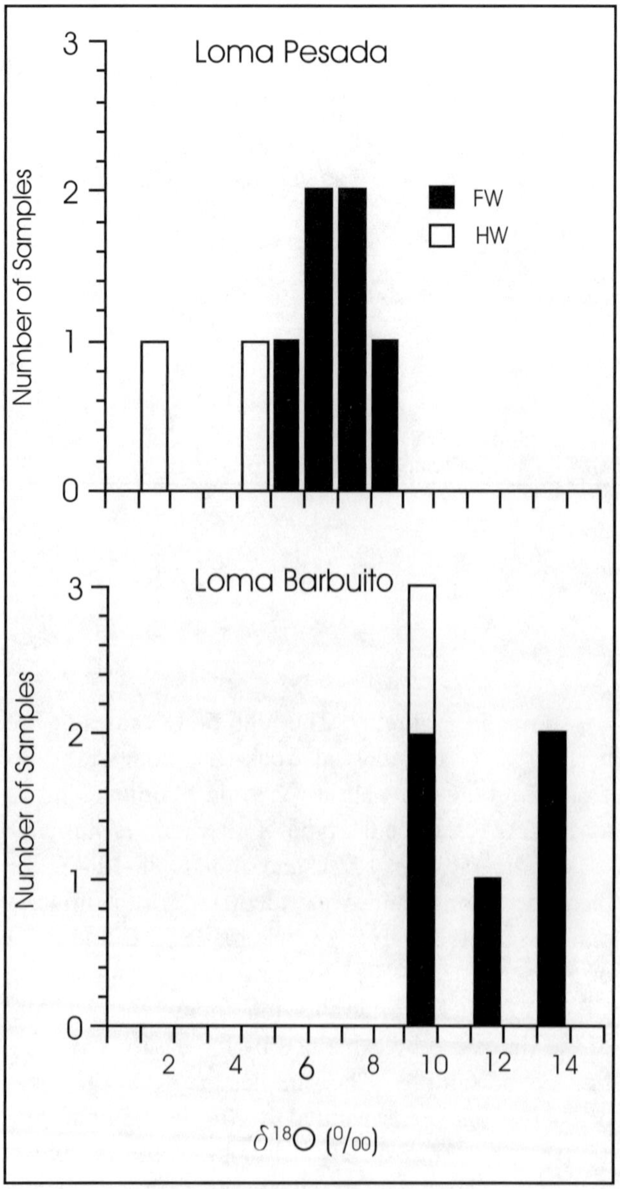

Figure 17. Histogram showing the distribution of whole rock $\delta^{18}O$ values for rocks from the Loma Pesada and Loma Barbuito deposits

eastern margin of the Maimon belt (Fig. 2). The geology of the area and details of the two massive sulphide bodies that have been drilled are discussed by Holbeck and Danbeny (2000 this volume).

The copper zinc massive sulphide body is thin but appears to occur over a wide area and in this and other respects the San Antonio deposits differs from the other Maimon deposits as the mineralization is mainly zinc-rich. The sulphides are laminated with zinc- and copper-rich bands and sulphide lenses are zoned from a pyrite-chalcopyrite base to a more zinc-rich top. Semi massive to massive barite occurs at San Antonio, a feature not reported from elsewhere in the Maimon Formation. Moderately extensive quartz-sericite-pyrite alteration is associated with the mineralization.

Notes on the geology and prospects at El Altar, Loma La Mina and Los Hojanchos

These three areas along the northern margin of the Maimon belt (Fig. 2) close to the Hatillo thrust, all show significant evidence at the surface of mineralization at depth. Limited amounts of drilling have been carried out in these three areas. The rocks in the three areas are little deformed for the most part except for local shearing. A feature common to all three areas, particularly at Los Hojanchos and Loma La Mina is the extent of the alteration at the surface. We consider that much of this near surface alteration is a secondary feature resulting from fracturing and mobilization of hydrothermal fluids related to the Hatillo thrust event. In several areas hydrothermal alteration is found to be directly associated with the Hatillo thrust but without signs of mineralization.

Sulphide mineralization, but with low base and precious metal values, has been intersected by drilling in all three areas. Evidence for massive sulphides in the form of massive pyrite was found at Loma La Mina and Los Hojanchos. By analogy with the findings at Loma Pesada and Barbuito, it is apparent that the drilling so far at Loma La Mina and Los Hojanchos has intersected the pyrite-rich sections of the massive sulphide orebody. Childe (2000) suggests that the near-surface oxide hosted copper and gold mineralization at Loma La Mina was largely sourced by the weathering of a high-grade massive sulphide section. The same ideas are applicable to El Altar and Los Hojanchos.

Four holes were drilled at El Altar and at Arroyo Loita, to the northwest of the El Altar holes. The drilling was based on the occurrence of abundant gossan rock and geophysical surveys. Although disseminated sulphide along with sericitic alteration was found at El Altar this occurs along a zone of shear. Drilling at Arroyo Laito found disseminated pyrite in

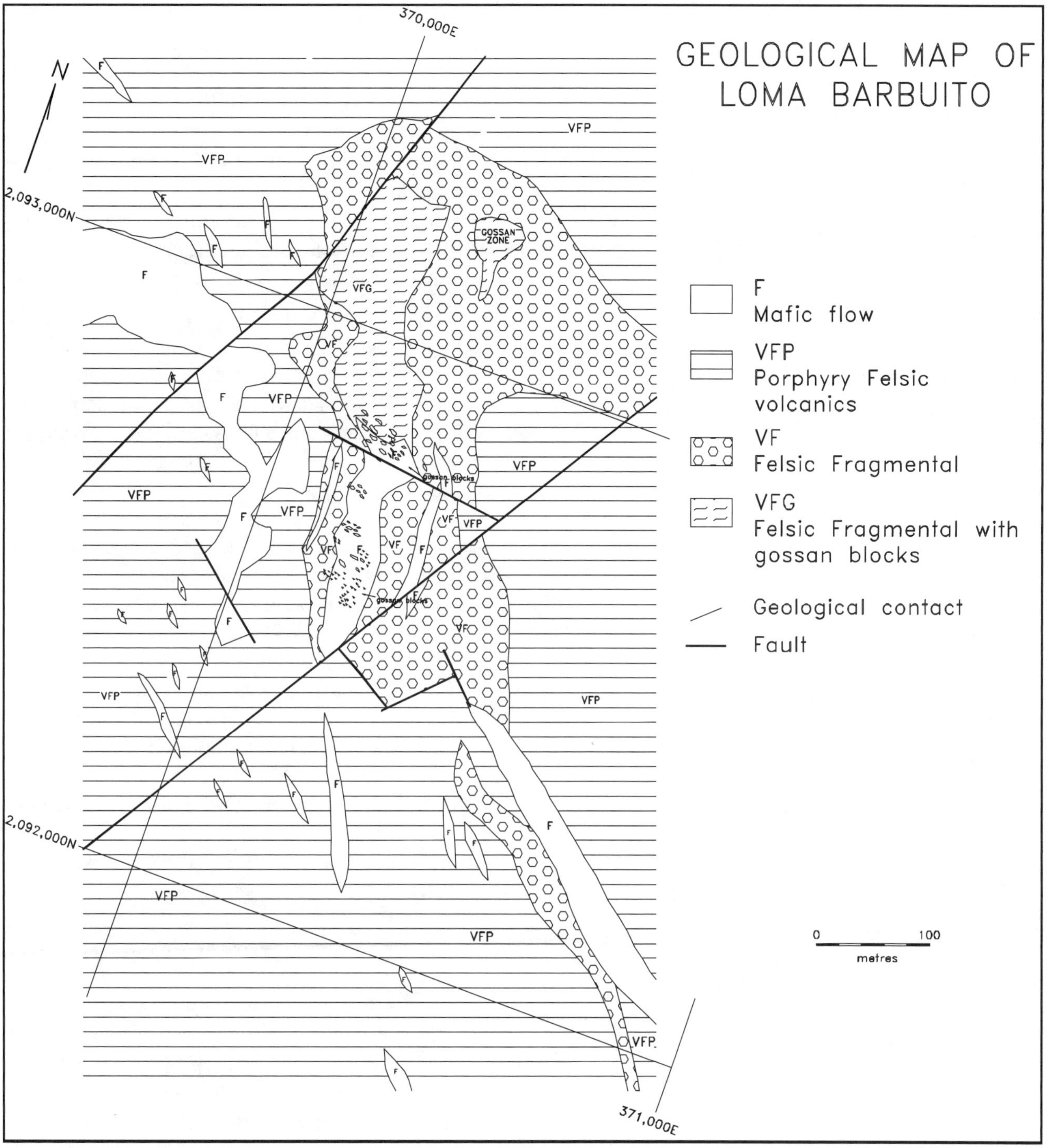

Figure 18. Geological map of the Loma Barbuito area.

carbonaceous shales. Thus the surface and near surface showings of mineralization in the El Altar area probably largely reflects weathering of primary sulphides as well as mobilized fluids related to later faulting

CONCLUSIONS

In an area like the Maimon Formation where hydrothermal alteration, metamorphism, deformation and weathering have largely obliterated the original

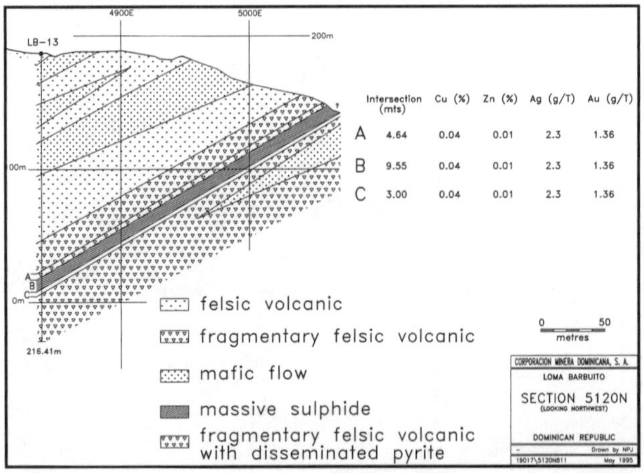

Figure 19(a). Cross sections through drill core LB-13 at Loma Barbuito.

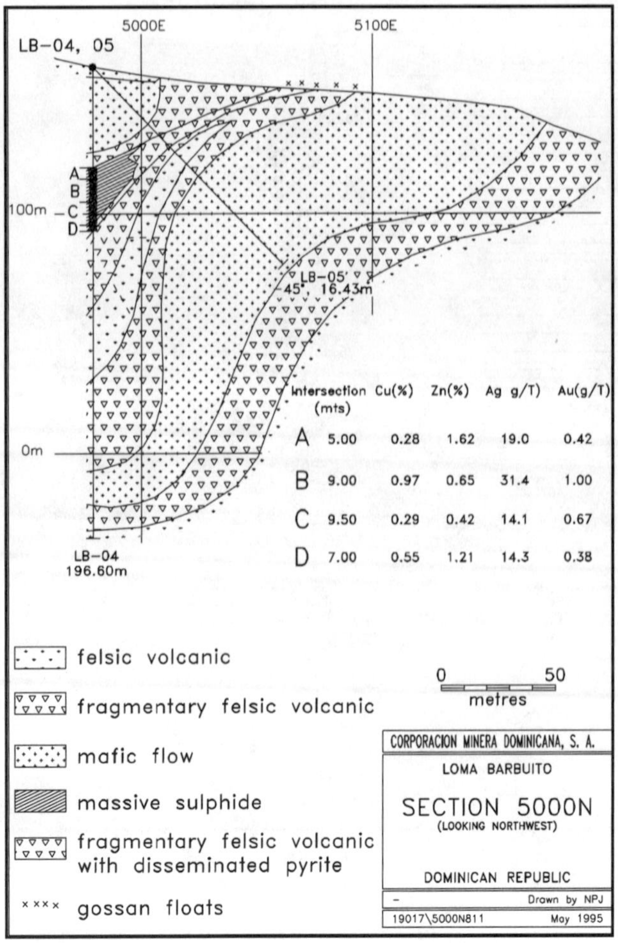

Figure 19 (b). Cross sections through drill cores LB-04 and LB-05 at Loma Babuito

chemistry and textural features of the rocks, it is difficult to determine the original nature of the rocks. Using petrographic and lithogeochemical techniques, combined with an oxygen isotope study it has been possible to determine the primary geochemical signatures in the rocks and obtain an understanding of the alteration trends.

As a result of these studies the following conclusions are made concerning the massive sulphide deposits and associated host rocks in the Maimon Formation.

(1) Although definite flow rocks have been identified, most of the sequence appears to be composed of volcaniclastic rocks. Compositional layering and laminations in the metamorphosed rocks are interpreted to represent relict bedding. The presence of pillow basalts, fossil-bearing limestones, cherts, carbonaceous shales and exhalites indicates that most, if not all, the sequence is submarine in origin.

(2) Although the analyzed rocks show a continuous range in chemical composition from basaltic to rhyolitic, the petrographic and chemical data indicate the primary magmatism is bimodal. Based on the composition of selected least altered rock samples, principally those from the Loma Pesada section, the rocks of the Maimon Formation consist of a spilite-keratophyre association.

(3) The Maimon Formation VMS deposits, as a whole, are best classified as the Zn + Cu-type with Cu:Zn~2:1 (Solomon, 1976; Franklin et al., 1981) but the pyrite-rich Loma Pesada body is the Cu-type.

(4) Although there is variation in the Cu:Zn ratio through the larger Cerro de Maimon massive sulphide body, zoning of metals is not observed in this deposit. At Loma Pesada fine-grained pyrite-chalcopyrite encloses a thick lens of coarse pyrite. At San Antonio sulphide lenses are zoned from pyrite-chalcopyrite at the base to a sphalerite-rich top (Holbeck and Danbeny, 2000, this volume).

(5) In terms of tonnage the Maimon deposits are small (1-3.5 million tons) compared with many other VMS deposits but the grade is higher than the mean grade of many deposits of the same

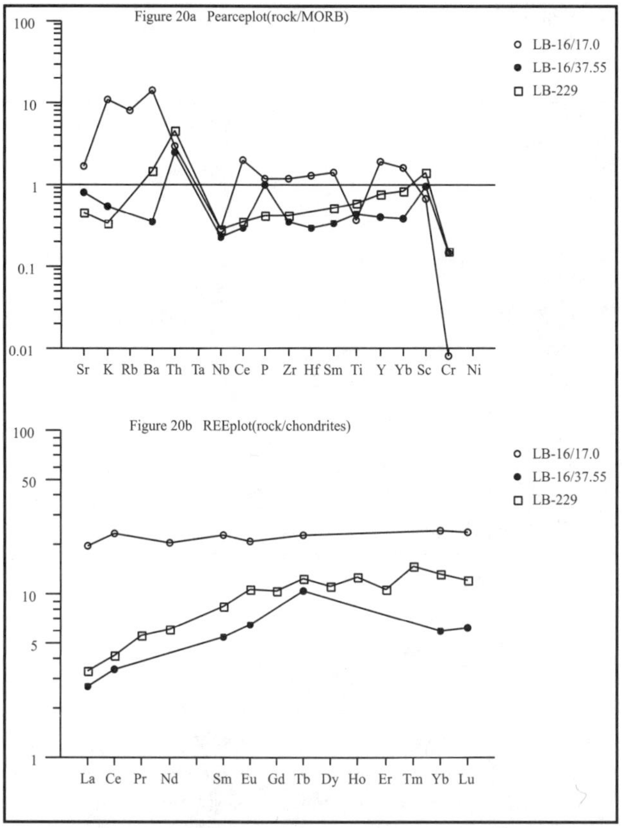

Figure 20(a). Multi-element plots (Pearce, 1983) normalized to N-type MORB of meta-mafic and intermediate rocks (LB-16/17.0) from Loma Barbuito.
Figure 20(b). REE plots normalized to chondrite of meta-mafic and intermediate rocks from Loma Barbuito.

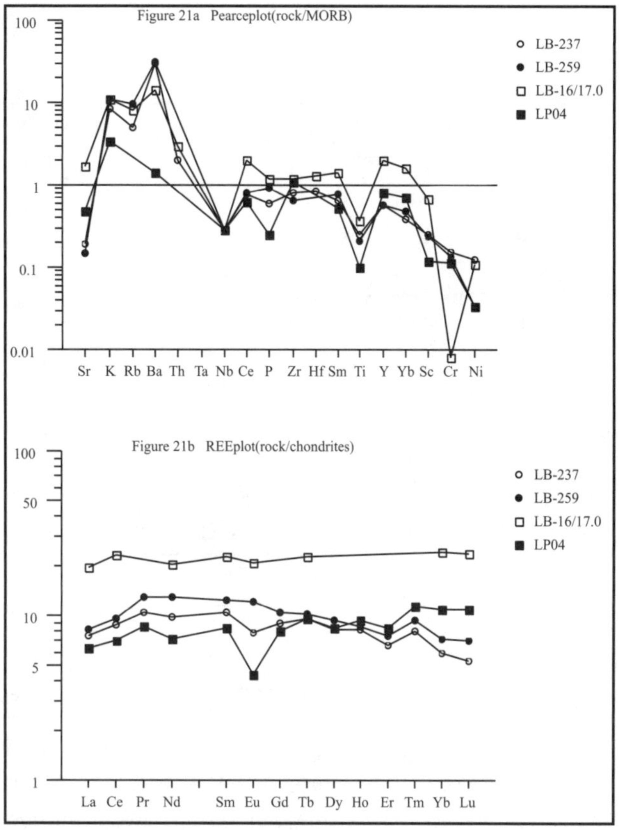

Figure 21(a). Multi-element plots (Pearce, 1983) normalized to N-type MORB of meta-felsic rocks from Loma Barbuito.
Figure 21(b). REE plots normalized to chondrite of meta-felsic rocks from Loma Barbuito. LB-16/17.0 is an andesite for comparison. LP04 is from Loma Pesada.

size (Table 2 in Large, 1992). The average grade for gold in the Cerro de Maimon deposit is 0.69 g/t. Thin lenses show Au values up to 16 g/t at San Antonio.

(6) Although the complete dimensions and shape of the massive sulphide bodies has not been sufficiently investigated all the bodies are stratiform lenses with a low aspect ratio as can be seen in the cross sections. It is possible that thin sheet-like bodies may extend over several hundreds of metres at San Antonio.

(7) Sodium and calcium depletion is a significant factor in the alteration to the footwall of the Maimon VMS deposits. Potassium and silica are usually added with the growth of sericite and quartz. The highest values for the alteration index $(MgO+K_2O)/(Na_2O+CaO+MgO+K_2O)$ are in the footwall rocks (Ishikawa et al., 1976).

(8) The high $\delta^{18}O$ values varying from 8.1 to 13.4‰ found in the footwall rocks at Cerro de Maimon and Loma Barbuito are considered to be directly related to the introduction of hydrothermal silica into the system along with an enriched $\delta^{18}O$ for the ore-forming fluids.

(9) The VMS deposits in the Maimon Formation were formed in a nascent primitive island arc, probably in the forearc area.

ACKNOWLEDGEMENTS

Many geologists have contributed to our present knowledge of the VMS deposits in the Maimon Formation particularly the Cerro de Maimon deposit. These include G. McVeigh, R. Moore, J.J. Watkins, T. Watts (Falconbridge Limited.), G. Bloise, S. Brouwer,

Table 5. Oxygen Isotope Values of Mineral Separates for Loma Pesada and Loma Barbuito

Sample #	$\delta^{18}O$ (‰) - Quartz	$\delta^{18}O$ (‰) - Sericite	T (°C)	$\delta^{18}O$ (‰) - H_2O
LP-05-120.4	8.4			
LP-05-144.5	9.0			
LP-07-125.4	8.9	2.1	117.9	-9.6
LP-10-141.9	8.4			
LB-16-77.3	12.7	6.9	152.2	-2.4
LB-16-82.9	12.1			
LB-16-106.5	10.8	7.7	351.7	5.5
Qtz-H_2O	3.34(106/T2) - 3.31	Matsuhisa et al (1979)		
Ser-H_2O	2.38(106/T2) - 3.89	Friedman and O'Neil (1977)		

LP=Loma Pesada; LB=Loma Barbuito

C. Chaves, E. Reyes (Falconbridge Dominicana) and graduate students S. L. Horan and V. A. Astacio. Most of the analytical work presented here was funded through a National Science Foundation grant to Lewis and by Falconbridge Dominicana and Falconbridge Limited. The oxygen isotope study was funded by Falconbridge Limited through a grant to A. Campbell and V. A. Astacio at New Mexico Institute of Mining and Technology.

REFERENCES

Arculus, R. J., Gust, D., and Kushiro, I., 1991, The evolution of Fuji and Hakone volcanoes, Honshu, Japan, National Geographic Research and Exploration, 7, 276 -309.

Astacio, V. A., 1997, Mineralogy, lithogeochemistry, and oxygen isotope study of the Cerro de Maimon massive sulfide deposit, Dominican Republic. Unpublished M.S. thesis, New Mexico Institute of Mining and Technology, 100 pages.

Astacio, V. A., Lewis, J. F., Campbell, A, and Espaillat, J., 2000, Oxygen isotope and alteration geochemistry of the Cerro de Maimon massive sulfide deposit, Dominican Republic. In Caribbean Geology in the New Millenium. Edited by T. Jackson, Transactions 15th Caribbean Geological Conference, Kingston, Jamaica (in press).

Beard, J. S. and Lofgren, G.G., 1991, Dehydration melting and water-saturated melting of basaltic and andesitic greenstones and amphibolites at 1,3 and 6,9 Kb. Journal of Petrology, 32, 365-401.

Bloomer, S. H., Taylor, B., Macleod, C. J., Stern, R. J., Fryer, P., Hawkins, J. W., Johnson, L., 1995. Early arc volcanism and the ophiolite problem: A perspective from drilling in the western Pacific in Active Margins and Marginal Basins of the Western Pacific. Edited by B. Taylor and J. H. Natland, American Geophysical Union Monograph 88, p. 1-30.

Bowin, C.O., 1966, Geology of the Central Dominican Republic, in Hess, H. H., editor, Caribbean geological investigations: Geological Society of America Memoir 98,11-98.

Childe, C., 2000, Geology and tectonic setting of the volcanogenic massive sulfide mineralization in the Greater Antilles. In VMS deposits of Latin America. Edited by R. Sherlock and A. Logan. Geological Association of Canada Special Publication,

Cumming, G.L. and Kesler, S.E., 1987, Lead isotopic composition of the oldest volcanic rocks of the eastern Greater Antilles island arc: Chemical Geology, 65, 15-23.

Draper, G. and Lewis, J.F., 1982, Petrology, deformation, and tectonic significance of the Amina Schist, northern Dominican Republic, In Transactions of the 9th Caribbean Geological Conference, Santo Domingo, Dominican Republic, Amigo del Hogar Publishers, 53-64.

Draper, G. and Lewis, J.F., 1991 Metamorphic belts of central Hispaniola, In Geological and tectonic development of the North American-Caribbean plate boundary in Hispaniola, Edited by P. Mann, G. Draper, and J. F. Lewis, Geological.. Society America, Special Paper 262, 29-45

Draper, G., GutiÈrrez, G. and Lewis, J.F., 1996, Thrust emplacement of the Hispaniola peridotite belt: Orogenic expression of the mid-Cretaceous Caribbean arc polarity reversal? Geology, 24, 1143-46.

Donnelly, T.W. and Rogers, J.J.W., 1978, The distribution of igneous rock suites throughout the Caribbean: Geologic en

Mijnbouw, 52, 151-162.

Franklin, J.M., Sangster, D.F. and Lyndon, J.W., 1981, Volcanic-associated massive sulfide deposits, Economic Geology, 75th Anniversary volume, 485-627.

Friedman, I., and O'Neil, J.R., 1977. Compilation of stable isotope fractionation factors of geochemical interest; in Data of Geochemistry, Sixth Edition, Edited by M. Fleisher. U.S. Geological Survey Professional Paper 440-KK, KK1-KK12.

Holbeck, P.M. and Danbery, P.H., 2000, Geology of the San Antonio Concession, Dominican Republic, In VMS Deposits of Latin America. Edited by R. Sherlock and A. Logan, Geological Association of Canada Special Publication.

Horan, S.L., 1995, The geochemistry and tectonic significance of the Maimon-Amina schists, Cordillera Central, Dominican Republic, Unpublished M.S. thesis, University of Florida, Gainesville, 172 pages.

Ishikawa, Y., Sawaguchi, T., Iwaya, S., and Horiuchi, M., 1976, Delineation of prospecting targets for Kuroko deposits based on modes of volcanism of underlying dacite and alteration haloes, Mining Geology, 26, 105-117 (in Japanese with English abstract).

Kesler, S., Russell E., N., Reyes, C., Santos, L., Rodriguez, A. and Fondeur, L., 1991, Geology of the Maimon Formation, Dominican Republic, In Geologic and tectonic development of the North American - Caribbean plate boundary in Hispaniola, Edited by P. Mann,, G. Draper, and J. F. Lewis,, Geological Society of America Special Paper 262, 173-185.

Large, R. R., 1992, Australian volcanic-hosted massive sulfide deposits, Features, styles, and genetic models, Economic Geology, 97, 471 - 510.

Lewis, J.F. and Draper, G., 1990 Geology and tectonic evolution of the northern Caribbean margin, In The Caribbean region, Edited by G. Dengo, and J. E. Case, Boulder, Colorado, Geological Society of America, The Geology of North America, H, 77-140.

Lewis, J.F., Perfit, M., Horan, S. and Diaz de Villavilla, L., 1995, Geochemistry and petrotectonic significance of early arc bimodal volcanism in the Greater Antilles arc, Abstracts with Programs, Annual Meeting Geological Society of America, New Orleans, A227.

Lewis, J. F., Astacio, T., and Espaillat, J., 1998, The Maimon Formation, in Mineral Deposits of the Dominican Republic. Edited by P.G Fiess, The Society of Economic Geologists, March 1998 Field Trip, Dominican Republic.

MacLean, W.H. and Barrett, T.J., 1993, Lithogeochemical techniques using immobile elements, Journal of Geochemical Exploration, 48, 109-133.

Mann, P., Draper, G. and Lewis, J.F., 1991, An overview of the geologic and tectonic evolution of Hispaniola. In Geological and tectonic development of the North American - Caribbean plate boundary in Hispaniola. Edited by P. Mann. G. Draper.and J.F.Lewis, Geological Society of America Special Paper 262, 1-28.

Matsuhisa, Y., Goldsmith, J.R. and Clayton, R.N., 1979. Oxygen isotopic fractionation in the system quartz-albite-anorthite-water, Geochemica et Cosmochimica Acta, 43, 1131-1140.

Pearce, J. A., 1983, Role of the subcontinental lithosphere in magma genesis at active continental margins. In Continental Basins and Mantle Xenoliths, Edited by C. J. Hawkesworth and M. J. Norry, Nantwich, Shiva, 230 - 249.

Pearce, J. A. and 7 others, 1992, Boninite and harzburgite from Leg 125 (Bonin-Mariana Fore-arc): A case study of magma genesis during the initial stages of subduction. In P. Fryer, Pearce, J. A., Stocking, L.B., et al., Proceedings Ocean Drilling Program, Scientific Results, 125, College Station, TX , 623-659.

Rodríguez Demorizi, E., 1965. Riqueza Mineria y Agricola de Santo Domingo. Academia Dominicana de la Historia. XX, Editores del Caribe C. por A.

Rosario Dominicana, S.A., 1985, Exploration Project in the Maimon Formation, Dominican Republic, Santo Domingo, Rosario Dominicana, S.A., 184 pages.

Solomon, M., 1976, "Volcanic" massive sulfide deposits and their host rocks — a reveiw and an explanation. In Handbook of strata-bound and stratiform ore deposits, II, Regional studies and specific deposits,.Edited by Wolf, K. A., Amsterdam, Elsevier, 21 - 50.

Watkins, J., 1990, Geologic Setting of the Cerro de Maimon Deposit, Dominican Republic, Geologic Report for Falconbridge Dominicana, C. por A., Santo Domingo, 43 pages.

VOLCANOGENIC MASSIVE SULPHIDE DEPOSITS OF CUBA

NORMAN RUSSELL
CaribGold Mines Inc., 1ra. Avenida No. 1410, Apto. 6, e/14 y 16, Miramar, Ciudad de La Habana, CP 11300, Cuba

JESÚS MOREIRA AND ROBERTO SÁNCHEZ
Instituto de Geología y Paleontología, Vía Blanca, San Miguel de Padrón, Ciudad de La Habana, CP 11000, Cuba

ABSTRACT

Although Cuba is rich in natural resources, there are few widely available reviews of Cuban mineral deposits. In this review we describe the tectonic setting of Cuban volcanogenic massive sulphide deposits and group them into the conventional Cyprus, Kuroko and Besshi classification.

The geological history of Cuba began with the breakup of Pangea and the formation of oceanic crust in Jurassic time. The Greater Antilles island arc was created when subduction began in Lower Cretaceous time and continued until mid-Eocene, when the Cuban portion of the arc collided with, and was attached to, the North American Plate.

The collision created three main tectonic belts. On the north side of Cuba, carbonate facies of the Bahamas Platform dominate. These are overthrust by a dissected ophiolitic assemblage of serpentinite, tholeiitic basalt and marine sedimentary rocks. In western Cuba, Cyprus type deposits occur in tholeiitic basalts and serpentinites of the ophiolite complex.

The Cuban ophiolites are in turn overthrust by volcanic rocks of the Cretaceous island arc. Kuroko type, or arc-related, massive sulphide deposits occur in the lower part of the arc. The host rocks are a Primitive Island Arc suite that has been described from other Greater Antilles islands. No Kuroko type deposit is known in the upper, calc-alkaline portion of the arc. The Paleogene arc, ocurring only in eastern Cuba, also hosts Kuroko type deposits, including El Cobre, the first copper mine discovered in the New World.

In western and central Cuba, blocks of metamorphosed volcanic and sedimentary rocks that are interpreted as fragments of the continental margin are host to volcanogenic massive sulphide deposits. In western Cuba massive sulphide deposits associated with intervals of basaltic to andesitic volcanism are considered to be Besshi type. In south-central Cuba the Escambray block of predominantly marble and schist, hosts deposits that are associated with ophiolitic assemblages in a major fault zone. They are described as tectonically emplaced Cyprus type deposits, although some Cuban geologists consider them to be Besshi type deposits similar to those in western Cuba.

Compared to other Greater Antilles islands, Cuba has a greater abundance of Cyprus and Besshi type deposits. The Besshi deposits are associated with Mesozoic continental fragments that are not preserved on other islands. Similarly, the collision of the Cuban portion of the Cretaceous arc with the Bahamas Platfom resulted in a greater proportion of outcropping ophiolitic rocks and associated Cyprus type deposits in Cuba.

INTRODUCTION

Cuba is the largest and most westerly island of the Greater Antilles. Although rich in natural resources and with a mining history dating back to the Spanish conquest, there have been few widely available reviews of Cuban mineral deposits. Kesler et al. (1990) included some Cuban deposits in their discussion of the metallogenic evolution of the Caribbean area but noted that the literature, then available, lacked the observations necessary to classify most deposits. Since then there has been a greater tendency by Cuban geologists to identify deposits by generally accepted types. In this review, with greater access to unpublished, or locally published work, we classify Cuban volcanogenic massive sulphide (VMS) deposits into the conventional types of Cyprus, Kuroko and Besshi and describe the geological setting of each group of deposits.

The base metal deposits of the Pinar del Rio region in western Cuba constitute the most important group economically. Individual deposits in this area, where previously described, have been classified as either sedimentary exhalative (SEDEX) or Besshi type (Kesler et al., 1996). Because of the loosely defined position of Besshi deposits in the spectrum from SEDEX to VMS deposits, we have included some of these deposits in this discussion, while acknowledging that they may lie outside some definitions of the VMS type. In the Escambray area in central Cuba the deposits are now recognized as volcanogenic massive sulphides, but there continues to be discussion among Cuban geologists as to whether they are of Cyprus or Besshi type.

Cuba is the most tectonically complex island of the Greater Antilles, due to its collision with, and attachment to, the North American Plate in Eocene time. Although the present geology is well understood (Fig. 1), there remain a number of unresolved problems related to the tectonic history of the Greater Antilles, in which the prevalent interpretation from one island conflicts with interpretations from another. The geological history of Cuba as described here, with emphasis on current local interpretation, is intended to provide a basic understanding of the origins of the various terranes in which the Cuban VMS deposits are located.

GEOLOGICAL SETTING

Tectonic Evolution of Cuba

Cuba is at the western end of the Greater Antilles island arc, which extends eastwards to the Virgin Islands. Volcanic rocks of similar ages and compositions have been described along the length of the arc and prior to the collision of Cuba with the Bahamas Platform in Eocene time, the islands of the Greater Antilles apparently shared a similar geologic history.

Caribbean geological history began with the break-up of Pangea and the creation of oceanic crust in Jurassic time (Fig. 2). Although the island arc assemblages formed mainly on a basement of ocean floor, fragments of continental crust as old as Proterozoic have been preserved in Cuba (Renne et al., 1989). Subduction began in Early Cretaceous time, creating the Greater Antilles arc, and continued to Middle Eocene, when a change in the tectonic regime of the area was brought about by collision of the arc with the Bahamas Platform. Initially the arc was aligned northwest-southeast and deformation was most intense at the western end of the arc, diminishing to the east. Thus, Cuba is the most severely deformed island of the Greater Antilles. Following

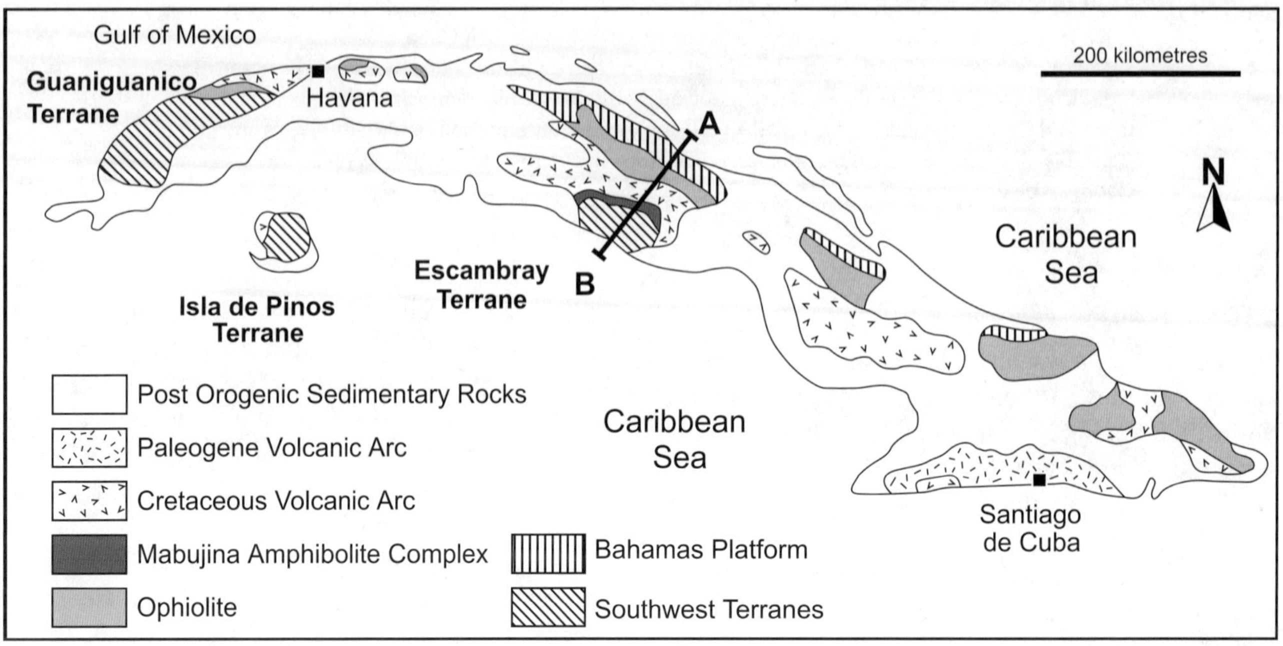

Figure 1. Generalized geologic map of Cuba. Modified from Lewis and Draper (1990) and Iturralde-Vinent (1994). See Figure 5 for section AB.

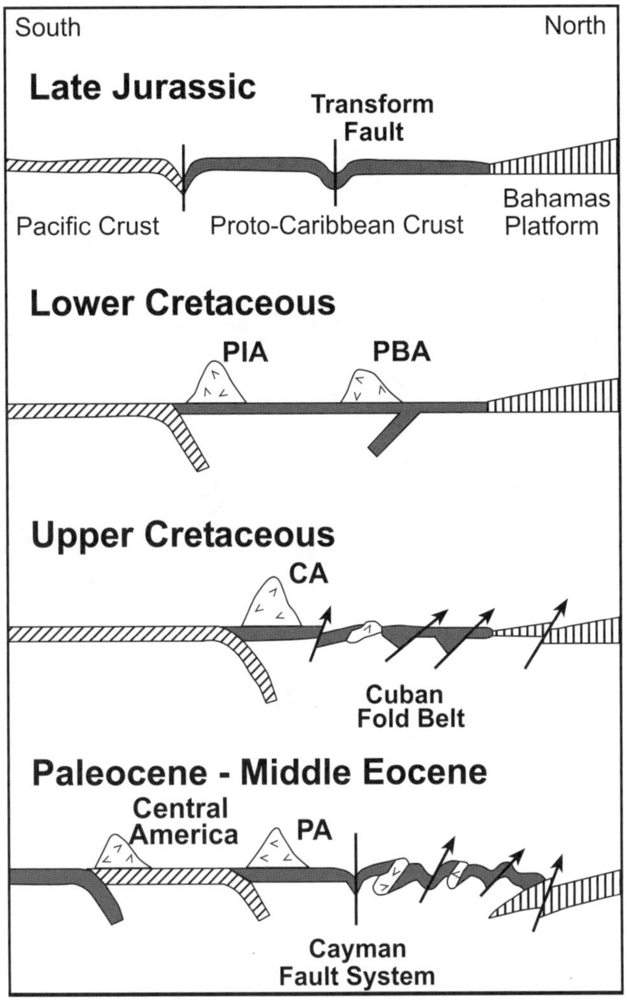

Figure 2. Cross sections showing the plate tectonic evolution of Cuba. Modified from Kerr et al. (1999). PIA – primitive island arc; PBA – primitive boninite arc; CA – calc-alkaline arc; PA – Paleogene arc.

collision, Cuba was attached to the North American Plate and has been essentially tectonically inactive, while the rest of the Greater Antilles remained part of the Caribbean Plate, with the plate boundary running parallel to the southeastern coast of Cuba as the Oriente, or Bartlett, strike-slip fault.

One of the major uncertainties in reconstructing the tectonic history of the Greater Antilles is the polarities of the Cretaceous and Paleogene volcanic arcs. Varied interpretations of Greater Antilles tectonic history postulate a south-facing arc on the North American Plate (Malfait and Dinkelman, 1972; Salvador and Green, 1980), a south-facing arc on Caribbean oceanic crust (Iturralde-Vinent, 1994; Kerr et al., 1999), a north-facing arc (White and Burke, 1980; Pindell and Dewey, 1982; Sykes et al., 1982; Coney, 1983) and an initially south-facing arc that changed to north-facing (Walper, 1980; Duncan and Hargraves, 1984; Pindell and Barrett, 1990). Pindell and Barrett (1990) provide a review of the previous interpretations and list the evidence for and against each. In a more recent discussion, Iturralde-Vinent (1994) proposed that geological relations in Cuba require a south-facing arc that developed on oceanic crust not far from its present position. Rosencrantz (1996) has interpreted the Camagüey Trench, a 6 km deep trench that dips northward beneath Cuba, as the remnant of a Cretaceous north-dipping subduction zone. Recent documentation of boninites in the ophiolitic rocks near Holguin in eastern Cuba (Kerr et al., 1999) suggests that a separate, short-lived primitive arc may have existed during Lower Cretaceous time (Fig. 2).

Iturralde-Vinent (1994) concludes that the Paleogene volcanic arc in eastern Cuba, which partly overlies the Cretaceous arc, was also south-facing, with subduction toward the north, citing the well preserved back-arc volcano-sedimentary stratigraphy on the north side of the volcanic arc. Although the subduction zone in the remainder of the Greater Antilles appears to have been in approximately the same position throughout the Cretaceous and Paleogene, volcanic activity and the arc complexes are superimposed and the subduction zone in the western Caribbean appears to have migrated to the south or southeast at the end of Cretaceous time (Fig. 2). This apparent relocation was accompanied by a change in arc orientation from northwest-southeast to east-west, although the reasons for the relocation have not been resolved (Iturralde-Vinent, 1994).

Cuban Geology

The present geology of Cuba was largely determined by the collision of the Cretaceous volcanic arc with the Bahamas Platform in Middle Eocene time. Northward-directed thrust faulting was most intense in western Cuba and diminished eastward. Three main geotectonic belts can be recognized, from north to south, parallel to the trend of the island: the carbonate and evaporite continental facies of the Bahamas

Platform, the Ophiolite Belt that is thrust over the Bahamas Platform rocks, and the Cretaceous-Paleogene island arcs that are in turn thrust over the ophiolites (Fig. 1, 5) (Iturralde-Vinent, 1996a). A fourth, fragmented belt, consists of three blocks of metamorphosed continental margin deposits: the Guaniguanico block at the western end of Cuba, the Isle of Youth (Pines) off the south coast, and the Escambray Massif on the south coast of central Cuba. Iturralde-Vinent (1994) has named them collectively as the Southwestern Cuban Terranes. VMS deposits occur in all belts, except the Bahamas Platform.

Following collision of Cuba with the Bahamas Platform and its attachment to the North American Plate, latest Eocene to Recent sedimentary rocks were deposited unconformably on the arc rocks and now represent about 60 % of the surface geology of the island (Fig 1).

Southwestern Cuban Terranes

The Southwestern Terranes have been largely ignored in most plate tectonic models. Iturralde-Vinent (1994) has proposed that they are parts of the Yucatan Block that became separated during intra-continental rifting in Late Jurassic time. Other authors consider them to be part of the Bahamas Platform (Khudoley and Meyerhoff, 1971). The largest block, Guaniguanico, at the western end of the island (Fig. 1), consists of low-grade metamorphosed siliclastic deposits of deltaic and shallow marine environments, overlain by conglomerates, sandstones, and limestones with intercalations of tholeiitic basalt. On the north side of the Guaniguanico block, the Cajálbana ophiolites consist mainly of tholeiitic pillow basalt with intercalated limestones, cherts, sandstones and rare serpentinites (Fig. 3). The geochemistry of the basalts is consistent with their formation during the rifting event between the Yucatan block and South America (Kerr et al., 1999). The terrane hosts a large number of massive sulphide deposits, most of which have been previously described as SEDEX, but some of which have been considered as Besshi-type (Simón Méndez, 1992; Kesler et al., 1996) (Fig. 3).

The Escambray massif contains high-pressure, low-temperature metamorphic rocks that include stratigraphic sections similar to the Guaniguanico block (Somin and Millán, 1981) and is interpreted by Iturralde-Vinent (1994) to be a fragment of the Yucatan block that was incorporated into the subduction zone beneath the Cretaceous volcanic arc. This interpretation is supported by Rosencrantz (1996), who interprets the contact between the metamorphosed Escambray Terrane and the Cretaceous arc rocks as the exposed westward continuation of the Camagüey Trench, although he notes that this interpretation assumes that the Escambray and Isle of Pines Terranes converged on the arc from the south, whereas the Guanicanico Terrane appears to have originated north of the arc. Massive sulphide deposits associated with ultramafic rocks are found in the Escambray Terrane (Fig. 4).

Ophiolite Belt

The main Cuban ophiolites crop out along almost the entire length of the island, on its north side. The outcrops cover an area of 1500 square kilometres and their total extent beneath the post-orogenic sediments could be over 15000 square kilometres (Lewis and Draper, 1990). They are disrupted, occurring as thrust slices and melanges with interspersed fault blocks of Cretaceous volcanic and sedimentary rocks. In spite of the deformation, all components of the ophiolite assemblage have been recognized in most localities. The age of the ophiolites is estimated, from their relations to other rocks, to be Jurassic to Early Cretaceous, (Iturralde-Vinent, 1996b) and although they appear to form a continuous belt, there are three distinct types of emplacement. Ophiolites west of Havana dip moderately to the north, are thrust over the Guaniguanico block, and are in turn overthrust by the Cretaceous volcanic arc. In contrast, the ophiolites of central Cuba dip steeply to the south, are thrust over rocks of the Bahamas Platform, and are themselves overthrust by the Cretaceous volcanic arc (Fig. 5). The ophiolites of both areas are considered to be derived from back-arc basins of a south-facing arc (Iturralde-Vinent, 1996b). In eastern Cuba the ophiolites are much less dismembered and form a large tabular, sub-horizontal thrust sheet from 800 to 1000 metres thick. They were thrust northward over metamorphosed and unmetamorphosed Cretaceous volcanic arc rocks and so are unlikely to have originated

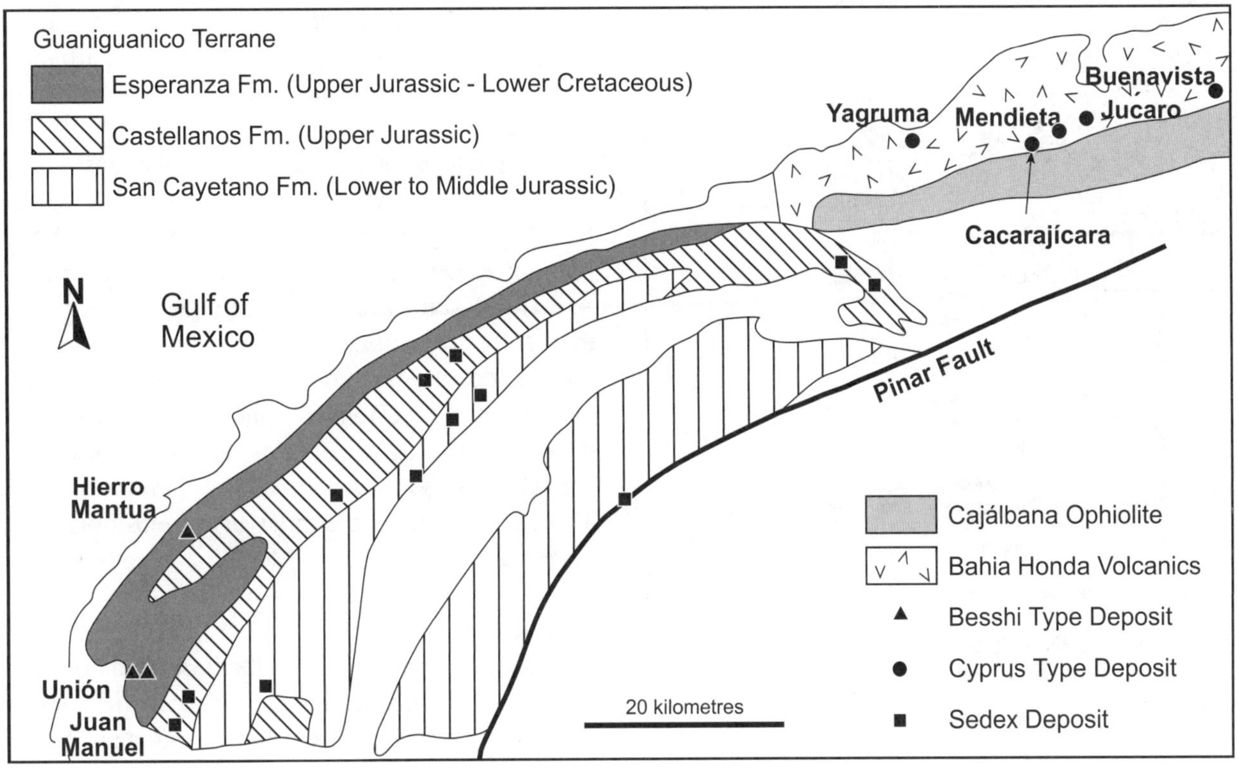

Figure 3. Geology and mineral deposits of western Cuba. Modified from Kesler et al. (1990) and Iturralde-Vinent (1996a).

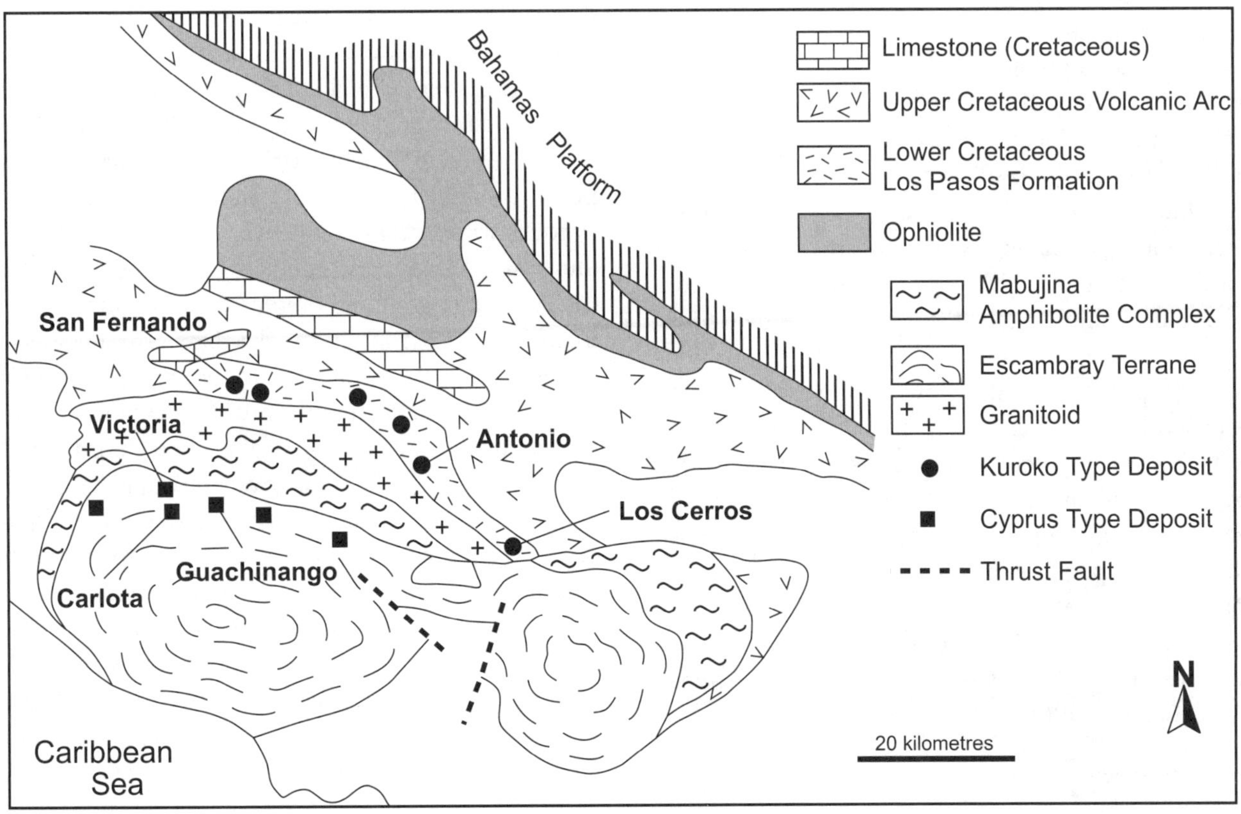

Figure 4. Geology and VMS deposits of central Cuba. Modified from Cabrera (1986).

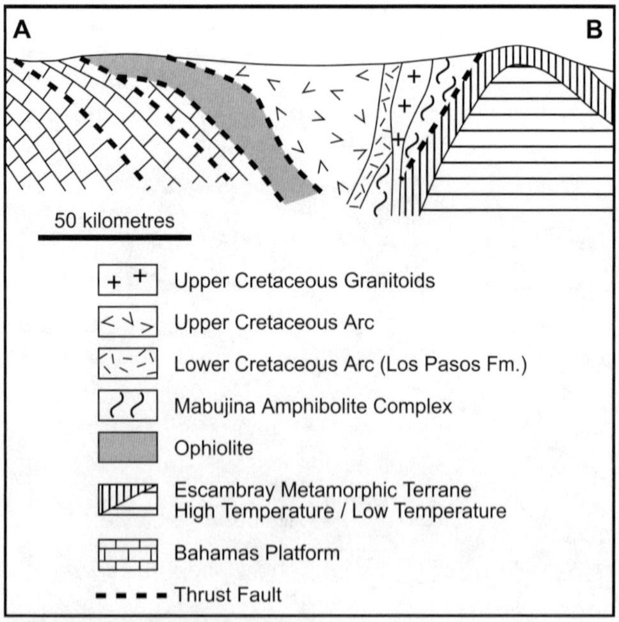

Figure 5. Generalized geological section through central Cuba. Modified from Iturralde-Vinent (1994). See Figure 1 for location.

in the back-arc basin. With their large area of exposure and tabular form, they are host to world-class nickel laterite deposits.

A distinct ophiolite-volcanic assemblage is the Mabujina amphibolite complex in central Cuba, on the south side of the Cretaceous arc (Fig. 4). It is in fault contact to the south with the Escambray metamorphic terrane and to the north with Lower Cretaceous volcanic rocks of the Los Pasos Formation. Somin and Millán (1976) originally considered the complex to be the oceanic basement to the Cretaceous arc, but more recently (1981) concluded that it is actually the lower part of the arc. Geochemical evidence (Kerr et al., 1999) also suggests that the amphibolites are derived from island arc tholeiites. Dublan et al. (1988) dated pollen fossils in the complex as Upper Jurassic to Lower Cretaceous. The high-temperature metamorphism of the Mabujina complex has been interpreted as evidence of the suture zone of the Cretaceous trench, formed when the Escambray block was subducted into the trench (Rosencrantz, 1996).

Volcanic Arcs

There are two main volcanic arcs in Cuba: the Cretaceous arc that runs almost the length of the island, parallel to its axis, and the east-west trending Paleogene arc that occurs only at the eastern end of the island (Fig. 1).

The Cretaceous arc rocks are located mostly to the south of the ophiolite belt, but because of the scale of thrust faulting, may also occur to the north of the ophiolites. During the last decade a Primitive Island Arc (PIA) suite has been recognized in Cuba, that may correlate with the PIA rocks that are thought to represent earliest arc volcanism in other islands of the Greater Antilles (Donnelly and Rogers, 1967). Díaz de Villalvilla (1988) has documented the rocks of the pre-Albian Los Pasos Formation in central Cuba (Fig. 4) as a bimodal suite similar in composition to PIA rocks, and the adjacent Mabujina complex to the south is also interpreted as composed of metamorphosed PIA rocks (Somin and Millán, 1981). Other possible PIA rocks occur at the base of the volcanic section in the Camagüey area and in the Havana-Matanzas area. However, Iturralde-Vinent (1996d) considers that these rocks have not yet been studied in sufficient detail to exclude the possibility that they are derived from oceanic crust and represent the basement of the Upper Cretaceous arc.

The Upper Cretaceous arc (Late Albian to Campanian) is predominantly calc-alkaline in composition. Iturralde-Vinent (1996c) distinguishes, from north to south: 1) a suite of epiclastic and sedimentary rocks with rare lavas, that were deposited in a back-arc basin, 2) an axial zone of lavas and tuffs, that includes large granitoid plutons, and 3) a suite of sedimentary and pyroclastic rocks that were chaotically deposited in deep water as a fore-arc accretionary prism. This last is found only as a window in the Paleogene volcanic arc rocks of eastern Cuba (Fig. 1).

The Paleogene arc crops out only in the eastern end of the island. The axial zone is present along the coast, with back-arc sediments present to the north. The presumed fore-arc portion is not represented in Cuba, where the arc is truncated by the Oriente, or Bartlett, Fault zone. The left-lateral movement on the fault suggests that the fore-arc portion of the Cuban Paleogene arc is present in western Hispaniola (Iturralde-Vinent, 1996e).

VOLCANOGENIC MASSIVE SULPHIDE DEPOSITS

Massive sulphide deposits that can be included in the VMS category are widespread throughout Cuba, but apart from El Cobre deposit in eastern Cuba, few have been mined successfully for their base metal content. The deposits occur in the Ophiolite Belt, the Southwestern Terranes, the lower part of the Cretaceous volcanic arc (PIA) and the Paleogene volcanic arc, but are notably absent in the Upper Cretaceous calc-alkaline part of the arc (Fig. 6). In the available literature many of the Cuban massive sulphide deposits have been described as other than VMS, and are usually considered to have formed in structural sites by replacement of the host rocks. Many of these are now recognized as probably of volcanogenic origin (Table 1).

Cyprus type deposits

Massive sulphide deposits of Cyprus type are best developed in the ophiolitic rocks to the west and east of Havana. West of Havana, the Encrucijada Formation of Albian-Cenomanian age is host to the deposits (Fig 3). The formation consists of pillowed basalts intercalated with calcareous mudstone, fine-grained limestone and radiolarian chert. Due to the complex tectonic history of the area the Encrucijada Formation is recognized in both the Bahía Honda volcanic arc rocks and as lenses in the Cajálbana ophiolites to the south (Iturralde-Vinent, 1996b). The host rocks of porphyritic basalt, basaltic tuff, tuffaceous mudstone and limestone, with porphyritic sills of basaltic and diabasic composition are considered by Iturralde-Vinent (1996b) to represent the effusive-sedimentary component of the ophiolite sequence.

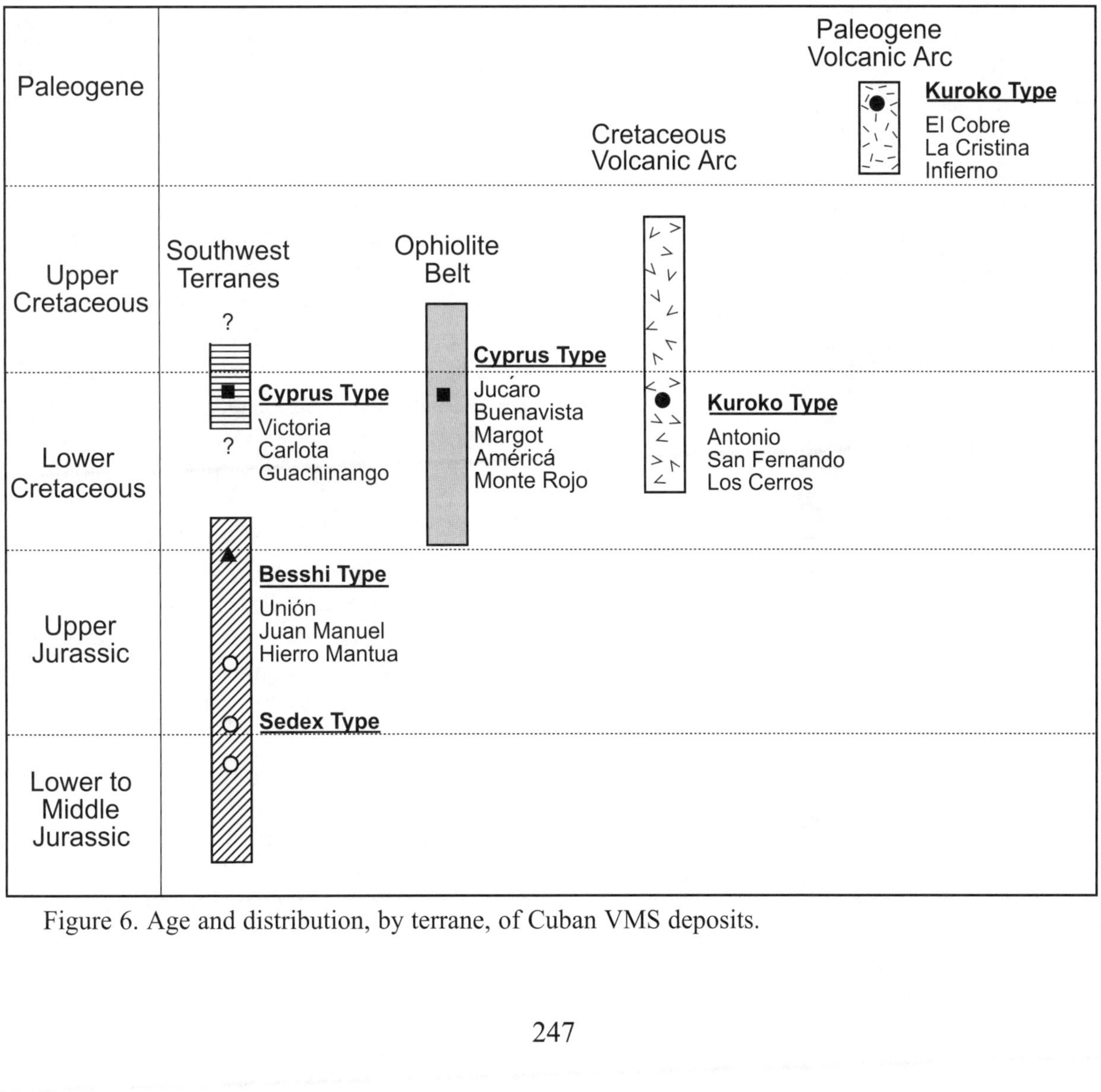

Figure 6. Age and distribution, by terrane, of Cuban VMS deposits.

The basalts are chemically similar to MORB (Cabrera et al., 1985), and were described by Daziano and Barbón (1998) as ocean-floor basalts, rich in MgO and with komatiite affinities. More recently, Kerr et al. (1999) have described them as geochemically akin to rift basalts.

The Júcaro (Fig. 7) and related deposits of Cacarajícara, Mendieta, Buenavista and Yagruma (Fig. 3) have the form of massive lenses that are clearly stratigraphically controlled, but vein and disseminated mineralization is also present. The ores consist of pyrite, chalcopyrite and sphalerite, with lesser marcasite, pyrrhotite, enargite and bornite. Three main mineral associations have been recognized: pyrite, pyrite-chalcopyrite-sphalerite-quartz and pyrite-quartz. Alteration minerals in the host rocks include quartz, epidote, sericite and chlorite. At Júcaro, chlorite is most evident beneath the massive sulphides (Cruz Gómez, 1993). Copper grades are highest in the Buenavista deposit (2.7 %) and zinc grades are always less than 1 % (Table 1).

East of Havana, in the most easterly of two small ophiolite occurrences, are two Cyprus type deposits in the Margot Formation (Fig. 1). The formation has a paleontologic age of Upper Albian-Cenomanian (Piotrowska et al., 1981) or Aptian-Albian (Fonseca et al., 1989). Basalts of the Margot Formation have a geochemistry consistent with that of oceanic tholeiites (Kerr et al., 1999). The ophiolites generally occur as a melange, along with slices of Bahamas Platform rocks, Cretaceous arc rocks and Campanian-Paleocene sedimentary rocks. Thrust faulting has emplaced serpentinites above gabbro, diabase and basalt. Although the ophiolites only crop out in small areas around the deposits, oil wells have shown the ophiolites to be over 4000 m thick (Wassal, 1956).

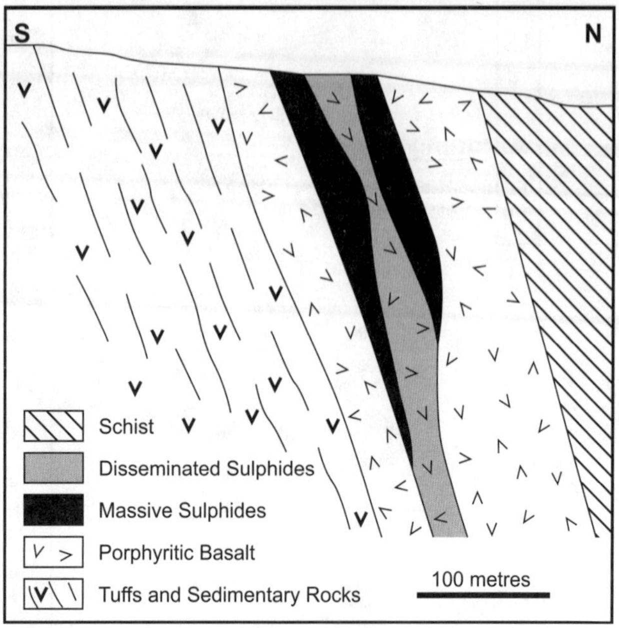

Figure 7. Geological section through the Júcaro Cyprus type VMS deposit. After Tolkunov et al.(1974b).

The deposits occur in flows and sedimentary rocks at the top of the ophiolite sequence, usually in tectonic contact with serpentinites. The Margot deposit (Linares and Lobachev, 1971) is 200 m long, up to 20 m thick and occurs in basalt, with tuff and limestone horizons. The massive sulphide body is elongated and appears to have been deposited, along with the basalt, tuff and limestone, in a narrow channel on top of serpentinite (Morales and Arzuaga, 1994). Meyerhoff et al. (1957) noted pillows in the basalt and intercalations of radiolarian chert. Mineralization consists of massive and disseminated pyrite, with minor chalcopyrite and sphalerite. The grade of hand samples is reported as up to 1.55 % Cu, with 1.17 g/t Au and 4.4 g/t Ag. Associated alteration minerals are chlorite, sericite, quartz and calcite. Mining ceased in 1957 when the pit collapsed during heavy rains. The nearby América deposit is a pyrite lens 50 m long and 15-20 m thick in serpentinite breccia. The lens contains up to 75 % pyrite with inclusions of pyrrhotite. Hand samples contain up to 0.52 % Cu in chalcopyrite. Silicification is the most common form of alteration around the deposit, with lesser amounts of chlorite and calcite.

Cyprus type deposits are also known in the Ophiolite Belt in eastern Cuba (Moreira et al., 1999). In general they are small deposits and have not been exploited. Near Holguín, the Monte Rojo deposit is a 2.5 m thick massive sulphide lens with a strike length of 550 m and a down-dip extension of more than 60 m. It occurs at the contact of serpentinite with gabbros and diabases of the cumulative phase (Penteleyi and García, 1990). Alteration surrounding the sulphides consists of silicification, chloritization and epidotization. An unusual feature of the deposit is an intrusion of trachyte that cuts the western end of the massive sulphides, contains up to 2 g/t Au and is considered a later superimposed event.

The Cuba Libre deposit, near Camagüey, is associated with sub-volcanic intrusions of gabbro and diabase that are in fault contact with serpentinites. Escobar (1994) describes the deposit as consisting of pyrite, chalcopyrite and pyrrhotite in quartz, surrounded by an alteration zone of quartz, chlorite and argillite. The deposit has been traced for 600 m along strike, 150 m downdip and is up to 40 m thick. Because of the lack of massive sulphides and basaltic flows, Escobar (1994) concludes that the deposit is not truly of Cyprus type, but probably formed a short distance beneath the sea floor, in feeder zones to a now-eroded Cyprus type deposit.

In Guantánamo Province, El Hoyo deposit occurs in tectonized serpentinite. Selected hand samples contain 0.5-7.12 % Cu and 0.1-11.75 % Zn (Nicolaiev et al., 1981). The body is 300 m long and 50 m wide with disseminated to massive pyrite. The Ventura body, with a strike length of 700 m and a thickness of 3-10 m, occurs in serpentinized peridotite and contains up to 0.4 % Cu and up to 1 g/t Au (Svoboda, 1966).

In the Escambray Terrane, a group of unusual, possible Cyprus type, deposits occurs on the northwest side of the metamorphic complex (Fig. 4). Although the host rocks are predominantly marbles and schistose limestones, the sulphide bodies are always closely associated with ultramafic and mafic rocks that occur locally along a 70 km fault zone. Tolkunov et al. (1974a) described the deposits as Cyprus type, but only on the basis of their mineralogical composition. They believed that they formed much later than the host rocks, by replacement along faults and they did not recognize the ophiolitic nature of the mafic and ultramafic rocks, which they considered to be Eocene intrusions in the Jurassic metamorphic rocks. Pardo et al. (1994) considered the deposits to be of sedimentary-exhalative origin, later modified by regional metamorphism.

Following the model of Iturralde-Vinent (1996b), it is suggested here that the ophiolitic rocks and associated massive sulphides are fragments of ocean floor that were emplaced in the Escambray Terrane at the time of its collision with the Cretaceous volcanic arc. This view differs from the current opinions of some Cuban geologists who have worked extensively in the Escambray metamorphic terrane. In the most recent discussion of the deposits, Alvarez et al. (1989) state that the deposits most closely resemble the Besshi type. In reviewing the information from other recent studies of these deposits (Dublan et al., 1986; Stanik et al., 1981; Millán and Somin, 1985) they conclude that the volcanic rocks with which the deposits are associated are not tectonic slices of ocean floor that were incorporated into the Escambray Terrane during its attempted subduction, but are original components of the metamorphosed terrane and have undergone the same degree of high pressure metamorphism. They consider the deposits to be syngenetic and more closely related in origin to the Besshi type deposits in the Guaniguanico terrane, that are described below. However, whether the massive sulphide mineralization was deposited syngenetically within the Escambray stratigraphy, or was emplaced tectonically at a later time, its undoubted association with ophiolitic rocks suggests a Cyprus type origin.

There are three main deposits: Carlota, Victoria and Guachinango, along with a number of smaller lenses. The three main deposits are separated by about 10 km along strike, but pyritic lenses are found over a distance of 40 km and all are closely associated with a major fault that dips moderately to the north. The Guachinango deposit, containing 5 Mt of 0.81 % Cu, is estimated to be 800 m long, 200 m down-dip and up to 31 m thick. It occurs as a concordant lens of banded and massive sulphides in schistose and marbleized limestone (Tolkunov et al., 1974a). Closely associated with the sulphides are altered peridotites and mafic volcanic rocks, as well as micaceous schists. The sulphides are almost exclusively pyrite, with minor pyrrhotite, chalcopyrite, sphalerite and galena. The base metals are concentrated in the hangingwall. The composition of the Carlota deposit is similar, with 1.13 % Cu and 0.28 % combined Pb and Zn (Table 1). The Victoria deposit (Fig. 8) has an estimated reserve of 0.54 Mt, averaging 0.86 % Cu and 0.39 % combined Pb and Zn (Table 1).

Kuroko type deposits

Kuroko type, or arc-related, massive sulphide deposits are known in the lower part of the Cretaceous

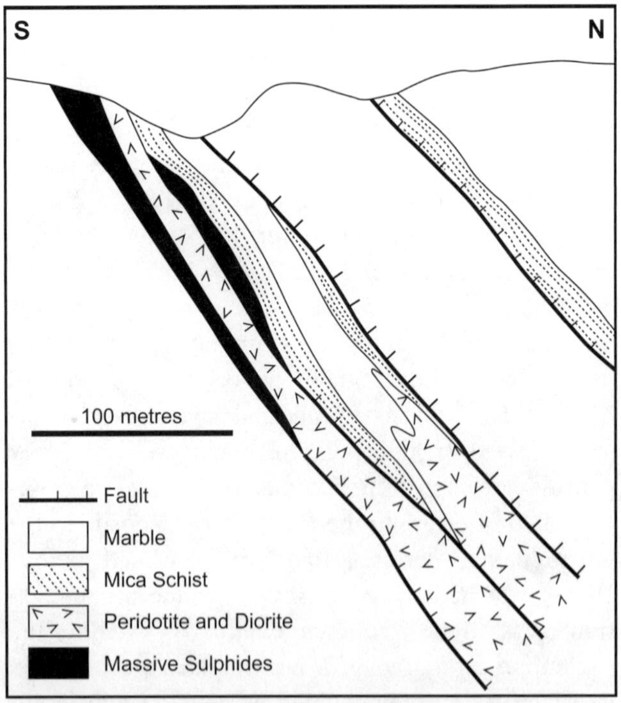

Figure 8. Geological section through the Victoria Cyprus type VMS deposit. After Tolkunov et al. (1974a).

arc in central Cuba and in the Paleogene arc in eastern Cuba (Fig. 6, Table 1). No deposit has been described from the Upper Cretaceous arc.

The Los Pasos Formation, in south central Cuba, is considered to represent a bimodal volcanic assemblage comparable to the PIA assemblages on other islands of the Greater Antilles (Donnelly and Rogers, 1967; Lebron and Perfit, 1993). Its extent in Cuba is limited, ocurring north of the Escambray Terrane and Mabujina amphibolite complex and south of the Upper Cretaceous arc rocks (Fig. 4). The formation consists of mafic volcanic rocks that are often spilitized, and felsic volcanic rocks (Díaz de Villalvilla, 1988). Its age is considered to be Neocomian and it is overlain by Aptian limestone that separates the formation from the overlying calc-alkaline arc rocks. This period of limestone deposition, between the PIA assemblage and the Upper Cretaceous calc-alkaline assemblage, may correlate with the Hatillo Limestone Formation in the Dominican Republic, which unconformably overlies the PIA rocks of the Los Ranchos Formation and represents a hiatus in volcanic activity (Russell and Kesler, 1991). Within the Los Pasos Formation are the massive sulphide deposits of Antonio, Los Cerros and Los Mangos-San Fernando (Fig. 4). The deposits appear to be at a similar stratigraphic level and are associated with felsic pyroclastic rocks (Bravo et al., 1989).

The Antonio deposit (Fig. 9), which is underlain by dacite tuff and overlain by dacite flows and lava-breccias (Tolkunov et al., 1974b) has dimensions of 450 m along strike, 340 m down-dip and a maximum thickness of 62 m (Gallardo et al., 1992). It was exploited intermittently for its enriched oxide zone. The massive sulphides consist mainly of pyrite, with minor chalcopyrite, sphalerite, sulphosalts, Ag-tellurides and electrum present in the upper part of the lens. Cu reserves of the Antonio deposit have been calculated at 1.7 Mt containing 0.52 % Cu (Table 1).

Los Cerros deposit was mined from 1954-57. It consists of steeply dipping quartz-sulphide lenses (Estrugo and Santa Cruz Pacheco, 1984), consisting mainly of pyrite, with lesser amounts of chalcopyrite and sphalerite. The felsic host rocks are altered to quartz, chlorite, epidote, sericite and albite. Metal contents are 0.38 % Cu, 0.49 % Zn and 0.09 % Pb, with 0.45 g/t Au and 0.8 g/t Ag.

The Los Mangos-San Fernando deposit occurs as massive to semi-massive sulphides in the upper part of a unit of felsic lapilli tuff and is overlain by basaltic lapillii tuff. The host unit is intensely altered to quartz-sericite-chlorite-biotite, whereas the overlying basaltic rocks are not altered (Bottrill et al., this volume). They conclude that the mineralization is exhalative, of Kuroko type, and was deposited in local depressions in the felsic tuff unit. Santa Cruz Pacheco et al. (1997) have distinguished sphalerite-rich (black) ore and chalcopyrite-rich (yellow) ore in the mineralization. Recent drilling has outlined a resource of 1 Mt grading 1.84 % Cu and 3.35 % Zn, with the possibility of another 1M tonnes downdip (Bottrill et al., this volume).

Kuroko type deposits are also known in the Paleogene arc of eastern Cuba (Fig. 10). El Cobre was the first copper mine in the New World and began operation in 1544. Mining continued intermittently until 1998 and it is estimated that more than 3 Mt have been mined at grades ranging from 2 to 20 % Cu. Current reserves are 1.55 Mt grading 2.2 % Cu (Table

Table 1. Cuban VMS deposits.
* proven + probable reserves and mineral grades. (Oficina Nacional de Recursos Minerales, 1998).
** Bottrill et al., this volume

Abbreviations: serp = serpentinite; py = pyrite; cpy = chalcopyrite; sph = sphalerite; po = pyrrhotite; gal = galena; qtz = quartz; chl = chlorite; ser = sericite; cal = calcite; epid = epidote.

Type	Deposit	Formation	Age	Host Rocks	Minerals	Alteration	Size(tonnes)	Cu %	Pb+Zn %	Au g/t	Ag g/t
CYPRUS	Júcaro	Encrucijada	Aptian-Albian	Tholeitic basalt	py, cpy, sph	qtz, chl, ser, cal, epid	589,760*	1.38	0.31		
	Cacarajícara	Encrucijada	Aptian-Albian	Tholeitic basalt	py, cpy, sph	qtz, chl, ser, cal, epid	616,800*	1.20			
	Mendieta	Encrucijada	Aptian-Albian	Tholeitic basalt	py, cpy, sph	qtz, chl, ser, cal, epid					
	Buenavista	Encrucijada	Aptian-Albian	Tholeitic basalt	py, cpy, sph	qtz, chl, ser, cal, epid	105,800*	2.58			
	Yagruma	Encrucijada	Aptian-Albian	Tholeitic basalt	py, cpy, sph	qtz, chl, ser, cal, epid		0.72	0.90		
	Margot	Margot	Aptian-Albian	Tholeitic basalt	py, cpy, sph	qtz, chl, ser, cal,		<1.55		<1.17	<4.4
	América	Margot	Aptian-Albian	Serp. Breccia, basalt	py, po, cpy	qtz, chl, cal	<0.52				
	Monte Rojo		Aptian-Albian?	Serp., gabbro		qtz, chl, epid					
	Cuba Libre		Aptian-Albian?	Serp., basalt, gabbro	py, po, cpy	qtz, chl, clays	1,000,000	1.00			
	Ventura		Aptian-Albian?	Serp.	py, cpy			<0.4		<1.0	
	El Hoyo		Aptian-Albian?	Serp.	py, cpy			0.5-7.12	0.1-11.75		
	Carlota		Jur.-Lr. Cret.	Peridotite, calc. schists	py, po, cpy, sph		2,352,000*	1.13	0.28		
	Guachinango		Jur.-Lr. Cret.	Peridotite, calc. schists	py, po, cpy, sph		5,005,000*	0.81			
	La Victoria		Jur.-Lr. Cret.	Peridotite, calc. schists	py, po, cpy, sph		536,000*	0.86	0.39		
KUROKO	Antonio	Los Pasos	Neocomian	Dacite breccia	py, cpy, sph		1,666,300*	0.52			
	San Fernando	Los Pasos	Neocomian	Felsic lapilli tuff	py, cpy, sph	qtz, chl, ser, barite	1,000,000**	1.84	3.35		
	Los Cerros	Los Pasos	Neocomian	Felsic pyroclastics	py, cpy, sph	qtz, chl, epid, ser		0.38	0.58		
	El Cobre	Hongolosongo	Lr. Pal.-Ur. Eoc .	Andesite lavas, tuffs	py, cpy, sph	qtz, ser, chl, clays	8,436,010*	1.83			
	La Cristina	El Cobre Group	Lr. Pal.-Ur. Eoc .	Andesite tuff		qtz, ser, chl, barite		0.8-8.0	0.5-3.0	1.0-6.0	
	Infierno	El Cobre Group	Lr. Eocene	Andesite-dacite tuff	py, cpy, sph, gal	qtz, ser,chl, cal,		0.6-1.41	0.3-38.2	0.5-4.19	10-121
BESSHI	Hierro Mantua	Esperanza	Ur. Jur.-Lr. Cret.	Porphyritic basalt	py, cpy, sph		11,389,000*	1.76			
	Hierro Mantua	Esperanza	Ur. Jur.-Lr. Cret.	Porphyritic basalt	py, cpy	qtz, cal, gossan zone	2,043,000*			1.44	11.65
	Unión	Esperanza	Ur. Jur.-Lr. Cret.	Diabase	py, cpy	qtz, cal		<0.5			
	Juan Manuel	Esperanza	Ur. Jur.-Lr. Cret.	Diabase	py, cpy	qtz, cal		<0.5			

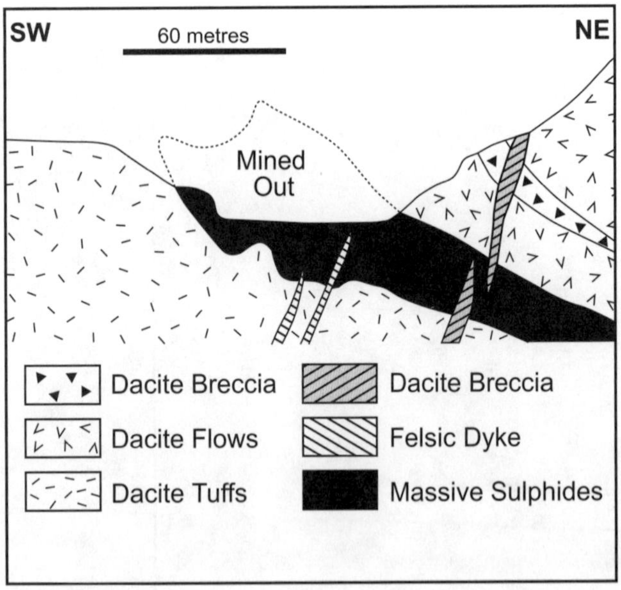

Figure 9. Geological section through the Antonio Kuroko type VMS deposit. After Tolkunov et al. (1974b).

1). Although almost all of the mined ore at El Cobre has come from a central cross-cutting vein system of pyrite and chalcopyrite, exploration in the area has demonstrated that there are a number of stratigraphically controlled sulphide lenses in El Cobre system (Fig. 11), which is considered to include both epithermal vein or stockwork mineralization and stratabound exhalative mineralization (Luna, 1994). The mine occurs in the Hongolosongo Formation of El Cobre Group, comprising Lower Paleocene to Upper Eocene andesitic agglomerates, tuffs and breccias. The stratabound lenses at El Cobre consist of Pb-Zn mineralization and are hosted by felsic ignimbrites. Luna et al. (1992) have noted that the sulphide lenses are present in the thinner parts of the ignimbrites, suggesting deposition in depressions on the sea floor. The sulphide lenses generally are copper-rich in their central parts, with zinc predominant on the flanks. Around the lenses Luna et al. (1992) have documented alter-

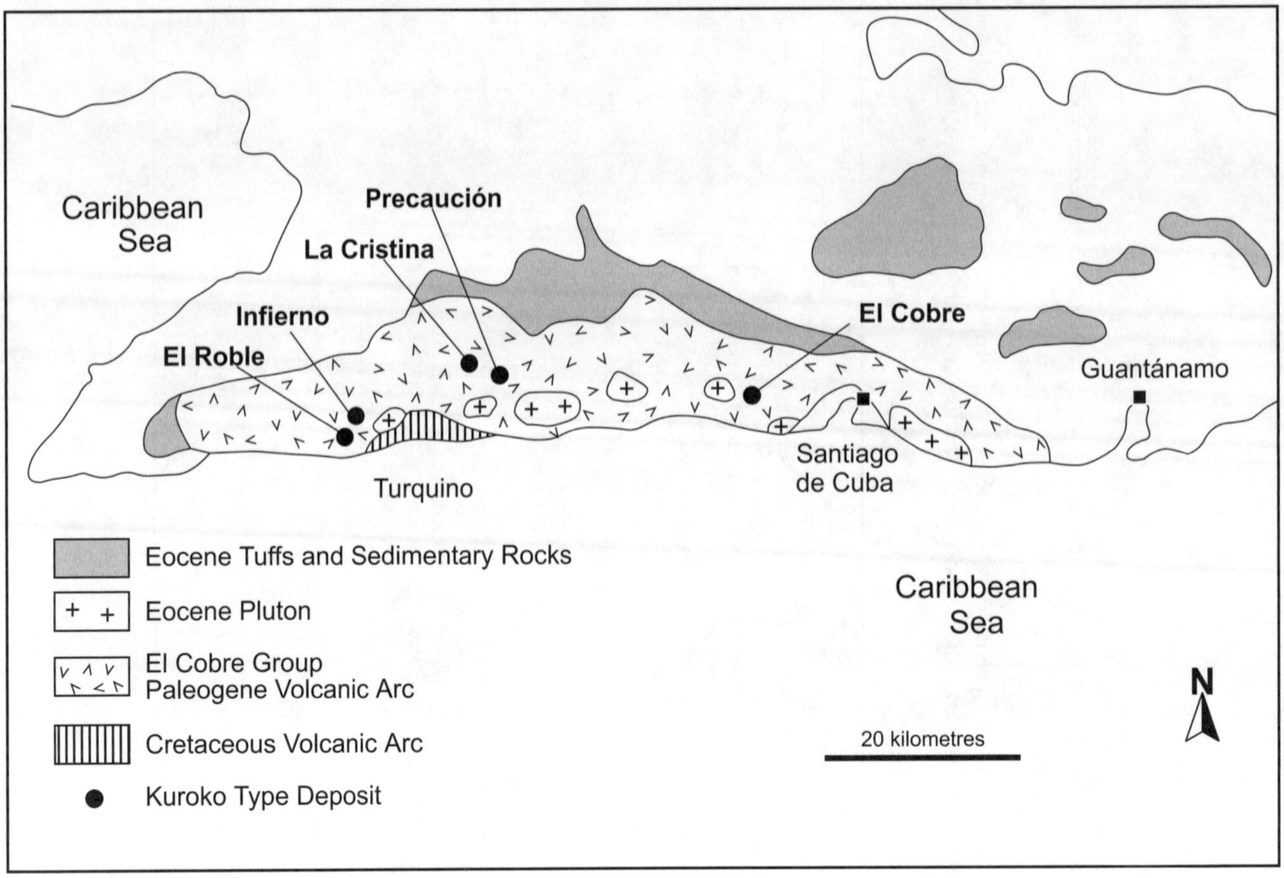

Figure 10. VMS deposits of eastern Cuba. Geology after Iturralde-Vinent (1996d).

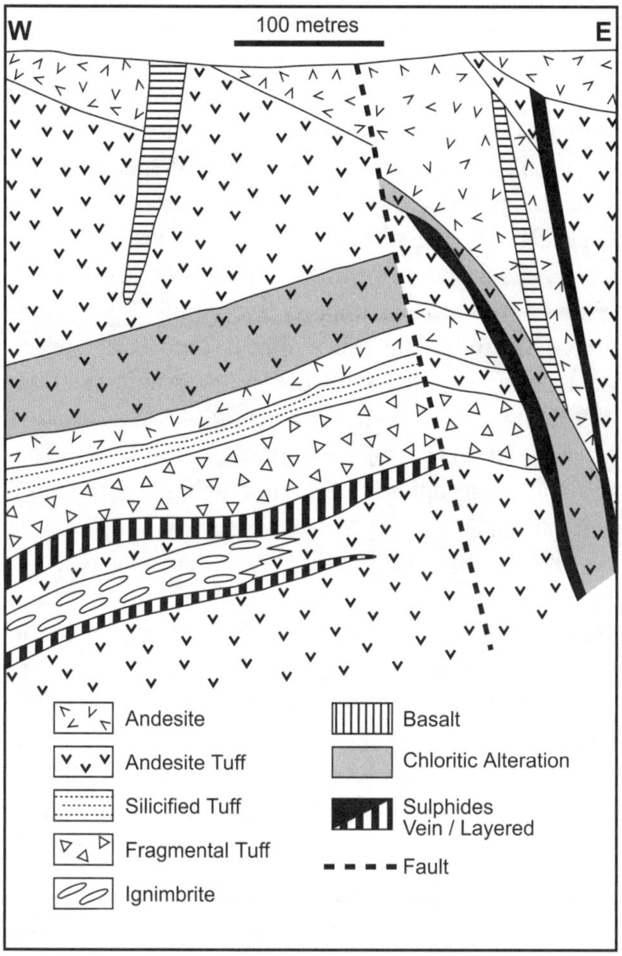

Figure 11. Geological section through El Cobre deposit, showing the main ore vein and stratigraphically controlled massive sulphide horizons. After Luna et al. (1992).

ation of the host rocks, which includes clays, micas, gypsum and anhydrite towards the centre and quartz, sericite and chlorite at the periphery. Fluid inclusion studies (Izquierdo et al., 1991) suggest vein formation temperatures of 100°-200°C. The North Zone is a stratiform body within intensely altered andesitic rocks. Silicification and sericitization are the principal alteration types. This zone has dimensions of 500 m along strike and is, on average, 5 m thick. It has been traced for 200 m down-dip. The sulphide minerals are pyrite, sphalerite, chalcopyrite and galena, with average grades of 0.13 % Cu, 3.18 % Zn and 0.79 % Pb, with 1-2 g/t Au.

In the western Sierra Maestra probable Kuroko type deposits occur at La Cristina and Infierno (Fig. 10). La Cristina (including the old Eureka mine, which was estimated in 1957 to contain 0.5 Mt of ore grading 2-3 % Cu) occurs in andesitic tuffs. In the disseminated and massive mineralization the copper content varies from 0.8 to 8 %, zinc from 0.5 to 3 % and gold from 1 to 6 g/t (Svoboda, 1966). The host rocks are altered to quartz, sericite, chlorite and rare barite. The nearby Precaución prospect consists of two massive sulphide lenses in an altered package of volcanic rocks, with selected samples containing up to 9.13 % Cu and 5.07 g/t Au (Joutel Resources Ltd. 1995).

The Infierno and related deposits (El Pino, El Roble) occur in andesite-basalt tuffs with intercalations of andesite-dacite. The immediate host rocks are andesite-dacite tuffs. The massive sulphide lenses are often accompanied by stockworks. The lenses vary from 7 to 30 m in thickness and are found in a zone of altered rocks with a strike length of over 2 km and a width of 100 m. The sulphides are represented by sphalerite, galena, chalcopyrite and pyrite, with lesser covellite, native gold, marcasite and barite in a quartz gangue. The mineralization is stratigraphically controlled and is underlain by a stockwork of disseminated sulphides and quartz (Porro, 1994). The principal alteration minerals in the host rocks are quartz, chlorite, calcite and albite, with chlorite concentrated beneath the massive sulphides and sericite above and on the flanks. In hand samples the zinc content ranges up to 38.2 %, lead to 28.8 %, copper to 1.41 %, gold to 4.19 g/t and silver to 121 g/t (Moreira et al., 1999).

Besshi type deposits

In the Guaniguanico block of western Cuba, SEDEX deposits are well-represented (Fig. 3). The large Matahambre mine produced copper for many years and the oxide cap of the Castellanos deposit, with reserves of 3.3 Mt grading 1.45 g/t Au is at present being mined (Oficina Nacional de Recursos Minerales, 1998). The known base metal deposits occur in three belts. In the south, Copper deposits, including Matahambre, occur in the San Cayetano Formation. Further north, in the Castellanos Formation of Late Jurassic to Early Cretaceous age, Zn and Pb-Zn deposits are present at Castellanos and Santa Lucia. In both belts mineralization is in carbonate-terrigenous sediments of the continental margin and their sedimentary-exhalative origin is widely accepted. The most northerly belt of mineralization is in the Esperanza Formation of Upper Jurassic to Lower Cretaceous age, and includes the Hierro Mantua orebody and the Juan Manuel - Unión deposits (Fig. 3). Copper is the principal base metal present in this belt and lead and zinc are insignificant. Although these deposits might also be included in the SEDEX category, they appear to be associated with volcanic horizons and have beeen classified as Besshi deposits (Kesler et al., 1996).

The mineral deposits occur in the middle part of the Esperanza Formation at the transition from terrigenous sediments below to carbonate-dominant above. The host rocks to the mineralization are limestone and calcareous schist, with intercalations of sandstone, mudstone and carbonaceous schist. Volcanic rocks are represented as concordant lenses of basaltic to andesitic composition (Lavandero et al., 1985). The sulphide mineralization consists of pyrite and pyrite-chalcopyrite, with minor pyrrhotite, magnetite and enargite and forms discontinuous conformable lenses over a strike length of 30 km (Feoktistov et al., 1983). Individual bodies range up to 1000 m long, 400 m downdip and 25 m thick. Outcropping mineralized zones have extensive gossan development, with secondary enrichment of gold and copper. The Hierro Mantua deposit (Fig. 12), with a strike length of 1300 m, occurs mainly in sedimentary rocks, but the mineralization itself is concordant with a unit of porphyritic basalt (Tolkunov et al., 1974b). The sulphide zone is composed of pyrite and chalcopyrite with minor sphalerite, galena, enargite and pyrrhotite and has a reserve of 11.3 Mt containing 1.76 % Cu. The oxidized zone is at present being mined for its gold content (Lavandero et al., 1997) and has a reported reserve of 2 Mt grading 1.44 g/t Au (Table 1). Tolkunov et al. (1974b) report that this zone also contains 50-60 g/t combined germanium and gallium.

The Unión and Juan Manuel deposits, west of Hierro Mantua, also consist mainly of pyrite and chalcopyrite, but with non-economic copper contents in the primary mineralization. Some small-scale mining of copper in the oxidised zone took place in the 19th century. The area contains more than twenty small concordant sulphide bodies over a strike length of 7 km, with dimensions ranging up to 1000 m along strike, 40-400 m downdip and 1-25 m thick. The sul-

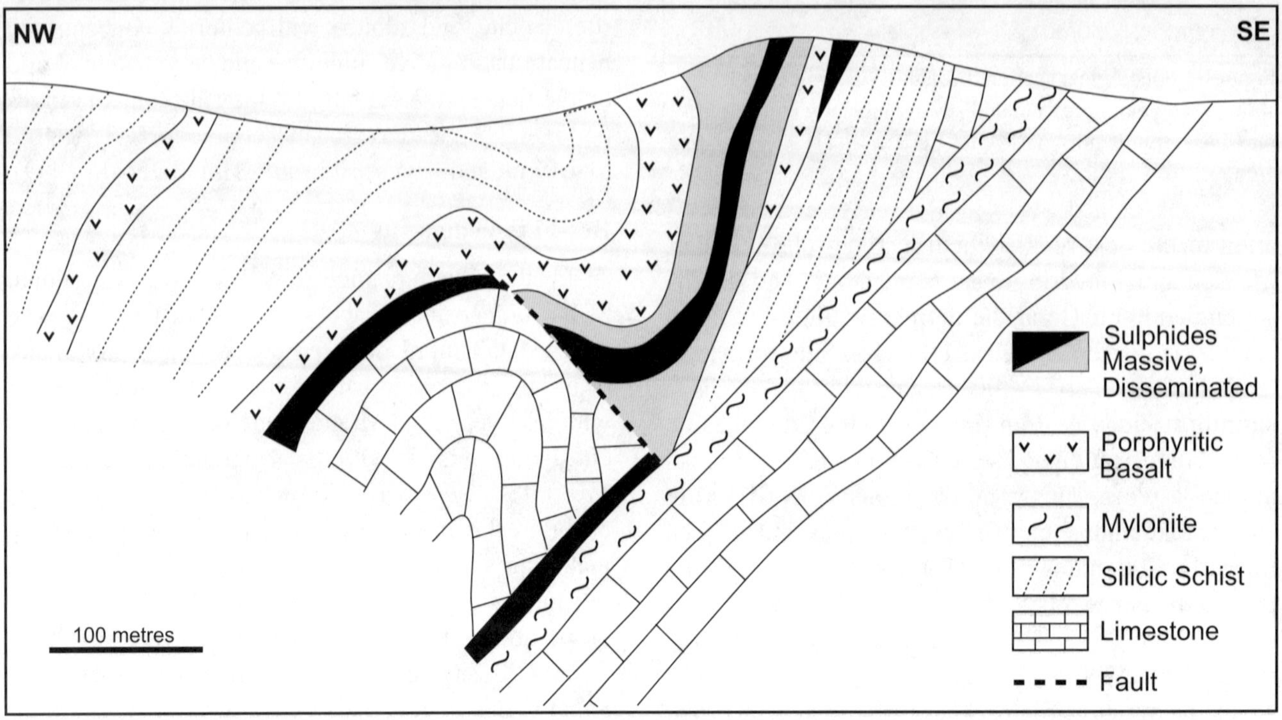

Figure12. Geological section through the Hierro Mantua Besshi type VMS deposit. After Tolkunov et al. (1974b).

phides are massive and locally banded and are always closely associated with horizons of diabase (Simón Méndez, 1992). The massive lenses consist mainly of pyrite, with minor chalcopyrite, marcasite, melnikovite, pyrrhotite, enargite and bornite. Silicification and carbonatization are the most common type of alteration of the host rocks.

CONCLUSIONS

Cuba appears to have a higher content of VMS deposits than other islands of the Greater Antilles, particularly of the Besshi and Cyprus types. The presence of Besshi type deposits, and the even more abundant SEDEX deposits, in the Southwestern Terranes, is related to the continental rifting of Pangea near the present site of western Cuba and the preservation of Mesozoic continental fragments alongside the Cretaceous volcanic arc rocks. In other islands of the Greater Antilles, where the arc formed farther from the continental margin, no such fragment is known.

Similarly, the collision of the Cuban portion of the Cretaceous volcanic arc with the Bahamas Platform, caused more intense tectonic compression there, compared to the eastern part of the arc. This resulted in a higher percentage of outcropping ophiolitic rocks in Cuba compared to other islands of the Greater Antilles, and therefore more exposure of Cyprus type deposits.

Kuroko type deposits, that are directly associated with arc development, are not particulary more abundant in the Cuban portion of the Greater Antilles volcanic arc. These deposits are present in the probable PIA rocks of Lower Cretaceous age in central Cuba and also in the Paleogene arc of eastern Cuba, but are not known in the Upper Cretaceous calc-alkaline portion of the arc. As a result of the attachment of Cuba to the North American Plate it is now much less tectonically active than other islands of the Greater Antilles and subsequently is much flatter due to erosion and lack of ongoing vertical uplift. In fact, the few mountainous areas that remain in Cuba, particularly the Guaniguanico Terrane, the Escambray Terrane and surrounding Lower Cretaceous PIA rocks, and the Sierra Maestra range of eastern Cuba, are the sites of nearly all of the known VMS deposits. The central part of the island, where Upper Cretaceous arc rocks crop out, is mainly of low elevation and much of the area is covered by flat-lying post-orogenic sediments. Even the areas shown as being underlain by Upper Cretaceous arc rocks (Fig. 1) are mapped from scattered outcrops in generally flat agricultural areas. Perhaps the apparent lack of VMS deposits in the Upper Cretaceous arc rocks is simply a consequence of the paucity of outcrop. It may also be significant that the largest preserved area of Upper Cretaceous arc rocks, in east-central Cuba, contains widespread epithermal mineralization (Simon et al., 1999), suggesting that the presently exposed rocks were deposited in shallow water or subaerial conditions and not in an environment that favoured formation of VMS deposits.

ACKNOWLEDGEMENTS

The authors are very grateful to Jesús Hernandez, Director of the Instituto de Geología y Paleontología, Havana, for permission to research the files of the Institute and have access to many unpublished documents. CaribGold Mines Inc. provided support during the preparation of the manuscript. We would like to thank to Ross Sherlock and Fiona Childe for their reviews and suggestions for improvement. Thanks also to Manuel Iturralde-Vinent, Guillermo Millán and Dr. Stephen E. Kesler for their useful comments and suggestions.

REFERENCES

Alvarez, H., Romero, O., Espinosa, A., Lavandero, R., Pérez, M., Alemán, L., Darias, J. and Zamora, L. 1989. Fundamentación de las perspectivas pronósticas para minerales sólidos en la Cúpula Trinidad, Macizo Metamórfico del Escambray. Tema Científico No. 27, Empresa Geominera, Santa Clara, Cuba. Unpublished.

Bottrill, T. J., Formel, F. and Raman, S. Los Mangos – San Fernando Deposit, Santa Clara, Cuba, Geology and Mineralization in a Cretaceous Volcanic Arc. This volume.

Bravo, F., Lavandero, R., Santa Cruz, M., Estrugo, M., Hanchivín, A. and Montenegro, J. 1989. Tipos geólogo-industriales y formaciones minerales de los yacimientos sulfurosos de plomo-zinc y cobre-zinc de Cuba y algunas interrogantes de su génesis. Ministerio de la Industria Básica, Serie Geológica, No. 2, pp. 63-79.

Cabrera, R., Malinovski, E. P., and Pantaleón, G. 1985. Texto explicativa para el mapa de yacimientos minerales, Escala 1:500,000. Instituto de Geología y Paleontología, Ciudad de La Habana, Cuba. Unpublished.

Cabrera, R. 1986. Geología y regularidades de la distribución de los yacimientos de cobre y oro de la región mineral de Las

Villas. Instituto de Geología y Paleontología, Academia de Ciencias de Cuba. 130 pp.

Coney, P. J. 1983. Un modelo tectónico de México y sus relaciones con América del Norte, América del Sur y el Caribe. Revista del Instituto Mexicano del Petróleo, v. 15, pp. 6-15.

Cruz Gómez, E. M. 1993. Papel del vulcanismo básico en la formación de los yacimientos cupro-piríticos de la zona estructuro-facial Bahía Honda, Pinar del Río. Ph.D. thesis, Centro Universitario de Pinar del Río, Cuba.

Daziano, C. O. and Barbón, R. 1998. Gequímica de lateritas del yacimiento Prado en la Caracterización Metalogénica y Potencialidad Económica de las rocas subyacentes, Provincia Pinar del Río, República de Cuba. IV Reunión de Mineralogía y Metalogenia, Universidad Nacional del Sur, MINMET '98, pp. 57-62.

Díaz de Villalvilla, L. 1988. Caracterización geológica y petrogeológica de las asociaciones vulcanógenas del Arco Insular Cretácico en Cuba central. Ph.D. thesis.

Donnelly, T. W. and Rogers, J. J. W. 1967. Crust vs. Mantle derivation of eastern Antillean igneous rocks [abs.]. EOS (American Geophysical Union Transactions), v. 48, p. 253.

Dublan, L., Alvarez, H., Milcoch, B., Molak, B., Vázquez, ., Santos, E., Soucek, J., Pérez, M., Mihalikova, A., Bernal, L., Zoubebek, J., Ordoñez, M., Lavandero, R., Lledías, J. P., Marouzek, K., Sbestka, J., Mandur, J., Marsal, W., Pérez, R., Gonzalez, E. and Rodriguez, R. 1986. Informe final del Levantamiento Geológico y Evaluación de los Minerales Utiles a escala 1:50,000 del polígono CAME-1, Zona Centro. Oficina Nacional de Recursos Minerales, Ministerio de la Industria Básica, Ciudad de La Habana, Cuba. Unpublished.

Dublan, L. P., Snopkova, P. and Alvarez-Sánchez, H. 1988. Datos preliminares sobre la edad de las anfibolitas del cinturón de Mabujina de Cuba central según el método paleobótanico. Boletín de Geociencias, v. 3(2), Pinar del Río, Cuba, pp. 48-56.

Duncan, R. A. and Hargraves, R. B. 1984. Plate tectonic evolution of the Caribbean region in the mantle reference frame. In The Caribbean-South American Plate Boundary and Regional Tectonics. Edited by W. E. Bonini, R. B. Hargraves and R.Shagam. Geological Society of America Memoir 162, pp. 81-93.

Escobar, E. 1994. Características geologícas del yacimiento "Cuba Libre". Unpublished report.

Estrugo, M. and Santa Cruz Pacheco, M. 1984. Yacimiento "Los Cerros", características mineralogeoquímicas y génesis. Serie geológica, Ministerio de la Indústria Básica, Cuba, No. 2, pp. 35-50.

Feoktistov, V. P., Aniyatov, I. A. and Norman, A. 1983. Metallogeny of western Cuba. International Geology Review, v. 25, No. 3, pp. 309-318.

Fonseca, E., González, R., Delgado, R. and Savicleva, G. 1989. Presencia de efusivos ofiolíticos y de boninitas en las provincias de La Habana y Matanzas. Boletín Tecnológica de Geología, No. 1, Ministerio de Indústria Básica, Cuba, pp. 1-9.

Gallardo, E., Delgado, S., Moya, R. and Romero, O. 1992. Características geológicas, geofísicas y geoquímicas del área Antonio-Independencia. Empresa Geominera del Centro, Villa Clara, Cuba. Unpublished report.

Iturralde-Vinent, M. A. 1994. Cuban Geology: a new Plate-tectonic Synthesis. Journal of Petroleum Geology, v.17(1), pp. 39-70.

Iturralde-Vinent, M. A. 1996a. Introduction to Cuban Geology and Geophysics. In Ofiolitas y Arcos Volcánicos de Cuba. Edited by M. A. Iturralde-Vinent. IUGS/UNESCO International Geological Correlation Programe, Project 364, Contribution No. 1, Chap. 1, pp. 3-35.

Iturralde-Vinent, M. A. 1996b. Geología de las Ofiolitas de Cuba. In Ofiolitas y Arcos Volcánicos de Cuba. Edited by M. A. Iturralde-Vinent. IUGS/UNESCO International Geological Correlation Programe, Project 364, Contribution No. 1, Chap. 2, pp. 83-120.

Iturralde-Vinent, M. A. 1996c. Cuba: El Arco de Islas Volcánicas del Cretácico. In Ofiolitas y Arcos Volcánicos de Cuba. Edited by M. A. Iturralde-Vinent. IUGS/UNESCO International Geological Correlation Programe, Project 364, Contribution No. 1, Chap. 3, pp. 179-189.

Iturralde-Vinent, M. A. 1996d. Evidencias de un arco primitivo (Cretácico Inferior) en Cuba. In Ofiolitas y Arcos Volcánicos de Cuba. Edited by M. A. Iturralde-Vinent. IUGS/UNESCO International Geological Correlation Programe, Project 364, Contribution No. 1, Chap. 3, pp. 227-230.

Iturralde-Vinent, M. A. 1996e. Cuba: El Archipiélago Volcánico Paleoceno-Eoceno Medio. In Ofiolitas y Arcos Volcánicos de Cuba. Edited by M. A. Iturralde-Vinent. IUGS/UNESCO International Geological Correlation Programe, Project 364, Contribution No. 1, Chap. 3, pp. 231-246.

Izquierdo, J. M., Shershniov, V., Escobar, E., Fernández, A., Sánchez, R., Donskij, V., Torres, M., Estrugo, M., Gentoiu, M., Rodriguez, J., Cobo, J. and Dieguez, H. 1991. Informe del tema 401.03, fundamentación de las direcciones de prospección preliminar y prospección detallada para cobre en la región del campo menífero El Cobre, incluyendo la cuantificación de recursos pronósticos. Instituto de Geología y Paleontología, La Habana, Cuba.

Joutel Resources Limited, Toronto, Canada. 1995. Annual Report, p. 5.

Kerr, A. C., Iturralde-Vinent, M. A., Saunders, A. D., Babbs, T. L. and Tarney, J. 1999. A new plate tectonic model of the Caribbean: Implications from a geochemical reconnaissance of Cuban Mesozoic volcanic rocks. Geological Society of America Bulletin, v. 111, no. 11, pp. 1581-1599.

Kesler, S.E., Levy, E. and Martin F. C. 1990. Metallogenic evolution of the Caribbean region. In The Caribbean Region. Edited by G. Dengo and J. E. Case. The Geological Society of America, The Geology of North America, v. H, Chapt. 18, pp. 459-482.

Kesler, S. E., Russell, N. and Bell, D. 1996. Gold-silver mineralization in Cuba and its geologic setting in the Greater Antilles. In Geology and Ore Deposits of the American Cordillera. Edited by A. R. Coyner and P. L. Fahey.

Geological Society of Nevada Symposium Proceedings, Reno/Sparks, Nevada, April 1995. Pp. 1433-1441.

Khudoley, K.M. and Meyerhoff, A.A. 1971. Paleogeography and geological history of Greater Antilles. Geological Society of America Memoir 129.

Lavandero, R., Bravo, F. and Pantaleón, G. 1997. Perspectivas metalíferas de la porción nor occidental de la provincia Pinar del Río, Instituto de Geología y Paleontología, Ciudad de La Habana, Cuba. Unpublished report.

Lavandero, R., Estrugo, M., Santa Cruz, M., Bravo, F., Melnikov, Q., Casañas, X., Aniatov, I., Krapiva, L., Bayarkhu, B., Carillo, D. and Altarriba, I. 1985. Sistematización y Generalización de los Yacimientos Minerales Metálicos. Instituto de Geología y Paleontología, Ciudad de La Habana, Cuba. Unpublished report.

Lebron, M. C. and Perfit, M. R. 1993. Stratigraphic and petrochemical data support subduction polarity reversal of the Cretaceous Caribbean island arc. Journal of Geology, No. 101, pp. 389-396.

Lewis, J. F. and Draper, G. 1990. Geology and tectonic evolution of the northern Caribbean margin. In The Caribbean Region. Edited by G. Dengo and J. E. Case. The Geological Society of America, The Geology of North America, v. H, Chapt. 4, pp. 77-140.

Linares, E. and Lobachev, A. 1971. Informe geológico sobre las investigaciones en la región Habana-Matanzas. Oficina Nacional de Recursos Minerales, La Habana, Cuba. Investigación 295. Unpublished.

Llanes Castro, A. I., Santa Cruz Pacheco, M., García Cádiz, I., Morales Quintana, A. and Palacio Alvarado, B. 1997. Petrología y mineralización de la asociación ofiolítica en la región Habana-Matanzas. Instituto de Geología y Paleontología, La Habana, Cuba. Unpublished.

Luna, J. A., Padró, T. and Geli, B. I. 1992. Informe Prospección Detallada, Cobre Zona Sur. Oficina Nacional de Recursos Minerales. Ministerio de Industria Básica, Ciudad de La Habana, Cuba. Unpublished.

Luna, J. A. 1994. Características del yacimiento El Cobre y su campo menífero. Programas y Resúmenes, Segundo Congreso Cubano de Geología y Minería, Santiago de Cuba. p. 104.

Malfait, B. T. And Dinkelman, M. G. 1972. Circum-Caribbean tectonic and igneous activity and the evolution of the Caribbean Plate. Geological Society of America Bulletin, v. 83, pp. 251-272.

Meyerhoff, A. A., Hatten, M. G. and Norton, P. 1957. Reporte sobre la mina Margot. Oficina Nacional de Recursos Minerales, La Habana, Cuba. Investigación 971. Unpublished.

Millán, G. and Somin, M. 1985. Contribución al conocimiento geológico de las metamorfitas del Escambray y Purial. Academia de Ciencias de Cuba, reporte de Investigación, No. 2, Ciudad de La Habana, Cuba. pp. 1-74.

Morales, A. and Arzuaga, H. 1994. Perspectivas Metalíferas de la Región Habana-Matanzas. Memorias del II Congreso Cubano de Geología y Minería, Santiago de Cuba. Pp. 1-10.

Moreira, J., Zafra, J. and Montano, J. 1999. Modelos de depósitos minerales existentes o inferidos de existir en la región Oriental de Cuba. Instituto de Geología y Paleontología, Ciudad de La Habana, Cuba. Unpublished.

Morris, A. E. L., Taner, I., Meyerhoff, H. A. and Meyerhoff, A. A. 1990. Tectonic evolution of the Carribbean region; Alternative hypothesis. In The Caribbean Region. Edited by G. Dengo and J. E. Case. The Geological Society of America, The Geology of North America, v. H, Chapt. 17, pp. 433-458.

Nicolaiev, A., Nuñez, A., Meretskov, S., Sánchez, R., Skorina, P., Cordovés, R., Demidov, V., Reborido, J. and Rosales, C. 1981. Sobre los resultados de los trabajos de búsqueda y levantamiento geológico en escala 1:100,000 en las montañas de Sierra de Purial, al norte de la provincia Guantánamo. Oficina Nacional de Recursos Minerales, Ministerio de la Industria Básica, Ciudad de La Habana, Cuba. Unpublished.

Oficina Nacional de Recursos Minerales. 1998. Balance Nacional de Reservas Minerales, Estado al 1-1-98, Metálicos. Ministerio de la Industria Básica, La Habana, Cuba.

Pardo, M., Millán, G., Alvarez, H., Rodriguez, A. and Lavandero, R. 1994. La Mineralización Endógena Asociada al Proceso Metamórfico del Macizo Escambray. Memorias del II Congreso Cubano de Geología y Minería, Santiago de Cuba, pp. 1-11.

Penteleyi, I. and García, A. 1990. Informe sobre los resultados del levantamiento geológico complejo, poligono IV CAME, Holguín, Cuba. Oficina Nacional de Recursos Minerales, Ministerio de la Industria Básica, Ciudad de La Habana, Cuba. Unpublished.

Pindell, J. L. and Dewey, J. F. 1982. Permo-Triassic reconstruction of western Pangea and the evolution of the Gulf of Mexico/Caribbean region. Tectonics, v. 1, pp. 179-211.

Pindell, J. L. and Barrett, S. F. 1990. Geological evolution of the Caribbean region; A plate-tectonic perspective. In The Caribbean Region. Edited by G. Dengo and J. E. Case. The Geological Society of America, The Geology of North America, v. H, Chapt. 16, pp. 405-432.

Piotrowska, K., Pszczolkowski, A., Piotrowski, J., Myczynski, R, Rudnicki, J., Kusniarski, N., Peñalver, L. L., Franco, G. L., Perez, N. and Albear, J. F. 1981. Texto explicativo del mapa geológico escala 1:250,000 de la provincia de Matanzas. Instituto de Geología y Paleontología, La Habana, Cuba. Investigación No. 536, Unpublished.

Porro, A. 1994. Geología del yacimiento de menas polimetálicas Infierno en la parte occidental de La Sierra Maestra. Programas y Resumenes, Segundo Congreso Cubano de Geología y Minería, Santiago de Cuba.

Renne, P. R., Matinson, J. M., Hatten, C. W., Somin, M., Onstott, T. C., Millán G. and Linares. E. 1989. 40Ar/39Ar and U-Pb evidence for Late Proterozoic (Grenville age) continental crust in North Central Cuba and regional tectonic implications. Precambrian Research, v. 42, pp. 325-341.

Rosencrantz, E. 1996. Basement structure and tectonics in the Yucatan basin. In Ofiolitas y Arcos Volcánicos de Cuba. Edited by M. A. Iturralde-Vinent. IUGS/UNESCA International Geological Correlation Programe, Project 364,

Contribution No. 1, Chap. 1, pp. 36-47.

Russell, N. and Kesler, S. E. 1991. Geology of the maar-diatreme complex hosting precious metal mineralization at Pueblo Viejo, Dominican Republic. In Geologic and Tectonic Development of the North America-Caribbean Plate Boundary in Hispaniola. Edited by P. Mann, G. Draper and J. F. Lewis. The Geological Society of America, Special Paper 262, pp. 203-215.

Salvador, A. and Green, A. G. 1980. Opening of the Caribbean Tethys, in Auboin, J., coordinator, Geology of the Alpine chains born of the Tethys. Bureau de recherches Géologiques et Miniéres, Memoire 115, pp. 224-229.

Santa Cruz Pacheco, M., Díaz de Villalvilla, L., Palacios, B., Pérez, M., Miliá, I. and Domínguez, E. 1997. Estudio mineralógico y petrográfico en la parte norte del sector "Los Mangos" del prospecto San Fernando, Provincia Villa Clara. Instituto de Geología y Paleontología, La Habana, Cuba. Unpublished.

Simon, G., Kesler, S. E., Russell, N., Hall, C. M., Bell, D. and Piñero, E. 1999. Epithermal Gold Mineralization in an old Volcanic Arc: The Jacinto Deposit, Camagüey District, Cuba. Economic Geology, v. 94, No. 4, pp. 487-506.

Simón Méndez, A. 1992. La evolución metalogénica del territorio cubano. Instituto de Geología y Paleontología, La Habana, Cuba. Unpublished manuscript.

Somin, M. L. and Millán, G. 1976. Some features of the structure of the metamorphic sequences of Cuba. Geotektonica, v. 5, pp. 270-275.

Somin, M. L. and Millán, G, 1981. Geology of the metamorphic complexes of Cuba (in Russian). Moscow, Nauka, 219p.

Stanik, E., Manour, J., Ching, R. and Vasquez, C. 1981. Informe de los levantamientos geológicos, geoquímicos y geofísicos realizados en la parte sur de Cuba Central en las provincias de Cienfuegos, Sancti Spiritus y Villa Clara. Oficina Nacional de Recursos Minerales, Ministerio de la Industria Básica, Ciudad de La Habana, Cuba. Unpublished.

Svoboda, V. 1966. Informe final sobre la búsqueda de yacimientos en la provincia de Oriente. Oficina Nacional de Recursos Minerales, Ministerio de la Industria Básica, Ciudad de La Habana, Cuba. Unpublished.

Sykes, L. R., McCann, W. R. and Kafka, A. L. 1982. Motion of the Caribbean plate during the last 7 million years and implications for earlier Cenozoic movements. Journal of geophysical Research, v. 87, pp. 656-676.

Tolkunov, A. E., Bolotin, Y. A., Cabrera, R., Maximov, A. and Zarianov, D. P. 1974a. Regularidades de la distribución y condiciones de formación de los yacimientos tipo "Lentes Piritosos" en el anticlinorio de Trinidad. In Geología de los yacimientos minerales útiles de Cuba, Academia de Ciencias de Cuba, Special Publication No. 3, pp. 62-81.

Tolkunov, A. E., Malinovski, E. P., Cabrera, R. and Carrassou, G. 1974b. Característcas comparativas de los yacimientos de cobre de Cuba. In Geología de los yacimientos minerales útiles de Cuba, Academia de Ciencias de Cuba, Special Publication No. 3, pp. 7-61.

Walper, J. L. 1980. The tectonic-sedimentary history of Caribbean basins and their hydrocarbon potential. Canadian Society of Petroleum Geologists, Memoir No. 6, pp. 887-911.

Wassal, H. 1956. Bacuranao and Cruz Verde oil fields. Oficina Nacional de Recursos Minerales, La Habana, Cuba. Investigación No. 851. Unpublished.

White, G. W. and Burke, K. 1980. Outline of the tectonic evolution of the Gulf of Mexico and the Caribbean region. Houston Geological Society Bulletin, v. 22, pp. 8-13.

LOS MANGOS - SAN FERNANDO DEPOSIT, SANTA CLARA, CUBA, GEOLOGY AND MINERALIZATION IN A CRETACEOUS VOLCANIC ARC

TERENCE J. BOTTRILL
Bottrill Geological Services, 192 Weldon Avenue, Oakville, Canada L6K 2H8 (botgeol@istar.ca)

FRANCISCO FORMELL CORTINA
GeoMinera, S.A., Havana , Cuba

K. SETHU RAMAN
Holmer Gold Mines Limited, 1103-121 Richmond Street West, Toronto, Ontario M5H 2K1 (info@holmergold.com)

ABSTRACT

Los Mangos - San Fernando is a volcanogenic massive sulphide deposit within the Cretaceous Los Pasos Formation, one of a series of similar deposits within the Manicaragua district. The host rocks are part of a volcanic arc which accreted with the southern margin of the North American continent in the Eocene. The deposit lies at the contact between a hangingwall basalt lapilli-tuff with sub-ordinate andesite-basalt flows and an underlying sequence of felsic lapilli-tuffs, ash-tuffs and minor mixed tuffs. There are other base and precious metal sulphide showings in the surrounding area which have similar characteristics to the Los Mangos - San Fernando deposit, but which have had only minor exploration. The volcanic sequence in the district centred on the deposit and enclosing these other showings is considerably thicker compared with sections along strike to both east and west, is intruded by a synvolcanic body of diorite and appears to have been deposited in a local constructional volcano. Regional metamorphism is of lower greenschist or sub-greenschist facies.

The Los Mangos - San Fernando deposit consists of at least five discrete horizons within a 50 metre thick, felsic lapilli-tuff which lies close to the contact with overlying basaltic lapilli-tuff and minor flows. The sulphides appear to have been deposited as exhalite concurrent with the felsic pyroclastic volcanism in local depressions between individual debris flows. Alternatively the mineralization may represent a form of sub-sea floor replacement as pore and clast boundary filling and glass replacement of essentially unconsolidated felsic ash-tuffs.

The footwall and mineralization hosting felsic tuffs are intensely altered to a mixture of quartz, sericite, chlorite, biotite, clay minerals and local andalusite with disseminated and veinlet pyrite, chalcopyrite and sphalerite. The hangingwall basalt unit is essentially unmineralized and unaltered except for widespread chlorite and biotite.

The deposit was mined at various times in the 19th Century and again in 1955-61 when it produced 400,000 tonnes at a grade of 2.75 % Cu, 7.0 % Zn, 3.0 g/t Au and 205 g/t Ag. There have been various phases of exploration in 1958-63, 1975-81, 1988-91 and by Holmer Gold Mines since 1994. Holmer's indicated resources have been estimated as 1,000,000 tonnes at a grade of 1.84 % Cu and 3.35 % Zn, with inferred resources of an additional 1,000,000 tonnes of similar grade.

INTRODUCTION

Los Mangos - San Fernando deposit is in the Manicaragua mineralized district, located in central Cuba, south of the city of Santa Clara, capital of Santa Clara (or Villa Clara) Province at 22° 12' 00" North and 80° 4' 30" West (Fig. 1). It is an area of rolling to locally steep hills at elevations of 85 to 245 metres above sea level. These are typically covered by dense vegetation, primarily the dry thorn maribu bush. The southern part of the area is flatter and agricultural, primarily in tobacco plantations and cattle ranching, and to the south there are small towns and agricultural villages.

Access to the district is by multi-lane paved highway from Havana to Santa Clara, along a paved road to the south to Manicaragua, to the east towards Cumanayagua and Cienfuegos and then limited to a few gravel and dirt roads to the historical Los Mangos - San Fernando mine site.

HISTORY

The Los Mangos - San Fernando deposits were discovered in 1827 and mined periodically until 1961. They were developed from a series of adits and twelve shafts, from San Fernando in the east, through Ceiba, Santa Isabela and Los Mangos to Arroyo Azul in the west, with mineralization developed down to 145 metres vertically and over a strike length of up to 200 metres east of the Los Mangos shaft on eight irregularly spaced levels mining various discrete mineralized bodies or lenses.

Past production records are incomplete, but production in 1840-1868, 1883-85 and 1942 is estimated at 15,000 tons of 17-20 % Cu, probably from supergene enriched near-surface mineralization or as hand-cobbed concentrate (Allende, 1925, 1927; Ansted, 1856; Bartlett, 1955, Bottrill, 1997; Castro, 1956, 1957; Constant, 1917; Long, et al., 1942, Pagliuchi, a, b, 1943; Pfeffer, a, b, c, 1958; Ramagosa, undated). Most of this production came from the upper levels on the south side near the Los Mangos and Santa Isabela shafts.

The property was examined and reported on favourably by many geologists in the late 1890's and early 1900's, including by E. G. Spilsbury (1884), N. S. Shaler (1903), M. B. Yung (1906), A. S. Dwight (1908), C. M. Weld (1916) and H. F. Henderson (1916). The mine was dewatered in 1903 and then again in 1915-1916, the latter involving re-opening 900 m of old workings and 150 m of new headings (Constant, 1917, Pagliuchi, 1943).

In 1942, the San Fernando shaft was explored to the 29.5 metre level, with drifts on the 15.8, 19.2, and 25 metre levels (Long, W., Seymour, O. G., 1942). The mine was visited by many geologists including Thayer, Giles, Hawkes, and C.F. Parks of the USGS. In 1943 the Santa Isabela shaft was dewatered in an unsuccessful attempt to find a nine metre thick shoot reported at the 58.5 metre level of an unidentified shaft.

Following a drill program in 1953, the Santa Isabela and Los Mangos workings were rehabilitated to a depth of 36.6 metres and new (unstated) reserves were discovered with average drill grades of 3.2 % Cu and 9.7 % Zn. A flotation plant of 50 tons per day was opened in 1955, increased later to 100 t/d (possibly in 1956) and to 300 t/d in 1958 and continued at this rate until the closure of the mine in 1961. There are no actual recorded final production figures but at full production of 350 days per year this would total 400,000 tons at grades of 2.5 to 3.0 % Cu, 6.0 to 8.0 % Zn, 2.0 to 4.0 g/t Au and 100 to 300 g/t Ag, with recoveries of 89 % Cu, 80 % Zn and 40 % Au and Ag. Total mined tonnage is not recorded but there were no mineable reserves left in 1961.

In 1958-63 a combined team from the Soviet Union and Cuba (Gorielov, 1964) carried out a program of underground drifting (667 m) and drilling (3,419 m) from the Los Mangos shaft as well as six surface diamond drill holes (1,175 m) in an attempt to locate reserves sufficient for a 90,000 t/y plant. They explored on the 66 metre level to the south with drilling towards the west and on the 170 metre level where they drifted to the east beneath the area of the historical Ceiba shaft to as far as the San Fernando shaft, with limited fan drilling from these headings. Although they concluded that they failed to find any mineralization, they in fact intersected the down-faulted northern extension of the mineralization from station C-1 to the north of the historical workings (Table 1). The majority of the development was in the barren footwall felsic pyroclastic unit and interbedded mafic units, and nowhere near what is now understood to be the stratigraphic horizon which hosts the bedded sulphide mineralization.

The area including the present project was explored as part of a joint Cuban-Czechoslovak 1:100,000 regional, geological and geochemical program from 1975 to 1981, which resulted in the identification of numerous anomalies in the larger region. The Cubans undertook a follow-up program in 1988 which resulted in the identification of various anomalous zones including San Joaquin, Santa Rosa and Loma Chivo (Fig. 2).

Further drilling in the area of the mine in 1988-1991 by a Cuban-Bulgarian joint-venture resulted in the calculation of a resource in the area of the historical deposit (Arcial, et al., 1991).

Since 1994, Holmer has undertaken an airborne magnetic and electromagnetic survey over the original concession from GeoMinera in February, 1994; completed ground geophysical surveys of 30 km of VLF-EM on eight grids and 4.775 km of induced polarisation-resistivity surveys on three grids in 1995; surveyed total field magnetics and MaxMin II horizontal loop electromagnetics ("HLEM") over 18 km on 24 lines in the Los Mangos - San Fernando area in November 1996 and April 1997; taken selected soil samples for geochemistry, primarily for gold, in 1995; and completed programs of diamond drilling totalling 4,040.9 metres in 26 holes (Arcial, 1995; Bottrill, 1995, 1996; Formell, 1997; Rodríguez, 1998; Santa Cruz, et al., 1997).

General geology of Cuba

The geology of Cuba is relatively simple (Fig. 1), as a volcanic island arc which accreted with the southern edge of the North American craton seen in five litho-stratigraphic belts, from north to south across the island (Iturralde-Vinent, a, b, c, 1996; Iturralde-Vinent, et al., 1996; Kerr, et al., 1999; Lewis and Draper, 1990; Pushcharovsky, 1989).

1. The north side of the island from the west of

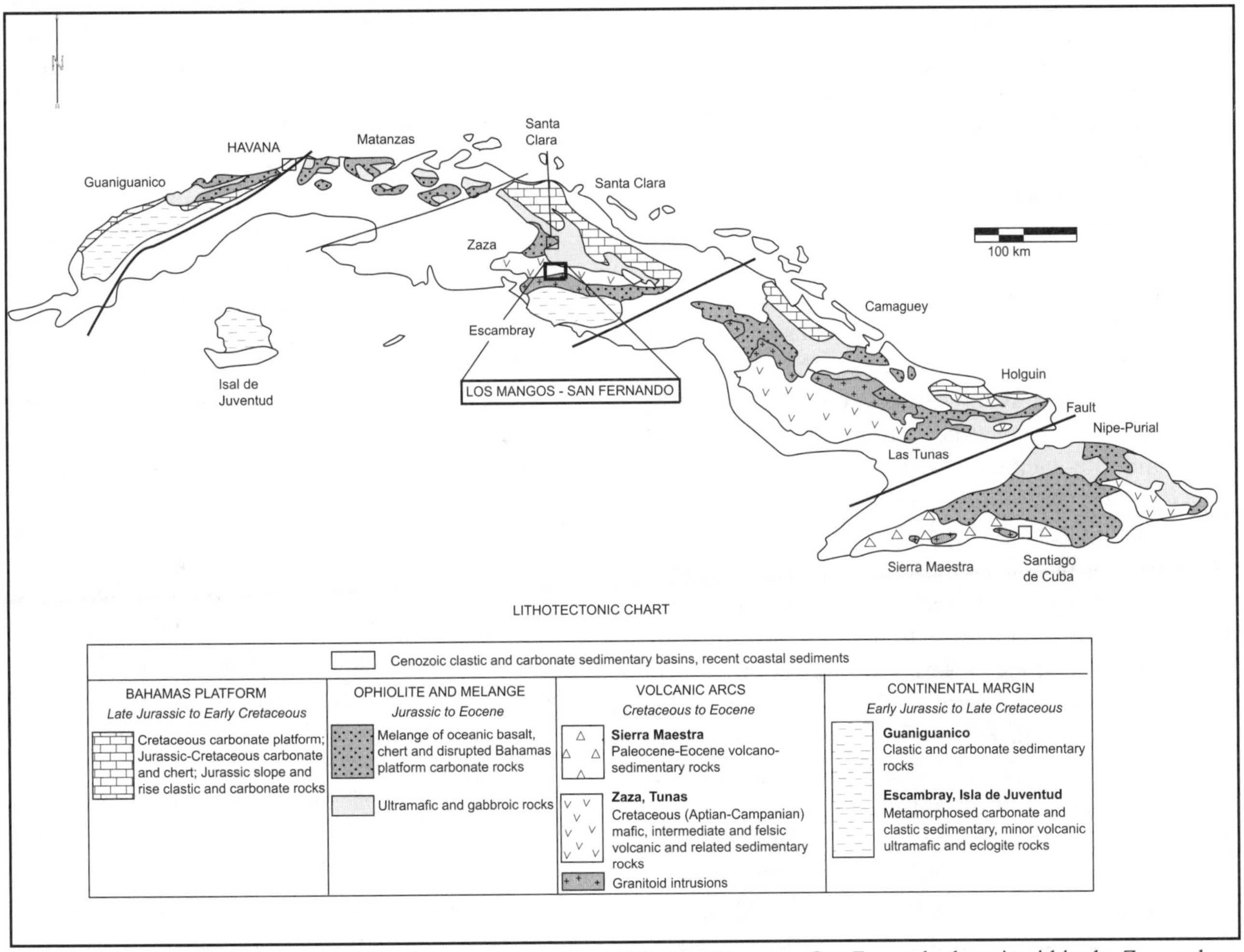

Figure 1. The general geology of Cuba showing the location of the Los Mangos - San Fernando deposit within the Zaza volcanic arc north of the Manicaragua batholith, within the lithotectonic framework for the island of the various litho-stratigraphic assemblages of the Bahamas Platform, the ophiolite and melange sequence, the Zaza and Sierra Maestra volcanic arcs and the exotic continental margin assemblage in the south and west.

Havana to about mid-way along the coast, exposes the edge of the North American craton in the Jurassic and Cretaceous carbonates of the Bahamas Platform. Three distinct zones are identified with progressively increasing chert and continental clastic rocks to the south which correspond to the shelf, slope and rise facies of the original continental margin sedimentary wedge. These are all overlain by Palaeocene and Eocene carbonate block olistostromes with accompanying ophiolite blocks.

2. Ophiolite melange sequences are exposed as south dipping wedges, with intervening bands of Bahamas platform carbonates, or as melanges or olistostromes and were probably obducted onto or are in strike-slip fault contact with the edge of the North American craton. They consist of dunite, harzburgite, gabbro and sheeted diabase dykes, with overlying tholeiitic basalts, cherts and abyssal sedimentary rocks. At the far east of the island they form shallow north dipping sheets or flat synclines which contain large lateritic nickel deposits.
3. Island-arc and back-arc sequences of Late to Early (Aptian-Campanian) Cretaceous calc-alkaline "Zaza Arc" volcanic rocks are exposed as tilted wedges younging to the north from basal mafic, basaltic-andesite flows and flow-breccias upwards through intermediate andesite-dacite, to local felsic dacite-rhyolites. The arc was formed above a north-dipping subduction zone in its present orientation during its formation somewhere in the original Cretaceous Caribbean plate to the south and was later brought into contact with North America along a series of transform faults, probably during anti-clockwise rotation of the Caribbean plate. An amphibolitic blueschist terrain, traditionally included as part of the Escambray metamorphic complex, underlies this Zaza arc. The arc volcanic rocks are intruded granite, quartz-diorite, tonalite and syenite batholiths. The intrusions in the Los Mangos - San Fernando area appear to under plate the volcanic sequence, intruding the Escambray blueschist terrain, whereas those further to the east in the Camagüey area cross-cut the marine volcanic stratigraphy and appear to be related to the later stages of evolution of the arc and are comagmatic with locally extensive felsic volcanic rocks.
4. Sequences of Jurassic and Cretaceous clastic and carbonate sedimentary rocks form the majority of the westernmost part of Cuba, the Isla de la Juventud and the Escambray Massif to the south of Los Mangos - San Fernando. These rocks are very similar to the Caracas Formation along the coast of Venezuela, and are possibly rifted sections of the margin of the South American craton. They have been subjected to high temperature-low pressure metamorphism on Isla de la Juventud, with evidence for a large underlying granitoid. In the Escambray Massif they are of high pressure, low temperature facies, as subduction wedges, and were probably metamorphosed in the north dipping subduction zone beneath the volcanic island arc. In the exposures close to the west end of the island these Mesozoic sedimentary sequences are intermediate pressure and temperature facies as slates and shales in a series of thrust fault slices, which host a variety of sedimentary-exhalative base metal deposits.
5. The Sierra Maestra, in the southeast of the island, is a Palaeocene volcanic island arc, with post-arc volcaniclastic and sedimentary rocks to the immediate north, intruded by Palaeocene granitoids.

These litho-stratigraphic belts are exposed in a series of tectonic blocks, separated by east-northeast striking faults which are overlain by thick, post orogenic, Cenozoic sedimentary basins (Fig. 1). Each tectonic block varies in its age of collision with the Bahamas platform, with the initial collision at the west end, and progressing to the east. This west to east progression in the timing of collision may be a reflection of anti-clockwise rotation of the Caribbean plate relative to the North American craton. The collision appears to have begun whilst the Zaza volcanic arc was still being actively developed along the corresponding subduction zone. The section at the west end is relatively incomplete as an arc, consisting mostly of basal mafic volcanic units, so that its formation appears to have been terminated by the early collision and truncation of the corresponding subduction zone. Those sections in the centre of the island in the Santa Clara block exposure a more completely developed arc including some relatively aerially restricted upper felsic units, co-magmatic batholiths intruding the deeper stratigraphic units at the base of the arc in the blueschist terrain of the Escambray Massif - and volcanogenic massive sulphide deposits. Those Zaza arc sections further to the east in the Camagüey-Holguin blocks are the most complete, including extensive younger felsic volcanic units, more extensive co-magmatic intrusions, extensive volcanic-derived sedimentary basins - and a spectrum of mineral deposits including representatives of porphyry-copper deposits, skarns and epithermal precious metal systems. The final collision was at the east end of the island with the youngest, and least deformed ocean floor sequence in the Nipe-Purial ophiolites and the youngest volcanic arc in the Sierra Maestra. There is a progression in styles of deformation from west to east, corresponding to the age of collision and the formation and preservation of more complete sections of the arc, with the most complex structures (primarily anastomosing thrust and strike slip fault duplexes) in the west, through relatively simple tilted homoclinal blocks with block-faulted basins in the centre, to essentially upright, weakly deformed sequences at the east end.

Local geology

The immediate area around the Los Mangos - San Fernando deposit is underlain predominantly by a north-dipping homoclinal sequence of Cretaceous marine volcanic rocks and their hypabyssal sub-volcanic intrusive equivalents of the Zaza volcanic arc, intruded along the south side by the Manicaragua batholith (Fig. 2). Outcrop is generally very poor although the soil cover is typically shallow. There is considerable difficulty in locating natural outcrops due to the dense thorn bush.

Stratigraphy

The volcanic rocks are part of the regional Mahagua Group of mafic to intermediate lavas and pyroclastic rocks, minor limestones and interbedded clastic and volcaniclastic sedimentary rocks. At a more local scale (Fig. 2) the sequence is divided into two formations. The lower is the Los Pasos Formation of bimodal marine felsic and mafic volcanic units with some evidence of subaerial input, which hosts the mineralization. The upper is the Relámpago Formation of dominantly mafic volcanic rocks, both flows and pyroclastics, with some interbedded clastic sedimentary rocks.

Within the Los Pasos Formation there are a series of distinct volcanic cycles from basal basalt flows, locally pillowed, through basaltic-andesites, as flows and pyroclastic rocks, into overlying felsic volcanic rocks, mostly pyroclastic. There are local felsic flows or rhyolite domes which appear to be flanked on their margins by coarse felsic debris flows. There are at least three mappable cycles in those areas where the stratigraphy has not been intensely altered or disrupted by faulting. Large areas within the district as shown on figure 2 are underlain by relatively homogeneous silicic-clay rich rocks from extensive re-charge hydrothermal silica and sericite alteration in the footwall of the various mineralized horizons, so that the individual volcanic units can no longer be distinguished.

In general the Los Pasos Formation thickens towards the centre of the area, as do individual mappable units, indicating deposition in an original volcanic constructional feature. It is not possible to determine whether this is a depositional basin or an original constructional strata-volcano.

In the immediate area of the Los Mangos - San Fernando deposit (Fig. 3) there are four main stratigraphic units from bottom to top:

a. A local basal unit of predominantly rhyolite and dacite lapilli tuff with abundant coarse ash lapilli tuffs and local coarse and fine ash tuffs at least 200 metres thick. This unit hosts only minor sulphides, mostly pyrite, accompanied by relatively weak hydrothermal alteration. These felsic units are interbedded with or intruded by minor predominantly porphyritic, but locally massive intermediate to mafic units as flows or sills, as well as heterogeneous intermediate tuff breccias, both in beds which are typically 10 to15 metres thick.
b. A distinct, mineralization-hosting unit, approx-

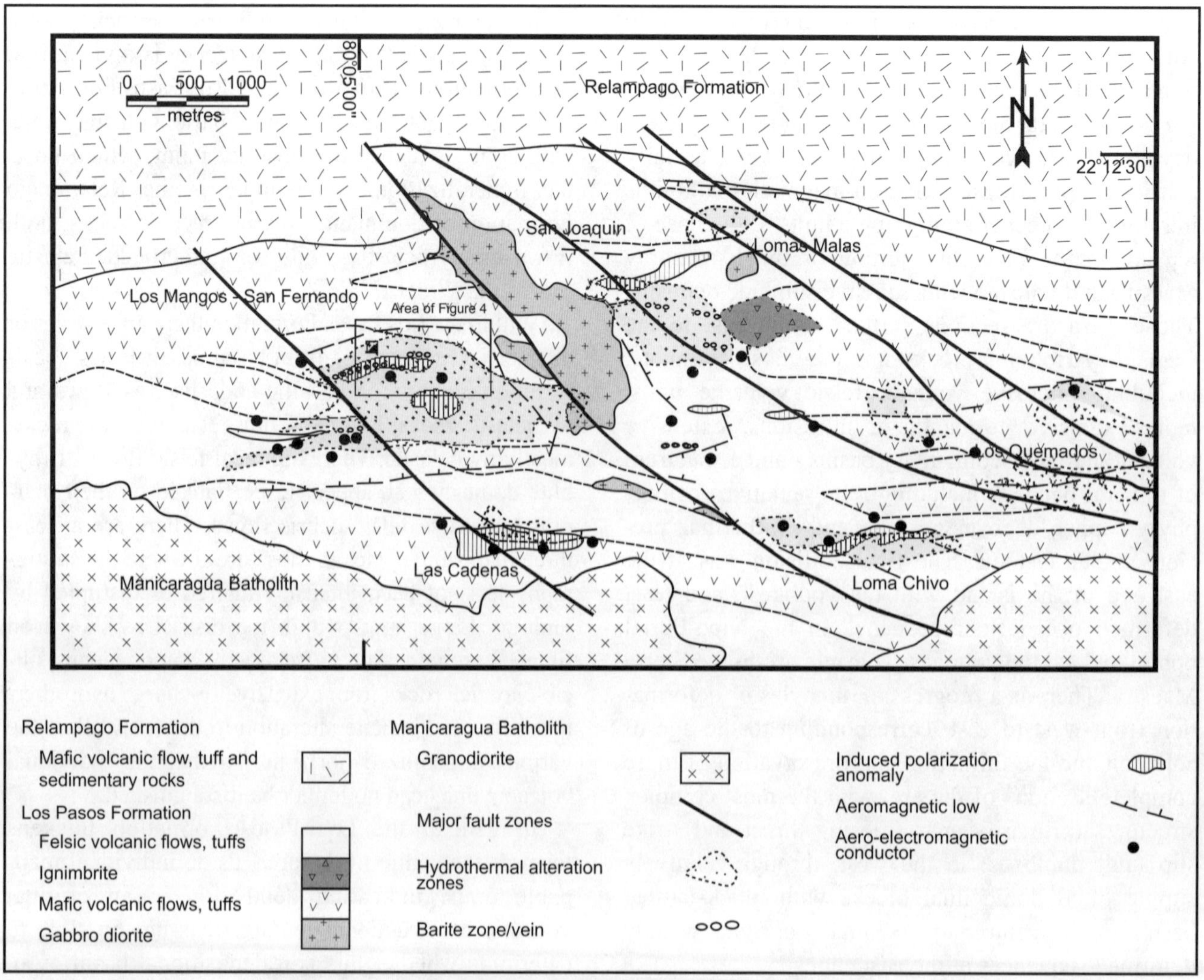

Figure 2. The geology, alteration zones, mineral occurrences and exploration features within the Los Mangos - San Fernando section of the Manicaragua district. The mineral showings are identified through a combination of their location at felsic to mafic volcanic contacts, together with associated alteration as described in the text, a general distribution within broad areas of low magnetic amplitude and localised induced polarisation anomalies.

imately 50 metres thick, consisting of beds similar to those in the underlying unit of coarse ash-lapilli rhyolites and dacites with minor finer ash tuffs and interbedded with thinner mafic flows or sills. The overall distribution of individual volcanic units appears to be more irregular with thinner and less extensive individual beds than in the underlying unit. No distinct cyclical arrangement can be established between either the coarse and fine felsic beds, or between them and the more mafic and mixed pyroclastic beds or layers. Rather they represent an almost random infilling of a local depositional feature from distinct sources, probably deposited at the same time as, or very shortly before, deposition of the sulphide mineralization.

c. A 15 to 30 metre thick rhyolite-dacite fine ash tuff overlying the mineralized unit, developed mostly down dip and towards the east.

d. An upper unit, at least 150 metres thick, of predominantly basalt to andesite-basalt lithic lapilli tuffs, with intercalations of fine grained basalt tuffs and minor basalt flows. This unit forms the majority of the outcrop in the area of

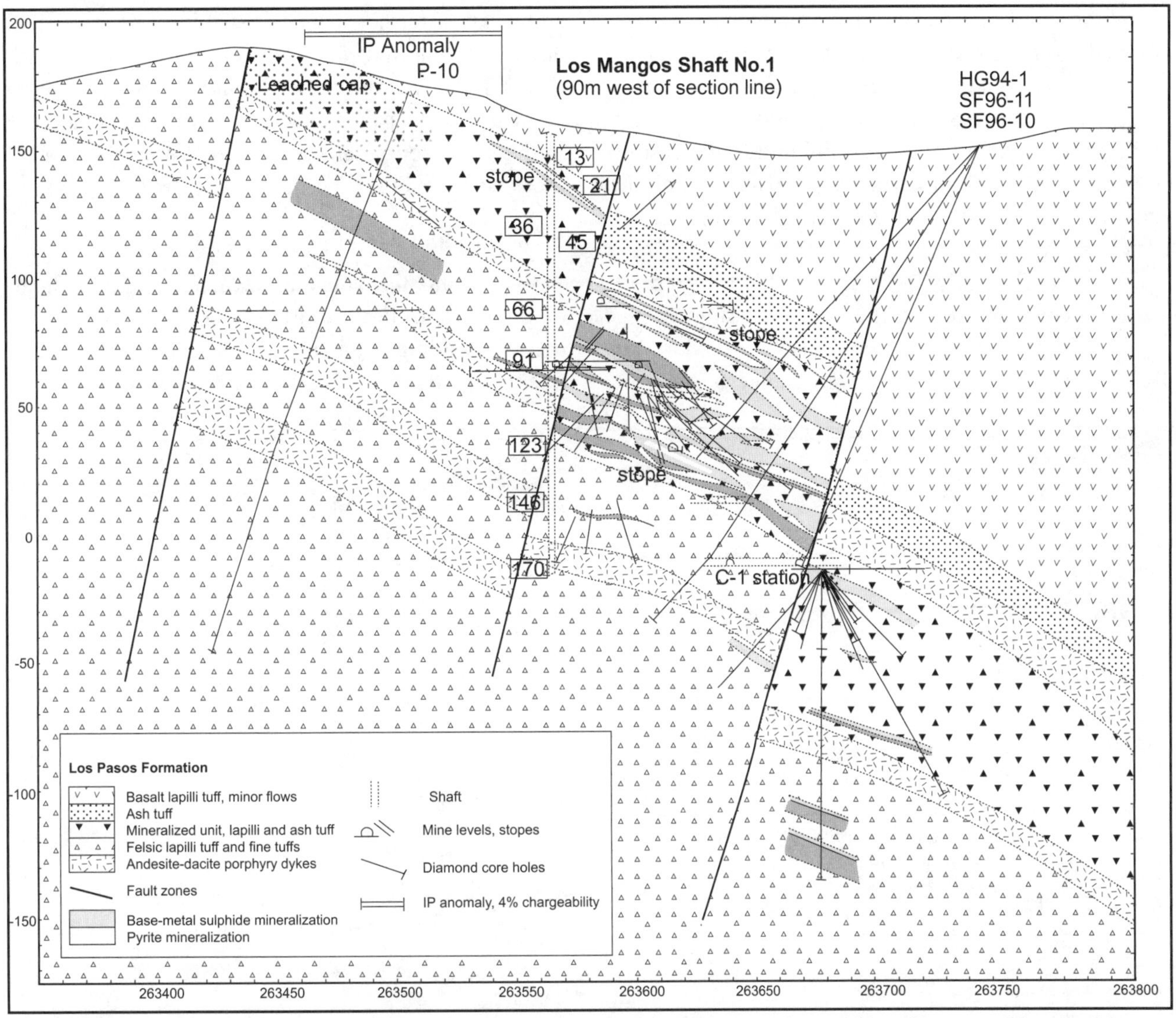

Figure 3. A typical cross-section along line 263,750 East. It is based on the intersections within a 30 metre wide strip, 15 metres on either side of the section line. The Los Mangos No. 1 shaft is 90 metres west of the section, with development on shallow levels (-13 to -45 m) to the south and at deeper levels (-66 to below the -123 m level) on either side of one of the steeply south dipping northwest striking faults. A third mineralized block extends north of a second, parallel fault and has been tested by historical underground drilling to a depth of 300 metres. The sulphide mineralization extends down dip from the leached-cap outcrop within the 50 metre thick uppermost felsic lapilli and ash tuff unit beneath the basalt lapilli tuff unit. While much of the sulphide mineralization is within small lenses these tend to lie on five main horizons with locally distinct pyrite bodies, typically in the footwall of the base metal sulphides. The three recent holes on this section cut various of these horizons down-dip of the historically exploited sulphide horizons.

the Los Mangos and San Fernando shafts. Much of it has the appearance of a mafic feldspar porphyry, similar to those intruding the basal felsic unit, but here these porphyritic bodies form a far larger proportion of the stratigraphic sequence as seen in the core intersections.

Intrusions

The south side of the volcanic sequence is in contact with the Manicaragua batholith, a composite Late Cretaceous granite, granodiorite, quartz-diorite and syenite pluton.

Within the Los Pasos Formation there are a series of small composite intrusions of gabbro and diorite, probable sub-volcanic and hypabyssal bodies related to the volcanic rocks which they intrude. The largest of these forms a northwest-striking unit to the east of the Los Mangos - San Fernando deposit, possibly in the centre of the original depositional basin or constructional volcano.

There are locally extensive dyke swarms of various compositions primarily intruding along the northwest fault set, possibly as feeders of Relámpago Formation. There are numerous north-south and north-northwest striking, near-vertical andesite-dacite porphyry dykes as well as basalt dykes in the area of the Los Mangos - San Fernando deposit. Most of these are relatively narrow and are individually too small to show on either the typical cross-section (Fig. 3) or the geology map (Fig. 4).

Structure and Metamorphism

In general the volcanic sequence is homoclinal, dipping to the north at 30° to 70°. There is no evidence of folding or any major stratigraphic repetitions due to thrusts.

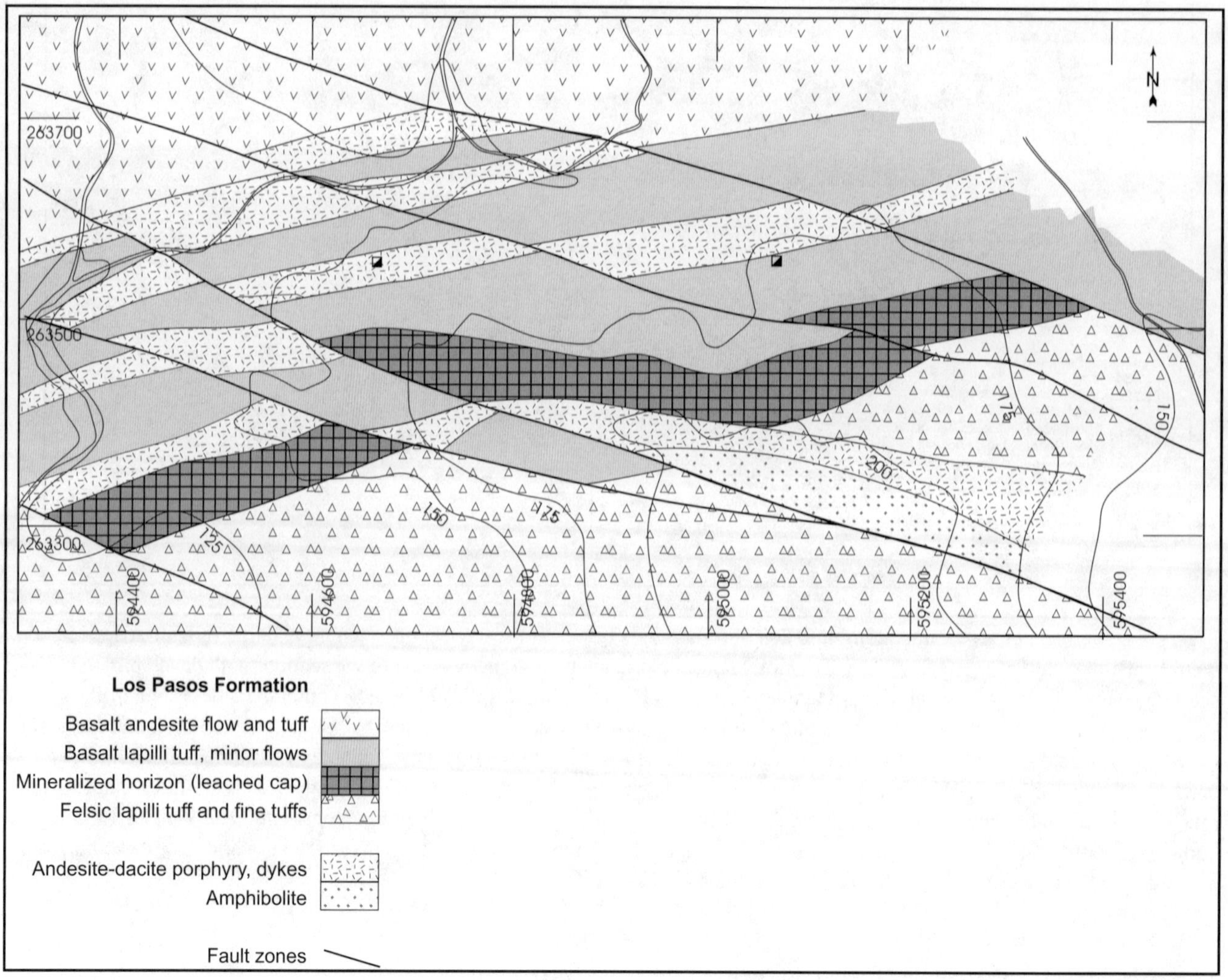

Figure 4. Interpreted distribution of the major lithological units in the Los Mangos - San Fernando deposit. The mineralized zone is seen at surface as a zone of deep iron oxide development or a leached cap, dipping to the north at shallow angles. It is underlain by a sequence of predominantly coarse felsic pyroclastic rocks and overlain immediately by basalt lapilli tuff with predominant flows and finer tuffs to the north. The entire sequence is separated by a series of northwest striking faults.

Both the volcanic and intrusive rocks are cut by a braided network of close-spaced faults and wider deformation zones, primarily striking northwest, with a less clearly defined northeast striking set. The predominant northwest striking set, known as the Cachimba faults, are nearly vertical, and appear to be curvilinear, concave to the southwest. These form areas of deformation and cataclastic fabrics which are difficult to distinguish from pyroclastic rocks due to the deep tropical weathering. Numerous other faults can be interpreted from a 1994 aeromagnetic survey.

There is a strong concentration of these Cachimba faults in the centre of the area from east of Los Mangos - San Fernando and east of the sub-volcanic gabbro-diorite body (Fig. 2), throughout the area underlain by most of the other mineral showings in the area. Off-sets appear to be both sinistral and dextral, compressional and extensional, and the net effect is neutral. In part, these northwest striking faults appear to be the result of the intrusion of the Manicaragua batholith into the base of the volcanic sequence where the Los Pasos Formation is at its thickest.

In the immediate area of Los Mangos - San Fernando these faults strike at 110°, and dip steeply at 80° to the southwest with an apparent reverse sense of motion, locally duplicating the host stratigraphy. The

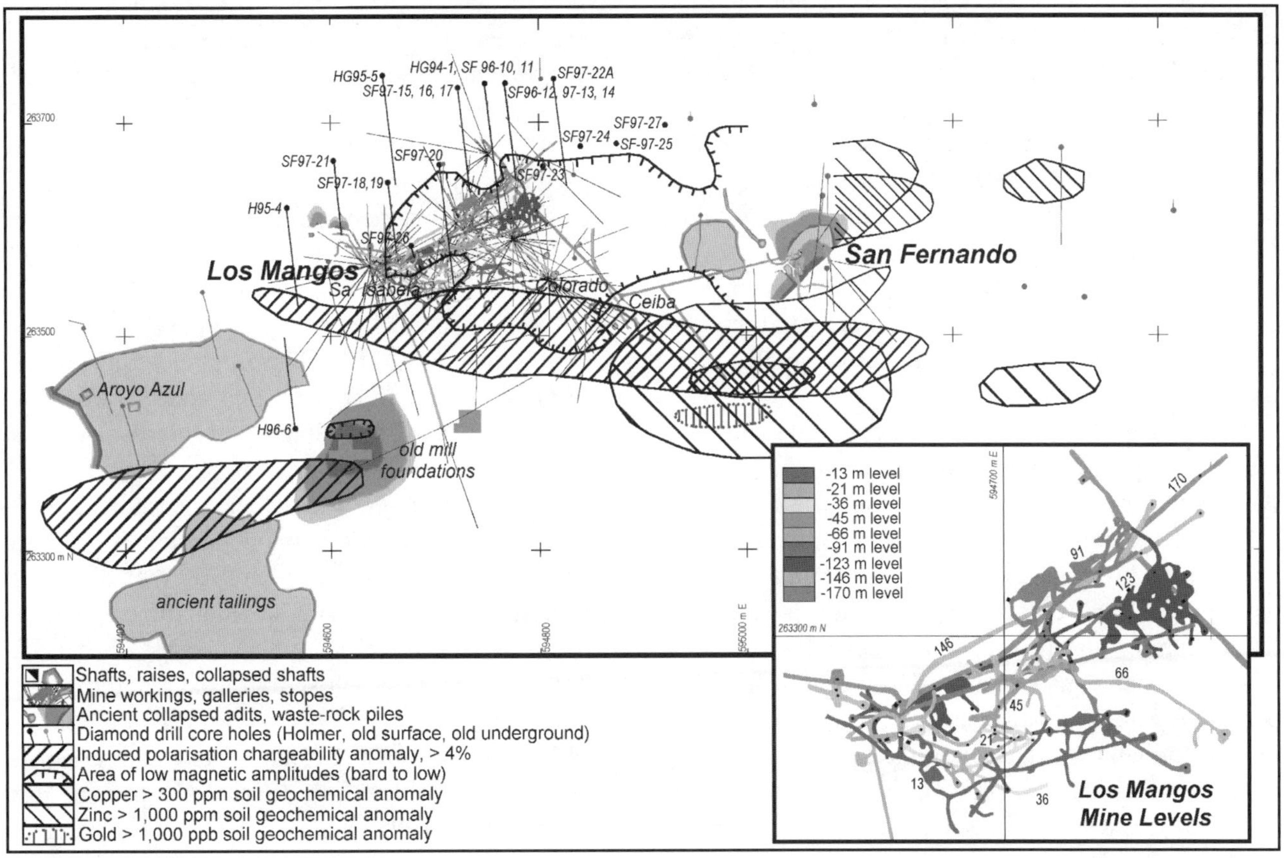

Figure 5. Distribution of the known historical mine workings and other exploration indicators in the Los Mangos - San Fernando deposit. The majority of the Los Mangos workings extend over a strike length of 200 metres and width of 100 metres and to a depth of 150 metres, with the smaller San Fernando workings a further 250 metres to the east. An exploration drive at the -170 metre level extends beneath the San Fernando workings in the footwall of the mineralized stratigraphy. The up-dip expression of the historical workings, seen as a leached cap on surface, locally corresponds with a coincident copper-zinc-gold soil geochemical anomalies. There are extensive induced-polarisation anomalies down-dip of the surface expression south of the old workings, as well as a distinct area of low magnetic amplitudes corresponding to the old workings extending to the east, open beyond the area surveyed to date and the trend of the mineralized intersections in the core drill holes.

effect of these faults on the local stratigraphy and distribution of the mineralization was not well recognised and led to an impression of a steeper apparent dip of 55° compared with the actual 30° north dips.

Although the mineralized areas contain both biotite and andalusite as alteration minerals, the majority of the area is only weakly metamorphosed, probably of sub-greenschist facies. Zeolites are observed in late stage extensional fractures.

EXPLORATION RESULTS

Geophysics

The Cuban-Bulgarian organisation completed an induced polarisation-resistivity survey over the entire concession in 1988 using unknown instruments and specifications. A series of anomalies were identified, which are summarised as metal factor and chargeability outlines for the Los Mangos - San Fernando mine area. The Cuban data indicate that different systems were used in different parts of the original survey area, with the more coherent and discrete anomalies corresponding to the area of highest potential including Los Mangos - San Fernando, San Joaquin and the northern part of Loma Chivo.

These IP anomalies appear to be discrete and correspond to specific stratigraphic targets, rather than to the areas of general pyritic alteration. The most significant IP anomaly at > 4 % chargeability lies just south of the historical Los Mangos and San Fernando workings and corresponds to the up-dip position of the main mineralized horizon, immediately down-dip of the near-surface leached cap and gossan zone (Fig. 5). A separate IP anomaly lies to the southwest, and may be the faulted extension of the same mineralized horizon, which does not outcrop in this area beneath historical waste and tailings and the river alluvium.

The Cuban-Bulgarian organisation also completed a down hole induced polarisation survey from hole 11 at depths of 52 and 92 metres, using unknown instruments, arrays or power sources. Distinct anomalies were identified to the north and south.

Holmer completed a Geoterrex fixed-wing airborne survey over the property in February 1994, collecting multi-frequency GEOTEM time-domain electromagnetic and magnetic data. The magnetic data indicate a series of east-west domains of higher magnetic amplitude, some of which correspond with mapped basalt units, as well as more irregular or elliptical highs which equate with synvolcanic gabbro bodies or with the possible rhyolite domes, with their high magnetite content. In general, it is possible to outline the individual stratigraphic units of different compositions within the magnetic data, especially from the calculated vertical gradient map. It is also possible to distinguish the numerous off-sets of these anomalies corresponding to the northwest striking faults, and other parallel lineaments.

Within the volcanic stratigraphy there are extensive areas within which the overall magnetic amplitude is substantially depressed, i.e. in which the magnetite content is reduced, possibly through alteration of magnetite to various sulphide minerals. Despite the overall lower amplitudes it is still possible to trace the individual stratigraphic units from adjacent zones of overall higher magnetic amplitude. Some of these areas of low magnetic amplitude correspond with known zones of extensive wall rock alteration, such as in the footwall of Los Mangos - San Fernando.

Numerous GEOTEM airborne electromagnetic (AEM) anomalies were identified and classified by Geoterrex as: narrow conductors of vertical extent; broad areas of shallow sources or flat lying conductive zones reflecting surface alteration and weathering; or, narrow sources of moderate amplitude and greater depth. It is typically anomalies of the latter type which correspond with sulphide mineralization. Some of the more significant AEM anomalies include those in an east-west belt south of the outcrop of the Los Mangos - San Fernando mineralized horizon.

A very low frequency electromagnetic (VLF-EM) survey was completed by Sagax Geophysics for Holmer early in 1995 over a series of connected grids covering parts of the San Fernando, San Joaquin, Santa Rosa and other unnamed targets. There is one strong anomaly which corresponds with the interpreted trace of the linear AEM conductor along the outcrop trace of the Los Mangos - San Fernando mineralized horizon.

In April 1995, JVX completed an induced polarisation-resistivity survey for Holmer covering three lines over Los Mangos, of which only the two outer lines extended to the south over the host stratigraphy. In general, the overall Los Mangos - San Fernando mineralized system is identified as a broad chargeability high and resistivity low.

In 1996-97 Holmer completed a Max-Min II and horizontal loop electromagnetic ("HLEM") and total field magnetic survey over 18 km on 24 lines in the Los Mangos - San Fernando area. The principal conductors correspond in part with the 110° striking faults which off-set the mineralized horizon. The magnetic data revealed the existence of a distinctive area of low magnetic amplitudes corresponding to the deeper part of the historical Los Mangos mine area and extending to the east towards San Fernando beyond which this anomaly is open. The magnetic low is also parallel to and down-dip from the large IP anomaly described above (Fig. 5).

Soil Geochemistry

In 1988 a Cuban-Bulgarian programme completed a soil geochemical survey which outlined significant, high amplitude anomalies in copper, zinc and barite, some of which correspond with known mineralization, and others which have no known sources. Prominent among these anomalies are those at Los Mangos - San Fernando, San Joaquin, Santa Rosa, Loma Chivo and Porfirio. Smaller anomalies include those at Las Cadenas, Loma Malas and unnamed anomalies to the east and west of Santa Rosa. The anomalies are shown as outlines at various contours of greater than 300 ppm Cu, 600 ppm Zn and 1,000 ppm Ba. Most of the significant anomalies are on or close to hill tops, and appear to be more-or-less in situ over their probable bedrock sources.

In 1995 Holmer completed limited soil sampling coverage on 100 metre spaced lines in the area south of the historical workings which outlined significant gold anomalies of 1 to 3 g/t Au as well as copper and zinc anomalies (at > 600 and >1,000 ppm, respectively) along the surface trace of the Los Mangos - San Fernando mineralized horizon (Fig. 5).

Diamond Drilling

Surface diamond drilling campaigns were completed in 1963, 1988 and 1991 by the various Cuban-Soviet, -Czechoslovakian and -Bulgarian organisations in the immediate area of the Los Mangos - San Fernando mine, totalling 6,145 metres in 25 holes. Historical drilling of 12,175 metres in 169 holes was completed in the late 1950's from underground on the 21, 66, 91 and 123 metre levels, mostly as fans of multiple holes in dip and azimuth from ten drill stations, which have proven to be difficult to interpret. During the 1958-63 program the Soviet-Cuban team completed and additional 52 underground holes totalling 3,420 metres from the drifts on the 66 and 170 metre levels. No core is available from any of the past drilling programs, which generally suffered from poor recoveries and selective assays of only the visually better mineralized intervals. The holes in the immediate area of the historical mine workings of approximately 800 metres in 46 holes formed the basis of the resource calculation using Soviet methods.

Holmer completed programs of diamond drilling totalling 4,040.9 metres in 26 holes in 1994 (1 hole), 1995 (7 holes), 1996 (3 holes), 1997 (15 holes), of which 3,337 metres in 22 holes were in the Los Mangos - San Fernando mine area (Fig. 5). The first hole (HG-94-01) was located to test the down-hole IP anomaly located north of the historical workings and intersected bedded massive to semi-massive sphalerite-rich, and locally chalcopyrite-rich mineralization on two horizons within the altered felsic lapilli tuff unit. Subsequent holes were drilled to the southwest of the historical mine; as 25 metre spaced step-outs, undercuts and over-cuts to HG-94-01, and to both the west and east along the down-dip projection of the mineralized horizon, those to the east being mostly vertical holes. The intersections to the west are mostly along the northern margin of the historical mine and intersected the extensions of the same mineralized horizons which were exploited historically. In most cases the holes were stopped within the felsic unit on entering the first one or two mineralized layers, based on the spatial relationship of the holes to the old stopes as then understood and the supposed steeper dip of the stratigraphy. Other holes entered dykes which were interpreted at the time to be a lower mafic unit stratigraphically below the felsic pyroclastic unit.

Table 1 Summary of Significant Drill Hole Intersections

Hole No.	Zone	Target	Depth (m)	Results				
				Cu %	Zn %	Ag, g/t	Au, g/t	Length,m
C-1-10	Los Mangos	170 m level	170	2.76	0.24	n/a	n/a	12.50
C-1-18	Los Mangos	170 m level	170	1.35	8.21	n/a	n/a	6.10
PE-6	Los Mangos	down hole IP	250	1.29	0.00	n/a	n/a	5.20
PE-7	Arroyo Azul	stratigraphy	185	0.18	3.33	n/a	n/a	10.00
P-5	Arroyo Azul	stratigraphy	60	0.59	13.86	n/a	n/a	1.50
P-8	Los Mangos	stratigraphy	105	2.11	0.19	n/a	n/a	1.30
		and	120	0.24	2.25	n/a	n/a	10.10
P-11A	Los Mangos	old mine	50	0.99	1.95	17.8	n/a	8.20
P-12	Los Mangos	down-dip	135	2.65	2.97	27.5	n/a	2.00
P-15	Los Mangos	down dip NE	115	0.10	1.14	<det.	n/a	3.00
P-21	San Fernando	old mine	25	1.10	0.85	13.3	n/a	8.40
P-27	San Fernando	geochem Zn	155	0.02	0.46	2.8	n/a	5.50
HG-94-01	Los Mangos	Down hole IP	130	0.97	14.40	286.5	1.60	2.75
			150	0.46	1.95	52.3	0.65	3.45
DDH-04	Los Mangos	IP anomaly	91	0.75	1.02	17.3	0.12	3.00
SF-96-10	Los Mangos	Overcut 94-01	125	3.80	12.10	104.2	0.96	4.00
SF-96-11	Los Mangos	Undercut 9401	160	1.44	1.57	33.8	0.40	4.00
SF-96-12	Los Mangos	East of 94-01	150	1.04	8.95	128.9	0.92	7.20
SF-97-13	Los Mangos	Undercut 9612	145	0.34	1.88	15.8	0.14	6.00
SF-97-15	Los Mangos	West of 94-01	140	0.04	3.42	167.5	0.77	2.00
SF-97-16	Los Mangos	Overcut 96-15	130	0.12	2.01	21.2	0.26	13.00
			145	0.77	2.30	21.0	0.37	4.00
			150	0.89	3.45	36.2	1.07	2.05
SF-97-17	Los Mangos	Undercut 9615	150	0.01	0.21	85.4	0.02	4.00
SF-97-18	Los Mangos	IP, HLEM	85	0.15	1.37	12.6	0.24	7.00
			100	0.13	1.02	34.1	0.26	15.00
SF-97-19	Los Mangos	IP, HLEM,	85	0.07	0.55	19.4	0.14	5.70
		100m west	90	0.97	1.08	30.0	0.28	2.00
		of	95	0.54	0.36	10.1	0.25	3.00
		HG-94-01	110	0.42	1.53	8.7	0.20	4.20
SF-97-20	Los Mangos	West of 94-01	80	0.15	1.81	44.2	3.05	1.90
SF-97-22A	Los Mangos	East of 94-01	130	4.83	3.84	85.4	0.81	18.50
SF-97-23	Los Mangos	East of 94-01	100	0.42	2.08	37.8	0.30	6.00
SF-97-24	Los Mangos	East of 94-01	105	9.97	8.78	214.5	1.82	3.00
SF-97-25	Los Mangos	East of 94-01	105	0.63	0.79	18.7	0.26	3.00

MINERAL DEPOSITS

Each of the mafic to felsic volcanic cycles of the Los Pasos Formation host massive sulphide mineralization zones, mostly as surface showings with the exception of those in the immediate Los Mangos - San Fernando area (Fig. 2). The lowermost cycle contains mineralization at its top in Las Cadenas and Loma Chivo zones. The most extensive middle cycle contains Los Mangos - San Fernando in the west, San Joaquin in the centre and the Santa Rosa and Los Quemados in the east. The immediate area around and to the southwest of Los Mangos - San Fernando contains two locally developed cycles which may be separate stratigraphic horizons or represent structural repetition of this middle cycle. The uppermost cycle contains Loma Malas at the top of the thickest section of the Los Pasos Formation.

The major deposit is in the area around the small, past-producing Los Mangos - San Fernando mine. This is a volcanogenic massive sulphide deposit in three distinct mineralogical facies of massive chalcopyrite, bedded, typically weakly to strongly disseminated sphalerite-pyrite-chalcopyrite and barren pyrite. The first two contain significant by-product silver and gold.

Mineralogy

The principal sulphide occurrences are as veins and disseminations, primarily as pyrite with locally predominant sphalerite and/or chalcopyrite, with local and rare tetrahedrite, galena, pyrrhotite, arsenopyrite and bornite. The gangue minerals are mainly quartz, sericite, and minor chlorite.

Three distinct sulphide assemblages have been recognized:

1. Massive, 30-70 % densely disseminated, veined and mottled chalcopyrite, 4-50 % pyrite, < 1 % tetrahedrite and <1 to 25 % sphalerite. The characteristic sulphide textures are anhedral-granular, corroded or as cement. The main gangue minerals are quartz, sericite and chlorite.
2. Grey or semi-black zones of sphalerite > pyrite > chalcopyrite with minor tetrahedrite - chalcopyrite - pyrrhotite - galena - bornite - arsenopyrite. They are densely disseminated, spotted and veined in the east, changing to principally disseminated mineralization toward the west. Sphalerite is the principal mineral at 12-60 % in the densely disseminated ores and much less (up to < 1 %) in the weaker disseminated zones. There is 2-48 % pyrite, 3-22 % chalcopyrite and rare grains up to < 1 % of galena; there are even rarer grains of tetrahedrite, arsenopyrite, pyrrhotite and bornite. The predominant sulphide textures are subhedral-granular, anhedral-granular and corroded. The principal gangue minerals are quartz, sericite and chlorite.
3. Pyrite » chalcopyrite » sphalerite, as disseminated to densely disseminated and veins of 2 to 80 % pyrite, rare marcasite and very rare sphalerite, chalcopyrite, tetrahedrite and galena. Textures are predominantly euhedral and anhedral-granular.

No distinguishable mineral zoning as in Cu:Zn ratios or chalcopyrite:sphalerite ratios can be established from the available data. Whereas individual samples or intersections represent close to end members of the chalcopyrite or sphalerite rich assemblages, most typically contain both. The pyrite mineralization is more extensive than either of the the base metal sulphide assemblages, either as discrete lenses with only minor and local zones of base metals, and more typically as a separate layer in the immediate footwall of the base metal sulphides. There is also significant widespread pyrite throughout the felsic rocks, in both the main mineralized unit and in the footwall felsic lapilli tuffs, as discrete semi-massive layers and as broad disseminations.

Alteration

There is a distinct propylitic facies of widespread chlorite, epidote and locally pyrite throughout the Los Pasos Formation and in parts of the overlying Relámpago Formation basalts. In the footwall felsic to mixed pyroclastic rocks in the immediate Los Mangos - San Fernando area there is a distinct zonal pattern of alteration with a central core, immediately southwest of the mine, of andalusite-sericite-quartz surrounded by a broad, stratabound sericite-quartz assemblage. To the south there is a cross-stratal zone of quartz-sericite-biotite alteration.

Broad areas are mapped as underlain by felsic pyroclastic rocks, but it is not clear to which extent these represent true felsic volcanics or are mafic units which have been extensively altered in a broad volcanic geothermal system.

There are also extensive areas with intense oxidation at surface and which probably correspond in large parts to the original distribution of more pyritic areas. These generally fall into two classes, the first of which are stratabound, primarily in the footwall of known volcanogenic massive sulphide occurrences, and the second which follow some of the major northwest striking faults.

Distinct barite horizons have been mapped, originally described as quartz-barite veins. Many of these correspond with stratabound barite anomalies in the areas of known volcanogenic massive sulphide mineralization, and others are associated with areas of alteration and geochemical and geophysical anomalies in exploration target areas.

Distribution of Mineralized Zones

The Los Mangos - San Fernando deposit has been traced on surface and to depth for three kilometres along strike, of which the major section from Los Mangos to San Fernando is 450 metres long and traced down dip from surface to 300 metres along the bedding plane or for 250 metres north and to a vertical depth of 230 metres to the base of the mineralized unit relative to the collar of the Los Mangos shaft.

The felsic-mafic contact and the mineralization dip to the north at an average of 30°, with a strike of approximately 075°. In the 200 metre strike extent of the original Los Mangos mine for which there are detailed level plans the deposit consists of a series of discrete lenses which reflect at least five separate stratigraphic horizons within the uppermost altered felsic lapilli tuff unit. The mineralization is also offset into separate blocks by the series of 110° striking steep reverse faults with the more northerly blocks progressively down-dropped to the north. More locally, the mineralized horizons are divided into discrete shoots by numerous, mostly north striking, post-mineral dykes.

The upper (13 to 45 metre) levels in the block from surface down to the first major 110° striking fault was mined in the 1800's primarily from a supergene enriched copper zone as chalcocite, covellite and bornite. There were at least two major mineralized horizons which were mined, one to the west, immediately adjacent to the Los Mangos and Santa Isabela shafts on the 13 to 45 metre levels, and a second some 100 metres further east on the 13 and 21 metre levels only.

This zone was later extended in the primary sulphides from the 45 to 146 m levels, in an area 105 m long by 25 m wide, within which there are a series of irregular to spherical ore shoots and steeply dipping lenses.

The deeper, northern block was mined from the 66 to the 146 metre levels on at least three separate horizons. Mineralized shoots were developed at the west end near the Los Mangos shaft on the 45, 66 and 123 metre levels, but the more extensive development was towards the east on the 91 and 123 m levels, with additional access from the 146 m level.The latter was mostly driven for development, but failed to locate any significant mineralization as the shallow dip and fault controls, although recognised by the consulting geologist at the time (Pfeffer, 1958), were not used to direct the location of the development headings.

The Soviet-Cuban drilling from the 170 metre level in 1958-63 located additional mineralization from the northernmost drill station (C-1) in the next fault block top the north. The down-dip potential of this zone is unknown, but open.

A series of historical shafts and extensive adits were developed midway between the Los Mangos and San Fernando zones in the area of the Ceiba and Colorado shafts (Fig. 5). These probably represent development on the up-dip extent of the deeper mineralized horizons than those exploited from the Los Mangos and Santa Isabela shafts.

The original San Fernando shaft area, is primarily a zinc zone, at depths of 12 to 25 metres in the shaft. Samples taken in 1917 (Constant) averaged 33.2 % Zn, 5.22 % Cu and 345 g/t Ag. Forty tons which were hand-picked to minimise the copper content assayed 41.0 % Zn, 2.72 % Pb, 1.51 % Cu, 8.6 g/t Au and 555 g/t Ag.

Four of the five holes drilled by Holmer to the east of the historical mine workings and north of the Soviet-Cuban underground development and drilling has intersected significant widths of locally high copper and zinc grade massive sulphides, while the fifth probably entered a near vertical feldspar porphyry dyke of unknown strike orientation.

The overall distribution of the mineralization as recorded appears to be relatively complex with a number of isolated ore lenses or bodies which form an irregular pattern in plan, cross-section and long-section. Part of this complexity is due to the local development of ore shoots on the five separate mineralized horizons within the overall 50 metre thick mineralized upper felsic lapilli tuff unit and the local limits of the mineralization on the post-mineral dykes. Part of the complexity may also be due to the mineralization event coinciding with active volcanism, with deposition of the sulphides upon and between separate pulses or layers of individual pyroclastic layers and mafic flows with irregular shapes and distribution. The sulphides may have been deposited in local pools between coarse felsic volcanic lobes or as replacement bodies between those semi-consolidated lobes within finer grained, glass-rich, ash units.

Resource Estimates

In late 1997 indicated resources were estimated by Holmer from twelve cross-sections, 25 m apart, and for 25 metres horizontally north and south along the sections in areas of widely spaced holes as 1,036,296 tonnes at a grade of 1.84 % Cu and 3.35 % Zn. The data included all surface and underground intersections using a cut-off of 1 % Cu, 1 % Zn or 20 g/t Ag, and averaged by incorporating all true thickness corrected intersections on each cross-section. The results were only calculated for Cu and Zn because of the lack of data on Ag or Au for most of the historical, pre-Holmer holes.

The data-base, both the actual distribution of the mineralization and the local grades, is highly restricted in the mine area. Most of the data in this area consists of underground holes which were drilled as fans in both azimuth and dip radiating from a few major set-ups, and are therefore everywhere oblique to both strike and dip. Even projections of 12.5 metres can create numerous false impressions of the distribution of the mineralization. The *in situ* density was calculated from the measured density of the host altered rock of 2.8 g/cc, and the average grades and known densities of the sulphide minerals in a combination of 30 % sulphide and 70 % gangue for an overall average of 3.43 g/cc.

Inferred resources were estimated extending for 200 metres on the dip and for 100 metres along strike, with an average thickness of 15 metres, for a total of 1,029,000 tonnes, with the same grades as above.

Conclusions

From the historical data and the more recent drilling it is apparent that the Los Mangos - San Fernando deposit is primarily stratabound massive to semi-massive sulphides of essentially volcanogenic character. Some of the features of the deposit are:

- It is hosted within a 50 metre thick altered, sericitic and andalusite bearing felsic lapilli tuff and ash tuff unit, underlain by similar felsic tuffs interbedded with heterogenous intermediate lapilli tuffs and mafic flows, immediately overlain by a thin, finer grained rhyolite-dacite tuff unit with a hangingwall unit of aerially extensive, largely unaltered unit of mafic flows and basalt-andesite lapilli-tuff.
- The overall zone has been traced for up to 3,000 metres along strike, for 300 metres down dip from surface along the bedding plane or for 250 metres north and to a vertical depth of 230 metres. Within this extensive area the base metal mineralization is restricted to a single stratigraphic unit up to 50 metre thick and in up to five separate stratigraphic horizons each up to eight metres thick, extending as more or less continuous sheets or as more discrete lenses as either base metal sulphides or separate pyrite rich bodies.
- There is little or no development of any cross-stratal mineralized stringer zone within either the felsic lapilli tuff or the interbedded heterogeneous lapilli tuffs.
- The detailed distribution of the mineralized horizons is controlled by the form and distribution of original felsic tuffs as various lobes, with local depressions or pools between them.
- The overall stratigraphic package, the host unit and the individual mineralized horizons strike at 075° and dip to the north at an average of 30°; the overall host unit is separated into distinct blocks by a series of evenly spaced, subparallel, 110° striking, 80° south dipping reverse faults.
- Individual ore-shoots are terminated against numerous, but volumetrically minor andesite-dacite porphyry and basalt dykes, possibly as feeders to the overlying mafic units within which the dykes are more abundant.
- The overall extent of the base metal mineralized system is open along strike and down-dip.

A idea of the overall size of the system is seen in the soil geochemical data (>1,000 ppb Au, > 300 ppm Cu and >1,000 ppm Zn) as well as the IP anomalies. The surface expression of the mineralized horizon is a leached cap lying well south of the old mine area, and is potentially overlying a supergene enriched zone similar to that originally developed in the older, shallower sections of the Los Mangos, La Ceiba and San Fernando shafts. The overall zone of potential extends for at least 1,000 metres along strike, and with a known down-dip extent of 300 metres, and open to depth down-dip.

ACKNOWLEDGEMENTS

This paper has been prepared by some of the team who have explored the area at various times since 1994 funded by Holmer Gold Mines Limited in a multi-year Economic Association Contract of exploration, development and mining with GeoMinera, S.A. the Cuban state mining agency. It incorporates the work of many other geologists who worked on the project including Sr. R. Rodríquez G., Mr. T. Neelands, the recent Exploration Manager and his predecessor Ing. Luis Igreda Coz, as well as from Ing. Florencio Arcial C., the original Cuban project geologist. Much of the geology is derived from a detailed petrological and mineralogical study completed for Holmer as part of their exploration programme by Ing. Maria Santa Cruz Pacheco et al. of the Cuban Instituto de Geologia y Paleontologia.

The section on the General geology of Cuba was developed by two of the authors (TJB, FFC) based on field work throughout the island and a thorough review of the published as well as much unpublished literature by Cuban authors and their associates from the former communist block in the CIS and Eastern Europe. The senior Cuban author (FFC) was the senior representative of the Cuban government during the development and publication in Moscow of the joint Cuban-USSR geology map of Cuba at 1:250,000 (Pushcharovsky, 1989) and was later the associate director and most senior mineral deposit geologist within the Cuban Instituto de Geologia y Paleontologia.

REFERENCES

Note: Most of these references as indicated by (*) are to documents in the historical archives of the Department of Industry in Havana, Cuba, observed and reviewed by the first listed author . There has been little published in the readily available literature for many years on the geology of Cuba or its mineral deposits.

Allende, Roque (a). 31 May, 1925. Finca San Joaquin: San Fernando, Sta Elena, Sta Isabel, San Jose, Minas de Santa Clara. (*); (b). 1927. Yacimientos Minerales de la Republica de Cuba, Monografia de Cobre, Boletin de Minas # 11. (*)

Ansted, D.N. 1856. Of the San Fernando Copper Lodes near Cienfuegos, in Cuba, Quarterly Journal of the Geological Society of London, vol XIII, p. 240-242.

Arcial, C., F. 1995. Informe de los trabajos realizados Enero-Agosto 1995; Internal report of Holmer Gold mines Limited, 8 p. (*)

Arcial, C. F., and Dundlov, T., et al. 1991. Informe prospecion detallada Cobre San Fernando, Empresa Geologo-Minera Santa Clara.

Bartlett, Charles E. May 6, 1955. Memorandum to Pedro Muniz, Operacion de la Mina San Fernando. (*)

Bottrill, T. J. (a) 1995. San Fernando Project, Santa Clara, Cuba; private report for Holmer Gold Mines Limited, November 8 1995, 26 p.; (b) 1996. Review of geology, mineralization and exploration programs on the San Fernando Project, Santa Clara, Cuba; private report for Holmer Gold Mines Limited, July 1996, 32 p.; (c) 1997. San Fernando Mine: history and geology of the mine as derived from review of the historical records in the archives of the Fondo Geologo, Minbas; private memorandum for Holmer Gold Mines Limited, January 26, 1997, 12 p.

Castro, Carlos and Muniz, Pedro. June 1956. Compañia Inspiracion de Cobre, Report to Dept Mines. (*)

Castro, Carlos. Feb, 1957. Report to Cuban Department of Mines. (*)

C. L. Constant Co., N.Y., N.Y. December 8, 1917. Report on the San Fernando Mine. (*)

Formell C., Francisco. October 1997. San Fernando Project, Manicaragua, Cuba, internal report for Holmer Gold Mines Limited, with December 1997 addendum.

Gorielov, V. 1964. Informe, San Fernando Cobre, sobre los trabajos de exploracion geologica, efectuados en 1961-1963 en el yacimiento de cobre "San Fernando" de la Provincia de Las Villas, Instituto Cubano de Recursos Minerals. (*)

Iturralde-Vinent, Manuel, A., 1996 (a). Ofiolitas y Arcos Volcanicos de Cuba (Cuban Ophiolites and Volcanic Arcs). IGCP, Working Group on Stratigraphic Correlation of Volcano-Sedimentary Sections, Project 364, Caribbean Ophiolites and Volcanic Arcs, Special Publication No. 1.

Iturralde-Vinent, M., A., 1996 (b). Introduction to Cuban Geology and Geophysics. In Iturralde-Vinent, Manuel, A., ed., Ofiolitas y Arcos Volcanicos de Cuba (Cuban Ophiolites and Volcanic Arcs). IGCP, Working Group on Stratigraphic Correlation of Volcano-Sedimentary Sections, Project 364, Caribbean Ophiolites and Volcanic Arcs, Special Publication No. 1, p. 3-35.

Iturralde-Vinent, M., A., 1996 (c). Cuba: El Arco de Islas Volcánicas del Cretácico. In Iturralde-Vinent, Manuel, A., ed., Ofiolitas y Arcos Volcanicos de Cuba (Cuban Ophiolites and Volcanic Arcs). IGCP, Working Group on Stratigraphic Correlation of Volcano-Sedimentary Sections, Project 364, Caribbean Ophiolites and Volcanic Arcs, Special Publication No. 1, p. 179-189.

Iturralde-Vinent, M., A., Millán, G., Korpás, L., Nagy, E., and Pajón, J., 1996. Geological Interpretation of the Cuban K-Ar Database. In Iturralde-Vinent, Manuel, A., ed., Ofiolitas y Arcos Volcanicos de Cuba (Cuban Ophiolites and Volcanic Arcs). IGCP, Working Group on Stratigraphic Correlation of Volcano-Sedimentary Sections, Project 364, Caribbean Ophiolites and Volcanic Arcs, Special Publication No. 1, p. 48-69.

Kerr, A. C., Iturralde-Vinent, M. A., Saunders, A. D., Babbs, T. L., Tarney, J. 1999. A new plate tectonic model of the Caribbean: Implications from a geochemical reconnaissance of Cuban Mesozoic volcanic rocks. Geological Society of America Bulletin, November 1999, v. 111, p. 1581-1599.

Lewis, J. F., and Draper, G. 1990. Geology and tectonic evolution of the northern Caribbean margin. In Dengo, G. and Case J. E., eds.., The Caribbean region: Boulder, Colorado, Geological Society of America, The Gseology of North America, V, H., p. 77-140.

Long, W., Seymour, O. G. 1942. Report on San Fernando Mine, Minas de Matahambre. (*)

Pagliuchi, F.D. (a) September 1943. Resumen of Various Reports on the San Fernando Mines. (*); (b) December 1943. Addendum to My Report (as above). (*)

Pfeffer, H. William. (a) November 21, 1958. Report on the Geology of the San Fernando Mine, Las Villas, Cuba for Cia. Inspiración Cuba de Cobre, S.A. (*); (b) November 18, s1958. Letter to Dr. Ernesto Ramagosa, Cia. Inspiracion Cuba de Cobre (re exploration opportunities in the Los Mangos mine). (*); (c) November 18, 1958. Report on Ore Reserves of the San Fernando Mine, letter to Cia. Inspiración Cuba de Cobre, S.A. (*)

Pushcharovsky, Yu. M. 1989. Geology of Cuba, Explanatory Note to the 1:250,000 Geological Map of Cuba. USSR Academy of Sciences Geological Institute Holding the Order of the Red Banner of Labour, and Cuban Academy of Sciences Institute of Geology and Palaeontology, Moscow 42 sheets.

Ramagosa, Ernesto. (undated). Compañia Inspiracion Cubana de Cobre. (*)

Rodríguez Ruiz, G. 1998. San Fernando Project, Los Mangos Deposit, Executive Summary, internal report for Holmer Gold Mines Limited.

Santa Cruz Pacheco, M., et al.1997. Estudio mineralogico y petrogafico en la parte norte del sector "Los Mangos" del prospecto San Fernando, Provincia Villa Clara; Instituto de Geologia y Paleontologia.

GEOLOGY AND GEOCHEMISTRY OF THE OXEC, CYPRUS-TYPE VMS DEPOSIT, GUATEMALA

Erich U. Petersen

Department of Geology and Geophysics, The University of Utah, 135 S. 1460 E., Room 719, Salt Lake City, UT 84105

Abstract

The Oxec copper deposit occurs in the northwest portion of a large ultramafic-mafic thrust sheet that constitutes the Sierra de Santa Cruz, Guatemala. The deposit formed in the proto-Caribbean ocean about 138-113 Ma. By late Campanian time (84-74.5 Ma) this slice of oceanic crust (Sierra de Santa Cruz ophiolite) and the deposit were obducted and slid to their current location on the Cretaceous Sepur Fm.

In the mine vicinity, the ultramafic-mafic complex consists of serpentinized peridotite (hartzburgite), massive gabbro, a sheeted dike complex, two pillow lava sequences, and overlying radiolarian chert. The copper ores are hosted by the lower pillow lava sequence. Intrusion of dikes that gave rise to stratigraphicaly higher lava units dissects the orebody. As a result the approximately 1 million ton orebody of 3 % Cu was disaggregated into numerous ore pods the largest of which are a few tens of metres in maximum dimension.

Whole rock chemical analyses indicated N-MORB affinity for the mafic rocks. The gabbros, and upper pillow basalts are pervasively altered to a chlorite-albite±epidote-actinolite-sphene assemblage. Mass transfer calculations demonstrate that these rocks are strongly enriched in Na_2O and H_2O, strongly depleted in CaO, and slightly depleted in FeO. The lower pillow basalts sequence and dikes intimately associated with the ore are strongly chloritized and silicified. They show strong leaching of Na_2O and CaO and strong enrichment in FeO and H_2O.

Pyrite, pyrrhotite and chalcopyrite are the dominant sulphides. A sulphide-basalt breccia occurs in the northern part of the deposit and is inferred to represent part of the feeder zone. Minor, paragenetically early phases include hematite, magnetite, and valleriite and indicate an early oxidizing hydrothermal environment. Reduced fluids displaced early oxidizing fluids precipitating pyrite followed by pyrrhotite and chalcopyrite.

Microthermometric measurements on mineralizing fluids trapped in vein quartz with pyrite indicate temperatures of 280 to 320°C (pressure adjusted). Chlorite geothemometry indicates that maximum temperatures of 327°C were reached in the strongly altered rocks and agree closely with homogenization temperatures. Chlorite compositions in weakly altered rocks indicate temperatures near 255°C. Fluid salinities range from 3 to 8 weight percent NaCl equivalent with an average of 4.9 percent. There is no correlation between temperature and salinity. Saline fluids probably originated by phase separation that occurred in the sub-seafloor hydrothermal system.

Introduction

The Oxec copper deposit is a Cyprus-type volcanogenic massive sulphide deposit (Petersen and Zantop 1980) located 140 km northeast of Guatemala City, Guatemala. It lies within a Cretaceous mafic-ultramafic complex first described as being a serpentinized harzburgite (Bonis, 1968). Wilson (1974) recognized that these rocks were an allochthonous unit and belonged to an ophiolite sequence. Regional reconnaissance mapping of the ophiolite by Rosenfeld (1981) identified the presence of radiolarian cherts, plagiogranites, massive and cumulate gabbros, and melange zones. Roberts and Irvine (1957) first examined the Oxec district. Petersen and Zantop (1980) provided a detailed description of the mineralization. Wilson and Petersen (1987) clarified the thermal history with a fluid inclusion study. The Oxec deposit produced just over 1 million tons of 3 % Cu copper ore for its productive life at the rate of approximately 400 tons of ore per day.

In this paper we summarize the geology of the Oxec district, describe the mineralization, and provide new data on the thermal history and present new mineral chemistry data on the magmatic and hydrothermal alteration minerals in Oxec ore system.

GEOLOGY

Regional Geology

The Polochic transform fault system, extends from Mexico in the west to the Caribbean in the East and forms an approximate boundary between metamorphosed Paleozoic rocks to the South and unmetamorphosed upper Paleozoic and younger rocks to the North (Fig. 1, Bonis, 1970). A series of mafic-ultramafic rocks occur on the northern side of the fault. The largest and eastern most sheet-like mafic-ultramafic complex is the Sierra de Santa Cruz ophiolite and it measures 15 km wide, 85 km long and up to 2 km thick. Well-developed nickel laterites occur along the southern margin of this ophiolite in the ultramafic portion of the complex. A slightly smaller mafic-ultramafic body is exposed 50 km to the west, and still another one is exposed another 50 km farther west. In the next 100 km along the fault and splays of the fault another 7 or 8 small slivers of mafic-ultramafic complex can be found.

All these mafic-ultramafic outcrops are believed to be fragments of oceanic crust (Wilson, 1974, Rosenfeld, 1980, 1981, 1990). Intra basalt chert nodules indicate that a spreading centre forming the proto-Caribbean ocean had been initiated by Valanginian time (138 to 131 Ma). Supra-basalt volcaniclastics indicate development of a primitive island arc during Aptian time (119-113 Ma.). The Jolomax Fm., a shaley argillite melange that underlies a large area in the core of the ophiolite, has been interpreted as an accretionary prism developed on the wall of a Cenomanian age (97.5-91 Ma.) trench. In late Campanian time (84-74.5 Ma) the Jolomax accretionary prism and a slab of

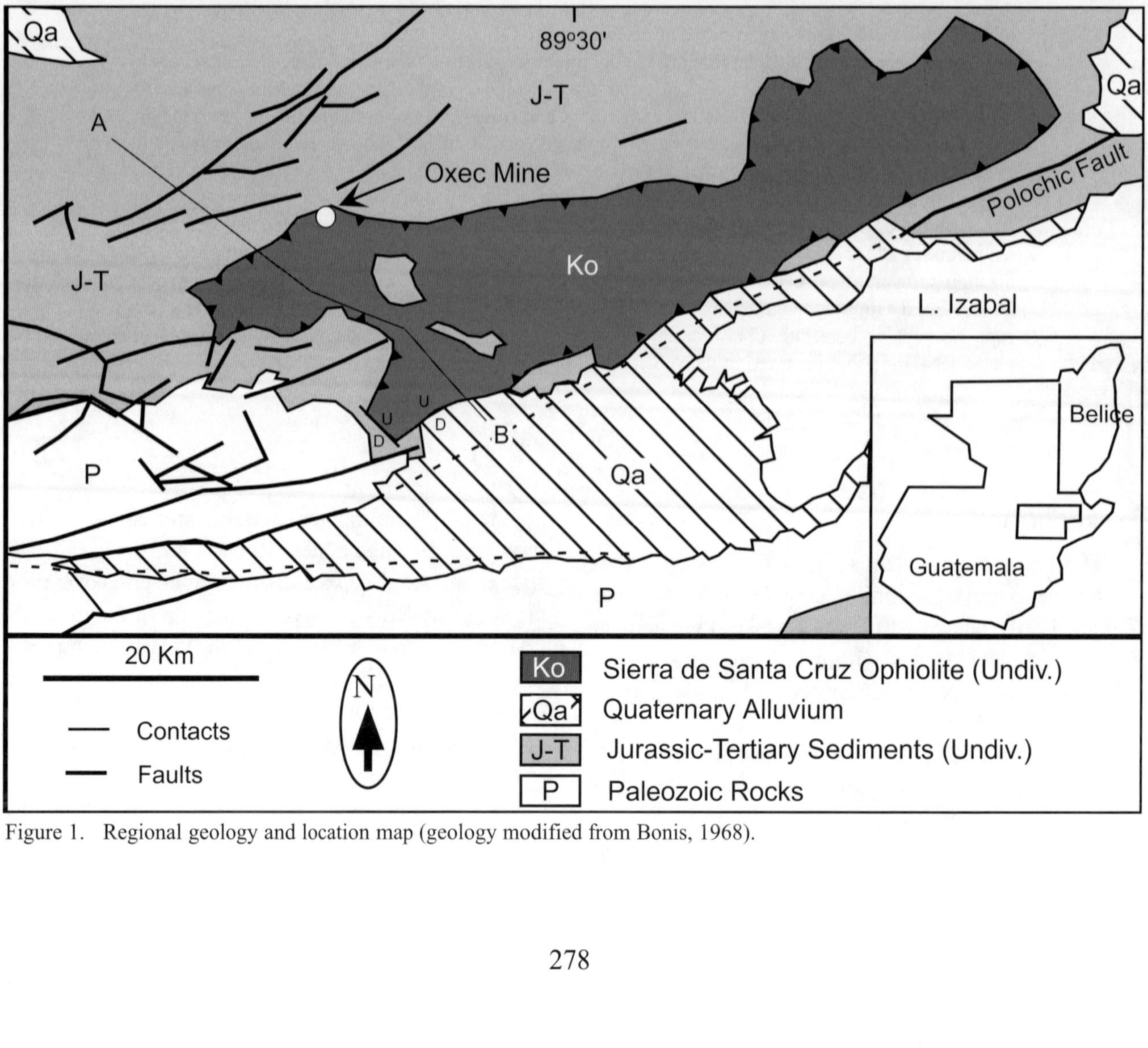

Figure 1. Regional geology and location map (geology modified from Bonis, 1968).

the proto Caribbean lithosphere were obducted onto the leading edge of the Yucatan. Gravity sliding then placed the allochton on the Sepur foreland basin (Fig. 2). Folding by transpression of the Chortis terrain against the southern margin of Yucatan took place in Paleocene times (Rosenfeld, 1990). Neogene strike-slip movement on the Polochic fault cut off and transported to the East the southern extension of the Santa Cruz Ophiolite (Fig. 2).

District Geology

The district geology summarized here is based on a detail description by Petersen and Zantop (1980). The Oxec copper mine, operated by Transmetales Ltd. in the late seventies, is located on the Oxec River. The deposit is situated in the northwest margin of a large mafic-ultramafic complex that makes up part of the Sierra de Santa Cruz (Fig. 1).

Three thrust faults occur in the immediate deposit area (Fig. 3). The Santa Cruz thrust fault defines the contact between the ophiolite suite and the overridden Cretaceous-Tertiary Sepur Fm. Sediments. The Oxec thrust fault juxtaposes mafic rocks (dike complex) with ultramafic rocks (serpentinite complex). Exposures are too poor to determine whether the contact between the lower pillow basalts and upper pillow basalts is tectonic or stratigraphic, however, a finely brecciated zone indicates that the upper pillow basalts are in tectonic contact with the sheeted dikes.

Three sets of normal faults are identified in the mine area. The El Poso fault (Fig. 3) strikes N 70ºW, dips steeply south, and displaces the Oxec fault in apparent left-lateral sense. Displaced pods of ore, however, suggest that the southern side was down-dropped slightly accounting for the apparent left-lateral surface displacement. Numerous offsets parallel to the El Pozo fault, also with apparent left-lateral offset, are observed within the mine.

A minor N10ºE fault system is parallel to the southern extension of the Oxec fault where it has a dominant strike-slip component. A N70º to 80ºE fault system is well developed underground, but has no surface expression.

A stratigraphic reconstruction of the rock units in the mine area is shown in figure 3. The lower-most unit is the Sepur Formation, a unit which in the mine area consists of a rhythmic sequence of thinly bedded shale and sandstone (Bonis, 1968). Overlying the Sepur Formation is the ophiolite that consists, from base to top, of the serpentinite complex, the dike complex, lower pillow basalts, upper pillow basalts, radiolarian chert. This is not a continuous section as the Oxec thrust juxtaposes the serpentinite and gabbro and the unnamed thrust juxtaposes the upper basalts and sheeted dike complex. The gabbro and the sedimentary cover units commonly associated with ophiolites are not exposed in the mine area but have been identified outside the map area (Rosenfeld, 1979).

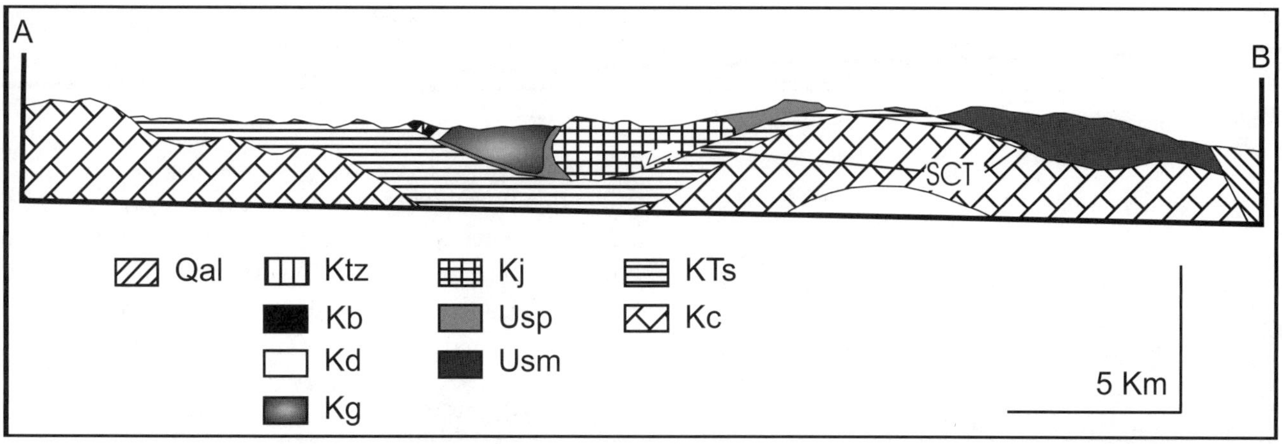

Figure 2. Northwest-southeast cross-section showing the ophiolite lithologies. Qal = Quaternary alluvium, Ktz = Tzumuy Fm., Kb = basalt, Kd = dike complex, Kg = massive gabbro, Kj = Jolomax Fm., Usp = serpentinite, Usm = serpentinite melange, KTs = Sepur Fm., Kc = Coban Fm. (after Rosenfeld, 1990).

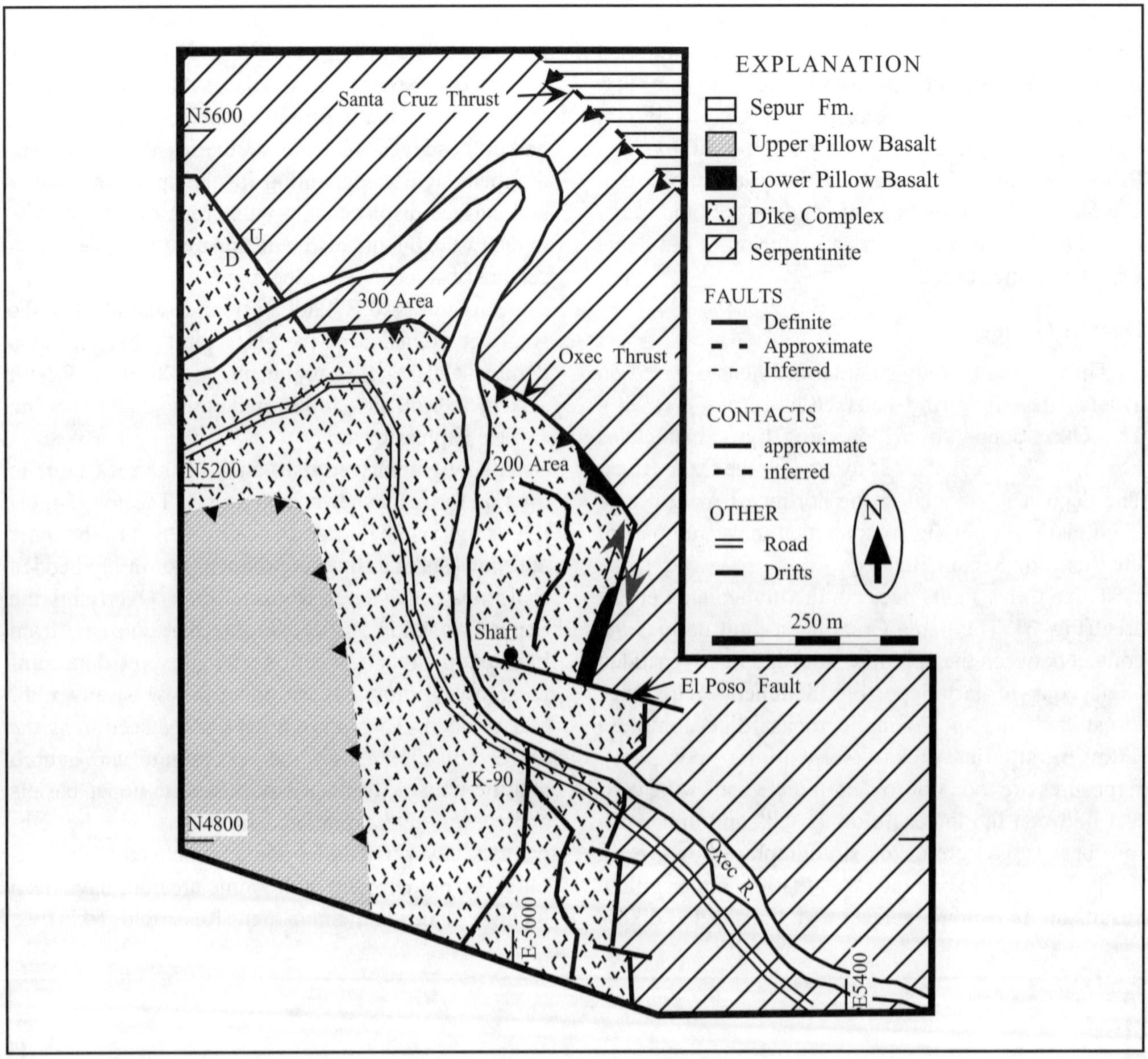

Figure 3. Surface geology of the Oxec mine area (after Petersen and Zantop, 1980).

Serpentinite complex

Volumetrically, the serpentinite is the largest unit in the mine area. It is extensively sheared and is locally intruded by gabbroic dikes that are commonly discontinuous, broken into short segments, pulled apart, and cut by younger dikes.

The serpentinite complex in the mine area consists of completely serpentinized hartzburgite. Weathering turns the surface of the rock into a whitish clay-like alteration product and etches out a gneissic-like foliation. Weathering of orthopyroxene crystals, 2 to 10 mm in diametre, give the exposed surface of the rock a hobnail appearance (Fig 5A). Extreme shearing and serpentinization have locally obliterated the original mineralogy and structures of the former hartzburgite.

Fresh serpentinite is very dark green and massive consisting of pseudomorphed orthopyroxene (16 %), olivine (82 %) and chromite (<2 %). In thin-section orthopyroxene appears uniform, whereas olivine has a net texture (Fig. 5B). Electron microprobe analyses show that the serpentine after orthopyroxene contains

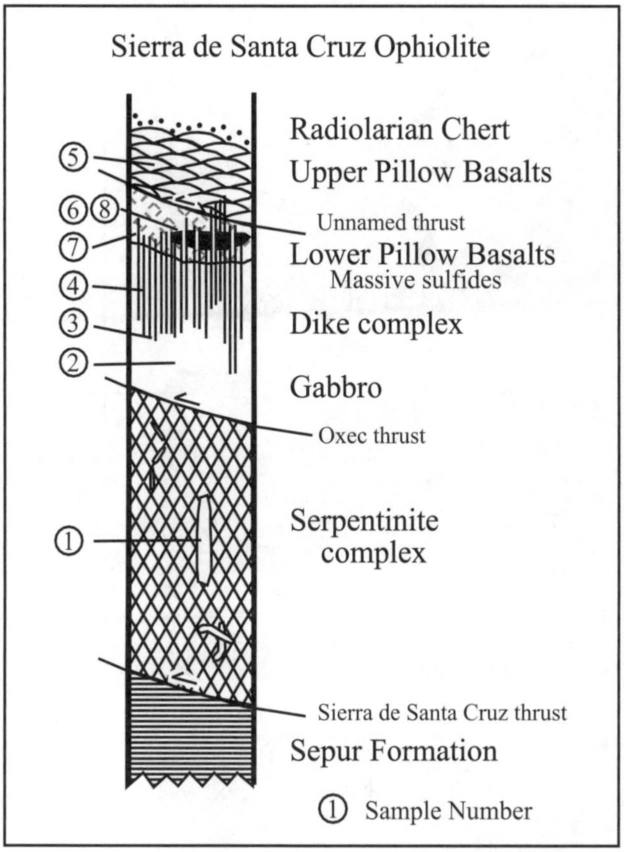

Figure 4. Generalized stratigraphic section in mine area (after Petersen and Zantop, 1980)

minor chromium whereas serpentine after olivine does not (Table 1). Electron microprobe analyses of chromite indicate that it is a Cr-, Fe-rich spinel of a composition typically associated with chromite from alpine peridotites (Steel et al., 1977).

Dike complex / Gabbro

The dike complex is well exposed in the mine area (Fig. 3). It forms a belt roughly 300 m wide separating the pillow basalts to the southwest from the serpentinite to the northeast. Contacts with footwall and hangingwall units are tectonic.

The lower part of the dike complex grades into massive gabbro. The gabbro consists of plagioclase (39 %), clinopyroxene (27 %), chlorite (23 %), epidote (2 %), with sphene and opaque minerals making up the remainder (Petersen and Zantop 1980). Electron microprobe analyses show that plagioclase is almost pure albite (An_2, Table 1), clinopyroxene is augite ($En_{45}Fs_{15}Wo_{40}$), chlorite is high-Fe, pycnochlorite (Hey, 1954), and epidote is Fe-rich (Ep_{60}-$_{80}Zo_{40}$-$_{20}$) (Table 1).

In the mine, where the upper portion of the complex is exposed, the dike density decreases and the proportion of inter-dike pillow basalt increases. Dikes and sills range in width from 5 cm to over 10 m and have well-developed chilled margins up to 1 cm wide. Intense faulting has broken the dikes to the degree that individual segments can rarely be correlated, giving the assemblage the appearance of a megabreccia. Late dikes intrude early ones and give rise to sills that, on the scale of the mine, prevent correlation of ore pods.

The dikes are subdivided into post-ore dikes, intensely hydrothermally altered dikes, and unclassified dikes. The multiple generations of dikes indicate almost continuous magmatic activity over a significant time interval. Post-ore dikes crosscut the ore and have developed chilled margins against the ore. They are light in colour and contain two varieties of pyroxenes in a fine-grained chlorite-plagioclase matrix: euhedral clinopyroxene with well-developed hourglass (Fig. 5C) and rapid chill textures, and pyroxenes that have been pseudomorphed by chlorite or a chlorite-actinolite intergrowth. Minor sulphides and disseminated secondary sphene are present.

Intensely hydrothermally altered dikes are recognized by their black colour and invariable association with the ore host rocks (lower pillow basalts). The contact between the two is usually tectonic, but in places it appears to be gradational. The altered dikes are highly chloritized and silicified. The common mineral assemblage is chlorite ± actinolite, plagioclase, quartz, epidote, sphene, and sulphides. Minute veinlets containing epidote, quartz, and zeolite (?) are dispersed throughout the rock. Euhedral augite phenocrysts are altered to a brown chlorite or to a green chlorite-actinolite intergrowth. Plagioclase is highly sericitized, and albite twinning is all but obliterated. Quartz is disseminated throughout the rock and commonly encloses other minerals, e.g., plagioclase with well-preserved twinning.

The unclassified dikes, volumetrically the largest group, are dikes whose age with respect to the ore cannot be determined because of the limited exposure and tectonic complexities. The oldest dikes show con-

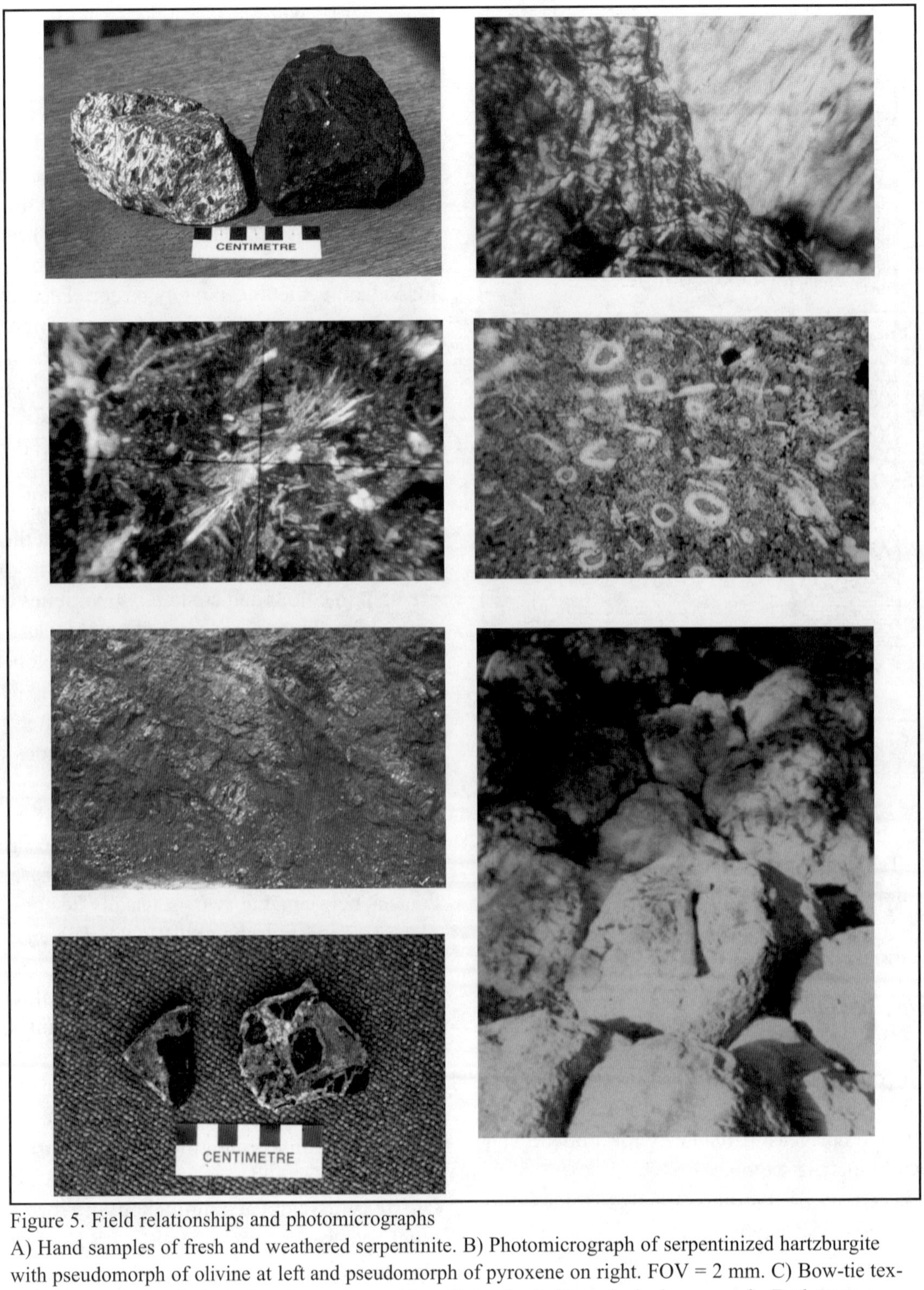

Figure 5. Field relationships and photomicrographs
A) Hand samples of fresh and weathered serpentinite. B) Photomicrograph of serpentinized hartzburgite with pseudomorph of olivine at left and pseudomorph of pyroxene on right. FOV = 2 mm. C) Bow-tie texture of pyroxene and plagioclase in massive gabbro. Note also hollow plagioclase crystals. Both textures indicated rapid cooling. FOV = 1 mm. D) Photomicrograph of vesicles in lower basalt filled with chlorite and quartz. All plagioclase has been silicified. FOV = 2 mm. E) Dikes cut and dissect orebody. 300 Area high-wall. D = dike, O = ore in the lower pillow basalt, and DOB = dike ore breccia. F) Pillow basalts in Oxec river. Hammer indicates scale. Photo by Rosenfeld. G) Brecciated ore from 300 Area feeder zone.

[a]Sample number as in Table 2. Notes: Analytical conditions: 15 KeV, 30nA, 15 sec/element, 10mm spot. Standards: fluorphlogopite for F, Si, Al, K, Mg, rhodonite for Mn, Binn ilmenite for Ti, ferrosillite95 for Fe, ON-70 for Cl. Normalization basis: chlorite- 10 cations, 18 O, 8 H; Chromite- 3 cations, 4 anions; plagioclase- 5 cations; serpentine- 5 cations 4 H; pyroxene- 4 cations; epidote- 7 cations, 11 H, 13 O.

Table 1. Electron microprobe analyses of chlorite (CHL), serpentine (SER), chromite (CHR), plagioclase (PL), pyroxene (PX) and epidote (EP).

Anal. No.	23	25	13	14	42	48	8	12	40	45	46	41	10	11	9	24
Mineral	CHL	CHL	CHL	CHL	CHR	CHR	PL	PL	SER	SER	SER	SER	PX	PX	EP	EP
Sample[a]	117	117	50	50	77	77	50	50	77 px	77 px	77 ol	77 ol	50	50	117	50
El. Wt. %																
K	0.02	0.00	0.01	0.01	0.01	0.00	0.04	0.04	0.02	0.00	0.03	0.02	0.01	0.01	0.02	0.02
Na	0.00	0.01	0.05	0.04	0.04	0.00	8.69	8.70	0.00	0.02	0.01	0.02	0.19	0.22	0.00	0.03
Ca	0.01	0.03	0.12	0.19	0.01	0.00	0.17	0.20	0.04	0.05	0.04	0.04	14.02	14.09	16.85	16.48
Mg	7.85	8.74	9.64	9.70	10.98	11.04	0.00	0.00	20.64	21.18	23.34	23.65	9.53	10.18	0.00	0.00
Fe^{2+}	21.96	20.67	19.05	18.90	6.61	6.68	0.03	0.08	3.80	3.74	2.09	1.39	7.39	6.32	0.00	0.00
Fe^{3+}	0.50	0.13	0.00	0.00	5.22	4.01									7.67	9.14
Mn	0.15	0.14	0.27	0.26	0.00	0.00	0.00	0.00	0.03	0.08	0.03	0.02	0.20	0.15	0.08	0.09
Ti	0.07	0.00	0.00	0.03	0.04	0.00	0.02	0.03	0.04	0.03	0.01	0.02	0.32	0.31	0.14	0.04
Cr	0.02	0.06	0.01	0.00	21.53	24.13	0.00	0.01	0.83	0.58	0.00	0.00	0.00	0.01	0.00	0.00
Al	9.84	9.76	8.79	8.61	17.57	16.54	9.97	9.98	1.22	0.98	0.19	0.10	1.01	1.06	12.59	11.69
Si	11.91	12.25	12.96	13.05	0.17	0.01	31.79	32.09	18.27	18.96	20.38	20.13	24.13	24.46	17.65	17.55
H	1.21	1.23	1.23	1.23					1.34	1.33	1.39	1.38			0.20	0.20
O	43.74	44.20	44.29	44.25	37.17	36.77	48.21	48.60	47.63	48.40	50.40	49.97	42.71	43.28	43.04	42.55
F	0.00	0.00	0.00	0.00	0.63	0.55	0.00	0.00	0.00	0.12	0.01	0.00	0.00	0.00	0.00	0.00
Cl	0.02	0.03	0.03	0.02	0.01	0.04	0.01	0.03	0.36	0.36	0.07	0.02	0.03	0.03	0.00	0.01
Sum	97.28	97.24	96.43	96.28	99.71	99.54	98.92	99.76	94.12	95.71	97.97	96.75	99.53	100.11	98.26	97.78
Atoms																
K	0.00	0.00	0.00	0.00	0.00	0.00	0.00	0.00	0.00	0.00	0.00	0.00	0.00	0.00	0.00	0.00
Na	0.00	0.00	0.01	0.01	0.00	0.00	1.00	1.00	0.00	0.00	0.00	0.00	0.02	0.02	0.00	0.01
Ca	0.00	0.01	0.02	0.03	0.00	0.00	0.01	0.01	0.00	0.00	0.00	0.00	0.78	0.78	2.03	2.01
Mg	2.13	2.34	2.58	2.60	0.78	0.79	0.00	0.00	2.60	2.62	2.77	2.83	0.88	0.92	0.00	0.00
Fe2+	2.59	2.41	2.22	2.21	0.20	0.21	0.00	0.00	0.21	0.20	0.11	0.07	0.30	0.25	0.00	0.00
Fe3+	0.06	0.01	0.00	0.00	0.16	0.13									0.66	0.80
Mn	0.02	0.02	0.03	0.03	0.00	0.00	0.00	0.00	0.00	0.00	0.00	0.00	0.01	0.01	0.01	0.01
Ti	0.01	0.00	0.00	0.00	0.00	0.00	0.00	0.00	0.00	0.00	0.00	0.00	0.01	0.01	0.01	0.00
Cr	0.00	0.01	0.00	0.00	0.71	0.81	0.00	0.00	0.05	0.03	0.00	0.00	0.00	0.00	0.00	0.00
Al	2.40	2.36	2.12	2.08	1.12	1.07	0.98	0.97	0.14	0.11	0.02	0.01	0.08	0.09	2.25	2.12
Si	2.79	2.84	3.01	3.03	0.01	0.00	3.00	3.01	1.99	2.03	2.09	2.08	1.92	1.92	3.03	3.05
H	8.00	8.00	8.00	8.00					4.10	4.00	4.00	4.00			0.96	0.98
O	18.00	18.00	18.03	18.04	4.01	4.00	7.99	8.00	9.12	9.08	9.09	9.07	5.97	5.97	12.98	13.00
F	0.00	0.00	0.00	0.00	0.06	0.05	0.00	0.00	0.00	0.02	0.00	0.00	0.00	0.00	0.00	0.00
Cl	0.00	0.00	0.00	0.00	0.00	0.00	0.00	0.00	0.03	0.03	0.01	0.00	0.00	0.00	0.00	0.00
A site	0.00	0.01	0.03	0.04	0.98	1.00	1.02	1.01	0.00	0.01	0.01	0.01	0.80	0.80	2.03	2.02
Al^{iv}	1.21	1.16	0.99	0.97			0.00		0.01				0.08	0.08		
Al^{vi}	1.19	1.20	1.13	1.11	0.29	0.19	0.98	0.98	0.13	0.14	0.11	0.09	0.00	0.01	2.28	2.17
XMg	0.45	0.49	0.54	0.54	0.79	0.79	0.00	0.00	0.93	0.93	0.96	0.98	0.75	0.79		
T(°C)	327	311	258	250												

Table 2. Chemical analyses for eight rocks from the Oxec Mine area (Oxides in weight percent, trace elements in ppm)

Analysis No.	1	2	3	4	5	6	7	8
Sample No.[a]	33	50	57	83	25	102	106	78
SiO_2	50.1	52.2	53.8	51.9	50.7	52.6	51.0	66.8
Al_2O_3	16.0	14.8	14.0	15.1	14.9	13.9	12.7	6.99
FeO[b]	7.73	9.31	9.02	7.70	8.30	16.9	17.9	14.3
Fe_2O_3[b]	8.59	10.3	10.0	8.56	9.22	18.8	19.9	15.9
MnO	0.14	0.17	0.15	0.14	0.16	0.13	0.13	0.11
MgO	7.23	5.56	8.17	5.91	7.89	6.01	9.17	3.39
CaO	10.4	6.82	8.66	9.71	7.30	2.63	2.45	0.61
Na_2O	3.36	5.77	5.04	4.80	5.37	1.20	0.46	0.06
K_2O	0.09	0.16	0.29	0.09	0.04	0.09	0.08	0.03
TiO_2	0.88	1.20	0.31	0.71	0.97	0.49	0.31	0.68
P_2O_5	0.07	0.12	0.01	0.06	0.08	0.03	0.01	0.02
LOI[c]	3.44	2.56	1.95	2.42	3.97	4.42	4.87	4.21
Total[d]	100.3	99.7	99.4	99.4	100.6	100.3	101.0	98.9
Cr	240	140	260	180	260	140	460	260
Co	2	23	11	19	22	30	42	78
Ni	17	15	30	31	62	31	78	1
Cu	57	81	2	89	86	7	5	2650
Zn	4	70	15	56	60	58	36	7
Pb		10						

[a]Sample number, x, in Gu/O-n-77. [b]Total Fe as FeO and as Fe_2O_3. [c]Loss on ignition (H_2O; $CO_2 < 0.2$ %). [d]SUM when total Fe is as Fe_2O_3*. nd, not determined; tr, trace.

Notes: Sample locations are as follows: (1) Dike completely enclosed in the serpentinite, about 4.5 km south of the mine; (2) Fresh pre-ore dike from the N-80 drift; (3) Pre-ore dike with hydrothermally altered margins from the K-90 drift; (4) Post-ore dike from the No. 12 stope; (5) Upper pillow lavas 0.9 km north of the mine; (6) Ore host rock, i.e., lower pillow lava from the 1-17 drift; (7) Highly altered syn-ore dike in DDH 70-54; (8) mineralized Lower pillow basalt from the 200 area. Mine coordinates for each sample are given in Petersen (1979).

siderable cataclasis. Even in the least altered and deformed of these dikes is extensively chloritized.

Compositions of chlorite in the most altered dikes are given in Table 1, and whole rock chemical compositions are given in Table 2. Chemically the chlorites are low-Fe, low-Si brunsvigite (Fig. 6, Hey, 1954).

Lower pillow basalts

The lower pillow basalts host the massive sulphide orebodies and are volumetrically the smallest unit. They are so altered and deformed that they are recognized as pillow lava from the vessicles seen in thin-section (Fig 5D). The rock is shiny, black, and massive and contains variable concentrations of disseminated and massive sulphides. Outcrops are commonly red due to the oxidation of the sulphides. Dikes feeding higher basalts and the upper basalts cut through the lower basalts and orebody partitioning them into small pods (Figs. 5E, 7). The pods have maximum dimensions of several tens of metres.

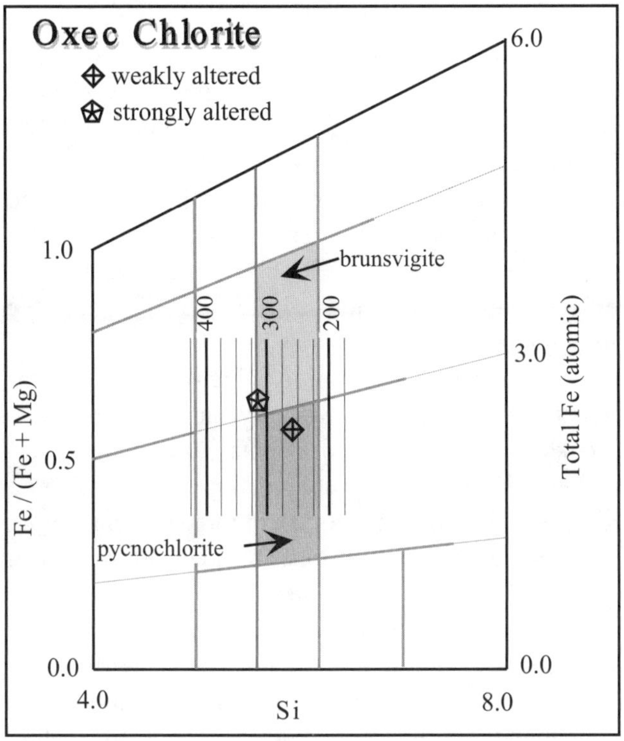

Figure 6. Chlorite compositions in weakly and strongly altered Oxec rocks. Chlorite fields from Hey (1954). Temperature contours (°C) calculated from Cathelineau (1988). Units are atomic proportions or absolute atoms calculated on a 20 cation basis.

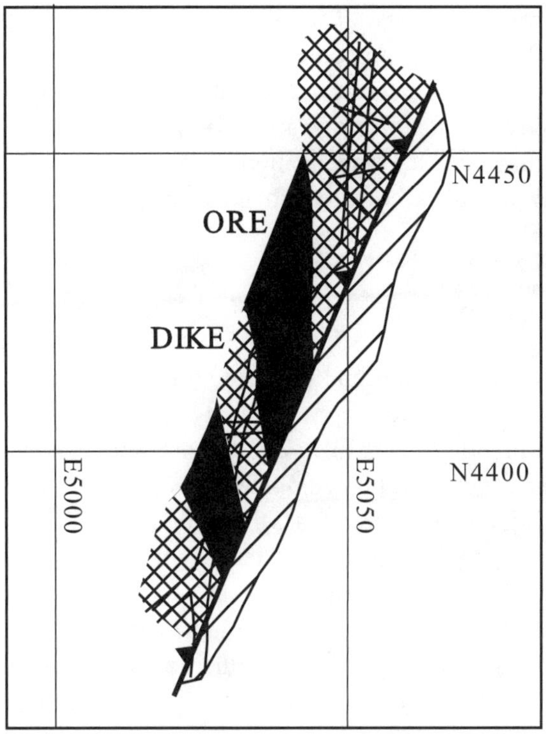

Figure 7. Geologic map of K-90 drift showing dissection of orebody by late dikes (after Petersen, 1979). Symbols: Cross-hached = dikes; shaded = ore; hached = serpentinite complex. The fault is the Oxec Thrust fault.

In sub-economic zones the lower pillow basalts are largely composed of a complex intergrowth of albite and chlorite and chlorite-replaced mafic phenocrysts. Plagioclase is largely sericitized and albitized, and the original albite twinning is poorly preserved. Epidote, sphene, and sulphides are minor components. Silicification is extensive.

Equivalent, considerably more altered rocks (Table 2) consist almost exclusively of quartz and chlorite. Quartz occurs as patches, as small laths, in veins, and in spherules (Fig. 5E). The quartz laths are silicified plagioclase and the spherules appear to be relict vesicles. These textures, relict "bow tie" texture, abundant chlorite, and late-quartz indicate that the rocks are highly chloritized and silicified pillow basalts.

Upper pillow basalts

The upper pillow basalts are exposed in the southwestern part of the mine area (Fig. 2). Aceituno (1971) and Rosenfeld (1981) indicate that this unit forms a relatively continuous belt 15 km long and 1 km wide, striking west-southwest. Rosenfeld (1990) divided this unit into an upper and lower series by on the basis of the local occurrence of the Tzumuy Fm. However, in the mine vicinity the absence of the Tzumuy Fm. makes it impossible to separate the two units and in figure 3 these units are simply identified as "upper basalts". This unit is strongly faulted and intensely weathered. Pillows rarely exceed 1 m in diametre (Fig. 5F). Hyaloclastite is abundant locally.

Pillow interiors are greenish gray and very fine-grained. Glomeroporphyritic textures and plagioclase-clinopyroxene bow-tie glomerocrysts typical of ocean-floor basalts (Frey et al., 1974) are well developed. Olivine microlites have been altered to chlorite with associated minute pyrite crystals. Minor pyrite occurs in the pillows. Pillow rinds are black, contain abundant light coloured variolites, and average about

8 mm in thickness. The pillow rinds consist of chlorite, skeletal amphibole (uralitized pyroxene), and albite. The skeletal texture of the uralitized pyroxene is a quench texture, typical of pyroxene in ocean-floor basalt rinds (T. Donnelly, oral commun.). Minor minerals include secondary sphene, calcite, and epidote.

The Oxec deposit

Structure

Dike intrusion and brittle deformation has disaggregated the Oxec deposit, which originally formed as one orebody (Figs. 5D, 7). The ore pods and additional sub-economic sulphide concentrations consist of a chaotic mixture of massive and disseminated iron and copper sulphides associated with the chloritized and silicified lower pillow basalt.

Ore pods vary greatly in volume and shape. Some are long and narrow whereas others are digitated, doubly convex, polygonal, pencil-like, or wedge-shaped. Large ore pods measure 2 to 30 m wide, 40 to 80 m long and 2 to 15 m high. Ore-grade mineralization is concentrated along an 800 m zone which is partly bounded on the east by the Oxec fault (Figs. 3, 7).

Mineralization and paragenesis

Copper and iron sulphide mineralization occurs as masses and lenses which vary in size from a few centimetres to several metres; as thin, sigmoidal stringers; in symmetrically zoned veinlets; and in quartz-basalt breccia. Large sulphide masses are aggregates of pyrite, pyrrhotite, and chalcopyrite. The sulphides are completely enclosed by chloritized and silicified basalt. Some hand specimens from the massive ores hint of centimetre-scale layering. The thin sigmoidal stringers of sulphides found throughout the mine, particularly in the K-90 drift (Fig. 7), are all that remains of sulphide coatings on pillows.

Sulphide-bearing veins with symmetrical alteration halos occur in three different rock types where they exhibit distinctive mineralogies and textures. First, in the K-90, drift, they are found within dikes in close proximity to the lower pillow basalts. Typically, the zoning sequence from the centre outward is pyrite ± epidote to quartz to highly chloritized dike and finally to unaltered dike. The veins contain euhedral pyrite crystals. Sulphide-bearing veins within the altered lower pillow basalts typically consist of a sulphide and epidote centre rimmed by quartz. Finally, quartz-lined, sulphide-filled veins are found in weakly altered basalt.

A sulphide-basalt-quartz breccia is well exposed in the 300 area (Fig. 3). There, massive quartz encloses angular fragments of highly altered basalt (Fig. 5G). Chalcopyrite and pyrite are disseminated throughout the breccia.

The copper mineralization is highly variable within and between ore pods. Usually, only pods that have blocks of massive sulphides contain ore-grade mineralization. Hand picking upgraded ore coming from a given stope to over an average of three percent copper on average. Numerous stopes yielded ore grades in excess of eleven percent copper.

The hydrothermal mineralogy of the Oxec deposit is relatively simple. Pyrrhotite, chalcopyrite, and pyrite are the dominant sulphides. Exceedingly minor constituents of the ore include hematite, magnetite, and valleriite. A paragenetic sequence is shown in figure 8. In the early stages, hematite formed, followed by magnetite, early pyrite, chalcopyrite and pyrrhotite. The formation of late pyrite, quartz, and calcite are at the end of the mineralizing cycle. Supergene minerals include native copper, chalcanthite, and malachite.

At least three types of pyrite are recognized and include early and late varieties as well as that replacing pyrrhotite. Early pyrite forms euhedral crystals up to 2 mm on edge and contains inclusions of magnetite ± hematite and chalcopyrite filled fractures. Late pyrite postdates formation of chalcopyrite as indicated by pyrite-bearing quartz veins which cut early pyrite crystals in chalcopyrite. Both early and late pyrite contain 0.5 to 0.15 weight percent cobolt (Petersen, 1979). Pyrite after pyrrhotite contains 0.6 to 0.7 weight percent cobalt.

Magnetite occurs as small, 10-μm irregular blebs randomly distributed in early pyrite, and very rarely in chalcopyrite. Hematite occurs only in the early pyrite and is always associated with magnetite. Magnetite usually encloses the hematite.

Chalcopyrite is the main copper-bearing sulphide at Oxec. It has a very uniform grain size and composition. It may occur as relatively pure masses, but more commonly it is associated with pyrrhotite and pyrite.

Magnetic pyrrhotite is an extremely widespread mineral at Oxec. It occurs as relatively pure masses with or without chalcopyrite, as blebs (200-500μm) in chalcopyrite, and as nuclei enclosed by pyrite. In most cases in which pyrrhotite and pyrite are intimately associated, the sulfidation of pyrrhotite to pyrite is evident. Pyrite first develops along the basal parting of the pyrrhotite; when the pyrrhotite is completely converted to pyrite, the resulting pyrite has a well-developed bird's-eye texture. Age relationships between the pyrrhotite and the chalcopyrite are impossible to establish. Each contains irregular inclusions of the other, pyrrhotite inclusions in chalcopyrite being more common than the converse. Pyrrhotite typically contains 0.3 to 0.5 weight percent cobolt and 0.1 weight percent nickel.

Valleriite occurs in trace amounts in both chalcopyrite and pyrrhotite. It occurs along pyrrhotite-chalcopyrite contacts, along microcracks in chalcopyrite, and apparent exsolution in the pyrrhotite.

Quartz occurs in thin veinlets that crosscut all sulphides and represents a late stage in the mineralizing process. In the 300 area, quartz is the dominant alteration phase and probably related to a feeder zone, as shown by enclosed basalt fragments, and patches and stringers of pyrite and chalcopyrite (Fig. 5G).

Calcite occurs locally in small patches and thin veinlets and is the last hydrothermal phase.

Early solutions were oxidized based on early presence of hematite and later magnetite (Fig. 6). Magnetite precipitated as local conditions became more reducing through increased discharge of reducing hydrothermal waters. fO_2 declined and fS_2 increased in later fluids and resulted in pyrite enclosing or replacing the earlier magnetite and hematite. Chalcopyrite and pyrrhotite formation suggests lower fS_2 than pyrite prevailed during main stage mineralization. In the waning stages of mineralization, pyrite again became dominant, along with quartz.

HYDROTHERMAL ALTERATION

Mass transfer

Eight samples from the dike and pillow basalt complexes were analyzed to provide an initial assessment of chemical changes during hydrothermal subseafloor alteration and mineralization (Fig. 4, Table 2). All rocks have undergone chemical changes as indicated by the mineralogical descriptions in the previous sections. None of the rocks analyzed from the mine area can be considered unaltered. Analyses 2, 3, 4, and 5 represent weakly altered rocks whereas analyses 6, 7, and 8 represent of highly altered rocks.

On the basis of relatively conserved elements Petersen and Zantop (1980) concluded that the basalt / gabbro suite were ocean floor basalts (N-MORB). Using the chemical data for average N-MORB of Wilson (1989) as an approximation for an unaltered parent it is possible to calculate chemical fluxes using the method of Grant (1986). In the absence of a large database of trace elements to assist in the identification of conserved elements, the calculations are based on conservation of aluminum (Fig. 9, Table 3).

Weakly altered rocks show small variable changes in Fe_2O_3 and MnO, weak gains in SiO_2, major gains in Na_2O and LOI and moderate losses in MgO and CaO. By comparison strongly altered rocks show weak gains in MnO, major gains in SiO_2, Fe_2O_3 and LOI, weak losses in MgO, and major losses in CaO

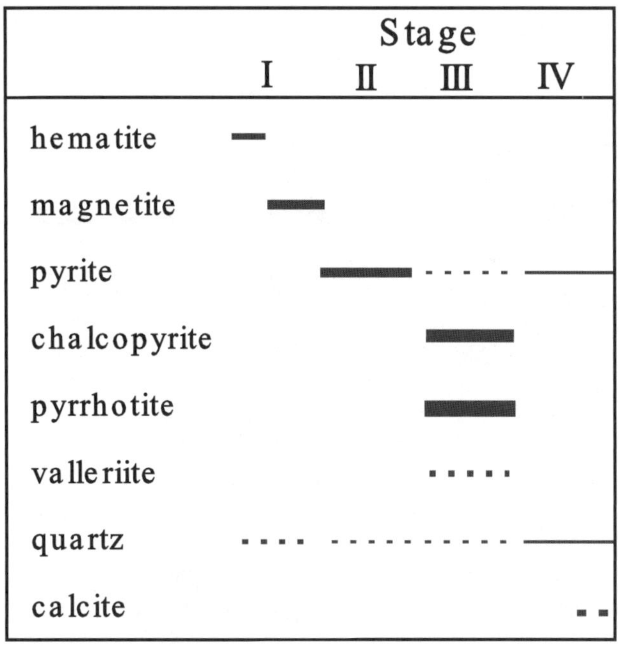

Figure 8. Paragenesis of sulphides and gangue minerals (after Petersen and Zantop, 1980).

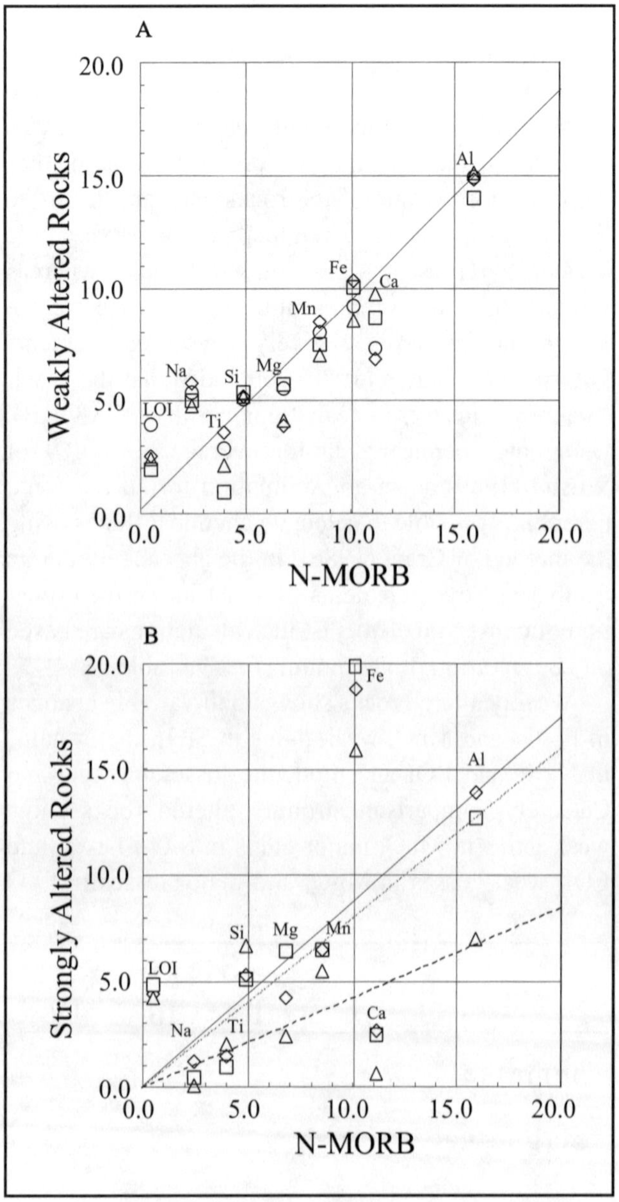

Figure 9. Isocon diagram showing mass transfer for alteration (scaled weight percent oxide). Scale factors are as follows: Si, 0.1; Mn, 50; Mg, 0.7; Ti, 3. N-MORB data from (Wilson, 1989). Sample numbers are as in Table 2. A. N-MORB parent vs weakly altered rocks. Sample symbols: Filled diamond = 2, open square = 3, open triangle = 4, open circle = 5. B. N-MORB parent vs. strongly altered rocks. Sample symbols: Filled diamond = 6, open square = 7, open triangle = 8; solid line is constant Al basis for sample 6, light-dotted line is constant Al basis for sample 7, and dashed line is constant Al basis for sample 6.

and Na_2O. These chemical changes clearly reflect the mineralogical changes. The strongly altered rocks are notably silicified, lack feldspar and contain abundant Fe-rich chlorite. The weakly altered rocks generally have no quartz, contain albite (An_2, Table 1) and contain moderate amounts of Mg-chlorite.

The direction and relative magnitude of the elemental fluxes observed in the weakly altered Oxec rocks are almost identical to those observed in the Reykjanes geothermal system (Tomasson and Kristmannsdottir, 1972), in basalt alteration studies (Humphris and Thompson, 1978), and in seawater/basalt interaction experiments (Hajash, 1975; Bischoff and Dickson, 1975; Mottl and Holland, 1978; Mottl et al., 1979). The chemical changes are consistent with alteration between 200 and 300ºC at low water/rock ratios (Mottl and Seyfried, 1977). The direction and magnitude of chemical changes in the strongly altered rocks are consistent with alteration over a similar temperature range at high water/rock ratios (Mottl and Seyfried, 1977).

THERMAL HISTORY OF MINERALIZATION

Geothermometry

Petersen and Zantop (1980) estimated temperatures for alteration to be in the range of 200ºC to 475ºC on the basis of silicate mineral assemblages. They estimated temperatures of mineralization near 300ºC on the basis of sulphide mineral relations. These temperature estimates were refined by fluid inclusion studies (Wilson and Petersen, 1980) and by chlorite thermometry as reported below.

Fluid inclusion thermometry

Wilson and Petersen (1989) examined the physical-chemical characteristics of Oxec hydrothermal fluids. Ninety-six paired salinity-temperature measurements were made in primary and pseudosecondary fluid inclusions in quartz from 6 samples from likely vent rocks. Secondary inclusions were not measured.

Average sample temperature ranges from 301 to 327ºC (adjusted for an assumed pressure of 250 bars, Styrt et al. 1981) and average salinity ranges from 3.7 to 7.4 NaCl equivalent weight percent (Table 4). No visual evidence for CO_2 or boiling was found. Little

Table 3. Elemental changes resulting from hydrothermal alteration. Mass gains and losses in percent.

Sample Oxide	1	2	3	4	5	6	7	8
SiO_2	2	15	25	12	11	24	31	212
Al_2O_3	0	0	0	0	0	0	0	0
Fe_2O_3	-16	10	13	-11	-3	114	146	259
MnO	-18	8	0	-13	0	-12	-4	47
MgO	-26	-38	-4	-36	-13	-29	19	-20
CaO	-8	-34	-42	-8	-30	-73	-73	-88
Na_2O	37	155	136	108	135	-43	-76	-94
TiO_2	-34	-3	-74	-44	-22	-58	-71	16
LOI	581	451	343	409	745	916	1118	1814

P_2O_5, K_2O not listed because their analytical totals are extremely low. Sample numbers as in Table 2.

Table 4. Summary of fluid inclusion data.

Sample	Salinity (NaCl Equiv. weight percent)		Pressure-corrected homogenization temperture (°C)	
60	4.7	(3.0-8.4)	304	(304-327)
46	6.8	(3.3-8.7)	319	(283-336)
49	7.4	(5.5-8.5)	310	(306-314)
103B	5.2	(4.3-5.8)	327	(239-347)
139A	3.7	(3.5-4.1)	322	(322-344)
96	3.7	(3.2-4.4)	301	(248-332)

Sample Gu/O-n-77; Sample location given in Wilson and Petersen (1989)

overall correlation between homogenization temperature and salinity exists at Oxec.

Chlorite thermometry

Chlorite geothermometry has been applied in a number of deposit settings to estimate thermal conditions attending mineralization (Larson, 1994; Braxton and Petersen, 1999). DeCaritat et al. (1993) provide a thorough review of the various approaches and calibrations comparing five different methods across a range of formation temperatures. Their study showed that no single method adequately predicts chlorite formation temperature in all environments owing to the limitations inherent in each approach. This study used the empirical temperature-composition relation reported by Cathelineau (1988) because it was calibrated in a geothermal field where chlorite was forming in mafic volcanic rocks. The relation T(°C) = - 61.92 + 321.98 Al^{iv} where Al^{iv} is the tetrahedral aluminum site occupancy in chlorite is used to calculate temperature.

Chlorite is a wide spread alteration mineral in Oxec rocks and has the potential of providing tighter constraints on temperature variations in this hydrothermal system. An average temperature of 255°C is calculated for chlorite in weakly altered rocks and an average temperature of 320°C is calculated for chlorite in strongly altered and mineralized rocks (Table 2). The 320°C temperature for the highly altered rocks is consistent with fluid inclusion temperatures in quartz from feeder zone rocks. This suggests that the pressure corrections applied by Wilson and Petersen (1989) were of the right order of magnitude. It is reasonable to postulate that temperatures would be lower in rocks distal to the feeder zone.

Discussion and summary

There are several easily measurable variations in the composition of chlorite from different parts of the hydrothermal system. Rocks that have higher percentages of chlorite have a greener cast, and those that are more altered have a deep green to black appearance. The colour of the chlorite is a function of the Mg/Fe ratio. The tetrahedral site occupancy varies as a function of temperature with the higher temperature chlorites containing higher amounts of tetrahedral Al. In Oxec rocks, higher temperatures correlate with samples that are mineralized and have experienced greater amounts of mass transfer (sample 117 vs 50). The number of samples in which the composition of chlorite was determined is inadequate establish a thermal zoning pattern that might be useful to exploration. Nevertheless, chlorite compositions may be useful in regional exploration to vector into regions of high fluid and heat flow because most of the gabbro and basalt would have similar pre-alteration compositions.

The coincidence of maximum temperatures arrived at from fluid inclusion studies and chlorite chemistry is remarkable. Maximum measured temperatures do not appear to have exceeded about 325°C. Considerably higher temperatures have been recorded at other Cyprus-type deposits (Spiess et al., 1980; Styrt et al., 1981). The relatively low temperatures at Oxec may indicate that the system was not very robust and may explain the small size of the deposit.

Salinities higher than seawater values in VMS deposits are common and indicate that magmatic waters may be involved in the mineralization or that phase separation has taken place in the sub-seafloor hydrothermal system (deRonde, 1995). If phase separation was an ongoing process in the Oxec hydrothermal system, the absence of low salinity fluids suggests that mineralization took place when moderate salinity fluids were exiting the vent. In the absence of additional chemical and isotopic data a magmatic contribution cannot be ruled out.

The Oxec deposit shares many characteristics with other Cyprus-type deposits such as association with basaltic host rocks, basalt host rocks that are part of an ophiolite sequence, copper mineralization as chalcopyrite, and alteration consisting of chloritization and silicification of host rocks and albitization of peripheral rocks. There are also some significant differences: pyrrhotite is a major component of the ores at Oxec, whereas in other Cyprus-type deposits it is only a variable constituent, usually at the top of the deposit (Constantinou and Govett, 1973).

One economically unfavorable characteristic at Oxec is that as a resulted from protracted magmatic activity at the site of mineralization the orebody was intruded by numerous dikes that partitioned it into a multitude of mineable ore pods and hundreds of non-mineable, sulphide-poor pods. Initial drilling results failed to recognize the significance of these dikes. The dilution effects became apparent as the ore zone was exposed underground. On the other hand, had the deposit not been covered, none of it may have survived.

ACKNOWLEDGEMENTS

Numerous individuals participated in the cumulative research efforts aimed at understanding the Oxec copper deposit — Drs. Half Zantop and Richard Stoiber, Peter Marsh, Ing. Cesar Recinos, Ing. Leo Piedmont, Dr. T. Donnelly, Joshua Rosenfeld, Paula Wilson, Stan J. Morrison, Michael DePangher and Dr. William T. Parry and their contributions are gratefully acknowledged. Transmetales, Ltd., Dartmouth College and the University of Utah Electron Microbeam Laboratory and the Fluid Inclusion Laboratory provided funding for these efforts. Reviews by Ross Sherlock and Ron Britten improved the manuscript and are gratefully acknowledged.

REFERENCES

Aceituno, M.A. 1971. Photogeologic map: Company files, Guatemala City, Transmetales LTDA.

Bischoff, J.L. and Dickson, F. W. 1975. Seawater-basalt interaction at 200°C and 500 bars: implications for origin of seafloor heavy metal deposits and regulation of seawater chemistry: Earth and Planetary Science Letters, 25: 838-897.

Bonis, S.B. 1968. Geologic reconnaissance of the Alta Verapaz fold belt, Guatemala. Unpub. Ph.D. thesis, Louisiana State University, Baton Rouge.

Bonis, S.B. 1970. Mapa Geologico de la Republica de Guatemala 1:500,000. Insituto Geographico Nacional. 4 sheets.

Braxton, D.P. and Petersen, E.U. 1999. Thermal auerols of fossil epithermal systems: A case study from the Calera Vein, Orcopampa, Peru. 75th Anniversary Volume. The Geological Society of Peru.

Cathelineau, M. 1988. Cation site occupancy in chlorites and illites as a function of temperature. Clay Mineralogy, 23: 471-485.

Constantinou, G. and Govett, G.J. S. 1973. Geology, geochemistry, and genesis of Cyprus sulfide deposits. Economic Geology, 68: 843-858.

DeCaritat, P., Hutcheon, I. and Walshe, J.L. 1993. Chlorite geothermometry: A review. Clay and Clay Minerals, 41: 2, 219-239.

deRonde, C.E.J. 1995. Fluid chemistry and isotopic characteristics of seafloor hydrothermal systems and associated VMS deposits: Potential for magmatic contributions. In MAC Short Course 23, Magmas, Fluids and Ore Deposits, Edited by J.F.H. Thompson. 479-509.

Frey, F.A., Bryan, W.B. and Thompson, G. 1974. Atlantic ocean-floor: geochemistry and petrology of basalts from legs 2 and 3 of the Deep Sea Drilling Project. Journal of Geophysical Research, 79: 5507-5527.

Grant 1986. The isocon diagram- A simple solution to Gresen's equation for metasomatic alteration. Economic Geology, 81: 1976-1982.

Hajash, A. 1975. Hydrothermal processes along mid-ocean ridges: an experimental investigation. Contributions to Mineralogy and Petrology, 53: 205-216.

Hey, M.H. 1954. A new review of the chlorites. Mineralogical Magazine. 30: 277.

Humphris, S.E. and Thompson, G. 1978. Hydrothermal alteration of oceanic basalts by seawater. Geochimica et Cosmochimica Acta, 42: 107-135.

Larson, P., Cunningham, C.G. and Naeser, C.W. 1994. Large-scale alteration effects in the Rico paleothermal anomaly, Southwest Colorado. Economic Geology, 89: 1769-1779.

Mottl, M.J. and Holland, H.D. 1978. Chemical exchange during hydrothermal alteration of basalt by seawater V. Experimental results for major and minor components of seawater. Geochimica et Cosmochimica Acta, 42: 1103-1105.

Mottl, M.J. and Seyfried, W.E. 1977. Experimental basalt-water interaction: rock versus seawater-dominated systems and the origin of submarine hydrothermal deposits. Geological Society of America Abstracts with Programs. 9: 1104-1105.

Mottl, M.J., Holland, H.D. and Corr, R.F. 1979. Chemical exchange during hydrothermal alteration of basalt by seawater-II. Experimental results for Fe, Mn, and sulfur species. Geochimica et Cosmochimica Acta, 43: 869-884.

Petersen, E.U. 1979. The Oxec copper deposit, Guatemala: An ophiolite copper occurrence. Unpub. M.A. thesis, Dartmouth College, Hanover.

Petersen, E.U. and Zantop, H. 1980. The Oxec deposit, Guatemala: An ophiolite copper occurrence. Economic Geology, 75: 1053-1065.

Roberts, R.J. and Irving, E.M. 1957. Mineral deposits of Central America. U. S. Geological Survey Bulletin, 1034: 57-58.

Rosenfeld, J.H. 1980. The Santa Cruz Ophiolite, Guatemala, Central America. In Conferencia Geologica del Caribe 9, Edited by L.C. Romeo, G.G. Nelson, S. Michael, T. Ivan and S. William. 2: 451-452.

Rosenfeld, J.H. 1981. Geology of the western Sierra de Santa Cruz, Guatemala, Central America: An ophiolite sequence. Unpbl. Ph.D. Thesis, State University of New York, Binghamton. 313 p.

Rosenfeld, J.H. 1990. Sedimentary rocks of the Santa Cruz Ophiolite, Guatemala; A proto-Caribbean history In Conferencia Geologica del Caribe 12, Edited by Larue, D.K. and G. Draper. 513-519.

Shido, F., Miyashiro, A. and Ewing, M. 1974. Compositional variation in pillow lavas from the Mid-Atlantic ridge. Marine Geology, 16: 177-190.

Spiess, F. N., MacDonald, K. C., Atwater, T., Ballard, R., Carranza, A., Cordoba, D., Cox, D., Diaz Garcia, V. M., Francheteau, J., Guerrero, J., Hawkins, J., Haymon, R., Hessier, R., Juteau, T., Kastner, M., Larson, R., Kuyendk, B., MacDougall, J. D., Miller, S., Normark, W., Orcutt, J. and Rangin, C. 1980. East Pacific Rise: hot springs and geophysical experiments. Science, 207, 1421-1432.

Steele, I.M., Bishop, F.C., Smith, J.V. and Windley, B.F. 1977. The Fiskenaesset Complex, West Greenland, Part III. Groenlands Geol. Unders. Bulletin. 124.

Styrt, M. M., Brackmann, A. J., Holland, H. D., Clark, B. C., Pisutha-Arnond, V., Eldrige, C. S. and Ohmoto, H. 1981. The mineralogy and the isotopic composition of sulfur in hydrothermal sulfide/sulfate deposits on the East Pacific Rise, 21oN latitude. Earth and Planetary Science Letters, 53, 282-290.

Tomasson, J. and Kristmannsdottir, H. 1972. High temperature alteration of minerals and thermal brines Reykjanes, Iceland. Contributions to Mineralogy and Petrology, 36: 123-134.

Wilson, H.H. 1974. Cretaceous sedimentation and orogeny in nuclear Central America. American Association of Petroloum Geologists Bulletin, 58: 1348-1396.

Wilson, M. 1989, Igneous Petrogenesis: A Global Tectonic Approach. Unwin-Hyman. London.

Wilson, P.N. and Petersen, E.U. 1989. Fluid inclusion evidence for fluid mixing in the Oxec Cyprus-type copper deposit, Guatemala. Economic Geology, 84: 444-449.

VOLCANOGENIC MASSIVE SULPHIDE OCCURRENCES AND POTENTIAL IN VENEZUELA, WITH EMPHASIS ON THE GUAYANA SHIELD

DOMINIC M. DER. CHANNER, PATRICK F. N. ANDERSON
Guaniamo Mining Company, Centro Gerencial Mohedano, Of.9D, Calle Los Chaguarramos, La Castellana, Caracas, Venezuela

ABSTRACT

The Venezuelan portion of the Guayana shield occupies an area of nearly 400,000 km^2 of which about 135,000 km^2 are occupied by volcano-sedimentary terrains, including granite - greenstone belts. In Venezuela the shield can be divided into four lithotectonic provinces (Imataca, Pastora, Cuchivero, and Roraima) and also the Amazonas territory. No volcanogenic massive sulphide mineral deposits, or even showings, have been reported. In contrast, a base metal exploration program in neighbouring Guyana in the 1960's found numerous showings. The Guyana greenstone belts are contiguous with those of eastern Venezuela. The geological characteristics of the Guayana shield greenstone belts are similar to those of other, well-known, Precambrian greenstone belts such as the Abitibi, which contain volcanogenic massive sulphide deposits.

The Pastora - Botanamo greenstone belt in the Pastora province has the highest potential to host Precambrian volcanogenic massive sulphide deposits. Exploration in this region has historically focussed on shear zone hosted gold deposits and volcanogenic massive sulphide deposits may have been bypassed. The Cuchivero province has lower potential for hosting volcanogenic massive sulphide deposits. This province is dominated by felsic volcanics but results of field studies suggest that much of the volcanism was subaerial. However, large areas of this province remain unmapped and it is possible that the oldest parts of the sequence were formed subaqueously. The Amazonas region consists of high grade gneisses and is of relatively unknown potential for sulphide ore deposits.

Phanerozoic Cu - Zn - Pb deposits and showings occur in northern Venezuela in a north - east trending branch of the Andean mountain range. The largest known deposit is the De Lima II, near Bailadores, with reserves of 2 Mt at 1.5 % Cu.

The Ministry of Mines conducted extensive regional studies throughout Bolivar state and the Amazonas territory during the 1970's and early 1980's. Exploration by mining companies in the 1990's has focussed on gold and diamonds, and most work has been in the greenstone belts. The main control on the location of volcanogenic massive sulphide deposits is intermediate to felsic subaqueous volcanism, and any regional exploration program must start from this premise, as was successfully done in Guyana.

INTRODUCTION

The Guayana shield occupies the whole of the southern part of Venezuela, with its northern edge roughly defined by the present course of the Orinoco river. The Venezuelan portion of the shield occupies an area of nearly 400,000 km^2 of which almost 60,000 km^2 is occupied by granite - greenstone belts, and about 75,000 km^2 by volcano-sedimentary belts, dominated by felsic volcanics. In Venezuela the shield can be divided into four lithotectonic provinces: Imataca, Pastora, Cuchivero, and Roraima (Menéndez, 1968; Martin-Bellizia, 1972; Gibbs and Barron, 1993), and also the undivided Amazonas territory (Fig. 1). Several authors have observed that a large proportion of this area is prospective for volcanogenic massive sulphide deposits, but that no deposits have yet been found (Gibbs and Barron, 1993; Sidder, 1995). Ally (1985) wrote on the potential for volcanogenic massive sulphide deposits in Guyana and cited several reasons for the relative lack of success in making a significant discovery. These reasons were: the lack of proper regional geophysical coverage at the required line spacing, the lack of modern exploration programs using recent exploration

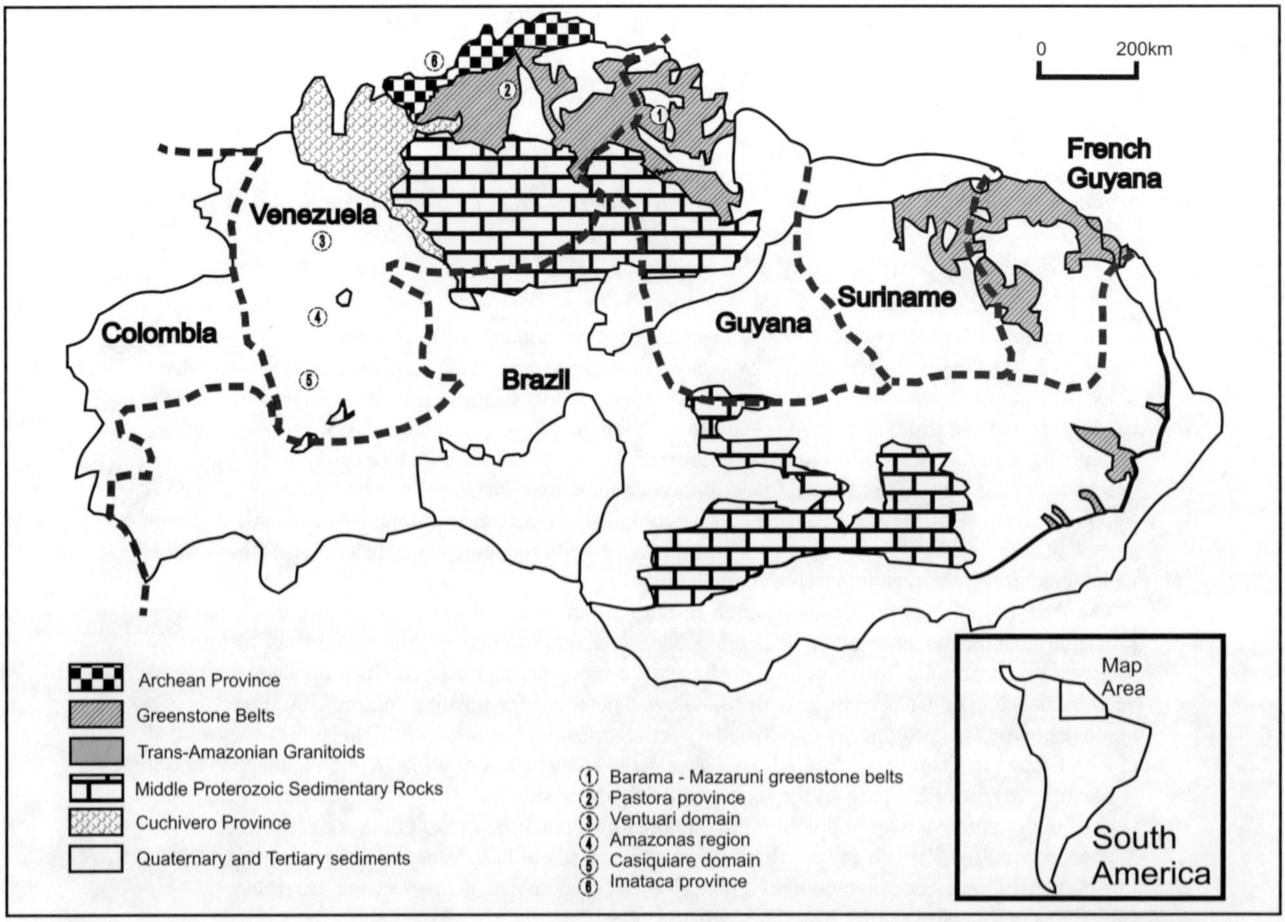

Figure 1. Locations of the Guayana shield and the principal lithotectonic provinces in Venezuela (after Ledru and Milési, 1995). Note that the Roraima province consists of the Mid Proterozoic sedimentary rocks in the south-eastern part of Venezuela.

models for volcanogenic massive sulphide deposits, and the lack of focus and exploration dollars from mining companies. Walrond (1985) described a metallogenic scheme for the Guayana shield in Guyana, Surinam, and French Guiana and observed that the difficulty of access to remote jungle areas, combined with the interpretive problems arising with remote sensing data in deeply weathered tropical terrains, had also contributed to the general lack of success in the location of bedrock ore deposits. These authors recognized the potential for volcanogenic massive sulphide deposits for geological and tectonic reasons. Venezuela, despite its potential, has been largely bypassed by the exploration boom in South America during the past ten years.

In this paper the volcanogenic massive sulphide potential in the Guayana shield of Venezuela is examined using the following approach. First, the key characteristics of Precambrian volcanogenic massive sulphide deposits are reviewed, then the general geology of the various provinces of the Guayana shield is summarized. Subsequently, the prospectivity of these provinces is assessed based on their geology and the presence or absence of the key characteristics of volcanogenic massive sulphide deposits from other Precambrian areas. Since no volcanogenic massive sulphide occurrences have been described from the Precambrian of Venezuela, particular attention is given to the descriptions by Ally (1985) of volcanogenic massive sulphide occurrences in Guyana. These occur in the Barama - Mazaruni greenstone belts, which are geologically continuous with those of the Pastora province in Venezuela (Fig. 1), and provide the strongest empirical evidence for the probable

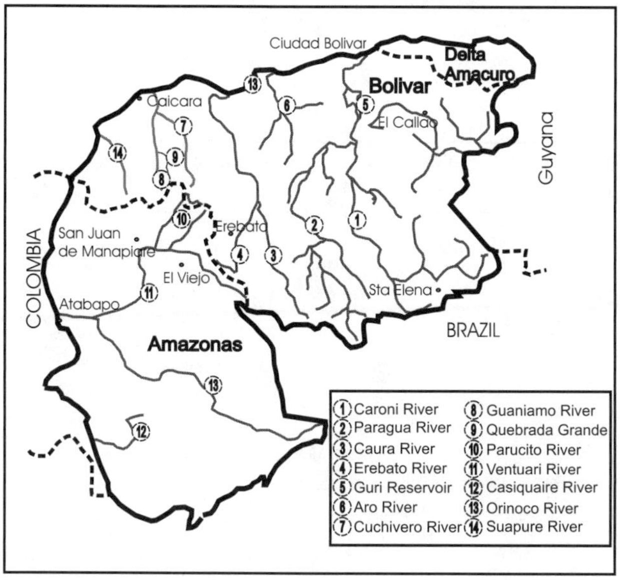

Figure 2. Geographical features (rivers and towns) mentioned in the text for the Venezuelan part of the Guayana shield

existence of volcanogenic massive sulphide deposits in the Venezuelan greenstone belts. In this article the Venezuelan spelling has been used for Guayana, with different spellings used only when referring to other countries such as Guyana. Geographical areas and location names used in the text are shown in Figure 2.

Venezuela has some recorded base metal production from Phanerozoic deposits in the north and west of the country. Although not the main focus of this article, we also summarize the deposits and occurrences.

KEY GEOLOGICAL FEATURES OF PRECAMBRIAN VOLCANOGENIC MASSIVE SULPHIDE DEPOSITS

The principal regional and local scale geological features of Precambrian massive sulphide deposits are reviewed in Table 1. In separate columns of Table 1, examples of these features are given for the Guyana and Venezuela portions of the Guayana shield. In Table 2 the principal features of numerous Precambrian greenstone belts are summarized and the presence or absence of volcanogenic massive sulphide mineralization is indicated.

Regional features include the lithotectonic association, the stratigraphic control, and the observed clustering of deposits into camps or districts within some of which a log normal size - frequency distribution has been measured (e.g., Ladysmith - Rhinelander district, Wisconsin - DeMatties, 1994). Local features include the facies association, characteristic alteration patterns, and fault control. Most Precambrian volcanogenic massive sulphide deposits are dominated by Cu - Zn ores (Franklin et al., 1981) and have been affected by deformation and metamorphism, causing changes to initial geometry and mineralogy (Sangster, 1972).

The lithotectonic association is the most important criterion in regional area selection for exploration. Volcanogenic massive sulphide deposits occur in greenstone belts of both Archean (e.g., Abitibi belt) and Proterozoic (e.g., North Wisconsin, Flin Flon - Snow Lake) ages (see Table 2). Relative proportions of mafic and felsic volcanic rocks vary widely from mafic - dominated belts (e.g., Abitibi, Flin Flon - Snow Lake) to felsic - dominated (e.g., Bergslagen; Table 2).

At the local scale, the most important criterion for area selection is the clear association between massive sulphide deposits and felsic volcanic centres. In fact, Ally (1985) observed that the best exploration strategy in Guyana was to explore in areas of known concentration of felsic volcanics, since the paucity of data prohibited any more detailed identification of favorable horizons or areas.

THE GEOLOGY OF THE VENEZUELAN PART OF THE GUAYANA SHIELD

The Venezuelan section of the Guayana shield includes ~25 % of the total shield area, which extends into Brazil, Colombia, Guyana, Surinam, and French Guyana (Gibbs and Barron, 1993). In Venezuela the shield can be divided into four lithotectonic provinces: Imataca, Pastora, Cuchivero, and Roraima (Menéndez, 1968; Martin-Bellizia, 1972; Gibbs and Barron, 1993). The Amazonas territory forms a fifth region, not yet identified as a separate province (Fig. 1). The Roraima province consists of mid - Proterozoic fluvio - lacustrine sediments and is not considered to be prospective for volcanogenic massive sulphide deposits. Comprehensive descriptions of the geology of the Venezuelan section of the Guayana shield are to be found in Gibbs and Barron (1983, 1993) and Sidder and Mendoza (1995), and much of the information summarized here is taken from these sources. The general geological sequence

Table 1. Key geological features of Precambrian volcanogenic massive sulphide deposits with examples from Guyana and Venezuela

REGIONAL FEATURES [a, b]	SPECIFIC FEATURE	COMMENTS	EXAMPLES FROM GUYANA [i]	EXAMPLES FROM VENEZUELA [j]
Greenstone belts	Age	Early Archean to Proterozoic	Barama - Mazaruni	Pastora - Botanamo
	% felsic rocks	5 to 50	8	20
	Area (km^2)	700 to 115,000	30,000	60,000
	Tectonic setting	Island arc to back arc; some at rifted continental margins	Ocean island arc to back arc	Ocean island arc to back arc
	District size (km)	15 to 50, clustering common	Groete Creek - Area 33 zone is 100 km long, but this may represent several districts	
Favorable horizons	Size distribution	Log normal [f]		
	Lithology and extent	Graphitic or chert horizons most common; occur on km - scale [f,g]	Carbonaceous horizons	
LOCAL FEATURES				
Facies	Felsic volcanic centre forming positive topographic feature [c,d]	Synvolcanic intrusion; associated dacite-rhyolite lava and debris flows with onlapping sediments	Supergroup rocks including Ianna and Yakishuru localities (Barama belt), Million Mount (Cuyuni belt),and Eagle Mountain - Mahdia area (Mazaruni belt)	Yuruari and Caballape formations
Alteration	Discharge zones	2 to 3 km wide; local pluton provides heat source	Alteration described at: Baramalli Creek, Area 33, Aranka	
	Recharge zones	Up to 30 km wide, hydrothermal cell may last for 10 Ma and penetrate to 8 km depth (e.g., Noranda district) [h]		
Local structure	Synvolcanic, extensional faults	Control location of discharge zones		
Metamorphism and Deformation	Change of primary mineralogy and deposit geometry [e]	Felsic and mafic host rocks form qz-fspr schists / gneisses and amphibolites, respectively. Minor deformation causes orebody parallel to foliation, major deformation causes a rod - like, sub-vertical body .	Greenschist to amphibolite facies metamorphism; folding and faulting have occurred	Greenschist to amphibolite facies metamorphism; folding and faulting have occurred

Notes: a - Franklin et al. 1981; b - Herrington et al. 1997; c - Binns and Scott, 1993; d - Fouquet et al. 1993; e - Sangster, 1972; f - DeMatties, 1994; g - Brauhart et al. 1998; h - Cathles, 1993; i - Ally, 1985; j - Gibbs and Barron, 1993.

Table 2. Comparison of Venezuelan and Guyanese greenstone belts with other Precambrian examples.

Location	Age (Ga)	Volcanic rock percentages				Stratigraphic thickness (km)	Area (sq. km)	Volcanic series	VMS mineralization	Reference
		ultramafic	*basalt*	*andesite*	*felsic*					
Venezuela greenstone belts (Pastora - Botanamo)	2.25 - 2.1	*2*	*73*	*17*	*8*	10	60,000	predominantly tholeiitic in lower part; increasingly calc-alkaline up-section. Oceanic island arc to back arc setting	no reported showings	Sidder and Mendoza (1995)
Guyana greenstone belts	2.2	2	50	28	20	9	30,000	predominantly tholeiitic in lower part; increasingly calc-alkaline up-section. Oceanic island arc to back arc setting	Occurrences and showings (e.g., Groete Creek Resource 33 Mt @ 0.25% Cu, 0.5 g/t Au)	Ally (1985)
Older greenstone belt sequence (Zimbabwe craton)	3.0 - 2.8	50		50		5 - 7	28,579 (23 greenstone belts)	Lower Bulawayan series. Continental rift environment.	none	Blenkinsop et al. (1997)
Younger greenstone belt sequence (Zimbabwe craton)	2.7	100		0		10		Upper Buluwayan series; greenstones in west have bimodal volcanism. Continental rift setting.	none	Blenkinsop et al. (1997)
Barberton belt (Kapvaal craton)	3.5 - 3.0	10	85		5	10	6,000	dominantly komatitic and some tholeiitic at base; tholeiitic up-section; calc alkaline rare. Oceanic back arc.	Bien Venue deposit (~300,000 t) (C. De Ronde: pers. comm.)	Brandl and de Wit, 1997
East Pilbara belt (Pilbara craton)	3.6 - 2.8	70			30	10	15,000	arc / back arc	Sulphur Springs (5.3 Mt @ 6.1% Zn 2.2% Cu); Kangaroo Caves (1.7 Mt @ 9.8% Zn 0.6% Cu)	Barley (1997); Brauhart et al. (1998)
Miagri belt (Tanzania craton)	3.0 - 2.5	0	20	30	50	10	1,000	no ultramafics; island arc	MacCalder mine - 2 Mt (Cu-Zn-Au-Ag)	Borg and Shackleton (1997)
Quadrilatero Ferrifero (Sao Francisco craton)	3.0 - 2.7	95			5	6	7,000	oceanic back arc basin	none	Baars (1997)
Murchison belt (Yilgarn craton)	3.0 - 2.8	78		2	20	15	120,000	rifting and intracratonic collisional	none	Myers and Swager (1997)
Kalgoorlie belt (Yilgarn craton)	2.7 - 2.68	50		50		7	25,000	amalgamated arc	none	Myers and Swager (1997)
Abitibi belt (Superior province)	2.76 - 2.67	93			7	12	115,000	predominantly tholeiitic in lower part increasingly cal-alkaline up section; volcanic arcs in microplate setting	major deposits - Kidd Creek (130 Mt @ 6.1% Zn, 2.9% Cu, 0.2% Pb, 85 g/t Ag), Louvicourt (24 Mt @ 2.0% Zn, 3.9% Cu, 31 g/t Ag, 1 g/t Au), Mattagami Lake (25.6 Mt @ 5.1% Zn, 0.42% Cu, 21.6 g/tAg, 0.3 g/t Au)	Stott (1997)
Point Lake belt (Slave province)	ca. 2.7	90		10		?	700	tholeiitic to calc-alkaline up section. Either rift basin margin within sialic basement, or oceanic crust	Significant VMS area (e.g., Izok Lake 9.8 Mt @ 14.4% Zn, 2.85% Cu, 1.46% Pb, 75.1 g/t Ag); numerous showings	King and Helmstaedt (1997)
Sukumuland belt (Tanzania craton)	2.8 - 2.5	0	40	30	20	7	20,000	no ultramafics; island arc	2 possible VMS deposits (Bulyanhulu, Samena)	Borg and Shackleton (1997)
Various greenstone belts (West Africa craton)	2.2 - 2.1	45		55		10	95,000 (12 belts)	bimodal volcanism; island arc	one deposit	Attoh and Ekwueme (1997)
Rio Itapicuru (Sao Francisco craton)	2.2 - 1.9	65		35		10	7,000	island arc tholeiites; calc-alkaline and pyroclastic felsic volcanics; back arc turbidites	none	Baars (1997)
Reindeer zone (South Trans - Hudson orogen)	1.91 - 1.76		85		15	10	12,000 (2 belts)	oceanic island arc	Major VMS area (e.g., Flin Flon 63 Mt @ 4.1% Zn, 2.2% Cu, 43.2 g/t Ag, 2.85 g/t Au)	Lewry and Stauffer (1997)
Ladysmith Rhinelander belt (Pembine - Wausau subterrane, N. Wisconsin)	1.88 - 1.76	75			25	?	15,000	volcanic arc and back arc	Major VMS area (e.g., Crandon 67.4 Mt @ 5.56% Zn, 1.04% Cu, 0.48% Pb, 38.8 g/t Ag, 1.1 g/t Au)	DeMatties (1994)
Bergslagen region (Baltic shield)	1.9 - 1.87		8	3	89	10	50,000	calc-alkaline, continental back arc; quartzite sediments at base of volcanic sequence and intercalated with rhyolite dominated volcanics	Major VMS area (e.g., Falun 28.1 Mt @ 4% Zn, 2-4% Cu, 1.5% Pb, 13-24 g/t Ag, 2-4 g/t Au)	Allen et al (1996)

of events in the shield is summarized in Table 3, modified from Sidder and Mendoza (1995). The geology of the Venezuelan part of the Guyana shield is illustrated in Figure 3.

Imataca Province

This province is located in the north - eastern part of Bolivar state, forming a NE - SW trending belt between 65 and 130 km wide, and some 500 km long. It extends from the Rio Caura in the west to the Delta Amacuro in the east, where it disappears beneath young sediments of the Orinoco delta (Fig. 1 & 2). The rocks consist of high grade metamorphic mafic (~15 %) and felsic (~80 %) gneisses, amphibolites, granitic bodies, and banded iron formations (Chase, 1965; Sosa, 1977). Metamorphic grade varies from granulite in the north-east to amphibolite in the south-west. The region is known for large deposits of iron, and also for lesser deposits of manganese, bauxite, and kaolin.

The structural framework of the Imataca province is highly complex, with large isoclinal folds later refolded by open folds. The fold axes trend north-west but swing to north-east orientations close to the Guri fault. The Guri fault system separates the Imataca province from the Pastora province to the south (Figs. 1, 3), and is high angle with a history of various movement directions in times as recent as the Cenozoic (Benaim and Rios, 1977). This fault system may be traced eastwards to the Orinoco delta and westwards to the Cuchivero province.

Existing radiometric age data implies that protoliths of the high grade metamorphic rocks are early Archean (Montgomery, 1979). Deformation and metamorphism occurred in the late Archean, forming the La Ceiba migmatites (2800 - 2700 Ma). Proterozoic high grade metamorphism occurred during the Transamazonian event at 2150 - 1960 Ma (the Encrucijada granite and Pueblito gneiss; Table 3).

Recent seismic surveying, along with gravity and magnetic data, (Castillo et al. 1999) indicates crustal thicknesses of 45 - 48 km and an average crustal velocity of 6.6 km/s. Sub - crustal velocities are 8.2 km/s. Preliminary analysis of the data suggests a general downward inclination of the Moho to the west, from the Imataca into the Cuchivero province.

Pastora province

This area is located directly to the south of the Imataca province, separated by the Guri fault (Fig. 3). It is characterised by a greenstone belt assemblage of basic and felsic volcanic rocks, related sedimentary rocks, and various igneous intrusives (Menéndez, 1968, 1972). The general geology of the province is illustrated in Figure 4. Metamorphic grade is generally low, approaching amphibolite in some places. The oldest rocks consist of mafic volcanics of the Carichapo group (El Callao and Cicapra formations), overlain by intermediate to felsic volcanics and tuffs of the Yuruari formation. These rocks together form the Pastora supergroup. Discordantly overlying these rocks are volcanics, gravels, and conglomerates of the Caballape and Los Caribes formations, together forming the Botanamo group (Table 3). Intrusive igneous rocks of the Supamo complex include granite domes, migmatite, diorite, quartz porphyry, gabbro, and diabase (Benaim and Rios, 1977). These igneous rocks divide the volcano - sedimentary rocks into arcuate belts. These greenstone belts were formed from 2250 - 2100 Ma, and the Supamo complex from 2230 - 2050 Ma (Table 3), and correlate with the Barama - Mazaruni greenstone belts in adjacent Guyana.

Pastora supergroup

El Callao formation. This is the oldest formation in the province and consists of ~3000 m of subaqueous basalts and andesites, which show pillow structures. Occasional ferruginous and manganiferous interflow sediments occur. The rocks are mostly at greenschist grade, increasing in grade towards granites of the Supamo complex.

Cicapra formation. This formation consists of ~2000 m of bedded andesite tuffs and turbidites. It thins out and disappears to the south of El Callao.

Yuruari formation. This formation is dominated by sedimentary rocks, but also contains some felsic volcanic rocks. Rocks consist mostly of mica schists, phyllites, and felsic tuffs. Locally there occur tuffaceous breccias, lava flows, and chert. Only rarely are these rocks intruded by rocks of the Supamo complex.

Deformation. Most rocks have been deformed through isoclinal folding, which is related to the granites of the Supamo complex. Foliation is typically

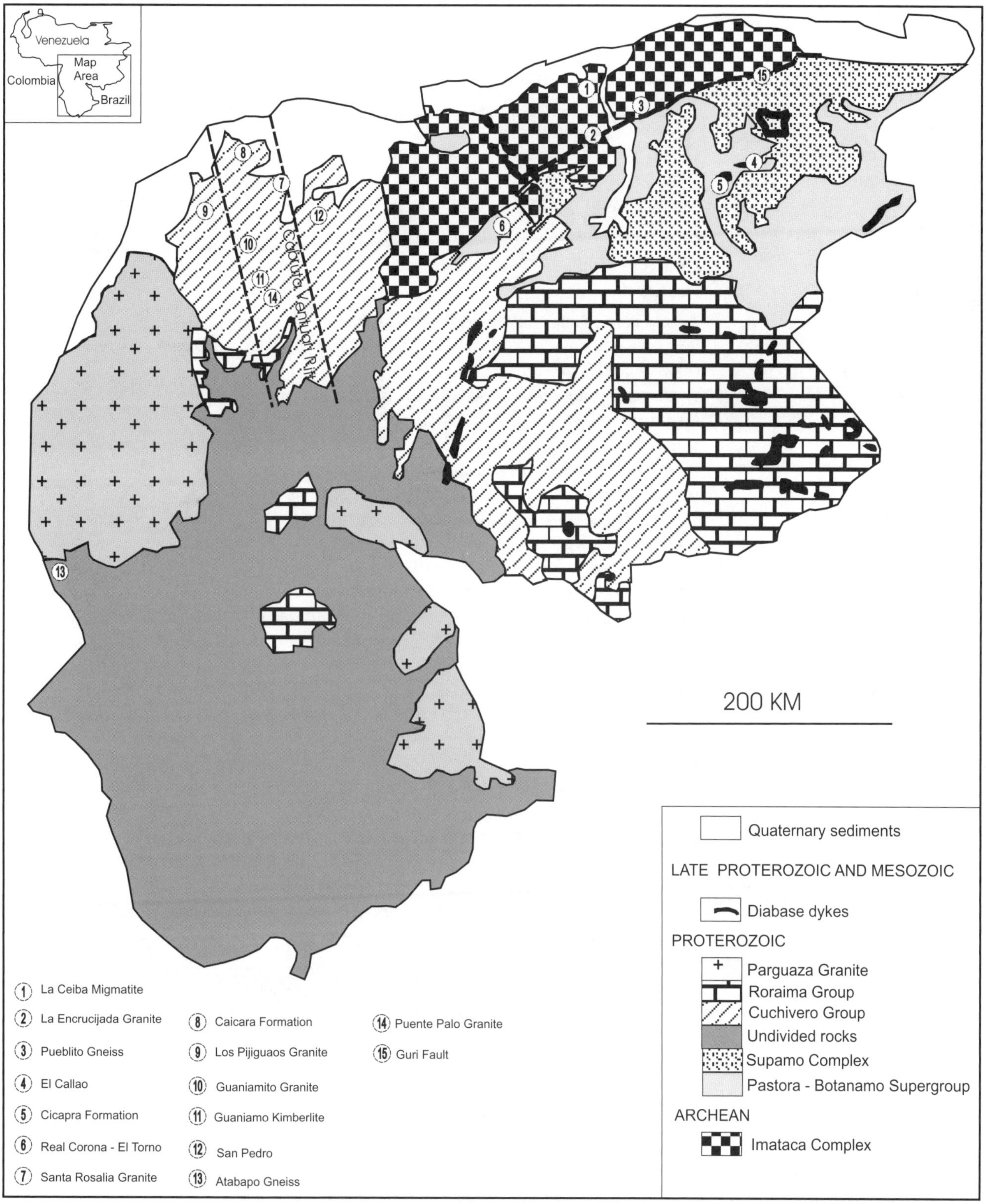

Figure 3. Geology of the Venezuelan part of the Guayana shield (after Sidder and Mendoza, 1995)

Table 3. Geological evolution of the Guyana shield[a]

Approximate age (Ma)	Event
Quaternary	Alluvium - *recent alluvial sediments*
Mesozoic - Cenozoic	Uplift, tilt, and formation of erosion surfaces
210 - 200	Diabase dikes - *tholeiitic*
600	Thermal event registered in isotopic systems in western part of Cuchivero province
710	Kimberlite - *large system of sills, Guaniamo area*[b]
850	Lamprophyre dikes - *Guaniamo area*[b]
1200	NICKERIE OROGENY
1425	Puente Palo granite - *massive, coarse grained, Guaniamo area*[b]
1545	Parguaza Granite - *massive, coarsely crystalline, porphyritic granite, commonly with rapakivi (wiborgite – type) texture*
1850 - 1650	Avanavero Suite - *continental tholeiitic dikes, sills, inclined sheets and small irregu lar intrusive bodies*
1900 - 1500	Roraima Group - *continental (fluvio – deltaic and lacustrine) quartz sandstone and pebble conglomerate with lesser arkose, siltstone, shale, jasper, chert, and interlayered felsic volcanic rocks; age of deposition decreases from east to west*
1860 - 1730	Undivided Proterozoic rocks - *Estado Amazonas only; synkinematic plutonic rocks (granite to tonalite and quartz diorite) and medium- to high-grade gneiss with both igneous and sedimentary protoliths*
1860 - 1730	UNNAMED OROGENY (Estado Amazonas)
1930 - 1790	Cuchivero Group - *thick sequence of felsic to intermediate, mostly subaerial, volcanic rocks (Caicara formation) and their associated granitic rocks (Guaniamito, San Pedro, and Santa Rosalia granites)*
2150 - 1960	TRANS-AMAZONIAN OROGENY
2230 - 2050	Supamo Complex - *gneiss, schist, migmatite, and granitic rocks such as trondhjemite, tonalite, granodiorite and quartz monzonite associated with the greenstone belt terrane*
2250 - 2100	Pastora Supergroup and Botanamo Group (Greenstone belt rocks) - *11,000 m thick volcano-sedimentary sequence consisting of: metamorphosed tholeiitic basalt and gabbro with interflow chemical and sedimentary rocks, in the lower part of the sequence (El Callao and Cicapra formations); interstratified sediments and calc-alka line, rhyolitic lava flows and tuffs in the middle part (Yuruari formation); and in the upper part, mafic to felsic lava flows, intercalated with volcaniclastic tuffaceous and turbiditic sediments (Caballape and Los Caribes formations). Also includes the Real Corona - El Torno assemblage*
2800 - 2700	PRE-TRANS-AMAZONIAN TECTONOMAGMATIC EVENT
From ~3500 to 2800	Imataca Complex - *amphibolite to granulite facies orthogneiss, paragneiss, charnockite, metamorphosed banded iron formation, and minor manganiferous metasedimentary rocks, dolomitic marble and anorthosite*

Notes. a - Modified from Sidder and Mendoza, 1995; b - Channer et al. 1998

strongest close to the granites. Subsequent deformation is related to major shear zones up to 1 km wide.

Botanamo group

Caballape formation. Rocks include mafic to felsic lava flows, pyroclastic flows, and turbidites. The

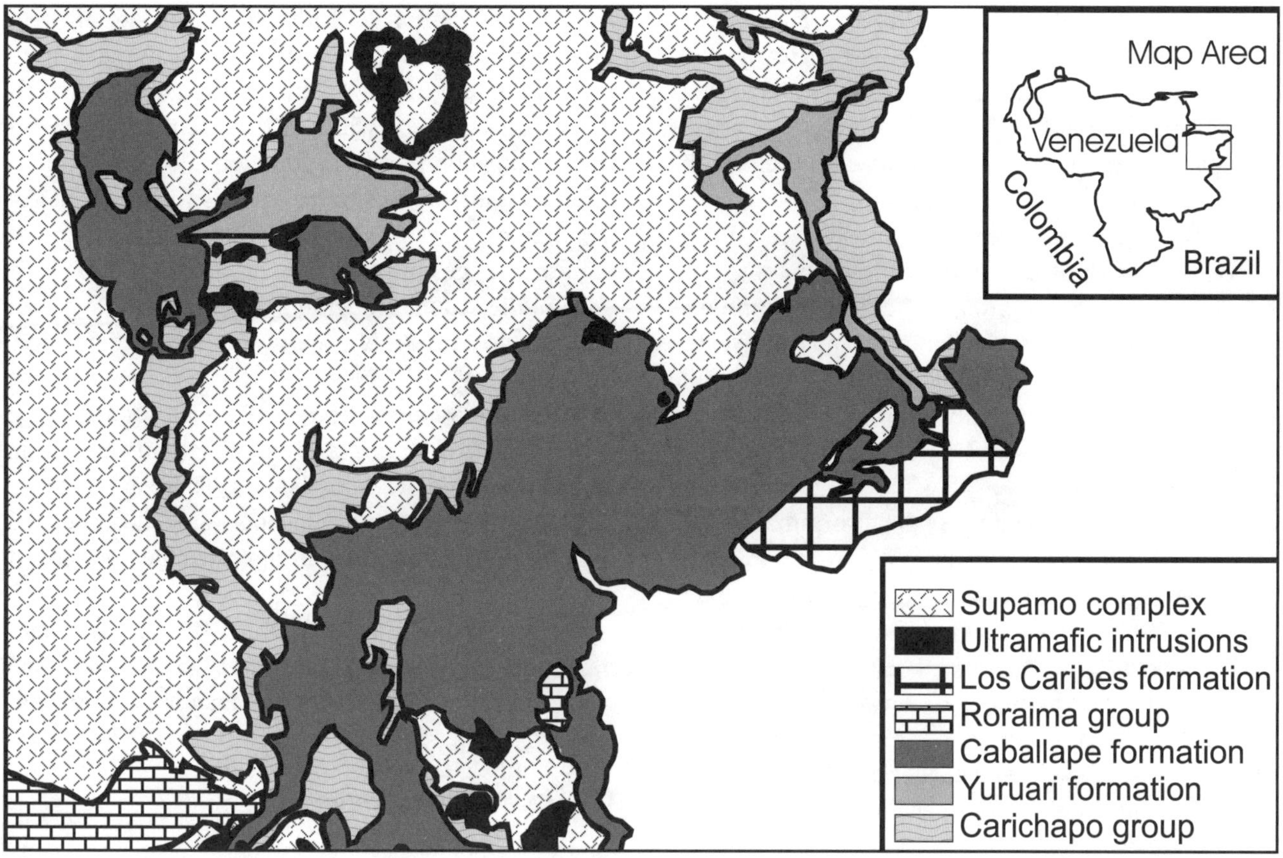

Figure 4. Geology of the central and eastern parts of the Pastora - Botanamo greenstone belt

formation is about 5000 m thick and is discordant on the Pastora supergroup. Metamorphic grade is no higher than greenschist and deformation is weak, with moderate folding.

Los Caribes formation. This contains red phyllite and sandstone, polymict conglomerate, siltstone, and minor felsic tuffs. The rocks are metamorphosed to greenschist facies and are folded.

Real Corona - El Torno assemblage

This is a separate area, 100 km south-west of Ciudad Bolivar, west of the Aro river (see Figs. 2, 3), consisting of a basin some 45 km by 16 km, containing basal quartzites, overlain by basalts, gabbro, and minor sediments. This assemblage is possibly part of the Pastora supergroup.

Tectonic environment

Geochemical studies have identified both tholeiitic and calc - alkaline differentiation trends. Tholeiitic, mafic to intermediate rocks are most abundant. Isotopic studies show that the volcanic rocks are mantle derived, with no component of Archean continental crust. It is thought that the Pastora province greenstone belts represent an evolution from immature oceanic island arcs to back arc marginal basin settings. The Transamazonian orogeny represents the accretion of these terranes to the Archean core of the shield.

Cuchivero province

This province occurs in the west and south of Bolivar State (Fig. 1) and consists of extrusive and intrusive felsic rocks. Rocks of the Cuchivero group occur in a zone from Santa Elena, through northern Brazil, northern Amazonas territory, and western Bolivar State over to the Caura river (Fig. 2). Lithologically the group consists of rhyolites, dacites, ignimbrites, high level granitic porphyries, granites, and lesser quantities of mafic rocks (Rios, 1969; Mendoza, 1972). In western Bolivar State the volcanic sequence has been denominated the Caicara formation and the intrusive units are known as the Guaniamito granite, the Santa Rosalia granite, and the San Pedro granite (Mendoza, 1972).

Rocks of the Cuchivero group extend east to the Suapure River (Figs. 2, 3), where they come into contact with the Suapure group. The Suapure group is younger and consists of granite intrusions, the Pijiguao granite and the Parguaza rapakivi granite (Mendoza, 1975). The combination of the Cuchivero and Suapure groups is known as the Cedeño supergroup. Discordantly overlying the Parguaza granite are stratified sediments of the Roraima group. However, Sidder and Mendoza (1995) report that conformable contacts between the Caicara formation and overlying Roraima sediments have been observed in southern areas.

Field and petrographic evidence suggest that rocks of the Cuchivero group are not regionally metamorphosed or deformed. Rather, there are local effects due to igneous intrusion or later shearing.

Caicara formation

The volcanic rocks of the Caicara formation consist of rhyolites, dacites, and associated volcaniclastic rocks. The felsic rocks consist of lavas, tuffs, and breccias of grey - green colour. The rocks clearly show their eruptive nature, with primary flow textures, porphyritic texture, and presence of clasts. Often, however, the rocks have been deformed and show zones of intense shearing, with abundant associated quartz veining and alteration.

Mendoza (1972, 1977) distinguished three distinct volcanic textures: rhyodacitic tuffaceous lavas with flow textures and phenocrysts, rhyodacitic welded tuffs or ignimbrites, and intrusive breccias with lithic fragments from 1 - 2 cm to 20 - 30 cm in size. The tuffaceous lavas are holocrystalline, massive to fluidal, and porphyritic. The matrix is fine grained with occasional mineral filled cavities. Ignimbrites of rhyolitic composition contain 20 - 50 % phenocrysts, and up to 20 % lithic fragments. The matrix is completely devitrified, and texturally modified by recrystallization. Original cooling fractures are filled with quartz, chlorite, and carbonate. Lithic fragments are of rhyolite composition and are difficult to distinguish from matrix, due to welding. They usually have finely disseminated opaques, which allow them to be identified. Compaction - related foliation is observed and is oriented north-west, similar to the structural trend of the Suapure area. These rocks are intruded by the granites, suggesting that they are the oldest exposed units in the group. Sidder and Mendoza (1995) report that the volcanic rocks were subaerially deposited. Moreno et al. (1985) found volcanic rocks of the Caicara formation in the Alto Paragua region: these rocks ranged from andesite to dacite and rhyolite in composition and are calc-alkaline. These authors also reported the presence of clastic sediments associated with the volcanic rocks, and suggested the presence of a local depositional basin.

Rb/Sr age determinations on these rocks give ages of ~1930 to 1790 Ma (Table 3). Geochemical data show that these rocks form a comagmatic calc-alkaline series (Mendoza, 1977).

Cuchivero group granites

Santa Rosalia granite. This granite is massive to foliated, and medium to coarse grained (Rios, 1969). It is intrusive into the volcanic rocks of the Caicara formation, although locally they may be in fault contact. Age determinations using Rb/Sr whole rock analysis have given a mean age of ~1880 +/- 88 Ma (Gaudette et al. 1978).

Guaniamito granite. The Guaniamito granite is generally foliated, and medium to coarse grained (Rios, 1969). Olmeta (1968) determined a whole rock K-Ar age of 1700 +/- 80 Ma for this granite.

Suapure group granites

San Pedro granite. The San Pedro granite is intrusive into the Caicara formation and contains xenoliths of metabasite. Mendoza (1972) suggests that it is of similar age to the Santa Rosalia granite.

Pijiguao granite. Mendoza (1972) describes the Pijiguao granite as a leucocratic rock of salmon pink colour, fine grained, equigranular, massive, and exposed below the Parguaza granite. The absolute age of this intrusion is unknown but it appears to be the immediate precursor of the Parguaza granite to which it is likely to be geochemically related.

Parguaza granite. The Parguaza granite is the largest known rapakivi granite intrusive in the world (~30,000 km^2). It is coarse grained, massive, inequigranular, and characterised by the rapakivi texture (Mendoza, 1975). The age of this intrusive complex is 1545 +/- 20 Ma (U/Pb zircon method; Gaudette et al, 1978). Mendoza (1975) suggested that the Parguaza granite formed due to extensive fractional crystallization of a tholeiitic magma. The age is very similar to that of the Roraima diabases (Gonzalez de Juana et al., 1980).

Puente Palo granite. This granite is unfoliated and occurs in the Quebrada Grande area, in the Guaniamo river basin. Single zircon U/Pb analysis of this rock gives an age of 1425 +/- 14 Ma (Channer et al., 1998).

Basic rocks

On the Rio Cuchivero (Fig. 2), Rios (1969) distinguished north to northwest trending amphibolite dykes, and northeast trending diabase dykes. These rocks intrude the Santa Rosalia and Guaniamito granites.

Mendoza (1972) suggested that the amphibolites correspond to the late stages of the Cuchivero volcanic cycle. Several stages of intrusion may have occurred before and after emplacement of the San Pedro granite. Abundant gabbro dykes occur within the Cuchivero province: these are probably part of the Avanavero suite (~1650 Ma) (Table 3).

Diabase dykes occur across the Guyana shield and within the Roraima formation. It is possible that some of these dykes are in fact Mesozoic in age, related to extension associated with opening of the Atlantic. Faulting associated with this phase of magmatic activity may have caused minor vertical movements within the shield.

Ultrabasic rocks

Diamondiferous kimberlite sills are present in the Quebrada Grande region (Nixon et al. 1992). These have been dated at 710 Ma by Rb-Sr analysis of single phlogopite crystals (Channer et al. 1998).

Tectonic environment

The Cuchivero province is bounded to the east by the Rio Caura and to the west by the Orinoco (Fig. 2). Both of these rivers are interpreted to approximately follow suture zones joining the Cuchivero province to other provinces in the Guyana shield.

Volcanic rocks show a primary vertical flow foliation oriented on 060º and two structural trends, 320º and 020º, with sub-vertical dips (Mendoza, 1972). Granitic rocks also show these foliation trends. Foliation is confined to discrete zones which also occur in younger lithologies. Regionally the NW trend is most common, although the NE trend is well developed, especially due to movement in the Nickerie orogeny (~1200 Ma; see Table 3). Various workers (e.g., Martin-Bellizia, 1972; Añez, 1985) have identified a rift valley, the Cabruta - Ventuari rift, which can be traced from the Orinoco in the Cabruta - Caicara area for more than 1000 km to the south - east into Brazil. Another zone of rifting is interpreted to lie along the present course of the Rio Suapure. Gaudette et al. (1978) suggest that extensive systems of horsts and grabens formed between 1500 Ma and 1600 Ma in response to shield scale extension. Associated with this extension was intensive mafic magmatic activity, with extreme fractionation giving rise to intrusions such as the Parguaza granite. In further development of this hypothesis, Gaudette and Olszewski (1985a,b) and Gibbs and Barron (1993) have suggested that a subduction zone lay along the present Orinoco river at the border with Colombia, and that the tectonic and magmatic activity was linked to subduction - related processes. Miron and Costanzo (1997) interpret the paleomagnetic characteristics of the Parguaza granite in terms of the horst and graben model of Gaudette et al. (1978). Sidder and Mendoza (1995), noting the lack of regional metamorphism and deformation in the Cuchivero group, define this group as post - orogenic and post - Transamazonian. Geochemical data for the Cuchivero group rocks suggests some crustal input to magmas and discrimination diagrams indicate that the granites are transitional from within plate to volcanic arc.

Amazonas province

This area is less well known than the Cuchivero province and most survey work has been conducted along river sections. Barrios et al. (1985) divided the region into the Ventuari dominion, lying north of the Orinoco, and the Casiquiare dominion, lying to the south (Fig. 1). Similar rocks on the Colombian side of the border are known as the Mitú migmatite complex (Priem et al. 1982). Rocks in the Casiquiare dominion consist of tonalite, trondhjemite, and granites, which show complex intrusive relations. Rocks in the Ventuari dominion include various volcanic units, which are probably equivalent to the Caicara formation, and granites equivalent to the Santa Rosalia granite (Mendoza et al. 1977).

Talukdar and Colvée (1975, 1977) studied the volcanic rocks (Yavi and El Viejo formations) in the El Viejo area and Parucito valley, in the Ventuari dominion. The volcanic rocks are intruded by synvolcanic granites, and are also in fault contact with later granites. The volcanics consist mostly of rhyolite and rhyodacite, with subsidiary dacite and andesite. All rocks are regionally metamorphosed to greenschist facies. The rhyolites are welded tuffs with disordered, discontinuous flow structures. The quantity, size, and type (pumice, crystal, lithic) of fragments is variable. Some lapilli tuffs are present. Many outcrops show well preserved flow structures, defined by glassy shards, while others are massive. Dacites occur in two types: one is porphyritic and appears to be a lava flow, the other is a lapilli tuff with abundant pumice fragments. Andesite also occurs in two types: one is porphyritic, while the other is massive and fine grained. Also, oligomictic conglomerate was found, containing rounded pebbles and boulders of volcanic rock and orthoquartzite. This indicates a subaqueous environment for this region. In the Atabapo region, further west of the Parucito valley, Barrios (1985) notes that volcanic rocks are interbedded with sedimentary strata. Geochemical analysis by the same author indicates a calc - alkaline trend for these rocks.

Gneisses in the Casiquiare dominion are known as the Atabapo, Minicia, and Macabana gneisses. Isotopic and geochronologic data suggest that igneous activity and metamorphism were contemporaneous between 1860 Ma and 1730 Ma (Gaudette et al. 1977; Olszewski et al. 1977; Gaudette and Olszewski, 1985a,b). Priem et al. (1982) determined that the granite gneiss basement in eastern Colombia had a minimum age of 1850 Ma, and that the Mitú migmatites formed between 1560 and 1450 Ma, at the same time as the Parguaza granite.

Regional geophysical studies (magnetic and radiometric aerial survey) were conducted in the Amazonas territory in the mid - 1970's. The line spacing was from 1 to 4 km, and altitudes of between 150 m to 300 m above the ground (Herrero, 1985). Large scale magnetic and radiometric anomalies were ground truthed by Mendoza et al. (1977), who reported diabase dykes, fault zones, and alkaline and mafic intrusives.

Tectonic environment

Gaudette and Olszewski (1985b) suggested that a tectonic boundary is present along the Orinoco and Ventuari rivers in the Amazonas province, forming the contact between the Ventuari and Casiquiare dominions. Regional gravity data (Perarnau and Graterol, 1985) show a strong gravity low along the Río Ventuari, in the area of the contact between the two dominions. It is possible that this area, along with the western side of the Cuchivero province further to the north, may have been a zone of NE - directed subduction over a long period of geological time, from 1900 Ma to about 1450 Ma (Priem et al. 1982; Barrios et al. 1985; Gaudette and Olszewski 1985b).

VOLCANOGENIC MASSIVE SULPHIDE POTENTIAL IN THE GUAYANA SHIELD

Imataca province

The Imataca province (Fig. 1) is of unknown potential for volcanogenic massive sulphide deposits. Any mineralization will have been strongly affected by the two episodes of high grade (upper amphibolite to granulite) metamorphism and deformation (Table 3).

Pastora province

The Pastora - Botanamo greenstone belt (Fig. 4) possesses many of the key elements of productive greenstone belt terranes, including a bimodal volcanic sequence with about 8 % felsic rocks (Table 2), and an interpreted oceanic arc to back arc tectonic setting.

Support for the prospectivity of the Pastora province comes from the documented massive sulphide showings in Guyana (Ally, 1985), which consist

Table 4. Description of the principal base metal showings in Guyana (after Ally, 1985)

Number[a]	Name of Occurrence	Local lithology	Description
1	Groete Creek	Basic schists	Some Fe-stained mica schists, also weak Cu staining. Drilling of coincident soil geochemical anomaly and TUREM anomaly found chalcopyrite - gold mineral ization. Resource of 33 million tonnes @ 0.25 % Cu and 0.5 g/t Au.
2	Tupuru - Mariwa Mountain - Sardine Hill	Intermediate volcanics	Alluvial gold area. Minor soil Cu anom alies. Geophysical anomalies drilled - no mineralization found.
3	Aremu	Intermediate volcanics, tuffs, and minor carbonaceous sediments	One horizon with disseminated pyrite - chalcopyrite mineralization (0.67 % Cu over 1.6 m along a strike length of 150 m.
4	Baramalli Creek	Intermediate - acid volcanics	Carbonate veining; weak disseminated pyrite - chalcopyrite mineralization (0.1 % Cu).
5	Mara-Mara river mouth	Acid - intermediate volcanics	Minor seams of pyrite - chalcopyrite mineralization.
6	Lower Kartuni river	Andesite	Outcrops are strongly pyritised. Soil Cu and Zn anom alies.
7	Area 33	Interbedded carbonaceous phyllites, tuffaceous greywackes; minor limestone lenses; also felsic volcanics	Volcanics are hydrothermally altered with values up to 400 ppm Cu and 1000 ppm Zn.
8	Popekai rapids (Cuyuni river)		Visible chalcopyrite. Soil Cu, Co, Ni anomalies.
9	Waikuri-Kutuau (Cuyuni river)	Phyllites and quartzites, .	Pyrite is common, along with disseminated chalcopy rite.
10	Haimaralli	Carbonaceous sediments	Cu staining at surface. Mineralization consists of: dis seminated pyrite, minor chalcopyrite, bornite, covel lite, and chalcocite. Drilling found 0.3 % Cu over 24 m, with highs of 1.3 % Cu and 1.2 % Zn.
11	Aranka	Intermediate to felsic lavas and tuffs	Mineralization consists of: thin stringers and veins of pyrite and chalcopyrite in a quartz - calcite gangue. Disseminated sulphides also present. Resource 2.4 million tonnes at 0.45 % Cu

Notes. a - Number corresponds with locations shown in Figure 5

of disseminated pyrite - chalcopyrite and are associated with felsic to intermediate volcanics, and clastic rocks, including carbonaceous horizons. Details of these showings are summarized in Table 4 and their locations are shown in Figure 5. The Barama - Mazaruni greenstone belts are contiguous with the Pastora - Botanamo greenstone belt (Fig. 1). In the Barama - Mazaruni greenstone belts the proportion of felsic rocks is higher at 20 %, than in the Pastora - Botanamo greenstone belt (see Tables 1, 2). In the Groete Creek - Area 33 belt, Ally (1985) reports six showings in a linear north - east zone some 100 km in length (Fig. 5): these showings are associated with sub-volcanic porphyry, coarse breccias, tuffs, and sulphide fragments. Walrond (1985) reports on earlier work by Hamilton that the Groete Creek deposit has a

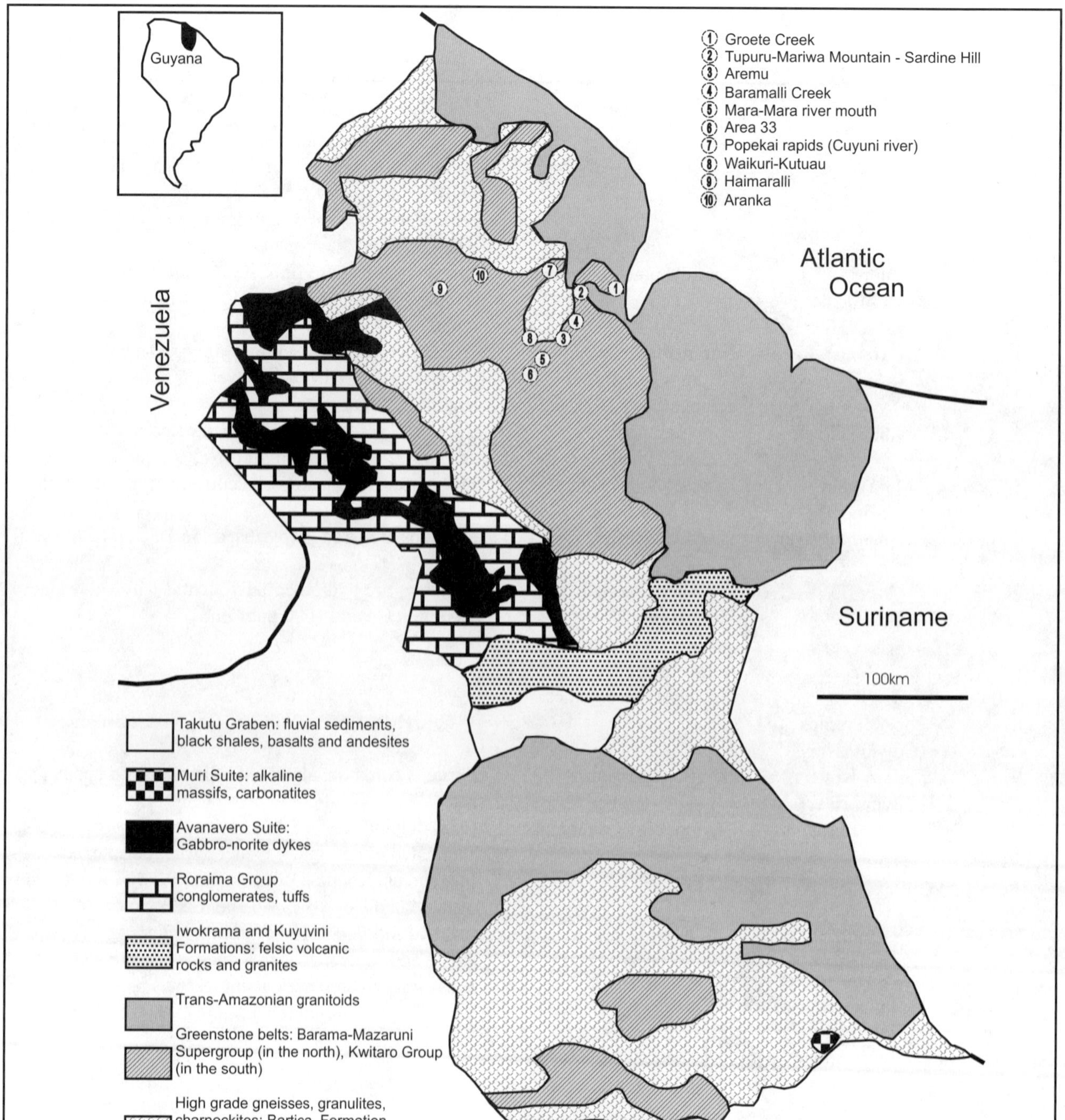

Figure 5. Geology of Guyana and locations of volcanogenic massive sulphide showings in the Barama - Mazaruni greenstone belt (after Voicu et al. 1999 and Ally, 1985)

strike length of 1525 m, a down dip extent of 410 m, and a mineralized width of 10 m at 0.6 % Cu, giving a resource of 16 million tonnes. The deposit contains a total resource of 33 million tonnes at 0.25 % Cu.

Even though no economic deposits were found, it is noteworthy that significant showings were found in some extremely remote areas, despite the relatively poor geophysical and geological understanding of massive sulphide deposits at the time, and the small investment made. The Barama - Mazaruni greenstone belts possess the key features associated with massive sulphide deposits (see Table 1) and their prospectivity for larger deposits is high.

In Table 1 the known key features of the Pastora - Botanamo greenstone belt are listed in comparison with the Barama - Mazaruni belts. In the Pastora province, felsic rocks occur in the Yuruari formation (Fig. 4), which is part of the Pastora supergroup, and in the Caballape formation, part of the Botanamo group, which is unconformable on the Pastora supergroup (Table 3). The Yuruari formation locally contains tuffaceous breccias, lava flows, and cherts, which suggest proximity to volcanic centres. Menéndez (1995) describes quartz - feldspar porphyry dikes and stocks intruding the Carichapo group in areas where lavas are developed in the Yuruari formation. Also, the Yuruari formation forms the upper part of a volcano-sedimentary cycle, when tectonic conditions may have been less active, thereby favoring accumulation and preservation of stratigraphic marker layers (e.g., chert layers) and sulphide mineralization.

Very limited exploration for massive sulphide deposits has been done in the Pastora province. Iturralde de Arozena et al. (1977) conducted ground follow up of anomalies identified from airborne electromagnetic surveys (Martínez, 1985; INPUT and TURAIR type). Soil sampling gave anomalous values for Co, Ni, Cu, and Zn but the authors determined that the conductors were caused by mineralized quartz veins. Note that regional aeromagnetic surveys have been conducted over the Venezuelan Guayana shield: details of these are summarized in the appendix to an article by Wynn et al. (1995).

Cuchivero province

Favorable features of the Cuchivero province include: the large area of felsic volcanic rocks, large scale Proterozoic rift systems implying extensional faulting, the calc-alkaline nature of the rocks, and the low degree of metamorphism and deformation. However, the large area covered by the felsic rocks of this group, and the difficulty of access, have limited volcanic facies mapping. In the areas which have been studied in the western part of the province (Suapure and Caicara regions), volcanic rocks have been interpreted as subaerial, an environment which is not conducive to formation of volcanogenic massive sulphide deposits. A good example of volcanogenic massive sulphide deposits occurring in a felsic volcanic dominated region is the Bergslagen district in Sweden (Allen et al. 1996). In Table 5, the principal features of the Cuchivero province are compared with those of the Bergslagen district. The data for Bergslagen show clearly that subaqueous felsic volcanism was an essential part of volcanogenic massive sulphide formation. The data presented in Table 5 also show that there are general similarities between the Cuchivero province, and the Bergslagen region (e.g., age, area, percentage of felsic rocks). Detailed studies of the Bergslagen district have shown that it formed in a back arc basin at an active continental margin. It is likely that the Cuchivero province (and Amazonas region) are related to a long lived subduction zone located on the western side of Venezuela, which became inactive during the Nickerie orogeny at ~1.3 to 1.0 Ga. The subduction environment would have favored ore deposit formation. The key to identifying prospective areas in the Cuchivero province is the location of areas of subaqueous volcanic activity and related sedimentation.

Although most areas described so far from the Cuchivero province consist of subaerial volcanics, Moreno et al. (1985) described intermediate to felsic volcanics intercalated with sediments in the upper Paragua river (Fig. 2). These observations indicate a subaqueous environment of formation. Moreno et al. (1985) also suggested that follow up work should be done in the vicinity of the mouth of the Río Carúm, a tributary of the Río Paragua, where andesites have potential for gold and copper mineralization. Sidder et

Table 5. Comparison of the principal geological features of the Cuchivero province (Guayana shield) and the Bergslagen district (Baltic shield)

Geological Features	Cuchivero Province [a,b,c]	Bergslagen District [d]
Age (Ma)	1900 to 1800	1900 to 1870
% felsic rocks	? > 85	89
Area (km^2)	75,000	50,000
Tectonic setting	? intraplate / continental volcanic arc	Extensional, back arc basin at active continental margin
District size (km)		20 to 100
Size distribution		Zinkgruvan (> 43 Mt) - Falun (28 Mt) - Uto (0.2 Mt)
Favorable horizons		Rhyolitic ash siltstone / limestone
Volcanic Facies	Rhyolitic tuffaceous lavas, welded tuffs, intrusive breccias; some areas with sediments	Felsic volcanic centres with vent, flank, and mar gin facies associations. Main facies is poorly welded pyroclastic flows and their resedimented equivalents; also subordinate dacite subvolcanic intrusions.
Alteration	e.g., Kakuri - Erebato, Amazonas region [e]	K, Si, and Mg metasomatism in footwall
Local structure	e.g., Caura - Erebato area - radial faults and circular anomalies f; Cabruta - Suapure rift valley - extensional tectonics	Early strong extension, declining with time; later compression
Metamorphism and Deformation	Minor metamorphism - thermal effects of granitic intrusions. Deformation also minor and confined to NW and NE directed shear zones	Lower to middle amphibolite facies. Strong defor mation with two phases of folding, shear zones, and brittle faults

Notes: a - Mendoza, 1972; b - Mendoza, 1975; c - Sidder and Mednoza, 1995; d - Allen et al. 1996; e - Mendoza et al. 1977; f - Herrero, 1985.

al. (1991) report that some areas of Caicara formation volcanics are strongly silicified with up to 10 % pyrite and trace chalcopyrite. Apart from volcanogenic massive sulphide deposits, epithermal gold deposits and Olympic Dam - type deposits type, are promising exploration targets in the Cuchivero province (Sidder and Mendoza, 1995).

Amazonas province

Favorable features of this region include: a large area of felsic rocks, some of which were formed subaqueously. From previous studies, numerous areas of possible economic significance were identified. In particular, to the south of San Juan de Manapiare, and also in the area between the Caura and Erebato rivers, large, circular anomalies were located: these anomalies are the foci of radial fault patterns and are suggested by Herrero (1985) as areas of potential sulphide occurrence (Table 5). Mendoza et al. (1977) reported on the economic potential of the different rock units, and identified the felsic volcanic units as having potential for sulphide mineralization. They noted some occurrences of disseminated sulphide mineralization with contents of 5 - 10 % in Kakuri - Erebato. This area shows strong hydrothermal alteration and is also a first priority aeromagnetic anomaly (Table 5).

Volcanogenic masive sulphide deposits and occurrences in northern Venezuela

Most deposits and showings of Cu - Zn - Pb in the northern part of Venezuela occur in the north - east trending mountain range which derives from the main

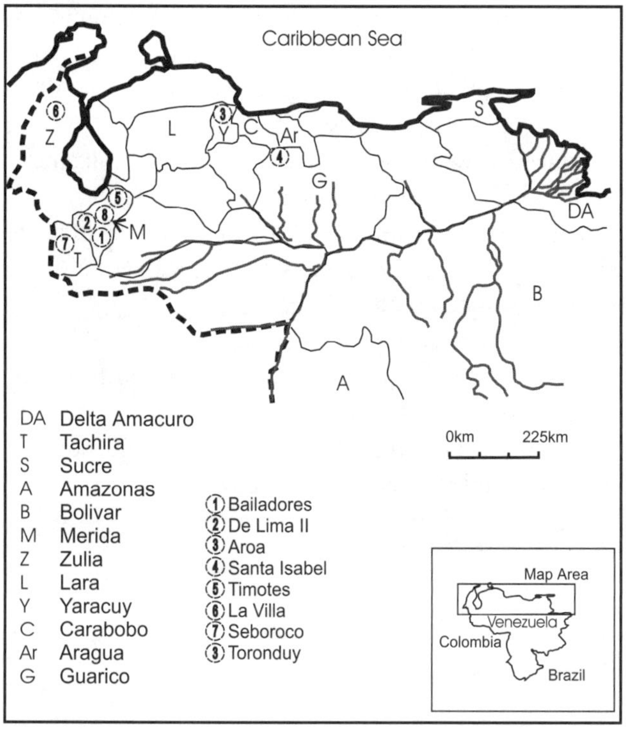

Figure 6. Locations of volcanogenic massive sulphide deposits and showings in the Phanerozoic rocks of Venezuela (after Rodriguez, 1986)

Andean chain in Colombia and trends through Táchira, Merida, Lara, and Yaracuy states, reaching the coast in Carabobo state. Here we summarize the published occurrences, using Rodriguez (1986) as a general reference. The Venezuelan ministry of mines conducted a mapping and exploration program in this area from 1969 to 1974, the results of which were summarized by Moya (1977). The locations of these showings are given in Figure 6.

Aragua - Guarico states

Volcanic rocks in the Villa de Cura group contain lenses and veins of chalcopyrite, pyrite, and sphalerite. Volcanic rocks consist of mafic to felsic compositions, with lavas, tuffs, and breccias. The principal area is known as Santa Isabel and was mined through underground workings until 1966. The mineralized zone trends east - west, following a fault zone. The strong faulting and folding in the area have separated what may have been larger sulphide accumulations into numerous small pods or lenses. The sulphide zones are surrounded by strong alteration, including sericitization and silicification (Rodriguez, 1977). Lenses of barite occur close to the sulphide pods. Grade data from Eda et al. (1967), reported in Rodriguez (1986) are 0.6 - 1.9 g/t Au, 33 - 156 g/t Ag, 1.04 - 2.14 % Cu, 0.1 - 0.6 % Pb, and 0.75 - 31.34 % Zn. In 1966, 96,000 tonnes of ore were processed. This mineralization appears to be syngenetic massive sulphide in origin (Rodriguez, 1977).

Yaracuy state

In this state copper mineralization occurs as hydrothermal veins but also as sulphide pods in areas of mafic volcanics and graphitic schists. The rocks are intensely deformed and the sulphides occur as numerous small pods. These deposits, known as the mines of Aroa, were found in 1609 and were exploited until 1963. Over 1,500,000 tonnes were mined at a grade of 8.4 % Cu. The pods occur parallel to stratigraphy and contain chalcopyrite and pyrite. Sphalerite and galena are rare. The deposits are interpreted as volcanogenic massive sulphide deposits. The complex stratigraphy and deformation in the area have prohibited further evaluation.

Merida state

The best known volcanogenic massive sulphide in Venezuela is the De Lima II deposit, some 10 km from the town of Bailadores. Studies by the Ministry of Mines from 1970 - 75 determined reserves of 4 million tonnes with Cu grades of 1.00 - 4.28 %. The lower section of the deposit is copper - rich, while sphalerite and galena occur in the upper section (Carlson, 1977). Sulphides are located in the lower part of the Mucuchachí formation, of upper Carboniferous age, along the contact of a basal pyroclastic unit with overlying black shales, the dominant lithology in the sequence. The pyroclastic unit has been altered to quartz - sericite. Sulphide minerals include sphalerite, pyrrhotite, galena, chalcopyrite, and lesser quantities of arsenopyrite and pyrite. Rocks in the area have been metamorphosed, thus the formation of pyrrhotite from pyrite. This deposit has been interpreted as a volcanogenic massive sulphide deposit due to the stratigraphic control on mineralization, the subaqueous volcano - sedimentary environment, the footwall alteration zone, and the general zonation from Cu - rich upwards to Pb - Zn - rich, typical of other massive sulphide deposits. The average grade of the deposit is 1.45 Mt, 26 % Zn, 7 % Pb, and 1.5 % Cu (Staargaard & Carlson, 2000. This volume).

Other regions

Various small hydrothermal base metal occurrences have been documented in Merida state (Timotes, Torondoy - both Cu), Zulia (La Villa - Pb), Lara (Pb), and Sucre (Pb). Stratiform sediment - hosted Cu deposits have been found in Táchira state in the Seboruco and El Cobre areas. Mineralization is hosted by the Triassic - Jurassic volcanic host rocks of the La Quinta formation (Moya, 1977). This area is thought to have significant potential (Rodriguez, 1986). Basic volcanic rocks in the Caño Tigre area of Zulia state contain native copper and other sulphides filling amygdales (Moya and Figueroa, 1977; Viteri, 1977a, 1977b). The copper mineralization occurred during low grade metamorphism of the Triassic - Jurassic volcanic host rocks of the La Quinta formation (Viteri, 1977b).

SUMMARY AND CONCLUSIONS

From this analysis of the potential for the existence of volcanogenic massive sulphide deposits in the Guayana shield of Venezuela, we conclude that the Pastora - Botanamo greenstone belt has the highest potential for such mineralization. In terms of area, relative proportions of mafic to felsic rocks, and tectonic setting it is comparable to greenstone belts such as the Archean Abitibi belt, host to the 141 million tonne Kidd Creek deposit and the Noranda camp, and the Proterozoic Reindeer zone in the south Trans - Hudson orogen, host to the 57.5 million tonne Flin Flon deposit. The Pastora - Botanamo greenstone belt is contiguous with the Barama - Mazaruni greenstone belts in Guyana, which contain a number of promising base metal occurrences. The Pastora - Botanamo greenstone belt has been explored for shear zone - related gold deposits but little attention has been paid to felsic volcanic centres, which may host massive sulphide deposits. Exploration should be directed at the Yuruari and Caballape formations, which contain the felsic volcanic rocks and related sediments.

The Cuchivero province and Ventuari dominion of the Amazonas region are felsic volcanic - dominated, but the small information base makes it difficult to assess their prospectivity. These areas show general similarities with the Proterozoic felsic volcanic - dominated Bergslagen district, host to the 28.1 million tonne Falun deposit. Previous studies indicate some areas of high prospectivity for massive sulphide deposits, especially the Erebato region.

The Venezuelan part of the Guayana shield is an underexplored region in comparison with other Precambrian shield areas. The geological characteristics of the Guayana shield suggest that volcanogenic massive sulphide deposits will be present.

ACKNOWLEDGEMENTS

We thank Dr. Cornel de Ronde, an anonymous reviewer, and Dr. Ross Sherlock for their constructive criticisms of the manuscript.

REFERENCES

Allen, R.L., Lundstrom, I., Ripa, M., Simeonov, A. and Christofferson, H. 1996. Facies analysis of a 1.9 Ga continental margin, back arc, felsic caldera province with diverse Zn-Pb-Ag-(Cu-Au) sulfide and fe oxide deposits, Bergslagen region, Sweden. Economic Geology, 91, 979-1008.

Ally, L. 1985. Volcanogenic massive sulphide potential in Northern Guayana. Memoria I, Simposium Amazonico, Boletin de Geología, Publicación Especial Nº 10, Ministerio de Energia y Minas. Dirección de Geología, 431-442.

Añez, G. 1985. Exploración y Evaluación de posibles depositos diamantiferos en el Distrito Cedeño del Estado Bolívar. Memoria I, Simposium Amazonico, Boletin de Geología, Publicación Especial Nº 10, Ministerio de Energia y Minas. Dirección de Geología, 443-463.

Attoh, K. and Ekwueme, B.N. 1997. The West African shield. In Greenstone Belts, Oxford Monographs on Geology and Geophysics 35. Edited by M.J. de Wit and L.D. Ashwal, Chapter 5.4, pp. 517-529.

Baars, F.J. 1997. The Sao Francisco craton. In Greenstone Belts, Oxford Monographs on Geology and Geophysics 35. Edited by M.J. de Wit and L.D. Ashwal, Chapter 5.5, pp. 529-557.

Barley, M.E. 1997. The Pilbara craton. In Greenstone Belts, Oxford Monographs on Geology and Geophysics 35. Edited by M.J. de Wit and L.D. Ashwal, Chapter 5.13, pp. 657-664.

Barrios, F. 1985. Geología de la sub - región Atabapo - Guarinuma, territorio Federal Amazonas. Memoria I, Simposium Amazonico, Boletin de Geología, Publicación Especial Nº 10, Ministerio de Energia y Minas. Dirección de Geología, 9-21.

Barrios, F., Rivas, G., Cordani, U. and Kawashita K. 1985. Caracterización geocronológica del Territorio Federal Amazonas, Venezuela. Memoria I, Simposium Amazonico, Boletin de Geología, Publicación Especial Nº 10, Ministerio de Energia y Minas. Dirección de Geología, 22-31.

Benaim, N. and Rios, J. 1977. Guia de la excursión Maiquetia - Ciudad Guayana - El Pao - Upata - Guasipati - Tumeremo- Sta. Elena De Uairen - Canaima - Maiquetia, V Congreso Geológico Venezuela, 77-124.

Binns, R.A. and Scott, S.D. 1993. Actively forming polymetallic sulfide deposits associated with felsic volcanic rocks in the eastern Manus back arc basin, Papua New Guinea. Economic Geology, 88, 2226-2236.

Blenkinsop, T., Martin, A. and Jelsma, H.A. 1997. The Zimbabwe craton. In Greenstone Belts, Oxford Monographs on Geology and Geophysics 35. Edited by M.J. de Wit and L.D. Ashwal, Chapter 5.7, pp. 567-580.

Borg, G. and Shackleton, R.M. 1997. The Tanzania and NE Zaire cratons. In Greenstone Belts, Oxford Monographs on Geology and Geophysics 35. Edited by M.J. de Wit and L.D. Ashwal, Chapter 5.9, pp. 608-619.

Brauhart, C.W., Groves, D.I. and Morant, P. 1998. Regional alteration systems associated with volcanogenic massive sulphide mineralization at Panorama, Pilbara, Western Australia. Economic Geology, 93, 292-302.

Brandl, G. and de Wit, M.J. 1997. The Kaapvaal craton. In Greenstone Belts, Oxford Monographs on Geology and Geophysics 35. Edited by M.J. de Wit and L.D. Ashwal, Chapter 5.8, pp. 581-607.

Carlson, G. 1977. Geology of the Bailadores, Venezuela, massive sulfide deposit. Economic Geology, 72, 1131-1142.

Castillo, J., Schmitz, M., Chalbaud, D., Izarra, C. and Lueth, S. 1999. The crustal structure of the Guayana shield, Southern Venezuela, obtained by seismic refraction, gravity and magnetic data. American Geophysical Union Spring meeting, Abstract, S215-S216.

Cathles, L.M. 1993. Oxygen isotope alteration in the Noranda mining district, Abitibi greenstone belt, Quebec. Economic Geology, 88, 1483-1511.

Channer, D.M.DeR., Cooper R.E. and Kaminsky, F.V. 1998. The Guaniamo diamond region, Bolivar State, Venezuela: A new kimberlite province. Extended Abstracts, 7th International Kimberlite Conference, Cape Town, South Africa, April 1998, 144-146.

Chase, R. L. 1965. El complejo de Imataca, la anfibolita de Panamo y la tronjemita de Guri: Rocas Precámbricas del cuadrilátero de las Adjuntas - Panamo, Edo. Bolívar, Venezuela, Boletin de Geología, Caracas, Vol.VII, Nº 13, 105-216.

DeMatties, T.A. 1994. Early Proterozoic Volcanogenic massive sulphide deposits in Wisconsin: an overview. Economic Geology, 89, 1122-1151.

Eda, Y., Hiroshi, H., Sasaki, D., Horita, A., Oshuga, A. and Iwase, Y. 1967. Report on geological development plan of Republic of Venezuela. MITI, Government of japan, Informe Interno M.M.H. Caracas.

Fouquet, Y., von Stackelburg, U., Charlou, J.L., Erzinger, J., Herzig, P.M., Muhe, R. and Wiedicke, M. 1993. Metallogenesis in back arc environments: the Lau basin example. Economic Geology, 88, 2154-2181.

Franklin, J.M., Lydon, J.W., and Sangster, D.F. 1981. Volcanic-associated massive sulfide deposits. Economic Geology, 75th Anniversary Volume, 485-627.

Gaudette, H.E., Olszewski, W.J. and Mendoza, V. 1977. U-Pb zircon ages of the Minicia and Macabana gneisses, Amazonas territory, Venezuela. V Congreso Geológico Venezolano, 527-536.

Gaudette, H.E., Mendoza, V., Hurley, P.M. and Fairburn, H.W. 1978. Geology and age of the Parguaza rapakivi granite, Venezuela. Geological Society of America Bulletin 89, 1335-1340.

Gaudette, H.E. and Olszewski, W.J. 1985a. Determination of radiometric ages, Amazonas territory, Venezuela. Memoria I Simposium Amazonico, Puerto Ayacucho, Venezuela. Boletin de Geología, Publicación Especial 10, 733-746.

Gaudette, H.E. and Olszewski, W.J. 1985b. Geochronolgy of the basement rocks, Amazonas territory, Venezuela, and the tectonic evolution of the western Guiana shield. Geologie en Mijnbouw 64, 131-143.

Gibbs, A. K. and Barron, C. N. 1983. The Guiana shield reviewed. Episodes, Vol. 1983, No. 2, 7-14.

Gibbs, A. K. and Barron, C. N. 1993. Geology of the Guiana shield, Oxford University Press, 246p.

Gonzalez de Juana, C., Iturralde de Arozena, J. and Picard, X. 1980. Geología de Venezuela y sus cuencas petrolíferas, tomo Y, Edición Foninves.

Herrero, E. 1985. Prospección geofísica aérea en el Territorio Federal Amazonas. Memoria I, Simposium Amazonico, Boletin de Geología, Publicación Especial Nº 10, Ministerio de Energia y Minas. Dirección de Geología, 373-383.

Herrington, R.J., Evans, D.M. and Buchanan D.L. 1997. Metallogenic aspects. In Greenstone Belts, Oxford Monographs on Geology and Geophysics 35. Edited by M.J. de Wit and L.D. Ashwal, Chapter 2.5, pp. 176-219.

Iturralde de Arozena, J.M., Pasquali, J. and Sifontes, R.S. 1977. Distribución de cobre, cinc, niquel, cobalto, manganeso, vanadio, titanio, y cromo en suelos desarollados sobre anomalias geofísicas en el sureste de Venezuela. V Congreso Geológico Venezolano, 893-904.

King, J. and Helmstaedt, H. 1997. The Slave Province, Northwest territories, Canada. In Greenstone Belts, Oxford Monographs on Geology and Geophysics 35. Edited by M.J. de Wit and L.D. Ashwal, Chapter 5.1, pp. 459-479.

Ledru, P. and Milési, J.P. 1995. Geology of Guyana and West Africa. Proceedings of III Simposio Internacional del Oro en Venezuela Asociación Venezolana del Oro, 77-89.

Lewry, J.F. and Stauffer, M.R. 1997. The Reindeer zone of the Trans - Hudson orogen, Canada. In Greenstone Belts, Oxford Monographs on Geology and Geophysics 35. Edited by M.J. de Wit and L.D. Ashwal, Chapter 6.1, pp. 739-746.

Martin-Bellizia, C. 1972. Paleotectónica del Escudo Guayana. IX Conferencia Geológica Inter - Guayanas, Ciudad Guayana, Venezuela, 1972. Boletin de Geología, Publicación Especial 6, 251-305.

Martínez, M. 1985. Investigación de anomalías E.M. INPUT en la Guayana Venezolana. Memoria I, Simposium Amazonico, Boletin de Geología, Publicación Especial Nº 10, Ministerio de Energia y Minas. Dirección de Geología, 398-399.

Mendoza, V. 1972. Geología del área del Río Suapure NW del Escudo de Guayana, parte noroccidental del escudo de Guayana, Edo. Bolívar, Venezuela (Informe de progreso). IX Conferencia Geológica Inter - Guayanas, Ciudad Guayana, Venezuela. Boletin de Geología, Publicación Especial 6, 306-338.Geología, Caracas, 10, No. 19, 309-338.

Menéndez, V. 1972. Geología de la Región de Guasipati, Guayana Venezolana. Proceedings of IV Congreso Geológico Venezolano, Boletin de Geología, Publicación Especial 5, 2001-2043.

Menéndez, V. 1995. Cinturones de rocas verdes del escudo de Guayana en Venezuela: revisión estratigráfica. Proceedings of III Simposio Internacional del Oro en Venezuela Asociación Venezolana del Oro, 123-139.

Miron, O.E. and Costanzo, V. 1997. Paleomagnetic and rock magnetic evidence for inverse zoning in the Parguaza batholith (southwestern Venezuela) and its implications about tectonics of the Guyana shield. Precambrian Research, 85, 1-25.

Montgomery, C.W. 1979. Uranium lead geochronology of the Archean Imataca series, Venezuelan Guayana shield. Contributions to Mineralogy and Petrology, 69, 167-176.

Moreno, L., Madrid, P.L. and Tylki, R. 1985. Reconocimiento geológico del alto Paragua. Memoria I, Simposium Amazonico, Boletin de Geología, Publicación Especial Nº 10, Ministerio de Energia y Minas. Dirección de Geología, 100-115.

Moya E. 1977. Aspectos metalogenicos de los Andes Venezolanos. V Congreso Geológico Venezolano, 1169-1179.

Moya E. and Figueroa C. 1977. Mineralizaciones cupriferas en la Sierra de Perija, Edo. Zulia. V Congreso Geológico Venezolano, 1119-1128.

Myers, J.S. and Swager, C. 1997. The Yilgarn craton. In Greenstone Belts, Oxford Monographs on Geology and Geophysics 35. Edited by M.J. de Wit and L.D. Ashwal, Chapter 5.12, pp. 640-656.

Nixon, P.H., Davies, G.R., Rex, D. and Gray, A. 1992. Venezuela kimberlites. Journal of Volcanology and Geothermal Research, 50, 101-115.

Olmeta, M.A. 1968. Determinación de edades radiométricas de rocas de Venezuela. Boletin de Geología, Caracas, 10, Nº 19.

Olszewski, W.J., Gaudette, H.E. and Mendoza, V. 1977. Rb-Sr geochronolgy of the basement rocks, Amazonas territory, Venezuela: a progress report. V Congreso Geológico Venezolano, 519-526.

Perarnau, A. and Graterol, V. 1985. Red Gravimétrica Amazonas. Memoria I, Simposium Amazonico, Boletin de Geología, Publicación Especial Nº 10, Ministerio de Energia y Minas. Dirección de Geología, 422-427.

Priem, H.N.A., Andriessen, P.A.M., Boelrijk, N.A.I.M., de Boorder, H., Hedeba, E.H., Huguett, A., Verdurmen, E.A. and Vershure, R.H. 1982. Geochronology of the Precambrian in the Amazonas region of southeastern Colombia (western Guiana shield). Geologie en Mijnbouw, 61, 229-242.

Ríos, J.H. 1969. Geología de la Región de Caicara, Edo. Bolívar. IV Congreso Geológico Venezolano, Boletin de Geología, Publicación Especial 5, 1759-1782.

Rodriguez, S.E. 1977. Halos de alteración asociados con sulfuros masivos tipo Zn-Cu-Ba ubicados en el complejo volcanico de Villa de Cura, Estados Guarico y Aragua. V Congreso Geológico Venezolano, 1083-1099.

Rodriguez, S.E. 1986. Recursos minerales de Venezuela. Ministerio de Energia y Minas Boletin de Geología, Volumen XV, Numero 27, 228 p.

Sangster, D.F. 1972. Precambrian volcanogenic massive sulfide deposits in Canada: a review. Canada Geological Survey Paper 72-22, 44p.

Sidder, G.B. 1995. Mineral deposits of the Venezuelan Guayana shield. U.S. Geological Survey Bulletin 2124, O1-O20.

Sidder, G.B., Brooks, W.E., Estanga, Y., Nuñez, F. and Garcia, A. 1991. Early to middle Proterozoic supracrustal rocks and mineralization of the southern Guayana shield, Venezuela. U.S. Geological Survey Circular 1062, p.69.

Sidder, G.B. and Mendoza, V. 1995. Geology of the Venezuelan Guayana shield and its relation to the geology of the entire Guayana shield. U.S. Geological Survey Bulletin 2124, B1-B41.

Staargaard, C.F. and Carlson, G.G. 2000. The Bailadores volcanogenic massive sulfide deposit Venezuela. In Volcanogenic Massive Sulfide Deposits of Latin America. Edited by R.L. Sherlock and M.A.V. Logan, Mineral Deposit Division, Geological Association of Canada Publication.

Sosa, C. 1977. Geología de la región El Pao - San Felix - Guri. V Congreso Geológico Venezolano, 289-314.

Stott, G.M. 1997. The Superior province, Canada. In Greenstone Belts, Oxford Monographs on Geology and Geophysics 35. Edited by M.J. de Wit and L.D. Ashwal, Chapter 5.2, pp. 480-507.

Talukdar, S.C. and Colvée, P.G. 1975. Geología y estratigrafía del área de la meseta de El Viejo - Cerro Danto, T.F. Amazonas. Sociedad Venezolano Geológico Boletin V, 201-220.

Talukdar, S.C. and Colvée, P.G. 1977. Implicaciones del estudio petrologico de las rocas volcanicas del valle del Parucito, T.F. Amazonas. V Congreso Geológico Venezolano, 591-610.

Viteri, E. 1977a. Mineralogía y paragenesis del yacimiento de cobre nativo de Caño Tigre, Sierra de Perija, Edo. Zulia. V Congreso Geológico Venezolano, 1129-1142.

Viteri, E. 1977b. Estudio de las características petrológicas y metalogénicas del yacimiento de cobre nativo de Caño Tigre, Sierra de Perija, Edo. Zulia. V Congreso Geológico Venezolano, 1143-1168.

Voicu, G., Bardoux, M., Jébrak. M. and Crépeau, R. 1999. Structural, mineralogical, and geochemical studies of the

Paleoproterozoic Omai gold deposit, Guyana. Economic Geology, 94, 1277-1304.

Walrond, G.W. 1985. A metallogenic scheme for the Guiana shield. Memoria I, Simposium Amazonico, Boletin de Geología, Publicación Especial Nº 10, Ministerio de Energia y Minas. Dirección de Geología, 609-624.

Wynn, J.C., McCafferty, A.E. and Salaxar, E. 1995. Analysis of aeromagnetic data to improve geologic maps of the Bochinche mining district, Estado Bolívar, Venezuela. U.S. Geological Survey Bulletin 2124, C1-C13.

THE BAILADORES VOLCANOGENIC MASSIVE SULPHIDE DEPOSIT, VENEZUELA

CHRISTIAAN F. STAARGAARD
Consulting Geologist, 912-510 West Hastings St., Vancouver, B.C., Canada V6B 1L8

GERALD G. CARLSON
Copper Ridge Explorations Inc, 500-625 Howe St., Vancouver, B.C., Canada V6C 2T6

ABSTRACT

The Bailadores base metal volcanogenic massive sulphide deposit is located in the Cordillera de Mérida in western Venezuela. It is hosted in a sequence of felsic pyroclastic rocks within the Devonian to Pennsylvanian Mucuchachí Formation, an unmetamorphosed to low grade marine sequence dominated by graphitic slates and phyllites. The Mucuchachí Formation is in turn part of a metamorphic core complex forming the backbone of the Cordillera de Mérida.

The deposit was investigated between 1967 and 1978, mainly by the Dirección de Geología of the Ministerio de Minas e Hidrocarburos of Venezuela which completed 56 diamond drill holes as well as two short adits and a variety of surface work. The last published resource estimate was stated as 1.45 million tonnes grading 26 percent zinc, 7 percent lead and 1.5 percent copper.

From bottom to top, the deposit sequence includes felsic lithic, lapilli, breccia and crystal tuffs, fine grained intermediate to felsic ash tuff and black phyllite with intercalations of felsic crystal and lithic tuffs. Massive to banded sphalerite and pyrrhotite with lesser galena and chalcopyrite and minor arsenopyrite occur in two slightly overlapping layers, each up to about 15 metres thick, at or near the contact zone between the felsic tuffs and the black phyllite.

The deposit is underlain by an alteration zone consisting of a core of massive chlorite-biotite-margarite successively enveloped by chlorite- and then sericite-dominant alteration. Neither the footwall alteration zone nor the minor stringer style chalcopyrite mineralization found within it have been completely delineated. Massive sulphides are open along strike and to depth.

INTRODUCTION

The Bailadores volcanogenic massive sulphide deposit, also known as the Las Tapias deposit, is located about seven kilometres south of the town of Bailadores in the Cordillera de Mérida in western Venezuela (Fig. 1). It is situated in mountainous terrain, at an elevation of between 2,400 and 3,000 metres above sea level. Large parts of the area are under small-scale cultivation but where original forest remains, it is dense. An access road leads from Bailadores through the deposit area and continues on into a national park at higher elevations.

The presence of mineralization has been known since colonial times, when a small amount of near surface, high-grade ore was mined by the Spanish. Between 1966 and 1978, the Venezuelan government completed 56 diamond drill holes and two short adits to evaluate the deposit. The last published resource estimate was stated as 1.45 million tonnes grading 26 percent zinc, 7 percent lead and 1.5 percent copper (converted here from the original Imperial units) (Mining Journal, 1976).

Numerous studies, both published and unpublished, have been carried out on the Bailadores deposit and region (Escarrachi, 1980; Nogueira et al, 1972; Sifontes and Garcia, 1975; Woznessensky, 1972; Graterol, 1972; Carlson, 1977; Staargaard, 1994a, b).

REGIONAL GEOLOGY

The Bailadores area is situated in the Venezuelan Andes, one of the extensions of the Cordillera Orientale also known as the Cordillera de Mérida. The latter consists of a complexly deformed core of Precambrian to Paleozoic metamorphic rocks, nonconformably overlain by mainly sedimentary cover

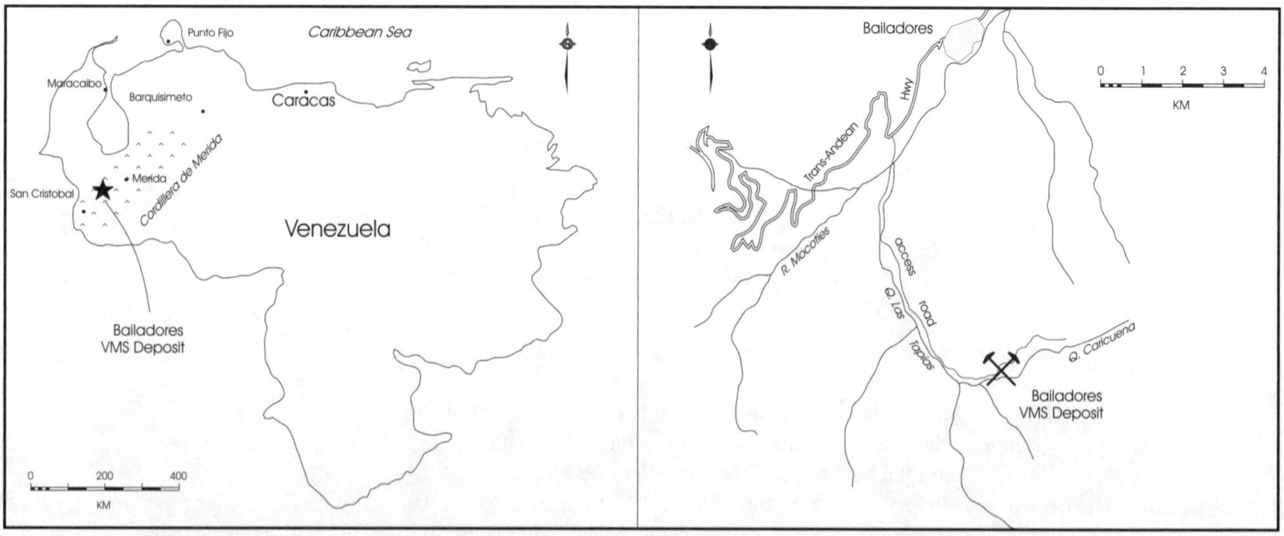

Figure 1. Location of Bailadores volcanogenic massive sulphide deposit.

ranging in age from Late Paleozoic to Tertiary (Fig. 2). It is distinct from most of the other South American Cordillera for the lack of younger volcanic rocks, its relief being entirely due to recent tectonic uplift (Giegengack, 1984). Numerous northeasterly trending faults, the largest of which is the seismically active Boconó fault zone, are present.

Geological contacts in the metamorphic core complex have been variously described as stratigraphic or as metamorphic isograds. The latest view is that the complex comprises a sequence of metamorphic facies and unmetamorphosed units of mainly Pennsylvanian and Permian age but locally as old as Precambrian (Case et al, 1990). Although a number of contacts are clearly isograds, the range of radiometric ages for granitic plutons (Late Precambrian to Early Triassic) enclosed within the complex suggests that some of the igneous-metamorphic associations must lie nonconformably on similar but older associations.

The oldest rocks have been grouped into the Sierra Nevada Formation and include medium grade quartzofeldspathic gneisses, schists, amphibolites and granitoid intrusives. Their age is believed to be as old as Precambrian although some portions may represent more strongly metamorphosed correlatives of Late Paleozoic units.

The Sierra Nevada Formation is overlain by the Mucuchachí Formation, an unmetamorphosed to low grade sequence of marine sedimentary deposits of Devonian to Pennsylvanian age. Up to 5,000 metres thick, it extends along almost the full length of the Cordillera de Mérida. It comprises mainly gray to black, often silty and/or graphite-bearing slates and phyllites along with locally developed lenses of limestone. A unit of felsic pyroclastic rocks, up to 2,000 metres thick, occurs at its base in the Bailadores area and hosts the Bailadores volcanogenic massive sulphide deposit.

The Mucuchachí Formation is overlain by the Pennsylvanian to Permian Sabaneta Formation, a sequence of continental sediments divided into a lower clastic member and an upper red bed member. It is in turn conformably overlain by the Permian Palmito Formation, an upwardly fining sequence of marine clastic sediments capped with limestone. The Tostosa greenschist, which is found mainly north of the Boconó fault, is thought to be at least partly correlative with the above Late Paleozoic section.

Other Paleozoic sediments overlying the core complex are mainly marine and include those of Ordovician, Silurian, and Carboniferous to Permian age. Mesozoic sedimentary strata of Triassic and Jurassic age are mainly continental while those of Cretaceous and Paleogene age are mainly marine. The youngest Neogene and Quaternary deposits are mostly continental.

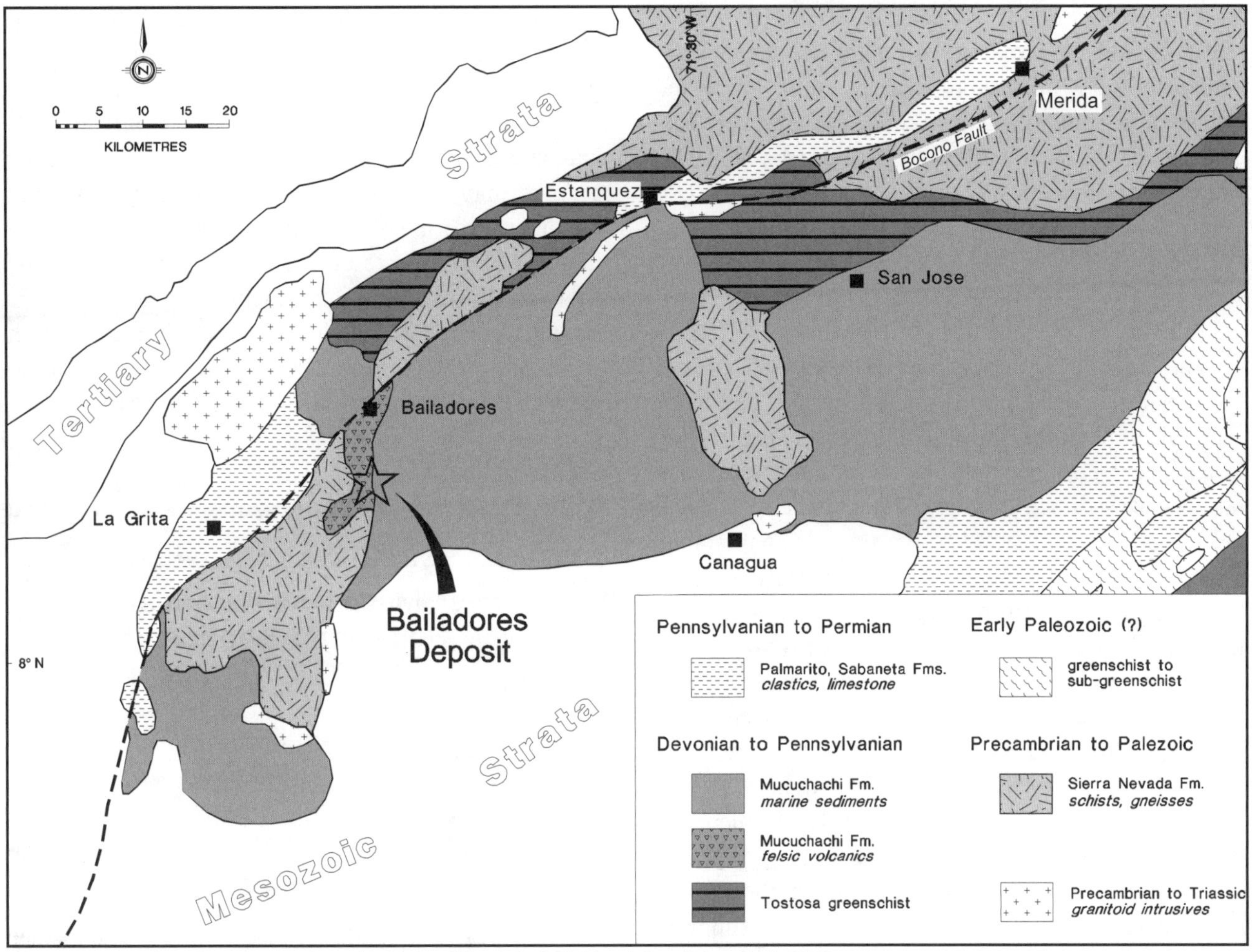

Figure 2. Regional geology of southern Cordillera de Mérida. After Case et al, 1990.

History of Exploration

Several old pits and adits as well as a small furnace in the deposit area date from small-scale mining in the Spanish colonial period, previous to 1800. An English company is said to have mined the deposit on a limited scale for copper and iron in the period from 1876 to 1881 (Ely, 1994). In 1954, the Compania Minera Occidental registered the "De Lima No. 2" concession with the objective of mining for copper and lead, however, a lack of funds and technical expertise together with insufficient exploration forced them to abandon this project and the property reverted to the government.

Between 1967 and 1970, the Dirección de Geología of the Ministerio de Minas e Hidrocarburos of Venezuela carried out a program of exploration and drilling that included 21 diamond drill holes over a strike length of about 400 metres. Two adits were driven and/or extended into mineralization for sampling and mapping. Another 35 diamond drill holes were completed between 1974 and 1976 and some metallurgical testwork was carried out.

At the end of 1976, bids were solicited from a number of foreign companies and consortia for the development of the Bailadores deposit. The foreign interest was to be 30 percent, the remaining 70 percent to be held by the government. Although one group was eventually selected, no development was ever carried out because of strong local opposition to mining and proximity to a national park. Since then, attempts by at least two other groups have failed for the same reasons.

The last records of physical work date from 1977 and 1978 and show that a small number of holes were drilled by the Ministerio to firm up the resource and that some ground magnetic and EM surveys were carried out to the north of the deposit (Martinez, 1977; Martinez and Garcia, 1978).

PROPERTY GEOLOGY

Stratigraphy and mineralization

The Bailadores deposit occurs along the contact between a sequence of felsic volcanic rocks and overlying black phyllites, the predominant lithology of the Mucuchachí Formation. Minor intercalations of various clastic sediments, amphibolite (mafic volcanics) and fossiliferous limestone (gastropods, tetracorals, crinoids) are also present in the area (Sifontes and Garcia, 1975). The felsic volcanics form a pile approximately 20 km long and up to 2,000 metres thick at the base of the Mucuchachí Formation where it lies unconformably on basement rocks. This is the only currently recognized occurrence of volcanic rocks within the regionally extensive Mucuchachí Formation.

The internal composition of the felsic sequence is not well understood because of a lack of regional mapping. The detailed stratigraphy over the 200 to 300 m section immediately hosting the sulphide deposit is much better known because of drilling and some underground openings. Figure 3 illustrates the stratigraphic section as it is currently understood. Unfortunately, only portions of the deposit area have been mapped at anything near a property scale. Figure 4 is taken from Carlson (1977) but is derived in part from earlier mapping by government workers (Sifontes and Garcia, 1973). Figure 5 illustrates several example cross-sections through the deposit area.

Footwall felsic fragmental

This is the lowermost unit known from drilling in the deposit area. It includes a variety of felsic crystal and lithic tuffs exposed in scattered, small outcrops on ridge tops and in creek beds. They range in composition from quartz-rich andesite to rhyolite and may include sub-volcanic intrusive equivalents. Thin layers of black phyllite are locally interbedded near the top of the sequence.

Chloritization, and to some extent sericitization, of this unit increase with proximity to the massive sulphide deposit. In places, a mottled texture suggests the presence of relatively sericitized, lapilli to breccia-sized felsic fragments in a more chloritic and finer grained matrix. In past work, the chloritized section has been described as a separate unit but it is likely that it actually represents footwall alteration of the footwall felsic fragmental rocks. The altered zone ranges from 100 to 300 m in thickness but not enough work has been carried out to determine its lateral extent beyond the deposit.

Massive sulphides

Semi-massive to massive sulphides occur in two

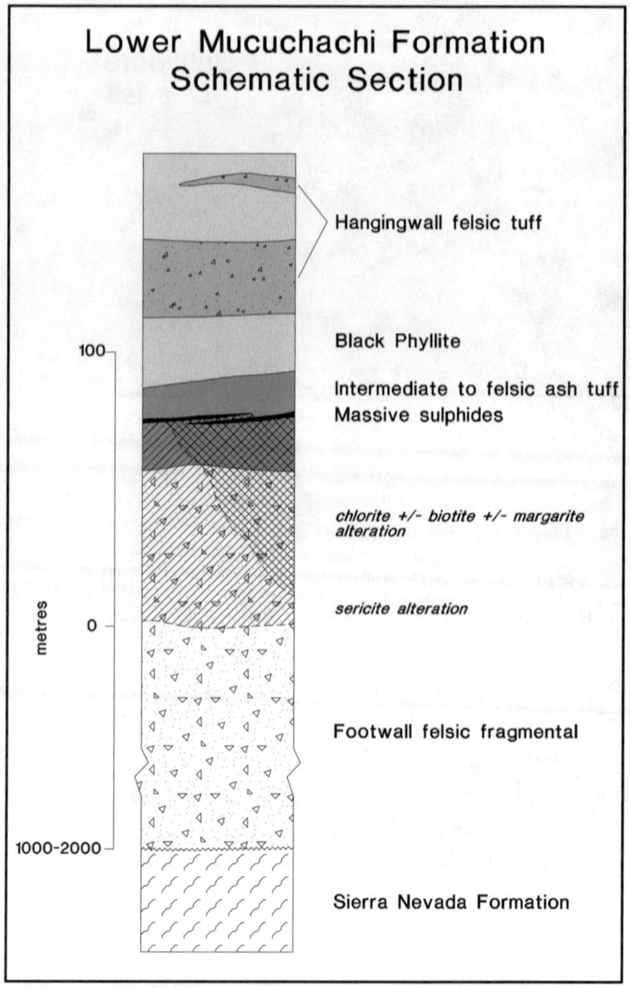

Figure 3. Schematic stratigraphic section, Lower Mucuchachí Formation (note scale change).

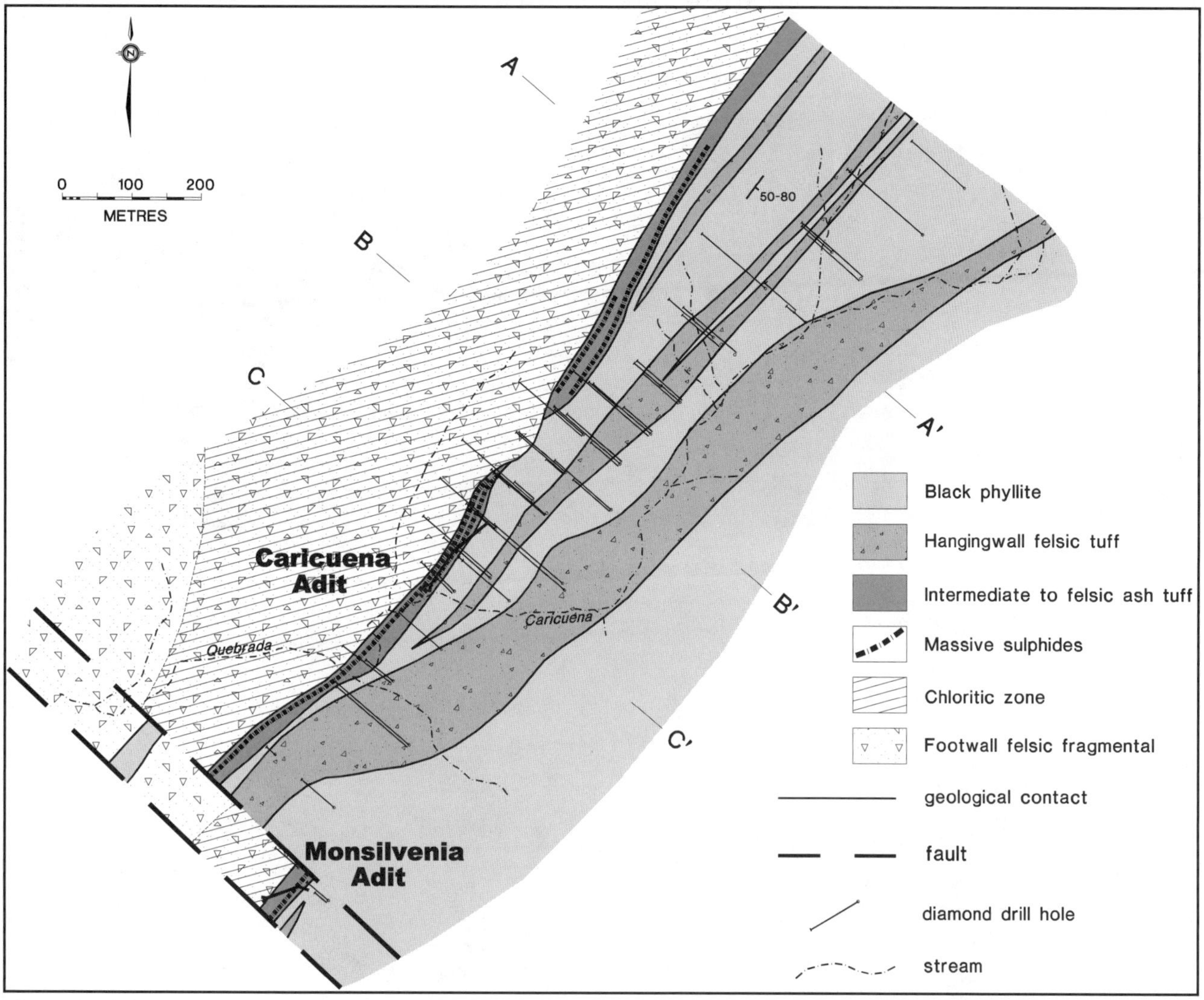

Figure 4. Schematic plan geology of the Bailadores deposit area.

main layers, generally separated by a few metres of ash tuff, that overlap near the centre of the deposit. Drilling has outlined the two zones along a strike length of approximately 1,150 m and from 70 to 250 m down dip. The lower and upper layers may reach thicknesses of up to 14.9 metres and 10.8 metres respectively (Staargaard, 1994b). Mineralization is open along strike and to depth.

The massive sulphides are quite uniform throughout the deposit and consist predominantly of sphalerite (+50 %) and pyrrhotite (15-25 %) with lesser galena (5-15 %), chalcopyrite (<10 %), arsenopyrite (<5 %) and pyrite (1 %). Gangue minerals comprise zero to 20 percent of the rock and consist mainly of quartz with lesser sericite, chlorite and biotite. In places, subangular quartz-rich fragments up to a few centimetres in size may represent metamorphosed chert fragments.

Sulphide layers are generally banded on a scale of 1 to 2 centimetres with respect to sphalerite-galena and pyrrhotite. Sphalerite grains are typically greater than 0.5 mm in diametre and are usually fractured. Pyrrhotite and galena are finer grained and, in sphalerite-rich layers, often interstitial. Within layered sulphides, chalcopyrite typically occurs as very fine grained inclusions in sphalerite grains. Arsenopyrite

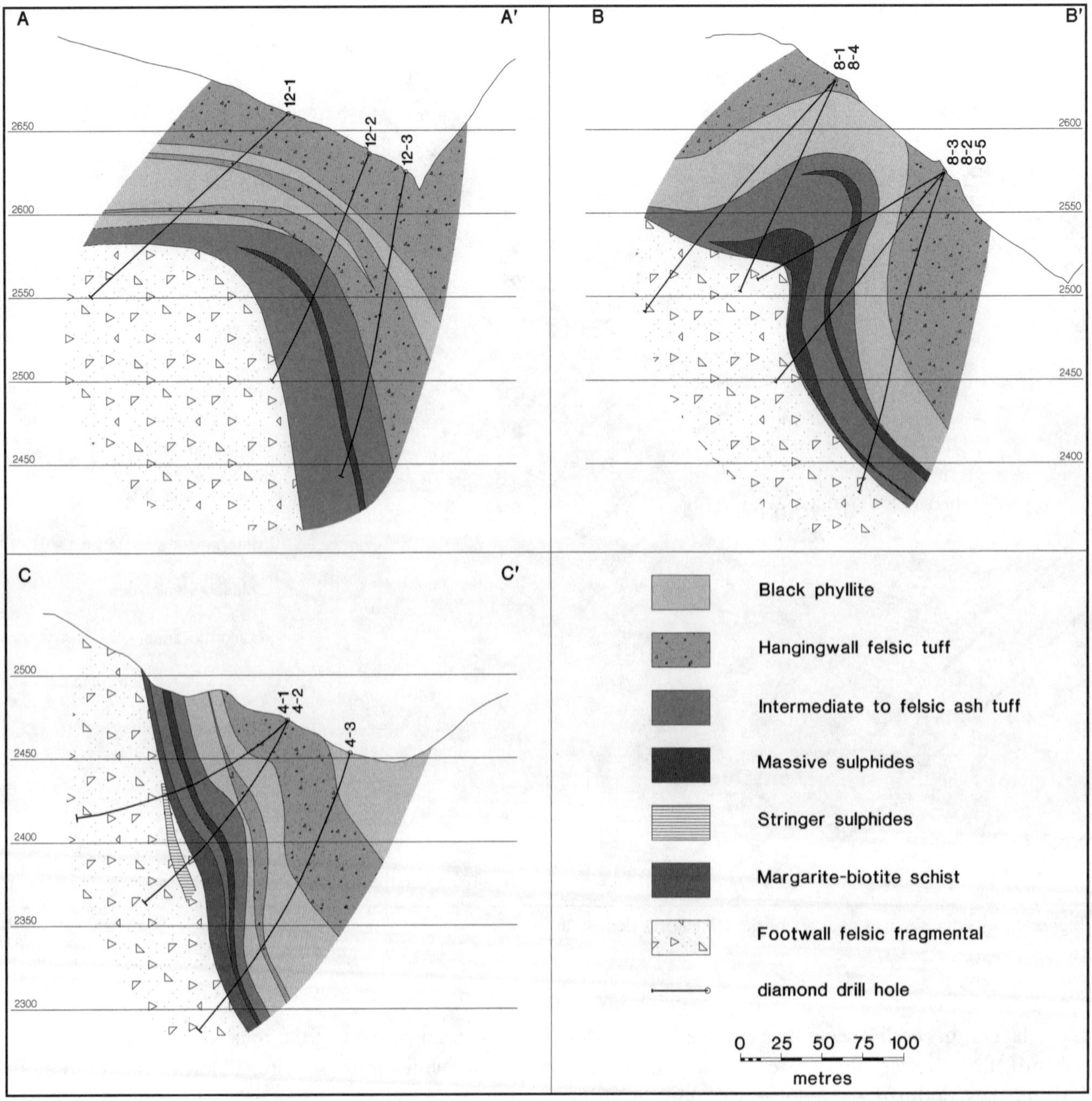

Figure 5. Selected cross-sections through the Bailadores deposit. See Figure 4 for locations.

is found as fine subhedral to euhedral grains, often in clusters, and frequently has the other sulphide minerals filling fractures within it.

Although a silver grade was not stated in the resource quoted earlier, inspection of drill hole intersections throughout the deposit indicates that silver values are generally in the range of 30 to 100 grams per tonne, in places reaching levels of several hundred grams per tonne (Staargaard, 1994b). ICP analysis of seven selected samples of massive sulphides collected from a dump near the Caricuena adit returned, in addition to high values in zinc, lead and copper, elevated levels of silver (53.6-88.5 ppm), gold (202-567 ppb), arsenic (237-1732 ppm), bismuth (85-489 ppm), cadmium (>100 ppm), antimony (188-222 ppm) and tungsten (425-1011 ppm). Values for barium (3-20 ppm) and gallium (1 ppm) were low (Staargaard, 1994a).

Intermediate to felsic ash tuff

This unit hosts the massive sulphide layers and consists of a light gray to tan- coloured, fine-grained, banded phyllitic rock composed mainly of quartz and sericite with minor chlorite and biotite. Small amounts of pyrrhotite are present as disseminated grains elongated parallel to foliation. Locally, more siliceous sections of this unit immediately overlying the main sulphide layers may contain thin layers and lenses of sphalerite and galena together with lesser pyrrhotite and occasional chalcopyrite.

Hangingwall felsic tuff

This unit consists of weakly sericitized, felsic lithic and crystal tuffs that occur in several layers ranging from less than one metre to more than 50 metres in thickness within the hangingwall black phyllites. Lower contacts tend to be sharp while upper contacts are more gradational with the black phyllite, suggesting sudden influxes of pyroclastic material that gradually waned. Plagioclase, which comprises 10 to 50 percent of the rock, occurs as variably sericitized crystals and crystal fragments up to 5 mm in length. The finer grained tuffs show evidence of shards and welding textures, although these have been typically obscured by subsequent metamorphism and deformation.

Black phyllite

The sequence in the deposit area is capped with fine-grained, black, phyllitic argillaceous rocks typical of the Mucuchachí Formation. These show a faint, delicate bedding defined by variations in grain size, quartz content or sulphide content. Petrographic work shows that they generally consist of quartz (20-50 %), sericite (≤70 %), chlorite (≤50 %) and biotite (15 %), with occasional small feldspar fragments. Disseminated pyrrhotite typically comprises three to five percent of the unit.

Footwall alteration and metal zoning

The Bailadores deposit is underlain by a relatively typical footwall alteration zone. Immediately below massive sulphides, the host ash tuff and underlying footwall felsic fragmental rocks have been intensely altered to a rock composed of up to 70 percent chlorite along with important amounts of biotite and margarite. With increasing distance both laterally and vertically from the deposit, margarite and biotite disappear, the intensity of chloritization decreases and sericitization becomes more obvious. The total extent of the footwall alteration zone is not known because of limited surface mapping and the confinement of drilling to the immediate deposit area. Limited whole rock analysis of diamond drill core by Escarrachi (1980) shows that values of Na_2O and CaO in the footwall rocks are generally less than 0.5 %, suggesting that they have been depleted.

Disseminated sulphides occur in both the hangingwall and the footwall of the massive sulphide horizons. In the immediate footwall of the deposit, the chloritic schist is variably mineralized with up to two percent pyrite and chalcopyrite. Stringer-style chalcopyrite-rich mineralization has been intersected in the footwall of the deposit in various drill holes although no clearly defined stringer zone has yet been outlined. On surface, mineralization and alteration are manifested in a broadly developed gossan in highly fractured felsic volcanic rocks. Portions of the gossan may represent a stockwork zone, although iron oxides have replaced all primary sulphides.

Metamorphism and structure

The deposit and host rocks have undergone low grade metamorphism. Case et al (1990) describe the results of regional mapping which show a metamorphic aureole within the Mucuchachí Formation centred on the Permian to Triassic Pueblo Hondo granite pluton about 15 km to the northwest of the deposit. The metamorphic effect appears to have been intensified locally in the vicinity of the Bailadores deposit, perhaps as a result of the altered bulk chemistry in this area due to hydrothermal alteration, as indicated by the local preponderance of pyrrhotite over pyrite within the Mucuchachí rocks. Annealing textures are present in some portions of the sulphide deposit and the sulphide minerals are relatively coarse grained (Escarrachi, 1980).

The deposit sequence strikes northeasterly and dips to the southeast at 45° to 80°. Although a weak northeasterly foliation with variable dip is present in the deposit area, margarite and biotite porphyroblasts in the footwall alteration zone rarely show preferred orientation, suggesting that metamorphism was largely thermal. Interpretation of diamond drill information suggests that the deposit and enclosing host rocks may have been deformed into an "S-fold" as shown in Figure 5 although this needs to be confirmed with systematic surface mapping. Small-scale drag folds have been observed in outcrop and in drill core.

Towards the southwest end of the deposit, a significant, northwest-trending left lateral fault has displaced the massive sulphide horizon by approximately 150 m (Fig. 4). The deposit is terminated at its southwestern end by a parallel fault and the offset portion has not yet been discovered. It is possible that other offsets occur within the deposit but they have not yet been recognized due to the wide spaced drilling pattern and lack of surface exposure.

DISCUSSION

The Bailadores deposit is a volcanogenic massive sulphide deposit of mid-Paleozoic age. Regionally, it is situated at the upper contact of a unit of felsic fragmental volcanic rocks constituting the base of a thick, weakly metamorphosed sequence of marine argillaceous to silty sediments. The deposit is zinc-rich, composed mainly of variably banded, stratiform pyrrhotite and sphalerite with lesser galena, chalcopyrite, pyrite and arsenopyrite. A copper-rich stockwork has been intersected in places below the layered sulphides but its full extent has not yet been determined. Footwall alteration is present, grading outwards from the strong development of chlorite, margarite and biotite immediately below the deposit to a chlorite-sericite assemblage and then a more diffuse zone of mainly sericitization. Limited lithogeochemical sampling suggests that Na_2O and CaO are relatively depleted in the footwall alteration zone. Based on the host rock association of felsic volcanic rocks in a largely clastic sedimentary sequence, the Bailadores deposit can be placed into the bimodal-siliciclastic category of Barrie and Hannington's (1999) VMS deposit classification.

This account of the geology of the Bailadores deposit has been largely descriptive, mainly because little modern research has been carried out on this interesting and relatively isolated example of mid-Paleozoic VMS mineralization. Of particular interest would be detailed studies of the full extent and character of alteration associated with the deposit as well as a more complete description of the stratigraphic section and tectonic history of the region. In addition to radiometric age-dating, the presence of well-preserved fossils in limestones within the Mucuchachí Formation in the immediate area might allow more precise constraints on the age and perhaps even the depth of formation of the deposit. Finally, and not least of all, further exploration is required to fully define the deposit itself, which remains open along strike and to depth, and to search for other deposits associated with the Mucuchachí Formation felsic volcanic rocks.

REFERENCES

Barrie, C.T. and Hannington, M.D., 1999. Classification of Volcanic-Associated Massive Sulfide Deposits Based on Host-Rock Composition. In Volcanic-Associated Massive Sulfide Deposits: Processes and Examples in Modern and Ancient Settings. Edited by C. Tucker Barrie and Mark D. Hannington. Society of Economic Geologists with the Mineral Deposits Division of the Geological Association of Canada, Reviews in Economic Geology, Volume 8, Chapter 1, pp.1-11.

Carlson, G.G., 1977. Geology of the Bailadores, Venezuela, Massive Sulfide Deposit. Economic Geology, 72: 1131-1141.

Case, J.E., Shagam, R. and Geigengack, R.F., 1990. Geology of the northern Andes; An overview. In The Geology of North America. Edited by G. Dengo and J.E. Case. Volume H, The Caribbean Region. The Geological Society of America, pp. 177-200.

Ely, R., 1994. Las Empresas y Los Grupos Ambientalistas: Una Advertencia para NAFTA. Paper presented at the Congreso Internacional AMEC in Mexico City. Asociación Mexicana de Estudios Canadienses. 16p.

Escarrachi M., R.A., 1980. Geología, Alteración, Mineralización, Geoquímica y Genesis del Yacimiento Volcanogénico de Sulfuros Masivos de Las Tapas, Estado Mérida, Venezuela. Ministerio de Energia y Minas de Venezuela report, 263p.

Giegengack, R., 1984. Late Cenozoic tectonic environments of the Central Venezuelan Andes. In The Caribbean-South American Plate Boundary and Regional Tectonics. Edited by

W.E. Bonini, R.B. Hargraves and R.B. Shagam. Geological Society of America Memoir 162, pp. 343-364.

Graterol, M., 1972. Mineralogía de la Mena del Yacimiento De Lima No. 2, Region de las Tapias, Bailadores, Estado Mérida. 4th Congreso Geologico Venezolano, Caracas, 1969. Boletin Geología Publicación Especial 5, pp. 2605-2613.

Martinez R., M. and Garcia G., L.S., 1978: Prospeccion Magnética y Electromagnética en el Yacimiento de Lima II, Bailadores, Estado Mérida. Ministerio de Energia y Minas report, 9p.

Martinez R., M., 1977: Estudio Geofisico Terrestre para la Localización y Cartografia de Vetas y Mineralizaciónes de Polisulfuros en el Yacimiento de Lima II-Bailadores, Estado Mérida - Mediante Calicatas Electromagnética s. Ministerio de Energia y Minas report, 58p.

Mining Journal, 1976.

Nogueira, A., Santana, A., Lavie, E. and Garcia D., E., 1972. El Yacimiento de Plomo, Zinc y Cobre de Bailadores, Estado Mérida. 4th Congreso Geológico Venezolano, Caracas, 1969. Boletin Geología Publicacion Especial 5, pp. 2728-2755.

Sifontes G., R.S. and Garcia D., E., 1973. Mapa geologico de la region Bailadores-Guaraque, Estado Mérida. Ministerio de Minas e Hidrocarburos preliminary map.

Sifontes G., R.S. and Garcia D., E., 1975. Prospeccion Geológico-Minera en la Region de Bailadores-Guaraque, Estado Mérida. Ministerio de Minas e Hidrocarburos report, 91p.

Staargaard, C.F., 1994a. Preliminary Evaluation of the Bailadores Polymetallic Massive Sulphide Deposit, Mérida State, Venezuela. Private report for client, 21p.

Staargaard, C.F., 1994b. Reconstruction of Historical Drilling on the Bailadores Polymetallic Massive Sulphide Deposit, Mérida State, Venezuela. Private report for client, 7p.

Woznessensky , B., 1972: Investigaciónes Metalogénicas en los Andes Venezolanos; 4th Congreso Geológico Venezolano, Caracas, 1969. Boletin Geología Publicación Especial 5, pp. 2827-2844.

GEOLOGICAL SETTING AND POTENTIAL OF VMS DEPOSITS IN COLOMBIA

LUIS JARAMILLO CORTES
Diagonal 103 no. 57ª-14, Ofic. 301, Bogota D.C. Colombia
jcle@multiphone,net.co

ABSTRACT

The Western Cordillera in Colombia represents an area of high potential for the discovery of volcanogenic massive sulphide deposits (VMS). Most of the cordillera is underlain by the Calima Terrain that consists of an ophiolitic sequence of Upper Cretaceous age, comprising basic to intermediate volcanic rocks and pelagic sediments.

To date, five VMS prospects have been discovered in the Western Cordillera. Their resources range from 0.1 to 4.8 million tonnes and grades from: 1.5-4 % Cu, 1-7 % Zn 0.5 % Pb, 2-3 g/t Au and 10-20 g/t Ag. Preliminary studies on these prospects suggest an affiliation with Kuroko type mineralization with the exception of the Sabanablanca deposit, which has a basalt association with high Cu values, characteristic of Cyprus type deposits.

Guadalupe, the only prospect located in the Central Cordillera, contains an indicated resources of about 28 million tonnes at 1.8 % Cu equivalent. The volcanic-sedimentary sequence hosting the mineral deposit is interpreted as an allochthonous block derived from the Western Cordillera. A Besshi type genetic model is suggested for this deposit.

Based on available information is difficult to establish any reliable differences in the genetic model of the deposits located in the Western and Central Cordilleras. In both cases the hosting rocks show evidences of syngenetic alteration associated with extrusion of lavas in a submarine environment and are affected by low grade metamorphism. Mineralization, usually related to hydrothermal alteration, displays similar paragenesis: Cu-Zn-Pb sulphides with variables amounts of Au-Ag. Considering that the favorable geological environment for the formation of massive sulphides occur along 800 km, the Western Cordillera of Colombia offers high potential for VMS exploration.

INTRODUCTION

In 1975 the Instituto de Investigaciones Geológico – Mineras de Colombia INGEOMINAS, (Geological Mining Investigations Institute of Colombia, INGEOMINAS), in cooperation with the United States Geological Service, initiated a metallogenic study in Colombia. The findings of this work highlighted the potential of the Western Cordillera for the occurrence of volcanogenic massive sulphide deposits (INGEOMINAS, 1986).

On the basis of these investigations, Colombian and foreign mining companies conducted regional exploration work that led to the identification and preliminary evaluation of selected VMS deposits. The information compiled to this date is preliminary and, in many cases, confidential which makes it impossible to carry out a detailed analysis of the metallogenic characteristics of the deposits and their economic potential. This paper presents a synthesis of the information available, mainly from INGEOMINAS and partly from company files.

TECTONIC SETTING

The geology of Colombia's Western Cordillera, from the Cretaceous to the Tertiary (Paleocene-Eocene) is dominated by the interaction of the Pacific, South American and Caribbean tectonic plates. In the Lower Cretaceous, along the western margin, submarine basalts are interbedded with deep water sediments which tends to host the VMS mineralization. During the Upper Cretaceous the "Calima Orogenisis" was developed (Barrero, 1979). This process caused the folding, faulting and thrusting of the volcano-sedimentary sequence that created the Western Cordillera (Calima Terrane, Fig. 1). This terrane, consists of oceanic material accreted to the Tahami terrane (Ta) which comprises continental material. The two terranes form the Central Cordillera of Colombia (Fig. 1). The tectonic contact between both terranes is known as the Romeral's Tectonic Belt. The subduction resulted in Upper Cretaceous calc-alkaline magmatism (Antioqueño and El Bosque batholiths). The accretion resulted in the tectonic juxtaposition of the oceanic allochtonous blocks (Calima Terrane), on the continental base of the Central Cordillera.

Geological Setting

The Western Cordillera is formed by Cretaceous volcano-sedimentary sequences, known as the Dagua Group and the Diabase Group (Nelson, 1962) and is correlated to the north with the Cañasgordas Group (Restrepo, J.J. and Tussaint, J.F., 1981). Locally, there are ultramafic and gabbro bodies, along the cordillera, suggesting an ophiolitic nature. During the Eocene, an insular arch was developed related with the subduction of the Pacific Plate under the Calima Terrane. This process is represented in calc-alkaline batholiths and stocks, which intrude the volcano-sedimentary sequence along the Western Cordillera. The porphyry copper deposits with variable contents of Cu, Mo, Au are associated with the more recent phases of this magmatism, consisting of subvolcanic andesitic and dacitic rocks.

In the Dagua, Diabasic and Cañasgordas groups, the volcanic rocks consist of basaltic lava, spilite and diabase, with interbedded tuff. In many cases, the lava shows pillow structures. In general, the basaltic lava have a tholeiitic affiliation with low contents of potassium. The associated sediments consist primarily of sandstone, siliceous lutites, cherts and limestone. In general the whole sequence shows low grade metamorphism.

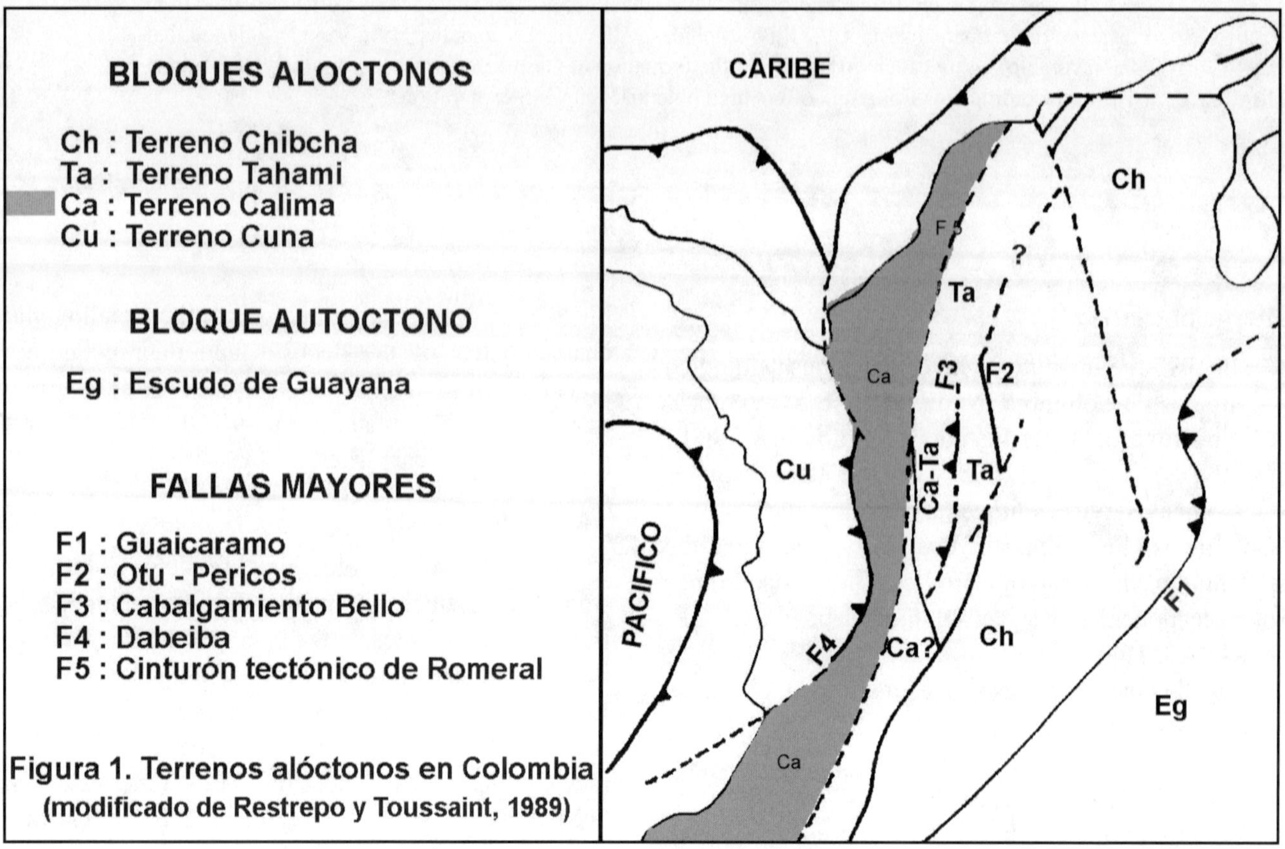

Figura 1. Terrenos alóctonos en Colombia (modificado de Restrepo y Toussaint, 1989)

Figure 1. Allochtonous terranes in Colombia (adapted from Restrepo and Toussaint, 1989).

Syngenetic Alteration

The spilite and pillow lavas show plagioclase albitization (originally An: 60-70), chloritized ferro-magnesian minerals, uralitization of the pyroxenes and the presence of epidote and carbonate. The mineralogical association, indicates an process of syngenetic alteration caused by the extrusion of lava in a marine environment. In general, the sequence shows an increase of Na and Mg and a decrease in K and Ca (Barrero, 1979).

The petrology and geochemistry of the volcano-sedimentary sequence shows similarities with rocks associated with Kuroko type deposits in Japan, in which the alteration was produced by the interaction of sea water with hot lava.

Metamorphism

The volcanic-sedimentary sequence shows variable degrees of metamorphism throughout the Western Cordillera, being in general lower at the north and then progressively increasing towards the south (INGEOMINAS, 1986). The sedimentary rocks in the middle part of the Cordillera were affected by three types of metamorphism (Barrero, 1979):

1) Low grade regional metamorphism represented by zeolites, prehnite-pumpelleite and green schists facies. The latter shows a higher aerial distribution and it is characterized by the presence of albite, muscovite, chlorite, biotite, epidote, calcite and quartz.
2) Contact metamorphism occurs locally in the aureola associated with the intrusive stocks.
3) Cataclastic metamorphism associated to the major faults.

In the two latter types of metamorphism, there was no important variation in the mineralogy generated by the regional metamorphism. The similarity between the mineralogical associations caused by the syngenetic, metamorphic and hydrothermal alteration makes it very difficult to differentiate between these processes.

Overall, the lithology, the type of alteration and the degree of metamorphism that characterizes the volcano-sedimentary sequence of Colombia's Cordillera Occidental, are similar to many other sequences that host volcanogenic massive sulphides in other parts of the world.

VMS potential

Although the exploration work in the western region of Colombia has been limited at best, six mineral deposits have been recognized that can be classified as VMS. Five of these deposits are located in the Western Cordillera and the other one in the Central Cordillera (Fig. 2). A synthesis of the geological indicators that characterize the deposits is shown in Table 1.

El Alacrán

This prospect is located in the Department of Cordoba, about 40 km SW of the Cerro Matoso, CMSA nickel deposit (Fig. 2). The sulphide deposit is hosted in a Cretaceous volcano-sedimentary complex. The sequence is underlain by siliceous pyroclastic rocks, which are overlain by sandstone, arkose, greywacke, limolites and chert, interbedded with porphyritic andesite, dacite and rhyodacitic which host the mineralization. Towards the west, on the top part of the complex is overlain by marine mafic volcanic rocks. The whole sequence has been intruded by quartz-dioritic rocks from the Tertiary (Eocene), that locally caused contact metamorphic effects. A closer look of the geology of the middle part of the deposit is shown in Figure 3. The two economically attractive mineralized horizons are located in the upper part of unit 2 and in the contact zone of units 4 and 5 (Vargas, 1999).

The prophylitic hydrothermal alteration is mainly in the mineralized areas, and consists of chlorite, epidote and carbonates. Sericitic alteration appears sporadically accompanied by silicification. The mineralogy of the deposit is characterized by an early magnetite associated with first generation pyrite, followed by calcite, pyrrhotite, chalcopyrite, pyrite and sphalerite. Calcite – aragonite, of later events, filled the faults.

The preliminary resource of this property on the basis of fifteen (15) test boreholes, leads us to estimate reserves in the order of 4.8 million tonnes with average grades of 1.4 % Cu, and 0.83 % Au. The oxide cap is estimated at 500,000 tonnes with an average grade of 2.5 g/t Au.

South of El Alacrán, approximately 3 km away,

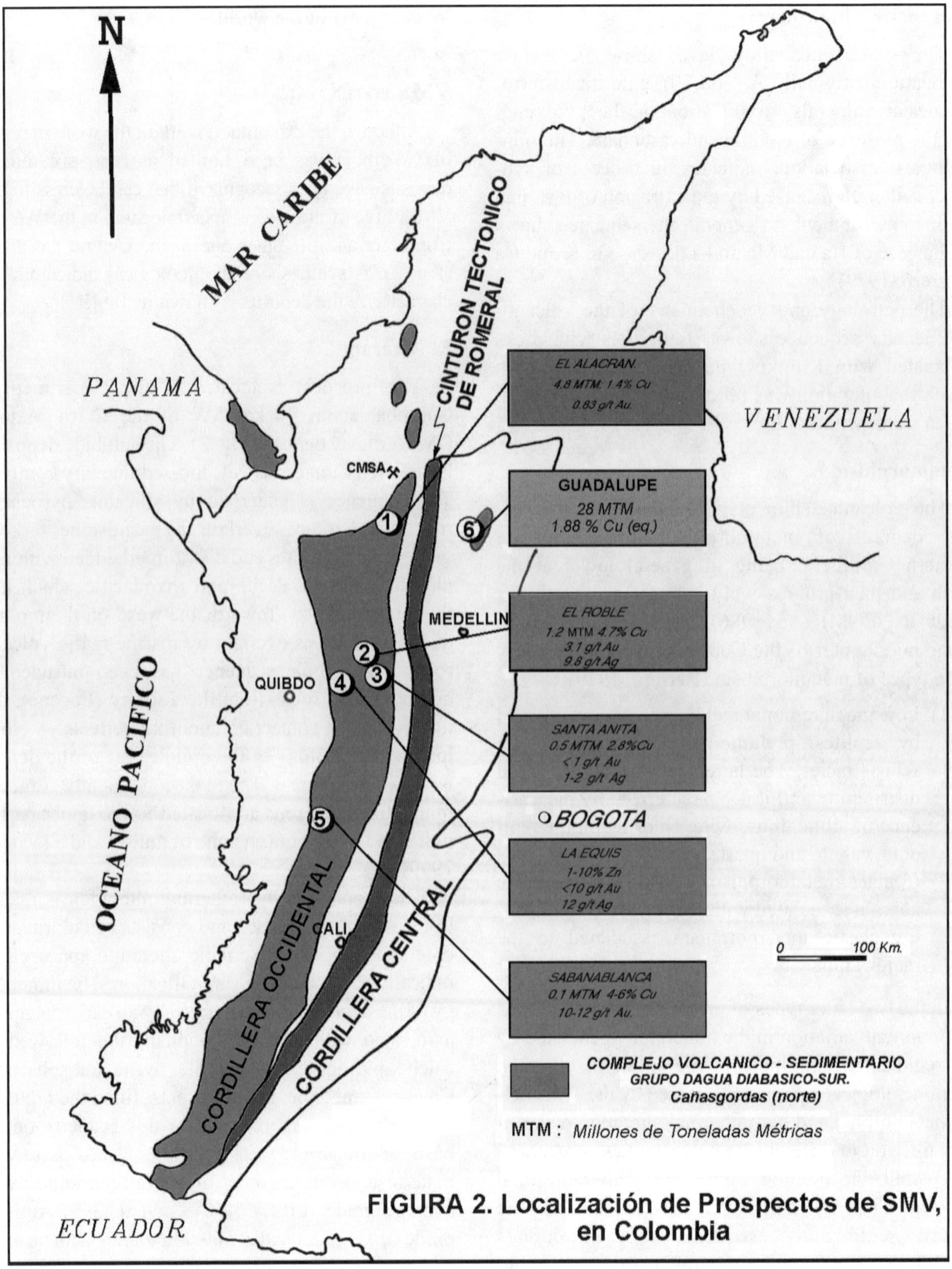

FIGURA 2. Localización de Prospectos de SMV, en Colombia

Figure 2. Location of VMS prospects in Colombia.

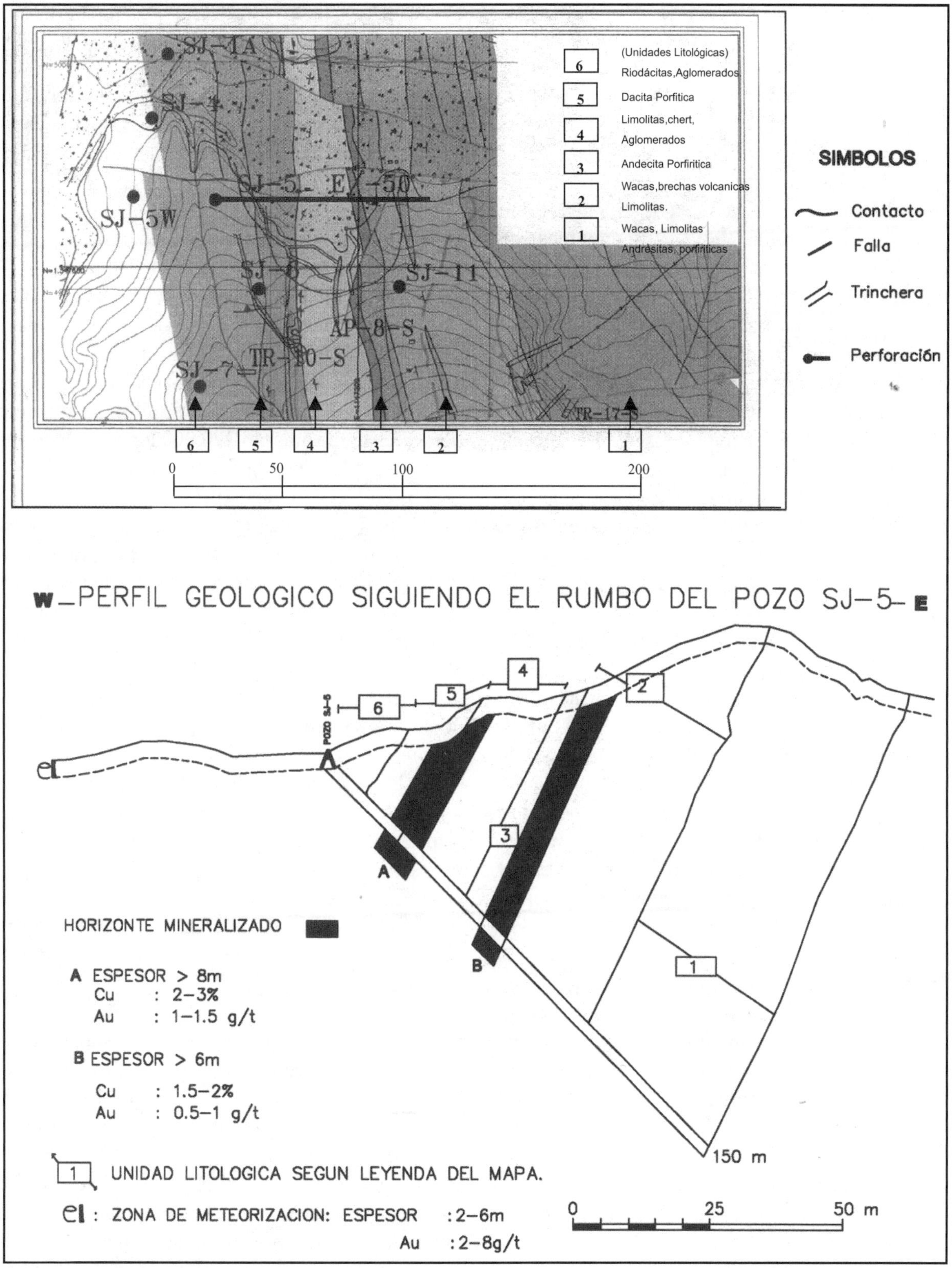

Figure 3. Site plan and geological profile of El Alacrán.

there is another property called Mina Ra, that although less important, it does demonstrate the potential of the volcano-sedimentary sequence for the exploration of the VMS.

El Roble

El Roble is located in the Department of Choco, 4 km north of the town Carmen de Atrato and 150 km SW of the city of Medellin (Fig. 2). The sulphide body is hosted in a sequence of diabase and andesites interbedded with cherts, clastic sediments (greywacke), some limestones and conglomerates of the Cretaceous Cañasgordas Group. Locally, the sequence is intruded by andesitic bodies in dykes and columns, probably associated with Tertiary magmatism.

The massive sulphides consist essentially of chalcopyrite, pyrite, pyrrhotite and some traces of sphalerite and galena with a quartz and carbonate gangue. The alteration of the host rock consists of chlorite, quartz and sericite (Calle and Salinas, 1983). The resource estimated by EERESA (Colombian-Japanese Consortium), were in the order of 1.2 million tonnes with average grades of 4.71 % Cu, 3.11 % g/t Au and 9.81 g/t Ag.

El Roble is the only VMS deposit that has been commercially mined in Colombia, for a period of 10 years, at an average rate of 300 tonnes per day and production of copper concentrate with economic gold and silver values. The concentrates were exported to Japan for refining. At the present time the mine is depleted and some exploration work is being carried out in its surrounding area, attempting to define additional mineralization.

Santa Anita

The Santa Anita prospect is located in the Department of Choco, approximately 140 km SW of Medellin (Fig. 2). The sulphide body is located very close to the contact between the Barroso and Penderisco formations of the Upper Cretaceous (Cañasgordas Group). The first of these formations is made up of basic volcanic rocks, tuffs and sedimentary rocks. The latter consists of lutites, cherts, greywacke, sandstone and conglomerates (Mazo and Gutierrez, 1971; INGEOMINAS, 1987).

The zone is extensively faulted and mineralization consists of chalcopyrite and pyrite in a quartz and calcite gangue. Approximately 500,000 tonnes are estimated with an average grade of 2.6 % Cu and traces of Au and Ag. This deposit has been the subject of a small scale mining producing copper concentrates. The operation has been inactive since 1976.

La Equis

La Equis is located in the Department of Choco, some 170 km SW of the city of Medellin (Fig. 2). The mineralized body is hosted in a pre-Eocene volcanic sequence of intermediate to felsic (andesites, dacites, rhyolites?) composition.. The mineralogy of the sulphide body consists of pyrite, chalcopyrite, galena, sphalerite, gold and silver in a milky quartz gangue. Reserves in the order of 120,000 tonnes were estimated with grades ranging from 8 to 12 % Zn, 0.8 to 1.5 % Pb, 12-15g/t Au, and 10-12 g/t Ag.

Calle and Salinas (1986) proposed two possible genetic models to explain the formation of the deposit. The first suggests an elongated structurally controlled sulphide body, produced by hydrothermal flows related to the intrusion of the Mande batholith. The second considers a VMS type mineralization, associated with the extrusion of the volcanic rocks in a submarine environment. It is interpreted as an incomplete section of a Kuroko type massive sulphide deposit. Based on the regional geological framework, the environment of formation and the metallogenic aspects, the author supports the second hypothesis.

Sabanablqnca

The Sabanablanca prospect is located in the Valle de Cauca Department, approximately 120 km NW of the city of Cali (Fig. 2). The Cretaceous volcano-sedimentary sequence consists of basalt, diabase and black lutites. Towards the east, there is a faulted contact with a metasedimentary sequence of phyllites and black schists (MINERALCO 1991). The mineralization is located in the northeast extension of the volcanic-sedimentary units (Kdb: basalts, diabase and pillow-like lava and Kdc: phyllites, shale and chert), defined by Barrero (1979). The massive sulphide deposits located close to the volcanic-sediment contact are made up of chalcopyrite, chalcocite (possibly secondary), pyrite and sphalerite. The gangue is composed essentially of quartz, carbonate and subordinate epidote. The alteration associated with the sulphides shows intense silicification (over 15 m) accompanied by subordinated chlorite. The estimated reserves up to now exceed 100,000 tonnes with an average grade of 6 % Cu and 12-13 g/t Au. Towards the north and south of the main zone, there are areas with alteration of oxides and copper carbonates which suggest a continuance of the mineralized zone.

Guadalupe

The Guadalupe prospect is located in the Department of Antioquia, approximately 140 km NE of the city of Medellin (Fig. 2). Guadalupe is the only VMS deposit discovered in the Central Cordillera. It is hosted in a Cretaceous sequence, called the San Pablo Formation, which consists of sediments and submarine basaltic volcanic rocks. The entire Cretaceous assemblage is interpreted as an allochthonous block derived from the oceanic domain of the Western Cordillera and tectonically juxtaposed.

The two mineralized intervals known as El Azufral and el Arroyo are interbedded in a sandstone, argillites and cornubians sedimentary sequence (Smith, 1998). Geophysical studies carried out by Val d'Or, Peru (1998) based on an electromagnetometric program (TME-MAG), confirmed the depth of the horizons discussed above and identified another two mineralized layers (Fig. 4).

The El Azufral strata has an average thickness of 9 m and can be followed along a strike of approximately 100 m. The main sulphides are pyrite, pyrrhotite, chalcopyrite and subordinated sphalerite. The oxidation zone shows secondary minerals, particularly limonite malachite and azurite. Ten (10) trench samples, taken from the sulphide body showed average grades of 2.03 % Cu, 0.3 % Zn, 0.13 ppm Au and 6.0 ppm Ag. The El Arroyo horizon to the south,

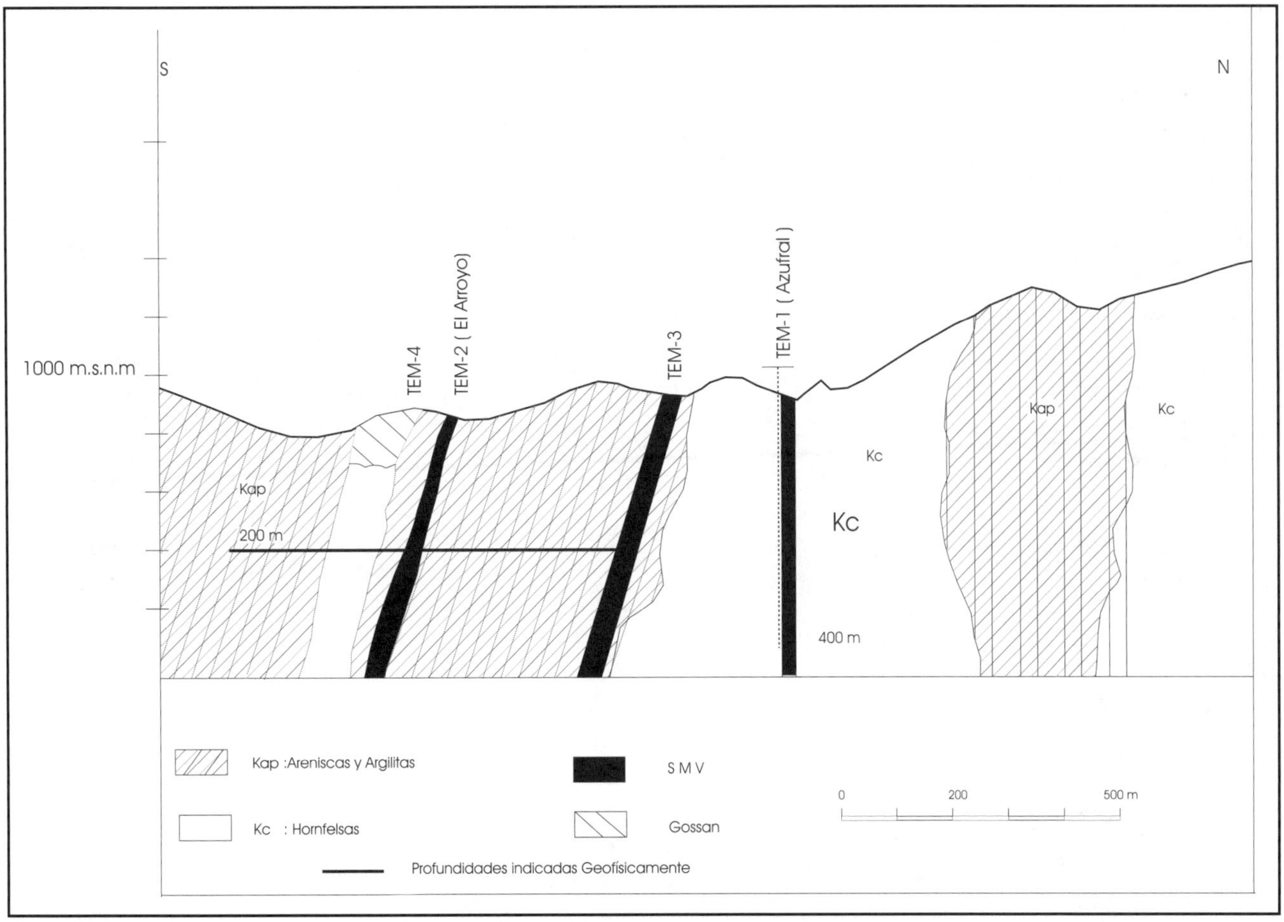

Figure 4. S-N profile of the Guadalupe VMS Prospect (adapted from Smith M, 1996).

shows the same mineral assemblage. Trench sampling resulted in average grades of 1.65 % Cu, 0.5 % Zn, 0.34 ppm Au and 18.5 ppm Ag. Since the sampling was done at surface for both zones, it is possible that the results obtained have been influenced by oxidation and do not correspond to the primary mineralization.

The main alteration assemblage is silicification, accompanied by the incipient development of sericite and chlorite. On the basis of the high proportion of Co + Ni / Cu and the low content of Pb, obtained in the geochemical canal samples, a Besshi type genetic model is suggested for Guadalupe. The results are very preliminary. The extension of the outcroppings of the mineralized horizons and their continuity at depth lead us to believe that there are inferred resources in the order of 28 million tons with 1.88 % Cu equivalent. The above comments, together with the excellent infrastructure of the area, confirm the great potential of this prospect.

Final considerations

VMS deposits in Colombia are associated with the submarine hydrothermal systems associated with Cretaceous ophiolitic sequences. In general, the mineralogical associations are rich in Cu and Zn with locally significant Au and Ag values. The Pb contents are minor with the exception of the Las Equis deposit where they reach values of up to 1.5 %.

The Western Cordillera (Calima Terrane) shows the greatest exploration potential for VMS deposits in Colombia. However, the Guadalupe deposit, located in the Central Cordillera, shows greater volume, although it should be noted that at the moment the reserves are only inferred.

Acknowledgements

The author would like to thank INGEOMINAS, Santa Gertrudis, SOM and the Grupo Bullet, SA, for providing the information which served as the basis for this paper.

(Translation. Original submitted in Spanish)

References

Barrero, D. 1979. Geology of the Central Western Cordillera, West of Buga and Roldanillo, Colombia. INGEOMINAS, Special Geological Publication, No. 4, 75 pp.

Calle, B. y Salinas, R. 1986. Geología y geoquímica de la plancha 165, Carmen de Atrato. Report, 1987. INGEOMINAS.140 pp.

INGEOMINAS,1987. Recursos minerales de Colombia. Second edition. Special Geological Publication. Vol. I. 564 pp.

INGEOMINAS - U.S.G.S., 1986. Map – Terrenos geológicos en Colombia. Special Geological Publication, No. 14-I, 235 pp.

INGEOMINAS - U.S.G.S., 1986. Evaluación de los recursos minerales no combustibles de Colombia. Special Geological Publication, No. 14-II, 55 pp.

Mazo, J. y Gutiérrez, N. 1971. Estudio geológico y de beneficio de mineral de cobre de la mina Santa Anita, Carmen de Atrato, Chocó. Ministerio de Minas y Petróleos. Zona minera de Medellín.

MINERALCO, 1991. Informe de comisión a la mina Sabanablanca, municipio de El Dovio. Internal Report, 9 pp.

Nelson H.W. 1962. Contribución al conocimiento de la Cordillera Occidental, sección Cali - Buenaventura. National Geological Service. Geological Bulletin 10. pp. 81-108.

Restrepo, J.J. y Toussaint,J.F., 1973. Obducción Cretácea en el Occidente Colombiano. Publicación Especial Geología. Universidad Nacional Medellín. pp 1-26.

Restrepo, J.J. y Toussaint, J.F.1989. Terrenos alóctonos en los Andes Colombianos, explicación de algunas paradojas geológicas. V Geological Congress of Colombia. Proceedings, Vol. I. pp 92-107

Smith, M.R. 1998. A major Besshi -type VMS Cu property in Colombia. Internal Report. Minerales Ensenada. 20 pp.

Val - D´OR, Perú. 1998. Geophysical report on Guadalupe VMS. Internal Report, Minerales Ensenada. 10 pp.

Vargas, H. 1999. Reservas y potencial en el proyecto El Alacrán, San Juan de Asís, Córdoba, Colombia. Internal Report. Santa Gertrudis, SOM - Río Quieto, B.V. 22 pp.

GOLD-RICH VHMS DEPOSITS OF THE WESTERN CORDILLERA OF ECUADOR: MINERALOGY, LEAD ISOTOPE AND METAL GEOCHEMISTRY

Massimo Chiaradia and Lluís Fontboté
Section des Sciences de la Terre, Rue des Maraîchers 13, CH-1211 Geneva 4, Switzerland

Abstract

The Western Cordillera of Ecuador hosts three Au-rich Cu-Zn VHMS deposits within an Early Tertiary island arc sequence, now accreted to the continent. The deposits are characterized by pyrite-chalcopyrite mineral parageneses including bornite, covellite, digenite, tennantite, and are affected by a quartz-sericite alteration. Lead isotope compositions are homogeneous within each deposit but differ significantly among the three orebodies, even if two of them are only 1.5 km apart. Lead isotope compositions of the orebodies overlap those of the volcanic host rocks and are consistent with lead derived from mixing of pelagic sediments, mantle and oceanic crust. Geological setting mineralogy, and gold grades of the VHMS deposits of the Western Cordillera of Ecuador bear some similarities to those of recent and present-day massive sulphides of the western Pacific.

Introduction

Gold-rich Cu-Zn VHMS deposits occur in the Western Cordillera of Ecuador within an Early Tertiary island arc sequence known as Macuchi Unit (BGS and CODIGEM, 1999; Chiaradia and Fontboté, submitted a and b). In this contribution we discuss geochemical and lead isotope data of these deposits (Macuchi, La Plata, El Patiño) and associated volcanic rocks focussing on (i) lead sources in the VHMS ores and host rocks, (ii) pyrite-chalcopyrite mineral assemblages, including bornite, covellite, digenite, tennatite, enargite, and (ii) the elevated gold grades (4.8 g/t at La Plata and 7.6 g/t at Macuchi) of the VHMS deposits.

Geological setting

The VHMS deposits studied are hosted by the Paleocene-Eocene Macuchi Unit, an intraoceanic island arc accreted to the continent during the Early Tertiary (Fig. 1: Cosma et al., 1998; Reynaud et al., 1999). The volcanic and volcaniclastic lithologies of the Unit are the result of submarine eruptions ranging from basalt to basaltic andesite, accompanied by lesser dacite and rhyolite, with tholeiitic to calc-alkaline affinity (BGS and CODIGEM, 1999). A lower sequence of Paleocene age (herein called Basal Macuchi), including primitive basaltic pillow lavas, and a more evolved upper sequence of Eocene age (herein called Main Macuchi), including basaltic andesite and andesitic pillow lavas, can be distinguished within the Macuchi Unit (Fig. 2; BGS and CODIGEM, 1999; Chiaradia and Fontboté, submitted a and b). The VHMS ore deposits are hosted at different levels of the Main Macuchi sequence (Fig. 2).

Results and discussion

Lead isotope geochemistry of the host sequence

Lead isotope compositions of the Basal and Main Macuchi volcanic rocks ($^{206}Pb/^{204}Pb$=18.66-19.09, $^{207}Pb/^{204}Pb$=15.53=15.67, $^{208}Pb/^{204}Pb$=38.20-39.00) define linear trends in conventional plots (Fig. 3), the Main Macuchi rocks being in general more radiogenic than the Basal Macuchi ones. The isotope trends indicate that lead in the Macuchi rocks derives from mixing of at least two different sources, which are isotopically homogeneous on a scale of 200 km, i.e., the distance across which samples have been collected (Fig. 1). Accepting the ensimatic nature of the Macuchi arc, the ^{207}Pb-rich source can only be represented by pelagic sediments (Chiaradia and Fontboté,

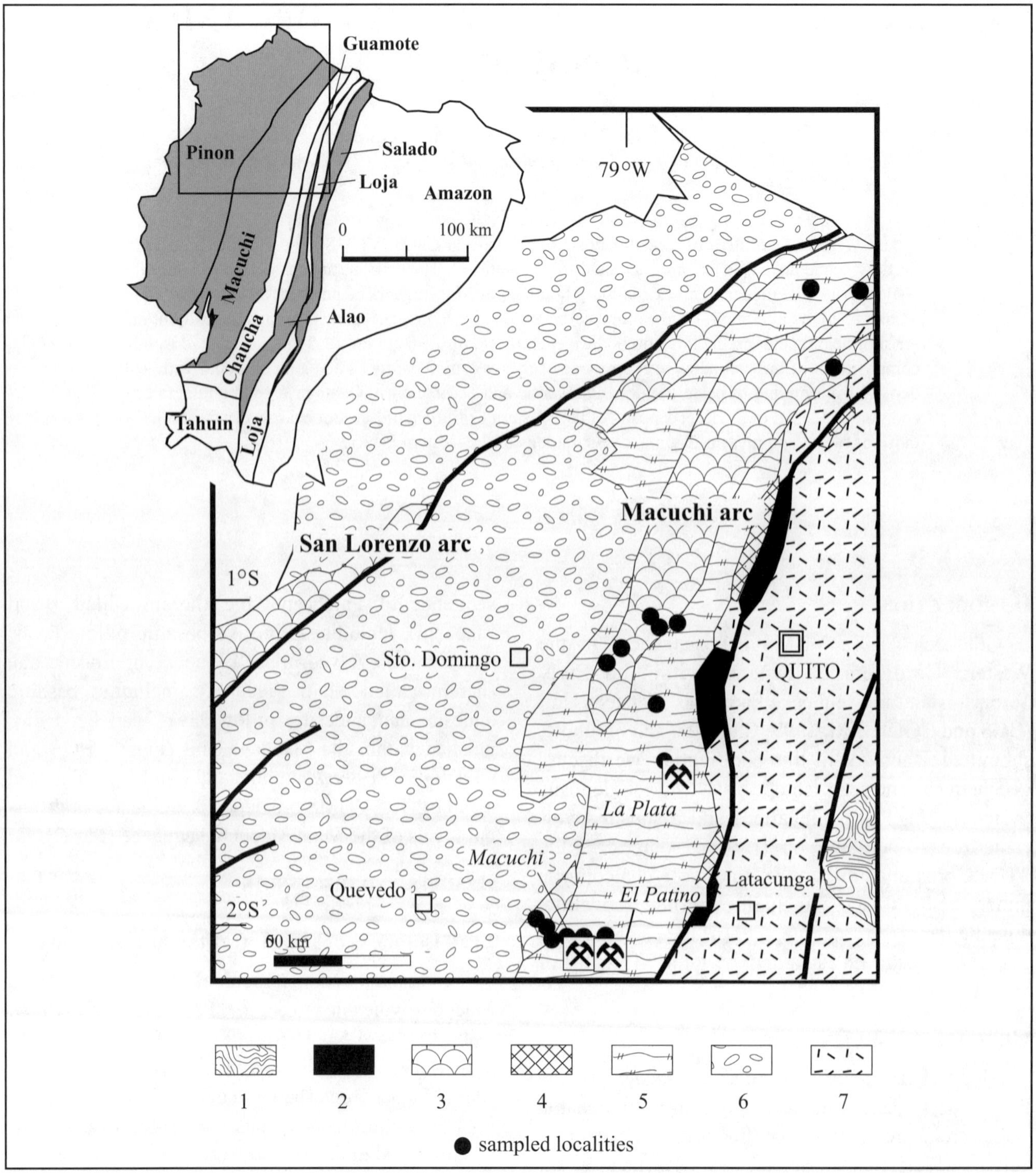

Figure. 1. Geological map of the Western Cordillera of Ecuador between 0° and 2°S showing the location of rock samples and VHMS deposits (modified from Cosma et al., 1998 and from BGS and CODIGEM, 1999). Legend: 1=pre-Cretaceous metamorphic basement rocks; 2=Cretaceous-Paleocene oceanic floor; 3=Cretaceous-Paleocene island arcs (including Paleocene Basal Macuchi); 4=Latest Cretaceous-Paleocene forearc; 5=Eocene island arc (Main Macuchi); 6=Tertiary-Quaternary forearc basins; 7=Tertiary-Quaternary continental arc. The thick lines represent terrane boundaries and major faults. The geotectonic map in the inset shows the main terranes of Ecuador (modified from Litherland et al., 1994). Grey=oceanic terranes; white=continental terranes.

submitted b). MORB-crust or San Juan oceanic plateau crust (proposed by Cosma et al., 1998, as the possible basement of the Macuchi arc) account for the ^{207}Pb-poor end-member (Fig. 3). Volcanic rocks of the Basal and Main Macuchi sequences display also positive correlations of the $^{207}Pb/^{204}Pb$ ratio with MgO and other fractionation indexes (Ni, V, Ti/Zr, etc.). This suggests their derivation from ^{207}Pb-rich parent magmas that have undergone fractional crystallization and assimilated low radiogenic Pb of MORB-crust or of the San Juan oceanic plateau at shallow levels. These correlations exclude assimilation of upper continental crust by the parent magmas reaffirming pelagic sediments as the only source of the radiogenic lead present in the Macuchi Unit (Chiaradia and Fontboté, submitted b).

Geology, mineralogy, metal and Pb isotope geochemistry of the VHMS deposits

La Plata, situated about 60 km SW of Quito (Fig. 1), is hosted by the upper part of the Main Macuchi sequence (Fig. 2). Lenses of massive and disseminated sulphides (several decimetres to a few metres thick and up to 100 m in extension, Lehne, 1990), as well as veinlets occur within bleached and sheared Na-depleted andesites that display silicification and sericitization. The ore lenses are zoned with a Cu-rich footwall and a Zn-rich hangingwall (Paladines, 1989; Lehne, 1990). A preliminary resource of 840,000 tonnes @ 4.8 g/t Au, 54 g/t Ag, 4.1 % Cu, 0.7 % Pb and 4.2 % Zn has been reported (Cambior Annual Report, 1998).

Macuchi, situated 70 km SSW of La Plata (Fig. 1), is hosted by the lower part of the Main Macuchi sequence (Fig. 2). The orebody is a lens of massive sulphides, 125 m long and up to 18 m thick, in a sequence of basaltic to basaltic andesite volcanic and volcaniclastic rocks with rarer felsic tuffs, porphyric andesites and dacites. The mineralization occurs as replacement, stockwork and layered sulphides. The main alteration assemblage is quartz-sericite, prevailing over quartz-chlorite. The Macuchi mine was exploited from 1941 to 1950 with an average ore grade of 5 % Cu, 7.6 g/t Au and 8.5 g/t Ag (Stoll, 1962).

El Patiño, a smaller pyritic orebody situated about 1.5 km NE of Macuchi, is found at a higher stratigraphic level than Macuchi (Fig. 2). The host basaltic andesites display a strong quartz-sericite alteration in proximity of the ore, similar to that observed at La Plata.

At La Plata and Macuchi the ore minerals display similar paragenetic sequences and define layered textures. The main ore minerals are early pyrite and chalcopyrite, the latter partly replacing pyrite. Chalcopyrite is in turn substituted by a bornite-pyrite association. At Macuchi bornite is replaced by covellite-digenite (the latter hosting rare enargite) and by idaite. Low-Fe sphalerite is coeval to or postdates bornite in both deposits. In general the paragenetic evolution of sulphides indicates a progressive increase in sulfidation conditions with time. Native gold forms blebs of few tens of microns inside early chalcopyrite (Macuchi: Figure 4) or is associated with bornite (Macuchi and La Plata). At La Plata gold has been also found in association with late galena.

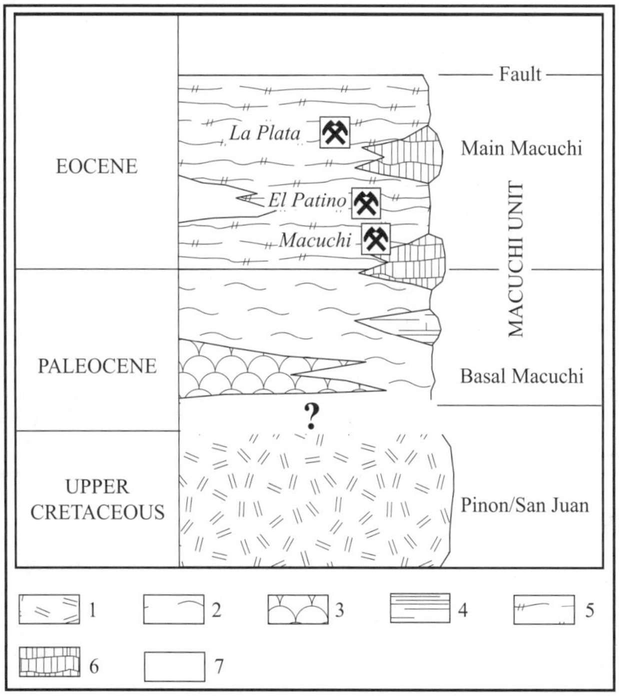

Figure. 2. Stratigraphic column of the occidental portion of the Western Cordillera of Ecuador at 1°S (modified from BGS and CODIGEM, 1999). Legend: 1=oceanic crust of the Piñon Formation or San Juan Complex; 2=undifferentiated volcanic and volcaniclastic rocks of the lower part of the Macuchi Unit (Basal Macuchi); 3=basaltic pillow lavas; 4=limestone; 5=undifferentiated volcanic and volcaniclastic rocks of the upper part of the Macuchi Unit (Main Macuchi) 6=basaltic andesite andesitic pillow lavas; 7=sandstones.

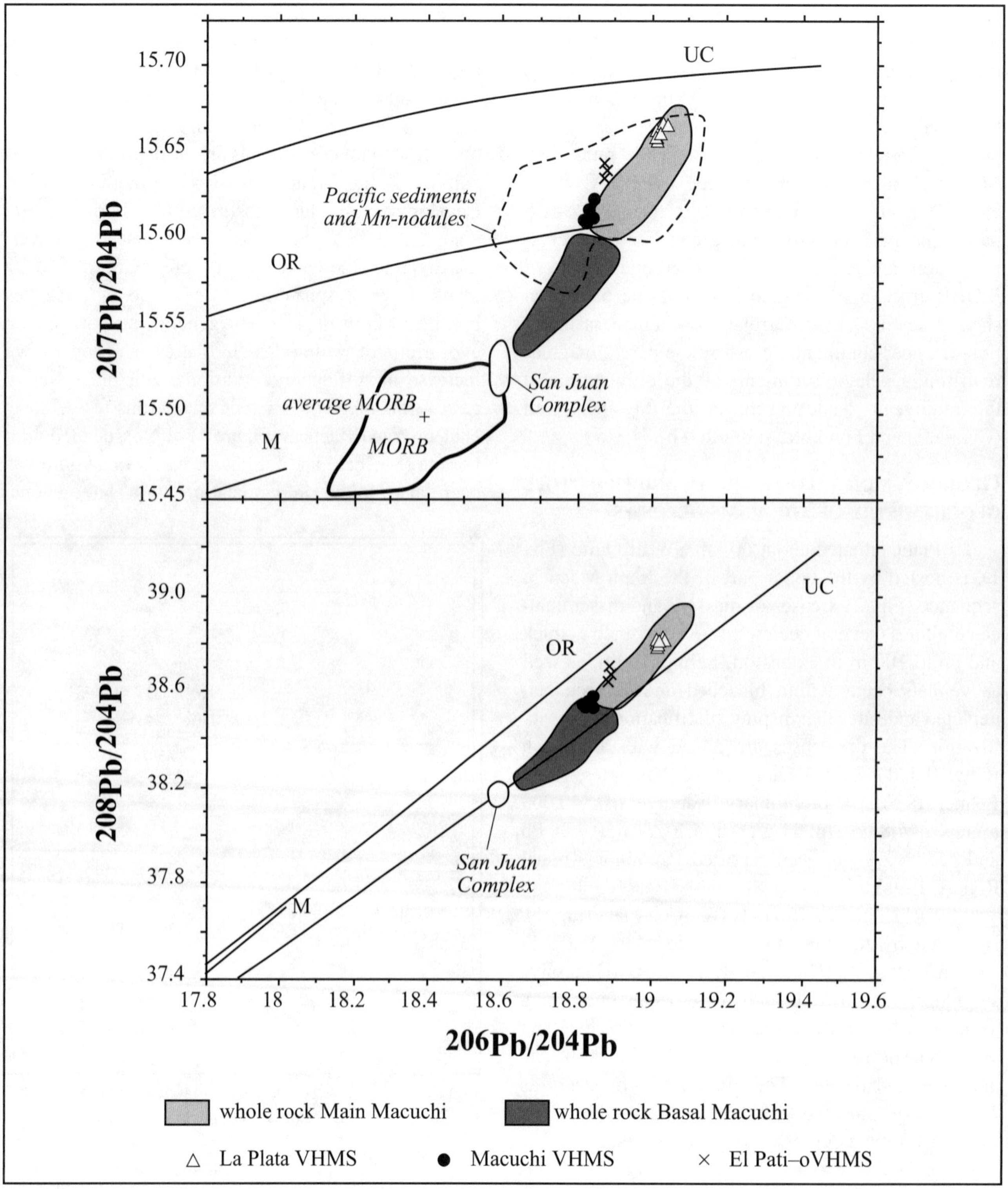

Figure 3. $^{207}Pb/^{204}Pb$ vs. $^{206}Pb/^{204}Pb$ and $^{208}Pb/^{204}Pb$ vs. $^{206}Pb/^{204}Pb$ plots showing the isotopic compositions of volcanic rocks and ore minerals of the Main Macuchi arc sequence. The source of data on Macuchi rocks and ores is Chiaradia and Fontboté (submitted a and b). The San Juan Complex isotopic compositions are from Mamberti et al. (1999). Sources of East Pacific MORB, Pacific pelagic sediments and Mn-nodules are various. Also shown for reference are the evolution curves of the upper crust (UC), orogen (OR) and mantle (M) (Zartman and Doe, 1981).

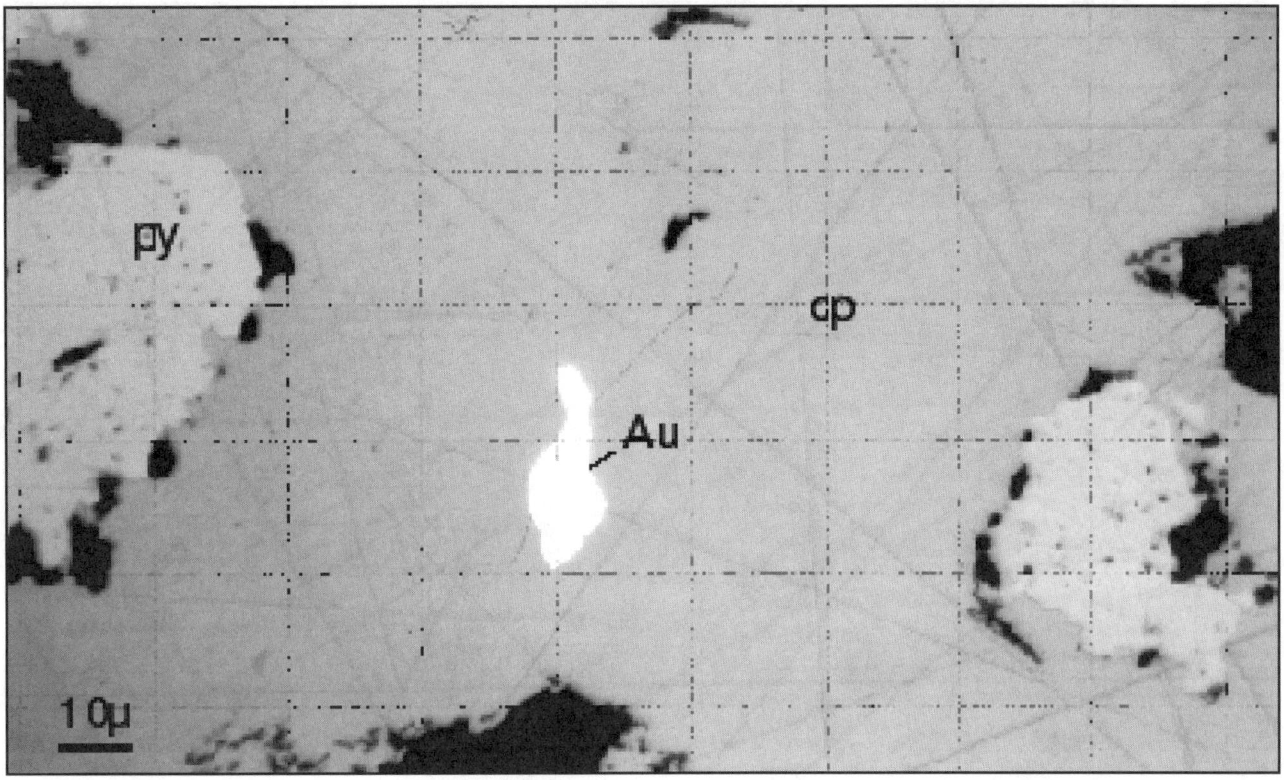

Figure 4. Microphotographs of ore minerals from the VHMS deposits of La Plata Abbreviations: Au=gold; cp=chalcopyrite; dg=digenite; py=pyrite.

Quartz, sericite, calcite, chlorite and barite are the gangue minerals.

Ore samples of La Plata, Macuchi and El Patiño display gold enrichments over silver and zinc when normalized to primitive mantle concentrations (Chiaradia and Fontboté, submitted a). Ore samples of the three deposits display also overall correlations of Au with Cu, Ag, As, Sb, Ba, and of Ag with As, Cu, Ba (Fig. 5).

The Pb isotope compositions of the three VHMS deposits fall along the trend defined by the volcanic arc rocks in conventional isotope diagrams and largely overlap the field defined by the Main Macuchi rocks (Fig. 3). Therefore, the VHMS deposits contain the same lead mixture of the volcanic rocks hosting them, i.e., MORB-type mantle enriched by pelagic sediments and either MORB-crust or oceanic plateau basaltic crust. The isotopic compositions are internally homogeneous within each of the three orebodies but vary significantly among the deposits, apparently in relation to their stratigraphic position (Figs. 2 and 3). The relatively low radiogenic signature of Macuchi, situated in the lowest part of the Main Macuchi sequence, suggests mixing of Pb of the Main and Basal Macuchi (Fig. 3) possibly due to hydrothermal convective cells straddling the two sequences. The same mechanism can explain the isotopic composition of El Patiño which, nevertheless, bears a larger component of Main Macuchi lead (Fig. 3) being situated at a higher stratigraphic level than Macuchi (Fig. 2). El Patiño requires perhaps a limited contribution from an additional source to explain its slightly lower $^{206}Pb/^{204}Pb$ ratios compared to the Main Macuchi rocks (Fig. 3).

CONCLUSIONS

The occurrence at Macuchi and La Plata of pyrite-chalcopyrite mineral assemblages, including covellite, bornite, digenite, idaite, tennantite, enargite may be typical of the high sulfidation VHMS type. However,

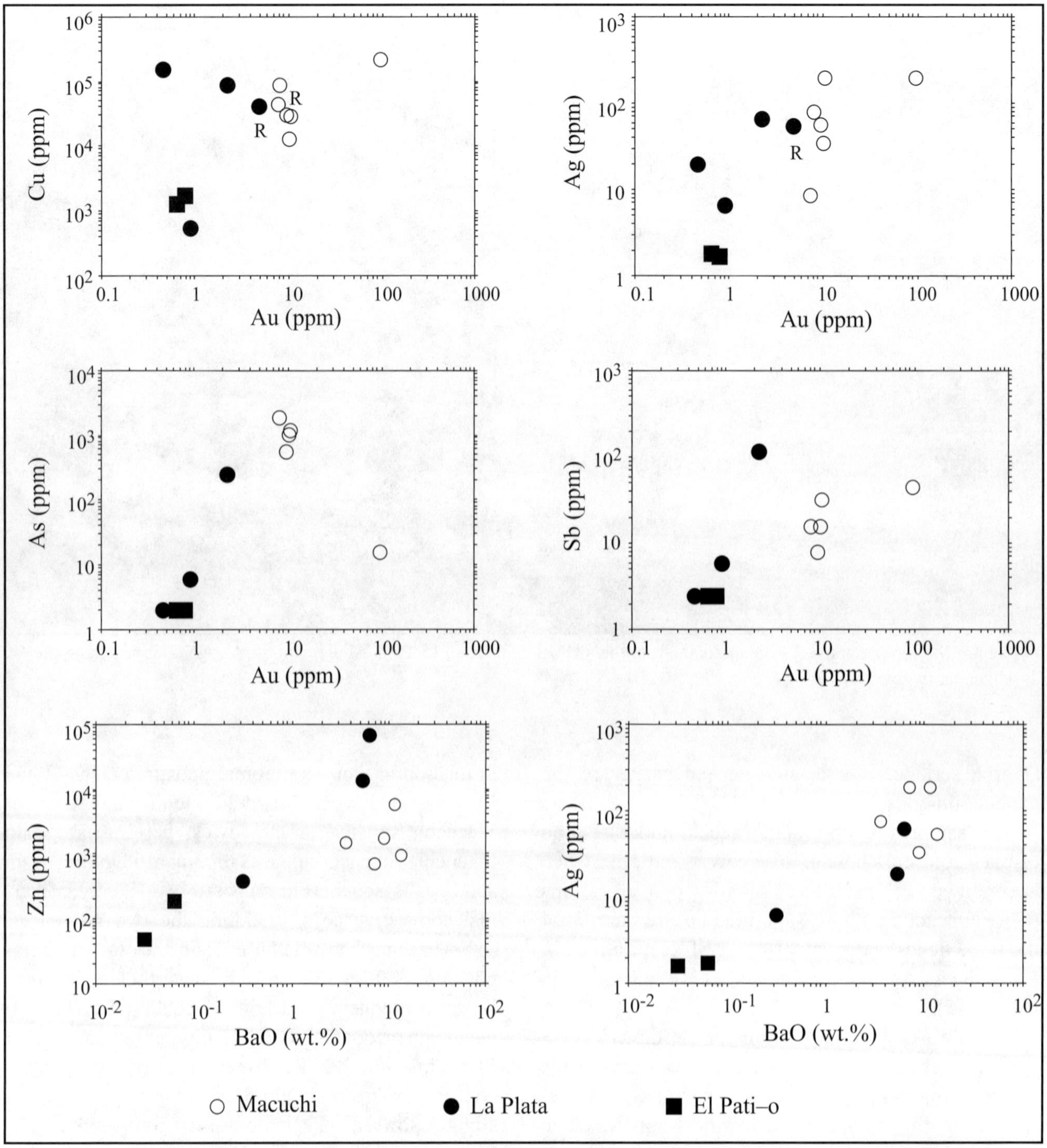

Figure 5. Element correlation diagrams for selected ore samples and reserves (R) of Macuchi, La Plata and El Patiño.

in contrast with the argillic or advanced argillic alteration commonly associated with high sulfidation VHMS deposits (Sillitoe et al., 1996), only sericitic alteration, indicative of slightly acidic conditions, has been observed. Also, different from typical Au-rich high sulfidation VHMS's (e.g., Sillitoe et al., 1993), La Plata and Macuchi occur in an arc sequence dominated by basic rather than by felsic magmatic rocks.

Lead isotope compositions indicate that lead (and by inference the other metals) of the VHMS ores is derived from the host volcanic rocks of the Main Macuchi sequence. As the latter, therefore, the VHMS ores contain radiogenic lead from pelagic sediments mixed with low radiogenic lead of MORB-type mantle and oceanic crust.

Lead isotope compositions of the three ore deposits investigated are internally homogeneous, but vary significantly among deposits. The isotopic difference between Macuchi and El Patiño, separated by 1.5 km, suggests a lack of homogenization at the hundreds of metre scale.

The gold enrichment over silver and zinc in the normalized spectra of ore samples as well as the significance of geochemical and isotopic compositions of the Main Macuchi rocks, host to the VHMS deposits, discussed in Chiaradia and Fontboté (submitted a), indicate a possible petrogenetic control on the high gold grades of these deposits.

Mineralogy, gold grades, metal association and possible petrogenetic control on gold enrichment of the Macuchi island arc VHMS deposits bear similarities with those described in recent Au-rich VHMS deposits from the western Pacific (Hannington et al., 1999).

ACKNOWLEDGEMENTS

We wish to thank Dr. Agustín Paladines (Universidad Central del Ecuador, Quito, Ecuador) for introducing us to the geology of the Western Cordillera of Ecuador. This study is funded by the Swiss National Foundation (grant # 2000-054150.98 to LF) and is a contribution to GEODE, a programme funded by the European Science Foundation.

REFERENCES

Aye, F., Cesbron, G. and Picot, P. (1983) Contribution de la pétrographie et dela minéralogie à la connaissance des indices à Au, Cu, Zn, Pb, Ba, de Macuchi (équateur). Note N. 924, Département Gîtes Minéraux, BRGM, Orléans, France, 16 p.

BGS and CODIGEM (1999) Mapa Geologico de la Cordillera Occidental del Ecuador entre 0°-1°S and 1°-2° S. Mision Britanica, CODIGEM, Quito, Ecuador.

Chiaradia, M. and Fontboté, L. (submitted a) Radiogenic lead signatures in Au-rich VHMS ores and associated volcanic rocks of the Early Tertiary Macuchi island arc (Western Cordillera of Ecuador). Submitted to Economic Geology.

Chiaradia, M. and Fontboté, L. (submitted b) Assimilation of oceanic crust lead by radiogenic magmas of the Early Tertiary Macuchi island arc (Western Cordillera of Ecuador). Submitted to Journal of Geophysical Research.

Cosma, L., LaPierre, H., Jaillard, E., Laubacher, G., Bosch, D., Desmet, A., Mamberti, M. and Gabriele, P. (1998) Pétrographie et géochimie des unités de la Cordillère occidentale d'équateur (0°30'S): implications tectoniques. Bulletin de la Société géologique de France, 169, 739-751.

Hannington, M.D., Poulsen, K.H., Thompson, J.F.H. and Sillitoe, R.H. (1999) Volcanogenic gold in the massive sulfide environment. In Barrie, C.T. and Hannington, M.D. (eds.) Volcanic-associated massive sulfide deposits: processes and examples in modern and ancient settings, Reviews in Economic Geology, 8, 325-356.

Lehne, R.W. (1990) The Cu-Zn-Au-Ag deposit of La Plata, Toachi), Ecuador. In Fontboté, L., Amstutz, G.C., Cardozo, M., Cedillo, E. and Frutos, J. (eds.) Stratabound ore deposits in the Andes. Special Publication of the Society for Geology Applied to Mineral Deposits 8, Springer-Verlag, 389-393.

Litherland, M., Aspden, J.A. and Jemielita, R.A. (1994) The metamorphic belts of Ecuador. Overseas Memoir 11, BGS, 147 p.

Mamberti, M., Bosch, D., LaPierre, H., Hernandez, J., Jaillard, E. and Polve, M. (1999) Petrology and geochemistry of Mg-rich basalts from Western Ecuador: remnants of the Late Cretaceous Caribbean plateau? In Extended Abstracts of the 4th International Symposium on Andean Geodynamics, ISAG99, 4-6 October 1999, Göttingen (Germany), Institut de Recherche pour le Développement.

Paladines, A. (1989) Zonificación geotectónica y metalogenia del Ecuador. Mañana Editores, Quito, Ecuador, 192 p.

Reynaud, C., Jaillard, E., LaPierre, H., Mamberti, M. and Mascle, G.H. (1999) Oceanic plateau and island arcs of southwestern Ecuador: their place in the geodynamic evolution of northwestern South America. Tectonophysics, 307, 235-254.

Sillitoe, R.H., Hannington, M.D. and Thompson, J.F.H. (1996) High-sulfidation deposits in the volcanogenic massive sulfide environment. Economic Geology, 91, 204-212.

Stoll, W.C. (1962) Notes on the mineral resources of Ecuador. Economic Geology, 57, 799-808.

Zartman, R.E. and Doe, B.R. (1981) Plumbotectonics - The model. Tectonophysics, 75, 135-162.

GEOLOGY AND VMS POTENTIAL OF BOLIVIA

OSVALDO ARCE-BURGOA
Senior Partner, Inproser S.A., Pasaje Villegas No. 1243, Casilla 22626, La Paz

HERNAN URIBE-ZEBALLOS
Coordinator Multi Andean Project (MAP), Servicio Geológico de Bolivia
(Sergeomin), F. Suazo No. 1673 ,La Paz

MANUEL MENACHO-LEON
Geologist, Servicio de Geología y Minería de Bolivia (Sergeomin), F. Suazo No. 1673 , la Paz

ABSTRACT

Bolivia is a land-locked country located in the central part of South America. It is recognized worldwide to have been a mining country since pre-colonial times. During the Spanish colonial period (1535-1825) Bolivia was a major silver producer. Bolivia became a world leader in tin production in the 20th century. A renewed effort of exploration and development began in the late 1980's and resulted in the discovery of bulk mineable deposits as Kori Kollo (Au-Ag), San Cristobal (Zn-Ag) and Don Mario (Au-Cu).

To date, little exploration has been directed towards volcanic-associated massive sulphide (VMS) deposits. However, there is evidence for this type of mineralization in two regions of Bolivia: in the Cordillera Real, northwestern Bolivia and in the Precambrian Shield in eastern Bolivia.

In the Cordillera Real, lenticular-shaped disseminated and massive sulphide mineralization of possible VMS-affinity is contained in Upper Ordovician sequences of pelites and psammites of the Amutara Formation. Also in Silurian and Devonian age rocks nearby Charazani and Akamani. The sulphides occur in stratabound/stratiform layers and consist mostly of pyrite with lesser amounts of pyrrhotite, galena, sphalerite and chalcopyrite. The layers of mineralization display anomalous gold, copper, lead and zinc values. A metre-thick layer of trachyandesite outcrops 200 m below the mineralization and suggests that there was volcanic activity during the Upper-Ordovician. Quartz-gold mantos and veins are located in sandstones about 500 m above the sulphide layers. These may be genetically related to the sulphides.

Potential VMS mineralization is contained in Proterozoic rocks of the San Ignacio Schist Super-Group of the Precambrian Shield in eastern Bolivia. The San Ignacio Schist Super-Group is composed of several individual schist belts, which include the Guarayos, Ñuflo de Chávez, San Ignacio and Cristal. The belts are made-up of sequences of quartzite, feldspathic metapsammites and micaceous schists and phyllites. Also included are subordinate ferruginous, calc-silicate, meta-volcanic and graphite-rich schists. Possible VMS mineralization occurs as thin seams of disseminated chalcopyrite and pyrite in amphibolite-grade schists. At Miguela, stratiform massive and disseminated sulphides occur closely associated with submarine felsic metavolcanic intrusions and lava flows.

A regional geochemical stream-sediment survey of the Precambrian rocks has identified copper anomalies within the San Ignacio Schist Super-Group. Sporadic associations of Zn-Cu-<Pb, Cu-<Pb<<Ag and Cu-Zn are seen in the Guarayos-Ñuflo de Chávez schist belts. In the Cristal schist belt, associations between Cu-Ba and Zn-Pb-Ag were respectively observed nearby and south of the Don Mario (Au-Ag-Cu) prospect.

A presence of disseminated and layered sulphide mineralization, geochemical anomalies and volcanic rock units suggest that parts of the Cordillera Real and Precambrian Shield in Bolivia may be favorable areas for the exploration for VMS-style deposits.

Chávez areas. In the Cristal schist belt, associations between Cu-Ba and Zn-Pb-Ag were observed nearby and south of the Don Mario prospect respectively.

It can be concluded that favourable environments for VMS mineralization were discovered in Bolivia worthy of additional and systematic exploration that would lead in the discovery of large VMS type ore-deposits.

INTRODUCTION

Bolivia is a land-locked territory and consists of six major geologic belts. From west to east these are: the Western Cordillera, the Altiplano, the Eastern Cordillera, the Subandean, the Chaco-Beni Plains and the Bolivian Precambrian Shield (Fig. 1).

Bolivia was an important producer of gold in pre-Spanish periods. Later, during the Spanish colonial time (1532 – 1825) it was one of the world's major silver producers. From the beginning of this century until 1952, when most of the private mines were nationalized, Bolivia became a world leader in tin production. It has also been a major producer of tungsten and antimony. The lifting of the fiscal reserve in 1986 enabled companies to start looking at non-traditional deposit types with modern geological models and mining technologies. Recent efforts have been directed towards exploration for bulk minable gold, silver and copper deposits in the Andes, and exploration of the Precambrian Shield in the jungles of Eastern Bolivia (Gustavson Associates, 1992).

The geology and mineralization of Bolivia are briefly described in the present paper with especial emphasis on the volcanic-associated massive sulphide (VMS) potential of the country, which to date, was subject of little exploration in Bolivia. Therefore, there is still incipient information on this type of deposits.

Previous work was mainly accomplished by Tanganika A.V.V. in early 1990's (Biste, 1985), which led to the discovery of VMS-mineralization at Miguela in 1994 (Heutschmidt, 1999).

OVERVIEW OF THE GEOLOGY AND MINERAL POTENTIAL OF BOLIVIA

Although Bolivia has long been known as a tin, silver, antimony and tungsten producer, in the last ten years several epithermal Au-Ag; sedimentary hosted gold; Mississippi Valley-Type Pb-Zn-Ag; VMS-style mineralization; etc. have been discovered. Good VMS potential exists in the Bolivian Precambrian Shield and evidences of this type of mineralization were recognized in the Cordillera Real of the Eastern Cordillera of the Andes.

The Western Cordillera

The Western Cordillera consists of late Miocene to Quaternary stratovolcanoes. The basement to the stratovolcanoes consists of eroded upper Tertiary stratovolcanoes, domes and stocks with volcanic and continental sedimentary sequences. The magmatism is dominantly andesitic to dacitic. The northern part is characterized by isolated and aligned volcanoes, while the southern part of the belt, in the Lipez region, is formed of a high altitude volcanic plateau over 4,500 m high. In the Western Cordillera of the Andes, there are numerous large volcanic centres, several of which have already shown the presence of anomalous gold and silver values. Several new large gold and copper mines have been discovered on the Peruvian, Chilean and Argentinian sides, relatively close to the Bolivian border. Since the geologic setting is similar, this suggests that there is potential on the Bolivian side. Additionally, there are several acid sulphate systems and high-purity sulphur deposits (Uribe, 1999).

The Altiplano

The Altiplano consists of a series of high, intermontane basins that formed primarily during the Andean cycle, apparently in response to folding and thrusting. An eastward underthrusting of the Proterozoic and Paleozoic basement of the Western Cordillera, concurrent with a westward overthrusting of the Paleozoic miogeosynclinal rocks of the Eastern Cordillera, resulted in continental foreland basins that received as much as 15,000 m. of sediment and interlayered volcanic rocks during the Cenozoic. During the main (Inca) pulse of Andean deformation, beginning in the Oligocene and continuing at least until the middle Miocene, a number of volcano-plutonic complexes were emplaced at several localities on the Altiplano, particularly along its eastern margin with the Eastern Cordillera Oriental, and to the south, in the Sud Lípez area. In Pleistocene time, large glacial lakes covered most of the Altiplano. The great salars of Uyuni and Coipasa are Holocene remnants of these lakes. The Salar of Uyuni has the largest lithium reserve in the world (Richter at al., 1992).

The most significant discovery to date in the Altiplano and perhaps in Bolivia, is the Kori Kollo gold-silver mine, which was the first open pit, heap leach operation in Bolivia. It has a resource of 65 million metric tonnes of ore with a grade of 2.33 grams

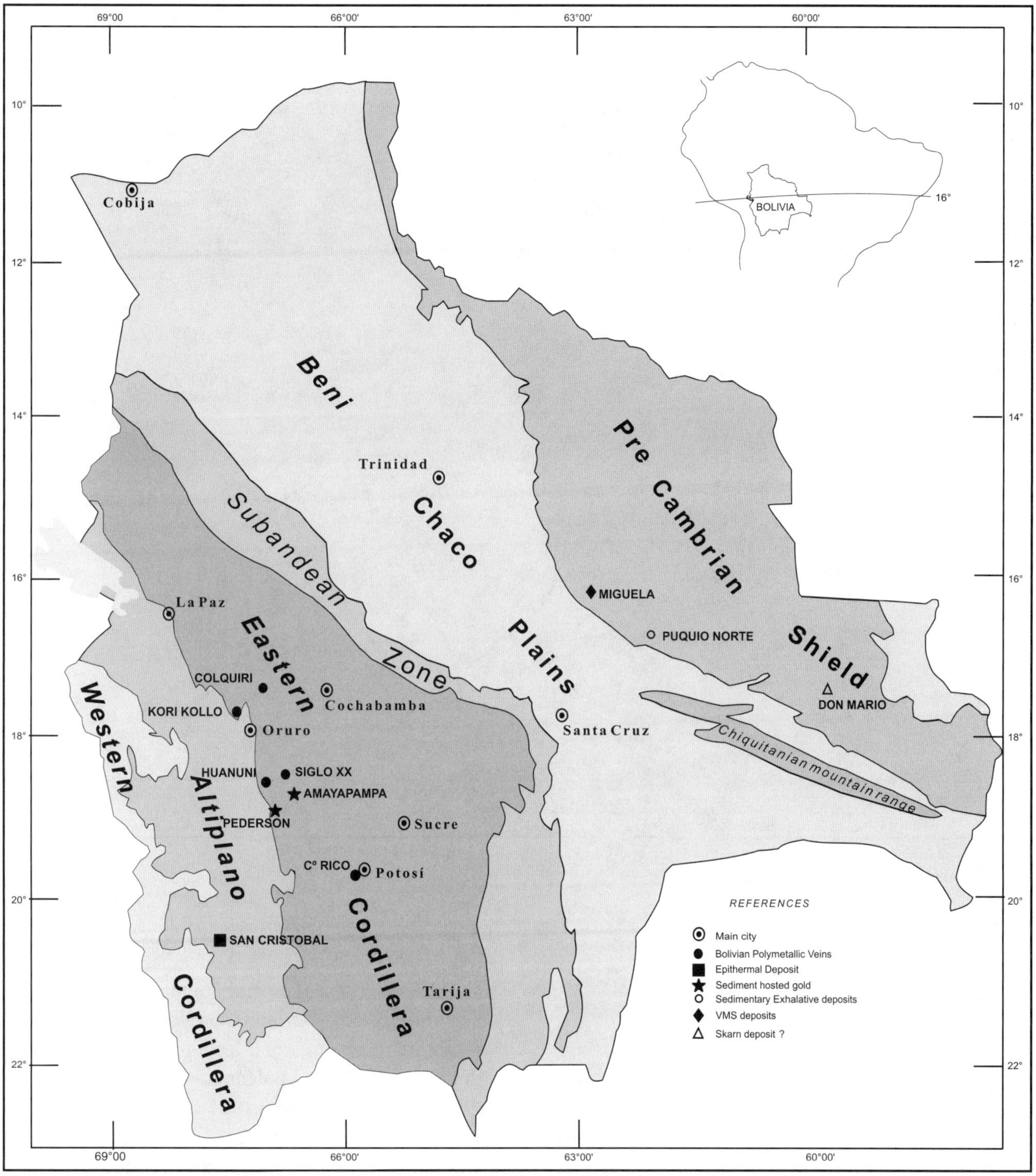

Figure 1. Geologic map and location of main mineral ocurrences in Bolivia.

of gold and 20 grams of silver. Gold production in 1999 was 256,000 ounces. The latest "discovery" in the southern Altiplano is the volcanic associated San Cristobal zinc, silver, lead deposit, whose proven and probable reserves total 259 million tonnes of ore grading 2.0 opt Ag, 1.57 % Zn and 0.55 % Pb (Apex Silver's press release, Oct. 1998).

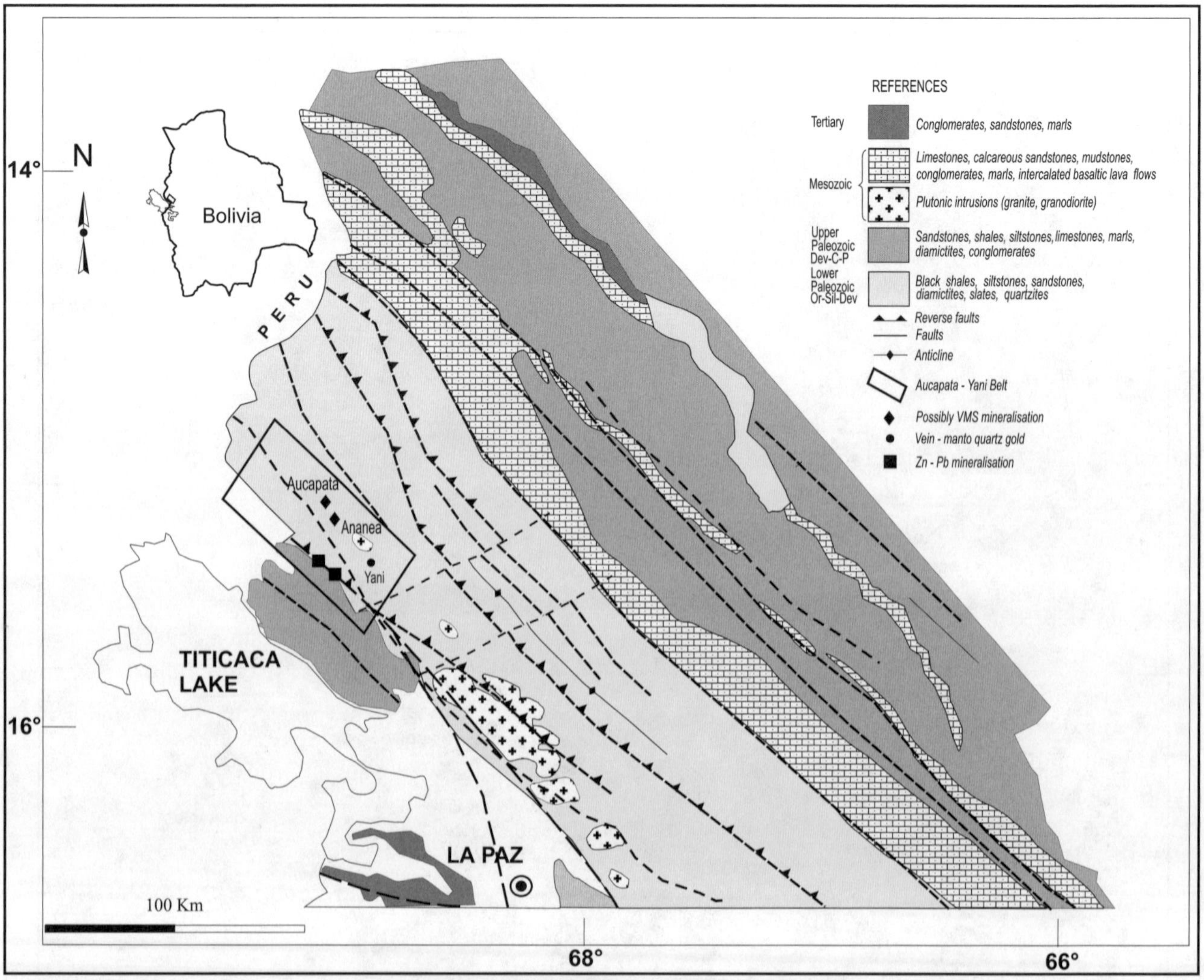

Figure 2. Geological map and favourable areas for VMS- mineralization in the Cordillera Real, Bolivia.

The Eastern Cordillera

The Eastern Cordillera mountain belt is about 1,000 km long and 150 to 400 km wide. It is formed of Paleozoic marine siliciclastic sediments, which comprise principally thick sequences of shales, siltstones and sandstones of Ordovician to Devonian age. There are infolded Upper Paleozoic shelf sediments and Cretaceous to Tertiary continental sediments. The sediments have been strongly folded, thrusted and locally intruded by dacitic-andesitic intrusives.

In the last decade during the exploration "boom", several sedimentary hosted vein-disseminated gold deposits were discovered in the Eastern Cordillera, from which the largest is Pederson with a resource of 2.3 M oz Au grading 1.4 g/t Au (Arce et al., 1995; Arce, 1999). Others are Amayapampa-Capacirca, Iroco, Rosario de Araca and Vinto. After a hundred years of extensive exploitation, polymetallic vein-type tin, tungsten and zinc-lead-silver mineralization still present additional potential.

The Cordillera Real in the northern part of the Eastern Cordillera (Aucapata-Yani belt) contains important gold placers, auriferous quartz veins and mantos associated with felsic plutons, and stratabound sulphide-gold mineralization.

Massive sulphide layers are distributed over more than 15 km in extent in the area NW of Yani. The lower level of the sequence contain coeval spilitized flows and volcanic sills. In addition, a trachyandesitic layer occurs at the base of the Caradocian Amutara formation, about 200 m below the massive sulphides. The sulphide mineralization, therefore appears to be close in age to that of the volcanic occurrences above mentioned and may be partly synvolcanic, i.e., suspected VMS-origin. Outcrops with massive sulphide polymetallic (Au, Cu, Fe, Sb, Ag, Pb, Zn) mineralization are common south of Ananea (Redwood, 1993). Furthermore, VMS-affinity mineralization occurs nearby Charazani and Akamani (SW of Yani)

The Subandean Zone

The Subandean Zone forms the foothills of the Andes and is the foreland of a fold-thrust belt formed of Paleozoic siliciclastic sediments and Mesozoic to Tertiary continental sediments. Well-vegetated mountain ridges and valleys characterize the region with the altitude varying between 2,000 and 500 m. The structures trend NW-SE in the northern part and N-S to the south of Santa Cruz. This orocline is variously known at the Santa Cruz Bend or Arica Elbow, after the location on the coast of northern Chile where the corresponding bend in the continental margin occurs. The Subandean zone has permissive areas for sizeable zinc-silver and copper of Mississippi Valley type mineralization in the Cuevo basin (south-central part of Bolivia).

The Beni-Chaco Lowlands

The Beni lowlands in the northern half consist of major rivers with tropical forest, lakes and wet savannas or swamplands. The Chaco lowlands, in the southern half, are dry savanna with scrub vegetation. The lowlands are covered by Holocene alluvial deposits, which overlie thick Tertiary redbed sediments (more than 6,000 m). The basement is Precambrian crystalline rocks, which outcrop in the Precambrian Shield to the east. The Serranías Chiquitanas are a 350 km long range of hills in the eastern Chaco lowlands, which trend WNW-ESE. These hills are formed of Silurian to Devonian marine shales and sandstones and red Cretaceous continental sandstones. The Beni-Chaco in its northern sector includes the Rio Madre de Dios and the Rio Beni, which has considerable potential alluvial gold, tin and other metals.

The Precambrian

The crystalline rocks of the Precambrian shield in the eastern part of Bolivia are the continuation of the Central Brazilian Shield, part of the Amazon Craton. It is equivalent to a dome planation surface laterized in the Tertiary and is buried by Quaternary alluvial basins at the margins. The Bolivian Precambrian comprises metamorphic and igneous rocks from the Proterozoic. It also includes a lesser proportion of sedimentary rocks from the Paleozoic and Mesozoic (Litherland et al., 1986) and intrusions of Mesozoic age (Fletcher and Litherland, 1981) (Table 1). The oldest rocks, underlying about half the area, are referred to as the Metamorphic Basement, which is of Lower to Middle Proterozoic age and comprises three metamorphic super-units, interpreted as a single metamorphic pile: the Lomas Maneches Granulite Complex, The Chiquitanía Gneiss Complex and the San Ignacio Schist Super-Group (Table 2). The main metallogenic feature of the metamorphic basement is late kinematic gold mineralization in the schist belts, which is typical of that found in greenstone belts. The Late Proterozoic Sunsas Orogenic Cycle (ca 1,280-950 Ma) marked the final stage of the cratonization of the shield.

In the Precambrian, the late kinematic gold mineralization includes BIF-hosted gold at "Puquio Norte" near San Ramón, which consists of widespread shear-zone hosted quartz-carbonate-gold veins. To date the open-pit operation produces 1,500 tpd of 1.8 g/t of gold. The region also includes the "Cristal" schist-belts, which contain the Don Mario a gold-silver-copper deposit with reserves of 1.5 Mt of 11.13 g/t Au; the San Javier belt, and the schist belts which host laterite hosted gold mineralization. The region includes BIF and PGM potential in the Rincón del Tigre.

VMS-style mineralization occurs mainly over the whole length of the Guarayos schist belt, but it may also exist in other areas within the San Ignacio Super-Group. The Precambrian's wealth extends to semi-precious stones as amethyst and bolivianite; a Mississippi Valley Type Pb-Zn-Ag mineralization and kimberlite pipes in the Tucavaca Trough. Finally, there is Olympic Dam type mineralization on the southern boundary of the Shield, iron at Mutún and tin in Rondonian-style granites.

Table 1. Main characteristics of the mineralization in the Cordillera Real, - Northeastern La Paz, Bolivia

Geology	Structure	Commodities & Mineralization	Metamorphic Grade	Age of host rocks	Orogeny
Meta-sandstone, black shale, pyritic shale	NW-SE megafracture	Au, Sn, Sb, Pb, Zn, Ag, Cu, U, quartz, pyrrhotite, galena, sphalerite, chalcopyrite, pyrite, stibnite	Sub-greenschist facies	Ordovician (Caradocian), Silurian and Devonian	Ocloyica orogeny (unconformity between Ordovician and Silurian) Upper Devonian Chanica orogeny, Kolla Phase and Quechua Phase

Volcanic-Associated Massive Sulphide (VMS) Mineralization in Bolivia

Volcanogenic massive sulphide mineralization in Bolivia is, to date, in an early exploration stage. Therefore, there is still a lack of complete information. However, suspected VMS mineralization occurs in the Ordovician sediment-rich sequences from the Cordillera Real in northwestern Bolivia, at the Yani-Aucapata belt, and evidences in the Precambrian schist belts in eastern Bolivia - notably at the Miguela prospect. The presence of massive sulphide mineralization in these two regions that they may contain other similar deposits and therefore they were selected for a more detailed assessment below:

GEOLOGY AND MINERALIZATION OF THE CORDILLERA REAL - NORTHWESTERN BOLIVIA

The Cordillera Real consists of some 10,000 m of Paleozoic marine sediments, which were folded and overprinted by low-grade regional metamorphism during the Variscan orogeny (Tistl, 1985). The continental sediments and volcanic rocks of Cretaceous age locally overlie Lower Devonian or Lower Silurian rocks which are composed of a monotonous sequence of pelitic and psammitic marine sediments. Small batholiths and related minor plutons in the axial zone of the chain were intruded during the Middle to Upper Triassic and the late Oligocene to early Miocene (McBride et al., 1983; and Avila, 1990).

SUSPECTED VOLCANIC-ASSOCIATED MASSIVE SULPHIDE (VMS) MINERALIZATION IN THE AUCAPATA-YANI BELT, CORDILLERA REAL

The Aucapata-Yani belt is underlain by an Upper-Ordovician volcano-sedimentary sequence of sandstones, quartzites and dark shales. Massive sulphide layers are distributed over more than 15 km in extent in the area NW of Yani. They are all of the same stratigraphic age and probably occur in other areas in the Cordillera Real. The sulphide layers are considered to be the source-bed of the gold-quartz mantos (Schneider, 1990).

The lower level of the sequence contains coeval spilitized flows and volcanic sills that are laterally associated with black shales, which in some cases are enriched in auriferous pyrite. In addition, a trachyandesitic lava layer occurs regionally at the base of the Caradocian Amutara formation, about 200 m below the massive sulphides. These evidences indicate volcanic activity during the Upper Ordovician, as has been reported from other areas of the Eastern Cordillera (Schneider, 1990).

The sulphide mineralization appears to be close in age to that of the volcanic occurrences above mentioned and may be partly synvolcanic. It is suggested that sedimentary strata overly a volcanic rock-dominated mineralization. Outcrops with polymetallic massive sulphide (Au, Cu, Fe, Sb, Ag, Pb, Zn) mineralization are common south of Ananea (Redwood, 1993).

Table 2. Chrono-Stratigraphy of the Bolivian Precambrian shield (after Litherland et al., 1986)

Period/Era	Orogenic Cycle	Groups	Rock Units	Intrusions
Quaternary	Hiatus			
Neogene	Hiatus	San Ignacio laterite		
Cretaceous		El Portón Group		Alkaline Complexes
Devonian		Santiago Group	Limoncito Siltstones Roboré Sandstones	
Silurian			El Carmen sandstones	
Neoproterozoic (1000 – 570 Ma)	Brasiliano (950 – 570 Ma)	Murciélago Group	Laminated and massive limestones	
		Tucavaca Group	Limestones,sandstones and shales	
		Boqui Group	Conglomerates and sandstones	
Mesoproterozoic (1600 – 1000Ma)	Sunsas (1280 – 950 Ma)	Vibosi Group	Sandstones and arkoses	Granites and granodior ites Granites & tonalites. Gabbros and diorites Rincon del Tigre Complex
		Sunsas Group	Conglomerates, sandstones, shales and quartzites	
	San Ignacio (1800 – 1280 Ma)	Metamorphic Basement: San Ignacio Supergroup	Schists and meta-psammites	Granites and tonalites Granites and granodior ites Gabbros and diorites Granophyric Complexes Meta-igneous mafic and ultramafic rocks
		Metamorphic Basement: Chiquitania Complex	Gneisses	
			Gneisses & migmatites	
Paleoproterozoic (2500 - 1600 Ma)		Metamorphic Basement: Lomas Maneches Complex	Gneisses and granulites	
	Transamazonic (2400 - 1800 Ma)	Metamorphic Basement: Lomas Maneches Massive	Leptites and granulites	

A summary of the main characteristics of suspected VMS deposits is shown In Table 1.

In the area gold-quartz veins, mantos and stockworks also occur. The mantos and veins are parallel to bedding and they commonly reach several kilometres in length and more than 500 m of vertical extent. Their thickness varies from few cm to 2 m. The gold content ranges from 10 ppb to 300 ppm Au, thus mining is very difficult. The mineral assemblage is simple, and composed of quartz, small amounts of pyrite, arsenopyrite, chlorite, scheelite, occasionally chalcopyrite, sphalerite, galena, pyrrhotite and albite. Structurally, many mantos are related to anticlines, other deposits are located near the junction of the NW -trending with a NNE - trending lineament (Fig. 3).

Vein-type sulphide Zn-Cu-Ag mineralization is hosted in Devonian pelites and psammites, in the lower plate of a regional thrust fault, which overlie Ordovician over Devonian rocks. These areas show similar fracture-fault-fold patterns as the Upper Ordovician (Fig. 3).

The uppermost parts of the Ordovician as well as parts of Lower Silurian are lacking in the entire Cordillera Real. Various authors interpret this regionally stratigraphic break as a result on the Ocloyica orogeny (Table 1) or of regional uplift (Fornari and Herail, 1991).

The tectonic style of the Cordillera Real is controlled by a general strike in the Andean direction (NW-SE), which predominates in Variscan (Chanica) orogeny's fold axes, foliation and lineaments. In temporal connection with the Variscan orogeny, a widespread contact metamorphism is developed linked to granitic intrusions. This observation is important for the genetic interpretation of the massive sulphide layers and gold-quartz mantos. The Andean (Kolla and Quechua Phases) Orogeny generated block tectonic movements and reactivation of faults (Schneider, 1990).

GEOLOGY AND MINERALIZATION OF THE SAN IGNACIO SCHIST SUPER-GROUP- SOUTHWESTERN PRECAMBRIAN

The San Ignacio schist Supergroup forms part of the Metamorphic Basement of the Bolivian Precambrian (Fig. 4). It crops out in the form of discrete belts composed of quartzites, feldspathic metapsammites and micaceous schists or phyllites with subordinate ferruginous, calc-silicate, metavolcanic and graphite-rich unit (Table 2). The San Ignacio Supergroup can be defined as: 'pre Sunsas Group schists and phyllites and other intercalated metasedimentary and meta-igneous rocks'.

Pelitic phyllites and schists are diagnostic of the schist belts and thus, by definition, the Schists Supergroup (Table 2). These belts are nor regarded as true analogues of the classic Archean greenstone belts (Windley, 1977), which are predominantly metavolcanic sequences, usually with distinct cuspate contacts with the surrounding granitoid rocks, their shapes being related to deformation around early plutonic bodies (Litherland, 1979). The Bolivian belts are almost certainly younger, mainly metasedimentary, and show a variety of individual forms believed to be due to the refolding of synformal cores during one or more orogenies. However, like the greenstone belts, gneisses generally surround them and granitoid rocks, and are favourable sites for mineralization (Litherland et al., 1986).

Bands rich in carbonaceous material are found in higher metamorphic grades in the form of graphitic phyllites or schists and, in places, as graphitic quartzites. Although laterisation processes produce superficial iron enrichment, especially in softer schists, primary iron concentrations in metapelites have been noted as ferruginous mudstones, phyllites and schists. Thin seams of conglomerates with a ferruginous matrix have also been reported. Within the southern arc of schist belt the somewhat monotonous pelite/psammite sequences are broken in places by outcrops of metamorphosed mafic or ultramafic intrusive rocks. The full sequence of Barrovian index minerals is represented in the metapelites: chlorite, biotite, garnet, staurolite, kyanite and sillimanite. Low grade, fine-grained, chlorite, chlorite-biotite or chlorite-muscovite phyllites are reported from several schist belts (Table 3).

Volcanic-associated massive sulphide (VMS) Mineralization in the Schist Belts of the Precambrian

At Miguela volcanogenic massive sulphides occur as three mineralized bodies hosted in a sequence of

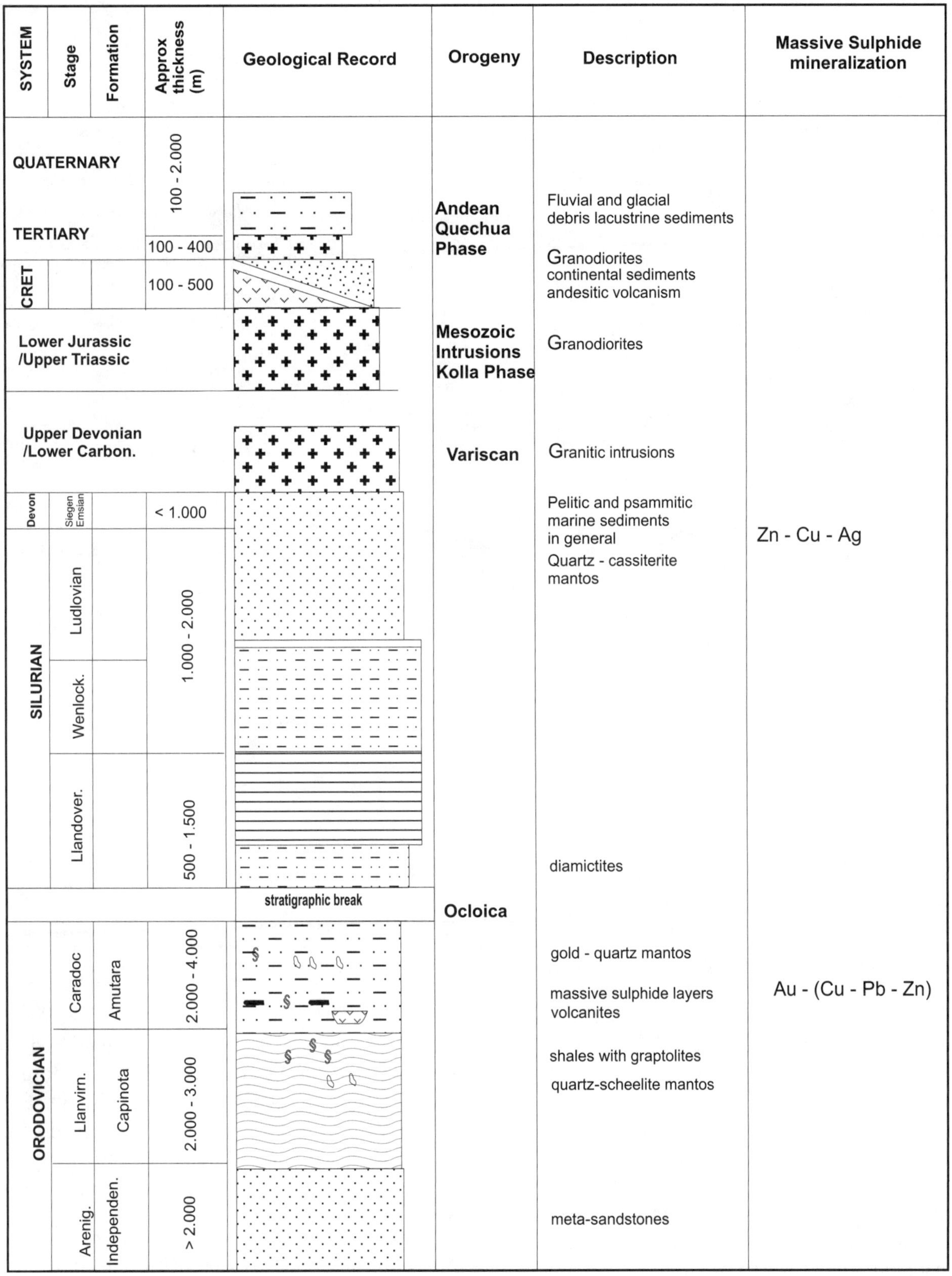

Figure 3. Stratigraphic sequence of the northern part of Cordillera Real

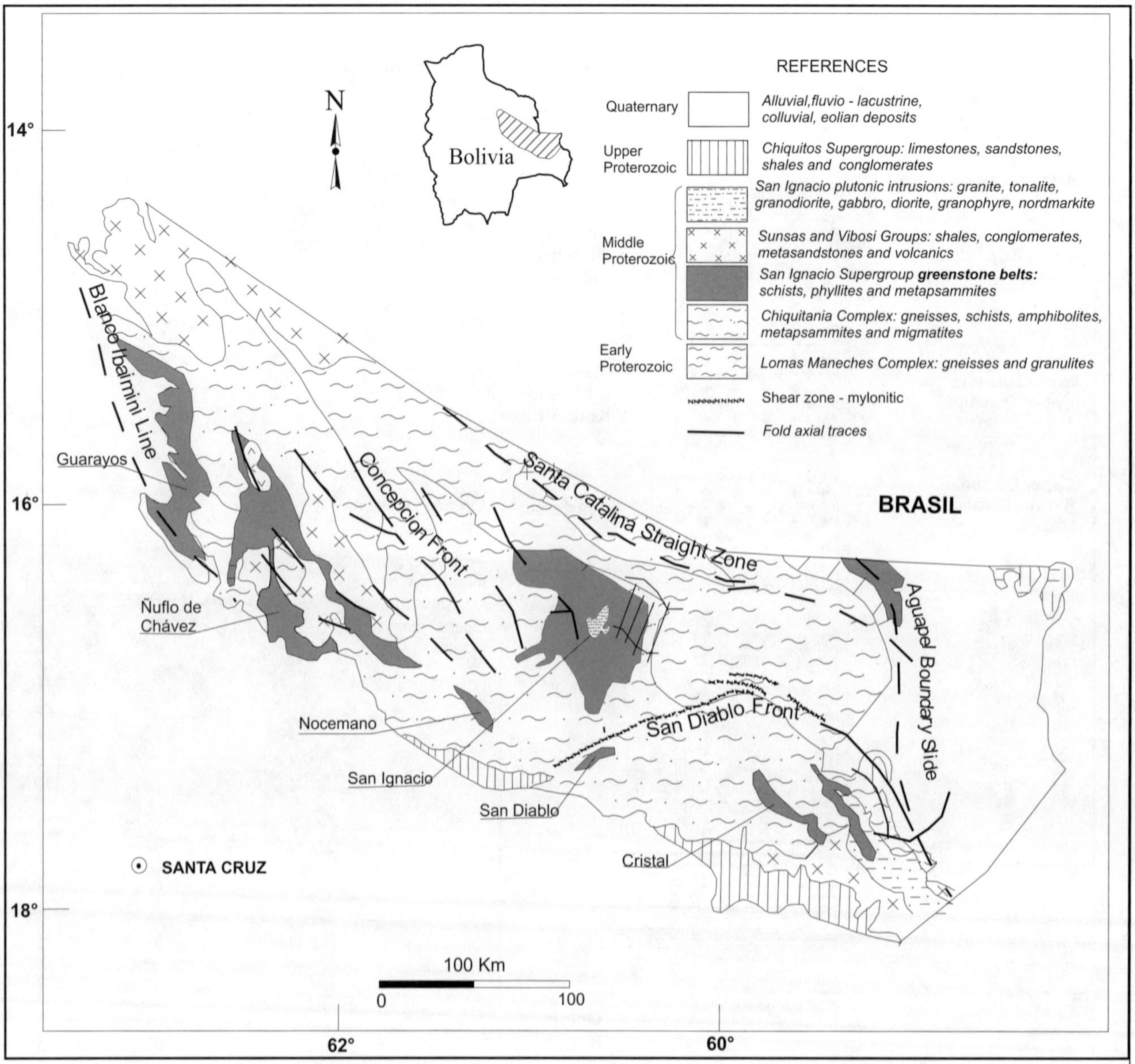

Figure 4. Geological map of the southwestern part (San Ignacio Schist Super Group) of the Bolivian Precambrian

volcano-sedimentary rocks. The main ore-body is tabular in shape and has about 500 m in strike length and a true thickness of about 20 m. Massive pyrite, chalcopyrite and minor sphalerite and galena (and rare magnetite and pyrrhotite) are hosted in a sequence of biotite-quartz schist, muscovite schist and overlain by amphibolitic andesite. All the gold and base metal geochemical anomalies are hosted in that lithology.

Possible evidences of VMS mineralization in the San Ignacio Super-Group are related to the occurrence of thin seams of sparsely disseminated chalcopyrite and pyrite in amphibolites. Moreover, prospectors have collected specimens of copper and silver sulphides and of massive pyrite allegedly found in the area (Appleton and Llanos, 1986).

Analysis of Available Information to Define New VMS targets

Summary of Structure and Mineralization

In order to define prospectivity of the schist belts,

the main characteristics from the schists belts from Guarayos, Ñuflo de Chávez, San José-San Diablo, San Ignacio and Cristal, are summarized in Table 4.

From Table 4, the schists from Guarayos, Ñuflo de Chávez, San Ignacio and Cristal present more consistent relationship between structure and mineralization. Therefore, they will be considered for further analysis.

The Guarayos and Ñuflo de Chávez schist belts show faulting-shearing trend between 115-140 degrees, which was developed during the Sunsas orogeny, coincident with the event of deformation Do3 from the San Ignacio orogeny. This resulted in a complex tectonic framework with a development of isoclinal folds, tight folds and upright open folds along several directions. Furthermore, at Miguela, several faults and fractures cross the area with 115° to 135° trend, which may correspond with the regional structural control of the VMS mineralization in that prospect area.

Folding during the Sunsas affected mostly the schists belts because of its ductility and correlates with an increase of the metamorphic grade towards the NE (Litherland et a., 1986). The Do3 fold parallels, on a wider arc, the Phanerozoic Arica elbow to the west against the Amazonic Craton. The inflexions in the fold are of 120°, ideal for continental break-up related to linking of triple-point fractures. A NNE-directed subduction zone could explain it and their Do3 overprinting by the change in strike from a NNW trending collision zone to the N-trending transform zones (Litherland et al., 1986).

The event of deformation Do3 can be preliminary defined as the main structural control of the suspected VMS mineralization in the San Ignacio Schist Super-Group.

Comparison of Lithologies Between Formations with known VMS Deposits to Those with Possible VMS Potential

An analysis of the lithology and petrology was carried out to determine additional areas for VMS mineralization in the Precambrian. The Quiser (Ñuflo de Chávez and Guarayos schists), Santa Rosa (Ñuflo de Chávez schist) , Guarayos (Guarayos schist) and Cristal (Cristal schist) Formations are known to host sulphide mineralization.

The methodoly used was simple and it consisted firstly on defining the lithologic controls of the sulphide mineralization on the four 'Guide Formations' mentioned above. Then, the identified lithologic and mineral components such as types of meta-sediments, meta-igneous sills, meta-volcanics and regional metamorphic minerals were used as guides to compare with all the formations in the San Ignacio schist Super-Group (Table 5).

As a result, quartzite. mica schist and graphitic units were identified as the more common meta-sediments in the schist belts; gabro/amphibolite and ultramafics as the usual meta-igneous sills; additional meta-volcanics (meta-tuffs and felsic) were seen in the Ñuflo de Chávez and Guarayos schists and finally the regional metamorphic minerals as hornblende/tremolite, muscovite/biotite and chlorite are widely distributed among most of the schist belts of the San Ignacio Super-Group.

Furthermore, eight additional formations within the San Ignacio schist Super-Group were defined as a permissive to host VMS-style mineralization. They are: Porvenir, La Honda, Zapocó; Páquio, Dolorida, Suriquizo; Motacú-Los Patos and Primavera (Table 5). They were classified by their host schist (Table 6), which have led to finally conclude that the Cristal, San Ignacio, Guarayos and Ñuflo de Chávez schist belts are permissive to host VMS-style mineralization in terms of lithology. As far as this analysis, the Ñuflo de Chávez schists would correspond to the more prospective lithologies for VMS-mineralization.

Geochemistry

One of the main objectives of the Proyécto Precámbrico carried out by the Servicio Geológico de Bolivia (formerly GEOBOL) and the British Geological Survey (1976-1982) was to identify mineral resources and areas of economic mineral potential (Litherland, 1986). One of the methods used was a reconnaissance geochemical surveys over the whole Precambrian Shield. Analyses for Ag, As, Co, Cu, Fe, Mn, Ni, Pb, Zn, B, Ba, Be, Cr, La, Li, Mo, Nb, Sn Sr, Y and Zr of stream sediment samples were carried out. Analytical methods used were atomic absorption spectrophotometry and colourimetry for certain element analysis and optical emission spectrography for

Table 3. Detailed lithological and petrological components of the formations present in all the schist-belts of the Bolivian Precambrian (Modified from Litherland et. al., 1986).

							Guarayos												
SCHIST BELT	Ñuflo de Chávez													Cristal			San Ignacio		
FORMATION	D	S	SR	ET	SQ	PQ	CN	CL	P	Q	H	ZP	G	CH	CR	PR	B	MP	SU
Meta-sediments																			
Quartzite				c			a	a	s	s	s				c	s	c	c	a
Meta-conglomerate				c			s	s									c		s
Feldspathic psammite	s	a				a	s	s	a			c	a			a	c		s
Phyllite/slate		c					s	s			a		s				s		a
Mica schist	a			c						a		a	s		a	s		a	
Graphitic units	s		a	s				s									s	c	s
Ferruginous units						s			s								s		
Calc-silicates	s					s			c							s		s	
Meta-Igneous Sills																			
Gabbro/ amphibolite					a							s	s	a				s	
Ultramafics					c					s	s	s	s						
Metavolcanics																			
Mafic meta-lavas										s									
Intermediate meta-lavas																(s)			
Felsic meta-lavas																			
Meta-tuffs									(s)	(c	(s)								
Primary Elements																			
Grain boundaries		s					a	a									a		
Volcaniclastics							c	a									a		
Cross/graded beds			c	s		c	a								s	a		s	
Igneous textures		s		a										a					

a = abundant c = common s = sparse ( ) = interpreted on composition

Formations

D (Dolorida)
S (Sutto)
SR (Santa Rosa)
ET (Ex-Tajibos)
SQ (Suriquizo)
PQ (Páquio)
CL (El Cielo)
P (Porvenir)
Q (Quiser)
H (La Honda)
ZP (Zapocó)
G (Guarayos)
CH (Chaquipoc)
CR (Cristal)
PR (Primavera)
B (Bonanza)
MP (Motacú/Patos)
SU (Suponema)

Table 4. Main characteristics of the schist belts in Southwestern Precambrian-Bolivia

Schist Belt	Formation	Structure	Sulphides	Sulphide Occurrence	Commodities	Soil	Metamorphic Grade	Age
Guarayos	Quiser, Guarayos	Regional faults and fractures with general trend 115 to 135°	Pyrite, chalcopyrite, <sphalerite, <galena, & << pyrrhotite	Stratiform, disseminated	Gold, copper, silver, zinc	Laterite	Amphibolite facies (low to medium)	Middle Proterozoic
Ñuflo de Chávez	Quiser, Santa Rosa	Regional faults & shear zones trending 130 to 140 °	Arsenopyrite, chalcopyrite, pyrite, sphalerite & pyrrhotite	Stratiform	Native gold	Unknown	Greenschist facies to amphibolite facies (low to medium)	Middle Proterozoic
San Ignacio	Not determined	Regional faults & shear zones with 35° & 115° & shear zn. 65°	Pyrite, pyrrhotite, chalcopyrite & stibnite	Not determined	Copper, tin, antimony	Extensive laterite	Amphibolite facies (low to medium)	Middle Proterozoic
Nocemano	Not determined	Regional lineament of 135°	Unknown	Not determined	unknown	Laterite	Amphibolite facies (low to medium)	Middle to Lower Proterozoic
San José-San Diablo	Not determined	Regional faults & shear zones trending from 45 to 120°	Pyrite, chalcopyrite?	Not determined	Gold, copper?(*)	Laterite	Amphibolite facies (low to medium) & skarn?	Middle to Lower Proterozoic
Cristal	Cristal	Regional lineament striking 315°, a syncline,horst & graben	Chalcopyrite, galena, pyrite, chalcocite, sphalerite & pyrrhotite	Skarn-type, disseminated & stratiform?	Gold, silver, copper	Extensive laterite	Amphibolite facies (low to medium) & skarn	Middle to Lower Proterozoic

(*) The San José-San Diablo schist belt might host Au-Cu mineralization since is affected by the Don Mario shear zone, the same at the Don Mario Prospect (Au-Cu).

Table 5. Comparison of lithological, petrological and mineralogical components between formations in the Precambrian.

Rocks and Minerals used for comparison purposes		Guide-Formation (with VMS-deposits)	Other formations that are geologically similar to the Guide-Formations
Meta-sediments	Quartzite	Quiser, Cristal	Porvenir, La Honda, Motacú-Patos, Primavera
	Feldspathic psammite	Guarayos	Primavera, Páquio
	Phyllite/slate	Guarayos	La Honda
	Mica schist	Quiser, Guarayos, Cristal	Dolorida, Motacú-Los Patos, Primavera, Zapocó
	Graphitic units	Santa Rosa	Dolorida, Motacú-Los Patos
Meta-igneous sills	Gabbro/amphibolite	Guarayos	Motacú-Los Patos, Suruquizo, Zapocó
	Ultramafics	Quiser, Guarayos	La Honda, Suruquizo, Zapocó
Meta-volcanics	Metatuffs	Quiser	Porvenir, La Honda
	Felsic meta-volcanics	Quiser, Santa Rosa?	Porvenir, La Honda
Regional metamorphic Minerals	Hornblende/tremolite	Quiser, Guarayos, Cristal	Porvenir, Dolorida, La Honda, Suruquizo, Primavera
	Muscovite/biotite	Quiser, Santa Rosa, Guarayos, Cristal	Porvenir, Dolorida, Motacú-Los Patos, Primavera, Zapocó
	Chlorites	Quiser, Guarayos	Porvenir, La Honda, Suriquizo,Primavera

others. It should be mentioned that gold was not analyzed during this survey.

In the present study, only samples from the San Ignacio schist Super-Group have been reviewed, due to reasons formerly explained. They consisted of about five thousand samples, which covered an area of 52,500 km^2. Moreover, distributions of Ag, Cu, Pb, Zn and Ba in the study area were depicted (Fig. 5). The threshold values used are: Ba = 681 ppm, Ag = 1.5 ppm, Zn = 51 ppm, Pb = 32 ppm and Cu = 19 ppm. Arsenic was not taken into account since the analytical methods used acused important changes in sensitivity.

The results obtained have revealed that stream sediment samples derived from the Ñuflo de Chavez schist belts have revealed anomalous arsenic, lead and zinc (Appleton and Llanos, 1985). Moreover, the Guarayos and the Ñuflo de Chávez schist belts have distinct geochemical distribution patterns (Fig. 5). The first is controlled by the Concepción Front to the east and the Blanco Ibaimini Line to the west (Figs. 4 and 5) and the second area is controlled by two regional structures as the Aguapei Line to the east and the San Diablo Shear zone to the southwest.

In the first area, a geochemical association between Zn-Cu-<Pb occurs nearby the Miguela prospect and Cu-<Pb<<Ag in the Puquio Norte area. A Cu-Zn association was seen northward of Miguela and eastward of Puquio Norte. Finally, a geochemical association between Zn and Ba bounds the copper (gold?) mineralization.

The second area shows a clear association between Cu and Ba nearby the Don Mario prospect; and a Zn-Pb-Ag was observed south of Don Mario (Fig. 5).

Table 6. Formations and Schist Belts permissive for VMS mineralization

Permissive Formations for VMS mineralization	Host Schist Belt
Primavera, Cristal	Cristal
Motacú-Los Patos	San Ignacio
Zapocó, Guarayos	Guarayos
Porvenir, La Honda, Quiser, Dolorida, Santa Rosa, Páquio, Suriquizo	Ñuflo de Chávez

The Miguela and Don Mario Prospects- Important Mineral Occurrences in the San Ignacio Schist Super-Group

Don Mario Prospect

The Don Mario prospect (Orvana Minerals) occurs on the extreme western border of the Archean age (2,800-3,000 yr-old) Brazilian Shield. It is found in supracrustal rocks of mid- to lower-Proterozoic age that are surrounded by variably migmatised and deformed micaceous quartz-feldspathic gneisses of the Chiquitania Complex. Syn- to late-kinematic granites, tonalities, trondhjemites, granophyres, and diorites intrude the Complex. The Complex and intrusions comprise the 1,280-1,600 M yr-old San Ignacio Orogeny.

Don Mario is hosted by metamorphosed and altered volcanic sequences –principally the Cristal schists, that consists of biotite-plagioclase gneisses. Rocks comprising Don Mario hill form an asymmetric synclinal-fold oriented N45°W –bearing fault. The mineralized body at Don Mario is oriented parallel to the regional fault. The faults have an eastward trend.

The host rock consist of meta-arenite, tremolite, green mica, and amphibolite. Sulphide oxidation and alteration products – limonite, malachite and azurite are found in the core zone of the mineralization. Primary sulphides include chalcopyrite, galena, pyrite, chalcocite, sphalerite and pyrrhotite. Copper and zinc sulphides formed concurrent with metamorphic tremolite and amphibolite. Don Mario has reserves of 1.5 Mt of 11.13 gm/ton Au. (Kempff, 1995).

Miguela Prospect

The Miguela prospect is situated on the western margin of the Bolivian Precambrian Shield. It is hosted in a Proterozoic schist belt metamorphosed to amphibolite facies. The main rock types are meta-rhyolite and quartz-muscovite-rich, silica and iron rich mudstone meta-sediments.

The mineralization occurs in three ore-bodies, which are related to two stratigraphic levels and related to a system of synvolcanic growth faults. The main ore-body is tabular in shape and has about 500 m in strike length and a true thickness of about 20 m. Massive pyrite, chalcopyrite and minor sphalerite and galena (and rare magnetite and pyrrhotite) are hosted in a sequence of biotite-quartz schist, muscovite schist and overlain by amphibolitic andesite. All the gold and base metal geochemical anomalies are hosted in that lithology. Miguela has a resource of 1.62 Mt of 3.76 % Cu, 1.26 g/t Au, 11.3 g/t Ag and 0.33 % Zn (Biste, 1999).

DISCUSSION

Bolivia has a long mining tradition, dating back to the pre-Spanish times, when gold, silver, tin and other metals were mined. For about four hundred years, during the Spanish colonial period, Bolivia was a major silver producer. The main silver district was Cerro Rico de Potosí as well other mines in the Andes region. Later, in the 20th century Bolivia became a world leader in tin production. Modern exploration started in late 1980's when companies started to look at non-traditional deposit types with new exploration techniques, after the lifting of the fiscal reserve. Since then, several bulk minable deposits such as Kori Kollo (Au-Ag), Pederson (Au-Sb), San Cristóbal (Zn-Ag), Don Mario (Au-Cu) and Puquio Norte (Au) were discovered (Fig.1).

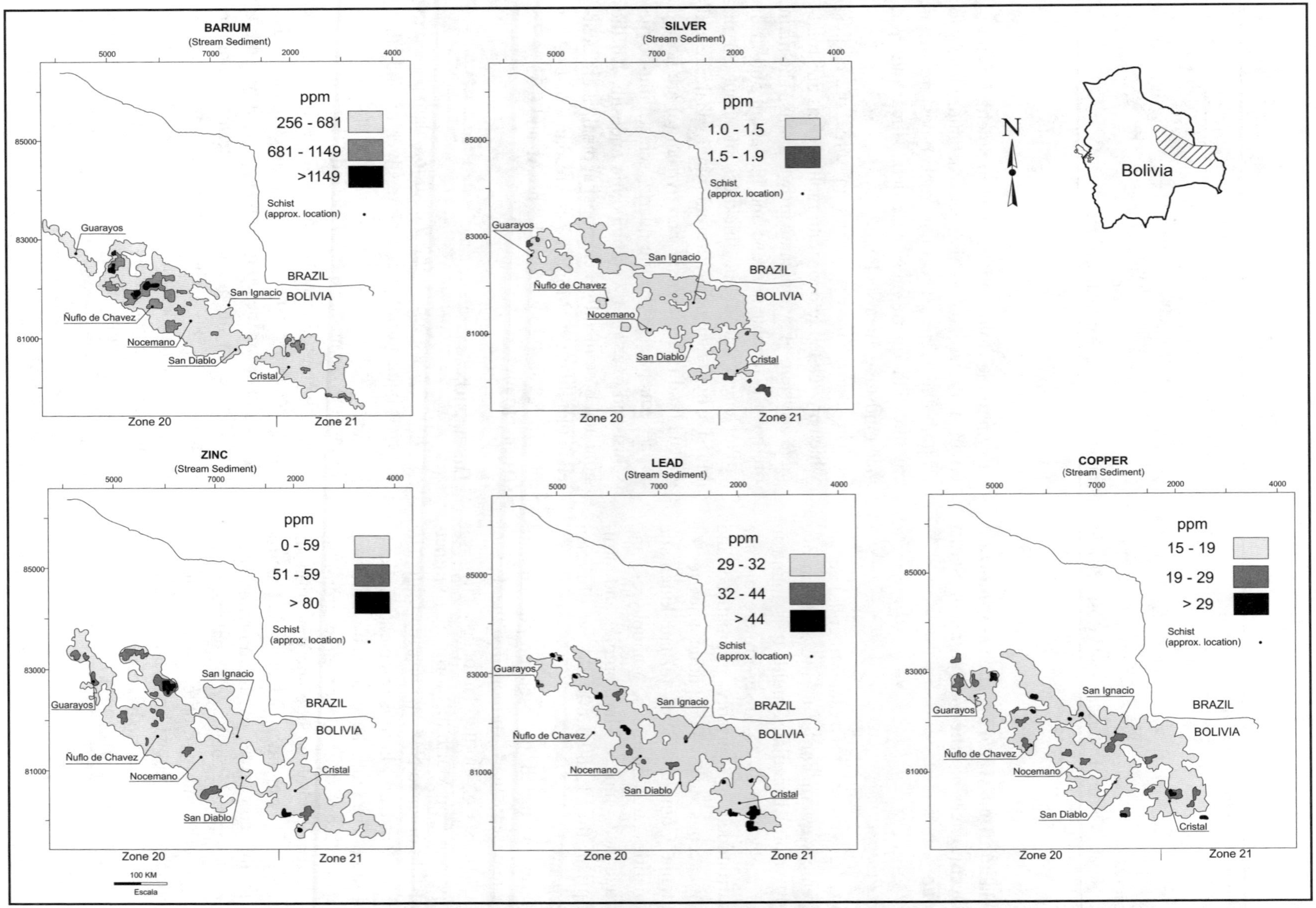

Figure 5. Geochemical anomalies of selected (Cu, Ag, Zn, Pb, Ba) elements in stream sediment samples in the southwestern part (San Ignacio Schist Super - Group) of the Bolivian Precambrian Shield (Appleton et al., 1985)

Volcanic massive sulphide (Au-Cu-Pb-Zn-Ag) mineralization occurs in two regions in Bolivia: northwestern Bolivia in the Cordillera Real in Ordovician sequences, and eastern Bolivia in Mid-Proterozoic schist belts of the Precambrian Shield.

In the Cordillera Real, stratabound/stratiform (lenticular-shaped) massive sulphide mineralization is contained in Upper Ordovician (Amutara Formation) and Devonian sequences of pelites and psammites (Figs. 2 and 3), which were affected by a low-grade (sub-greenschist facies) regional metamorphism. The sulphide layers consist largely of pyrite and lesser pyrrhotite, galena, sphalerite and chalcopyrite. They show anomalous gold, copper, lead and zinc values. Evidence for volcanic activity is provided by a metre-thick layer of trachyandesite, which outcrops 200 m below the massive sulphides in the base of the Amutara Formation. Quartz-gold mantos and veins are located in sandstones about 500 m above the sulphide layers.

The schist belts from the Bolivian Precambrian (San Ignacio Schist Super-Group), comprise sequences of quartzites, feldspathic metapsammites and micaceous schists or phyllites with subordinate ferruginous, calc-silicate, metavolcanic, graphite-rich units and metamorphosed mafic igneous rocks (Tables 2 and 3). These rocks were faulted and sheared and metamorphosed to amphibolite facies during the San Ignacio orogeny. Later they were affected by the Sunsas orogeny. These schist belts show a variety of structural forms believed to be due to the refolding of synformal cores during the orogenies. They have received local names, and the main schist belts are Guarayos, Ñuflo de Chávez, San Ignacio and Cristal (Fig. 3).

An analysis of the lithology and petrology to determine additional areas for VMS mineralization in the Precambrian were carried out. Known sulphide host formations as Quiser (Ñuflo de Chávez and Guarayos schists), Santa Rosa (Ñuflo de Chávez schist) , Guarayos (Guarayos schist) and Cristal (Cristal schist) were used on that purpose.

Quartzite. mica schist and graphitic units were identified as the more common meta-sediments in the schist belts; gabro/amphibolite and ultramafics as the usual meta-igneous sills; meta-tuffs and felsic are the meta-volcanics, the common regional metamorphic minerals are hornblende/tremolite, muscovite/biotite and chlorite, which are widely distributed among the schist belts of the San Ignacio Super-Group.

Eight additional formations within the San Ignacio schist Super-Group were defined as a permissive to host VMS-style mineralization. They are: Porvenir, La Honda, Zapocó; Páquio, Dolorida, Suriquizo; Motacú-Los Patos and Primavera (Table 5). They were classified by their host schist (Table 6), which have led to finally conclude that the Cristal, San Ignacio, Guarayos and Ñuflo de Chávez schist belts are permissive to host VMS-style mineralization in terms of lithology. The Ñuflo de Chávez schists seems to be the more prospective lithologies for this type of mineralization.

Geochemically, two areas with distinct geochemical distribution patterns were defined. The first include the Guarayos and the Ñuflo de Chávez schist belts. A geochemical association between Zn-Cu-<Pb occurs near the Miguela prospect and Cu-<Pb<<Ag in the Puquio Norte area. A Cu-Zn association was seen northward of Miguela and eastward of Puquio Norte. A geochemical association between Zn and Ba bounds the copper (gold?) mineralization. The second area includes the San Ignacio and Cristal schist belts, where the association Cu-Ba and Zn-Pb-Ag were observed nearby and south of the Don Mario prospect respectively (Fig. 5).

As a result of the present study, it can be concluded that favourable environments for VMS mineralization are located in the Yani-Aucapata belt within the Cordillera Real (NW part of Bolivia), and principally the Ñuflo de Chávez schist belt in the Precambrian. The the Guarayos schist (that hosts the Miguela prospect), the the San Ignacio schist ane the Cristal schist (which includes the Don Mario prospect) are also favourable areas. All these regions are worthy of additional and systematic exploration that could lead to the discovery of large VMS-type ore-deposits.

ACKNOWLEDGEMENTS

We wish to thank Marcelo Claure Zapata, Executive Director of the Servicio de Geología y Minería de Bolivia (SERGEOMIN), for his invaluable support and facilities given to the preparation of this paper. To Nicolás Calderón who assisted in the preparation of figures. Many thanks to Carlos Riera for his kind support and to Jaime Guzmán, Chris Picken and GAC reviewers for their suggestions to improve the manuscript.

REFERENCES

Appleton, J. D. and Llanos, A., 1986: Geochemical atlas of eastern Bolivia: Keyworth, British Geological Survey; La Paz, Servicio Geológico de Bolivia.

Arce, O., Villaroel, L., & Thompson, I., 1995: Mineralización aurífera en sedimentos en el Altiplano Central, Bolivia. Prospecto Nobel e Isvaya, nuevos ejemplos. E. M. Altiplano - Orvana Mineral. In Bolivia Mining 1995, La Paz, 11 p.

Arce, O., 1999: Geología y exploración en el Yacimiento Auro-antimonífero de San Bernardino (Pederson) Bolivia. In Bolivia Mining 1999, 14 p. Santa Cruz, 1999.

Avila, W., 1990: Tin Bearing granites from the Cordillera Real, Bolivia; Petrological and geochemical review. Geological Society of America, Special Paper 241, p. 145 – 159.

Biste, M., 1985: Strata-bound gold mineralization in the Precambrian basement of eastern Bolivia and the Rondonia/Para region (Brazil). Monograph. Ser.on Min. Deposits, v. 25, pp.137-150, Gebrüder Brontraeger, Berlin-Stuttgart.

Biste, M., 1999: The Miguela Copper Gold discovery in the Precambrian. Presentation in the Mining and Construction Conference Bolivia 99, Santa Cruz, Bolivia.

Fletcher, C. J. N. and Litherland, M., 1981: The geology and tectonic setting of the Velasco alkaline province, eastern Bolivia: London J. geol Soc. V. 138, p. 541-548.

Fornari, M., Herail, G., 1991: Lower Paleozoic gold occurrences, in the "Eastern Cordillera" of southern Perú and Northern Bolivia: a genetic model, In: Ladeira E., A., (ed.) Proceeding Sympsium Brazil Gold 91. Belo Horizonte, Brazil, 13 - 17 May 1992. A. A. Balkema, Rotterdam, p. 135 - 147.

Gustavson Associates, Baker and McKenzie , Mintec & GEOBOL, 1992: Compendio de Geología Económica de Bolivia. Ministerio de Minería y Metalurgia. La Paz.

Heuschmidt, B., Miranda, V., 1999: Mapa Metalogénico de Bolivia Esc. 1:1.000.000. Boletín SERGEOMIN, 19. La Paz 50 p.

Kempff, O., 1995: Don Mario, una ocurrencia precámbrica de cobre-oro, Departamento de Santa Cruz. La Paz, Conferencia Bolivia Mining '95.

Litherland, M. V., 1979: La geología y potencial de minerales del área de San Ignacio de Velasco (Quad. SE 20-4: Santa Cruz, Proyecto Precámbrico, IGS/GEOBOL, Informe Nº 3 (open file), 123 p.

Litherland, M., Annells, R. N., Appleton, J. D., Berrangé, J. P., Bloomfield K., Burton, C. C. J., Darbyshire, D. P. F., Fletcher, C. J. N., Hawkins, M. P., Klinck, B. A., Llanos, A., Mitchell, W. I., O'Connor, E. A., Pitfield, P. E. J., Power, G. and Webb, B. C.,: 1986, The geology and mineral resources of the Bolivian Precambrian Shield: British Geological Survey, Overseas Memoir 9, 153 p, incluye mapa geológico del área del Proyecto Precámbrico, escala 1:1.000.000.

McBride, S., L., Robertson, R.,C.R,., Clark, A., H. & Farrar, E., 1983: Magmatic and metallogenetic episodes in the northern tin belt, Cordillera Real, Bolivia. Geol. Rundsch., 72; p. 685 - 713.

Redwood, S., 1993: The Metallogeny of the Bolivian Andes. Mineral Research Unit, Short Course No. 15. UBC, Vancouver, B.C., Canada, 59p.

Richter, D., H., Ludington S., & Soria-Escalante, E., 1992: Geologic setting, in Geology and mineral resources of the Altiplano and Cordillera Occidental, Bolivia: U.S. Geological Survey Bulletin 1975, p. 14 - 24.

Schneider, H., J., 1990: Gold deposits in Lower Paleozoic sediments of the Cordillera Real, Bolivia. In Fontboté et al., (eds). P. 137 - 146.

Tistl, M., & Schneider, H., J., 1985: The Variscan thermometamorphism and its relations to gold-quartz mineralization in the NE Cordillera Real., Bolivia, 2Bl. Geol. Paläont., Teil 1, p. 1579 - 1589.

Uribe - Zeballos, H., 1997: Mineralogy and Fluid inclusions of the Polymetallic veins in the Escala District South Altiplano - Bolivia. MSc Thesis 102 p. Imperial College of Science, Technology and Medicine. London, 1997.

Windley, B.F., 1977: The evolving continents 385pp. (new York: John Wiley).

GEOLOGY AND SETTING OF THE MIGUELA A-ZONE, GUARAYOS GREENSTONE BELT, EASTERN BOLIVIA

MICHAEL BISTE
Essex Resource Incorporated - Bolivia, Calle Aruma No 10/11, Urbari, Casilla 2341

ANDREW W. GOURLAY
Essex Resource Corporation, Suite 1220 - 800 West Pender Street, Vancouver, B.C., Canada, V6C 2V6

ABSTRACT

The Miguela A-Zone volcanogenic massive sulphide (VMS) deposit is located at the western border of the Precambrian shield of eastern Bolivia, hosted in a Proterozoic greenstone belt and metamorphosed to amphibolite facies. The mineralization occurs in a 400 m thick felsic interval within a thicker succession of tholeiitic mafic volcanic rocks. The main rock types are meta-rhyolite and quartz-muscovite-rich meta-sediments in the footwall to the VMS mineralization, and silica and iron-rich mudstone and siltstone, magnetite or pyrrhotite-rich banded iron-formation in the hangingwall and lateral to the known VMS mineralization. This lithofacies is informally known as the "La Pastora" formation and can be traced for at least 28 km of strike length. All important geochemical and geophysical anomalies and gold and base metal showings are hosted in this formation.

The mineralization occurs in three lenses, is confined to two different stratigraphic levels, and is related to a system of synvolcanic growth faults. The lowermost A-3 lens is underlain and laterally surrounded by a zone of hydrothermal alteration, intense pyritization and sodium depletion. The main A-1 lens has been the focus of exploration. It is tabular in shape, dips 45°, has a true thickness between 12 and 23 m and is capped by a quartz-rich layer enriched in barium. It is continuous for 450 m in strike, 350 metres down-dip, with an inferred resource of 1.62 Mt grading 3.76 % Cu, 1.26 g/t Au, 11.3 g/t Ag and 0.33 % Zn, although the deposit remains to be fully defined.

The A-Zone is deeply weathered due to the intensive lateritization of the regolith since the Miocene. A 45 m thick supergene chalcocite and a 40 m thick oxide zone overlie the primary sulphide mineralization. The oxide zone is enriched in gold and depleted in base metals and silver, whereas copper is strongly enriched in the supergene zone.

Routine geochemical and geophysical surveys, commonly used in massive sulphide exploration in Canada and elsewhere, have proved effective in the deeply laterized Bolivian Shield. Exploration on the Miguela and El Porvenir concessions have identified several targets with geochemical and geophysical signatures comparable to the A-Zone, which remain to be drill tested. Further exploration of the remainder of the Guarayos Greenstone Belt is a priority. Given the exploration success in a short period of time, the Guarayos Greenstone Belt has excellent potential to host world class deposits.

INTRODUCTION

The Precambrian of eastern Bolivia is the southwestern extension of the Brazilian Shield, which is host to large primary gold and base metal deposits in Brazil. Exploration in Bolivia commenced relatively late after the lifting of the fiscal reserve in 1986, when a few small exploration companies started exploring for primary gold mineralization in areas of old alluvial gold workings (Biste et al., 1991). In the early 1990's Rio Tinto Zinc and COMSUR started to explore the layered ultra-mafic intrusion Rincon del Tigre for nickel and platinum. Exploration for volcanogenic massive sulphide (VMS) mineralization was initiated by Tanganika A.V.V. in 1993 (Biste & Matthews, 1995, 1996a and 1996b), and since 1996 Essex Resource Corporation and Tanganika have jointly explored for VMS deposits in eastern Bolivia. Exploration has focused on the Miguela and El Porvenir concessions where VMS mineralization was discovered at the A-Zone, within a sequence favourable for the deposition of volcanogenic massive sulphides. This publication describes the discovery, the geological setting and potential of this new mineral district.

GENENERAL INFORMATION

Location, Access and Topography

The Miguela Concession is located at the south-western edge of the Precambrian shield of Central South America, about 230 km to the north of the city of Santa Cruz de la Sierra in the Guarayos Province of eastern Bolivia, at 63° 08' West and 15° 98' South (Fig. 1). Access is via vehicle from Santa Cruz de la Sierra to Ascension de Guarayos, which are connected by a 275 km asphalt road. From Guarayos the property is accessed by 15 km of secondary dirt road and five kilometres of rehabilitated timber track, which is readily accessible during the dry season. The journey takes about four hours from Santa Cruz to Ascension de Guarayos, and a further ½ hour to the property.

The Miguela Concession, and the adjoining El Porvenir Property, also controlled by Essex, covers a gently undulating lateritic surface at an average elevation of approximately 275 metres above sea level. Locally, isolated hills reach an elevation of 400 m above sea level. Tropical forests with limited areas of slash-and-burn agriculture cover the entire area. Most of the marketable timber has been already harvested.

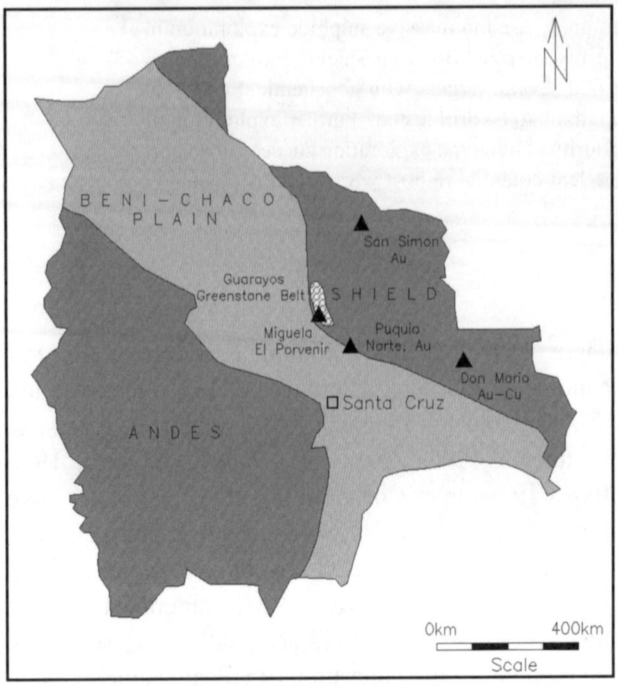

Figure 1. Location map of the Guarayos Greenstone Belt and the Miguela and El Porvenir concessions.

Previous Mining and Exploration

The Guarayos and the adjacent Ñuflo de Chavez provinces have a long history of small-scale gold mining (Biste, 1985; Biste et al., 1991). Exploitation by Jesuits in the 17th century, a rush on small alluvial placer deposits during the 1880's and another between 1980 and 1982 are the most notable mining events. Some placers around San Ramon, east of Ascensión de Guarayos, and of the Serrania San Simon close to the border with Brazil are still worked on a small scale. Between 1975 and 1983 the Bolivian shield was mapped jointly by the British and Bolivian Geological Surveys, which produced the first geological maps and the first inventory of mineral potential (Litherland et al., 1986). At least 50 percent of the total area has never been ground surveyed due to difficult or non-existent access. In 1991 and 1992, an airborne magnetic and radiometric test survey was carried out in Ñuflo de Chavez province and portions of Guarayos Province over an area of 13,000 square kilometres. The resulting maps are useful for interpreting the highly tectonized southwest margin of the shield and for the delimitation of greenstone belts (Witchard et al., 1993).

The San Ramon greenstone belt, located approximately 100 km to the southeast of the Miguela concession, outcrops over a 40 km strike length and is the best known and most accessible area. The most advanced project in this belt is COMSUR's "Puquio Norte" gold deposit (Fig. 2), which has an indicated mineral resource of 4 million tonnes with a gold content of about 2.4 g/t. Open-pit/heap leaching commenced during 1997. In recent years, there has been small-scale exploitation of alluvial and colluvial placer deposits west of the Miguela concession. A privately owned Bolivian exploration company EMSA LTDA. investigated the alluvial gold potential of the area between 1986 and1989 (Bufler et. al, 1990; Biste et al., 1991). The state-owned mining company Corporacion Minera De Bolivia ("COMIBOL") staked the El Porvenir claim in 1989 and other companies followed, staking the remaining claims between 1994 and 1996. Several small miners

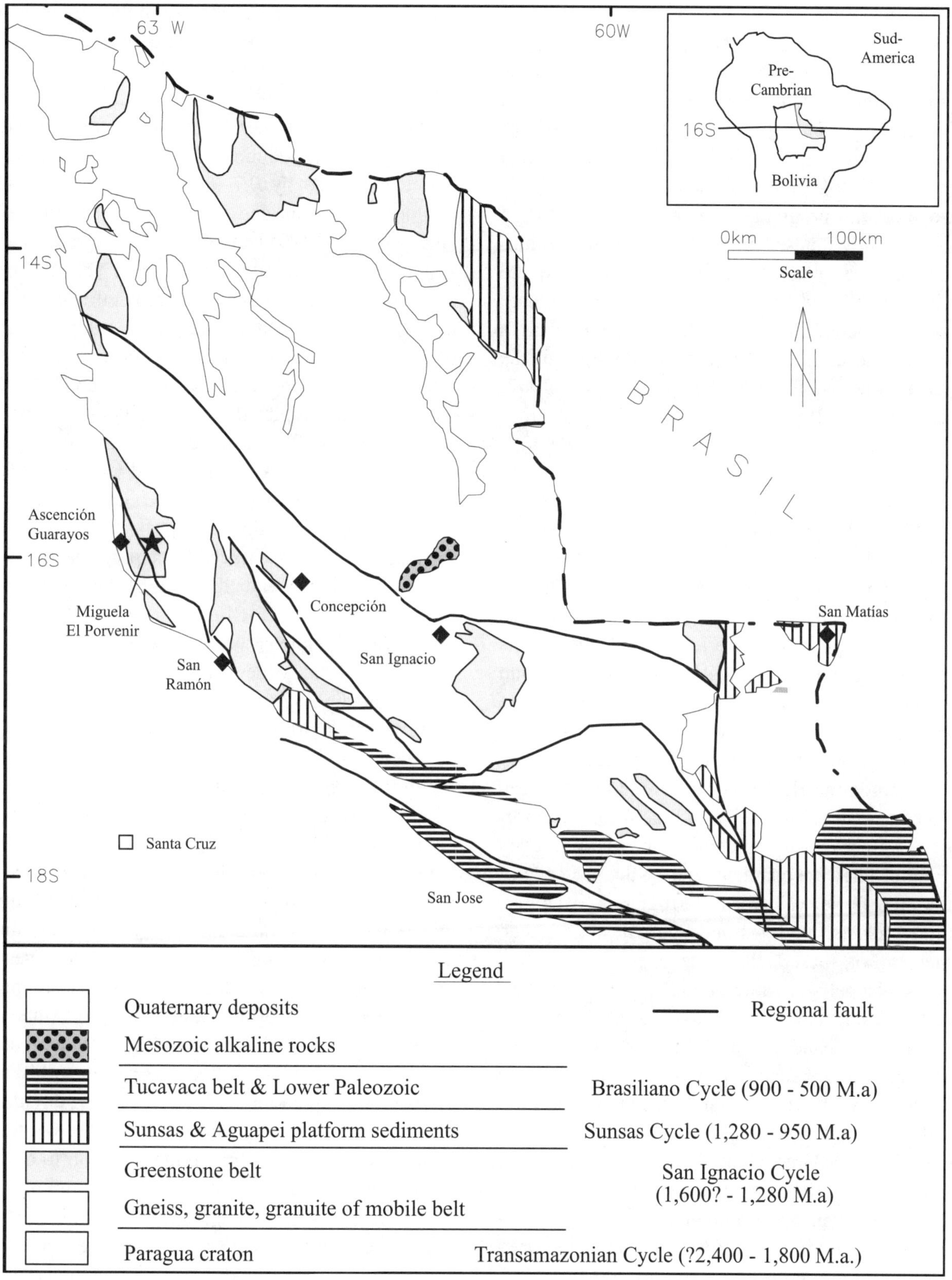

Figure 2. Simplified geological map of the western border of the Precambrian shield of eastern Bolivia.

(garimpeiros) have exploited the gold placer deposits "La Pampa" and "Iyozar" since 1994, producing a total of approximately 300 kilograms of gold. These activities were suspended at the end of 1997 due to the declining gold price and the depletion of resources. The exploration companies Tanganika A.V.V. and EMSU S.R.L. started an extensive grass root exploration program on the Miguela concession in 1993, mainly focused on gold and base metal mineralization in a volcano-sedimentary belt (Biste and Matthews, 1995 and 1996a). In 1995, Essex Resource Corporation acquired a 100 % interest in Tanganika A.V.V. and accelerated systematic exploration of the Miguela concession (Biste and Matthews, 1997; Biste, 1998a and 1998 b).

GEOLOGY

Regional Setting

The Precambrian of eastern Bolivia is an uplifted Tertiary laterized plain buried by Quaternary alluvial sediments at its margins (Fig. 2). Three well-defined Proterozoic tectonic belts are recognized; these belts are essentially sub-parallel and decrease in width and metamorphic grade from north to south. These are known as the Parana Craton and the Sunsas and Tucavaca/Aquapei tectonic belts (Litherland et al., 1986). Approximately 10 percent of the Precambrian shield consist of "schist belts", which were metamorphosed to greenschist/amphibolite facies and intruded by granite. They are characterized by the presence of mafic and felsic volcanics, ferruginous exhalites, graphitic schists, phyllites and quartzites. Less than 30 percent of these belts have been investigated. These "schist belts" are interpreted to represent greenstone belts, and have excellent geological potential for auriferous banded iron-formation, shear zone related gold mineralization, volcanogenic massive sulphide (VMS) deposits and secondary laterite hosted gold mineralization.

The Guarayos Greenstone Belt is host of the VMS mineralization of the Miguela concession. It comprises supracrustal volcano-sedimentary rocks of amphibolitic metamorphic grade, overlying an older crystalline basement and has been affected by the 1,400 Ma Mid-Proterozoic San Ignacio Orogeny. Rock outcrops are rare, and most of the area is flat and deeply laterized to a depth of up to 40 m.

Discovery and Exploration

The A-Zone mineralization was discovered in 1994 by stream sediment and soil sampling, which delineated a 2.0 by 0.7 km gold anomaly close to boulders of gossan and iron-stained quartzite (Biste and Matthews, 1995). A trenching program in 1995 and 1996 confirmed the presence of volcanic rocks and a strata-bound gossan formation enriched in gold in the 1 to 70 gram/tonne range and with peak values of up to 250,000 gram/tonne (Biste and Matthews, 1996a). Induced polarization and ground magnetic surveys were completed at a regional scale across the Miguela and El Porvenir concessions with detailed surveys over the A-Zone (Val d'Or, 1997, Biste 1998a). This work identified a favourable stratigraphic sequence, informally known as the "La Pastora" formation, which was traced for approximately 12 km across the Miguela and adjoining El Porvenir concessions. During 1996 2,464 m of diamond drilling in 19 holes were completed at the A-Zone, and two holes totalling 434 m wide drilled at El Porvenir. The drilling at the A-Zone intersected VMS mineralization below a 40 m thick oxide zone (Biste and Matthews, 1997). A subsequent Horizontal Loop Electromagnetic ("HLEM") survey confirmed successfully the extensions of three individual massive conductors (Val d'Or, 1998).

A 4,000 m diamond-drilling program was carried out in 1997 to explore the continuity of VMS mineralization of the A-Zone. It delineated an upper mineralized level extending 350 m down-dip to a vertical depth of approximately 240 m, and traced the mineralization for over 550 m of strike length. Three diamond holes were drilled north of the A-zone in the El Bagre Zone to explore the extension of the VMS mineralization. In parallel 3,399 m of reverse circulation drilling was carried out to investigate the weathered zone on top of the A-Zone mineralization to a depth of 80 m below surface. Follow up soil sampling, geological mapping, trenching, trench sampling, test pitting, auger drilling, HLEM, ground magnetic and IP surveys have been completed at the Miguela and El Porvenir concessions. This work has been concentrated in the central and southern part of the area to explore the continuation of the prospective La Pastora formation (Biste, 1999a and 1999b).

An 800 m reconnaissance drilling program was completed in 1998 in the southern central part of the El Porvenir concession (Biste 1998a). The soil base metal anomalies and electromagnetic conductors defined on this concession are related to a sulphide and magnetite-bearing banded iron-formation with anomalous base metal content.

Property Geology

The geology of the area has been derived from a synthesis of geological surface mapping, interpretation of geophysical airborne and ground surveys, and logging of soil, auger, trench, reverse and diamond drill samples (Fig. 3). A gneiss-granite basement complex borders the eastern side of the Miguela claim. The major part of the area consists of mafic, intermediate and felsic volcanic rocks, tuff and clastic sediments, and a exhalitic facies consisting of chert and banded iron formation. An oval shaped mafic body occurs in the centre of the Miguela claim, which represents a younger intrusion of probable Upper Proterozoic age.

The stratigraphic relations between the different sites is not clearly understood due to the absence of rock outcrops and the presence of complex tectonic structures. It is assumed that the rock sequence of the A-Zone mineralization is in a normal position, striking 40 degrees and dipping between 40 and 60 degrees northwest. The VMS mineralization is confined to a

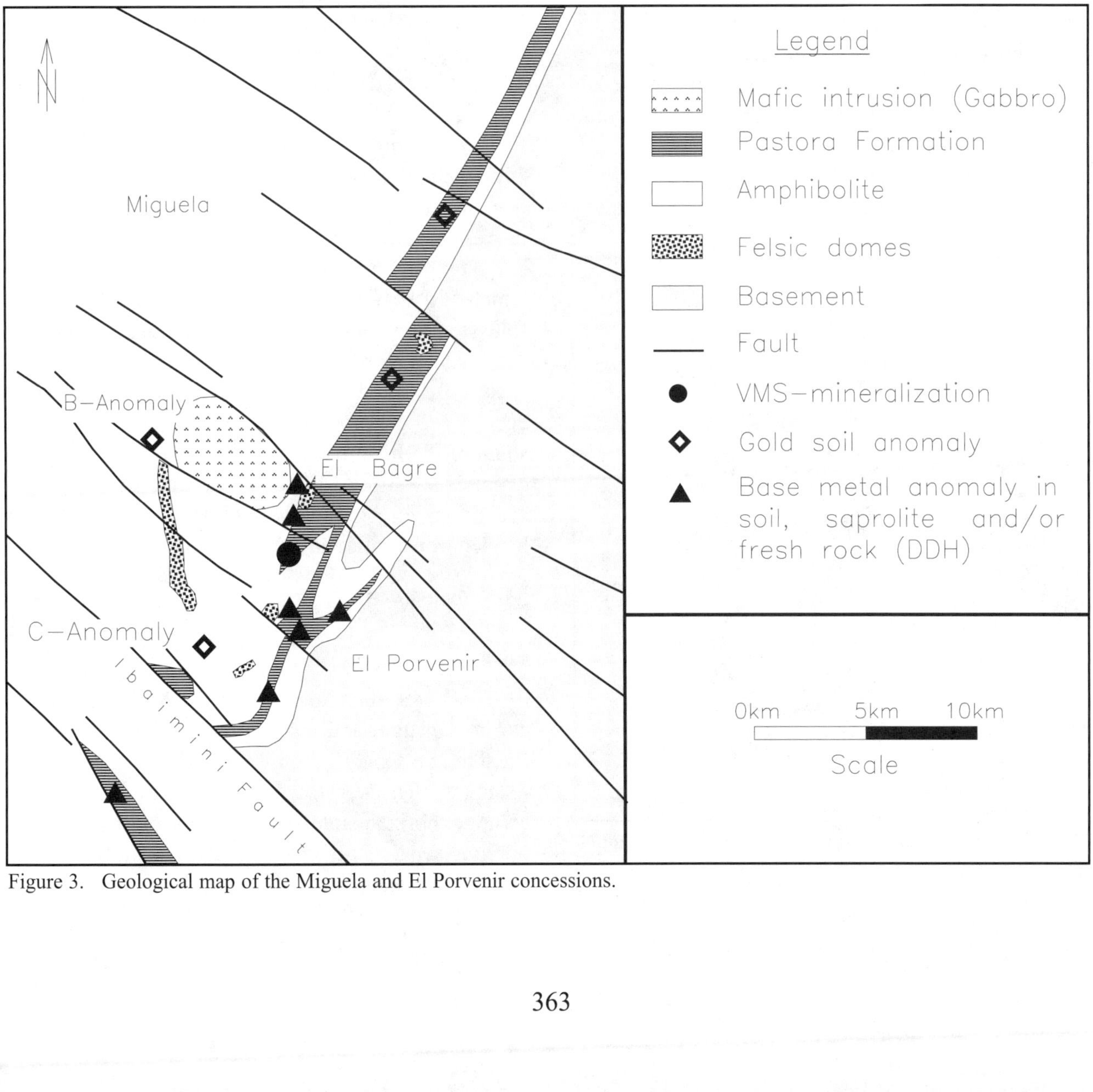

Figure 3. Geological map of the Miguela and El Porvenir concessions.

400 m thick felsic sequence, which is composed of intermediate to rhyolitic volcanic rocks, quartz-muscovite-rich sediments with thin layers of mafic material (Fig. 4). The hanging and the footwall of this felsic unit consist mainly of massive fine-grained amphibolite. The felsic rocks diminish along strike to the south of the A-Zone, due to the presence of a synvolcanic growth fault, and are replaced completely by amphibolitic andesite.

The lithological units of the El Porvenir claim trend 40 degrees and dip 45 to 55 degrees to the northwest. The western part of the claim consists of deeply laterized amphibolite with minor inclusions of felsic volcanic rocks. These are overlain by the "La Pastora" formation, which consists of silica, and iron-rich metamorphosed mudstone and siltstone, thin layers of felsic tuff and tuffite, and a magnetite or pyhrrotite-rich banded iron-formation, which covers approximately 20 percent of the claim. It is assumed that this formation forms the hangingwall and the lateral equivalents of the A-Zone mineralization and other inferred ore bodies.

Felsic dome structures occur about 2 km north of the A-Zone in the El Bagre area and in the footwall of

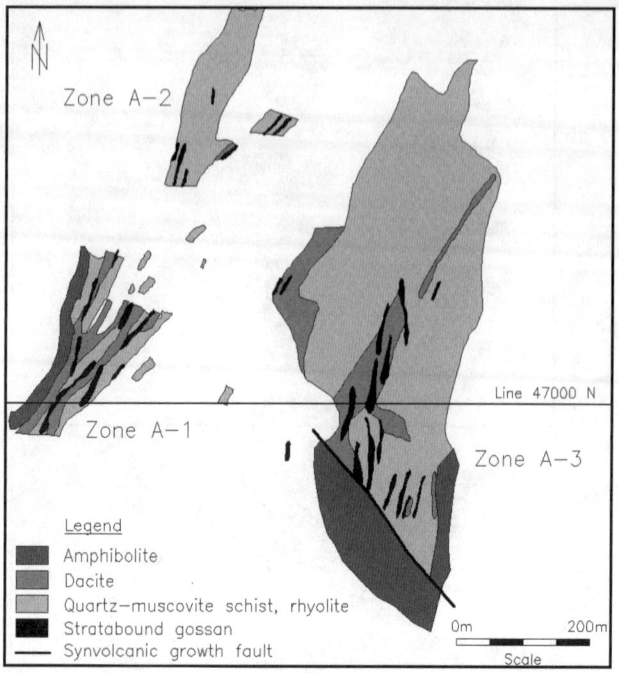

Figure 4 Detailed geological map of the VMS mineralization of the Miguela A-Zone

the La Pastora formation in the southern part of the El Porvenir claim. A major, six kilometre long, north-south striking elongated felsic lens exists in the central part of the Miguela claim about 5 km west of the A-Zone (Fig. 4). These bodies consist mainly of massive recrystallized quartz-rich granofels and are sandwiched in the less competent country rocks, similar to large scale boudins.

Structure

The contact zone between the local basement and the described supracrustal rock sequence is not exposed. Most of the rock types are highly foliated. Only the massive felsic and quartz-rich units form bodies of competent lithologies up to several kilometres length. Several regional-scale faults and fractures cross the area trending 115 to 135 degrees (Fig. 4). They are parallel to the shape of a seven by three kilometre large elongated magnetic anomaly in the centre of the Miguela claim and are of Upper Proterozoic age. The most important lineament is the Ibaimini fault, which divides the area in two parts with different structural regimes. The lithological units north of the fault trend 25 to 40 degrees and dip 45 to 75 degrees northwest. The Pastora formation forms a complex tectonic structure in the El Porvenir claims, which is "V"-shaped, forming overturned isoclinal fold structures with axial planes dipping northwest. The strike of the "La Pastora" formation turns to the west close to the Ibaimini fault, indicating the presence of a "U"-shaped large scale structure. The rocks south of the Ibaimini fault are outside of the Miguela claim. They strike 140 degrees, are vertical and consist principally of pelitic sediments, thin layers of banded iron-formation and mafic material.

MINERALIZATION

Form and Shape

The VMS mineralization of the Miguela A-Zone consists of three individual mineralized bodies, confined to two separate stratigraphical levels, within the felsic unit. The western A-1 and A-2 bodies occur in an upper horizon and the eastern A-3 body in a lower horizon, separated by a 300 m thick sequence of volcano-sedimentary rocks (Fig. 5). Massive sulphides predominate in the A-1, semi-massive to disseminated in the A-2 and thin, massive to semi-massive sulphide layers and a large strata-bound pyrite dissemination in the A-3 body. The main A-1 body is the best explored lense. It is tabular in shape, dips 45 degrees northwest and exhibits a true thickness between 12 and 23 m along the drilled section (Fig. 6). It is continuous for 450 m along strike, 350 metres down-dip and remains open to depth and along strike. The mineralization is hosted in a sequence of biotite-quartz schist, muscovite schist and rhyolite and overlain by amphibolitic andesite. The direct hangingwall of the VMS layer is a quartz-rich rock, which exhibits high barium values of up to 7,199 ppm, equivalent to 1.3 weight % of barite. There is evidence of pillow structures and volcanic agglomerate (Figs. 7 and 8) in the andesite and rhyolite, respectively.

Ore Mineralogy and Fabric

The VMS mineralization contains only a restricted range of opaque minerals. The most important primary minerals are pyrite and chalcopyrite with minor amounts of sphalerite and galena in places. Magnetite and pyrrhotite are rare in the A-Zone but are very abundant in the El Bagre and El Porvenir zones. No arsenopyrite is present. The dominant nonsulphide oxide gangue minerals are sericite/muscovite, biotite, quartz and minor chlorite and carbonate. North and south of the A-Zone, stratabound calcsilicate minerals such as garnet, actinolite and diopside are abundant.

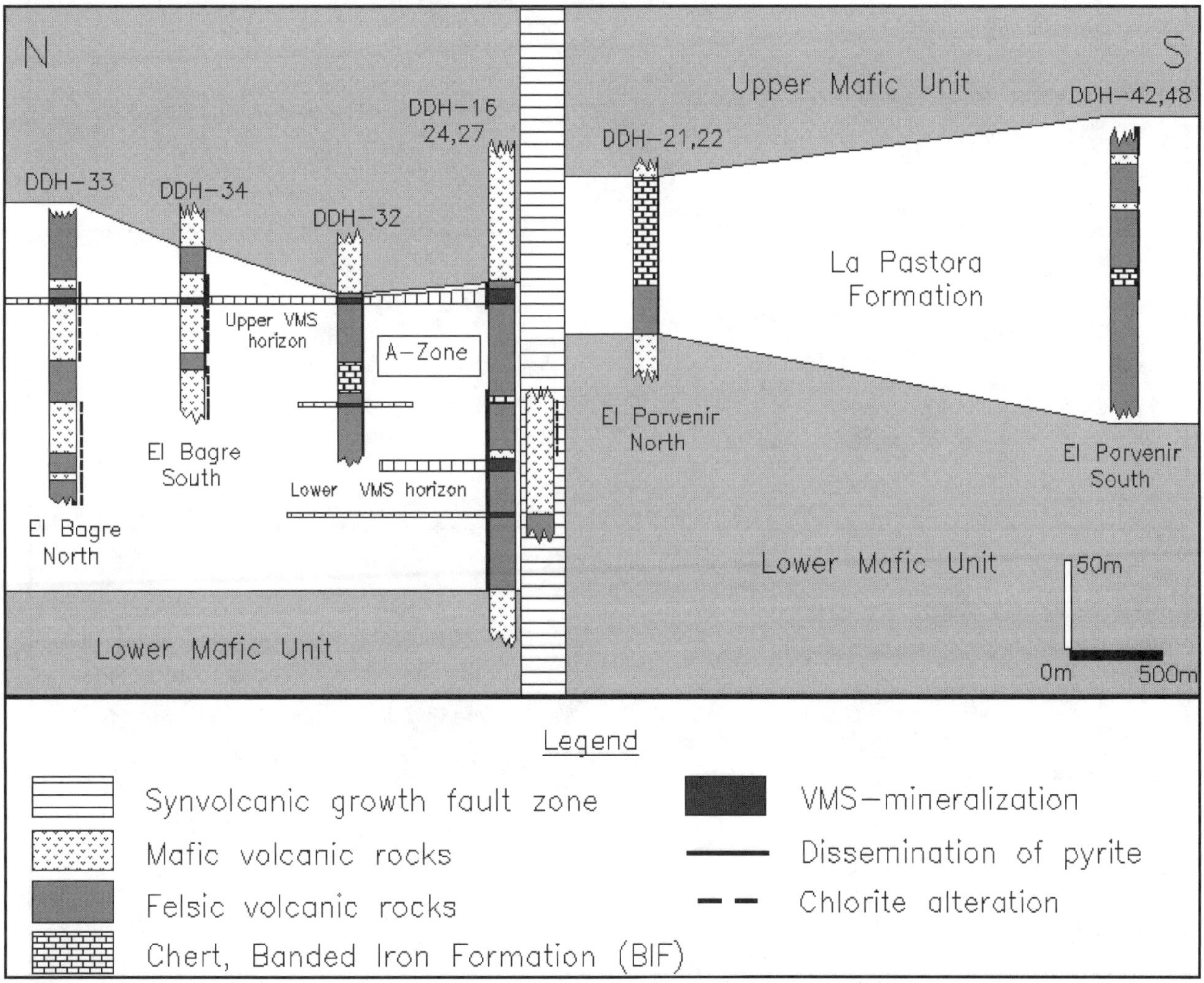

Figure 5. Schematic cross section through the Miguela/El Porvenir stratigraphy.

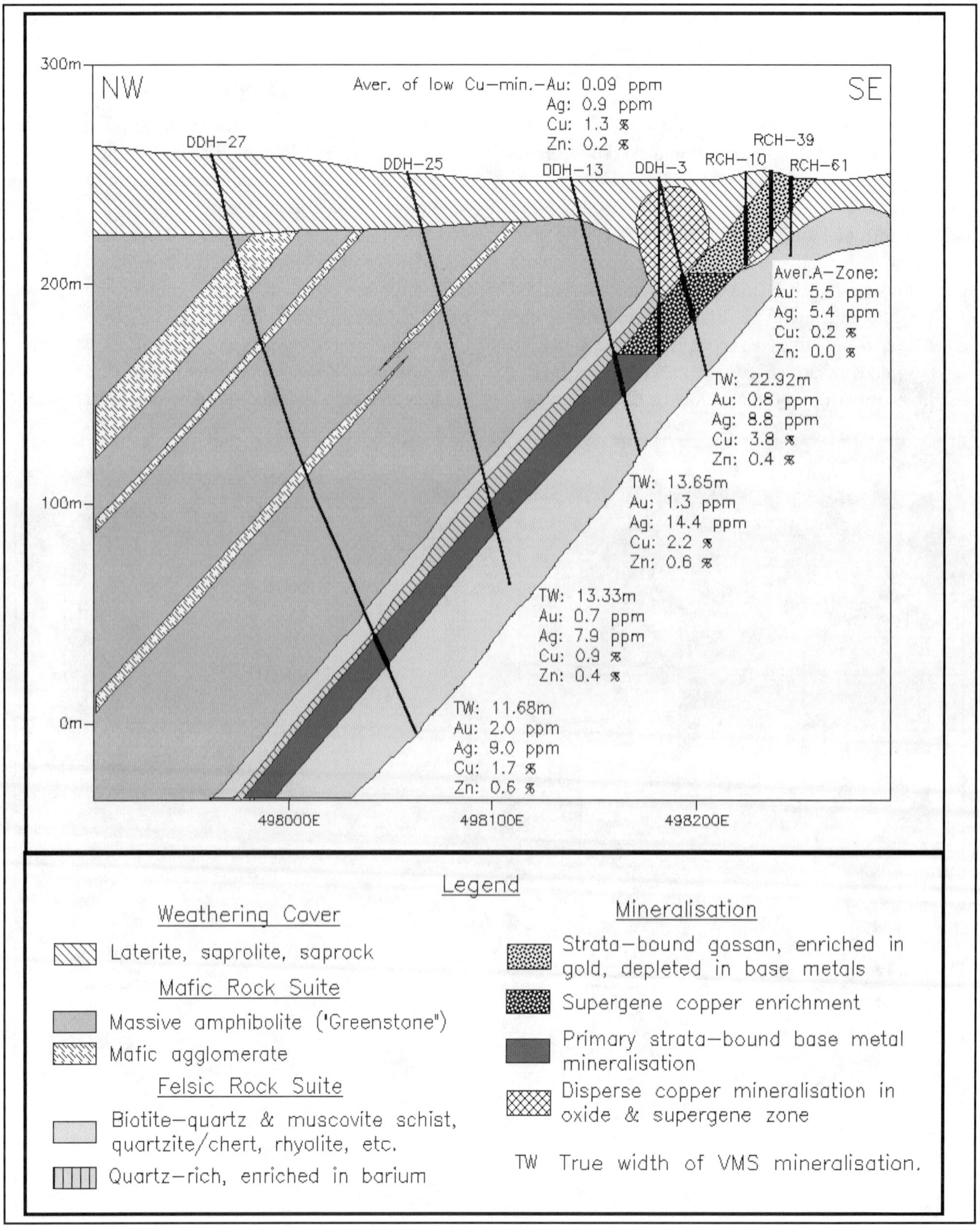

Figure 6. Geological NW-SE cross section of the Miguela A-1 zone.

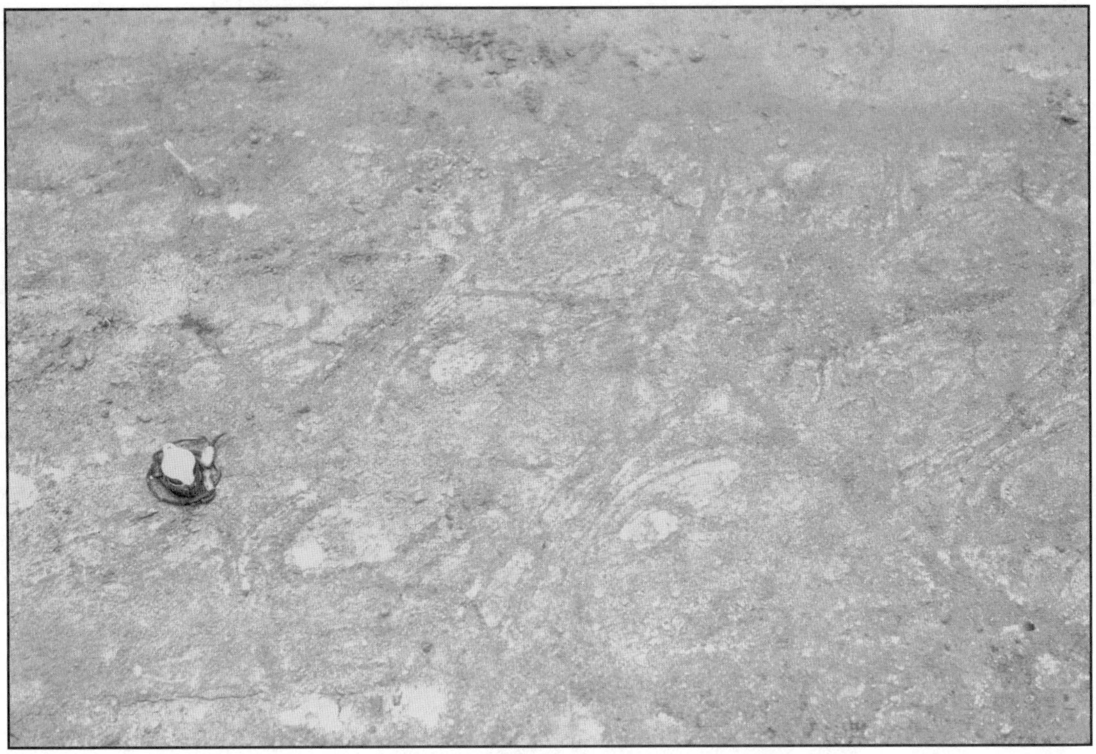

Figure 7. Pillowed meta-volcanic rock of intermediate composition of Miguela A-3 zone.

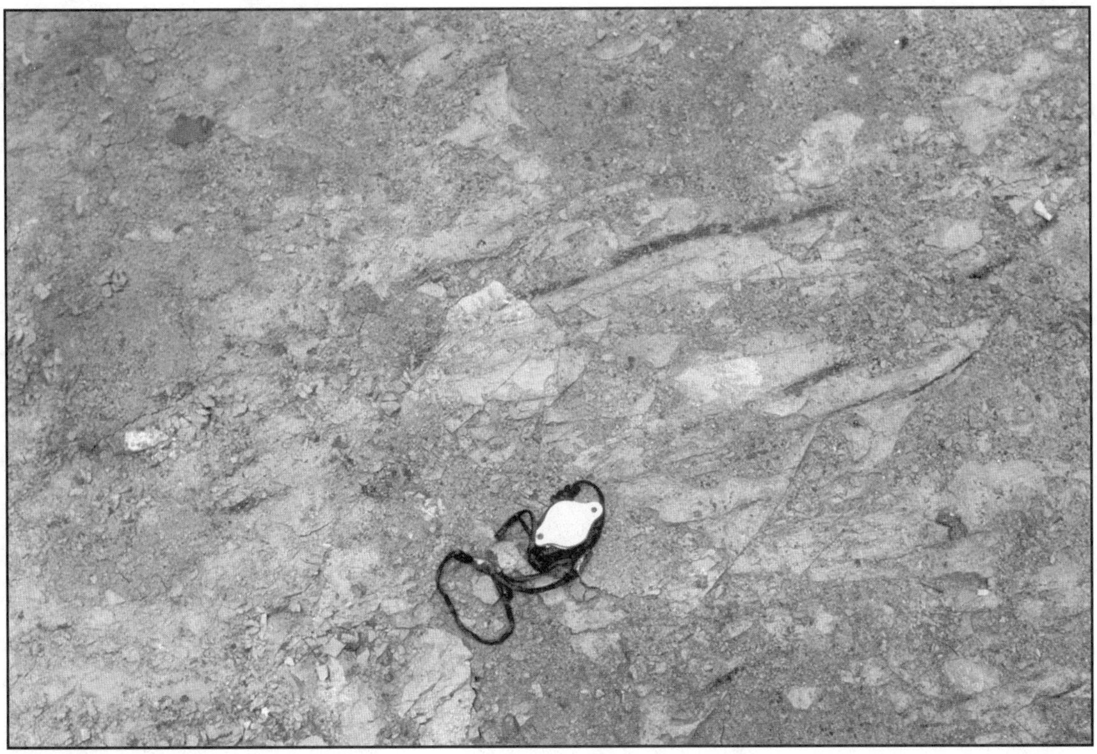

Figure 8. Meta-agglomerate of intermediate composition of Miguela A-3 zone.

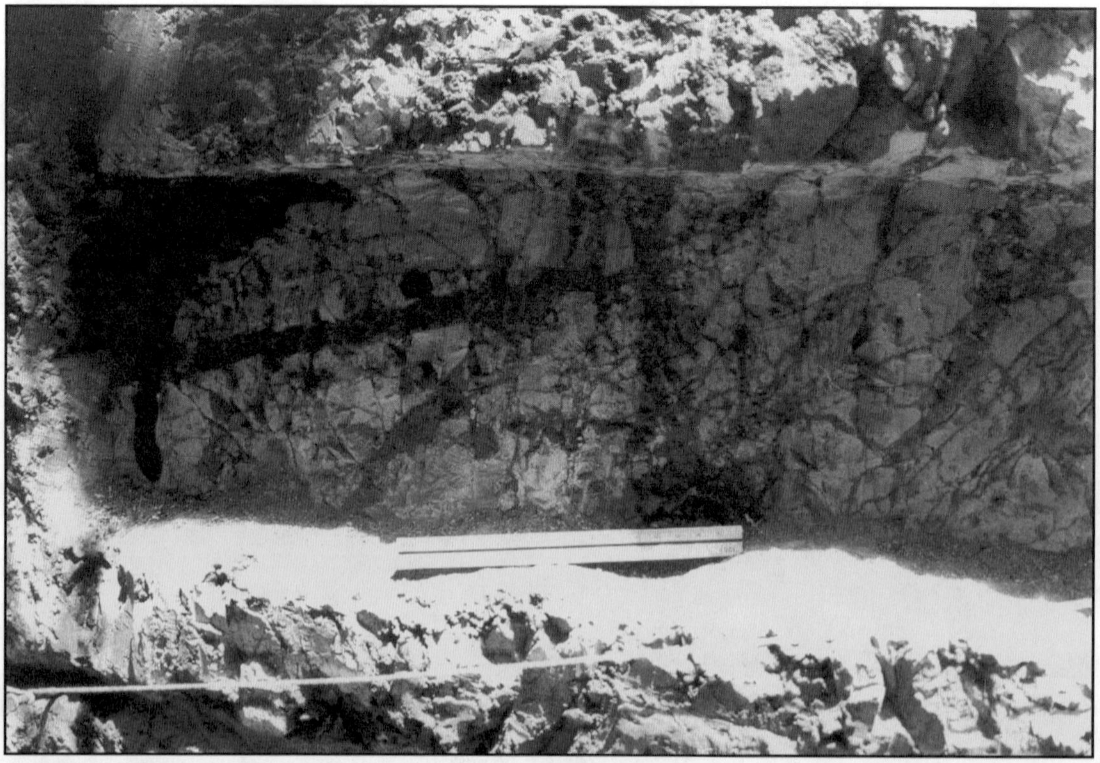

Figure 9. Stockwork mineralization of altered meta-volcanic rock of intermediate composition, Miguela A-3 zone.

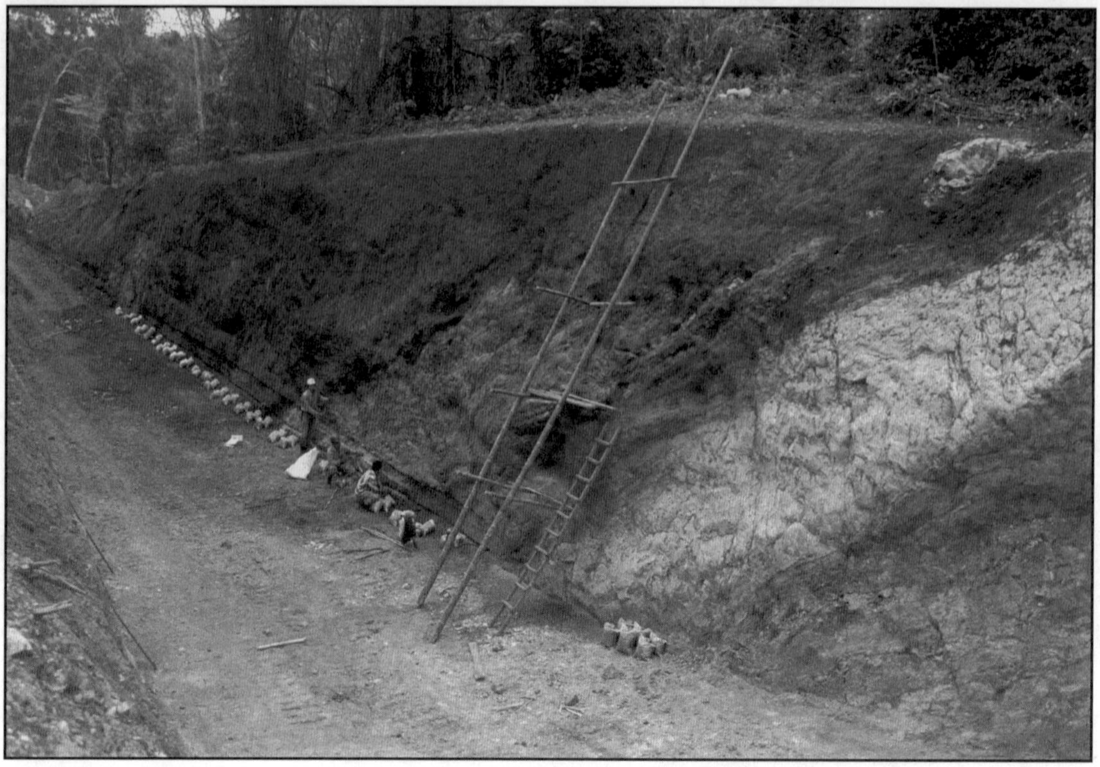

Figure 10. Oxide Zone on top of the Miguela A-1 ore body of deep trench at line 47,000 N.

The sulphide minerals are mostly coarse grained due to strong recrystallization by metamorphism and deformation. For this reason, primary sulphide bedding is rarely preserved, but bedding between sulphide layers and volcanic material is quite common. Stockwork (Fig. 9) mineralization is less frequent, but occurs in the lowermost A-3 body where massive sulphide layers are in contact with andesitic layers.

Hydrothermal Alteration

Hydrothermal alteration occurs both stratabound and semiconformably in the footwall, and laterally to the known VMS mineralization. The alteration assemblage consists of pyrite, muscovite, silica and lesser tourmaline, carbonate and chlorite. The alteration is most intense in the footwall and laterally adjacent to the A-3 lens, and can be traced at least two kilometres to the north within the favourable horizon. The southern limit of the A-Zone is marked by a fault zone, interpreted as synvolcanic, which on local scale has controlled the geometry of the sulphide mineralization and hydrothermal alteration (Fig. 14). The felsic rocks disappear abruptly south of this fault and are replaced by amphibolitic andesite and the serizite/muscovite and pyrite alteration by chlorite and carbonate.

Weathering Zone

The VMS mineralization of the A-Zone exhibits a deep weathering profile, which is due to the lateritization of the regolith since the Miocene. The primary sulphide mineralization is overlain by up to 45 m thick supergene chalcocite and 40 m thick oxide zones. The latter consists of iron-silica-rich rocks and a strata-bound gossan formation with a strong enrichment of gold (Fig. 10). Copper is also enriched in the hangingwall of the strata-bound A-1 Zone mineralization forming a halo of dispersed native copper, chrysocolla, malachite and azurite, and secondary chalcocite averaging 1.12 % copper (Fig. 6).

Metal Distribution

The A-Zone plots in the ternary Zn-Cu-Zn diagram in the field of copper-rich VMS mineralization. Average grades of the diamond drill core samples are set out in Table 1.

Most of the gold and silver is concentrated in the strata-bound massive pyrite-chalcopyrite mineralization reaching maximum values of 8.25 g/t gold and 162 g/t silver respectively. The alteration zone in the footwall of the A-3 zone is highly anomalous in gold but of uneconomic grade. As a rule the gold distribution is erratic and no correlation with any mineralogical parameters can be recognized. The width of the massive and semi-massive sulphide layers diminishes north of the A-Zone and the mineralization becomes richer in zinc, lead and silver.

The drilling at the El Bagre Zone intersected a 340 m thick zone of pyrite/pyrrhotite mineralization, an extensive zone of chloritization and a thin massive pyrite layer with highly anomalous cobalt (411 to 680 ppm). Sulphide mineralization south of the A-Zone is only moderately developed. It is confined to the exhalitic sediments of the "La Pastora" formation and consists of disseminated and well-laminated pyrrhotite, minor pyrite, and traces of sphalerite and chalcopyrite. The base metal content is anomalous, but subeconomic and reaches the highest abundance levels in the southern part of the El Porvenir claim.

Gold is enriched in the oxide zone, where base metals are leached away from the parent rock by deep weathering (Table 2). Copper is highly concentrated in the supergene zone, where gold and base metals are depleted. The best element correlation exists in the primary mineralization, where gold correlates well with silver and copper, and copper with silver. In the oxide and supergene zone gold correlates only with lead (Biste, 1999c).

LITHOCHEMISTRY

The volcanic rocks of the Guarayos greenstone belt were deposited in a subaqueous environment, having been affected by hydrothermal alteration processes during the formation of the VMS mineralization and by regional metamorphism under amphibolitic conditions. For that reason, least altered rock samples were used for a rock classification based on lithochemical composition. Major and minor element analyses were performed by X-Ray-Fluorescence analysis, and trace elements by Atomic Absorption Spectroscopy; both at the laboratory of Bondar Clegg/Inchcape Testing Services of Canada.

Table 1. Average grade of base and precious metals of the different primary mineralization types of the Miguela A-1 zone.

Type of Mineralization	Gold (g/t)	Silver (g/t)	Copper (%)	Zinc (%)	Lead(%)
Massive	1.28	12	3.15	0.55	0.05
Banded	0.27	3	0.30	0.08	0.01
Disseminated	0.01	2	0.08	0.04	0.02

Table 2. Average grade of base and precious metals of the oxide, supergene and primary mineralization of the Miguela A-1 zone.

Type of Mineralization	Gold (g/t)	Silver (g/t)	Copper(%)	Zinc(%)	Lead (%)
Oxide zone, enriched in gold	4.7	7.18	0.14	0.00	0.09
Oxide zone, enriched in copper	0.06	1.30	1.12	0.14	0.00
Supergene zone	0.68	7.54	2.63	0.06	0.01
Primary VMS Mineralization	1.53	13.93	2.29	0.50	0.14

Table 3. Chemical whole rock composition of diamond drill core samples of the Miguela A-1 zone. Reported are average values of individual samples.

Rock Type	n	SiO_2	TiO_2	Al_2O_3	Fe_2O_3	MnO	MgO	CaO	Na_2O	K2O	P_2O_5	Cr	Ba	Sr	Y	Nb	Zr	Rb
Rhyolite	30	76.92	0.29	7.52	6.00	0.01	0.25	0.19	0.26	1.56	0.10	600	216	67	9	19	104	50
Dacite	31	66.25	0.36	14.69	4.39	0.05	1.70	2.36	1.40	2.36	0.11	300	547	173	17	18	153	67
Andesite	19	61.08	0.33	14.93	8.19	0.06	3.49	1.49	0.83	2.56	0.09	500	521	73	12	10	116	59
Gabbro	16	54.76	0.96	18.42	8.26	0.12	3.63	7.68	3.22	1.45	0.20	300	439	297	31	7	198	62
Dacite	11	65.03	0.40	15.38	4.95	0.06	2.36	1.86	5.39	1.61	0.12	200	424	184	21	18	149	62
Agglomerate	64	61.18	0.38	14.67	7.45	0.09	4.04	3.99	1.66	1.81	0.12	300	457	132	15	11	118	61
Tholeiitic Basalt	89	53.77	0.55	14.87	12.46	0.18	5.05	7.91	2.00	0.59	0.11	200	327	185	13	6	109	26

Table 4. Summary of the gold and base metal data used in the resource estimate of the Miguela A-1 zone.

Hole	Width (m)	% Cu	Au g/t	Ag g/t	Zn %
96-3	9.56	6.71	1.07	14.10	0.12
96-4	6.60	7.62	1.49	14.87	0.37
96-5	5.64	3.36	0.46	6.40	0.18
96-13	5.33	3.23	2.29	24.22	0.98
97-25	3.90	1.93	0.93	13.16	0.47
97-26	3.45	3.29	1.35	12.10	0.14
97-27	10.05	1.94	2.47	9.70	0.71
97-28	3.05	1.33	0.77	4.29	0.15

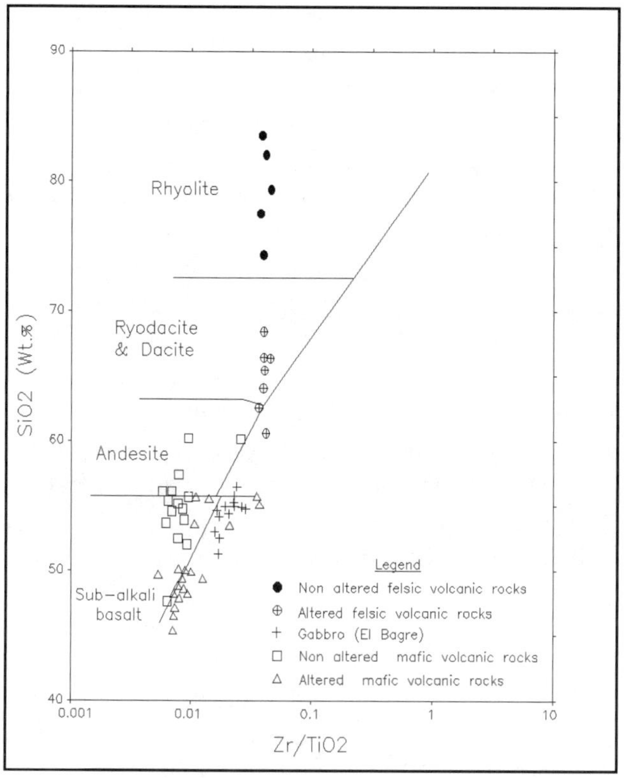

Figure 11. Geochemical Discrimination diagram SiO_2-Zr/TiO_2 of least altered mafic and felsic rocks of the Miguela A-Zone

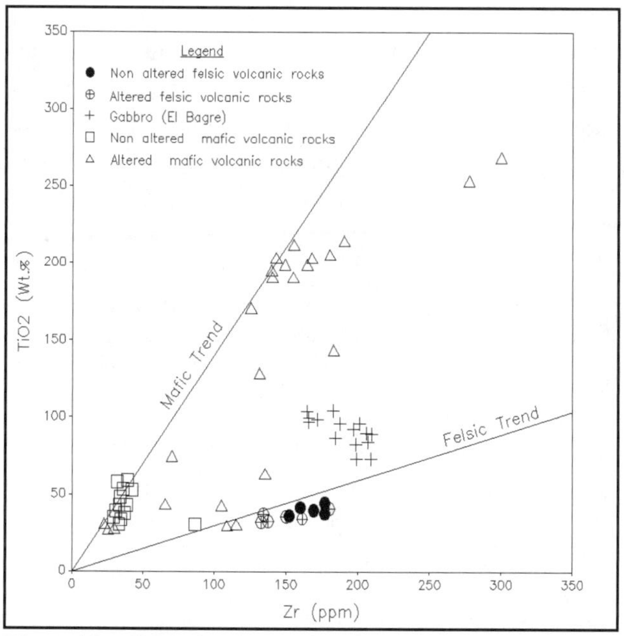

Figure 12. The volcanic rocks of the Miguela A-Zone in the Zr vs. TiO_2 variation diagram

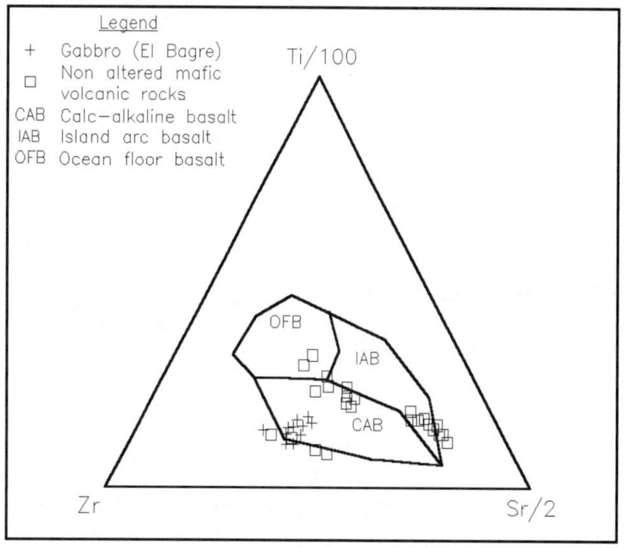

Figure 13. The Miguela greenstone samples in the ternary Ti/100-Zr-Sr/2 diagram

The rocks represent a wide compositional range from basalt to rhyolite. The more mafic varieties contain actinolitic hornblende, tremolite, actinolite, plagioclase, minor biotite, chlorite and epidote plus accessory magnetite, ilmenite, sphene and apatite, and the felsic rocks mainly quartz, plagioclase, muscovite and minor biotite (Craig, 1996, 1997a and 1997b). The SiO_2-Zr/TiO_2 diagram (Winchester and Floyd, 1977) confirms that the host lithology of the Miguela VMS mineralization is andesitic and rhyolitic in composition (Fig. 11). Drill cores, logged as hydrothermically altered, plot in the field of rhyodacite/dacite. The mafic and felsic trend is clearly established in the plot of TiO_2 versus Zr (Fig. 12). The magmatic affinity is tholeiitic according the Y versus Zr diagram. Least-altered mafic rocks plot into the three fields of ocean floor, island arc and calc-alkaline basalts of the Zr-Ti/100-Sr/2 ternary diagram (Fig. 13).

The hydrothermal alteration in the footwall of the A-3 lens mineralization is characterized by sodium depletion of rocks of rhyolitic composition. The material on top of the A-1 lense is quartz rich and carries high barium values of up to 7,199 ppm in a lense of several metres thickness. The chromium content of quartz-rich schist ranges from 200 to 1,300 ppm indicating a possible derivation from mafic to ultramafic material.

RESOURCE ESTIMATE

A preliminary resource estimate has been carried out for the best investigated A-1 lense by an independent consulting geologist (McNamee, 1997). Eight diamond drill holes placed in a small area of the southwestern portion of the upper mineralized level have demonstrated continuity of mineralization in three dimensions. The assay results from these eight drill holes on three section lines were used in the calculation of an Inferred Mineral Resource by application of the following criteria (Table 4).

- The mineralization has a down-dip length of 350 m.
- No projection has been made down-dip beyond the deepest intersection.
- The mineralization has an indicated strike length of 210 m using a projection of 50 m to the north and 50 m to the south of the three section lines.
- The specific gravity of the massive sulphide mineralization is 4.5.

Based on these assumptions, an Inferred Resource of 1,620,000 tonnes has been calculated with weighted average grades of 3.76 % Cu, 1.27 g/t Au, 11.27 g/t Ag and 0.33 % Zn. Assuming that the A-1 lense mineralization is continuous over 450 m of strike length and down-dip for 450 m, it has the potential to host about 4.25 million tonnes of a gold-bearing copper-rich base metal mineralization.

DISCUSSION

The discovery of VMS mineralization at the Miguela A-Zone is a very significant development in the exploration of the Bolivian Shield. The mineralization is hosted in a bimodal tholeiitic metavolcanic sequence of the Guarayos greenstone belt which extends over a distance of about 100 km parallel to the western border of the shield area (Litherland and al., 1996). This belt appears to be of a comparable age of the greenstone belts of the Canadian shield, which host many bodies of VMS mineralization in similar geological conditions. The Miguela VMS mineralization is confined to a felsic unit, informally known as "La Pastora" formation, which has been traced for at least 28 km of strike length, but its limits have not yet been defined. It may extend over the whole length of the Guarayos greenstone belt.

The VMS mineralization of the Miguela A-Zone occurs in three lenses related to two different stratigraphical levels. The mineralization is copper-gold-rich and its formation has probably been controlled by a synvolcanic growth fault system (Fig. 14). The ore bodies are stratabound and no stringer zone has been observed so far. The copper-zinc metal zonation expected in a VMS deposit is not well defined at the A-1 Horizon. However, the drill holes completed north of the A-Zone intersected significant zinc and lead grades. The ore lenses represent sea-floor precipitates and/or a near-sea-floor replacement mineralization within permeable host lithologies of the felsic unit (Large, 1992; Galley et al., 1995; Zalesky and Peterson, 1995). The geological resource potential of the A-1 lens is estimated at over 4 million tonnes. This size compares well with deposits of other VMS districts and places the A-1 resource in the median size category of VMS deposits of Canada and Australia (Large, 1992; Franklin, 1997).

Precambrian VMS deposits are known to occur in clusters and the recognition of three massive sulphide lenses at the A-Zone, and various other significant showings along the strike of the favourable horizon, is an extremely positive development at such an early exploration stage. The presence of known anomalies with geochemical and geophysical signatures comparable to the A-Zone is most encouraging, and provides ample evidence that the Guarayos greenstone belt may have the potential to host a significant VMS camp.

ACKNOWLEDGEMENTS

This paper is the result of an intensive exploration program, which was financed by Tanganika A.V.V. and Essex Resource Corporation. The authors give thank to the Bolivian colleagues and employees of Essex's Santa Cruz office who made with their qualified work an important contribution to this publication. Critical comments by two GAC reviewers were very helpful in refining the manuscript.

BIBLIOGRAPHY

Biste, M.H. 1985. Stata-bound Gold Mineralization in the Precambrian Basement of Eastern Bolivia and the Rondonia/Pará Region (Brazil). In Monograph Series of

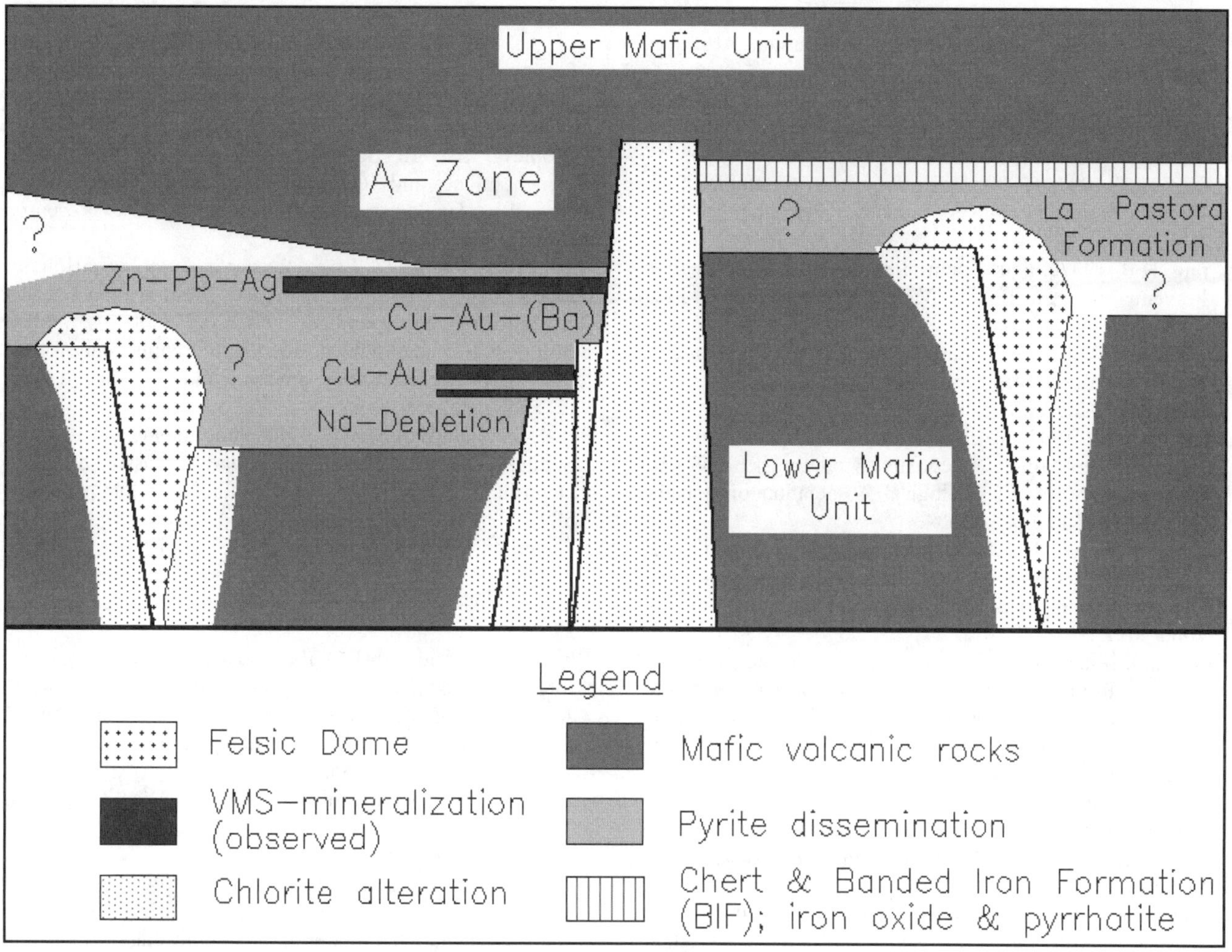

Figure 14 Schematic representation of the VMS mineralization of the Miguela A-Zone

Mineral Deposits 25: 137-150; Gebrüder Borntraeger, Berlin-Stuttgart, 1985.

Biste, M.H., Bufler R. and Friedrich, G. 1991. Geology and Exploration of Gold Placer Deposits of the Pre-Cambrian Shield of Eastern Bolivia. In Gisements Alluviaux d'Or, Alluvial Gold Placer, Yacimientos Aluviales de Oro. Edited by Gérard Hérail et Michel Fonari. Editions de l'ORSTORM, La Paz 1991, pp. 145-158.

Biste, M.H. and Matthews, M.J. 1995. Report on the First Year of Geological Exploration in the Pre-Cambrian Claims of Tanganika A.V.V, Eastern Bolivia. Internal Exploration Report, 17 p.

Biste, M.H. and Matthews, M.J. 1996a. Tanganika A.V.V. - 1995 Work Progress Report and 1996 Work Program and Budget. Internal Exploration Report, 32 p.

Biste, M.H. and Matthews, M.J 1996b. Essex Resource Corporation - 1996 Work Program and Budget for Geological Exploration of the Bolivian Pre-Cambrian Projects. Internal Exploration Report, 11 p.

Biste, M.H. and Matthews, M.J. 1997. Essex Resource Incorporated Bolivia. 1996 Work Progress and 1997 Work Program and Budget. Internal Exploration Report, 36 p.

Biste, M.H. 1998a. Essex Resource Incorporated Bolivia. Results of Geological Exploration. First Phase from 1995 to 1998. El Porvenir Joint Venture COMIBOL - ESSEX, Final Exploration Report, Volume 1 to 10.

Biste, M.H 1998b. Summary Report. The Guarayos VMS-Belt and Its Exploration Potential, Private Consulting Report, 16 p.

Biste, M.H. 1999a. Essex Resource Incorporated Bolivia. 1997 Work Progress and 1998 Work Program and Budget. Internal exploration report, 51 p.

Biste, M.H 1999b. Essex Resource Incorporated Bolivia. Results of Test-Pitting Program, Miguela Zone A, 1998. Internal Exploration Report, 9 p.

Biste, M.H 1999c. Essex Resource Incorporated Bolivia. Miguela Zone A-1. Preliminary Report on Estimation of Mineral Resources as of January 01, 1998. Internal Exploration Report, 18 p.

Bufler, R., Friedrich, G. and Biste, M.H. 1990. Supergene gold enrichment in laterites of the Ascensión de Guarayos area, eastern Bolivia. In Lateinamerika Koloquium, Abstracts, München.

Craig, H.B. 1996. Petrographic Report. 20 Samples from DDH Program, Miguela Concession, Eastern Bolivia. Vancouver Petrographics Ltd., 29 p.

Craig, H.B. 1997a. Petrographic Report on 6 Samples from Miguela Project in Bolivia. Vancouver Petrographics Ltd., 10 p.

Craig, H.B. 1997b. Petrographic Report on 12 Samples from Porvenir Project in Bolivia. Vancouver Petrographics Ltd., 19 p.

DeMatties, T.A. 1994. Early Proterozoic Volcanogenic Massive Sulfide Deposits in Wisconsin: An Overview. Economic Geology, 89: 1122-1151.

Franklin, J.M. 1997. Volcanic-associated Massive Sulphide Deposits. In Mineral Deposits Modeling, Edited by Kirkham, R.V. et al., Geological Association of Canada, Special Paper 40, pp. 315-334.

Galley, A. G. et al. 1995. The Subsea-Floor Formation of Volcanic-Hosted Massive Sulphide: Evidence from the Ansil Deposit, Rouyn-Noranda, Canada. Economic Geology, 90: 2006-2017.

Gibson, H.L. and Kerr, D.J. 1993. Giant volcanic-associated massive sulfide deposits: with emphasis on Archean examples. In Giant Ore Deposits. Edited by Whiting B.H. et al., Special Publication, Number 2, Society of Economic Geologists, pp. 319-348.

Large, R.R. et al. 1989. Gold Distribution and Genesis in Australian Volcanogenic Massive Sulfide Deposits and Their Significance for Gold Transport Models. Economic Geology, 67:520-536.

Large, R.R. 1992. Australian Volcanic-Hosted Massive Sulfide Deposits: Features, Styles, and Genetic Models. Economic Geology, 87: 471-510.

Litherland, M. et al. 1986. The geology and mineral resources of the Bolivian Pre-Cambrian shield. British Geological Survey, Natural Environment Research Council, Overseas Memoir 9, London, Her Majesty's Stationary Office, 153 p.

McNamee, J.A., 1996. Geological Report on the El Porvenir Property, Eastern Bolivia and Review of Preliminary Geochemical and Geophysical Results, Independent Consulting Geologist's Report prepared for Essex Resource Corporation.

McNamee, J.A., 1997. Essex Resource CorporationBolivia, Independent Consulting Geologist's Report prepared for Essex Resource Corporation

Setmin 1999. Leader in the positioning of mining concessions. State of the art technology, precision and efficiency, technical and legal security. 28 p.

Syme, E. C. and Bailes, A. H. 1993. Stratigraphic and Tectonic Setting of early Proterozoic Volcanogenic Massive Sulphide Deposits, Flin Flon, Manitoba, Economic Geology, 88: 566-589.

Winchester, J.A. and Floyd, P.A. 1977. Geochemical discrimination of different magma series and their differentiation products using immobile elements. Chemical Geology, 20: 325-343.

Witchard, F. et al. 1993. Airborne Geophysical Survey and Interpretations of Remote Sensing in the San Ramon Area. Assessment of Mineral Resources of the Pre-Cambrian of Bolivia, Part 1. Boletin del Servicio Geologico de Bolivia, No.2 (Especial), 1993, 55p.

Val d'Or 1997. Geophysical Report. Volume 1 to 3. Empresa Minera Suruqui S.R.L., Miguela Project, Department of Santa Cruz, Bolivia.

Zalesky, E. and Peterson, V.L. 1995. Depositional Setting and Deformation of Massive Sulfide Deposits, Iron Formation, and Associated Alteration in the Manitouwadge Greenstone Belt, Superior province, Ontario. Economic geology, 90: 2244-2261.

REGIONAL SETTING, STRATIGRAPHY, ALTERATION AND MINERALIZATION OF THE TAMBO GRANDE VMS DISTRICT, PIURA DEPARTMENT, NORTHERN PERU

Peter Tegart, Gordon Allen, Andrew Carstensen
Manhattan Minerals Corp., Vancouver, British Columbia, Canada

Abstract

Precious metal-bearing, volcanogenic massive sulphide deposits in the Tambo Grande region of northern Peru rank among the largest of all VMS occurrences in the world. To date, three sulphide deposits are known, and geologic and geophysical data imply that additional occurrences remain to be found. The TG1 deposit, the best known of the three, contains an inferred resource of 64 million tonnes grading 1.7 % Cu, 1.4 % Zn, 0.7g/t Au and 31g/t Ag. A barite oxide cap overlying the sulphides contains an additional resource of 8.2 million tonnes grading 5.2g/t Au and 48g/t Ag. The TG3 deposit, 500 metres south of TG1, contains a resource of 110 million tonnes grading 0.7 % Cu, 1.0 % Zn, 0.7 g/t Au and 19g/t Ag. The deposits, including the newly discovered B5 deposit, 11 km south of TG3, lie proximal to dacite domes emplaced in pre-mid-Cretaceous, tholeiitic-subalkaline basalt flows of the Ereo Formation, a basal member within the northeasterly oriented Lancones Basin. The basin formed within a rifted marine continental margin, between the coastal Amotape ranges and the continental Olmos Massif. Rifting was likely the product of northwesterly directed extensional tectonism as part of the continued continental break-up of Laurentia from Gondwana which began in Middle Jurassic time. Secondary grabens and locally developed Tertiary sub-basins, within the Lancones Basin, are characterized by basalt horsts, dacite domes, flanking volcanic breccias, volcanic conglomerates adjacent to synvolcanic faults and overlying locally derived heterolithic debris flows. Massive sulphides lie within sub-basins. Sulphides filled a deep northwesterly oriented, in part structurally bounded trough at TG1, whereas, TG3 sulphides filled northwesterly elongated basins proximal to a central dacite dome emplaced over a basalt horst. The B5 deposit appears to have a similar setting to the TG1 and TG3 deposits, although the details are as yet unknown. The region has undergone negligible post-mineral tectonism and magmatism, and the deposits are relatively pristine with volcanic and mineralogic textures being well preserved.

The deposits display all the classic characteristics of VMS deposits. These characteristics include a distinct lithologic break from footwall to hangingwall, basal quartz-chlorite stockwork zones and sulphide zoning within the mounds, including barren pyrite cores, basal chalcopyrite replacement, and peripheral zones with mixed chalcopyrite-sphalerite and locally tennantite. Metal contents are similar to compositions of "typical" VMS deposits in bimodal mafic sequences, although the median gold content is higher. The deposits are flat lying and unusually thick, attributable to long-lived hydrothermal systems. The deposits have many similarities, but also significant differences to the well known ancient VMS deposits in the Flin Flon and Noranda camps. The notable differences are in TG1 where late stage supergene copper enrichment in the form of chalcocite and digenite formed a zone at the top and margins of the sulphide pile. Another relatively unusual feature at TG1 is the presence of a late stage auriferous sulphate that overlies the sulphides in the form of a barite cap. Similar deposits are actively being formed in arc and spreading-centre environments on the modern day sea floor in the western Pacific, Juan de Fuca and mid-Atlantic ridges.

Introduction

The newly emerging, world-class volcanogenic massive sulphide (VMS) district at Tambo Grande is located in the Piura River valley at the northern edge of the Sechura coastal plain in northern Peru (Fig. 1). Minimal outcrop occurs in the area and the topography is relatively flat, with elevations ranging from 60 m to 200 m above sea level. Present economic activity in the area is agriculturally based, centered on the town of Tambogrande, 100 km east of the deep-sea port of Paita on the Pacific. Access by paved highways and secondary roads is excellent.

The base-metal potential of the area was recognized in the mid 1970's by the French state-owned mineral exploration and research group, Le Bureau de Recherches, Geologiques et Minieres (BRGM), in cooperation with the Instituto Geologico Minero y Metalurgico (INGEMMET), the state geological agency of Peru. Following up on iron oxide occurences documented in the Boletin de la Sociedad Geologica Del Peru (1904), BRGM collected rock samples in the town of Tambogrande that returned weakly anomalous base metal and silver values. Drilling of a self-potential geophysical anomaly by BRGM in 1978 resulted in the discovery of base metal massive sulphides in the TG1 deposit. Later detailed gravity surveys of TG1 defined a positive surface anomaly outlining the deposit. Based on 21 drill holes to the end of 1981, an inferred resource of 42.3 million tonnes grading 2.04 % Cu, 1.45 % Zn, 0.35 % Pb and 38.4 g/t Ag was outlined (BRGM, 1981). Injoque et al (1979) and Pouit (1981) describe

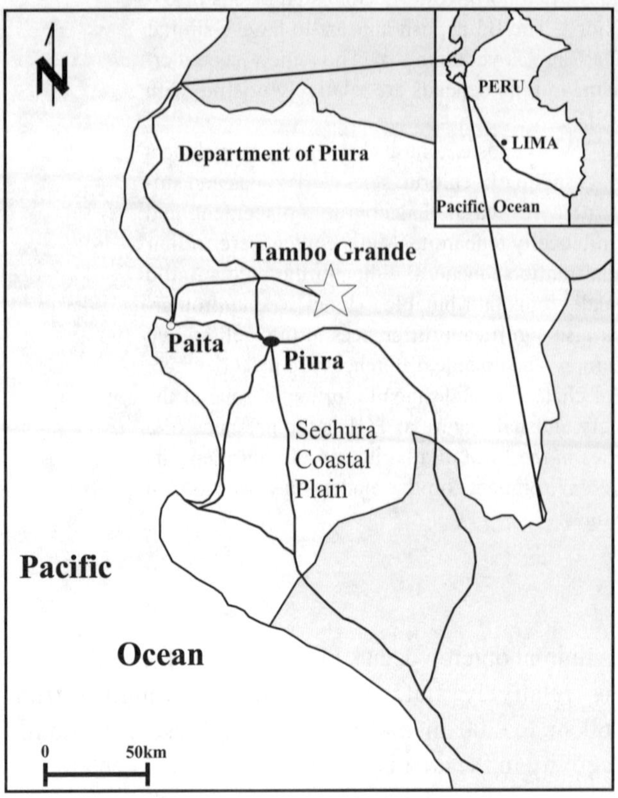

Figure 1. Location map of the Tambo Grande VMS district.

previous geological investigations of the deposit. Further exploration of the property was curtailed until May 1999 when Manhattan Minerals Corp. completed an agreement with the Peruvian government to explore and develop the resources of the area.

The ongoing diamond drilling program by Manhattan has partially defined two distinct separate deposits by diamond drilling and a third has recently been discovered. The deposits, TG1, TG3 and B5 (named after their associated gravity anomalies) are unusually thick, flat lying and, except for B5, near surface. The occurrences display typical characteristics of VMS deposits, including a distinct break in lithology from footwall to hangingwall, an oxide "cap" (TG1), a zinc-rich upper and distal zone, and increasing copper near the base. Chalcopyrite-sphalerite mineralogic zoning in the two deposits is similar, but at TG1 an upper and peripheral chalcocite-digenite enriched zone and a gold-barite-oxide cap occur. The deposits formed concomitantly with volcanism of the Ereo Formation, a pre-Albian, dominantly mafic volcanic assemblage deposited in the early stage of development of the Lancones Basin. The deposits are relatively unmetamorphosed with most volcanic and mineralogic textures being well preserved.

The TG1 sulphide deposit, measuring 950 m long, 350 m wide and ranging to over 200 m thick, occupies a northwesterly-elongated intra-basin graben. The inferred sulphide resource at TG1 is 64.2 million tonnes grading 1.7 % Cu, 1.4 % Zn, 0.7 g/t Au, and 31 g/t Ag contained within a larger 100 million tonne pyrite body. A flat-lying sequence of exhalative auriferous barite units, grading upwards to goethite precipitate or replacement deposit, directly overlies and extends beyond the limits of the sulphides. The barite gold resource lies under an average of 15 m of sand and gravel and contains an inferred resource of 8.2 million tonnes grading 5.2 g/t Au and 48 g/t Ag .

The TG3 deposits, 500 m south of the southern margin of the TG1 deposit, consist of multiple stacked sulphide lenses flanking a dacite dome. The deposits are overlain by volcanic debris flows and basalt which together have an average thickness of 120 m. Sulphides are contained in two mounds, one of which measures up to 300 m thick and 500 m across. The inferred sulphide resource at TG3 is 110 million tonnes grading 0.7 % Cu, 1.0 % Zn, 0.7 g/t Au and 19 g/t Ag .

A third massive sulphide body associated with the B5 gravity anomaly, 11 km south of TG3, was discovered in January 2000. Although little is known about the deposit, 280 m of massive sulphides were intersected and appear similar to mineralization at TG1 and TG3.

Manhattan Minerals' exploration and feasibility studies through June, 2000, consisted of gravity, magnetometer and electro-magnetic geophysical surveys, and detailed logging of more than 70,000 m of core in over 400 holes. Gravity, magnetic and in part electromagnetic surveys were interpreted by correlating the geophysical response to specific gravity, magnetic susceptibility, and rock conductivity measurements from core samples. The interpretive geophysics was used to define district geologic trends. The studies summarized here draw on results from approximately 16,000 sulphide core samples analysed for base and precious metal content, trace-element analyses, and 150 polish- thin sections. A preliminary set of 72 lithogeochemical and whole-rock analyses, in addition to thin sections of volcanic host rocks is described and interpreted together with petrographic observations of primary volcanic and secondary alteration textures. The overall paleo-tectonic setting of the deposits is interpreted relative to the regional geologic setting in the Lancones Basin as described by Reyes and Caldas (1987), Chaez et al. (1991), Morris and Aleman (1975) and its relationship to the geodynamic evolution of northern Peru (Mourier et al,1988; Jaillard et al, 1990; Macellari, 1988; Mitouard et al, 1990). The deposit settings are compared on the basis of chemistry to modern marine volcanic systems and some ancient VMS deposits.

REGIONAL GEOLOGIC SETTING

Stratigraphy

The Tambo Grande massive sulphide district in northern Peru formed contemporaneously with a pre-Albian (Mid Cretaceous) marine rift known as the Lancones Basin (Fig. 2). Mafic and less common silicic volcanic and volcaniclastic rocks, from stratigraphic lowest to highest, of the Ereo and La Bocana Formations filled the basin (Reyes and Caldas, 1987). These rocks are exposed in a 40 km wide by 80 km long northeasterly plunging anticline located along the southeastern side of the basin. The southwestward extent of the volcanic sequence is not known because Tertiary continental sedimentary rocks of the Sechura Basin cover the Lancones Basin.

The Ereo Formation consists of 500 m or more of basalt pillow lava flows intercalated with hyaloclastic breccias, minor dacite flows and tuff beds, and lesser volcaniclastic strata. Dykes of basaltic and possibly andesitic composition intrude them. Preliminary rock geochemical data from the Ereo Formation (Table 1) have tholeiitic to sub-alkaline affinities, similar to volcanic rocks erupted in marine or oceanic back-arc settings. The base of the Ereo Formation has not been observed. The basal Ereo is unconformably overlain by 250 m of Upper Albian agglomeratic andesite and dacite interbedded with calcareous arenite, impure limestone, greywacke, tuff and ignimbrite of the La Bocana Formation. Approximately 1500 m of the Lancones Formation lies conformably on the La Bocana on the east and west flank of the anticline, but is absent along the anticlinal crest. On the eastern flank of the anticline, the Lancones Formation is composed primarily of massive andesitic pyroclastic rocks, whereas the western flank is composed of grey-green to grey-violet andesitic pyroclastic rocks and interbedded sedimentary layers of calcareous arenites and greywacke. Numerous minor base-metal and barite occurrences are also found in the La Bocana Formation. The basin extends north into Ecuador where volcanism, coeval with Lancones Basin basal sequences, is represented by andesitic flows and volcaniclastic rocks of the Celica and Macuchi Formations (Macellari, 1988). These rocks also host volcanogenic massive sulphide occurrences.

The depocenter of the Lancones Basin shifted westward in Cenomanian time with deposition of the Copa Sombrero Formation consisting of flysch successions up to 3700 m thick (Fig. 2). The formation is represented in the lower units by debris flows, turbiditic sandstone and breccias intruded by igneous sills and dykes. Up-section the stratigraphic sequence changes to a finer turbidite facies consisting of rhythmically interbedded black shale and greywacke

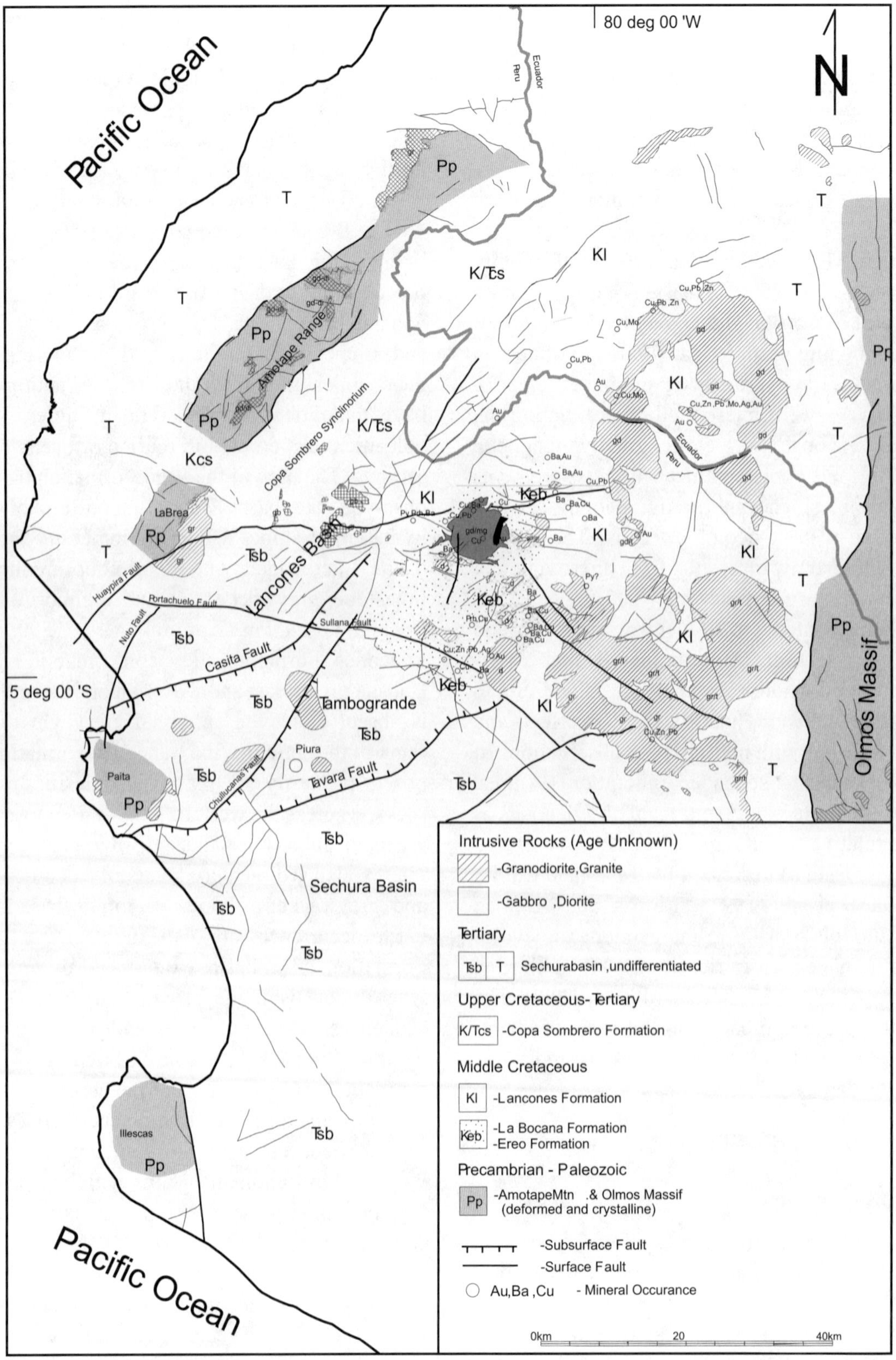

Figure 2. Simplified regional geology of the Lancones Basin (modified after Reves and Caldas. 1987: Petro Peru-unpublished reports).

Table 1. Chemical composition of representative volcanic rocks from the TG1 and TG3 deposits.

Sample ID	SiO2	TiO2	Al2O3	Fe2O3	MnO	MgO	CaO	Na2O	K2O	P2O5	LOI	Total	Cr2O3	Ba	Sr	Y	Nb	Zr	Rb
80TG1-019-170.60	73.88	0.21	10.37	2.41	0.04	1.44	1.50	0.19	2.95	0.05	3.01	99.60	0.07	10000	142	31	8	125	63
80TG1-010-126.40	71.68	0.27	13.26	1.41	0.05	0.43	2.42	5.96	0.71	0.06	2.64	99.05	0.03	961	72	54	18	175	41
79TG1-008-198.20	71.37	0.17	8.60	8.06	0.08	5.51	0.30	0.09	0.51	0.01	4.24	99.08	0.02	988	-5	36	15	132	26
79TG1-009-180.80	69.52	0.17	8.57	9.13	0.07	6.62	0.05	0.09	0.12	0.02	4.70	99.11	0.01	187	-5	30	13	128	17
80TG1-012-104.00	67.71	0.30	13.86	4.94	0.08	1.80	1.53	3.52	1.65	0.06	3.31	99.03	0.02	2119	73	59	11	181	63
80TG1-013-111.90	62.25	0.37	17.85	5.50	0.07	2.81	0.48	2.23	3.11	0.06	4.26	99.25	0.02	1967	48	71	11	270	93
80TG1-016-146.40	68.77	0.35	10.37	7.54	0.03	0.79	0.74	0.20	2.60	0.06	6.59	98.42	0.14	2217	13	34	9	96	67
80TG1-002-107.70	68.41	0.25	11.72	5.75	0.05	2.70	0.92	2.55	1.55	0.05	4.64	98.83	0.03	1718	147	53	13	174	51
80TG1-010-143.30	71.24	0.22	11.66	4.09	0.05	0.99	1.59	5.49	0.40	0.05	2.73	98.65	0.05	659	88	40	14	140	33
80TG1-012-112.60	71.74	0.24	11.97	3.08	0.04	1.10	2.13	5.84	0.08	0.05	2.55	98.93	0.04	383	90	59	19	163	22
80TG1-002-103.40	67.20	0.25	12.44	8.15	0.02	0.93	0.06	0.12	3.02	0.02	6.43	98.91	0.05	1878	8	52	12	175	62
99TG1-061-371.05	68.85	0.21	11.35	6.30	0.08	5.55	0.23	0.41	1.07	0.04	4.36	98.57	0.01	798	40	8	153	41	
79TG1-003-250.50	63.23	0.18	9.44	12.04	0.08	7.72	0.08	0.05	0.06	0.02	5.84	98.79	0.01	134	-5	25	6	124	14
79TG1-007-215.90	71.97	0.19	8.29	9.38	0.07	4.29	0.14	0.14	0.47	0.04	3.98	99.04	0.02	445	-5	24	9	110	21
80TG1-015-103.15	66.52	0.23	11.77	9.66	0.12	1.65	0.31	0.44	1.79	0.05	5.36	98.46	0.02	5128	50	39	7	165	48
79TG1-005-89.00	64.87	0.38	15.30	6.36	0.08	2.83	0.37	5.66	0.36	0.08	2.57	99.04	0.03	1166	64	64	16	213	33
79TG1-004-169.20	46.26	0.69	14.96	11.85	0.21	14.10	0.29	2.22	0.03	0.07	8.64	99.38	0.03	196	22	17	6	36	20
80TG1-002-55.50	50.25	0.87	16.75	10.81	0.12	8.17	3.50	3.03	1.10	0.05	4.77	99.84	0.02	3579	333	16	5	54	26
80TG1-012-56.40	49.44	0.80	15.50	11.66	0.17	6.80	3.90	5.20	0.04	0.13	5.53	99.26	0.01	525	104	19	6	40	13
80TG1-020-87.60	43.79	1.28	16.37	14.00	0.35	9.93	1.09	2.41	1.05	0.18	8.58	99.12	0.01	472	106	16	1	61	24
99TG1-062-148.30	47.24	0.66	15.39	7.58	0.15	13.13	2.71	2.12	0.50	0.06	8.35	98.15	0.04	1980	19	1	43	28	
99TG1-062-175.20	48.31	0.80	16.60	8.86	0.30	11.86	1.59	3.36	0.06	0.07	6.50	98.36	0.01	246	20	1	48	11	
99TG1-059-83.50	47.25	0.86	15.87	10.76	0.10	8.47	4.59	4.37	0.10	0.06	5.78	98.25	-0.01	187	16	1	36	12	
99TG1-059-100.40	49.09	1.09	15.77	10.81	0.07	8.97	3.48	1.92	0.53	0.12	7.15	99.06	0.01	256	18	1	57	22	
80TG1-013-117.10	44.65	0.84	15.19	9.97	0.21	10.05	8.32	1.58	0.39	0.17	8.13	99.63	0.05	401	254	17	7	63	20
80TG1-016-161.20	42.35	0.87	14.78	9.25	0.12	5.94	13.77	1.98	0.43	0.19	9.51	99.33	0.05	472	343	16	1	74	21
79TG1-006-94.00	59.65	0.97	15.96	7.55	0.12	2.97	5.07	5.00	0.07	0.22	2.29	99.95	0.02	231	230	29	9	128	21
79TG1-007-110.20	61.01	0.78	15.45	6.27	0.13	2.75	3.50	3.69	0.99	0.20	4.37	99.37	0.01	1736	166	36	8	147	40
79TG1-004-162.40	51.31	0.88	18.69	8.23	0.21	3.19	4.51	4.19	1.60	0.35	6.33	99.63	-0.01	819	376	25	9	87	55
80TG1-020-90.80	48.31	0.78	19.21	7.74	0.19	3.40	5.65	4.01	1.98	0.27	7.94	99.60	-0.01	801	255	26	10	76	57
80TG1-019-87.80	61.48	0.73	14.11	6.36	0.26	3.56	2.39	0.39	3.57	0.19	3.64	99.74	0.02	10000	225	29	1	130	61
80TG1-019-155.50	82.31	0.84	0.42	4.67	-0.01	0.07	0.15	0.08	0.04	0.03	6.83	98.45	0.06	10000	228	5	7	47	17
79TG1-005-76.70	97.75	0.29	0.21	0.49	-0.01	0.05	0.06	0.02	0.02	0.02	0.35	99.33	0.03	-50	40	42	17	216	31
79TG1-009-40.60	93.86	2.61	0.24	0.56	-0.01	0.06	0.05	0.02	0.02	0.02	1.53	99.79	0.03	7522	132	15	23	128	26
80TG1-020-59.40	92.43	1.63	0.45	1.44	-0.01	0.05	0.07	0.07	0.06	0.03	0.89	100.80	0.05	10000	211	15	15	196	25
79TG1-007-99.15	93.05	0.97	0.27	0.64	-0.01	0.03	0.09	0.01	0.05	0.02	4.54	99.72	0.02	-50	48	30	25	189	31
79TG1-007-84.00	95.54	0.81	0.26	1.32	-0.01	0.01	0.05	0.01	0.05	0.02	1.47	99.66	0.09	-50	59	17	22	160	31
79TG1-009-52.20	92.15	0.30	0.39	3.02	-0.01	0.05	0.08	-0.01	0.08	0.01	2.19	98.34	0.03	-50	73	22	16	193	25
79TG1-009-66.00	94.55	0.46	0.82	0.67	-0.01	0.09	0.10	0.11	0.11	0.02	0.84	100.01	0.06	10000	146	30	18	261	24
80TG1-016-78.70	93.76	0.38	0.72	1.10	-0.01	0.06	0.06	0.10	0.15	0.01	1.17	99.29	0.06	10000	124	19	19	199	34
80TG1-019-70.40	86.38	0.43	0.42	3.76	-0.01	0.05	0.06	0.08	0.06	0.01	3.21	99.57	0.11	10000	97	19	8	184	19

Table 1. Chemical composition of representative volcanic rocks from the TG1 and TG3 deposits (continued).

SampleID	SiO2	TiO2.1	Al2O3	Fe2O3	MnO	MgO	CaO	Na2O	K2O	P2O5	LOI	Total	Cr2O3	Ba	Sr	Y	Nb	Zr	Rb
99TG3-001-140.50	51.69	0.79	14.95	5.90	0.14	3.07	7.41	4.93	0.41	0.14	9.13	98.64	0.01	404	79	29	-5	89	19
99TG3-011-198.5	61.05	0.76	14.83	7.14	0.15	2.65	4.63	4.65	0.24	0.16	2.63	98.98	0.02	246	192	38	8	132	24
99TG3-003-109.40	45.39	0.87	16.34	8.31	0.20	5.66	9.18	4.63	0.04	0.17	8.45	99.29	0.01	112	81	20	-5	55	10
99TG3-001-71.40	58.37	0.84	15.42	8.07	0.14	3.66	2.38	5.55	0.16	0.10	4.06	98.79	0.02	99	88	27	7	76	11
99TG3-001-119.10	56.42	0.77	14.79	7.95	0.16	2.94	4.26	4.20	0.93	0.09	5.97	98.57	0.01	473	52	28	5	103	41
99TG3-002-63.09	55.81	0.85	15.97	9.43	0.15	3.22	8.22	2.62	0.04	0.10	2.88	99.35	0.02	89	207	26	-5	80	9
99TG3-002-111.86	61.54	0.74	14.71	6.93	0.12	2.84	5.36	4.12	0.11	0.10	2.90	99.52	0.02	89	159	30	6	90	16
99TG3-015-192	51.94	0.77	14.30	12.76	0.17	3.68	6.01	3.87	0.09	0.08	5.23	99.21	0.03	2690	123	19	-5	67	9
99TG3-003-32.50	44.54	0.99	16.68	12.31	0.18	8.20	6.77	2.66	0.67	0.13	6.70	99.92	0.02	414	188	16	-5	44	15
99TG3-003-86.40	48.67	0.97	16.51	10.65	0.14	7.00	8.98	1.85	0.58	0.09	4.61	100.15	0.02	246	400	10	-5	59	17
99TG3-002-49.20	46.92	0.88	14.86	11.05	0.19	8.35	7.86	3.67	0.39	0.19	4.50	98.96	0.02	217	328	15	-5	49	21
99TG3-003-77.50	45.33	1.12	15.65	10.41	0.15	6.31	8.02	4.53	0.25	0.16	7.45	99.44	0.01	207	126	20	-5	47	12
99TG3-003-191.90	47.77	1.01	15.85	9.03	0.17	8.64	4.85	1.40	0.77	0.18	9.09	98.95	0.04	1300	119	19	6	61	30
99TG3-013-63.75	46.35	0.94	15.11	8.15	0.17	10.25	9.24	1.59	1.39	0.19	5.85	99.40	0.09	463	190	16	-5	70	47
99TG3-001-58.30	47.39	1.37	15.71	9.14	0.18	7.53	5.58	4.32	0.12	0.25	7.28	98.96	0.05	177	112	23	-5	101	10
99TG3-001-90.80	44.29	1.22	16.89	9.17	0.23	8.27	4.91	2.73	2.12	0.22	8.06	98.36	0.05	1572	269	25	-5	110	41
99TG3-002-150.00	49.90	0.88	15.58	9.91	0.12	5.49	10.23	4.36	0.06	0.24	3.37	100.20	0.02	158	102	23	-5	47	19
99TG3-003-26.61	47.58	1.05	16.75	9.98	0.18	8.84	5.77	4.15	0.51	0.18	4.58	99.67	0.04	286	271	21	-5	73	24
99TG3-011-230.73	46.62	1.24	14.88	8.23	0.15	9.29	7.08	2.80	0.40	0.22	8.04	99.14	0.05	946	349	23	6	102	16
99TG3-002-80.60	46.02	0.89	15.14	10.09	0.17	6.78	12.85	2.03	0.69	0.21	4.21	99.18	0.01	414	336	9	-5	55	29
99TG3-013-174.9	72.14	0.29	12.09	2.16	0.06	0.69	2.45	5.33	0.57	0.05	3.12	99.19	0.02	1852	103	51	9	192	41
99TG3-002-187.30	72.63	0.16	10.56	2.49	0.05	0.55	4.17	0.22	2.64	0.03	5.24	98.97	0.04	1468	34	47	12	175	68
99TG3-013-206	68.95	0.34	12.78	4.02	0.09	1.03	2.63	3.96	1.27	0.06	3.73	98.96	0.02	325	78	51	10	212	56
99TG3-015-300	71.24	0.22	10.23	3.31	0.10	0.78	4.05	3.52	0.80	0.05	4.36	99.24	0.03	5143	140	49	8	163	35
99TG3-001-243.00	71.48	0.32	13.02	2.64	0.04	0.81	1.67	5.80	0.41	0.07	2.40	98.73	0.01	148	42	53	15	207	31
99TG3-002-228.30	68.59	0.26	14.29	3.21	0.04	0.78	1.80	7.56	0.08	0.05	2.58	99.29	0.01	69	56	42	16	176	29
99TG3-008-170.3	60.37	0.45	15.46	5.35	0.02	1.09	1.96	1.74	3.32	0.11	6.52	97.47	-0.01	10000	213	66	-5	219	92
99TG3-011-319.13	75.21	0.23	10.74	3.22	0.04	0.50	1.32	4.45	0.61	0.05	2.65	99.11	0.03	266	68	50	11	147	31
Cerro 1	65.74	0.54	13.89	3.48	0.11	0.73	4.89	4.81	1.01	0.15	3.94	99.41	0.02	481	233	45	18	138	39
Cerro 2	66.23	0.41	12.52	5.46	0.09	1.14	3.46	5.31	0.52	0.10	3.97	99.30	0.03	285	64	50	14	155	32
9TG3-011-242.93	74.22	0.23	12.03	2.68	0.04	0.47	1.19	4.06	1.21	0.03	2.23	98.54	0.04	778	112	59	17	209	53
99TG3-003-314.2	70.85	0.34	12.01	5.23	0.07	3.45	0.28	0.11	2.30	0.08	3.90	98.81	0.02	1429	-5	49	11	170	66
Cerro 3	78.07	0.20	10.93	1.24	0.02	0.27	0.73	4.65	0.88	0.05	1.47	98.60	0.04	187	30	49	15	167	64

sandstone. Uplift and erosion of the La Brea-Amotape Mountains to the west provided Paleozoic metamorphic clasts found along the western margin of the basin in the Copa Sombrero Formation. Paleocurrent data from these members have an average azimuth orientation of 40 degrees indicating a northeastward basinal paleoslope, likely resulting from an emerging paleo-high located to the southwest (Iddings and Olsson, 1928; Kennerly, 1973; Morris and Aleman, 1975; Reyes and Caldas, 1987; Chavez and Nunez del Prado, 1991). Present day Paleozoic exposures at La Brea, Paita, Illescas and Lobos de Tierra, and the absence of Mesozoic strata in the subsurface south of present day Piura city (Alencastre, 1980), suggest the Lancones depositional basin was bordered on the southwest by paleo-highs much as it is today. The Basin extended northward into Ecuador where deposition, equivalent to the Copa Sombrero Formation, is contained in the Napo Formation (Macellari, 1988).

Intrusive stocks within the Lancones Basin form part of the Upper Mesozoic and Cenozoic Coastal Batholith that stretches the length of western Peru (Reyes and Caldas, 1987). Within the Lacones Basin, the intrusions are composed entirely of gabbro and diorite, and are confined to a relatively small area north of Tambogrande. The small gabbro stocks are dominated by augite–orthopyroxene porphyries, but some contain olivine with ophilitic and metamorphic textures. The diorite ranges from fine to medium-grained, with grey-green zoned plagioclase, hornblende and accessory biotite. The age of these intrusions has not been determined, but chemically they are similar to the basal mafic volcanic series in the Lancones Basin (Ereo Fm), and therefore, these intrusions may be the subvolcanic equivalent of the volcanics. Peripheral to the basic intrusions are granodiorite and monzonite stocks, analogous to the Western Peruvian batholiths. These are found around the margin of the basin (Reyes and Caldas, 1987).

At the end of the Cretaceous, the tectonic setting of the northern Andean Cordillera changed. As a result, a thick sequence of Tertiary, continentally derived, marine sediments and local felsic volcanic units (Alencastre, 1980) was deposited on the southern portion of the Lancones Basin, and northern part of the younger, continental Sechura Basin that lies to the south. The Piura river in the Tambogrande area coincides with the present day northern limit of the continental basin. The stratigraphic sequence is characterized by intercalated grey-green-maroon marine lutite, poorly consolidated sandy layers, pebble conglomerate cemented with calcite, white friable marl, evaporite, and containing carbonaceous fragments. South of the Piura river, up to 100 m of Pleistocene sand with minor caliche deposits and coarse-pebble conglomerate cemented with calcite covers the Tertiary sequence. Water from wells drilled in this strata is typically salty. The thick accumulation of Tertiary sedimentary rocks and Pleistocene aeolian sand deposits that overlie the VMS deposits hosted in Cretaceous volcanics south of Tambogrande have made exploration challenging.

Structure

The Lancones Basin developed as a northeast-trending marginal continental graben formed by rifting along the northwestern coast of South America during the late stages of Gondwana breakup in Upper Jurassic and Cretaceous time. The basin lies within the coastal area of the Andes in the Huancabamba deflection, a major change in the orogen strike. A complete hiatus of post-Permian and pre-Albian deposition characterize the region, although the basal Ereo Formation has not been dated. The rift basin is located east of the Devonian miogeoclinal carbonate rocks, which unconformably overlie polyphased metamorphic rocks of Precambrian age of the Amotape Mountains, and west of the Olmos Massif, the continental-equivalent assemblage. Significant crustal thinning likely occured within the basin and oceanic rocks probably underlie the entire area as evidenced by a strong (100 mgal) positive Bouguer gravity anomaly coincident with the Amotape Range and Lancones Basin (Braban, 1987; Mourier et al, 1988).

The subsurface features of the Sechura Basin, south of the Lancones Basin, are documented in well logs from oil exploration (Alencaste, 1980; Petro Peru, unpublished well logs). Faults in the underlying Paleozoic sedimentary rocks and the distribution of Cretaceous volcanic rocks in the subsurface indicate that the Lancones Basin is a major first-order graben. Northeasterly trending faults within underlying older rocks do not cut unconformably overlying Tertiary strata. The faults can be projected from the Paita paleo-high to the Ereo volcanic terrain south of Tambogrande (Fig. 2). These faults also correlate with mapped sites in the Lancones Basin north of Tambogrande. All outcrop of Cretaceous volcanics in the Basin are contained within the projected northeast-trending Casita, Chulucanas and Tavara Faults (Tavara Fault inferred from gravity data). In addition, most basic intrusions, as well as all the copper, zinc and barite occurrences lie between these fault projections.

In plan view, an arcuate set of easterly striking faults is observed to cut Lower Cretaceous basin rocks and influence deposition of overlying Tertiary sedimentary rocks. Cretaceous volcanic rocks on the north side of these faults are consistently down dropped. The faults become tangential to the dominant northwesterly Andean trend east of the basin. These faults are also observed in well drilling (Petro Peru, unpublished reports), and seismic profiles exhibit northerly dips and normal movement with north side down (Fig. 2). The Huaypira, Portachuela and Sullana faults are mappable (Reyes and Caldas, 1987), whereas others are visible on satellite images. Government magnetometer and gravity surveys (Alencastre, 1980), and recent geophysical surveys in the area by Manhattan Minerals substantiate the projection of these faults.

Tectonic and depositional model - Lancones Basin

The Lancones Basin resulted from northwestward extension. Basalt, andesite and volcaniclastic sedimentary rocks were deposited prior to Middle Cretaceous time and filled a northeasterly oriented graben bounded by the Casita fault on the northwest and the projected Tavara fault on the southeast. Over 1000 m of volcanic flows and sedimentary derivatives were deposited in this restricted basin. Considering that the base of the Ereo volcanics is unknown, the volcanic sequence is likely much thicker and could have commenced deposition as early as Upper Jurassic time. The proposed graben and subsequent development of the Lancones Basin resulting from northwestward extension produced a northeasterly trending rift separating the Amotape Paleozoic shelf carbonates from their continental equivalent to the east. The resultant thinning of continental crust behind the Amotape Mountains was extreme, and allowed basaltic magma to penetrate and erupt undiluted within the Lancones Basin. Mourier et al, (1988) concluded from paleomagnetic measurements that Devonian strata in the Amotape Mountains underwent clockwise rotation from the main Andean trend. This is consistent with a northwest extensional environment and resulting northeasterly oriented graben-bounding faults.

The southwesterly extension of the Lancones Basin is restricted by the Illescas, Paita and La Brea paleo-highs. Cretaceous lithologies are also absent under Tertiary sedimentary rocks as recorded in oil well logs drilled as far northeast the city of Piura. Northeasterly directed paleo-currents recorded in the Copa Sombrero Formation also suggest development of a paleo-high, southwest of the Lancones Basin in Cretaceous time.

Jaillard et al (1990) proposed that during Early to Middle Mesozoic times the sedimentary and magmatic history of the north-northeast-trending Colombian-Ecuadorian Andes and the northwest-trending Peruvian coastal Andes exhibited a spatially contrasting evolution involving several successive tectonic and geodynamic settings. The Lancones Basin is situated near the junction of these contrasting western Andean continental margins at 5 degrees south latitude in what has been called the Huancabamba deflection. A geodynamic reconstruction of the Caribbean region (Pindell and Dewey, 1982; Klitgord and Schouten, 1986; Ross and Scotese, 1988) assumes a continuous western margin from northern Mexico to northern Peru in Early-Mesozoic times. During Early to Middle Jurassic times rifting, due to the northwestward shift of North America which began in the central Atlantic in western Gondwana during late Triassic times, created an oceanic embayment along northwest South America. Subduction beneath northwest South America started and resulted in emplacement of Mid to Late Jurassic calc-alkaline arc magmas along the Colombian-Ecuadorian Andes. Spreading along the oceanic ridges between South America and paleo-Mexican margins produced an extensional regime throughout the northern Andean region as well as sinistral transform offset along the southwest-facing

Peruvian margin. This extensional tectonic regime likely continued in northernmost Peru into the Cretaceous as evidenced by the structural and stratigraphic setting of the Lancones Basin. During the Middle Cretaceous, spreading along these ridges decreased, and was slowly replaced by Pacific spreading centres. As a result, oblique northeastward-directed subduction under South America commenced along northwestern Peru, resulting in southwestward extension, westerly oriented normal faulting and intrusion of Cretaceous-Tertiary plutons (Mitouard, 1990).

The Sechura, Paita and Illescas paleo-highs represent microcontinental remnants isolated by sinistral movement along the southwest-facing coast of northern Peru. Evidence for this proposed left-lateral movement is found in oil well logs as stratigraphic off-sets below the Tertiary sediments, paleomagnetic measurements of Paleozoic rocks in the Basin, and present-day Paleozoic geometry along the northwestern coast of Peru. The best candidate to account for this apparent sinistral movement is its relationship to Tethyan spreading along northwest South America, documented to have lasted until the Middle Jurassic. No plutonism older than Cretaceous has been recorded south of the Huacabamba flexure in northern Peru suggesting subduction under northern Peru caused by spreading in the southwest Pacific, didn't commence until at least Middle Cretaceous times. The model can best be explained by a series of diagrams exhibiting the stectonic events and volcanic deposition in the Lancones Basin in Cretaceous times and post depositional events influencing the basin in Tertiary times (Fig. 3).

SETTING OF THE DEPOSITS

The Ereo Formation mafic volcanic rocks form the core of a broad anticline that extends northeasterly where it plunges gently under the overlying Lancones Formation. South of Piura river Tertiary sedimentary rocks of the Sechura Basin cover the volcanic rocks. In this area of covered terrain, geophysical data define the structural model for the district. Air-borne magnetic surveys and ground gravity surveys combined with structural and stratigraphic interpretation of drill data from the TG1 and TG3 deposits and TG6, TG7 and TG8 anomalies suggest that secondary structural basins within the regional graben were sites for sulphide accumulation (Fig. 4).

The TG1 and TG3 deposits and TG8 and TG7 anomalies lie within a 7 km northerly oriented 2 milligal gravity anomaly (Tambo Graben Trend) that exhibits a chevron shape in plan view (Fig. 4). A 10 km gravity trend (West Graben Trend), and its extension to the south, contains the TG4, TG5 and TG6 anomalies and the B5 sulphide deposit. The gravity response is attributed to high specific gravity rocks (basalt, barite and sulphides). On the Tambo Graben Trend magnetic results mimic the gravity trends and display a linear dipole configuration similar to the gravity trend. Magnetic susceptibility testing of the core and three dimension modeling of magnetic data indicate that high susceptibilities result from basalt domes or horsts lying adjacent to and in part underlying massive sulphide accumulations. In the case of the Tambo Graben Trend, massive sulphides have been found to correlate with gravity anomalies with flanking areas of high magnetic susceptibility. The favourable geologic trends to massive sulphides dominantly contain mafic flows and locally intercalated dacite, volcanic breccia, locally prominent heterolithic volcanic conglomerates near faults, heterolithic volcanic debris flows and stratigraphically truncating synvolcanic faults dominate these trends geologically.

The west boundary of the northern portion of sulphides at TG1 is defined by a steeply dipping predepositional fault that strikes southerly, parallel to the west boundary of the Tambo gravity trend. Refer to the plan map of the TG1 and TG3 deposits related to the gravity response (Fig. 5). This fault appears to have been re-activated late in the development of the sulphide pile and forms a discontinuous sheared margin to the deposit. The TG1 sulphides fill a deep, northwesterly-oriented fault-bounded and dacite-lined trough, obliquely oriented at 35 degrees to the Tambo second-order graben (Fig. 6). Sulphide accumulations at TG3 fill elongated troughs on the flanks of a dacite dome overlying a northwesterly elongated elongated basalt high, similar to the TG1 structural orientation (Fig. 7). A thick volcanic debris flow covers the top of the TG3 deposit suggesting the presence of a paleo-horst to the west.

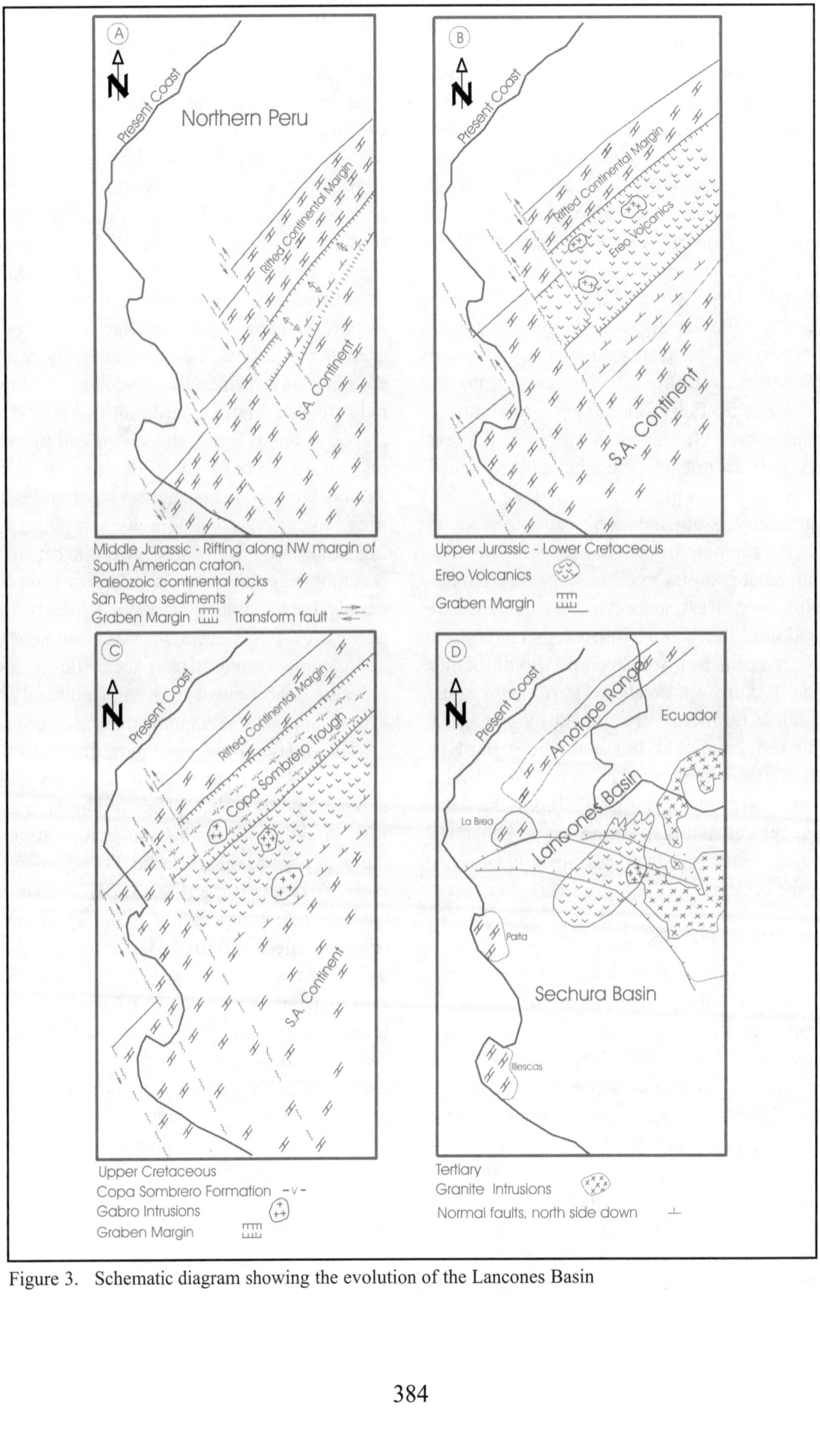

Figure 3. Schematic diagram showing the evolution of the Lancones Basin

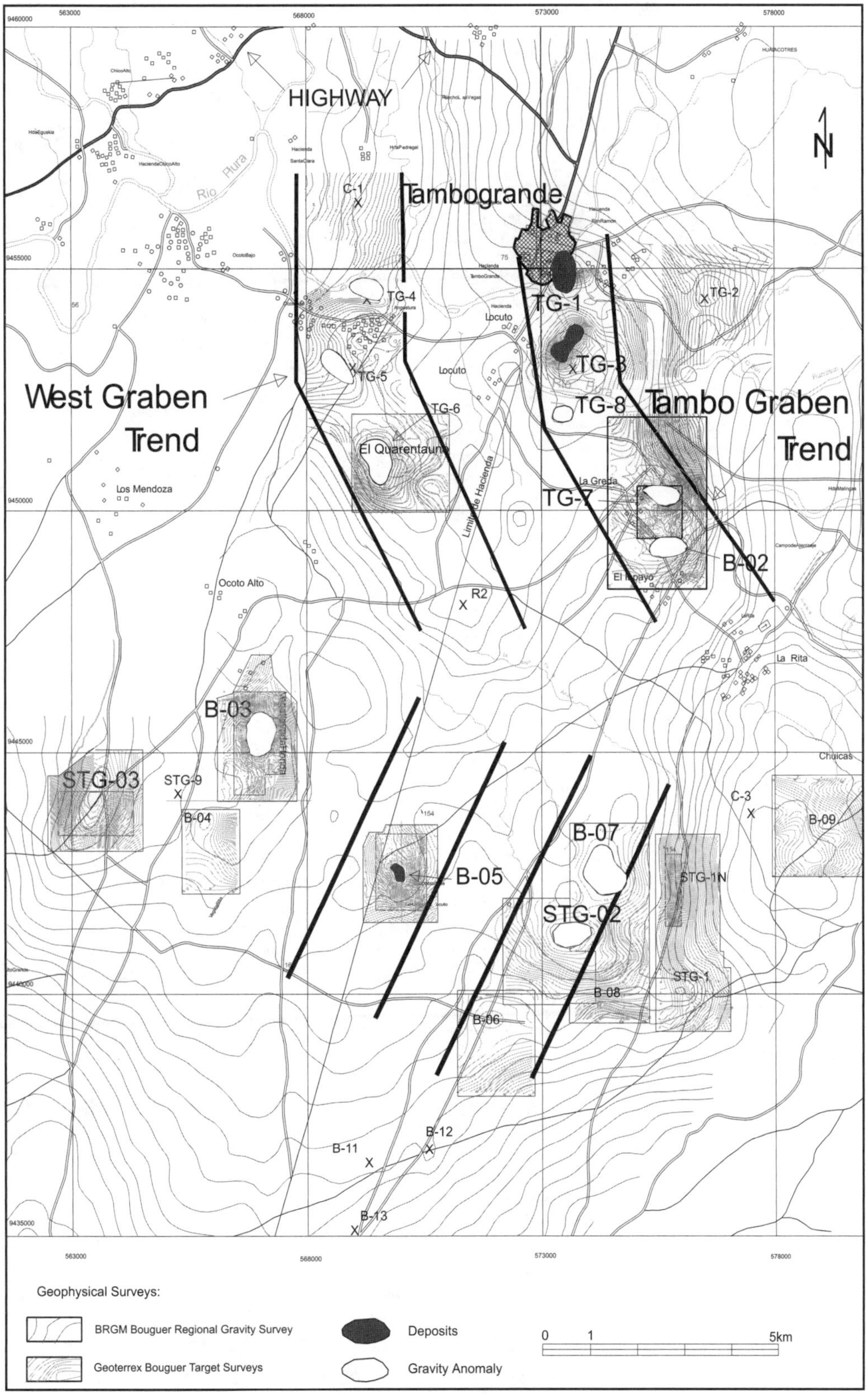

Figure 4. Simplified gravity map of the Tambo Grande District, showing the relationship of known deposits, gravity response and projected second order grabens

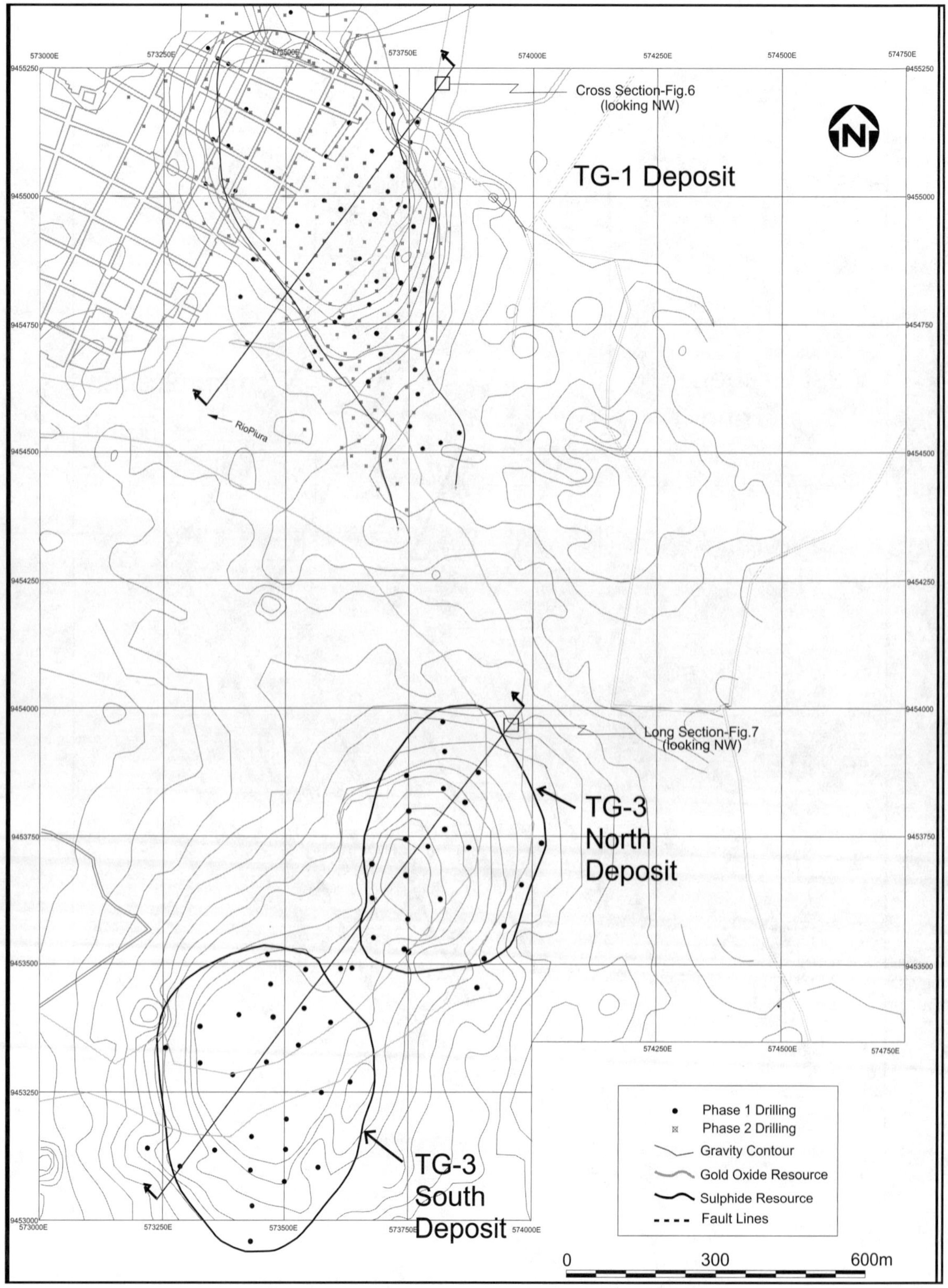

Figure 5. Plan map of the TG1 and TG3 deposits showing relationship of gravity response to deposits.

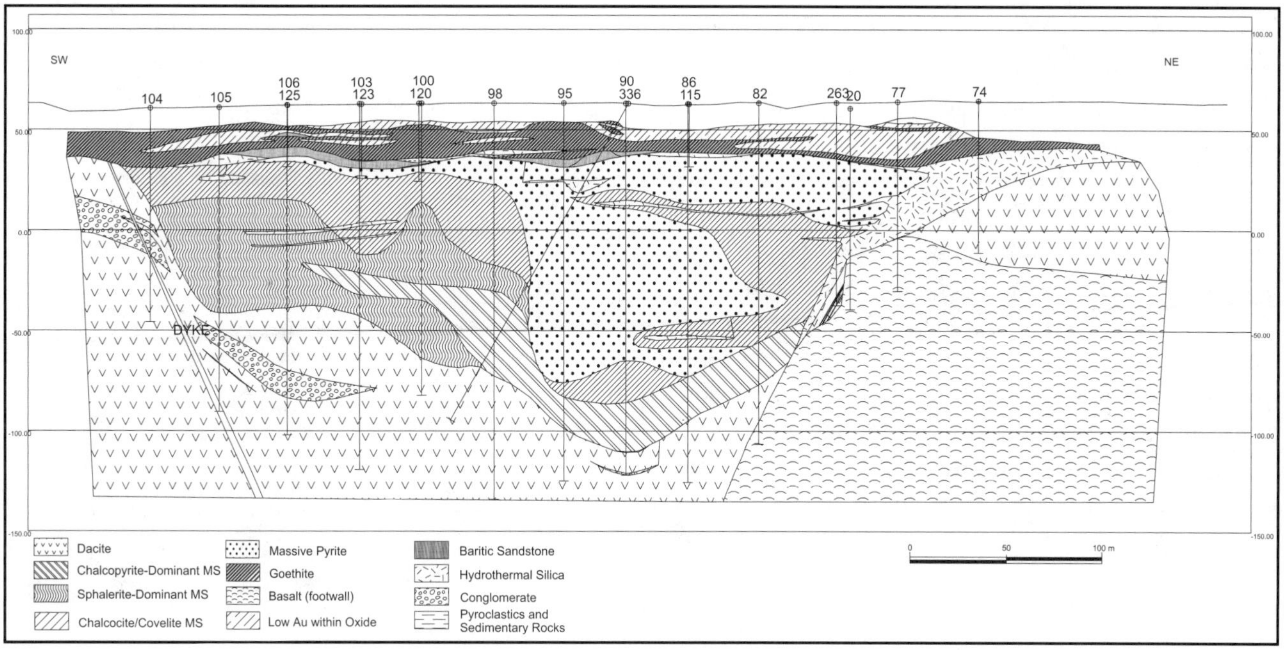

Figure 6. TG1 Section 1385W: Looking North-West (trace shown in Figure 5)

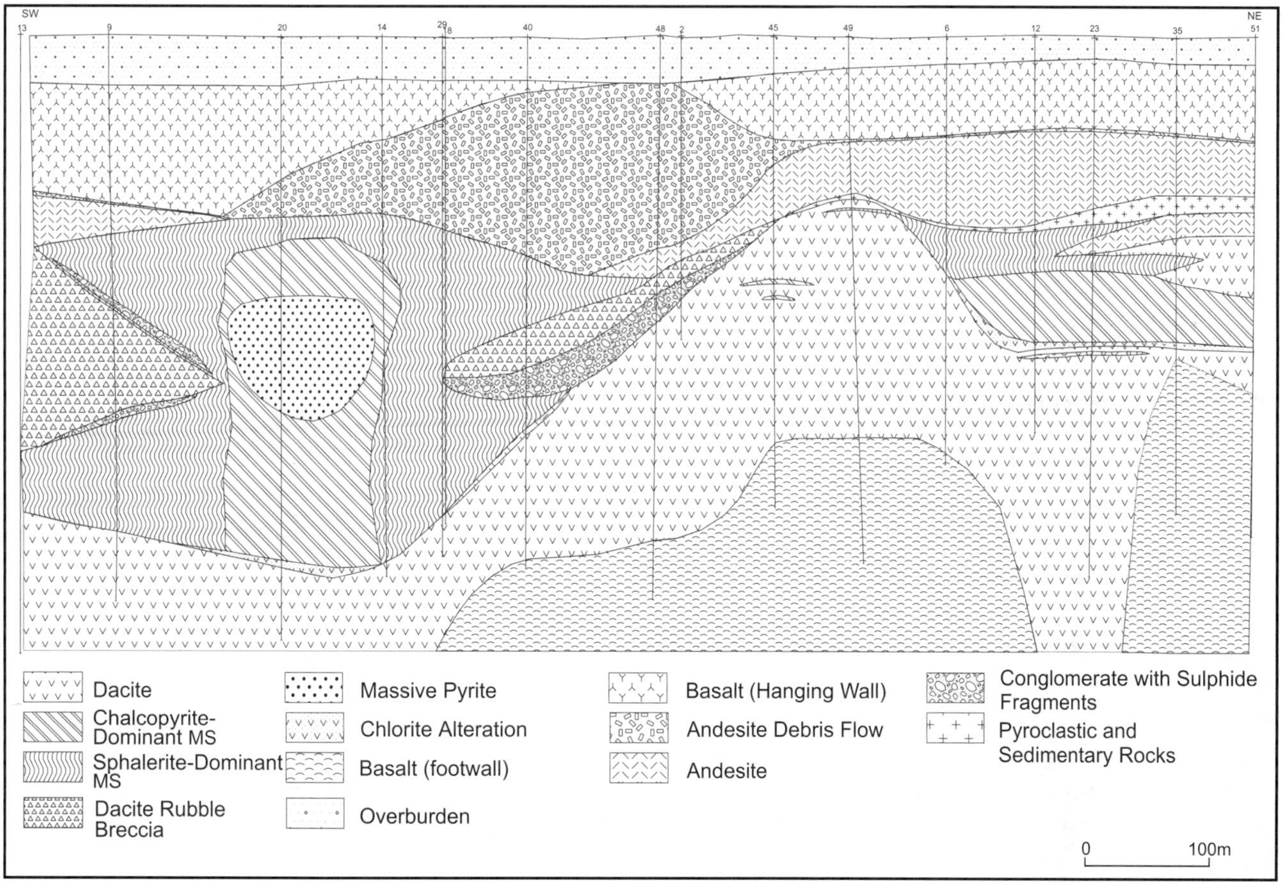

Figure 7. TG3 deposit long section looking North-West (trace shown in Figure 5).

STRATIGRAPHY AND PETROGRAPHY -TG 3 DEPOSIT

The most complete section of volcanic strata of the Ereo Formation is observed in drilling at the TG3 deposits. These deposits occur as two separate sulphide mounds (TG3 North and TG3 South) located in topographic basins underlain by massive dacitic flows and flow breccias on the flank of a dacite dome (Fig. 7). The dacite dome formed on top of a basalt paleo-high or horst in the floor of the Tambo secondary graben. Sulphide mound development was constrained laterally by fragmental dacitic rocks. Andesitic flows and volcaniclastic rocks overlay the sulphide deposits. At TG3 South, a thick andesitic debris flow appeared to have rapidly buried and in part, eroded the sulphide mound. Ultimately a thick sequence of basalt flows and flow breccias covered most of the older stratigraphy. The depositional sequence is presented in a generalized stratigraphic column of the TG3 deposit (Fig. 8), and lithologic units are described below.

The *footwall basalts* are a mix of massive amygdaloidal flows and flow breccias, generally aphanitic, dark greenish-grey, and moderately magnetic. Chemically they are tholeiitic-sub-alkaline in composition. Amygdules are typically spherical to ellipsoidal, averaging 2 to 3 mm, comprised of white calcite with lesser amounts of chlorite and/or epidote, and constituting between 5 to 30 percent of the rock. Basalt breccias are probably hyaloclastites.

Footwall dacites overlay and probably cut the footwall basalts. They underlie the deepest parts of the deposit and consist of massive flows and flow breccias indistinguishable from footwall dacites of the TG1 deposit. They are typically light to dark grey, massive and aphanitic to porphyritic with 3 to 5 percent lath-shaped euhedral plagioclase phenocrysts up to 2 mm long. Flow banding is common in both the aphanitic and porphyritic varieties. Dacite breccias generally have angular fragments averaging 2 to 4 cm in diameter in a fine-grained fragmental matrix. Fragments typically have curved surfaces, and commonly have "jigsaw fit" textures. These breccia textures suggest fragmented flows rather than a volcaniclastic origin (Fig. 9a).

The central *dacite dome* consists of massive flow

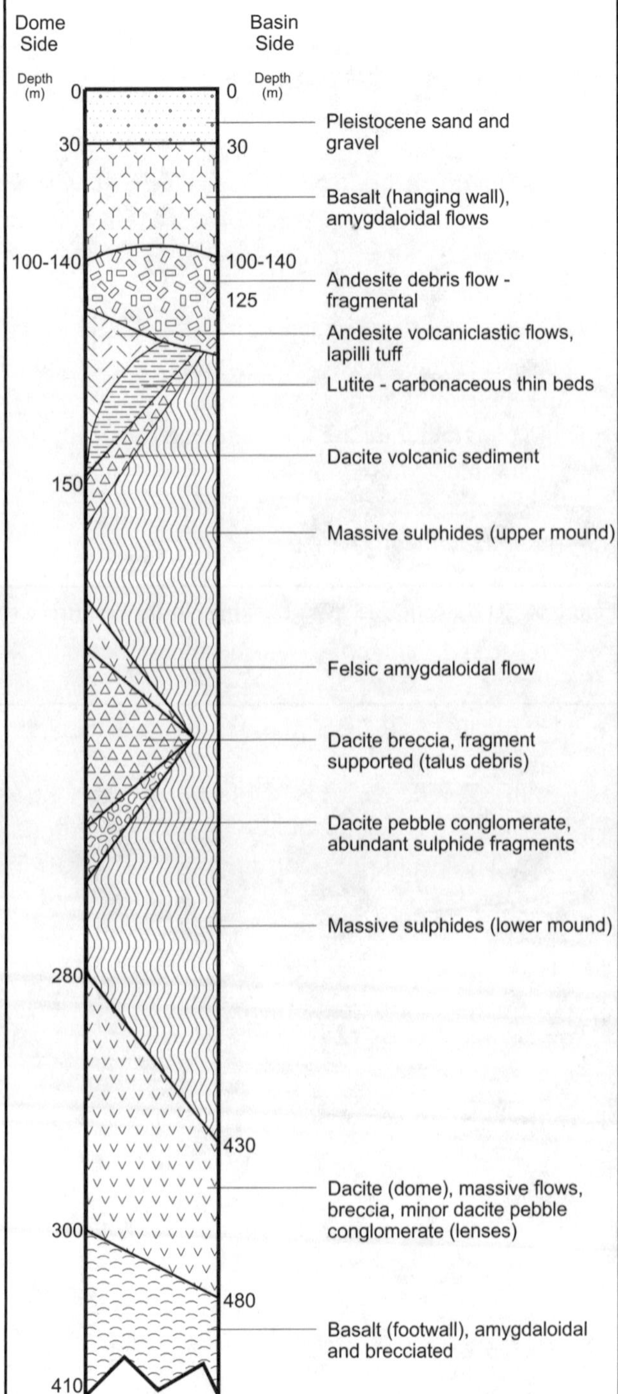

Figure 8. Generalized stratigraphic column of the TG3 South deposit

rocks and flow breccia located between the TG3 North and South sulphide basins. The dacites are typically light to dark grey and aphanitic to fine-grained feldspar phyric. Chlorite alteration of the breccia matrix is common. The TG3 North deposit sits directly on the flank of the domal dacites. In contrast at TG3 South, the dacite-basin margins, and the floor to a lesser extent, are partially filled with a thin sequence of intercalated volcanic-derived sediments, conglomerates and dacite rubble sloughing off the dome flank. These units may have acted as a seal to further focus hydrothermal solutions into the central part of the basin. Several thin discontinuous layers of dacitic pebble conglomerate are also intercalated at the base of the sulphides on the flank of the dacite-dome complex. Conglomerates are heterolithic with subangular to rounded aphanitic to porphyritic dacite pebbles averaging 1 to 2 cm in diameter. Other clast types include amygdaloidal basalt, chloritic altered basalt and felsic dyke material. The northeast flank of the dome formed a more pronounced steep-sided basin wall compared to the southwest flank of the dome.

The *sulphide mound* at TG3 South is a stacked series of sulphide lenses. Each lens has a dacite pebble breccia at its margin and is overlain by dacite flow breccia. The pebble breccia units are wedge-shaped and thickest near the steepest part of the mound. These epiclastic rocks are similar to those observed at the TG1 deposit and in the footwall of TG3 North deposit. Close to the base of these units they locally contain abundant rip-up sulphide fragments where the debris flows passed over the sulphide mounds (Fig. 9b). Rounded to subangular pyrite (some with minor base metal and barite) fragments up to 3 cm in diameter constitute up to 50 percent of the rock. These units formed down slope from the sulphide mound and provide good exploration indicators for nearby sulphide accumulations.

The inter-sulphide-lens pebble breccias are typically overlain by a *dacite rubble breccia* that in some places reaches a thickness of over 150 m. This unit partly overlays the flanks of the lower sulphide lens at TG3 South. It restricted subsequent sulphide deposition to a 150 m wide zone in the central part of the sulphide mound but did not completely bury the sulphide pile. The dacite breccia is a distinctive clastic rock consisting of angular, chloritic-altered, flow banded dacite fragments in a matrix of very fine-grained quartz and chlorite. Fragments make up 70 to 80 percent of the rock. The fragments are angular to subrounded and range up to 10 cm in diameter. Chlorite alteration is ubiquitous, but strongest in the matrix. This unit likely formed as talus wedges originating from the central dacite dome, and a dome developed southwest of the TG3 South deposit.

A distinctive felsic amygdaloidal flow unit occurs in the upper part of the dacite sequence. It is typically a medium grey to pinkish-grey, siliceous, aphanitic to fine-grained feldspar phyric or massive felsic rock. Amygdules consisting of calcite cores with chlorite rims can make up to 10 percent of the rock and form elongated tube-like bodies up to 1.5 cm long. The unit is noted in roughly the same stratigraphic location on both the north and south flanks of the TG3 South deposit. The distribution of this unusual unit suggests both the central and southern domes had similar eruptive histories and were fed from the same magma chamber.

The dacite dome and sulphides at both the TG3 North and South deposits are roughly stratigraphically equivalent. A thin discontinuous layer of lutite and/or conglomerate with sulphide fragments overlies both sulphides and dacites. At TG3 North, an approximately 15 m thick sequence of intercalated dacite lapilli tuff, dacite tuff, and lesser amounts of siltstone and lutite overlies the sulphides and is in turn overlain by andesites. The base of the sequence has a thin unit of chalcopyrite and sphalerite-bearing massive sulphides that correlates with the top of the TG3 North sulphide mound as well as the top of the TG1 deposit. It appears to be the last episode of felsic volcanism and associated sulphide deposition before the basin was filled with more mafic rocks.

A sequence of *andesite* volcaniclastic and flow rocks with minor intercalated fine-grained sedimentary rocks overlies the dacites and sulphides where the sediments are absent (Fig. 7). These andesitic rocks are typically medium to dark greenish-grey, aphanitic to fine-grained feldspar phyric, and amygdaloidal. They dip gently to the west in the TG3 North mound area, and range from a few metres to over 150 m in thickness. Much of the sequence is composed of homogeneous andesite lapilli tuff and massive aphanitic amygdaloidal flows with calcite and chlorite-filled amygdules averaging 1-2 mm in diameter. There are, however, a few unusual units within the sequence. Several flow units have distinctive large elongated amygdules (Fig. 9c). These units are generally aphanitic, massive, and have a medium greenish-grey to blue-green colour.

Distinctive, thin andesite breccia units (not shown on Fig. 7) commonly overlie the large-amygdule andesites. These units have pale to medium greenish-grey to blue-green, angular to subangular fragments ranging up to 10 cm in diameter and constitute 20 percent of the volume. Fragments typically have curved surfaces and, less commonly, delicate sharp points which suggest they are hyaloclastites. The andesite breccia is commonly located between sedimentary rocks (siltstones and/or lutites) above, and massive andesite flows below. They have the appearance of flow-top breccias that were subsequently buried by fine sediments.

An unusual appearing mafic fragmental rock containing sporadic amygdules may be a welded tuff. This unit is typically a light greenish-grey colour overall, but is mottled light to dark greenish-grey at the decimetric scale. The rock is aphanitic to fine- to medium-grained feldspar phyric. The rock appears to be a semi-welded lapilli tuff which had gas trapped in the matrix between fragments, giving the pockets an irregular shape.

Andesite tuff breccias make up a relatively minor part of the andesite package. The breccias consist of dark green to grey-brown elongated aphanitic amygdaloidal fragments up to 10 cm in diameter in a chloritic lapilli tuff matrix. The large fragments have calcite amygdules that are larger, up to 5 mm, near the fragment selvages giving them the appearance of bombs.

In the TG3 South area, part of the sulphide deposit is directly overlain by an andesite *debris flow* up to 100 m thick (Figs. 7 and 9d). In some places this unit overlays conglomerate above the sulphides. In other places it overlays and may be intercalated with the andesite sequence. The unit appears to be restricted to the south side of the dacite dome separating the TG3 North and South deposits and it tapers rapidly to the south pinching out near the centre of the TG3 South sulphide mound. The three dimensional shape of the unit is still not well understood, but the source appears to be from the west. The debris flow has no evident stratification and occupies a prominent basin between the underlying andesitic rocks. The unit appears to have been deposited rapidly, causing catastrophic in-fill of the sedimentary basin possibly due to collapse of a fault scarp. Two distinct types of andesite debris flow rocks have been noted. The most abundant type is a mottled light to medium greenish-grey fragmental rock with a sporadically siliceous quartz-epidote and chlorite-altered sandy matrix. Also present but less abundant are light to medium grey, aphanitic, siliceous dacite fragments and distinctive rounded to subangular jasper fragments. The second type of debris flow is darker-coloured than the epidote material described above. This unit has a mottled dark greenish to maroon-brown colour due to fine-grained disseminated hematite and is generally sporadically to moderately magnetic.

A series of dark coloured *basaltic rocks* overlies part of the andesite sequence and andesite debris flow unit. They consist of intercalated amygdaloidal flows, flow breccias and tuff breccias filling a basin up to 100 m thick. The flow rocks are dark green and generally massive and aphanitic (Fig. 9e). The basalt breccia generally consists of dark green aphanitic fragments with small chlorite amygdules in a matrix of massive chlorite or fine-grained chloritic fragmental material.

Basalt tuff-breccias consist of tightly packed flattened amygdaloidal fragments up to 5 cm wide in a lapilli-tuff matrix. This basalt commonly has sporadic quartz-epidote alteration, with irregular epidote patches up to 10 cm in diameter. This alteration is similar to that of the mafic flow rocks intercalated with the sulphides at TG1. Both rock types have the same chemistry and may be the same unit.

Mafic intrusions are more common than felsic or intermediate lithologies. Several types of mafic dykes cut the entire stratigraphic sequence from the footwall to the hangingwall, including the massive sulphides. Variations in the mafic dykes are considerable, but may simply be textural. Mafic dykes are most commonly a medium greenish-grey fine-grained

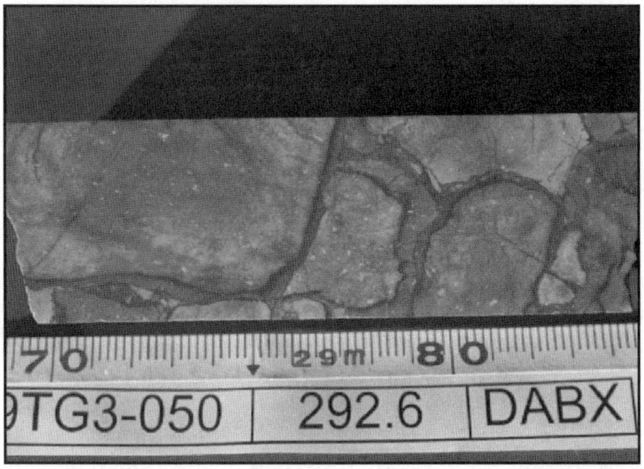

Figure 9a. Photo 99TG3-050, 292.60m; M9-14 Dacite flow breccia

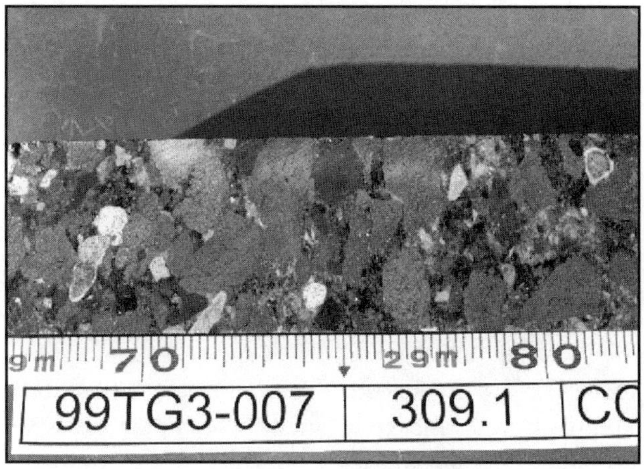

Figure 9b. Photo 99TG3-007, 309.10m; M9-5 Type 1 conglomerate with sulphide rip-up fragments

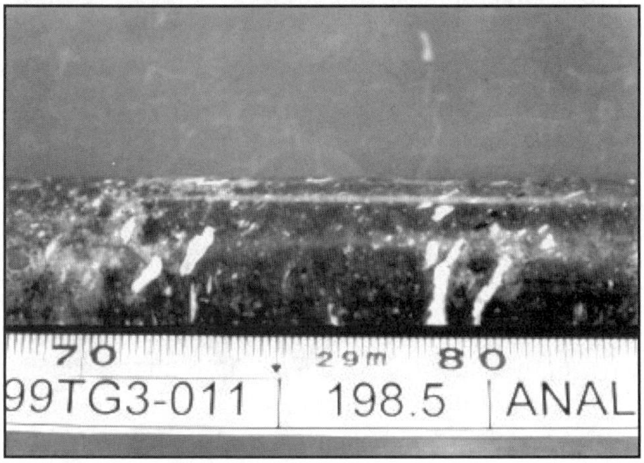

Figure 9c. 99TG3-011, 198.5m; M8-14 Amygdaloidal andesite with large amygdules (ANAL)

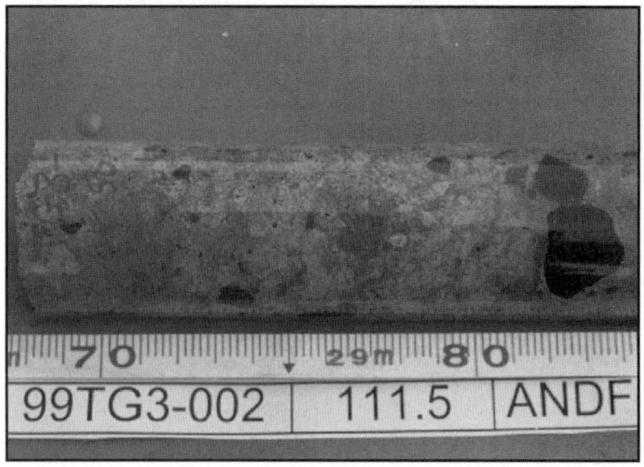

Figure 9d. Photo 99TG3-002, 111.50m; M8-29 Andesite debris flow(ANDF)

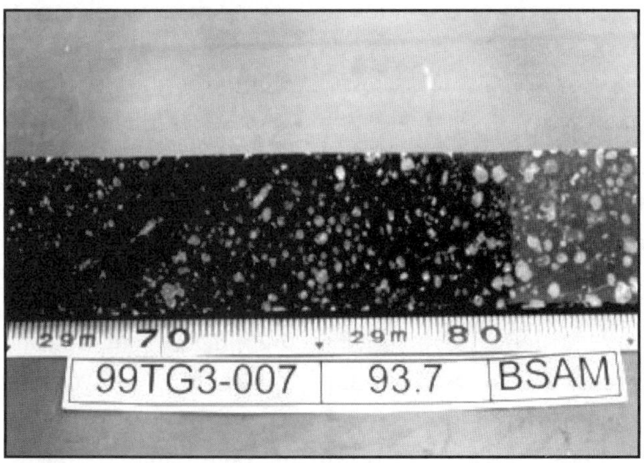

Figure 9e. 99TG3-007, 93.7; M8-11 Amygdaloidal basalt flow (BSAM)

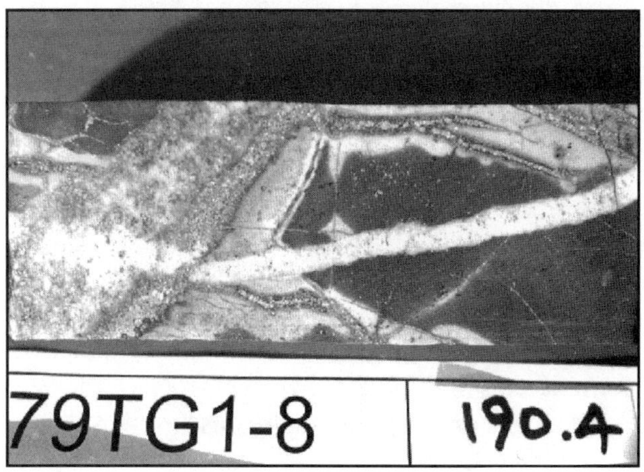

Figure 9f. Photo 79TG1-008, 190.40m; M2-23 Multiphase stockwork in the footwall of the TG1 deposit

crystalline aggregate of feldspar and chlorite with up to 15 percent fine-grained chloritic clots after mafic phenocrysts. The rock is generally very weakly magnetic. Preliminary chemical data (Table 1) suggests a sub-alkaline composition. These dykes or sills are common in the footwall and hangingwall of the TG3 deposit, but less abundant in the sulphides. They are common to both the TG1 and TG3 deposits. Rhyodacite intrusions identical to those noted in the TG1 deposit are observed cutting dacite southwest of the TG3 South deposit. These intrusions are light greenish-grey, massive, medium-grained feldspar porphyry and occur near the core of the southern dacite dome.

STRATIGRAPHY AND PETROGRAPHY - TG1 DEPOSIT

The *footwall and lateral host rocks* of the TG1 deposit appear to have the same volcanic lithologies as TG3, off-set by normal faulting during the formation of a northwesterly oriented, stepped graben (Fig. 6). Footwall rocks beneath the sulphides also contain intercalated breccias, most likely reflecting collapse of nearby fault scarps.

The *basal basalt* consists of dark greenish-grey massive aphanitic amygdaloidal to porphyritic flows or hyaloclastite breccias, and lesser amounts of tuff to lapilli tuff. They generally contain abundant sub-millimetric chlorite amygdules. These basalts probably represent the original seafloor.

The *dacite* flows and breccias, underlain on the east side of the graben by basalt found in the deeper holes, are most abundant in the immediate footwall of the TG1 deposit. Visually they are pale to medium grey porphyritic dacite flows or hypabyssal intrusions with 5 percent distinctive white euhedral plagioclase phenocrysts up to 4 mm long in an aphanitic, siliceous, commonly flow-banded matrix. Dacite breccias are also common and exhibit hyaloclastite textures. Volcaniclastic rocks (dacite tuff and lapilli tuff) are less common. Preliminary lithological data from samples of these felsic volcanic rocks indicate a rhyodacite composition analogous to the dacite domes at TG3.

The *conglomerate* units are heterolithic with an overall medium greenish-grey colour. Fragments are generally rounded to subangular, tightly packed, and average 1-2 cm in diameter. The most abundant fragments are fine-grained dacite or dacite porphyry. Other fragments consist of fine-grained, dark green crystalline andesite, amygdaloidal andesite or basalt with chlorite amygdules, dark green to black chlorite (plus or minus disseminated pyrite), and rarely fine-grained crystalline felsic material (aplite). These heterolithic conglomerates which invariably underlie the sulphides are found basin-ward at the base of projected normal faults on the flank of the sulphides.

Several layers of *felsic tuff* to lapilli tuff are intercalated and more numerous within the upper part of the sulphide pile. They are generally less than 2 m thick and form continuous to discontinuous flat-lying horizons. These felsic rocks consist of a white, massive, fine-grained, siliceous cherty material with ghost anhedral feldspar phenocrysts. In many cases they appear as thinly laminated fine-grained tuffaceous sediments. Rarely, quartz eyes are observed suggesting rhyolite compositions. These stratagraphic horizons in the central part of the deposit are commonly intensely altered to vuggy silica.

Amygdaloidal *basalt flows* are interbedded with sulphides principally along the southern and northeast sides of the deposit. The southern flow attains a thickness of more than 50 m. These rocks are a medium greenish-grey, medium hard, aphanitic to fine-grained crystalline aggregate of feldspar, chlorite and epidote with up to 10 percent amygdules of chlorite, calcite, and pyrite.

Intrusive rocks in the TG1 area are relatively common and many types noted in the logging may be largely textural variations. Preliminary lithogeochemical analyses indicate four types of intrusions. One intermediate and two mafic varieties form generally thin and discontinuous dykes and sills in footwall rocks and the sulphide pile. Rhyodacite forms irregular plugs in both the footwall and lateral host rocks to the sulphide deposit.

Mafic dykes and sills are the most abundant intrusions. They most commonly consist of massive dark greenish-grey to black aphanitic to fine-grained crystalline aggregates with or without small chloritic and/or rare calcite amygdules. Intermediate intrusions are either feldspar porphyries or melanocratic fine to medium-grained crystalline aggregates. These mafic and intermediate intrusive rocks are most abundant in the immediate footwall to the sulphide pile where they appear to be sill-like bodies deflected along the base of the sulphides. In some locations, however, these intrusions cut through the massive sulphides as northwest trending, near vertical dykes and form 2 to 10 m thick sills above the lower sulphide lens. Volumetrically these intrusions do not occupy a significant part of the sulphide body.

The mafic dykes may have been feeders to the amygdaloidal basalt flows observed intercalated with the sulphides in the southern part of the deposit. Dykes and sills are rare in the upper part of the sulphide pile suggesting that the upper sulphides may postdate the intrusions.

"Rhyodacite" intrusions are light greenish-grey massive, homogeneous feldspar porphyries. The groundmass consists of fine-grained crystalline feldspar, sericite and quartz, and hosts 15-20 percent stubby, euhedral to subhedral, prism-shaped white feldspar phenocrysts to 5 mm long (average 2-3 mm). Chemically, the intrusions are dacitic in composition and may be late stage intrusions related to the dacite domes and flank the sulphide body. Morphology of these intrusions is not well defined, but they occur as a northwest-trending series of irregular plugs and dykes up to 50 m wide in the footwall and along the western flank of the deposit.

Alteration

The footwall of the TG1 deposit is largely composed of ubiquitous quartz-sericite altered dacite. These rocks range from soft, sericite dominant, to hard, silicified dominant. Alteration intensity is generally greatest in the vicinity of the quartz-pyrite stockwork zones where original textures are commonly obscured. The alteration is caused by sodium depletion of the feldspars in the dacite footwall rocks (Table 1). The footwall stringer zone exhibits massive silicification. In thin section these rocks have remnant volcanic textures with phenocrysts and lithic fragments in a groundmass of very fine-grained sericite, plagioclase, quartz, plus or minus chlorite. Stringer zones in the dacite beneath the central part of the sulphide pile commonly have narrow, (less than a few metres wide) envelopes of dark green to black chlorite. This presumably iron rich chlorite is sporadically distributed in the immediate footwall to the sulphides and is likely related to hydrothermal solutions. Peripheral to the sulphide deposit, the quartz-sericite alteration is overprinted by sporadic light to medium green chlorite alteration. This probable magnesium-rich chlorite commonly occurs as rims around breccia fragments and likely formed as the result of contact with seawater. Alteration in footwall rocks in the TG1 deposit is most intense under the thickest part of the sulphides. Footwall alteration in the TG3 deposit area is identical to the TG1 deposit. The ultimate size and distribution of this alteration zone in TG3 is not known, but in a northeast direction exceeds 800 m in width.

Mineralization

Stockwork Zone

The stockwork zones in the TG3 and TG1 deposits are restricted to the footwall usually beneath the central and deepest parts of the sulphide mounds, where they cut all rock types. Stockwork zones do not extend to the limits of the sulphides indicating that sulphides were deposited above central vents and spread laterally onto structurally unfractured ocean floor. The most common stockwork zone consists of a quartz-sericite altered dacite host with up to 80 percent, generally less than 1 cm wide fine-grained crystalline pyrite stringers. Chalcopyrite-filled stringers are generally spatially limited to within a few metres of the base of the massive sulphides. Quartz is the most common gangue mineral, although chlorite, calcite and barite are also noted. In some locations the stringers are clearly multiphase. In hole 79TG1-008 medium-grained pyrite stringers with minor amounts of quartz and chlorite gangue initially cut dark greenish-grey dacite (Fig. 9f). The host rock was bleached to light yellowish-grey along the stringer selvages. A second phase of predominantly quartz stringers was developed within the cores of the pyrite stringers, but also crosscut the host volcanic material with no associated significant visible alteration haloes.

The stockwork zones at TG3 contain stringers and veins averaging 1 to 2 cm in width, composed of pyrite, quartz and rarely chalcopyrite. Some zones consist of a breccia matix flooded by silica in place of discrete stringers. Ore-grade intersections of stockwork are rare, and are generally restricted to the first few metres directly beneath the massive sulphides. The TG3 North deposit contains more intense chalcopyrite filled stockwork than the South mound. The dacite rubble breccia lying between the sulphide lenses at TG3 South contain only a few minor stockwork zones, suggesting that fluid movement was restricted to the central part of the sulphide pile and sulphides spread laterally onto the flanking dacite mounds.

Sulphide Zone

The TG1 and TG3 massive sulphide deposits consist of 85 to 99 percent pyrite, up to 15 percent barite, on average 5 percent combined chalcopyrite and sphalerite, and small amounts of quartz and calcite. The TG1 deposit contains more than 100 million tonnes and the TG3 deposit more than 110 million tonnes of massive sulphides. They can be divided into zones based on base metal mineralogy, gangue mineralogy and texture. Base metal mineral zones are the more consistent, predictable and understandable of the three.

Base metal sulphide mineral zones within the TG1 and TG3 deposits are spatially distinct within the sulphide piles (Figs. 6, 7). Sulphide zonation is similar in both deposits. In general, the central core of the deposits is composed largely of massive pyrite with little or insignificant base metal content. A basal chalcopyrite (plus or minus magnetite) rich zone, up to 50 m thick, developed along the base and margins of the TG1 and TG3 sulphide deposits. The chalcopyrite zone occupies the lower portions of TG1 and does not extend south where the deposit thins. This mineral zone constitutes approximately 15 percent of the TG1 deposit. In both deposits, a zone of chalcopyrite-sphalerite is distributed around the pyrite core lying above the basal chalcopyrite and extending to the margins of the deposit on all sides. This mineral zone is restricted to depths below 50 m from the top of the sulphides at TG1, but at TG3 the zone extends to the top and lateral fringes of the sulphide pile. At TG1, this zone occupies about 30 percent of the deposit and contains the major portion of the sulpho-salt mineralogy, principally as tennantite. A fourth mineralogical zone containing chalcocite, digenite and covelite, with little or no zinc occurs at TG1 above the chalcopyrite-sphalerite zone and along the margins of the deposit near the basin walls. This zone constitutes approximately 20 percent of the sulphides at TG1 but is absent at TG3. The top part of the sulphide pile at TG1 is composed largely of barren pyrite.

Gangue mineralogy consists largely of barite, calcite and minor quartz, all of which occur as a matrix interstitial to pyrite grains. The gangue matrix may be absent, or make up to 20 percent of the rock. Typically, barite and/or calcite constitute between 2 to 10 percent by volume of the rock. Distribution of the gangue minerals is not well documented to date, but initial observations indicate that barite is the dominant gangue mineral in the upper central part of the deposits. Chalcopyrite and sphalerite, are commonly but not invariably associated with a barite matrix. With depth at TG3, calcite becomes more abundant and eventually dominant. With depth at TG1 the matrix shifts from barite to quartz dominant. In the margins of the deposits the sulphides are more tightly packed and contain less gangue. In rare instances, the barite matrix and fine-grained loosely packed pyrite is observed merging with small barite stringers cutting more compacted pyrite masses, or possibly fragments. All textural evidence indicates that barite, quartz, and calcite were deposited relatively late in the formation of the deposit.

The sulphides at TG1 and TG3 exhibit a variety of textures. The most common textures are massive crystalline sulphides. that range from very fine to coarse grained. Very fine-grained pyrite (plus or minus base metal sulphides) is generally compact with little or no non-sulphide matrix. The crystalline sulphides have a conchoidal fracture and appear almost porcelain. Very coarse-grained pyrite can have crystal sizes in excess of 1 cm in diameter, and have up to 5 percent open pore space interstitial to the pyrite grains probably initially occupied by anhydrite which was dissolved by cooling fluids. Far more abundant than either of the extremes noted, however, is a fine-grained, crystalline pyrite aggregate with crystal sizes generally less than 0.5 mm in diameter. This material can be compact, or have up to 15 percent barite (plus or minus lesser amounts of quartz and/or calcite) as a matrix.

Relatively common features of the massive crystalline sulphides are very fine-grained porous zones with indistinct selvages within more compact coarser-grained sulphides (Fig. 9g). Pore spaces may be partially or completely filled with late stage barite, chalcopyrite, and sphalerite (Fig. 9h). Pyrite within these zones may be massive, colliform, or have an unusual bladed texture and, in many cases, pyrite grains are rimmed with sphalerite and barite. The porous zones are thought to be paleosolution channels. Colloform sphalerite formed peripheral to these channels as a result of cooling as fluids moved away from the hot conduit and into cooler marginal sulphides.

The second most common texture within the sulphides is a distinctive breccia with large sulphide fragments supported within a matrix of smaller sulphide fragments and barite. Fragments are generally rounded and range up to 5 cm in diameter. The rock has the appearance of a sulphide conglomerate (Fig. 9i), and is thought to be a slump breccia where a portion of the sulphide pile collapsed and was transported down the flanks of the mound due to anhydrite dissolution or earthquake activity. Fragments within these breccias can contain pyrite, chalcopyrite and sphalerite. Barite forms the matrix. In-situ fragmental rocks are distinctive from the sulphide slump breccias, but in most cases the two textural types grade from one to the other.

The southeast area of the TG1 deposit and the top of the north side of the TG3 deposit contain thinly laminated pyrite plus or minus chalcopyrite and/or sphalerite within lutites, siltstones, and fine-grained sandstones. They constitute a minor portion of the total sulphide deposit. It is unclear if these "bedded" sulphides are precipitates, reworked clastic sulphide sediments, or in-situ replacements. Some coarser-grained fragmental sulphide horizons have graded bedding and scour marks, and are heterolithic with a mix of pyrite, chalcopyrite and sphalerite (Fig. 9j).

Base metal sulphides formed interstially to the pyrite in both massive crystalline and fragmental varieties. Chalcopyrite and sphalerite occur separately or together, typically as fine-grained masses within a barite matrix. Sphalerite also occurs as irregular replacement masses up to 10 cm in diameter (Fig. 9k) at the extremities of the deposit. Chalcopyrite can be massive across several metres, invariably near or at the base of the sulphide pile. Disseminated magnetite is a significant constituent of the chalcopyrite rich basal zone.

Near the top of TG1, sooty black chalcocite is present as fracture coatings and pore space fillings. With depth, the sooty material changes to fine crystaline metallic chalcocite and/or digenite, with lesser amounts of covelite, and rare bornite. Secondary copper minerals occur interstitial to pyrite, along narrow stringers to depths of 60 to 80 m below the top of the sulphide system. Below the secondary copper zone chalcocite is observed rimming chalcopyrite grains over a few metre transition zone. Below this, chalcopyrite becomes the dominant copper mineral and secondary copper is restricted to isolated disseminated grains that can persist to the base of the sulphide pile. TG3 does not contain any secondary copper minerals.

Oxide Zone

At TG1 an oxide zone forms a continuous unit overlying and extending beyond the limits of the sulphide body. It outcrops in the north part of the deposit area, and in the southern part of the deposit along the Piura river. In most areas, however, it is overlain by consolidated sand and gravel. The oxide-sulphide contact is sharp. Pyrite is not observed in the oxide cap, and oxidized pyrite is only rarely observed in the main sulphide body. Baritic sandstone or felsic volcaniclastic rocks generally separate the sulphides from the iron oxides. The oxide zone is complex; appearing to be a mix of rhyolite tuff, volcanic sedimentary rocks, iron and barite-rich exhalatites, andesite, and weathered, compacted products of the above. The sequence of depositional events in the oxide cap is relatively consistent across the deposit, although all members of the zone are not present in all locations. A generalized stratigraphic column of the oxide zone is presented in Figure 10.

The top of the sulphides is commonly, but not continuously, capped with a thin, 1 to 10 cm horizon of amorphous, texturally vuggy silica precipitate below the oxides. The silica could be a bacterially-produced rind. At the base of the oxide zone, and commonly immediately overlying sulphides or the vuggy silica,

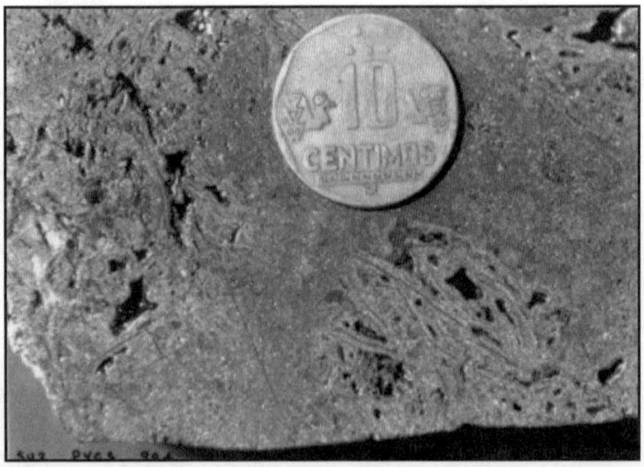

Figure 9g. Photo 79TG1-002, 72.80m; M0-27 Possible solution channelway within massive pyrite

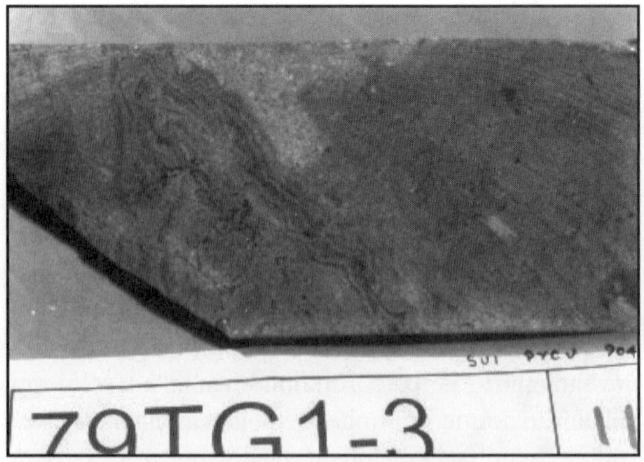

Figure 9h. Photo 79TG1-003, 110.80, M2-3 Coloform pyrite-sphalerite around fluid conduit in pyrite

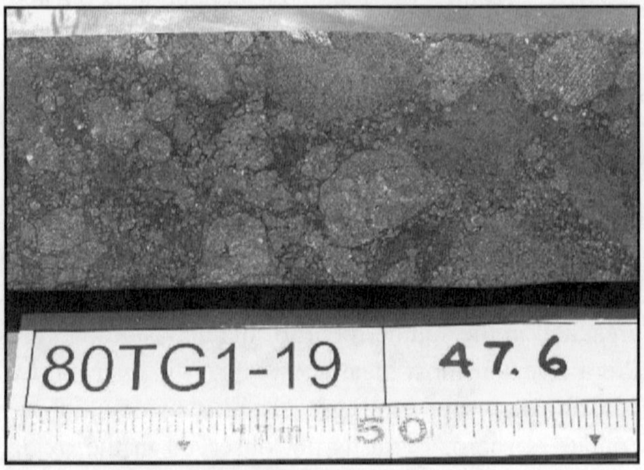

Figure 9i. Photo 80TG1-019, 47.6m; M3-1 Pyrite and sphalerite frgments

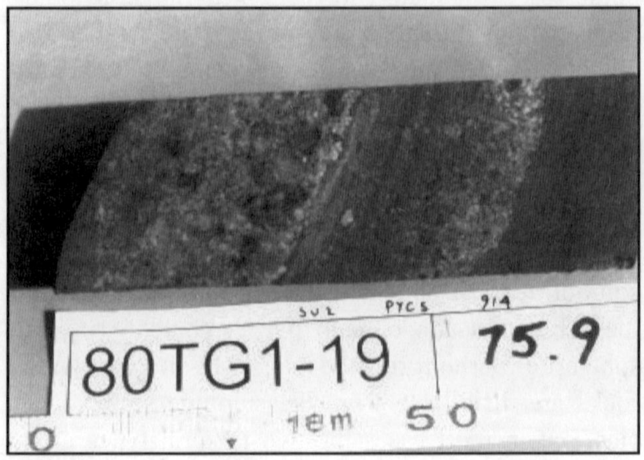

Figure 9j. Photo 80TG1-019, 75.9m (M3-20). Coarse-grained heterolithic fragmental sulphides with probable scour

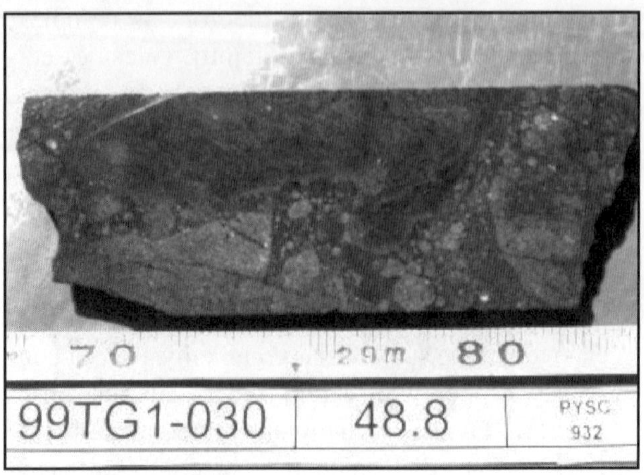

Figure 9k. Photo 99TG1-030, 48.80m, M7-3 Massive sphalerite replacing fragmental pyrite

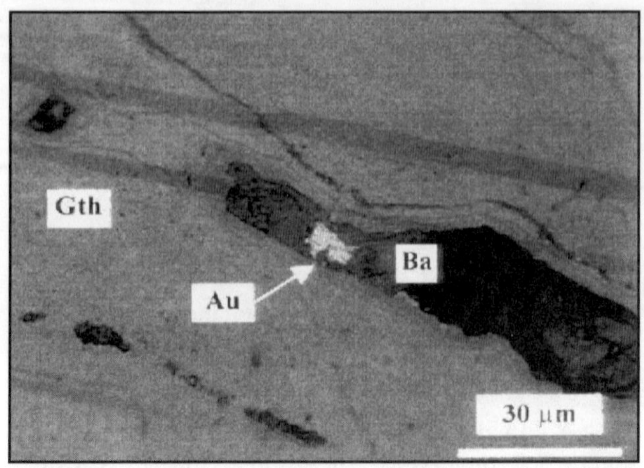

Figure 9l. Lakefield Research Laboratory, Sample 010516 - Gold grain encapsulated in barite within goethite

is a felsic volcanic sandstone or volcaniclastic unit, generally less than two metres in thickness. This unit is typically a distinctive breccia with a red hematitic matrix. Breccia fragments are angular to sub-rounded and range in diameter up to 15 cm. Fragments consist of aphanitic, massive to flow banded felsic volcanic flow rock, vuggy silica, and less commonly, felsic tuff. The matrix is generally a quartz-rich sandstone or reworked tuff with a mix of fine to coarse-grained, milky to vitreous angular quartz and barite grains in a hematite-rich silica (plus or minus) clay cement. Vuggy silica varieties of this unit are also common. Rarely, the stratigraphic position of the felsic fragmental unit is occupied by a rhyolite flow or flow breccia.

The felsic breccia unit is commonly intercalated with, and subsequently overlain by, baritic sandstone. The unit is probably a baritic precipitate or a reworked equivalent. It is typically fine to medium-grained, friable and composed predominantly of barite and milky to glassy quartz grains. Barite content can range from trace to over 70 percent. The colour of the unit varies from brick red to mottled grey and pinkish grey, but a pale to medium orange-brown colour is most typical. Crude bedding can be observed in most core. Both the sandy felsic breccia and the baritic sandstone units are generally gold enriched. Native gold most commonly occurs encapsulated within barite (Fig. 91).

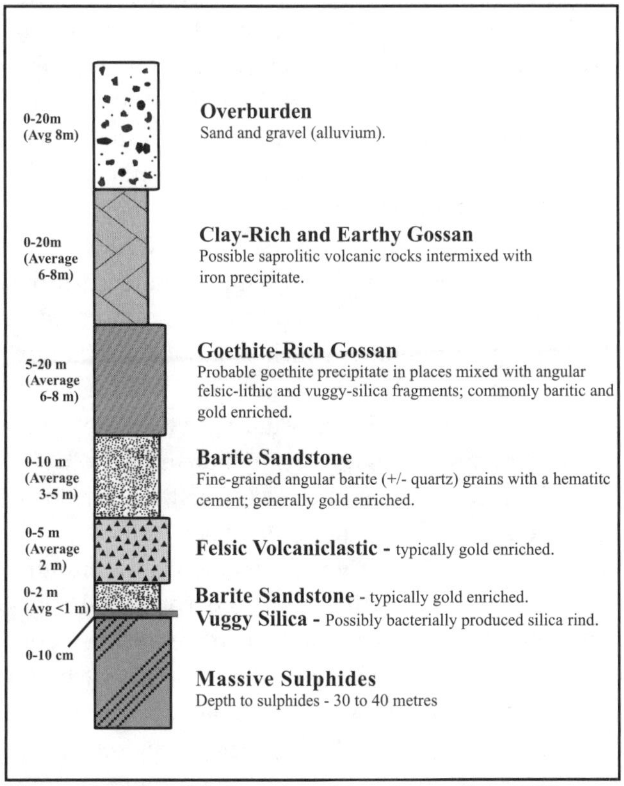

Figure 10. Simplified stratigraphic column of the TG1 oxide zone.

Overlying and in part intercalated with the felsic breccia and sandy baritic units are a variety of goethite-rich gossanous units. These goethite units have an overall dark red-brown colour but normally consist of a mix of mottled dark brown to almost black (goethite), dark red-brown (hematite) and dark yellow-brown (limonite) material. Significant variations in composition and textures occur within this unit. The most typical rock is a breccia with 1 to 3 cm angular to rounded, massive to thinly laminated, goethite fragments in a sandy to massive botroyoidal goethite matrix. Rare elongated barite crystal or fragments occur in the breccias. These may have formed in situ as barium-bearing fluids moved upward through the pile and encountered oxygenated seawater.

The upper part of the oxide zone is generally a mix of hematitic, earthy, and clay-rich gossan. Some parts are friable masses of hematite and limonite with fragments or zones of indurated goethite. The friable parts may have a clay component and hence are earthy in nature. The clay-rich gossan can vary in colour from white to grey to orange-brown, and is a mix of kaolinite and various iron hydroxides and oxides. In some places remnant feldspar phenocrysts are apparent, indicating that the protolith was a volcanic rock, probably an andesite or a dacite. Barite and associated gold can also be a significant constituents of the clay-rich and earthy gossans, indicating that in some places hydrothermal fluids permeated to the uppermost parts of the oxide zone.

LITHOGEOCHEMISTRY

A preliminary suite of samples from Tambo Grande has been analyzed for major oxides and trace elements at ITS-Bondar Clegg by borate fusion extraction and X-ray fluorescence methods. Representative analyses are given in Table 1. A total of 74 samples are included here; 41 from TG1 and 33 from TG3. These almost exclusively unweathered samples from drill core range from strongly altered quartz-chlorite-sericite-pyrite assemblages to relatively unaltered rocks. The samples are from the hangingwall and footwall volcanic strata close to the TG1 and TG3 deposits.

Immobile element data, for least altered samples, broadly display a bimodal distribution as shown on a Nb/Y and Zr/TiO_2 plot of Winchester and Floyd (1977) where the data cluster around basaltic andesite and rhyodacitic compositions (Figs. 11a and b). Zr/Y ratios vary between 2 and 7 suggesting a tholeiitic to transitional affinity for both the mafic and felsic lithologies.

Immobile element binary plots of Al_2O_3 - TiO_2 (Figs. 11c and d) can be used to distinguish lithologies, particularly where the rocks are strongly altered. Ideally an alteration line results from the alteration of a single precursor lithology with the spread of sample points along the line resulting from the net mass change of mobile elements (MacLean and Kranidiotis, 1987). This initial data set suggests there are three distinct geochemical types at TG1 and two of these types present at TG3. The best-developed alteration line is for felsic rocks at TG1, which shows a linear relationship in Al_2O_3 - TiO_2 ratios (Fig. 11c), suggesting a consistent precursor composition. Felsic rocks from TG3 plot around the alteration line established for TG1 suggesting similar compositions (Fig. 11d). The plots also, however, show increased scatter in the ratios indicating the presence of different felsic subtypes. The mafic rocks at both TG1 and TG3 show similar distribution of Al_2O_3 - TiO_2 ratios with some scatter, suggesting that there may be more than one-precursor composition for the mafic lithologies. Some TG1 rocks show an unusual lithology characterized by very high silica contents (greater than 90 % SiO_2) and relatively low Zr/TiO_2 ratios. These rocks are likely highly silicified mafics.

Chemical alteration features are exceptionally obvious in the preliminary data set (Table 1). Strong Na depletion and Si enrichment seem to characterize much of the alteration. A preliminary review of Na, K and Ba contents in rocks with corundum contents greater than five percent suggests that the rocks are highly altered. Any samples with less than one percent Na are considered an altered population and plot on the sections within the footwall dacites of TG1 and TG3. Samples with greater than 0.2 percent K form a distinct population and are probably altered. Most of these samples are mafic rocks that would not be expected to have such high K values. Their distribution correlates with dacite units stratigraphically. Barium values greater than 1100 ppm form a distinct population and are considered anomalous and correlate to sulphide horizons. Alteration generally appears to be characterized by a loss of Na and Ca, and gains in Fe, Mg, K and Si. This likely reflects destruction of feldspar and formation of chlorite-sericite and hydrothermal silica.

DISCUSSION

Geological setting and deposition of sulphides

The TG1 and TG3 deposits, and possibly the B5 deposit, are hosted in north trending, chevron shaped, second order grabens. These grabens formed obliquely to the northeast trend of the Lancones Basin as a result of a northwest oriented extensional tectonic regime which could have commenced as early as Upper Jurassic time (Fig. 3). Such geometry is relatively common to active seafloor volcanic extensional regimes such as the Sumisu rift, Izu-Bonin arc that resulted from conjugate oblique faulting within a larger extending basin (Okamura and Murakami, 1991). Within the Tambo Trend second order graben, TG1 and TG3 sulphides were deposited in conjugate subbasins initiated by northwest oriented horst and graben development in basal basalt. Faulted margins of the second order basin have not been observed in the drilling, but evidence such as a thick debris flow over top of the TG3 deposit indicates that there was significant relief in the area during, and shortly following, the formation of the sulphide mounds.

Geological settings of the TG1 and TG3 deposits are similar and they appear to have formed in the same manner. Dacitic volcanism, probably erupting along northwest trending, third order graben-bounding faults, modified the seafloor topography by covering vent areas near the margins and tops of basalt horsts. These multiple event dacite domes in part filled graben basins with dacite flows and epiclastic derivatives. Continued rifting and block faulting within the larger second order graben likely contributed to

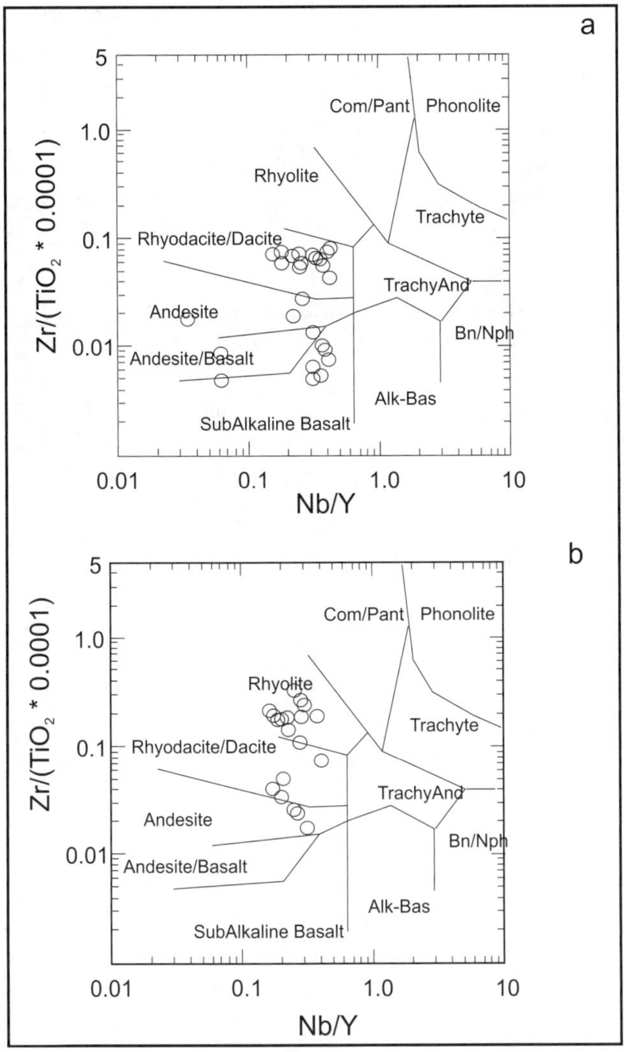

Figures 11a & b. Immobile element plots for least altered samples. for a) TG1 and b) TG3 (Winchester and Floyd, 1977).

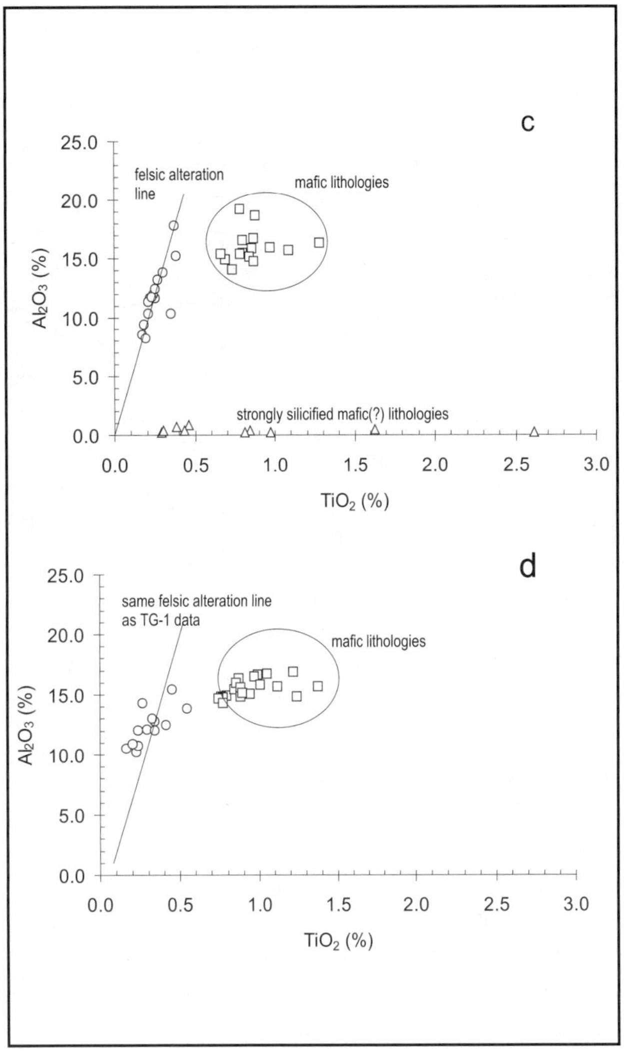

Figures 11c & d. Immobile element plots for dacite and basalt, c) TG1 and d) TG3.

this multi-episodic volcanic development. Hydrothermal fluids were localized along the original structures within the basal basalt. Sulphide mounds developed in basins adjacent to the dacite domes.

The *TG1 sulphides* are contained within a 1000 m long by 500 m wide northwest-oriented basin that slopes to the north. The shape and orientation of the basin was initiated by graben development in the basalt ocean floor. Subsequently, multi-episodic dacite domes grew on the basin margins and partially filled the basin with dacite flows. Dacite breccia spalling off of the dome flanks (carapace or rubble breccia) intermittently covered the basin floor. The basin was also partially filled with heterolithic epiclastics termed conglomerate or dacite debris flow. These epiclastic units contain both basalt and dacite fragments suggesting that the source material could have come from as far away as the inferred fault scarps of the second order graben. As the dacite domes grew, possibly with contemporaneous subsidence of the basin floor due to continued rifting, the conglomerate units were warped steeply up the basin walls.

The pyrite plus or minus base metal mineral stockwork that underlies the northern and deepest part of the basin, suggests sulphide accumulation started in this area and spread south onto unfractured ocean floor.

Thin horizons of felsic volcaniclastic or perhaps epiclastic material are sporadically intercalated with the sulphides and primarily have lateral continuity across the entire width of the deposit. The felsites are commonly altered to vuggy silica in the central part of the pile coincident with the barren pyrite core. Vuggy silica is likely a product of alteration due to continued hot upwelling fluids. The source for these felsic layers is still uncertain. They typically extend to the deposit margins where they appear to merge with more massive wedges of intense hydrothermally altered, silicified, and brecciated felsic volcanics up to 50 m thick. These felsic wedges have been logged as rhyolite but appear to be un-rooted and may simply be altered dacites where hydrothermal solutions migrated up the deposit margins. On the other hand, they could represent phreatomagmatic eruptions along the graben margins that may have been violent enough to broadcast debris across the entire width of the basin.

Part way through the deposition of sulphides at TG1, basalt flows entered the basin from the north and south, partially burying the sulphides. The largest of these flows, in the south part of the basin, reaches a thickness of over 50 m. Sulphide deposition continued after this volcanism, eventually completely burying the basalts. Similarities in chemistry and lithology between these mafic flows and the hangingwall basalt in TG3 suggest that TG1 is the younger of the two deposits.

The final depositional stages in the formation of the TG1 deposit are not well understood. A period of felsic volcanism likely immediately followed or occurred contemporaneously with the end of sulphide deposition. The eruptive centre was probably located near the eastern flank of the basin and not within the sulphide pile. The product of this volcanism, a quartz-rich sandy breccia (or possibly tuff), sporadically covers the sulphides in thin layers. The clastic component of this group of rocks may have eroded from a felsic eruptive centre, or may be reworked felsic tuff. In either case, it is predominantly an immature sediment appearing to fill shallow basins on a gently undulating sulphide mound. The discontinuous baritic sandstone overlies the sulphides and felsic clastic material in topographic highs and lows suggesting that it is a direct precipitate from hydrothermal solutions escaping from the sulphide pile below. The barite-bearing sandstone commonly contains milky to glassy quartz and indicates mixing and reworking by normal sedimentary processes occurred contemporaneously with the precipitation of exhalative barite.

The iron hydroxide (goethite predominant) precipitate or replacement deposit overlies the baritic units and extends well beyond the limits of the sulphides, suggesting that the hydrothermal system remained active after dacite volcanism ended. This unit is barium and gold enhanced above the sulphide deposit. Vuggy silica fragments incorporated within this iron cap may represent layers of silica sinter or possibly felsic tuff that broke up as the pile compacted. The top of the oxide sequence, dominated by clay with sporadic iron staining and goethitic fragments, may be a mix of volcanic tuffs or flows that were saturated with iron-rich solutions, and subsequently altered to clay by weathering or acidic hydrothermal fluid action. Some parts of the oxide cap are ultimately covered by saprolitic, hematite-altered andesite (or possibly dacite) porphyry. The lack of oxidation in sulphides below the felsic-barite units suggests the sulphides were protected from oxidation during uplift.

The *TG3 sulphide* deposits occupy basins marginal to dacite domes, similar to the setting of the TG1 deposit. A central multi-episodoic dacite dome developed on a horst of basalt prior to the deposition of the TG3 North and South sulphides (Fig. 12b). Dacite rubble breccia southwest of TG3 South and dacite flows northeast of TG3 North suggest that dacite domes also formed in these areas. Dome development in the graben was critical to the creation of third order intra-dome basins which host sulphides at TG3.

The depositional history of the TG3 sulphides started in the South deposit (Fig. 12b). Sulphides filled a roughly 400 m wide, symmetrical bowl-shaped basin to a depth of approximately 100 m. The upper surface of the sulphide pile at this point had a slight positive relief. A short hiatus in sulphide deposition allowed dacite conglomerate (or volcanic-derived debris-flow) units to accumulate along the flanks of the mound (Fig. 12c). Renewed dacite volcanism occurred simultaneously in the central and southern dacite domes (Fig. 12d). Chloritic-altered flow banded fragmental dacitic material (dacite rubble breccia) spalled off of the flanks of the domes and buried the margins of the initial sulphide mound on all sides. Massive sulphides in the TG3 North deposit commenced accumulating on the north flank of the central dacite dome at this time. Sulphide deposition continued in the central part of the TG3 South pile, keeping pace with the accumulation of dacitic debris from the flanking domes (Fig. 12e). Eventually the dacitic volcanism waned, and another set of conglomerates was deposited on both sides of the TG3 South deposit. Continued growth of the TG3 South deposit caused sulphides to on-lap the dacite rubble and conglomerate units adjacent the central and south domes. A third cycle of volcanism renewed growth of the central dacite dome and appears to have initiated the development of a third dome north of the TG3 North deposit. This dome buried the initial TG3 North deposit and forced the focus of deposition to the south, between the north and central domes. Late in the last felsic eruptive cycle dacite material in the central dome outpaced sulphide development and partly buried the flanks of both the TG3 North and South deposits. Dacite volcanism and sulphide deposition appear to have ended at approximately the same time.

The chemistry of the magmas that were erupted into the basin changed abruptly at the end of the sulphide-dacite depositional cycle. A sequence of andesite tuffs and flows covered the TG3 North deposit, dacitic rocks, and part of the TG3 South deposit (Figs. 12f and g). The reason for the discontinuous distribution of the andesites is unclear. The reason could be multiple sporadically located eruptive centres, or possibly due to erosion. Whatever the cause, it appears that a valley perhaps as much as 100 m deep was filled with an andesite debris flow from the north or northwest (Fig. 12h). Such a catastrophic depositional event suggests that the area had significant relief. The debris flow may have been derived from fault scarp failure on the western margin of the second order graben. The entire sequence was then partially covered with a series of amygdaloidal basalt flows and flow breccias. These basalts may be equivalent to the mafic flows intercalated with the TG1 sulphide deposit, suggesting that mineralization at TG1 continued after the TG3 deposits were buried.

Mineralization

The *stringer zones* beneath the sulphide mounds contain significant pyrite-chalcopyrite and, occasionally, minor sphalerite concentrations for a few metres below the massive sulphides. More commonly however, the stringer zones lack base metals. This suggests that, with local exceptions, fluid temperatures were too high for base metal deposition. The associated dark chlorite alteration envelopes in the barren stringer zones presumably developed in the areas of highest temperatures and fluid flow.

Within the *sulphide piles* the base metal mineral assemblages vary relative to the proximity of the hydrothermal conduits represented by the stringer zones in the footwall volcanic rocks. In general terms, the central core consists of massive pyrite with little or insignificant base metal content and presumably overlies the main hydrothermal conduit. The core was leached of base metals by continuous flooding with high temperature fluids. Base metals (copper and zinc) were transported to the cooler margins of the sulphide pile where they precipitated as chalcopyrite or sphalerite interstitial to crystalline pyrite. On the outer fringes of the sulphide piles, pore spaces between fragments, possibly formed due to anhydrite dissolution, provided paleo-channelways for hydrothermal solutions. Colliform sphalerite textures, observed peripheral to fluid conduits, are small-scale equivalents to sphalerite precipitation on the outer fringes of the pile, due to decrease of fluid temperatures. Sphalerite fragments near the margins of the pile may be the products of chimney collapse on the basin margins. A chalcopyrite (plus or minus magnetite) rich zone developed along the base of the deposit probably resulted from late stage hot hydrothermal fluids percolating into the base of a cooling sulphide pile.

Stratified sulphides within the fine-grained siltstones and lutites on the top and margins of the deposit are commonly thinly laminated. They have rare graded beds, scour marks, soft sediment slump folds, and syndepositional microfaults. Some coarser-grained fragmental sulphide horizons have a heterolithic mix of pyrite, chalcopyrite and sphalerite grains. These sulphide textural features could conceivably have formed either by epiclastic deposition

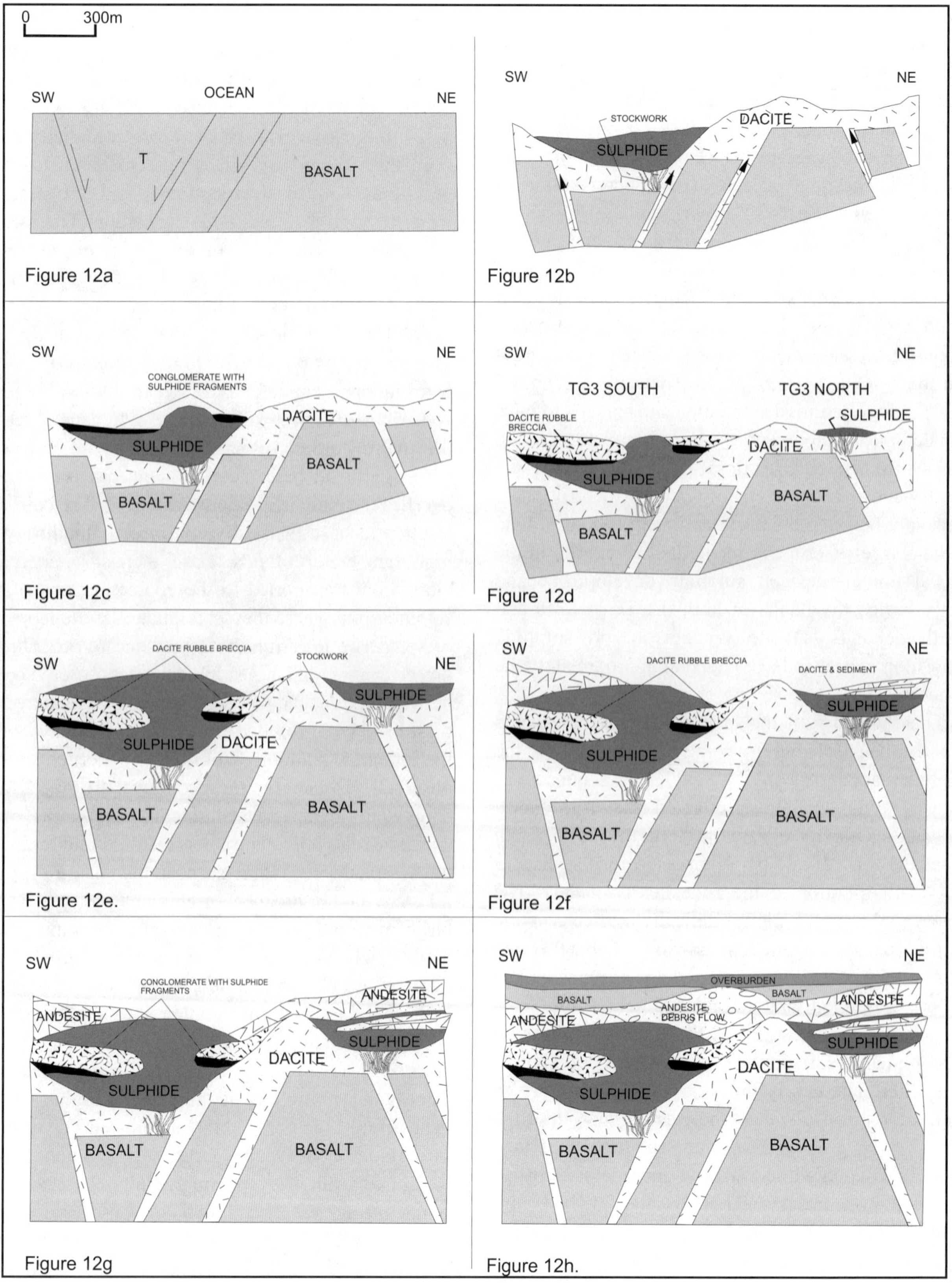

Figure 12. Schematic development of the TG3 deposits (looking Northwest).

sulphides, or by replacement of favorable permeable stratigraphy by hydrothermal fluids. Vent-related bedded sulphides are unlikely to form on the sea floor due to rapid oxidation of the fine-grained sulphide particles. It is more likely that hydrothermal fluids permeated soft carbonaceous sediments on the sea floor, cooled rapidly over short distances below the water interface and precipitated sulphides.

Gold deposition in the TG1 *oxide zone* is associated with barite. Both gold and barite are generally most abundant near the base of the oxide zone, specifically in the felsic fragmental and baritic sandstone units. Barite presumably formed when barium-bearing solutions contacted sulphate ions (SO_4) derived from seawater. Barite precipitates are most abundant immediately above the sulphide pile where solutions first came into contact with cold oxygenated seawater. Tabular barite crystals continued to grow in the base of the oxide zone as seawater continued to enter the pile and contact with the hydrothermal fluids.

The brecciated nature of the overlying *goethite* unit was caused by collapse of the pile, perhaps during simple compaction. Anhydrite could have been incorporated in the pile and later dissolved allowing the material to collapse. The argillic-altered volcanic flows and/or tuffs, intercalated with iron hydroxide precipitates that cover the deposit, are the product of continued hot spring activity.

Metal Transport Model

The TG deposits best fit a depositional model that is similar to most Cu-Zn deposits in a bimodal, mafic-dominated deep water suite. The deposits have little lead (typical of deposition from high temperature solutions i.e. ~350°C from a fluid that formed in equilibrium with basalt). Such precipitation usually coincides with chalcopyrite deposition (but not chalcocite-covellite), and occurred as the fluids cooled through ~280°C. The deposits however, have higher gold than some in this classification, and although not shown on the figures, the gold spacially correlates with zinc, lead, and barium. The gold is most abundant in sulphides and baritic oxides at the top of the deposit. The gold was more likely deposited (or re-deposited) from a lower temperature fluid, dominated by bi-sulphide transport and precipitation due to oxidation. TG3 is most representative of the bi-modal, mafic dominated deep-water suite. TG1 and to a lesser extent TG3 have been modified by a late stage, lower temperature event. Supergene copper developed in the upper part of the base-metal rich periphery to the TG1 deposit. The barite and gold-rich exhalite at the top make TG1 unique.

TG1 likely underwent significant modification due to the circulation of local seawater. Water was drawn through the massive sulphides by convection as has been observed at several scales in modern systems. At the TAG field at the Mid-Atlantic Ridge this type of remobilization was observed at both the deposit scale (Hannington, 1995) and at the chimney scale (Tivey and McDuff, 1990). In this case the altering fluid was modified seawater. Under slightly reducing, near-neutral pH conditions, the dominant transporting agent would be HS-.

This convective fluid model explains all the features noted at TG1. Key to this model is the dominance of bi-sulphide transport, which has been demonstrated in several places. Copper shows an unusual solubility relationship under these conditions. Virtually all copper precipitates as chalcopyrite on cooling to ~280°C. As a bisulphide however, copper is soluble at low temperatures and thus may be redistributed in significant quantities. Lydon pointed out that copper has a solubility "minimum"; it drops out from the primary Cl- dominated hydrothermal fluid at 280°C, but can be re-dissolved as a bisulphide at ~200°C (Franklin et al 1981). It then can be re-precipitated at about 50°C, as low temperature copper phases. Gold is also exceptionally soluble at low temperatures as a bisulphide. Thus a locally advecting, near-neutral, sulphur-saturated fluid would carry significant copper and gold. The copper would precipitate at low temperature in the upper and marginal part of the orebody as chalcocite and covellite. Gold would not precipitate until the bisulphide complex contacted an oxidizing zone (i.e. seawater). Upon oxidation, all of the gold would precipitate quickly and efficiently. This sequence of events could produce low-temperature copper zones near the top of the sulphides and a gold zone above the deposit at the seawater interface.

SUMMARY AND CONCLUSIONS

The Tambo Grande district, precious metal-bearing, volcanogenic massive sulphide deposits occur in pre-Albian, subalkaline-tholeiitic volcanic flows and associated dacite of the Ereo Formation. These rocks and the overlying thick succession of volcaniclastic and flysch sequences were deposited in the northeasterly oriented Lancones Basin. The Basin formed in a rifted continental margin between the coastal Amotape Range and Olmos Massif during continental separation of Laurentia from Gonwanda commencing in Middle Jurassic time. Since then, the deposits and enclosing volcanic stratigraphy have undergone negligible post-mineral tectonism and magmatism, allowing them to remain relatively pristine. Many of the textures recognized in modern seafloor massive sulphide systems, are preserved in the Tambo Grande deposits.

Although the Ereo Formation within the Lancones Basin is almost completely covered by Tertiary and Pleistocene sediments, indirect exploration techniques such as gravity, magnetics and, to a lesser degree, conductivity surveys, effectively outline the geology and hidden massive sulphide deposits. The relatively flat terrain and undisturbed nature of the deposits make the geophysical signature of the subsurface geology and associated deposits relatively easy to interpret. Geophysical interpretation has provided significant added insight to a geologic model that otherwise would be difficult to obtain in this buried terrain.

Second order structural grabens, filled by basaltic rocks and intercalated dacite domes and volcanic breccias host the massive sulphide basins and mounds. Sulphides filled a deep, northwesterly oriented fault and dacite dome-bounded trough, obliquely oriented to a second order graben. One kilometre south, TG3 sulphides filled northwesterly elongate basins proximal to a central dacite dome built on a basalt horst. The B5 deposit appears to have a similar setting, although it needs to be confirmed.

The deposits are flat-lying and unusually thick (300m for TG3 South), constrained laterally by either synvolcanic faults or coeval volcanism. They display virtually all the classic characteristics of VMS deposits including a distinct lithologic break from footwall to hangingwall, and zoned massive sulphides with zinc-rich distal phases, and increased copper concentrations at the base. Metal contents are similar to "typical" VMS deposits in bimodal, mafic-dominated sequences although the gold content is higher (Franklin, personal communication). The deposits have many similarities to the Flin Flon or Noranda camps. The unusual thickness of the deposits is attributable to the anomalous heat flows generated by episodic volcanism that provided a thermal recharge of the hydrothermal system. The conversion of the sulphide pile at TG1 from high temperature sulphide deposition to low temperature copper sulphides and barite precipitation is attributable to seawater being drawn into the deposit, driven by convective heat flows generated by the hot sulphides. This fluid then remobilized both copper and gold. Copper substantially dropped out as low-temperature sulphides in the upper and distal parts of the sulphide zone, and gold continued to move up and out of the sulphide body. Gold then precipitated at the sulphide-seawater interface due to interaction with oxygen-rich bottom waters.

The most striking similarity between the TG1 and TG3 deposits is the association with dacite volcanism. Sulphide and gangue mineral assemblages are essentially identical, indicating that the source fluids had similar compositions. In contrast, gold-bearing barite did not precipitate over top of the TG3 deposit, presumably because TG3 was buried before the oxide phase had a chance to form. Burial of the TG3 deposit also prevented the development of a secondary copper zone.

ACKNOWLEDGMENTS

This paper was made possible by the generous support of Manhattan Minerals Corp. which supplied the data and allowed the personnel time for research and writing.

A number of geologists not referenced in this text made important contributions to the development of the current level of understanding of the geology and to the success of the exploration program. These include Cristian Soux and his field geologists Miguel Jimenez and Jose Dilas who provided daily coordination for as many as six drills. The geological core logging crew consisted of Brian Thurston, Konstantin

Lesnikov, Sefika Lesnikov, Arturo Cordova, Juan Quiroga, Luis Aviles Rolando Cruzado, Segundo Castro, Juan Carlos Merino and Edward Lyons whose detailed observations form the backbone of this report. The geotechnical team headed by Brian Thurston consisted of Arturo Bulnes, Edwin Sandoval, Segundo Estrada, Jose Chang, Segundo Lopez and Jose Canales who logged the physical characteristics of the core that was then correlated to the geophysical surveys for on-going exploration. James Franklin's insight and knowledge provided valuable guides to interpreting the volcanic sequences as well as providing a petrochemical review of the rocks and comparisons to modern VMS systems. Ross Sherlock provided added guides to the whole rock and lithogeochemical signature of the volcanic stratigraphy. Richard Tosdal reviewed the paper and in particular criticized the proposed regional setting of the district which lead to many useful discussions. There are many others not mentioned who contributed, not the least of which was Steve Haras who put the figures together.

REFERENCES

Chavez, A., Nunez Del Prado, S.H., 1991. Evolucion Vertical de Facies de la Serie Turbiditica Cretacea (Grupo Copa Sombrero) en el perfil tipo Huasimal- Encuentros (Cuenca Lancones en el Noreste del Peru). Boletin de la Sociedad del Peru, V. 82, p.5-21

Fischer, A.G., 1956. Desarrollo geologico del Noroeste Peruano durante el Mesozoico. Sociedad Geologia del Peru, v.30, p 177-190

Hannington, M.D., Jonasson, I.R., Herzig, P.M., Peterson, S., 1995. Physical and chemical processes of seafloor mineralization at Mid-ocean Ridges: In Seafloor Hydrothermal systems. Physical, Chemical, Biological and Geological Interactions, Geophysical Monograph 91, American Geophysical Union, p. 115-157

Franklin, J.M., Lydon J.W., Sangster, D.F., 1981. Volcanic-associated massive sulphide deposits. Economic Geology 75 anniversary volume, p. 485-627

Injoque, J., Miranda C., Duninn-Borkowski E., 1979. Estudio De La Genesis Del Yacimiento de Tambo Grande y Sus Implicancias. Boletin de la Sociedad del Peru, v. 64, p. 73-99

Jaillard, E., Soler, P., Carier G., Mourier, T., 1990. Geodynamic evolution of the northern and central Andes during early to middle Mesozoic times: a Tethyan model. Journal of the Geological Society, London, v. 147, p. 1009-1022

MacLean, W.H. and Kranidiotis, P., 1987. Immobile elements as monitors of mass transfer in hydrothermal alteration: Phelps Dodge massive sulfide deposit, Matagami, Quebec. Economic Geology, v. 82, p. 951-962

MaLellari, C. E., 1988. Cretaceous paleogeography and depositional cycles of western South America. Journal of South America Earth Sciences, v. I, p. 373-418

Mitouard, P., Kissel C., Laj, C., 1990. Post-Oligocene rotatons in southern Ecuador and northern Peru and the formation of the Huacabamba deflection in the Andean Cordillera. Earth and Planatary Science Letters, v. II, p2, p. 329-339

Morris, R.C., and Aleman, A.R., 1975. Sedimentation and tcctonics of the middle Cretaceous Copa Sombrero formation in Northwest Peru. Boletin de la Sociedad Geologca del Peru, v. 48, p 49-64

Mourier, T., Laj C., Megard, F., Roperch, P., Mitouard, P., Farfau Medrano, A., 1988. An Accreted continental terrane in northwestern Peru. Earth and Planatary Science Letters, v. I, P1, p182-192

Ochoa Alencstre, A., 1980. Evaluacion hidrocarburifera de la Cuenca Sechura. Boletin de la Sociedad del Peru, v.67, p. 133-152

Palacios Moncaya, O. 1994. Geologia de los Cuadrangulos de Paita, Piura, Talara, Sullana, Lobitos y Zarumila. Instituto Geologico Minero y Metalurgio, Bul. 54, Serie A

Reyes,L. R., Caldas J. Y., (1987) Geologia de los Cuadranglos de las Playas, La Tina, Las Lomas, Ayabaca, San Antonio, Instituto Geologico Minero y Metalurgio, Bul. 49

Taylor, B., Klaus, A., Brown, G. R., Moore, G. F., Okamura, Y., Murakami, F., 1991. Structural development of Sumisu rift, Izu-Bonin Arc. Journal of Geophysical Research, v. 96, NO. B.10, p. 16,113-16,129

Winchester, J.A., and Floyd, P.A., 1977. Geochemical discrimination of different magma series and their differentiation products using immobile elements. Chemical Geology, 20, p. 325-343

CERRO LINDO PROJECT

Pedro Ly Zevallos
Manager, P.L. GEOEXPLOMIN E.I.R.L., Av. Del Parque Norte 643 - Lima 27 – Perú
Tel: (511) 224 –2693 Fax: (511) 225-3617 E-mail: geoexplo@si.com.pe & coriri@si.com.pe

Abstract

Cerro Lindo is a volcanogenic massive sulphide deposit with Zn-Cu-Ag mineralization, hosted in a sequence of sedimentary and volcanic rocks (Huaranguillo Formation) which has been intruded by granodiorites and tonalites of the Coastal Batholith. The volcanic-sedimentary sequence is metamorphosed, faulted and folded, forming a NW-SE belt approximately 9 km long. In addition to Cerro Lindo, there are 9 prospects, marked by colour anomalies with geochemicaly anomalous concentrations of Ag, Cu, Pb, Zn and Ba.

Initially four pyritic bodies (lenses 1, 2, 3 and 4) were identified; however, subsequent studies indicated that bodies one to three are dismembered portions of an originally single body, called the Main Lens, while the fourth lens is separate and located about 200 m to the northeast. The pyritic bodies have disseminated and layers of Zn-Cu-Ag mineralization and are cross-cut by veins containing similar mineralogy as well as andesitic porphyry dykes. The Main Lens is folded and faulted, forming an antiform with a thickness of 50 to 180 m. Lens 4, is highly faulted and disturbed by the dykes, with a thickness of 10 to 30 m.

In Lens 4, the footwall shows a silicified stockwork with pyrite veins and stringer mineralization which gradually increases the pyrite content until it contains rounded fragments of pyritized and silicified rock in a granular pyrite matrix. It also shows pyrite bands alternating with sphalerite, galena and chalcopyrite bands.

In Lens 2, the host footwall shows pyrite dissemination, veins and veinlets which grades into the pyritic body. The barite content increases towards the margins and there is a predominance of zinc at the top of the pyritic body while copper dominates towards the bottom. These findings lead us to the conclusion that the eastern sector of the footwall is almost vertical to the northeast of the pyritic bodies, while, in the western sector, the footwall is found below the pyritic bodies.

Phelps Dodge estimated 75 million tonnes classified as "Geological Resources" grading 0.89 % Cu, 3.28 % Zn and 50.7 g/t Ag.

Introduction

Cerro Lindo is located at 13°05' – 75°59', in the Chavin district, province of Chicha, department of Ica at 1,850 metres above sea level (Fig. 1). Cerro Lindo is a volcanogenic massive sulphide (VMS) deposit with Zn-Cu-Ag mineralization, hosted by metamorphosed volcanic and sedimentary rocks. The deposit is within an important 8 km lineament distinguished by yellow and white colour anomalies caused by the presence of jarosites and clays overlying the known sulphide bodies and a reddish colour caused by the hematite in the oxidized halo around the mineralized bodies.

From the metallogenic perspective, Cerro Lindo is part of a sedimentary-volcanic belt that outcrops from the south of Lima to the border with Ecuador. This belt includes deposits such as Perubar (Leonila Graciela), María Teresa, Raúl, Condestable and Palma and projects such as Tambogrande, and properties in the exploration stage such as Totoral, Potrobayo, Aurora Augusta, Budeku, Balducho, Los Icas, etc. (Vidal 1980, 1987; Chacón 1989). During the Albian-Cenomanian, the sedimentary volcanic sequence was deposited in a fault-bounded basin in an Andean orientation (NW-SE; Figure 2).

The history of Cerro Lindo is not well known; the available information goes back to the seventies when the deposit belonged to SMRL Cerro Lindo de Ica.

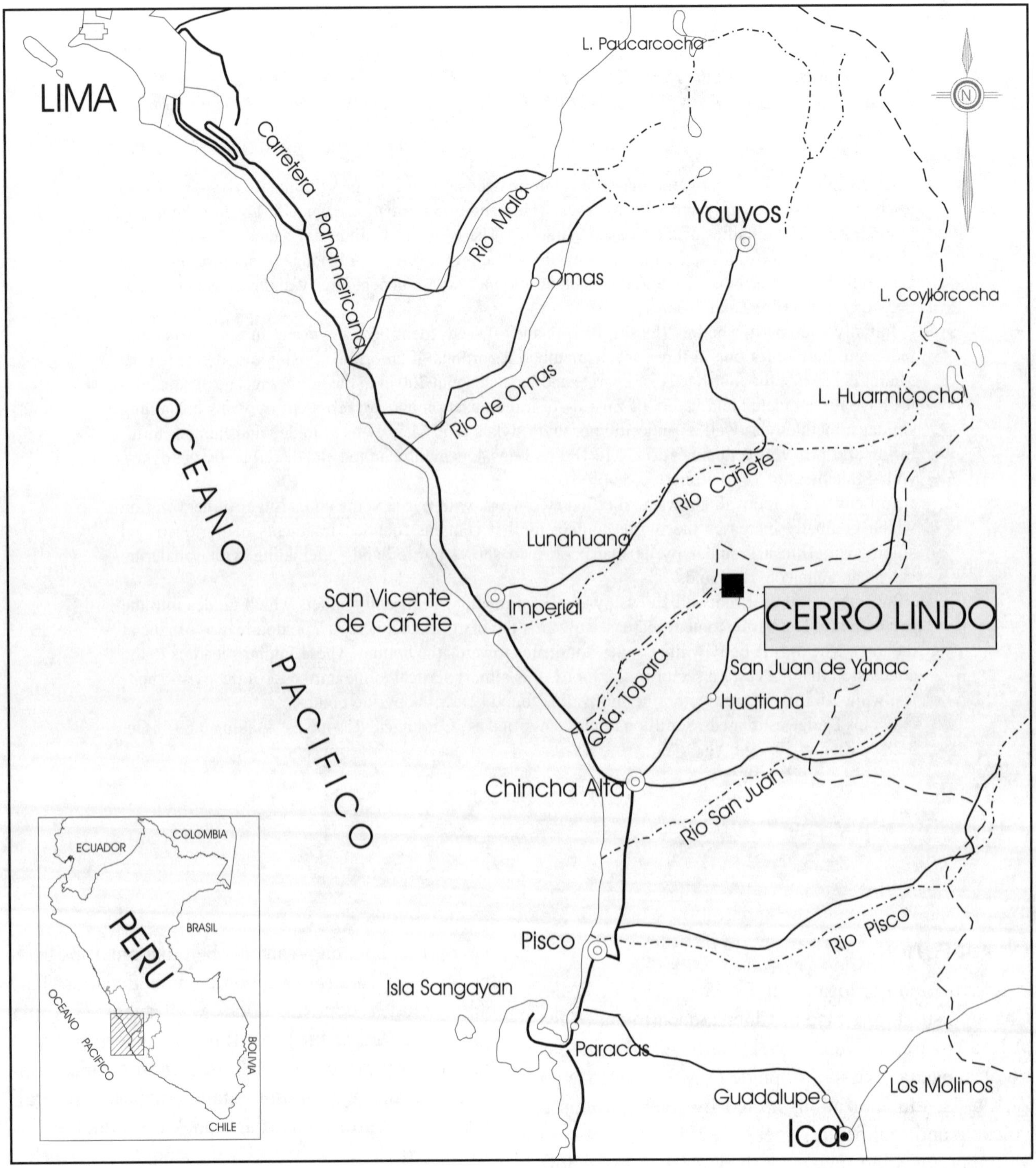

Figure 1. Location and access

The main shareholder was Mr. Luis Sulay, who tried to mine a barite outcropping. At that time, an induced polarization survey was carried out, which indicated there were 5 anomalies and the potential of sulphide resource at depth (Arce, 1973). The efforts to continue with the operation were abandoned when the price of barite dropped.

A short time afterwards this project was taken over by Minera BTX who found Ag anomalies of up to 1,500 g/t Ag in barite outcrops. A pyritic body was also found, as well as the presence of oxides and copper and zinc sulphates and sulphides in the bed of the Topara River.

In 1982 the project was purchased by Compañía Minera Milpo, S.A. who filed for new mining rights covering all the colour anomalies located within the lineament. In 1987 Milpo started a systematic exploration campaign carrying out detailed topographical-geological surveys, sampling of outcroppings and tunneling some 150 m in two galleries at 1,850 and 1,860 metres above sea level, called A and B respectively. The objective was to determine the distribution of barite and Ag below the outcroppings. The results showed 17.1 g/t in Gallery A and 602 g/t Ag in Gallery B. In 1992 Milpo completed a rough access road, 15 km of trenches, systematic sampling of benches, 3,000 m of underground workings and 3,557 m of drilling. On the basis of the information obtained from this work, it was determined that there were 4 massive sulphide bodies.

In 1995 Milpo formed a joint venture with Phelps Dodge, who continued the exploration work in Cerro Lindo, with 6,725 m of diamond drilling in 19 holes. As a result of this work, 75 million metric tonnes of mineral classified as "Geological Resources" were estimated, grading 0.89 % Cu, 0.36 % Pb, 3.28 % Zn and 50.7 g/t Ag. The mineralization towards the north, east south and in depth is still to be determined. At the present time Milpo has resumed exploration work with the intent of going into production.

GEOLOGY

Very little has been written on the geology of Cerro Lindo; although the area is included in the geological survey at scale 1/100,000 carried out by INGEMMET (Salazar and Landa, 1993).

Regional Framework

The deposit is located within a sequence of metamorphosed volcanic-sedimentary rocks of the Huaranguillo Formation (Middle to Upper Cretaceous), which is found as an enclave on the Coastal Batholith (Upper Cretaceous to Lower Tertiary) Figure 4.

The Huaranquillo Formation is the eastern facies of the Quilmana Formation which is dominated by sedimentary rocks in contrast to the western side where the volcanic rocks are dominant (INGEMMET – Bulletin 44, National Geological Mapping Series). Stratigraphically, the Quilmana Formation is located in the upper member of the Casma Group. Two members of the Huaranquillo Formation can be distinguished in this area (Salazar and Landa, 1993), the lower one contains laminated shaly lutites, lutities and volcanic ash alternating with andesitic and metavolcanic layers and occasionally with finely stratified limestone. The upper member has thin layers of limestone interbedded with laminar shaly lutites and volcanic beds.

The Coastal Batholith consists of several intrusions, the oldest and most widely distributed is tonalite and diorite, followed by subsequent intrusions of monzonite and granodiorite. This intrusive complex outcrops to the northeast and southwest of Cerro Lindo and caused the contact metamorphism, thrusting, faulting and deformation of the Huaranguillo volcanic – sedimentary sequence.

Local Geology

Hornfels have been detected in the area where the exploration work is being carried out, as well as nodular schists, interbedding of andesites and dacite-rhyolites, forming a thick package in contact with the intrusives of the Coastal Batholith. Both units were intersected by andesitic porphyry dykes and irregular, discontinuous pegmatitic veins (Ly, 1982, 1994). Figure 5.

Hornfels

Hornfels are located in direct contact with the massive sulphide bodies both at the hangingwall as well as at the footwall. Their texture is granoblastic, porphyroblastic and rarely lepidoblastic; colour may

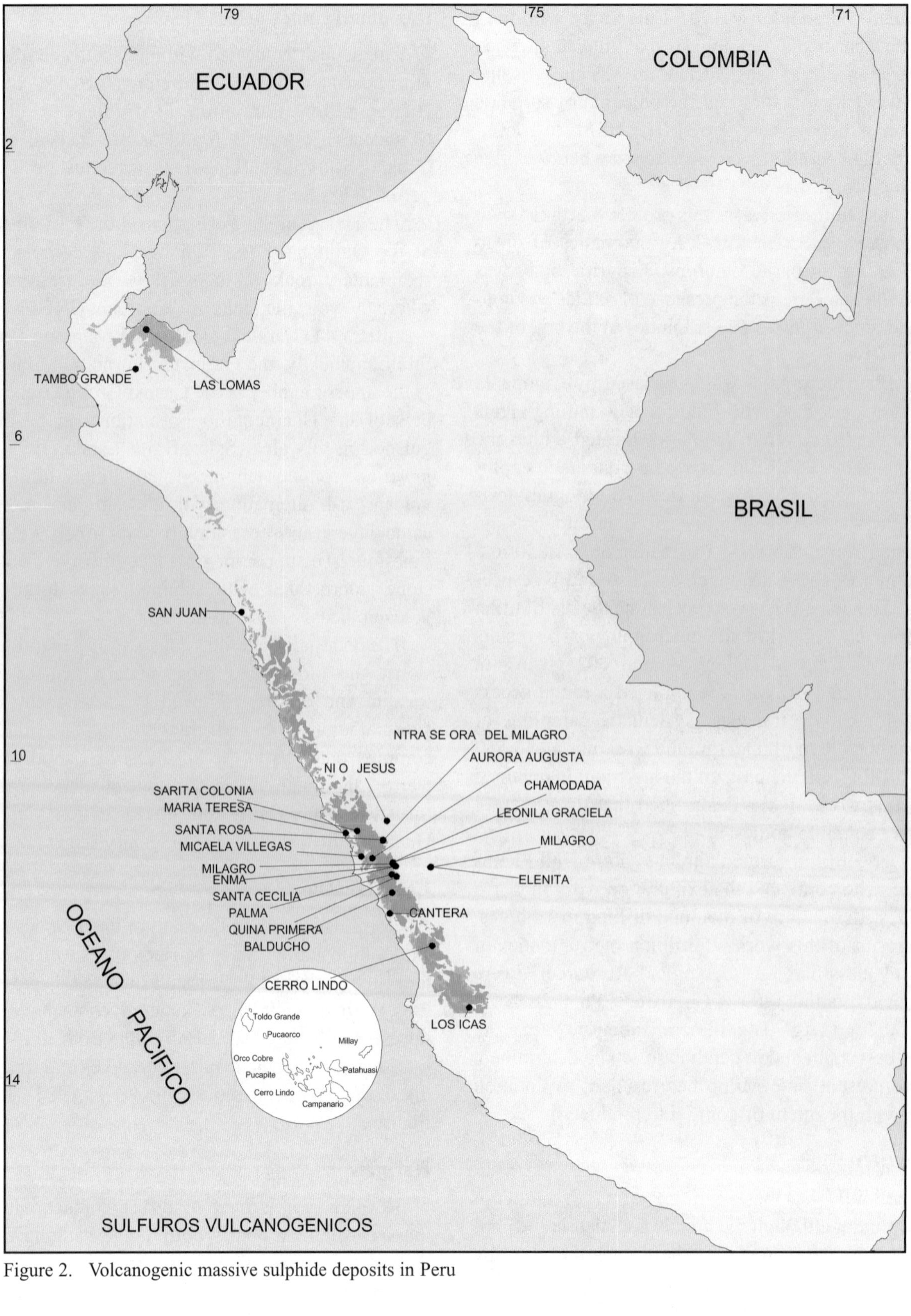

Figure 2. Volcanogenic massive sulphide deposits in Peru

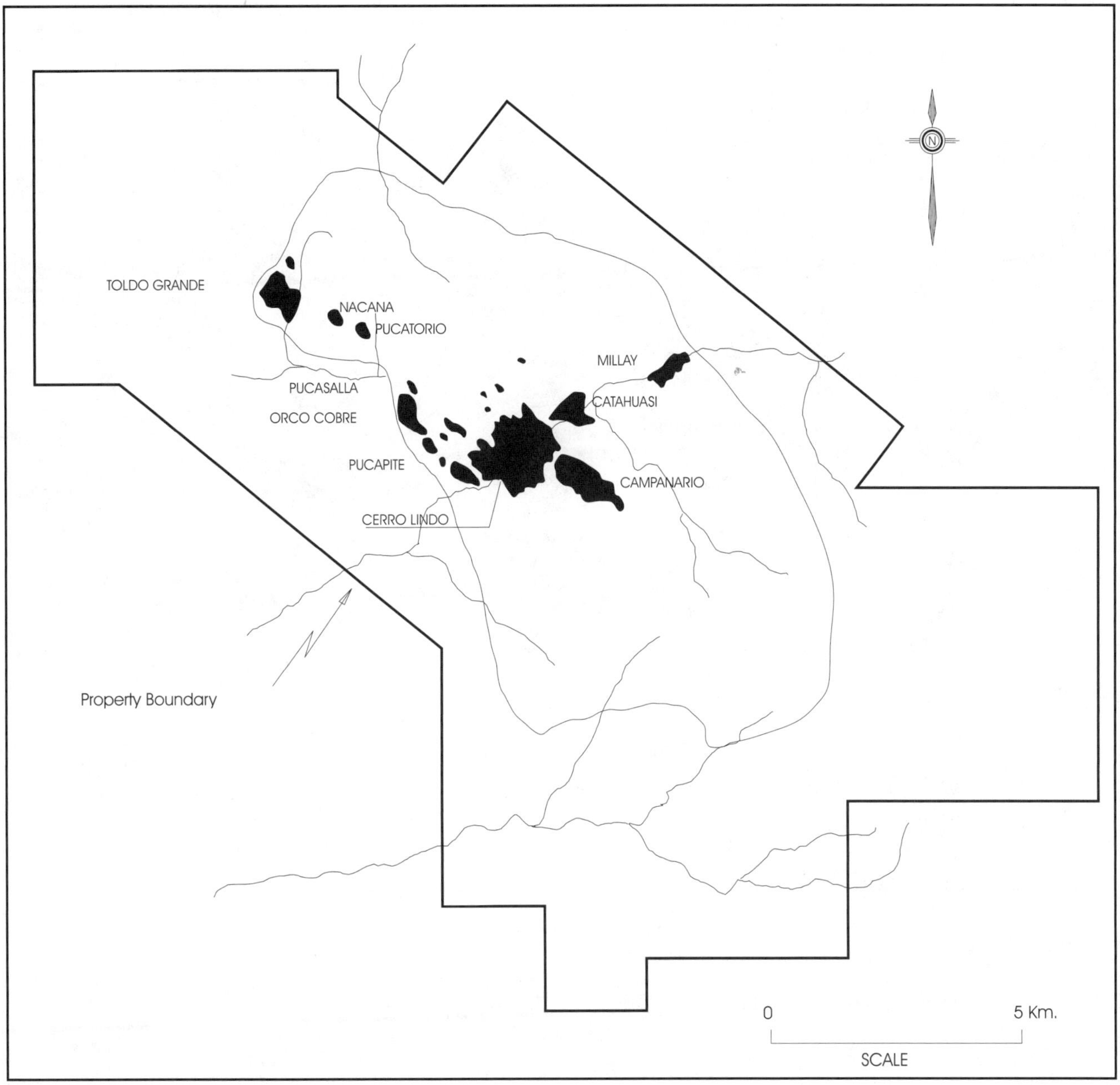

Figure 3. Geochemical anomalies of Cerro Lindo and surrounding area.

be light gray, brownish grey or yellowish on the surface. Quartz, muscovite (sericite), andalusite, biotite and feldspar assemblages make up the hangingwall with sporadic contents of barite, calcite and disseminated pyrite. In the footwall, an assemblage of quartz, muscovite (sericite), andalusite, potash feldspar, disseminated pyrite and granular pyrite veins. The hornfels probably originated from the contact metamorphism process starting from the sedimentary volcanic sequence integrated by the lutite, shaly lutite, sandstone and dacitic to rhyolitic tuff, with occasional interbedding of calcareous lutites.

Hornfels-Nodular Schist

This type of rock has been observed interbedded in the hornfels of the wall rock in Body 1 and consists

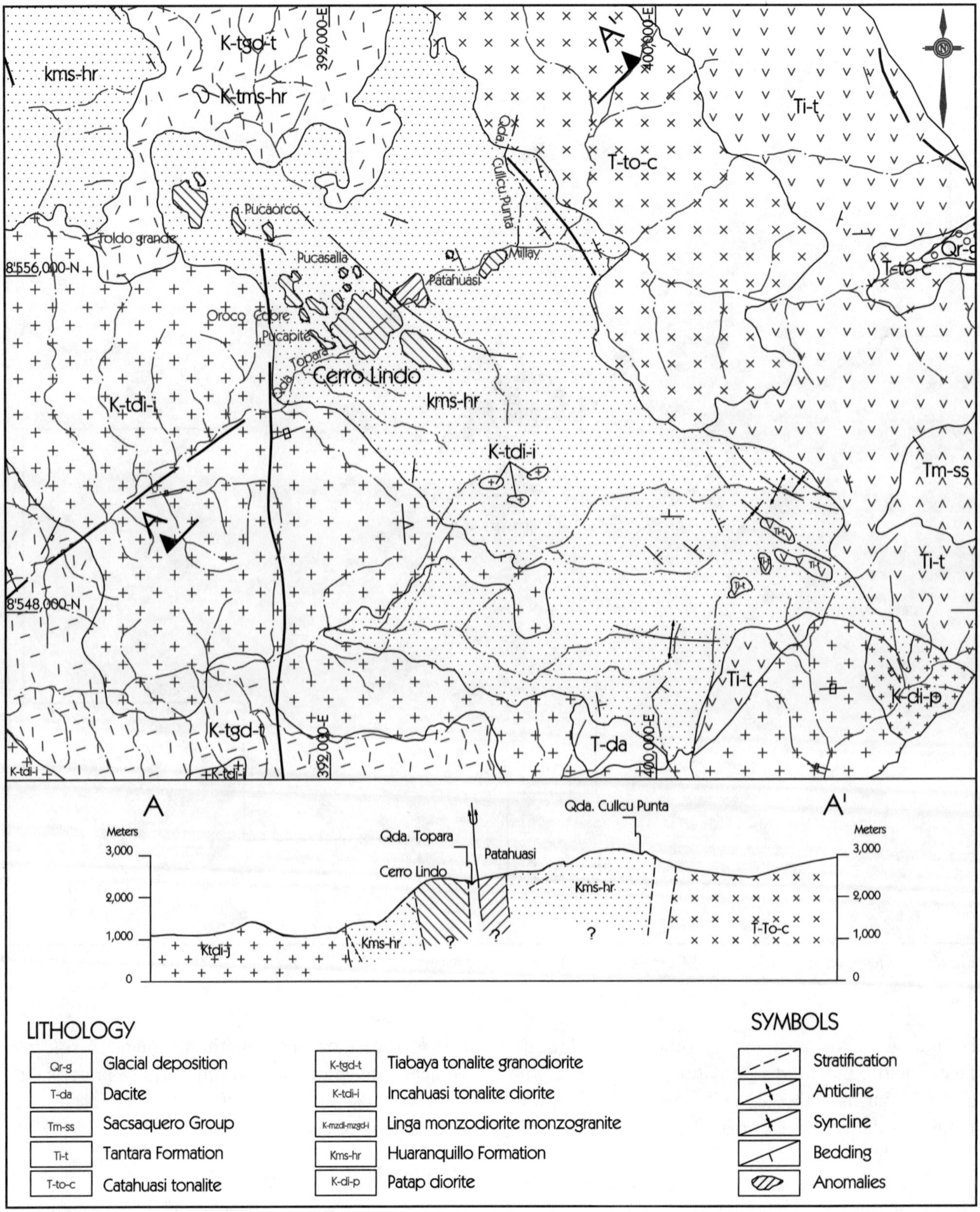

Figure 4. District geology around Cerro Lindo.

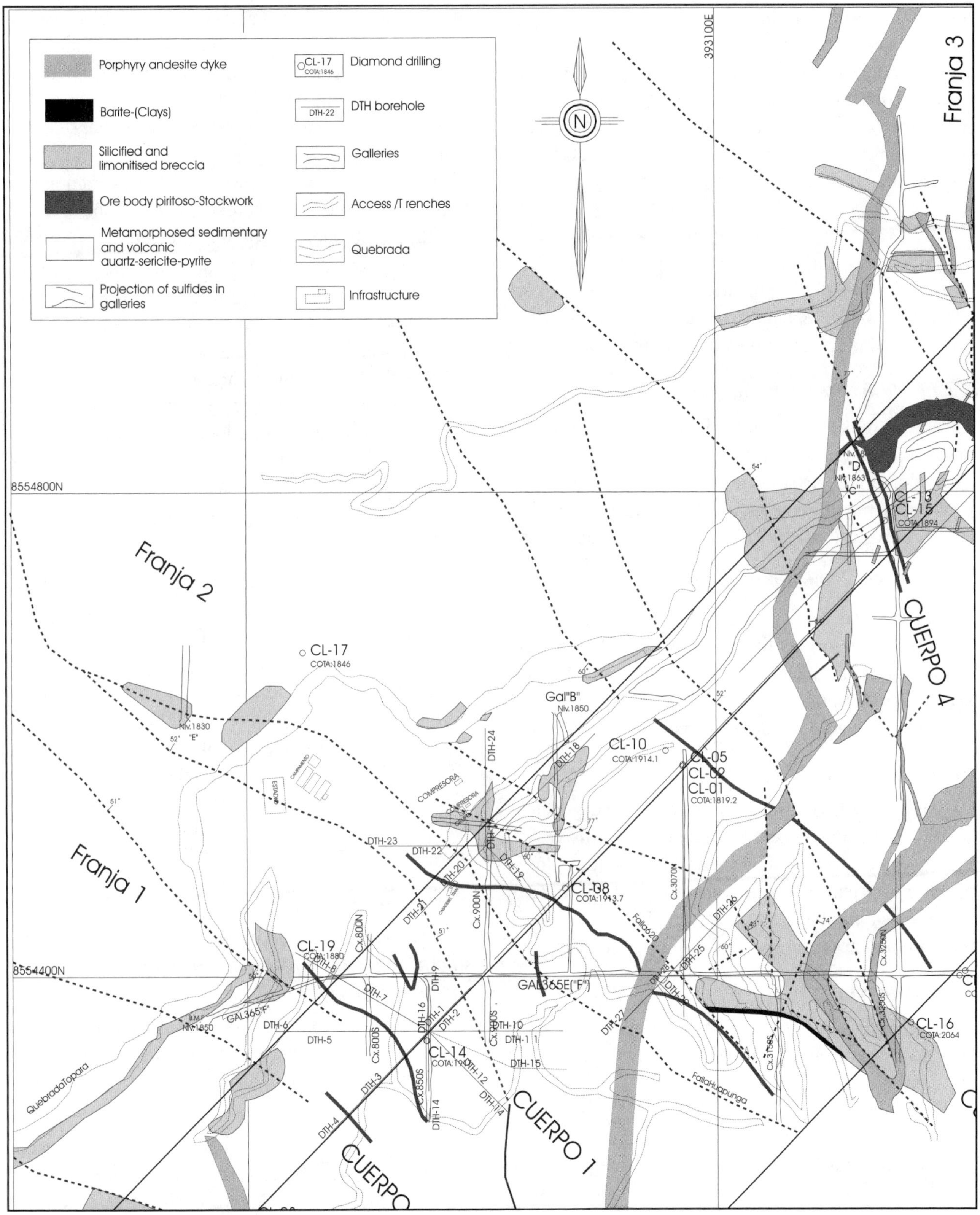

Figure 5. Local geology of Cerro Lindo ore body.

initially of spotted hornfels that due to a variation in the intensity of the metamorphism results in a schist with grey nodules encapsulated in a clear, creamy, fine matrix, composed of quartz, muscovite, and biotite with varying contents of andalusite, rutile and opaques (pyrite). The spotted hornfels would correspond to the areas which have a lower metamorphic grade.

Andesite

Andesite is found as interbedding in the sequence of hornfels, with an aphanitic texture, dark grey to greenish colour; aphanitic matrix and moderately propylitized plagioclase phenocrysts and biotite.

Dacite – Rhyolite

These rocks are found interbedded with the andesites within the hornfels and schist sequence. Their colour ranges from light grey to whitish with pyrite dissemination and veinlets, large quartz grains and biotite or chlorite caused by a subsequent alteration.

Granodiorite – Tonalite – Monzonite

These intrusives, belonging to the Coastal Batholith, outcrop to the southeast, northwest and northeast of the deposit and are responsible for the actual distribution, metamorphism, faulting and folding of the volcanic sedimentary sequence.

Andesitic porphyry dykes

These dykes intrude the volcanic sedimentary sequence, the mineralized bodies and the intrusives of the Coastal Batholith. They are a greenish-grey colour, porphyritic texture with euhedral and subhedral feldspar and hornblende phenocrysts. They reach up to 60 m in thickness and several kilometres in length.

Pegmatitic veins

Pegmatitic veins are of an irregular thickness, have sinuous shapes and lack longitudinal continuity.

SURFACE EXPRESSION OF MINERALIZATION

The surface geological survey identified the existence of siliceous breccia belts or strips with an abundance of limonites, kaolin, manganese oxide and sulphur, associated to granular and massive barite.

The siliceous breccia contains angular fragments of silicified, limonitized and sericitized rocks measuring from decimetres to millimetres, leached and consolidated by oxides (limonite, jarosite and goethite), sulphates and silicates. This breccia was generated by oxidation of the massive sulphides and collapse of the country rock.

Three main belts were identified containing a limonitized siliceous breccia on which benches or trenches were opened with a bulldozer.

1) Belt 1, 150 m wide, runs along the cut of the benches with a NW-SE strike. It is not possible to find out if it continues on the surface because it is covered with quaternary material.
2) Belt 2, Ranging from 30 to 200 metres wide, runs along the cut of the benches, with a NW-SE strike and a total length of 550 metres.
3) Belt 3, 200 metres wide, total length 350 metres, N-S strike, outcrops at both margins of the Topara quebrada.

Greenish copper sulphates outcrop at the bed of the Topara quebrada plus some white outcroppings with an occasional content of sphalerite and chalcopyrite associated with silicified outcroppings with dissemination of pyrite.

At the bottom of the quebrada (Belt 3) there is pyritic body outcropping with highly silicified rock fragments with pyrite dissemination and stringers. Towards the east, the pyrite fills the fractures within a stockwork, the content of pyrite increases towards the east until it engulfs the silicified rock blocks and forms a banded sulphide body.

Alterations

The alteration found in these colour anomalies are silicification, argillization, pyritization, sericitization and propylitization.

- Silicification: Affects leached breccia, the pyritic body that outcrops at the bottom of the quebrada within Belt 3 and, to a lesser extent, the country rock.
- Argillization: Associated to the leached breccia, decreases towards the periphery. Some kaolin has been identified in some sectors of the leached breccia.

- Pyritization: Affects all the rocks of the project, and increases more towards the silicified leached breccia, even forming a pyritic body that engulfs silicified and pyritized rocks in Belt 3. A large quantity of oxides (limonite, goethite and jarosite) within the breccia belts, and to a lesser extent, in its surroundings, is a product of this alteration.
- Sericitization: Similarly to the pyritization, it affects all the country rock, together with the pyritization and argillization determine the anomalous colouring that characterizes the project.
- Propylitization: Found surrounding the coloured anomaly, but it has been identified also within some other sectors of the project, limited to small areas.

Bench sampling

A total of 970 samples were collected from 5 to 10 m trench samples in the different benches and outcroppings. The pertinent statistical data resulted in the parameters shown in Table 1. The average of the analyses carried out with samples taken in some sections of the benches developed in the main belts, are shown in Table 2.

Geochemical maps of Ag, Cu, Pb and Zn indicate that the geochemical anomalies of silver and lead are located at the topographic highs while Cu and Zn anomalies are found at the topographic lows.

GEOLOGY OF THE DEPOSIT

Two types of mineralization were determined on the basis of mine workings and drill core: Massive sulphide bodies with Zn-Cu-Ag mineralization with development of a secondary enrichment horizon; and irregular Pb-Ag-Cu-Zn veins.

Zn-Cu-Ag massive sulphides

Portions of the massive sulphide bodies are banded structure, but there are also sections without banding with a coarse, brittle, granular pyrite. Associated with these bodies are semimassive sulphides, stockworks with sulphide disseminations and veinlets in the footwall.

Four pyritic lenses were explored during an exploration campaign which included galleries and diamond drilling. The diamond drilling program and the subsequent geological interpretation of Cerro Lindo's sections (Fig. 7) suggests that: lenses 1, 2 and 3 are actually a structurally dismembered lense and lense 4 was initially a separate body. For the purposes of this report, we shall continue using the initial classification because of the differences in comparing the thickness of lens 1, 2 and 3. In general, the bodies are near surface or outcrop in topographically high areas and are found down to 170 metres below surface towards the bed of the quebrada.

The dimensions of the bodies are not completely defined, since according to the boreholes and drifts, the continuity still has to be explored to the southeast, northwest, west and in depth.

Based on the results of the geological exploration, Phelps Dodge estimated the following resource of 75 million tonnes at 50.7 g/t Cu, Pb, Zn and Ag, 0.89 % Cu, 0.36 % Pb, 3.28 % Zn.

Mineralogy of the bodies

The ratio of pyrite with respect to the rest of the sulphides is about 85 to 15. The second most important mineral is sphalerite, followed by chalcopyrite and galena. The main supergenic enrichment minerals are covellite, chalcocite and bornite surrounding the upper parts of the bodies.

Pyrite occurs as bands and also with a coarse

Table 1. Geochemical Parameters of Surface Sampling.

	oz Ag/st	% Cu	% Pb	% Zn
Average	0.81	0.05	0.18	0.38
Standard deviation	1.27	0.20	0.59	0.48
Maximum value	18.20	3.90	8.00	9.60

Table 2. The above average values were obtained from samples taken from the benches and outcroppings.

	Length	oz Ag/tc	% Cu	% Pb	% Zn	Location
Belt 1	26.50	1.29	0.02	0.14	0.67	Southern slope
	10.50	1.01	0.00	0.00	0.33	Southern slope
	48.60	1.00	0.00	0.06	0.25	Southern slope
Belt 2	19.00	2.63	0.00	0.85	0.30	Southern slope
	20.80	1.47	0.01	0.56	0.00	Southern slope
	10.00	2.12	0.00	0.10	0.40	Southern slope
	14.60	2.51	0.03	1.17	0.02	Southern slope
	20.00	2.43	0.01	0.19	0.03	Southern slope
Belt 3	68.70	1.72	0.06	0.17	0.13	Southern slope
	10.00	0.56	1.27	0.10	1.01	Quebrada
	54.40	2.16	0.00	0.15	0.49	Northern slope
	14.50	6.55	0.01	3.86	0.45	Northern slope
	22.15	1.65	0.00	0.13	0.63	Northern slope

granular texture. Banding is defined by alternating thin layers of silica, barite, sphalerite, chalcopyrite and galena; but in highly pyritic sections, the banding is defined by the difference in the particle size which ranges from fine to medium. These textures are likely metamorphic in origin and do not reflect primary banding. The coarse grained nature of the sulphides are favourable for releasing minerals during the metallurgical process.

The most important non-metallic mineral is barite which can be found in granular form and mixed with clays and oxides (jarosite – hematite) in the different outcroppings. Inside the mine it occurs in a nodular, banded form combined with the sulphides.

Pyrrhotite has also been identified associated with the base of the massive sulphides, filling small veins associated with pyrite and chalcopyrite in the footwall and also disseminated in the lower levels of the massive sulphide body.

The study of polished sections recognized the occurrence of molydenite, arsenopyrite and tetrahedrite: the molybdenite and the arsenopyrite are associated to chalcopyrite and pyrite. Tetrahedrite occurs associated to sphalerite and galena, and as a filling in sphalerite microfractures (Aranda, 1996).

Paragenesis

Petrographic studies from different parts of the deposit were used to gain a better understanding of the paragenesis in Cerro Lindo (Aranda, 1996). There are several variants on the depositional sequence, but there is a general trend that indicates that the possible sequence of the formation, from the oldest to the most recent, would be as follows:

Pyrite
Sphalerite
Chalcopyrite – pyrrhotite
Galena
Barite
Quartz

Although this sequence describes the formation of the massive sulphide bodies, within the bodies themselves, textures of later replacements and fractures filled with pyrite, quartz, chalcopyrite and sphalerite have been observed that correspond to subsequent mineralization stages.

Zoning from footwall to hangingwall

The best preserved bodies are lenses 4 and 2. The different zones described in the following paragraphs have been recognized in these bodies.

Lens 4

This body outcrops at the bottom of the quebrada, 600 metres upstream from the campsite. The

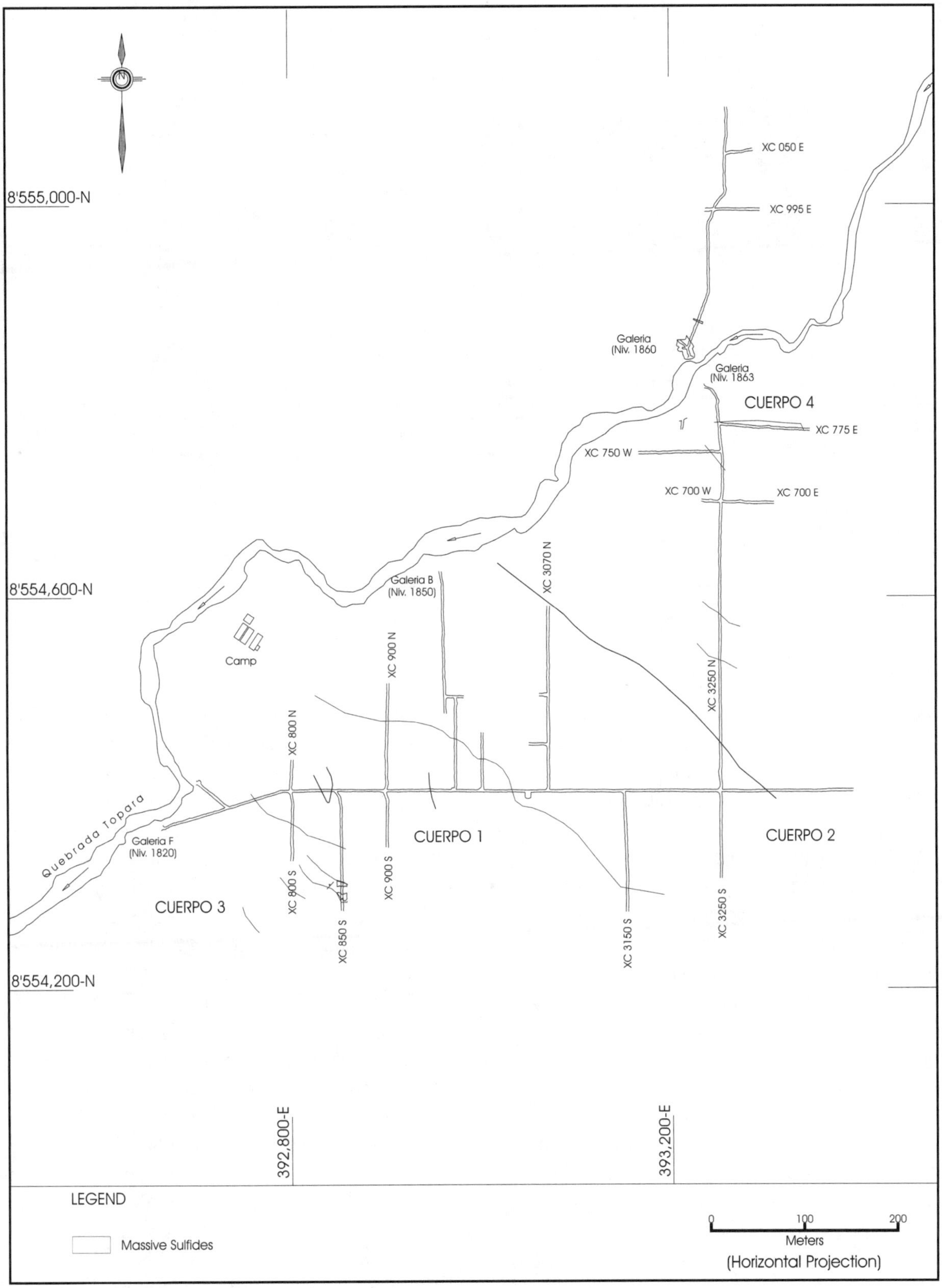

Figure 6. Cerro Lindo Project. Massive sulphide bodies (horizontal projection).

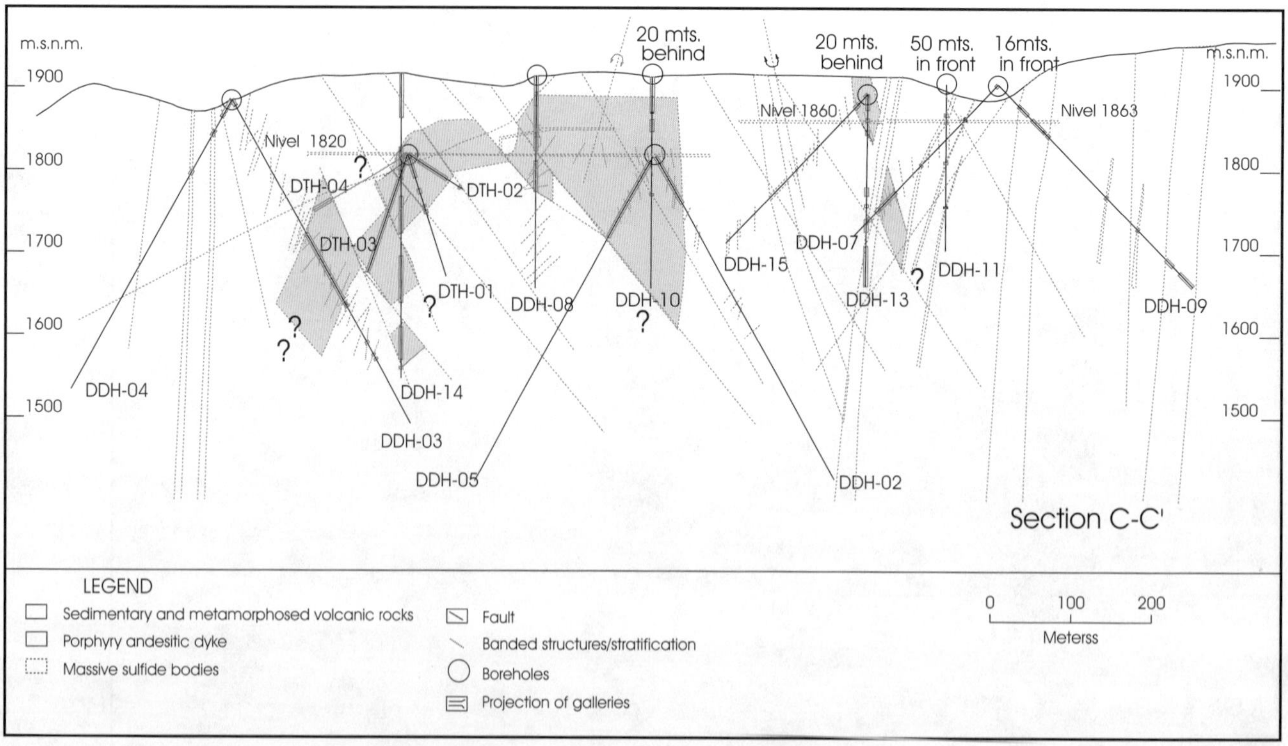

Figure 7. Cerro Lindo Project. Section facing NW.

sequence described below starts 100 metres upstream from the outcropping of the body and ends in the andesitic porphyry dyke, 25 metres downstream from the body. The different zones are illustrated in Figure 8.

Footwall consisting of very hard siliceous hornfels with white and pink spots and pyrite (5 %) in veins and disseminated, as an assemblage of sericite, quartz, andalusite and potash feldspar locally with biotite, rutile and zircon, which may have corresponded to a rhyolitic porphyry.

Gradually the rock appears more silicified and forms large stockworks with pyrite dissemination, small veins, and stringers; initially found in sporadic fractures (from 0.3 to 10 mm thick) filled with pyrite, but as it gets closer to the body, a stockwork defined with pyrite small veins and stringers can be recognized as well as the increased dissemination of pyrite in the rock.

The stockwork intensifies, the blocks of rock become smaller and the pyritic matrix increases until it forms 70 % of the outcropping. Initially, the fragments are silicified, show granular pyrite dissemination and appear rounded and aligned with a N 05°W strike; the matrix is coarse pyrite with a final filling of silica and fine pyrite. Almost at the top of this sequence there is a section of approximately 2 metres where the pyrite content increases in such a way that the blocks are surrounded by pyrite. The microscopic study of a rounded fragment surrounded by pyrite identified an assemblage of quartz, sericite and feldspar with pyrite (5 %), andalusite (5 %), rutile and apatite, which may have originated as a rhyolitic porphyry.

The size of the blocks decreases rapidly into the sedimentary part of this deposit, which consists of over 90 % sulphides, mainly pyrite with galena, sphalerite and chalcopyrite and presents a banding parallel to the alignment of the rock fragments. The grain size is between 0.5 and 1.5 mm and the bands do not exceed 2 mm in thickness; when the banding is solely pyrite, the bands are defined as a function of the particle size.

The configuration of the stockwork and the aligned blocks surrounded by pyrite would indicate

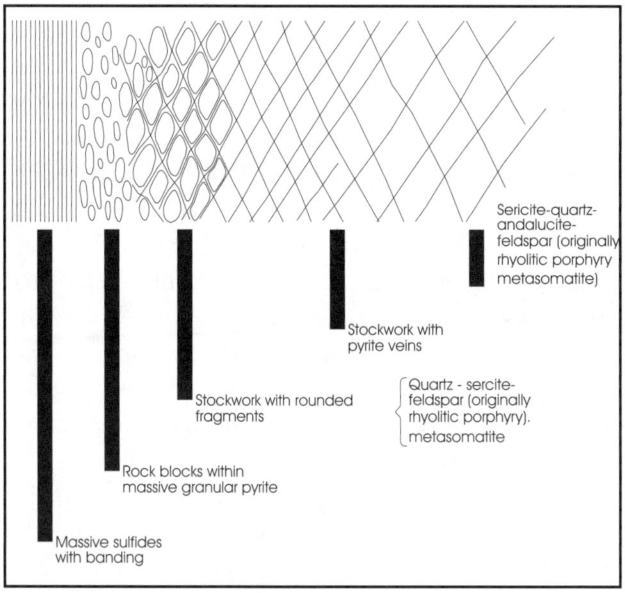

Figure 8. Zoning from footwall to hangingwall.

that this sequence is found in the periphery of the stringer or supply source; where the lateral flow of the hydrothermal solutions would have predominated.

It was not possible to distinguish the metallic zoning of the massive sulphide body, since it is affected by the supergene process that disturbs any primary zoning.

Lens 2

The best preserved segment of this body would be the final section of Gallery F.

A siliceous hornfels is an assemblage of quartz, sericite and pyrite with pyrite veinlets and dissemination.

Gradually it changes to a stockwork zone with pyrite veinlets, small veins and veins that intersect the host footwall in different directions. At the footwall itself, the disseminated pyrite content increases. This area is dominated by an assemblage of quartz and muscovite, with pyrite (30 %), clays (5 %) and andalusite (1 %) which originally corresponded to pelitic sandstone.

The stockwork zone is gradational to a massive sulphide zone with banding made up of pyrite, chalcopyrite and some sections of sphalerite surrounding blocks larger than 2 m long. Initially those blocks lie parallel to the strike and pitch of the massive sulphide banding, but afterwards they appear in a haphazard manner.

Finally, towards the hangingwall, the massive sulphides are in contact with the siliceous hornfels that, in some sections, appear chloritized. The samples taken in this sector are an assemblage of quartz, chlorite and sericite with quartz, feldspar, sericite and chlorites and andalusite, plagioclase, biotite, calcite, pyrite, rutile and zircon. Petrology suggests that they were originally rhyolitic-dacitic porphyries.

An increase of barite towards the hangingwall could be seen in Lens 2. Sections of barite were found only at the surface and in Gallery B at the top of the massive sulphides. Two samples taken from the outcropping of Body 2 contain 87 % and 96 % barite, with quartz, celestine ($SrS0_4$), benitoite ($BaTiSi_30_9$), pyrite and limonite.

Mineral Zoning in the Massive Sulphide Bodies

An analysis of the samples taken from the walls of the galleries shows us the distribution of chalcopyrite, galena and sphalerite within a pyritic mass, contributing to the determination of the spatial distribution of the bodies.

The following metallic zoning has been determined: the footwall starts with a belt approx. 35 metres with a noticeable predominance of copper values, followed by another 30 meter belt principally zinc, again a 10 m copper belt and towards the hangingwall a 30 meter zinc belt; between these belts there are others measuring approximately 5 metres with low values of both metals (Fig. 13). According to this zoning, the footwall is located to the northeast and the hangingwall to the southwest, coinciding with the geological showings and representing a typical characteristic of the massive sulphide deposits.

Secondary Enrichment

A top layer of barite and oxides can be seen in the outcropping bodies, then a practically all oxide strip and finally the sulphides. The oxidation zone in some cases, such as in Body 1, is approximately 80 metres and in Body 2, approximately 50 metres, affecting the barite zone.

The section with secondary enrichment that can be seen best is found at the entrance of Gallery F, where chalcocite and covellite are accompanied (at the present time) of calcanite and other sulphates. Gallery F intersects this horizon for 45 metres, which would represent between 20 and 25 metres vertically; the copper content varies between 1.5 and 20.0 % and the average of the sampling is 85.7 g/t Ag, 4.1 % Cu, 0.2 % Pb and 0.8 % Zn. On the surface, the secondary enrichment is represented by an outcropping of hematite, goethite and jarosite with spectacular reddish brown to yellow colours.

Another place where the secondary enrichment was intersected was in vertical borehole CL-08, which reached 10 metres vertically with copper values of 0.9 to 2.2 % Cu and average of 11.7 g/t Ag, 1.82 % Cu, 0.26 % Pb and 1.54 % Zn.

TYPE OF DEPOSIT

Cerro Lindo is classified as a massive sulphide volcanogenic deposit on the basis of the following features (Franklin et al, 1981; Lydon, 1990), Figure 9:

- Development of pyritic bodies where the sulphides of a granular texture and sections with banding can be seen.
- Presence of structures typical of volcanogenic deposits such as an area of stockwork in silicified rock with faults and veins filed with pyrite at the base, gradation to a zone comprising mainly granular pyrite with silicified and pyritized fragments and the final development of the massive sulphides with the presence of banding at the top.
- Massive pyrite with a predominance of chalcopyrite at the base of the massive sulphides and sphalerite and galena (to a lesser extent) to the top, also concentrations of barite to the top.
- Increase in the size of the grain associated to the metamorphism of the host volcanic sedimentary sequence.

The magnitude of the volcanogenic massive sulphide deposits generally present tonnages that do not exceed 10 million tonnes. It is possible that the volume found in Cerro Lindo represents a larger time of deposition of minerals or overlying of depositional events.

DISCUSSION OF RESULTS

As a result of all the exploration work carried out, Phelps Dodge was able to estimate the existence of mineral reserves, classified as "geological resources": 75 million tonnes grading 0.89 % Cu, 0.36 % Pb, 3.28 % Zn, 50.7 g/t Ag.

There is still a lot of work to do in the "known" bodies to better define lateral continuity, depth and spatial location. Likewise, there is still exploration work to be carried out in the other geochemical and geophysical anomalies, particularly on those located to the NW of Cerro Lindo, where there is a strong probability that there will be positive results.

In spite of the fact that the potential of major reserves has been confirmed, at the present time, the depressed price of metals coupled with the heavy taxation system, would mean that from an economic point of view , that the value of the mineral would result in a break-even underground operation. However, the situation could be reversed if the current conditions were to improve, or if the cut-off grade could be reduced by increasing the production rate, seeking to achieve a balance between investment and profitability.

There is a possibility to exploit part of the deposit by open pit. This would lower the initial operating costs and the profits obtained could be used to finance the underground mining operation. It would be necessary to undertake a study to determine the feasibility of carrying out an open pit mining operation.

ACKNOWLEDGEMENTS

The author would like to express his appreciation to Mr. Isaac Cruz, Eng., Manager of Compañía Minera Milpo S.A. for his permission to publish this paper; to the many other professionals who contributed to the development of the Cerro Lindo Project; to engineers Samuel Cayo and Jorge Hinostroza for their important collaboration in the preparation of the paper, and to the geologists who visited the project and contributed their ideas and experience providing us valuable information, among them, Darryl Drummond, Bruce A. Youngman, James L. Oliver, César Vidal, Neville Rhoden and Peter Tegart for their enthusiasm and support during the preparation and publication of this paper.

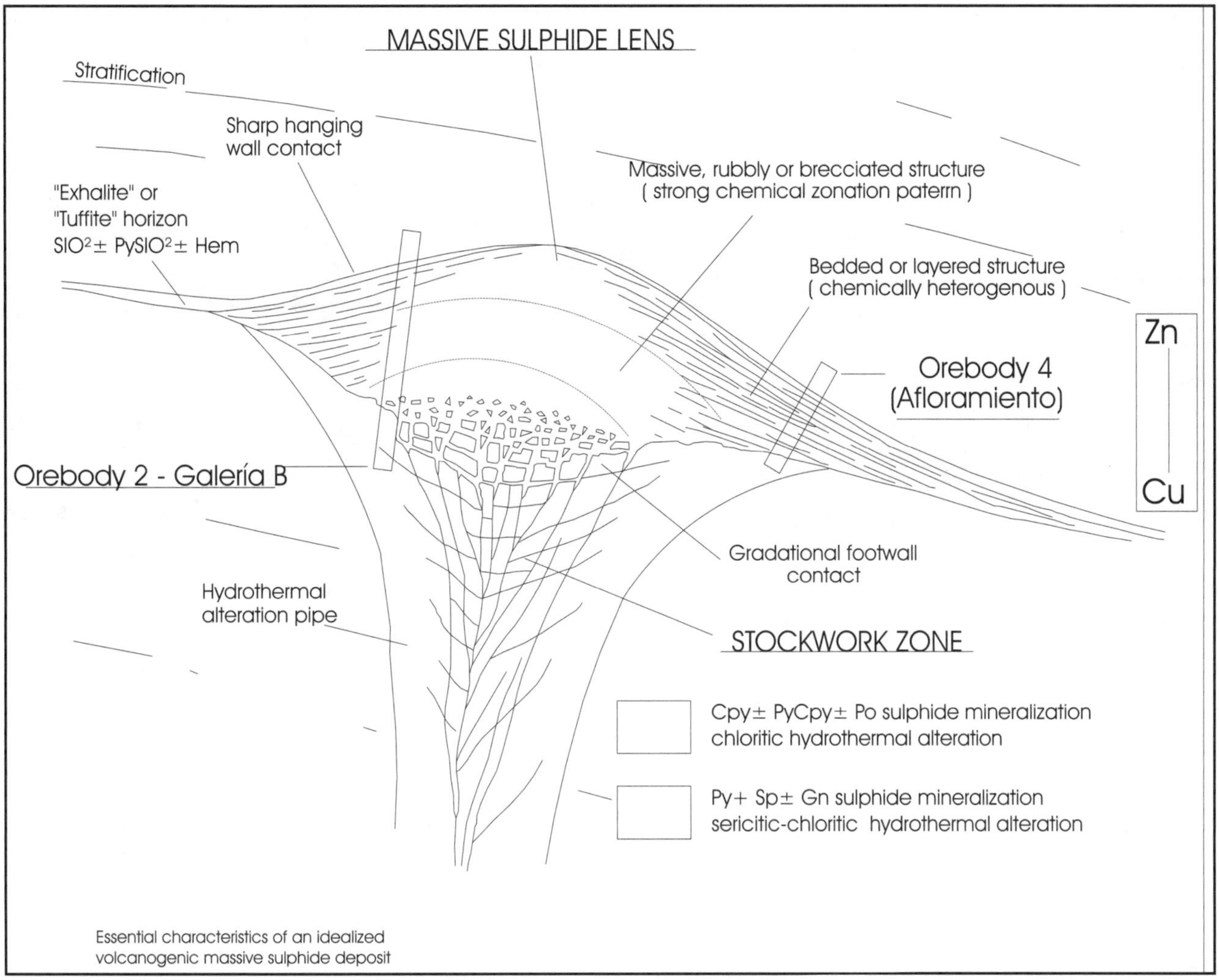

Figure 13. Similarity with the typical VMS model.

(Translated. Original submitted in Spanish).

REFERENCES

Aranda, A. 1996. Estudio Petromineralógico de 8 muestras. Private report.

Arce J.E. 1973. Estudio Geofísico de Polarización Inducida. Private report

Canchaya S. 1992. Estudio Microscópico de 8 muestras. Private report

Chacón N. 1989. Metalogenia del Eugeosinclinal Albiano-Cenoniano en la Cuenca Nor-Occidental del Perú. Thesis, Universidad Nacional Mayor de San Marcos, 180 p.

Chappuis M. 1996. Cerro Lindo Project - Quick Evaluation. Private Report

Franklin, J. M., Lydon, J. W. and Sangster, D. F. 1981. Volcanic-Associated Massive Sulfide Deposits: Economic Geology, 75th Anniversary Volume, p. 485-627

Ly P. 1982. Informe de los trabajos en el Prospecto Agatha. Private report

Ly P. 1994. Resumen de Operaciones 1993. Private report.

Lydon, J.W. 1990. Volcanogenic Massive Sulphide Deposits, Part 1: A Descriptive Model. Ore Deposit Models, Geoscience Canada reprint series; 3, p. 145-154

Lydon, J.W. 1990. Volcanogenic Massive Sulphide Deposits, Part 2: Genetic Models. Ore Deposit Models, Geoscience Canada reprint series; 3, p. 155-182

OMNI Microscopia Electronica. 1999. Estudio Petrográfico de 6 Secciones Delgadas. Private report.

Salazar H., Landa C. 1993. Geología de los Cuadrángulos de Mala, Lunahuana, Tupe, Conayca, Chincha, Tantará y Castrovirreyna. INGEMMET.

Salinas C. 1994-1995. Reportes Geológicos Mensuales. Private report.

Schuh, W. 1996. Executive Report for the period of August

through December 1996. Private Report.
Vidal C. 1980. Mineral deposits associated with the Coastal Batholith and its volcanic country rock. Thesis, Liverpool University, 239 p.
Vidal C. 1987. Kuroko-type deposits in the Middle Cretaceous marginal basin of central Peru: Economic Geology, p. 1409-1430

VOLCANOGENIC MASSIVE SULPHIDE DEPOSITS IN PERU

KLAUS STEINMÜLLER
Instituto Geológico Minero y Metalúrgico (INGEMMET), Av. Canadá N° 1470, Lima 41, Perú
Fax: 0051 14 672915 E-mail: steinmul@chavin.rcp.net.pe

NESTOR CHACÓN ABAD
U.N.M. de San Marcos, Unidad de Post Grado, Pabellón de Geología, Ciudad Universitaria, Lima-Perú
Fax: 0051 14 528945 E-mail: chaconabadl@mixmail.com

BRIAN GRANT
PO Box 8076, Victoria, BC, Canada, V8W 3R7
E-mail: dbgrant@hotmail.com

ABSTRACT

Volcanogenic massive sulphide deposits (VMS) have been mined in Peru for over half a century for their lead, zinc and barite resources. Currently, VMS deposits account for about 3 % of the annual base metal production in Peru and are therefore a significant component of the country's mining industry.

VMS deposits are known within the northern and central coastal belt, which forms part of the western flank of the Peruvian Andes. This portion of the Andes consists of rocks deposited in an aborted, Late Jurassic to Late Cretaceous back-arc basin. The VMS deposits are located within the Lancones, Huarmey and Cañete basins, which make up the volcanic, western part of this back-arc basin.

The VMS deposits can be divided into four groups:

- Cu-Zn deposits hosted by basaltic and andesitic rocks and locally felsic volcanic strata similar to deposits in bimodal mafic sequences;
- Cu-Zn deposits within basalt and andesite similar to the Besshi-type;
- Zn-Ba deposits associated with altered felsic domes of the Kuroko type; and,
- Zn-Ba deposits hosted by black shales and dark carbonate rocks and transitional between VMS and SEDEX-type deposits.

Host rocks to the VMS deposits are Early Cretaceous volcano-sedimentary strata. Only two VMS deposits are known within the Lancones and Huarmey basins: the Tambo Grande Cu-Zn deposit in the former, and the María Teresa Zn-Ba deposit in the latter. Basaltic and andesitic lava, volcaniclastic rocks and locally dacitic strata host the Tambo Grande, whereas María Teresa is associated with an altered and silicified complex within basaltic and andesitic lavas. The majority of VMS discoveries in Peru are located within the Cañete basin, where two main deposit types are distinguished. The copper deposits such as Raúl and Condestable represent the first type. They are hosted by basaltic and andesitic lava, volcaniclastic rocks, sandstone and limestone. The second type includes the zinc-barite deposits such as Perubar and Palma, which are hosted by black shales and dark carbonate rock, intercalated with basaltic and andesitic lava and volcaniclastic rocks.

An Early Cretaceous age is indicated for these VMS deposits based on K-Ar age determinations on alteration minerals, and other geological evidence, such as facies analyses suggest a shallow marine environment for ore deposition. Fluid inclusion and physicochemical evidence indicate formation temperatures for the copper ores between 340° and 350°C, and for the zinc-barite ores between 200° and 250°C. Stable isotope data indicates a mixture of heated seawater and magmatic fluids made up the ore fluids.

Exploration for VMS deposits should be directed to Cretaceous volcano-sedimentary environments (Lancones, Huarmey and Cañete basins), and should take into account both volcanic terranes and the transitional zones between sedimentary and volcanic terranes. Regional ore guides are abrupt facies changes and thickness differences in volcano-sedimentary strata, altered and silicified complexes within basic and intermediate volcanic rocks, and black shales and dark carbonate rocks intercalated with basic and intermediate volcanic and volcaniclastic rocks. In addition to these Cretaceous environments, Early to Late Jurassic volcano-sedimentary series, most probably formed in an arc-related marine environment, may also have good potential for VMS deposits.

INTRODUCTION

Volcanogenic massive sulphide deposits (VMS) have been mined in Peru for over half a century for their lead, zinc and barite resources. In 1948, barite was recovered for use as a component of drilling mud within the petroleum industry. Copper was produced from VMS deposits by 1960, and zinc was produced from the same deposits by 1980. Currently, mining of VMS deposits contributes 5 % to the zinc, 3 % to the copper, and 2 % to the lead production of Peru (Cardozo, 1996). Research within Peru on this class of deposits started in 1980 and academic interest was high until 1990 (Vidal 1980; Cardozo 1983; Steinmüller 1987; Chacón 1988). However, since then research has declined sharply. Growing interest by national and international exploration companies is expected to trigger renewed interest in Peruvian VMS deposits.

GEOTECTONIC SETTING OF VMS DEPOSITS

The geotectonic setting of the western flank of the Peruvian Andes has been characterized, since the Jurassic, by an active continental margin consisting of a magmatic arc and a back-arc basin, both formed on continental crust (Atherton et al. 1983). Stable continental foreland, comprising metamorphic rocks of Precambrian and Paleozoic age, bound the back-arc basin to the east. These zones are the Olmos Complex in northern, and the Marañón Complex in central Peru.

The magmatic arc back-arc basin couple was related to the subduction of the Farallon plate beneath the South American continent. The back-arc basin formed contemporaneous with an extensional tectonic regime and a steeply dipping position of the Farallon plate, which was connected to a spreading centre in the South Pacific (Soler and Bonhomme, 1990). Modelling gravity data from across the Peruvian Andes (Wilson 1985; Feininger 1987) suggests the emplacement of a dense mass of basic, mantle-derived rock within the continental crust during the Cretaceous. This emplacement was a consequence of the back-arc extension and caused an increase in the geothermal gradient (Aguirre and Offler 1985), and the thinning of the continental crust. However, the continental crust did not split up and no oceanic crust was created. Only small basic intrusions, with characteristics of mantle-derived material (Atherton et al. 1985; Musaka and Tilton 1985), were emplaced into the thinned continental crust. The back-arc basin is therefore considered to be of an "aborted" type (Aguirre and Offler 1985).

Marine deposition within the back-arc basin began in the Late Jurassic and continued until the Late Cretaceous. The depositional environment of the western part of the back-arc basin was strongly influenced by volcanism and an increased geothermal gradient, leading to the hydrothermal-burial metamorphism of its volcano-sedimentary fill (Aguirre and Offler 1985). In contrast, the eastern part of the back-arc basin generally lacks volcanic activity and is characterized by siliciclastic and carbonate platform sedimentation (Cobbing 1978). In the western part of the back-arc basin, the depositional environment for VMS deposits, three distinct but interconnected subbasins were formed during extension (Fig. 1). North to south these subbasins are known as the Lancones basin between Piura and Tumbes, the Huarmey basin between Trujillo and Lima, and the Cañete basin between Lima and Ica (Cobbing 1978). The basins are separated by zones between Piura and Trujillo and in the area of Lima, which have little or no volcanic component but consist of sequences of sedimentary rocks. These zones indicate that the magmatic arc was locally interrupted along the active continental margin during the Cretaceous.

GEOLOGICAL EVOLUTION OF THE VMS DISTRICTS

Lancones basin

Marine deposition within the Lancones basin started during the Early Cretaceous (Albian) and continued until the end of the Santonian (Caldas and Farfán 1997). The volcano-sedimentary pile was then deformed and the Lancones basin uplifted (Jaillard et al. 1997). A generalized northwest-southeast stratigraphic section through the Lancones basin is shown in Figure 2.

The northwestern margin of the Lancones basin is comprised of about 50 metres of bioclastic limestones, locally developed as reef limestones, and limy sandstones of the early Albian Pananga Formation. In addition, there is 300 metres of limy shales, dark

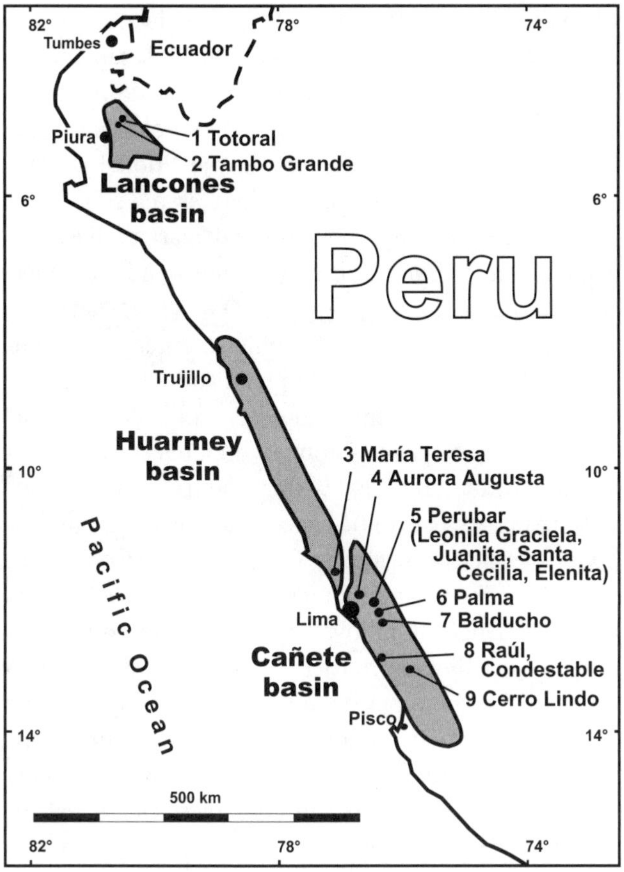

Figure 1. Location of the Cretaceous, Lancones, Huarmey and Cañete volcano-sedimentary basins. The locations of known VMS deposits within these basins are identified.

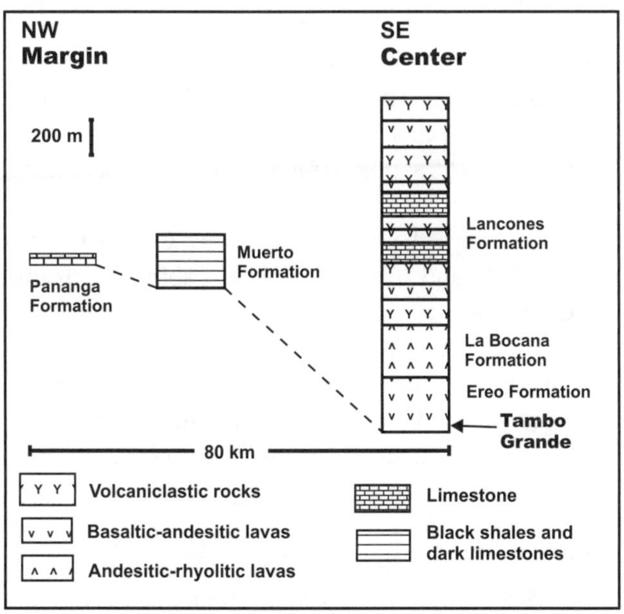

Figure 2. Generalized stratigraphy of the Lancones basin.

shales and black bituminous limestones of the middle to late Albian Muerto Formation. Towards the centre of the basin the sedimentary rocks interfinger with about 2000 metres of volcano-sedimentary rocks of the Lower to Upper Albian Ereo, La Bocana and Lancones formations. The oldest volcano-sedimentary rocks belong to the Ereo Formation and consist of basaltic-andesitic and andesitic lavas that locally exhibit pillow structures. Andesitic, dacitic and rhyolitic lavas intercalated with volcaniclastic rocks and sandstones of the La Bocana Formation overlie the Ereo Formation. The later is succeeded by the Lancones Formation, consisting of volcaniclastic rocks and andesitic lavas intercalated with bituminous limestone and limy sandstone. Based on the lithologies of the Pananga and Muerto formations, it is assumed that the southwestern margin was characterized by platform sedimentation which, towards the basin centre, passed gradationally into oxygen deficient conditions. The basinal volcano-sedimentary deposition, comprising the Ereo, La Bocana and Lancones formations, was fed by growing volcanoes (Caldas and Farfán 1997). Based on stratigraphic records Injoque et al. (1979) conclude that initially volcanic rocks were formed exclusively in a submarine environment, whereas later, subaerial volcanic deposition also took place.

The Late Cretaceous rocks of the Lancones basin consist of the Copa Sombrero Group (Cenomanian-Santonian), overlying the Pananga, Muerto and Lancones formations. The Copa Sombrero Group consists of 3700 metres of monotonous turbidites composed of greywacke sandstones, shales and volcaniclastic rocks, supplied almost entirely by a volcanic arc located northwest of the basin (Morris and Aleman 1975).

Contemporaneous with deposition of the volcano-sedimentary sequences, were subvolcanic stocks and dikes, consisting of microgabbros, andesites and dacites (Caldas and Farfán 1997). These subvolcanic bodies are considered to be early granodiorite and tonalite intrusions of the Coastal Batholith, which intruded into the southeastern part of the Lancones basin during Late Cretaceous to Paleocene time.

Huarmey basin

Marine deposition of volcano-sedimentary rocks (Cobbing et al. 1981) in the Huarmey basin lasted from the Late Jurassic (Tithonian) through to the Early Cretaceous (Albian). Prior to the end of Albian time the basin was uplifted and deformed during the Mochica orogenic phase at about 105 Ma (Megard 1984). Later, during the Late Cretaceous to Paleocene, the volcano-sedimentary basin fill was intruded by stocks of the Coastal Batholith. The generalized stratigraphy of the Huarmey basin showing west-to-east facies changes is presented in Figure 3.

The oldest rocks within the Huarmey basin outcrop along the southern margin, in the area of Lima, and belong to Puente Piedra Group (Tithonian-Berriasian), comprising 2000 metres of pillow lavas and volcaniclastic rocks with intercalations of limestone and shale (Rivera et al. 1975; Fig. 3). The basalts and basaltic andesites have both within-plate and island arc characteristics (Atherton et al. 1985), which are consistent with their formation during the initial stage of back-arc spreading.

About 500 metres of deltaic and fluviatile sandstones and shales of the Morro Solar Group (Valanginian) overly the Puente Piedra Group. Based

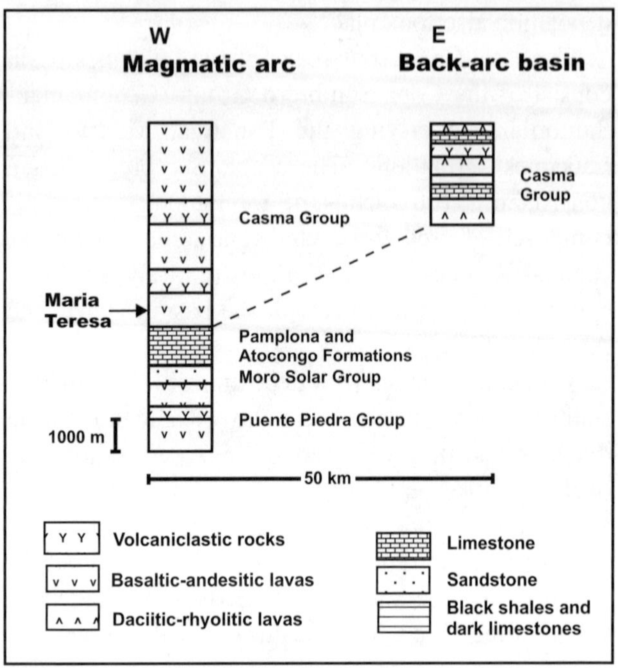

Figure 3. Generalized stratigraphy of the Huarmey basin.

on sedimentology, Wilson (1963) concluded that the Morro Solar rocks were deposited in an isolated basin separated from the ocean by a land mass to the west, which was the main source for the siliciclastic sedimentary rocks. Overlying and in transitional contact with the Morro Solar Group there is a 1200 metre thick succession of limestone and marl of the Late Valanginian to Early Albian Pamplona and Atocongo formations. According to Rivera et al. (1975), the carbonate rocks contain a peculiar indigenous fauna, which indicates that the Pamplona and Atocongo formations were also deposited within an isolated basin.

The Albian Casma Group, which overlies the carbonate rocks, outcrops within the Huarmey basin, only in the area north of Lima. The Casma Group has a well-defined west to east facies change (Cobbing et al. 1981). The western facies is a 6000 to 9000 metre thick sequence of pillow lavas, volcaniclastic rocks and minor sedimentary rocks. Eastward, the sequence decreases to about 3000 metres, and the proportion of sedimentary rocks, mainly shales and limestones, increases. Geochemical studies (Atherton et al. 1985) reveal that the volcanics of the western facies are mainly basalts and basaltic andesites, whereas those of the eastern facies consist mainly of dacites and rhyolites. Webb (1976) interpreted that the volcanic rocks of the western Casma facies were formed in relatively deep waters by fissure eruptions, whereas the easternmost volcanic rocks are products of stratovolcanos, which developed under shallow marine to subaerial conditions. The basic volcanic rocks have both island arc and ocean floor basalt characteristics, indicating their formation within a back-arc spreading zone (Saunders and Tarney, 1984).

Coeval with the formation of the Casma Group, basaltic sills and dikes as well as gabbro intrusions were emplaced into the volcanic rocks of the Huarmey basin. The basic intrusives belong to the early Patap-Superunit of the Coastal Batholith. They have geochemical patterns similar to the basalts of the Casma Group and are therefore interpreted as the plutonic equivalent of the volcanic rocks (Regan 1985).

Cañete basin

Cardozo (1990) reviewed the geological history of the Cañete basin. Marine deposition started in the

Late Jurassic (Tithonian) and terminated in the Early Cretaceous (Albian), accumulating mainly volcano-sedimentary rocks. Towards the end of Albian time, the basin was uplifted and deformed during the Mochica orogenic phase (around 105 Ma). During the Late Cretaceous to Paleocene, the volcano-sedimentary strata were intruded by the Coastal Batholith. The generalized stratigraphy of the Cañete basin, with west-to-east and north-to-south facies changes is shown in Figure 4.

The earliest rocks within the Cañete basin are basic volcanic and sedimentary rocks of the Puente Piedra Group (Tithonian-Berriasian), which outcrop from Lima southward as far as Ica. As mentioned above, the Puente Piedra rocks were probably formed during the early stage of back-arc spreading. The Morro Solar Group (Valanginian) which is made up of deltaic and fluviatile sandstones and shales, and which can also be traced from Lima to Ica succeeds the Puente Piedra Group. In the Lima area the siliciclastic rocks of the Morro Solar Group grade transitionally into the carbonate rocks of the Pamplona and Atocongo formations (Hauterivian to Aptian). South of Lima, the carbonate rocks change gradationally to basaltic and andesitic lavas and volcaniclastic rocks

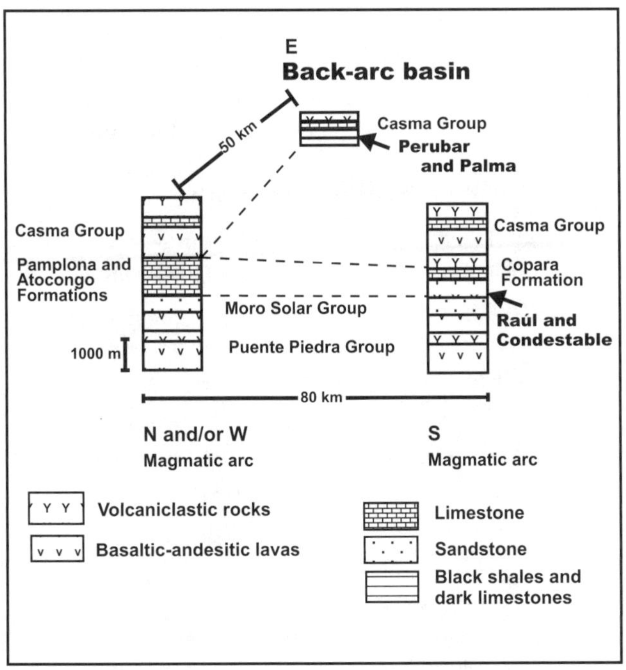

Figure 4. Generalized stratigraphy of the Cañete basin.

intercalated with bioclastic limestones and limy sandstones of the Copara Formation. According to Ostermann et al. (1983), the stratigraphic record of the Copara Formation reveals the presence of volcanic centres, locally surrounded by platform sedimentation with reef development.

Above the carbonates of the Pamplona and Atocongo Formations, and/or the volcano-sedimentary rocks of the Copara Formation, lie rocks of the Casma Group. The Casma Group also shows a west to east facies change (Ostermann et al. 1983; Steinmüller, 1987). The western facies consists of lavas intercalated with limestone and siltstone, whereas the eastern facies is made up of lava, volcaniclastic rock, bituminous shale, dark limestone as well as bioclastic limestone. Cardozo (1990) believes that the volcanic rocks of the western facies are products of fissure eruption, whereas the eastern Casma rocks are mainly subaerial with the local development of shallow marine basins (Steinmüller 1987). Wauschkuhn et al. (1986) and Steinmüller (1987) found that geochemically there are similarities to the volcanic rocks of the Huarmey basin, basalts and basaltic andesites with back-arc characteristics. However, a more felsic eastern facies with dacites and rhyolites, as recorded in the Huarmey basin, is not present in the Cañete basin.

In summary, it is concluded that the connection to the paleo-Pacific ocean was interrupted after the deposition of the Puente Piedra Group. In the southern Huarmey basin and the northern Cañete basin, this interruption prevailed during the sedimentation of the siliciclastic Morro Solar Group and the carbonatic Pamplona and Atocongo formations until the end of the Aptian. In the southern parts of the Cañete basin the interruption was terminated earlier, after the sedimentation of the Morro Solar Group in the Valanginian. The isolation from the paleo-Pacific ocean may be explained by a slowing of back-arc spreading, which triggered uplift in the late Berriasian. Cardozo (1990) suggests that this uplifted area was the northern extension of the Arequipa Massif, which bordered the Cañete basin to the south. The disappearance of the land mass and the reconnection of the Cañete basin to the paleo-Pacific ocean was caused by the intensification of back-arc spreading (Cardozo 1990).

VMS DEPOSITS

VMS deposits and occurrences are found within the Lancones basin, the Huarmey basin and the Cañete basin (Fig. 1). These basins are host to volcanic or volcano-sedimentary rocks of the Early Cretaceous. A list of all the known VMS deposits, their location, host rocks, type of deposits, commodities, tonnage and grades are presented in Table 1.

Deposits and occurrences within the Lancones basin

Tambo Grande is the only known VMS deposit within the Lancones basin (Injoque et al. 1979; Pouit 1987). However, throughout the basin there are a number of areas which have the potential to contain additional volcanogenic massive sulphide deposits. The most encouraging is the Totoral area (Chacón 1988).

Tambo Grande

The Tambo Grande, TG-1 deposit is located about 40 km northeast of Piura. For a long time it was considered an iron-ore deposit, primarily due to the high proportion of pyritic sulphides. The massive sulphides of the TG-1 occurrence were discovered in 1976 as a result of a joint exploration program of the French agency BRGM and INGEMMET. From 1978 to 1980, Tambo Grande TG-1 was drilled and a prefeasibility study conducted, which established the presence of a 700 metre long, northwest striking sulphide body, averaging 150 metres thick. Exploration during 1999 indicated that the TG-1 includes a near-surface gold-rich, flat lying oxide zone containing an estimated 8 million tonnes grading 5.2 g/t Au and 48 g/t Ag.

Underlying this oxide zone the TG-1 is estimated to contain in excess of 64.2 million tonnes of massive sulphides with 1.7 % Cu, 1.4 % Zn, 0.7 g/t Au and 31 g/t Ag (Manhattan Minerals, 1999).

In the area in the immediate vicinity of the original Tambo Grande VMS discovery (TG-1) are about 15 geophysical anomalies within favourable geology which have the potential to be additional VMS occurrences. Drilling of some these anomalies has encountered additional massive sulphide bodies, notably the TG-3 deposit. Ongoing exploration is resulting in additional sulphide intersections and an improved understanding of the local geology (Mining Journal, 1999).

Basaltic and andesitic lavas and volcaniclastic rocks, with locally dacitic strata, of the Ereo Formation host the Tambo Grande deposits. Volcanic rocks in contact with massive sulphides are hydrothermally altered and contain stockwork pyrite and chalcopyrite. The Tambo Grande TG-1 massive sulphide body consists mainly of pyrite with a chalcopyrite rich footwall and chalcopyrite-sphalerite in the margins. Gangue minerals are quartz, carbonate minerals and barite. The upper part of the economic zone consists of pyritic ore rich in secondary copper minerals such as digenite, chalcocite and covellite, that is topped by an oxide cap, comprising iron hydroxides, chert and barite (Pouit, 1987) which is enriched in gold.

Totoral

The Totoral occurrence is about 65 km northeast of Piura, roughly 25 km northeast of the Tambo Grande deposit (Fig 1). Chacón (1988) reported that gossanous rocks are associated with the Ereo and Lancones formations which underlie the area. The most promising site for VMS potential is believed to be Cerro Colorado, which consists of andesitic and basaltic lavas as well as volcaniclastic rocks of the Ereo Formation. The gossanous outcrop at Cerro Colorado is about 350 by 150 metres, and consists of silicified breccia with limonite and barite, and contains anomalous values in copper, zinc, lead and silver.

Deposits within the Huarmey basin

María Teresa is the only known VMS deposit within the Huarmey basin between Lima and Trujillo (Vidal 1980, 1987; Chacón 1988).

María Teresa

María Teresa is situated about 6 km west of Huaral. The deposit has been mined for barite and polymetallic ores on a small scale since 1973. Maria Teresa has estimated resources of about 1 million tonnes containing an average 4 % Zn, 1.3 % Pb, 0.3 % Cu and 100 g/t Ag.

Volcanic rocks of the western facies of the Casma Group host the deposit. The base of the deposit is sericitized and strongly silicified, containing dissemi-

Table 1. Characteristics of early Cretaceous VMS deposits and occurences in Peru.

Name	Longitude	Latitude	Host rocks	Type of Deposits	Commodity	Resource: Tonnage*	Resource: Average Grades	Ref
Tambo Grande	80-10-00	04-55-00	andesitic lavas and volcaniclastic rocks of the Ereo Formation	massive sulphide ore with m\arginal stockwork ore	Cu, Zn, Ag	64.2 million tonnes	1.7% Cu, 1.4% Zn, 0.7 g/t Au, 31 g/t Ag	Manhattan Minerals, 1999
					Au	8 million tonnes	5.2 g/t Au, 48 g/t Ag	N Miner 11/17/99
María Teresa	77-08-25	11-21-45	silicified complexes within basaltic and andesitic lavas of the western facies of the Casma Group	massive sulphide ore and barite lenses underlain by stockwork ore	Zn, Pb, Cu, Ag, Ba	1 million tons	4% Zn, 1.3% Pb, 0.3% Cu 100 g/t Ag	MEM 1998
Aurora Augusta	76-52-03	11-50-33	silicified complexes within andesitic lavas and volcaniclastic rocks of the western facies of the Casma Group	massive barite lenses	Ba	not known	87% BaSO4	BMP 1977
Perubar	76-35-00	11-54-30	Leonila Graciela, Juanita, Santa Cecilia: black shales and dark carbonate rocks intercalated with basaltic and andesitic lavas and volcaniclastic rocks of the eastern facies of the Casma Group	Leonila Graciela, Juanita, Santa Cecilia: massive sulphide ore and barite lenses underlain by stockwork ore	Zn, Pb, Ag, Ba	Leonila Graciela, Juanita, Santa Cecilia: 4 million tons of barite, 2.5 million tons of sulphide ore	Leonila Graciela, Juanita, Santa Cecilia: 80% BaSO4, 12% Zn, 0.7% Pb, 30 g/t Ag	Vidal 1987
			Elenita: breccia pipe emplaced into basaltic and andesitic lavas and volcaniclastic rocks of the eastern facies of the Casma Group	Elenita: massive sulphide-barite ore with marginal stockwork ore	Zn, Pb, Ag, Ba	Elenita: not known	Elenita: 7% Zn, 2% Pb, 110 g/t Ag	Vidal 1987
Palma	76-35-20	4/12/15	black shales and dark carbonate rocks intercalated with basaltic and andesitic lavas and volcaniclastic rocks of the eastern facies of the Casma Group	massive sulphide ore and barite lenses	Zn, Pb, Ag, Ba	not known	12% Zn, 3.8% Pb, 45 g/t Ag	MEM 1989
Balducho	76-34-37	12-19-34	contact metamorphosed rocks of the eastern facies of the Casma Group?	barite lenses, massive sulphide ore and stockwork ore	Ba, Zn	not known	not known	INGEMMET 1982
Raúl & Condestable	76-37-21 76-35-00	12-41-53 12-42-00	basaltic and andesitic lavas and volcaniclastic rocks intercalated with sandstones and limestones of the Copara Formation	massive sulphide ore, disseminated ore and stockwork ore	Cu	40 million tons	Raul: 1.35% Cu Condestable: 1.25 % Cu	Cardozo 1983
Cerro Lindo	75-53-48	6/13/26	contact metamorphosed andesitic lavas,volcaniclastic and clastic rocks of the eastern facies of the Casma Group	massive sulphide ore and barite lenses	Cu, Zn, (Pb,Ag), Ba	27 million tons	2.5% Zn, 1.2% Cu, 26 g/t Ag	Minas y Petroleo, 1999

* includes reserves and past production

nations and veinlets of pyrite and traces of sphalerite, chalcopyrite and galena. Near the hangingwall the silicified rock grades into an irregularly shaped, 20-metre thick, argillic alteration zone. The argillic zone consists of quartz, pyrite, clay minerals, iron oxides and jarosite, with anomalous lead and silver (Chacón 1988). Several subhorizontal barite lenses occur in the upper margins of this zone. The barite is fine grained and banded on a centimetre scale. The banding is defined by grain size differences, oxidation and intercalations of chert layers. In the deeper parts of the argillized zone diamond drilling confirmed the presence of massive sulphide ores made up of sphalerite, galena and chalcopyrite. Basaltic and andesitic lavas conformably overlie the argillized ore zone.

Deposits and occurrences within the Cañete basin

The majority of Peruvian volcanogenic massive sulphide deposits discovered to date are located within the Cañete basin. According to Cardozo and Vidal (1981), the deposits can be divided into two main types: copper deposits hosted by the Copara Formation and zinc-barite deposits hosted by the Casma Group. The Raúl and Condestable deposits comprise the first type (Wauschkuhn 1979a; Wauschkuhn and Thum 1982; Cardozo 1983, 1990; Cardozo and Wauschkuhn 1984). Aurora Augusta, Perubar (Leonila Graciela, Juanita, Santa Cecilia, Elenita), Palma, Balducho and Cerro Lindo comprise the second type (Vidal 1980,1987; Steinmüller 1987; Steinmüller and Wauschkuhn 1987,1990; Ly 1998). The copper deposits Raúl and Condestable are not universally accepted as VMS deposits. Injoque (1985), Vidal et al. (1990) and Injoque (1997) interpreted Raúl and Condestable as skarn-type deposits.

Raúl and Condestable

The Raúl and Condestable deposits are located 90 km south of Lima (Fig. 1), near Mala. The two are neighbouring and form a single economic entity. Mining at Raúl and Condestable started in 1960 and 1964, respectively. Total combined tonnage for the deposits is estimated at about 40 million tonnes with an average grade of 1.3 % Cu. Currently, mining at Raúl and Condestable is suspended due to low metal prices.

The host rocks of the deposits belong to the Copara Formation and comprise basaltic and andesitic lavas and volcaniclastic rocks intercalated with sandstones and bioclastic limestones. According to Cardozo and Wauschkuhn (1984) these rocks are products of a stratovolcano, which developed, partially subaerial, on a shallow marine platform. Caldera subsidence and the emplacement of a dacitic subvolcanic intrusion characterized the final development stage of the volcano.

Economic mineralization at Raúl and Condestable occurs both in volcanic and volcaniclastic rocks, occurring as stratabound disseminations, stringers and breccias in the former, and as stratiform bodies in the latter. The ore is predominantly pyrite and chalcopyrite, with minor pyrrhotite, marcasite and magnetite. Gangue minerals are actinolite, tremolite, clinozoisite, chlorite and prehnite, which indicate a "greenschist-like" alteration of the Raúl and Condestable ores (Cardozo 1990). It is believed that this peculiar alteration was created by hydrothermal alteration of rocks affected by burial metamorphism prior to ore formation (Injoque, 1999). Vein mineralization plays a subordinate role, but is relatively common in the Raúl deposit, where it appears in both northeast and east-trending systems. The northeast-trending veins are mineralogically very similar to the stratabound ores, whereas the east-trending veins contain major amounts of quartz, calcite and sphalerite. Geochronologic (K-Ar) data indicate that mineralization, as well as the alteration of the host rocks, took place simultaneously at around 128 Ma, during the deposition of the Copara Formation (Vidal et al. 1990).

Aurora Augusta

This deposit is located about 50 km northeast of Lima (Fig. 1), near Jicamarca. Aurora Augusta is a small-scale barite mine, which first produced in 1975.

Volcanic rocks of the western facies of the Casma Group host the deposit. The ore of Aurora Augusta occurs as irregular shaped, tabular bodies at the top of a funnel-shaped complex, with quartz-sericite-pyrite alteration. Potassium-argon dating suggests a formation age for the alteration between 116 and 106 Ma (Vidal 1987), which is coeval with the deposition of the Casma rocks. The ore consists mainly of monomineralic, fine-grained barite. Sulphide-rich zones are scarce. Volcaniclastic rocks and lavas constitute the hangingwall of the mineralized zone and the contact between these overlying volcanic rocks and the orebody is abrupt and largely concordant.

Perubar (Leonila Graciela, Juanita, Santa Cecilia, Elenita)

These mineral deposits are located 50 km east of Lima, near Cocachacra in the Río Rímac valley (Fig. 1). Mining operations began in 1950 with barite production from the Leonila Graciela deposit. Later, sulphide ores with high zinc concentrations were discovered at Leonila Graciela and Juanita leading to the start of zinc production in 1980. The Leonila Graciela, Juanita and Santa Cecilia deposits form a single, tectonically disrupted orebody with a combined tonnage of about 6.5 million tonnes of sulphide-barite ore, grading 80 % $BaSO_4$, 12 % Zn, 0.7 % Pb and 30 g/t Ag. The ore of the Elenita deposit grades about 7 % Zn, 2 % Pb and 110 g/t Ag (Vidal 1987).

All of these mineral deposits occur within a roof pendant of the eastern facies of the Casma Group intruded by Late Cretaceous granitoids of the Coastal Batholith. The Casma rocks are folded, with the northwest-striking fold axes plunging northwest. The most significant faults in the area trend north-northwest. Due to the emplacement of the intrusives, the mineral deposits and their host rocks are commonly affected by hornblende-hornfels facies, contact metamorphism (Vidal 1987). Mapping within areas not affected by contact metamorphism indicates that the Casma Group, in the mining area, consists of volcaniclastic rocks and basaltic and andesitic lavas, intercalated with dark shales and micritic limestones. These rocks locally contain algal mats and bioclastic debris and are products of a subaerial volcanism interrupted locally by deposition under shallow marine conditions (Steinmüller, 1987).

The Leonila Graciela, Juanita and Santa Cecilia deposits occur along a northwest trending fault trace. These orebodies are hosted by black shales and dark micritic limestones and consist of stratiform massive sulphide-barite zones underlain by stockwork ore. The stockwork ore is strongly silicified and principally made up of pyrite and sphalerite veinlets and disseminations; chalcopyrite, galena, pyrrhotite and magnetite are minor constituents. The massive sulphide-barite ore is banded and composed of pyrite, pyrrhotite and sphalerite with increasing barite concentration towards the top; chalcopyrite, galena and magnetite are subordinate. Both ore types have a contact metamorphic overprint. They are coarse-grained with granoblastic and lepidoplastic intergrowth of sulphides and barite. Also, the pyrrhotite is exclusively hexagonal (Vidal 1987).

The Elenita deposit is associated with a breccia pipe and consists of irregular, massive ore zones, grading outwards into stockwork ore. The massive sulphides are composed of pyrite, sphalerite and barite with minor chalcopyrite, galena, marcasite, pyrrhotite, jamesonite and sphalerite. The stockwork zone consists of quartz, pyrite and sphalerite.

Palma

The Palma deposit is located 55 km southeast of Lima in the Río Lurín valley (Fig. 1). Although mining at Palma began at a small scale in 1985, the deposit is incompletely explored and no reserve data are available. The ores grade 10 % Zn, 2 % Pb and 45 g/t Ag.

The deposit at Palma is hosted by rocks of the eastern facies of the Casma Group, consisting of basaltic and andesitic lavas and volcaniclastic rocks intercalated with black shales and dark micritic limestones with bioclastic layers. These were deposited by subaerial volcanic activity, which in places was interrupted by deposition in shallow marine environments (Steinmüller 1987). Structurally northwest trending and southeast plunging fold axes are characteristic in the area.

The Palma ore is on the eastern limb of an open, drag-folded anticline, within black shales and dark carbonate rocks. It is stratiform and consists, in its lower parts, of laminated bituminous shales with layers of pyrite and pyrrhotite and small amounts of sphalerite and chalcopyrite. The pyrrhotite is mainly monoclinic and is associated with Fe-rich sphalerite (Steinmüller 1987). Towards the higher parts of the mineralized zone, the pyrrhotite content diminishes and the sulphides are composed of thin layers of pyrite, sphalerite and galena. The top of the mineralized zone consists of barite lenses. The Palma ore is strongly deformed, generally fine-grained and reveals both brittle and plastic deformation textures. In spite of the tectonic overprint, sedimentary structures such as framboidal pyrite can still be identified within the black shales at the base of the orebody (Steinmüller and Wauschkuhn, 1987).

Balducho

The Balducho deposit is located 40 km northeast of Pucusana within the Rio Chilca valley (Fig. 1). Although it has been mined intermittently over the years, neither grade and tonnage, nor mineral production data are available.

The deposit is hosted by the near vertical, metamorphosed pelites, intruded by granodioritic intrusives of the Tiabaya Superunit of the Coastal Batholith (Vidal, 1987). The economic mineralization consists of stratiform barite and massive sulphide lenses and an adjacent stockwork sulphide zone. The maximum width of the zone of economic ore minerals is about 300 metres. Massive sulphides consist of pyrite and sphalerite, while the stockwork zone contains chalcopyrite. Due to the contact metamorphic overprint, the sulphides are coarse grained and exhibit granoblastic textures.

FORMATION OF THE VMS DEPOSITS

It is generally agreed that submarine volcanic processes formed the known VMS deposits in Peru, however, there has been relatively little research on these deposits. Detailed studies of ore formation have been conducted on the Raúl and Condestable (Ripley and Ohmoto,1977, 1979; Cardozo, 1983; Cardozo and Wauschkuhn, 1984), and the Leonila Graciela, Juanita, Santa Cecilia, Elenita and Palma deposits (Steinmüller, 1987, 1988). Also, there is recent and ongoing evaluation regarding the formation of the Tambo Grande ores (Franklin, 1999).

Tambo Grande

Geochemical evidence indicates that the volcanic host rocks of the Tambo Grande deposits formed in a back-arc setting (Franklin, 1999). The sulphides accumulated in a well confined rift basin, controlled by synvolcanic faults, which served as vents for the ore fluids. Based on physicochemical considerations, Franklin (1999) believes that ore deposition took place in water depths of about 1300 to 1500 metres. The chalcocite and digenite bearing upper part of the TG-1 orebody is believed to be a product of post-depositional remobilization processes. Oxidized seawater leached the chalcopyrite-rich lower part of the orebody, thereby dissolving copper and reprecipitating it at higher, cooler levels as chalcocite and digenite. The enrichment of gold in the oxide cap is also explained by diagenetic remobilization processes, which are summarized by Hutchison (1990). It is believed that the gold was leached out of the sulphides by convecting seawater and tranported as bisulphide complexes to higher levels where it precipitated under oxidizing conditions.

Raul and Condestable

Based on paleogeographical reconstruction, Cardozo (1983) assumes that the formation of the Raúl and Condestable deposits was related to submarine caldera subsidence. Sulphide deposition occurred under shallow marine conditions within a geothermal environment. Lead isotope analysis on sulphide minerals from Raúl and Condestable, indicates a mantle source for the lead (Gunnesch et al. 1990). Stratiform mineralization is believed to represent submarine hot spring deposition on the sea floor, whereas disseminations, stringers and breccias may result from impregnation and open space filling of volcanic rocks immediately beneath the sea floor. Fluid inclusion fillings and thermochemical evidence of coexisting sulphides suggest ore formation temperatures between 340° and 350°C (Ripley and Ohmoto 1977). Based on sulphur, oxygen and hydrogen isotope data, these authors suggest that the hydrothermal fluids were principally heated seawater, which was enriched in metals and reduced sulphur by circulation through the volcanic-sedimntary sequence. This modified seawater is believed to have been the source of the sulphides and, caused the "greenschist-like" alteration of the host rocks (Ripley and Ohmoto 1977, 1979). Heat was most probably derived from subvolcanic intrusions. On the other hand, Cardozo (1983), advocates a magmatic origin for the hydrothermal fluids based

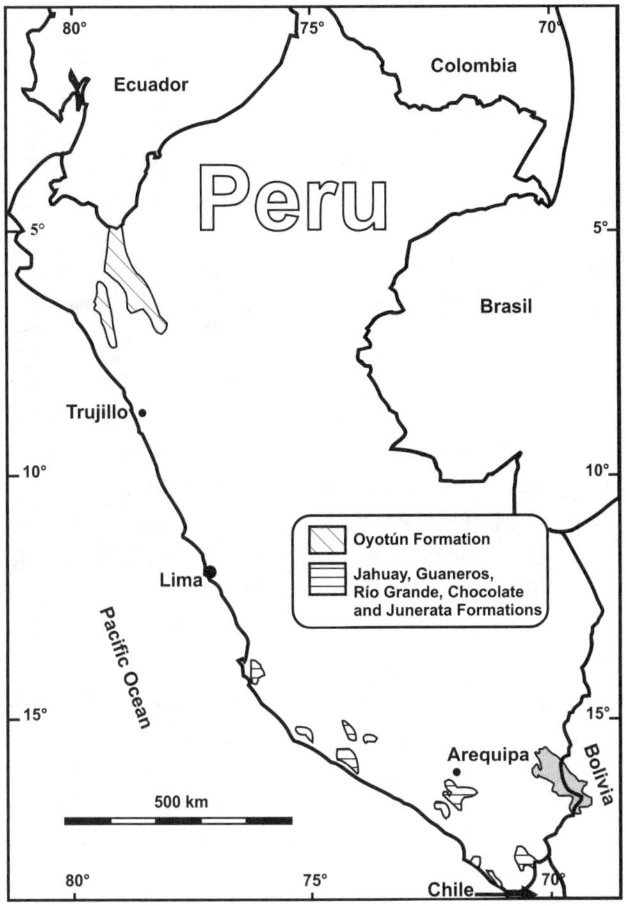

Figure 5. Exposures of Jurassic volcano-sedimentary environments in Peru.

on studies of sulphide deposition in volcanic lakes by Wauschkuhn (1979b).

As mentioned earlier, a submarine hot spring origin for Raúl and Condestable is not generally accepted. In particular, Vidal et al. (1990) and Injoque (1997) classify these deposits as amphibolitic Cu-Fe skarns. However, they agree that Raúl and Condestable were formed in a submarine geothermal environment by fluids derived mainly from seawater. However, they also point out that the mineralogical and geometric features are more characteristic of skarn than VMS-type deposits. These authors believe ore formation was essentially an endogenous process with little or no hot-spring associations on the sea floor.

Whether VMS deposits form on and/or beneath the seafloor is principally governed by water depth (Finlow-Bates, 1980). A copper-rich ore fluid hotter than 300°C needs a seawater depth of more than 1500 metres to reach the seafloor. If the sea water is shallower, the ore fluid will boil and chalcopyrite will precipitate at sub-seafloor level. As ore deposition at Raúl and Condestable occurred under shallow marine conditions, it is not surprising that most of their chalcopyrite-rich ores formed as replacement beneath the seafloor. Endogenous processes which are brought forward against the VMS model are therefore compatible with submarine volcanogenic ore deposition. For this reason, we support a volcanogenic origin of Raúl and Condestable.

Perubar (Leonila Graciela, Juanita, Santa Cecilia, Elenita) and Palma

Facies analyses suggest that the stratiform orebodies of Leonila Graciela, Juanita, Santa Cecilia and Palma were formed in anaerobic shallow marine basins subjected to extension along a northwestern trend (Steinmüller 1987). Steinmüller (1987) believes that the hydrothermal fluids responsible for sulphide deposition had a low pH, high chloride content, and temperatures between 200 and 250°C, based on the mineralogical and chemical composition of the sulphides. The fluids were discharged onto the seafloor through feeder channels evidenced by the stockwork sulphides below the stratiform, massive sulphide bodies. Accumulation of the sulphides probably took place within brine pools formed by the mixing of hydrothermal fluids with seawater. The zonation of the sulphide bodies is a result of decreasing temperature as well as increasing pH and oxygen fugacity during sulphide deposition.

As the mineralogy and chemistry of these stratiform sulphides and the Elenita sulphide breccia is similar, Steinmüller (1987) assumes that the hydrothermal fluids which formed the Elenita sulphides had physiochemical characteristics similar to the fluids responsible for the formation of the stratiform mineralization. Paleoenvironmental reconstruction and sulphur isotopes indicate that the Elenita deposit was not formed on the seafloor but under subaerial conditions and probably by phreatic eruptions. The sulphur of the hydrothermal fluids involved in the formation of the Elenita sulphide breccia and the stockwork mineralization beneath the stratiform sulphides, was of magmatic origin. However the sulphur involved in the formation of the stratiform sulphides appears to have been derived principally from bacterial reduction of seawater (Steinmüller, 1988). Lead isotope analyses by Gunnesch et al. (1990) revealed that the lead involved in sulphide formation is a mixture of a mantle derived component with a crustal component.

VMS DEPOSIT CLASSIFICATION

In summary, and in keeping with their metal content and their geological setting, the known Peruvian VMS deposits are divided into four distinct types:

- Cu-Zn deposits hosted by basaltic and andesitic rocks with locally dacitic strata (Tambo Grande) similar to deposits in bimodal mafic sequences;
- Cu-Zn deposits within basalt and andesite (Raúl, Condestable) similar to Besshi-type deposits;
- Zn-Ba deposits associated with altered felsic domes (María Teresa) similar to Kuroko-type deposits; and,
- Zn-Ba deposits hosted by black shales and dark carbonate rocks (Leonila Graciela, Juanita, Santa Cecilia, Palma) transitional between VMS and SEDEX-type deposits.

It is not easy to classify the known Peruvian VMS deposits based on the classification schemes for massive sulphide deposits proposed by authors such as Solomon 1976, Sawkins 1976, Hutchison 1980, Klau and Large 1980. Most of these deposits exhibit characteristics that match more than one deposit-type, and are therefore considered transitional between the end members.

In the case of Tambo Grande, Pouit (1987) sees similarities with deposits of the Cyprus type. However, the Tambo Grande is not associated with ophiolite sequences typical of Cyprus-type deposits, but is hosted by basalt and andesite with locally dacitic rocks and has a zinc-rich ore body. The Besshi-type classification for Tambo Grande, as proposed by Valdivia and Torres (1995) also has deficiencies; the host rocks of Grande are devoid of continental derived sedimentary rocks, typical of Besshi-type deposits (Fox, 1984). Finally, based on the geological setting and the metal content, Franklin (1999) describes Tambo Grande as being similar to deposits in bimodal mafic sequences (e.g., Noranda and Kidd Creek).

Cardozo (1983) points out that the Raúl and Condestable deposits are within the same geotectonic setting and have similar host rocks as Besshi-type deposits, but they contain much less zinc.

Vidal (1987) states that the deposits within the Casma Group belong to the Kuroko-type, but this has to be revised as Kuroko-type is only justified for deposits within the western facies of the Casma Group (María Teresa and Aurora Augusta). They are associated with silicified and brecciated bodies that have similarities with the rhyolite domes typical of Kuroko deposits. Black shales and dark carbonate rocks host all the deposits within the eastern facies of the Casma Group. They are surrounded exclusively by basic and intermediate volcanic rocks, which is not typical of Kuroko-type deposits. Based on the geological environment, the mineral zonation of the orebodies and the metal content, Steinmüller (1987) suggested these deposits are transitional between the VMS and SEDEX type deposits described by Large (1980, 1983). The intermediate character of the deposits is explained by their geological setting within the transitional zone between the western volcanic and the eastern sedimentary facies of the back-arc basin.

POTENTIAL FOR VMS DISCOVERIES IN PERU

Geological environments with good potential for hosting VMS deposits certainly include the Lancones, Huarmey and Cañete basins. The geological setting and history of these basins is well studied and understood. However, along the coastal belt of Peru there exist additional volcano-sedimentary strata, which may also prove to be suitable hosts for VMS deposits. In the north these comprise the Oyotún Formation and in the south the Jahuay, the Guaneros, the Río Grande, the Chocolate and the Junerata formations (Fig. 5). Unfortunately, the geological setting of these volcano-sedimentary sequences is not well understood.

It is concluded that the Lancones basin, due to extensive Early Cretaceous volcano-sedimentary sequences, gentle topography and good access, represents the most promising target area for new VMS discoveries. At present VMS deposits and occurrences are known only within the intermediate to basic volcanic rocks of the Ereo Formation. However, in light of the geological setting of the zinc-rich deposits within the eastern Casma facies of the Cañete basin, further exploration in the Lancones basin should include not only investigation of the volcanic terranes but also the transitional zones between sedimentary and volcanic facies. Particularly, those areas with black shales and dark carbonate rocks are considered highly prospective.

Due to the emplacement of the Coastal Batholith, outcrops of Early Cretaceous volcano-sedimentary stratigraphy within the Huarmey and Cañete basins are limited. Also, the terrane is rougher and access difficult. The setting for VMS deposits within these two basins, however, suggests that undiscovered Cu-Zn deposits, such as Raúl and Condestable, could occur with the Copara Formation between Lima and Ica. As these deposits are related to volcanic centres, detailed evaluation of the stratigraphy is strongly recommended for any exploration program (Cardozo 1983). Guides to finding new mineral resources are abrupt facies changes or variations in the thickness of the volcano-sedimentary Copara Formation. In addition, the western facies of the Casma Group within the Huarmey basin is prospective for Zn-Ba deposits such as María Teresa, in particular where there are altered and silicified complexes within intermediate volcanic rocks. Finally, the eastern facies of the Casma rocks in the Cañete basin offers good potential for Zn-Ba deposits, such as those at Perubar. Prospective sequences are black shales and dark carbonate rocks intercalated with intermediate volcanic and volcaniclastic rocks.

Jurassic rocks of the Oyotún, Río Grande, Jahuay, Chocolate, Junerata and Guaneros formations consist of dacitic to andesitic volcanic rocks intercalated with shallow water sedimentary rocks (INGEMMET, 1995). The volcano-sedimentary rocks were deposited in a marine arc environment situated to the west of a shallow marine platform, which is considered to be a precursor to the Cretaceous back-arc basin (Fontboté, 1990; Rosas et al, 1996). In this context, and in the absence of geochemical studies, one could speculate that the rocks of the Oyotún, Río Grande, Jahuay, Chocolate, and the Junerata and Guaneros formations indicate the start of the Mesozoic magmatic arc. Although, most of the Jurassic volcanic rocks have limited outcrops, the Oyotún Formation crops out quite extensively in the north of Peru (Fig. 5) and hosts mineralization which could belong to the VMS type; the best known examples are the Linderos prospect (INGEMMET, 1994) and the prospects of Compuerta-Nueva Arica (Torres, 1994).

We conclude that the Oyotún Formation as well as the Lancones, Huarmey and Cañete basins, have good potential for the discovery of new VMS deposits in Peru. Considering the gold association found at Tambo Grande, these have become much more attractive as exploration targets.

REFERENCES

Aguirre, L. and Offler, R. 1985. Burial metamorphism in the Western Peruvian Trough: its relation to Andean magmatism and tectonics. In Magmatism at a plate edge. The Peruvian Andes. Edited by W.S. Pitcher; M.P. Atherton, E.J. Cobbing and R.D. Beckinsale. Glasgow, pp. 59-71.

Atherton, M.P.; Warden, V. and Sanderson, L.M. 1983. The Mesozoic marginal basin of Central Peru. Nature, 305: 303-306.

Atherton, M.P.; Warden, V. and Sanderson, L.M. 1985. The Mesozoic marginal basin of Central Peru: a geochemical study of within-plate-edge volcanism. In Magmatism at a plate edge. The Peruvian Andes. Edited by W.S. Pitcher; M.P. Atherton, E.J. Cobbing and R.D. Beckinsale. Glasgow, pp. 47-58.

BMP 1977. Informe N 03/77-DPM. Mina "Aurora Augusta I", Lima.

Caldas, J. and Farfán, C. 1997. Tectonismo, magmatismo y sedimentación en la cuenca Lancones. Resúmenes Extendidos, IX Congreso Peruano de Geología, pp. 249-253.

Cardozo, M. 1983. Raúl als Beispiel vulkanogener Kupferlagerstätten im Copara-Metallotekt, Zentralperu. Ph. D. thesis, Universität Heidelberg, Germany.

Cardozo, M. 1990. The Copara metallotect in Central Peru: Geologic evolution and ore formation. In Stratabound ore deposits in the Andes. Edited by L. Fontboté, G.C. Amstutz, M. Cardozo, E. Cedillo and J. Frutos. Berlin. pp. 395-412.

Cardozo, M. 1996. El futuro de la minería polimetálica en el Perú, Mundo Minero, 170: 32-38.

Cardozo, M. and Vidal, C. 1981. Metalogénesis y magmatismo en el flanco occidental de los Andes Centrales: Revisión. Boletín de la Sociedad Geológica del Perú, 68: 13-24.

Cardozo, M. and Wauschkuhn, A. 1984. The Copara and the Patap metallotects of Western Peru. In Syngenesis and epigenesis in the formation of mineral deposits. Edited by A.

Wauschkuhn.; C. Kluth and R.A. Zimmermann. Berlin, pp. 616-646.

Chacón, N. 1988. Metalogenia del Eugeosinclinal Albiano-Cenomaniano de la Cuenca Noroccidental del Perú, Ph. D. thesis, Universidad Nacional Mayor de San Marcos, Lima, Perú.

Cobbing, E.J. 1978. The Andean geosyncline in Peru and its distinction from Alpine geosynclines. Journal of the Geological Society of London, 135: 207-218.

Cobbing, E.J. 1985. The tectonic setting of the Peruvian Andes. In Magmatism at a plate edge. The Peruvian Andes. Edited by W.S. Pitcher; M.P. Atherton, E.J. Cobbing and R.D. Beckinsale. Glasgow, pp. 3-12.

Cobbing, E.J.; Pitcher, W.S.; Wilson, J.; Baldock, J.; Taylor, W; McCourt, W. and Snelling, N.J. 1981. Estudio geológico de la Cordillera Occidental del Norte del Perú. Estudios Especiales, Serie D, Boletín N° 10, Instituto Geológico Minero y Metalúrgico.

Feininger, T. 1987. Allochthonous terranes in the Andes of Ecuador and northwestern Peru. Canadian Journal of Earth Sciences, 24: 266-278.

Finlow-Bates. T. 1980. The chemical and physical controls on the genesis of submarine exhalative orebodies and their implications for formulating exploration concepts. A review. Geologisches Jahrbuch, D40: 131-168.

Fontboté, L. 1990. Stratabound ore deposits in the Andes: a review and a classification according to their geotectonic setting. In Stratabound ore deposits in the Andes. Edited by L. Fontboté, G.C. Amstutz, M. Cardozo, E. Cedillo and J. Frutos. Berlin, 79-110.

Fox, J.S. 1984. Besshi-type volcanogenic sulphide deposits-a review. Bulletin of the Canadian Institute of Mining and Metallurgy, 77: 57-68.

Franklin, J.M. 1999. Notes on the geology and mineral potential of the Tambo Grande VMS discovery. Manhattan Minerals Corporation, 13 p.

Grant, B. 1996. Peru, a new millennium. The Gangue, issue 54, 7-18.

Gunnesch, K.A.; Baumann, A. and Gunnesch, M. 1990. Lead isotope variations across the Central Peruvian Andes. Economic Geology, 85: 1384-1401.

Hutchison, R.W. 1980. Massive base metal sulphide deposits as guides to tectonic evolution. In The continental crust and its mineral deposits. Edited by D.W. Strangway. Special Paper of the Geological Association of Canada, 20, pp. 659-684.

Hutchison, R.W. 1990. Precious metals in massive base metal sulfide deposits. Geologische Rundschau, 79: 241-263.

INGEMMET 1982. Inventario nacional de sustancias no metálicas, Lima.

INGEMMET 1994. Proyecto Linderos (San Ignacio - Cajamarca). Estudio geológico-geoquímico y geofísico, area Cerro Coyota, Lima.

INGEMMET 1995. Geología del Perú, Boletin N° 55, Serie A, 177 p.

Injoque, J. 1985. Geochemistry of Cu-Fe-amphibole skarn deposits of the Peruvian Central Coast. Ph. D. thesis, University of Nottingham, U.K.

Injoque, J. 1997. Yacimientos de Cu tipo manto: mineralizaciones económicas producto de sistemas geotermales mesozoicos andinos, relacionadas al metamorfismo regional, volcanismo y ambiente geotectonico. IX Congreso Peruano de Geología, Resúmenes extendidos, 45-49.

Injoque, J.; Miranda, C. and Dunin-Borkowski, E. 1979. Estudio de la génesis del yacimiento Tambo Grande y sus implicancias. Boletín de la Sociedad Geológica del Perú, 67: 73-99.

Injoque, J. 1999. The location and extent of volcanic massive sulphide and manto-type copper deposits in the Cretaceous volcanic arcs in the Peruvian Andes. Paper presented at PACRIM 99 Conference, Bali, Indonesia, 16 p.

Jaillard, E.; Bengston, P.; Dhondt, A.; Laubacher, G.; Bulot, L.G. and Robert, E. 1997. Revisión estratigráfica del Cretaceo superior del noroeste peruano, datos preliminares, consecuencias tectónicas. Resumenes Extendidos, IX Congreso Peruano de Geología, pp. 327-330.

Klau, W. and Large, D.E. 1980. Submarine exhalative Cu-Pb-Zn-deposits, a discussion of their classification and metallogenesis. Geologisches Jahrbuch, D40: 13-58.

Large, D.E. 1980. Geological parameters associated with sediment-hosted submarine exhalative Pb-Zn deposits: an empirical model for mineral exploration. Geologisches Jahrbuch, D40: 59-129.

Large, D.E. 1983. Sediment-hosted massive sulphide lead-zinc deposits: an empirical model. In Sediment-hosted stratiform lead-zinc deposits: Edited by D.F. Sangster. Mineralogical Association of Canada, Short Course Handbook Volume 8: 1-30.

Ly, P. 1998. Proyecto Cerro Lindo. P.L. Geoexplomin E.I.R.L., Lima.

Manhattan Minerals Corporation. 1999. Tambo Grande project update, TG-1 Resource Model and Phase II exploration program. New Releases for November 15, INTERNET, 2 p.

Mégard, F. 1984. The Andean orogenic period and its major structures in Central and Northern Peru. Journal of the Geological Society of London, 141: 893-900.

MEM 1989. Declaración jurada de reservas y producción Mina “Palma”, Lima.

MEM 1998. Informe técnico Mina “María Teresa”, Lima.

Minas y Petroleo. 1999. Prometedoras resultados en yacimiento polimetálico “Cerro Lindo”. 25 de Noviembre, Lima, p. 4.

Mining Journal 1999. Gold find at Tambo Grande. July 23, London, p. 56.

Morris, R.C. and Alemán, A. 1975. Sedimentation and tectonics of the middle Cretaceous Copa Sombrero Formation in northwest Peru. Boletín de la Sociedad Geológica del Perú, 48: 49-64.

Musaka, S.B. and Tilton, G.R. 1985. Pb isotope systematics as a guide to crustal involvement in the generation of the Coastal Batholith, Peru. In Magmatism at a plate edge. The Peruvian Andes. Edited by W.S. Pitcher; M.P. Atherton, E.J. Cobbing and R.D. Beckinsale. Halsted Press, Glasgow, 235-240.

Ostermann, G., Cardozo, M. and Wauschkuhn, A. 1983.

Descripción y correlación de los depósitos volcano-sedimentarios del Cretácico inferior en la región Lima-Cañete. Boletín de la Sociedad Geológica del Perú, 70: 35-45.

Pouit, G. 1987. L' amás sulfuré a Cu (Zn) de Tambo Grande dans le Crétacé du Nord Perou. Chronique de la Recherche Miniere, 489: 43-49.

Regan, P.F. 1985. The early basic intrusions. In Magmatism at a plate edge. The Peruvian Andes. Edited by W.S. Pitcher; M.P. Atherton, E.J. Cobbing and R.D. Beckinsale. Glasgow, 72-89.

Ripley, E.M. and Ohmoto, H. 1977. Mineralogic, sulfur isotope and fluid inclusion studies of the stratabound copper deposits at the Raul mine, Peru. Economic Geology, 72: 1017-1041.

Ripley, E.M. and Ohmoto, H. 1979. Oxygen and hydrogen isotope studies of ore deposition and metamorphism at the Raul mine, Peru. Geochimica et Cosmochimica Acta, 43: 1633-1643.

Rivera, R.; Petersen, G. and Rivera, M. 1975. Estratigrafía de la costa de Lima. Boletín de la Sociedad Geológica del Perú, 48: 159-186.

Rosas, S., Fontboté, L. and Morche, W. 1996. Within-plate volcanism in Upper Triassic to Lower Jurassic Pucará Group carbonates (Central Peru). In Third International Symposium on Andean Geodynamics. Edited by ORSTOM, Paris, 641-644.

Saunders, A.D. and Tarney, J. 1984. Geochemical characteristics of basaltic volcanism within back arc basins. In Marginal basin geology: Edited by B.P. Kokelaar and M.F. Howells. London, 59-76.

Sawkins, F.J. 1976. Massive sulphide deposits in relation to geotectonics. In Metallogeny and plate tectonics. Edited by D.F. Strong. Special Papers of the Geological Association of Canada, 14, 221-240.

Soler, P. and Bonhomme, M.G. 1990. Relation of magmatic activity to plate dynamics in Central Peru from Late Cretaceous to present. In Plutonism from Antarctica to Alaska: Edited by S.M. Kay and C.W. Rapela. Geological Society of America Special Paper 241, 173-192.

Solomon, M. 1976. Volcanic massive sulphide deposits and their host rocks: a review and an explanation. In Handbook of stratabound and stratiform ore deposits, 6. Edited by K.H. Wolf. Amsterdam, 21-53.

Steinmüller, K. and Wauschkuhn, A. 1987. Geology and mineralogy of the barite-sulfide deposits in the Eastern Casma Group of Central Peru. Zentralblatt für Geologie und Paläontologie, 7/8: 995-1005.

Steinmüller, K. and Wauschkuhn, A. 1990. Palma: A non-metamorphic stratabound massive Zn-Ba occurrence in the Eastern Casma Group of Central Peru. In Stratabound ore deposits in the Andes. Edited by L. Fontboté, G.C. Amstutz, M. Cardozo, E. Cedillo and J. Frutos. Berlin, 413-420.

Steinmüller, K. 1987. Beiträge zur Metallogenese der Baryt-Sulfid-Lagerstätten in der östlichen Casma-Gruppe Zentralperus. Ph. D. thesis, Universität Heidelberg, Germany.

Steinmüller, K. 1988. Geologische, mineralogische und geochemische Untersuchungen in den Baryt-Sulfid Lagerstätten der mesozoischen Casma-Gruppe, Zentralperu. Final Report, DFG-Research Projects Wa299/11-1/2 and Am23/69-4.

Valdivia, J. and Torres, A. 1995. Evolución estratigráfico-estructural en relación con la ocurrencia de mineralización volcanogénica en la cuenca de Lancones-Piura. Boletín de la Sociedad Geológica del Perú, Volumen Jubilar A. Benavides, 327-335.

Vidal, C. 1980. Mineral deposits associated with the Peruvian Coastal Batholith and its volcanic country rocks. Ph. D. thesis, University of Liverpool, U.K.

Vidal, C. 1987. Kuroko-type deposits in the middle Cretaceous marginal basin of Central Peru. Economic Geology, 82: 1409-1430.

Vidal, C.; Injoque, J.; Sidder, G.B. and Musaka, S.B. 1990. Amphibolitic Cu-Fe skarn deposits in the Central Coast of Peru. Economic Geology, 85: 1447-1461.

Wauschkuhn, A. 1979a. Geology, mineralogy and geochemistry of the stratabound Cu-deposits in the Mesozoic coastal belt of Peru. Boletín de la Sociedad Geológica del Perú, 62: 161-192.

Wauschkuhn, A. 1979b. Untersuchungen in rezenten vulkanisch-exhalativen Ablagerungsräumen und fossilen vulkanisch-exhalativen Sulfidlagerstätten. Ein Beitrag zur Genese dieses Lagerstättentyps. Habilitationsschrift, Universität Heidelberg, Germany.

Wauschkuhn, A.; Ohnsmann, M. and Pernicka, E. 1986. Geochemistry of the Mesozoic volcanic rocks in Central Peru and their plate tectonic position. Berliner Geowissenschaftliche Abhandlungen, A Sonderband: 29-31.

Wauschkuhn, A. and Thum, R. 1982. The Condestable mine, a volcano-exhalative deposit in the Mesozoic coastal belt of Central Peru. In Ore genesis. The state of the art. Edited by G.C. Amstutz, A. El Goresy, G. Frenzel, C. Kluth, G. Moh, A. Wauschkuhn and R.A. Zimmermann. Berlin, 174-188.

Webb, S.E. 1976. The volcanic envelope of the Coastal Batholith in Lima and Ancash, Peru. Ph.D. thesis, University of Liverpool, U.K.

Wilson, J.J. 1963. Cretaceous stratigraphy of the Central Andes of Peru. American Association of Petroleum Geologists Bulletin, 47: 1-34.

Wilson, D.V. 1985. The deeper structure of the Central Andes and some geophysical constraints. In Magmatism at a plate edge. The Peruvian Andes. Edited by W.S. Pitcher; M.P. Atherton, E.J. Cobbing and R.D. Beckinsale. Glasgow, 13-18.

THE PERUBAR BA-PB-ZN VHMS DEPOSIT, CENTRAL PERU

MARC POLLIAND AND LLUÍS FONTBOTÉ
Section des Sciences de la Terre, Rue des Maraîchers 13, CH-1211 Geneva 4, Switzerland

ABSTRACT

The mid-Cretaceous volcano-sedimentary sequences of the Casma Group in Central Peru hosts several Volcanic Hosted Massive Sulphide (VHMS) deposits. The main mine is on the Perubar Ba-Zn-Pb VHMS deposit, formed by the Graciela, Juanita, Cecilia Norte and Cecilia Sur massive sulphide (±barite) bodies. The stratigraphy of the Casma Group at Perubar consists of four units, mainly composed of submarine volcanic rocks and pyroclastic deposits ranging from basaltic-andesitic to rhyodacitic composition, intercalated with volcaniclastic sandstones, tuffaceous mudstones, siltstones, and impure limestones. The massive sulphide lenses are found on top of an impure limestone interval and in close spatial association with andesitic to rhyodacitic lavas, hyaloclastites and pyroclastic rocks. The Perubar deposit was strongly dislocated shortly after its deposition following an active fault-block subsidence event. Massive sulphide lenses were separated from their main feeder zones and partly mobilized along the margin of deeply subsiding blocks. Once put back in its original position the Perubar VHMS deposit presents a typical proximal-to-distal zonation, from: (i) pyrite-pyrrhotite-sphalerite (+ rare chalcopyrite) stockwork, (ii) massive pyrite-pyrrhotite-magnetite, (iii) massive Zn, (Fe>Pb) sulphides (±barite), (iv) banded barite and Zn, (Fe>Pb) sulphides, and (v) banded barite-pyrite. Typical footwall hydrothermal alteration zones have been recognized and range from a strongly chloritized-sericitized core to a peripheral extensive quartz-sericite alteration zone. The geological evolution recorded in the Casma rocks of the Cocachacra district suggest the existence of a local submarine caldera system at Perubar. The deposit probably formed at shallow water depth (<500 m?), as indicated by the presence of limestones in the basin at the time of mineralization.

INTRODUCTION

The mid-Cretaceous volcano-sedimentary sequences of the Casma Group in Central Peru (Fig. 1) hosts several Volcanic Hosted Massive Sulphide (VHMS) deposits (Vidal, 1987). The main mine is on the Perubar Ba-Zn-Pb VHMS deposit (Polliand et al., 1999, Vidal, 1987), mainly formed by the Graciela, Juanita, Cecilia North and Cecilia South massive sulphide (± barite) bodies (Fig. 2). The mine, which is owned by Perubar S.A. (Glencore), is situated in the Cocachacra mining district (11°55'S 76°34'W), 50 km east of Lima (Fig. 2). From 1978 to 1999, 5.6 million tonnes of massive sulphide ore have been extracted from the four main orebodies, with an average grade of 9.9 % Zn and 1.4 % Pb. Previously, about 10 million tonnes of barite ore were mined.

In this communication, we present partial results of an ongoing project at the University of Geneva, and mainly focus on the tectonic, volcanic and sedimentary environment that prevailed during formation of the Perubar deposit as an example of Mesozoic VHMS deposits in an ensialic back-arc marginal basin in the Central Andes.

GEOLOGICAL AND SEDIMENTOLOGICAL SETTING

The mid-Cretaceous Casma Group was deposited during the development of the Peruvian Huarmey-Cañete extensional marginal basin (Benavides, 1999; Atherton and Webb, 1989) during Aptian to Middle Albian times. According to these authors, the basin is floored by mantle material. This is in agreement with the 3.0 g/cm^3 arch-like structure found beneath the basin and considered by Couch et al. (1981) to be due to fracturing and insertion of material from the mantle. From its central part to the east, the Casma basin shows a marked polarity: a deep, mainly basaltic

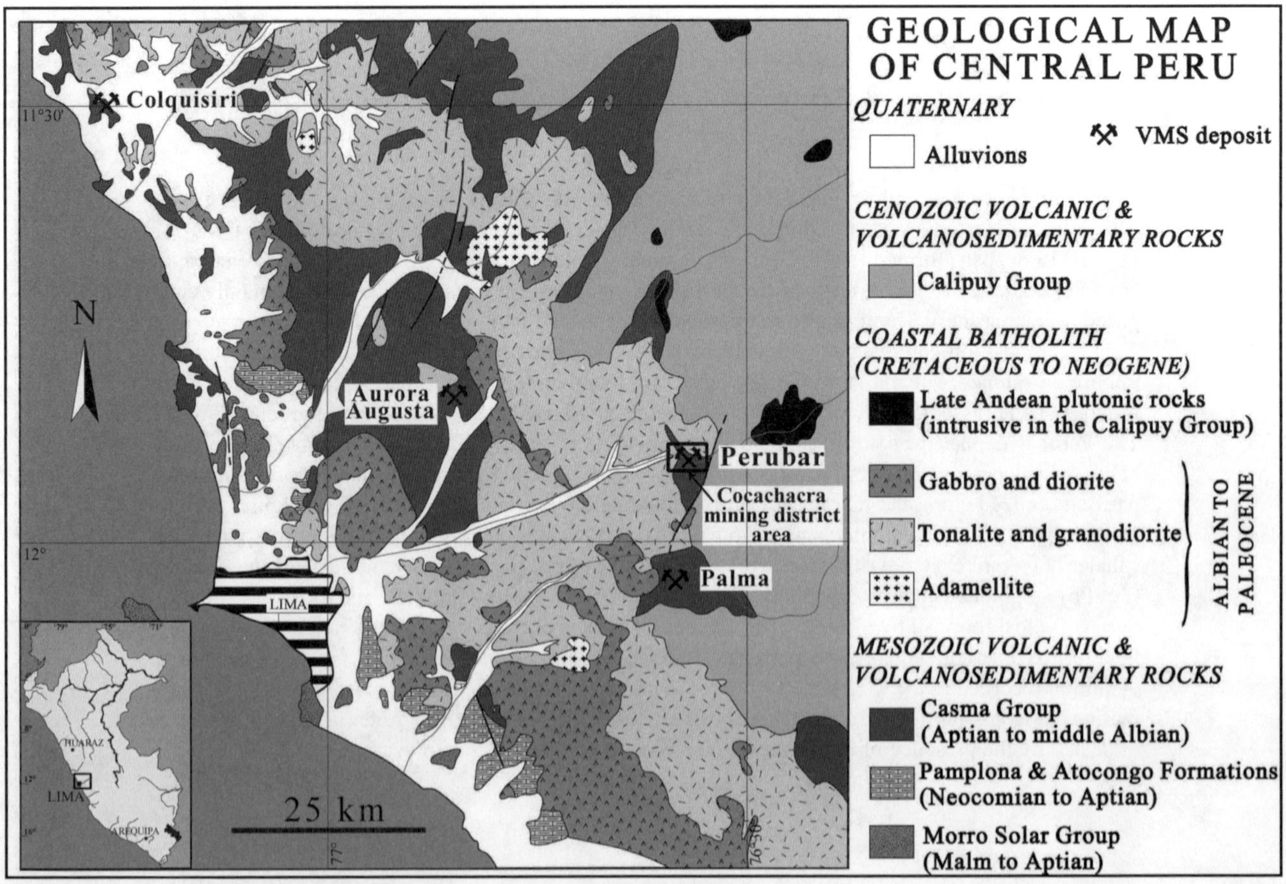

Figure. 1. Geological map of central Peru, modified from Mégard (1978).

central facies grading progressively to a shallower, more acidic, and generally more pyroclastic eastern facies (Atherton and Webb, 1989). The rocks of the western part of the basin are not exposed. The Casma rocks outcroping at Perubar are considered to be part of the eastern facies

The stratigraphy of the VHMS hosting Casma Group at Perubar consists of four main units (Fig. 3 and 4). The Footwall Unit (1) consists of a thick sequence (> 2km) of interbedded marine volcanogenic mudstones, siltstones and sandstones intercalated with submarine tuffs and basaltic to andesitic lava horizons with calc-alkaline and tholeiitic affinities. Towards the top of this unit, basaltic and andesitic lavas, hyaloclastite breccias and peperites become more predominant and indicate an increasing and more proximal volcanic activity. In addition, a dense network of gabbroic to dioritic sills intruded the Footwall Unit (Fig. 3). The overlying 100 to 150 m thick Prospective Unit (2) is characterised by the onset of bimodal volcanism and consists of submarine volcanic rocks and pyroclastic deposits ranging from basaltic-andesitic to rhyodacitic composition intercalated with volcaniclastic sandstones, tuffaceous mudstones, siltstones, and impure limestones. The massive sulphide lenses are found in this unit, at about 80 to 100 m above the last encountered sill of the Footwall Unit, just on top of an impure limestone horizon and in close spatial association with andesitic to rhyodacitic lavas, hyaloclastites and pyroclastic rocks (Fig. 3 and 4). The 50 to 100 m thick overlying Hangingwall Unit (3) consists of similar assemblages than found in the underlying Prospective Unit, but contains more abundant felsic volcanic rocks and is characterized by extensive mass flows, slumps, and polymictic breccias. The Upper Unit (4) consists of more than 200 m of relatively shallow marine volcanic and pyroclastic rocks possibly representing

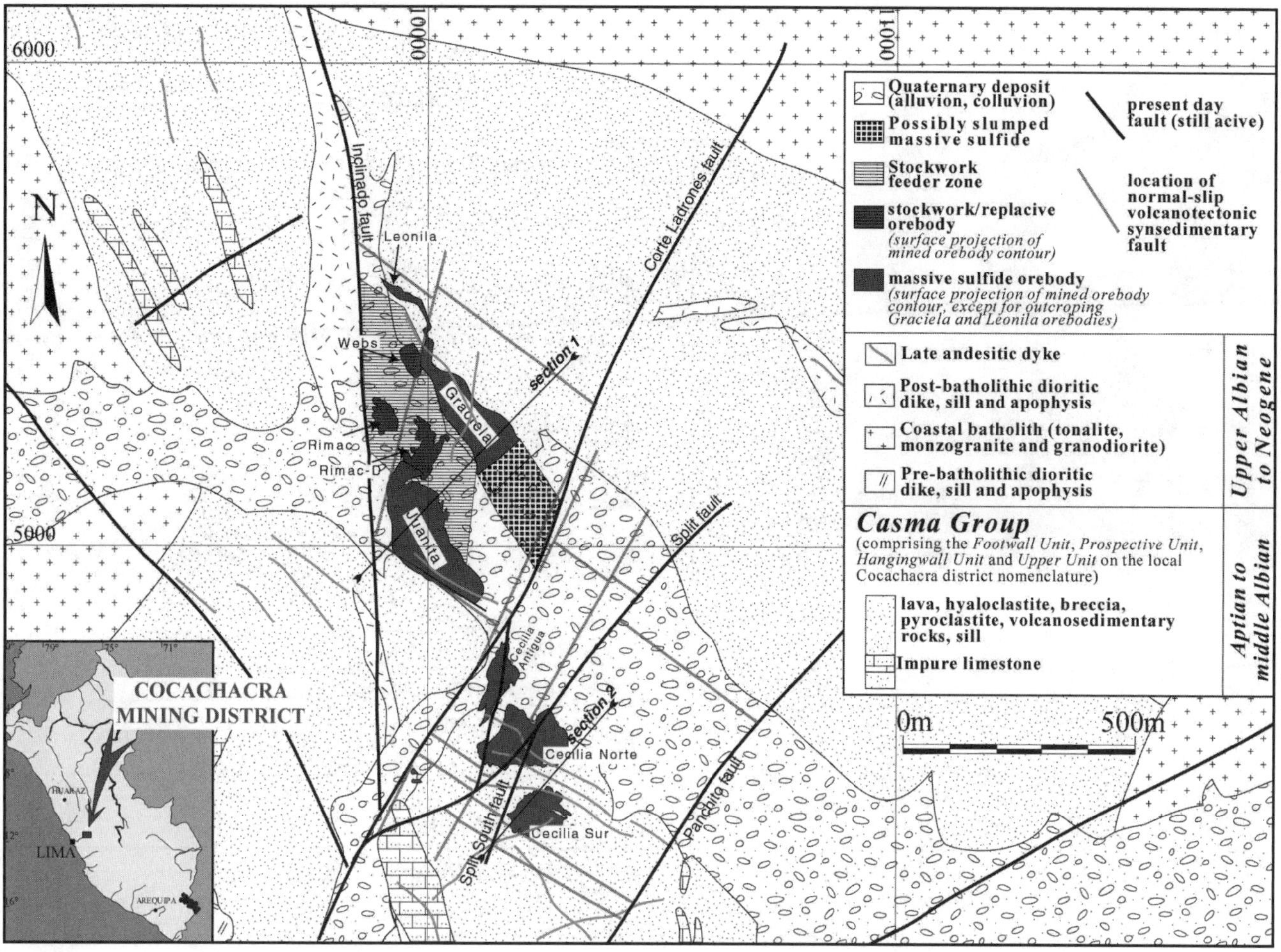

Figure. 2. Perubar deposit geological map, Cocachacra mining district (largely modified from Perubar staff maps).

debris flow deposits.

From Upper Cretaceous to Eocene, the Huarmey-Cañete marginal basin underwent compressive tectonic episodes and intrusion of the Peruvian Coastal Batholith, resulting in a progressive uplift and folding of the basin and development of contact metamoprhism aureoles in the vicinity of intrusive contacts.

The Casma rocks in the Cocachacra mining district are located in a roof pendant (Fig. 1) intruded by two granodioritic plutons of the Peruvian Coastal Batholith and underwent contact metamorphism up to amphibole (volcanics), biotite-sillimanite (volcaniclastic mudstones and sandstones) and pyroxene-garnet-calcosilicate (calcareous sediments) hornfels facies. Pyrite-pyrrhotite-magnetite assemblages formed in iron-rich massive sulphide zones. Whole-rock geochemistry of the volcanic host rocks did not significantly change since the VHMS hydrothermal event, as also confirmed by sulphur isotope data showing that closed system conditions prevailed during contact metamorphism (Polliand et al., 1999). From Oligocene to Pliocene, the Perubar deposit underwent successive Andean orogenic pulses, generating dextral normal-slip faults mainly activated along corridors corresponding to pre-existing NNE-SSW trending crustal-penetrating discontinuities. It resulted mainly to dextral translations along the NNE-SSW trending Corte Ladrones and Split faults (Fig. 2).

ORE SETTING

The massive sulphide orebodies at Perubar were strongly dislocated shortly after their deposition

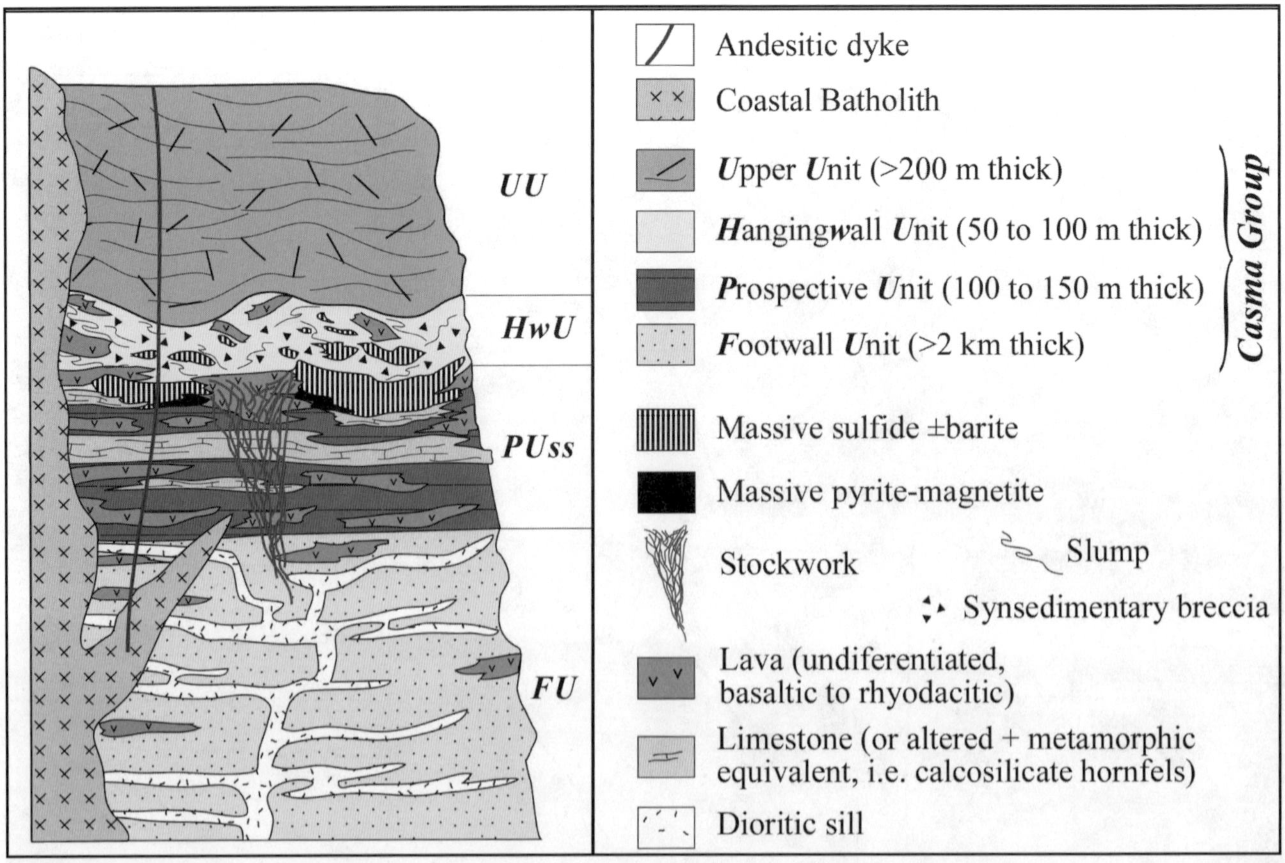

Figuer. 3. Stratigraphic column of the Casma Group outcroping in the Cocachacra mining district area.

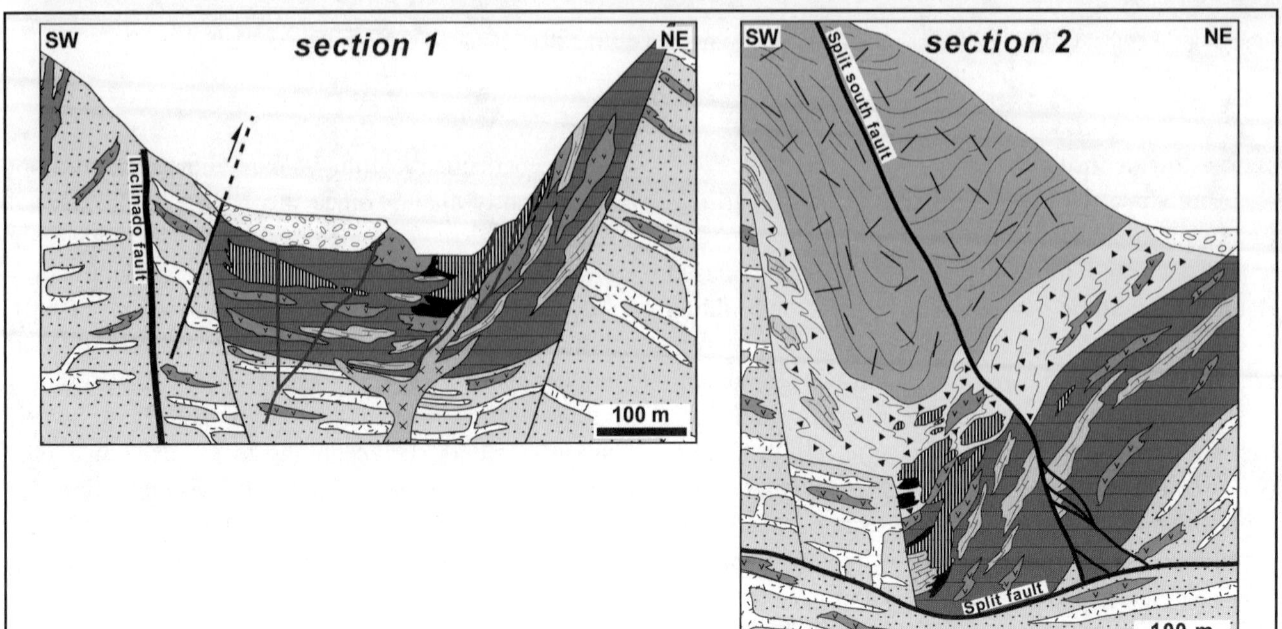

Figure. 4. Cross sections of the Perubar deposit. Note the deeply synsedimentary subsided blocks. For cross section location, see Figure. 2.

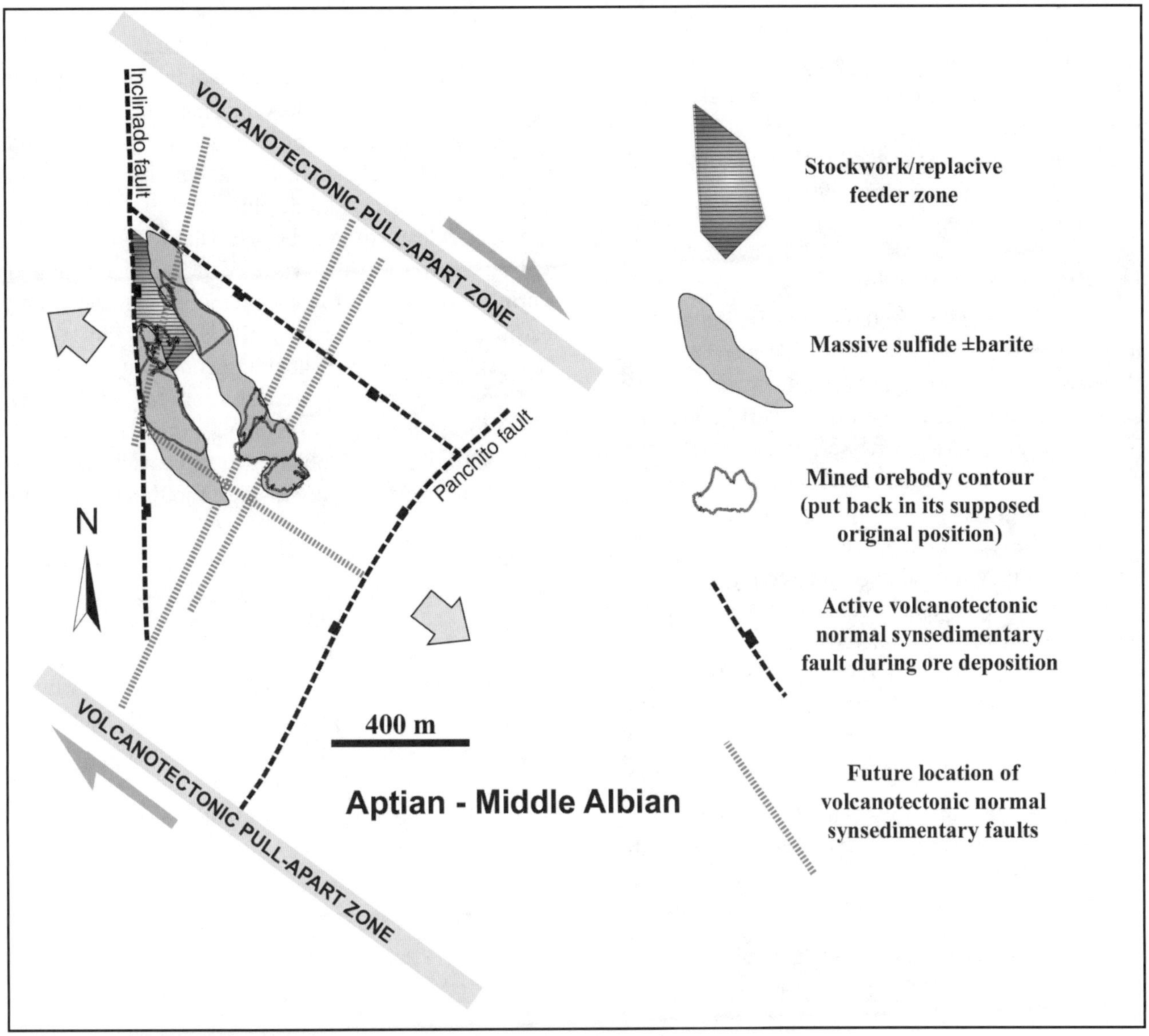

Figure. 5. Aptian-middle Albian schematic reconstitution of the Perubar deposit in its supposed original setting. Compare the outlines of the mined orebodies with those shown in Fig. 2.

following an active fault-block subsidence event. Massive sulphide lenses were separated from their main feeder zones and partly mobilized along the margin of subsiding blocks, producing massive sulphide slumping and brecciation. Figure 2 shows the present-day setting of the different massive sulphide and stockwork bodies of the Perubar deposit and Figure 5 an Aptian-middle Albian reconstitution of the deposit in its supposed original setting. Once put back in its original position (Fig. 5), the Perubar VHMS deposit presents the following zonation: (i) a central pyrite-pyrrhotite-sphalerite (+ rare chalcopyrite) feeder zone represented by the Webs and Rimac stockwork orebodies (Fig. 2); (ii) a transition zone, grading from stockwork-ore to more replacive-ore, mainly following impure limestone horizons and corresponding to the sphalerite and calcite-rich Rimac-D orebody (Fig. 2); (iii) massive sulphide (± barite) lenses (i.e. Leonila-Graciela, Juanita, Cecilia Norte and Cecilia Sur, Fig. 2). In addition, the massive sulphide lenses comprise a typical proximal-to-distal internal zonation, grading from: (i) massive pyrite-pyrrhotite-magnetite; (ii) massive Zn, (Fe>Pb) sulphides (± barite); (iii) banded barite and Zn, (Fe>Pb) sulphides; (iv) banded barite-pyrite. Copper is almost absent in the system.

HYDROTHERMAL ALTERATION

Typical footwall hydrothermal alteration zones (or their metamorphic equivalents) have been recognized (Polliand et al., 2000). They range from a strongly chloritized-sericitized core (stockwork zone) to a peripheral extensive quartz-sericite alteration zone, characterized by strong silicification, strong Na-depletion, and Ba and K-enrichment (Table 1). At the scale of the district, footwall rocks present wide-spread silicification and pyrite disseminations.

In addition, regional scale Na-metasomatism is recognized in the least altered mafic volcanic rocks (e.g., samples 2 and 4 in Table 1) and represents the background alteration at Perubar, attributed to early and/or late hydrothermal processes perhaps related to regional-scale burial metamorphism.

GEOLOGICAL EVOLUTION

In the Cocachacra district, at the end of the relatively deep marine sedimentation of the Footwall Unit formed during a main subsiding phase, carbonate sedimentation started abruptly, indicating a very rapid uplift to a relatively shallow-water environment. This dynamic uplift was rapidly followed by the onset of bimodal volcanism together with an increment of the volcanic activity. The Perubar VHMS deposit formed during this period of coeval bimodal volcanism and carbonate sedimentation, while the tectonic regime returned to (incipient) subsiding conditions.

Almost contemporaneously (slightly before or after) to the deposition of the ore, a dioritic sill-like stock intruded the footwall sequence. Gibson et al. (1999) interprete large, sill-like, multiphase subvolcanic intrusions which are formed in several VHMS environments as the intrusive equivalent of deeper magma chambers that fed the volcanic succession. Thus, the dioritic subvolcanic stock observed at Perubar may suggest the presence of a relatively high crustal magma chamber at the time of mineralization, which could have generated the local heat flow necessary to activate a seawater convection cell into

Table 1. Typical whole-rock geochemistry for footwall volcanic rocks. Samples 1, 3 and 5 are strongly altered samples. Samples 2, 4 and 6 are weakly altered samples (but ± regional Na-metasomatism).

		1 Subalkaline basalt	2 Subalkaline basalt	3 Andesite	4 Andesite	5 Rhyodacite	6 Rhyodacite
SiO_2	%	50.56	51.19	55.7	58.09	67.12	69.42
TiO_2	%	0.88	1.16	0.82	1.1	0.55	0.23
Al_2O_3	%	17.7	18.86	16.5	17.32	10.5	14.9
Fe_2O_3	%	4.22	10.79	4.31	6.77	4.32	2.25
MnO	%	0.16	0.19	0.19	0.2	0.09	0.05
MgO	%	2.38	3.33	3.18	2.66	0.94	0.82
CaO	%	8.36	7.1	4.01	5.6	2.73	2.23
Na_2O	%	0.74	5.05	0.99	6.66	0.91	4.84
K_2O	%	7.22	1.06	8.84	0.52	4.27	3.18
P_2O_5	%	0.15	0.27	0.21	0.2	0.15	0.09
LOI	%	2.35	0.4	3.11	0.66	1.14	0.71
Cr_2O_3	%	0.02	0	0.01	0.01	0.02	0.01
Ba	ppm	33200	966	25100	521	47600	2433

the footwall volcano-sedimentary pile.

Shortly after the VHMS mineralizing event, an abrupt and chaotic subsidence regime started, spliting the seafloor into deeply subsiding small sub-basins delimited by volcano-tectonic faults spaced commomly at less than 500 m. It resulted in the downward translation, slumping and brecciation of the Perubar VHMS deposit and emplacement of the chaotic Hangingwall Unit (Fig. 4). Together with this ongoing strong fault-block subsidence, volcanic activity became more and more predominant. Subsequently, a major eruptive event probably was responsible for the deposition of the Upper Unit volcanic/pyroclastic debris flow-like sequence.

CONCLUSION

Within the regional context of the Peruvian Huarmey-Cañete extensional marginal basin, the complex sedimentary and volcanic evolution recorded in the Casma rocks of the Cocachacra district, together with evidences of rapid uplift followed by abrupt fault-block subsidence suggest the existence of a local submarine caldera system at Perubar. According to Ohmoto (1996), the formation of submarine calderas played a key role in the genesis of VHMS deposits in the Japanese Hokuroku district. Under extensional basin settings, it is more likely to develop piecemeal caldera collapse rather than piston-like subsidence, as mentioned by Kokelaar (1992). The chaotic fault-block subsidence recorded in the Hangingwall Unit could correspond to such a piecemeal caldera collapse. The VHMS mineralization at Perubar most likely was emplaced in an intracaldera incipient depression, prior to the main caldera collapse. This situation differs slightly from the postcaldera collapse emplacement generally observed in Kuroko deposits. The narrow collapsing sub-basins at Perubar probably developed in fault-splays above steep, crustal-penetrating discontinuities that focused plumbing of magmas, basement fracturing and hydrothermal fluid discharges at these sites

Therefore, considering the Perubar deposit massive sulphide mineralogy, footwall alteration characteristics, volcanic environment and tectonic setting, the denomination of Kuroko-type deposit seems to be appropriate for this Andean VHMS mineralization. However, it most likely formed at shallow seawater depth (<500 m?), as indicated by the presence of limestones in the basin at the time of mineralization. Moreover, the general low Copper content at Perubar suggests that the temperature of the system was lower than for most Kuroko deposits, as the hydrothermal fluid did not effectively transport this element. Considering a fluid temperature <300°C with a salinity higher than that of normal seawater, the hydrostatic condition required for the formation of a Zn-rich and Cu-poor VHMS deposit like Perubar might have been attained at a seawater depth <500 m.

ACKNOWLEDGEMENTS

This work is part of an ongoing PhD thesis project at the University of Geneva supported by the Swiss National Science Foundation grant FN 2000-54150.98 and is a contribution to the Europe Science Foundation GEODE programme. We gratefully acknowledge W. Mueller and L. Oldham who instigated this project and transmitted us their knowledge of the deposit, the geologists and staff of the Perubar mine for their help during the field work periods, especially R. Egoavil and C. Zumarán, and the geologists from Glencore Peru, M. Steinmann and S. Bureau, for logistical support during the project.

REFERENCES

Atherton, M. P. and Webb, S. 1989. Volcanic facies, structure, and geochemistry of the marginal basin rocks of central Peru; Journal of South American Earth Sciences, v. 2, no 3, p. 241-261.

Benavides, V. 1999. Orogenic evolution of the Peruvian Andes: The Andean Cycle. Geology and ore deposits of the Central Andes, SEG Spec. Pub., v. 7, p. 61-107.

Couch, R., Whitsett, R., Huehn, B. and Briceño-Guarupe, L. 1981. Structures of the continental margin in Peru and Chile, in Kulm et al., eds., Nazca plate: Crustal formation and Andean convergence: Geological Society of America Memoir 154, p. 703-726.

Gibons, H. L., Morton, R. L. and Hudak, G. J. 1999. Submarine volcanic processes, deposits, and environments favorable for the location of volcanic-associated massive sulfide deposits, Reviews in Economic Geology, v. 8, p. 13-51.

Kokelaar, P. 1992. Ordovician volcanic and sedimentary record of rifting and volcanotectonism: Snowdon, Wales, United Kingdom, Geological Society of America Bulletin, v. 104, p 1433-1455.

Mégard, F. 1978. Etude géologique des Andes du Pérou central, Mémoires ORSTOM, Paris, v. 86, 310 p.

Ohmoto, H. 1996. Formation of volcanogenic massive sulfide deposits: The Kuroko perspective, Ore Geology Reviews, 10: 135-177.

Polliand, M., Fontboté, L., Bureau, S., Steinmann, M. and Egoavil, R. 2000. Ore setting and hydrothermal alteration at the Perubar VMS deposit, X Congreso Peruano de Geología, Resúmenes, Sociedad Geológica del Perú Eds., Lima, p. 233.

Polliand, M., Fontboté L. and Spangenberg, J. 1999. Tracing back sulfur isotope reequilibration due to contact metamorphism: A case study from the Perubar VMS deposit, Central Peru. Mineral Deposits: Process to Processing, Stanley et al. (eds), Balkema, Rotterdam, v. 2, p. 967-970.

Vidal, C. E., 1987, Kuroko-Type Deposits in the Middle Cretaceous Marginal Basin of Central Peru, Econ. Geol., v. 82, p. 1409-1430.

VOLCANOGENIC MASSIVE SULPHIDE MINERALIZATION IN THE ARIPUANÃ DISTRICT OF MATO GROSSO, BRAZIL

Staff of Anglo American Brasil, and David Kerr*
* *Present address: Department of Geology, Queens University, Kingston, Ontario*

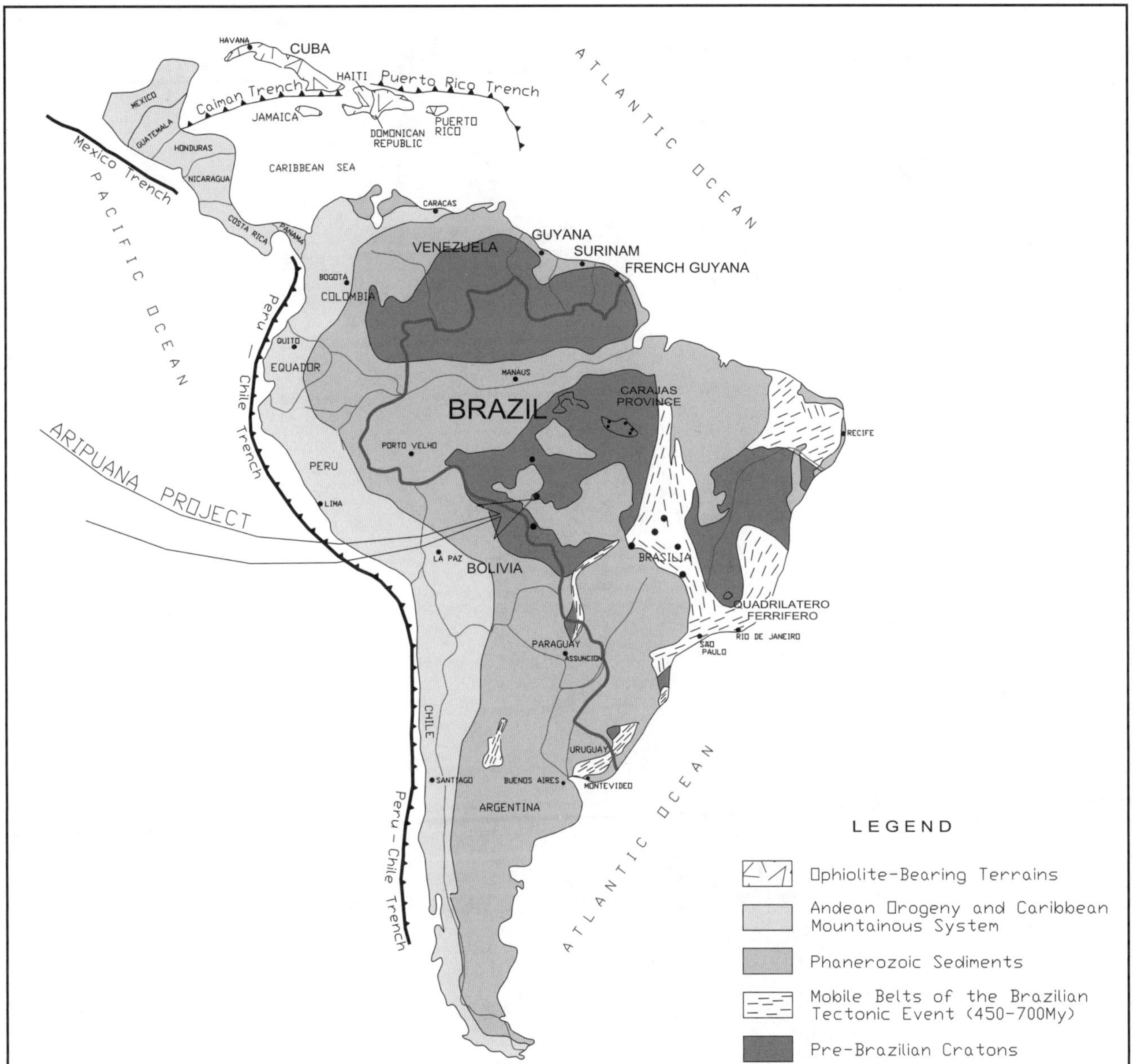

Figure 1. Generalized geology map of South America showing teh location of the Aripuanã project.

Introduction

Local prospectors found gold in stream alluvium and outcrop to the north of the town of Aripuanã, in western Mato Grosso State, in the 1980´s. Follow-up of these occurrences by mining companies in the early 1990's led to the discovery of oxide copper

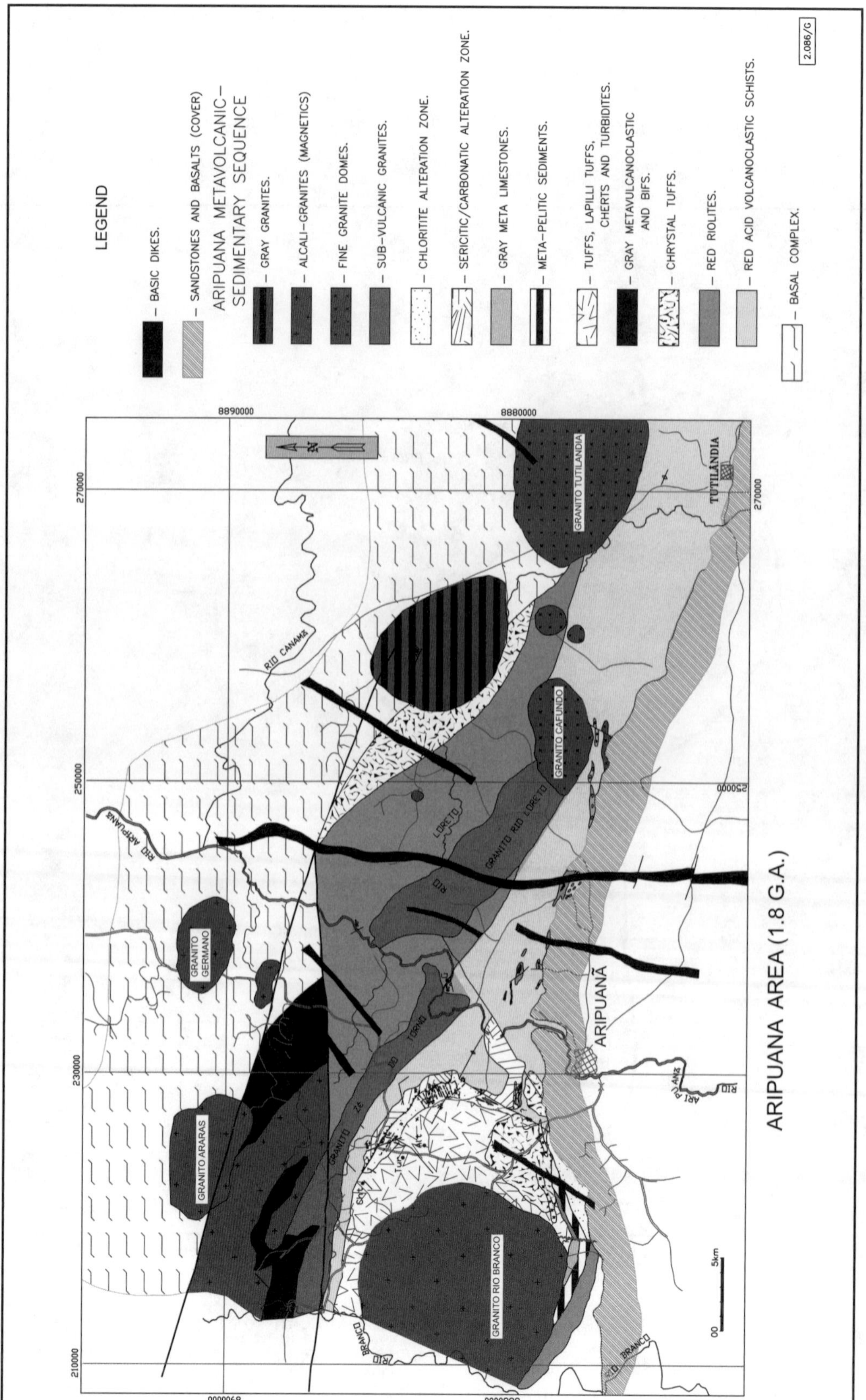

Figure 2. Geology map of the Aripuanã project.

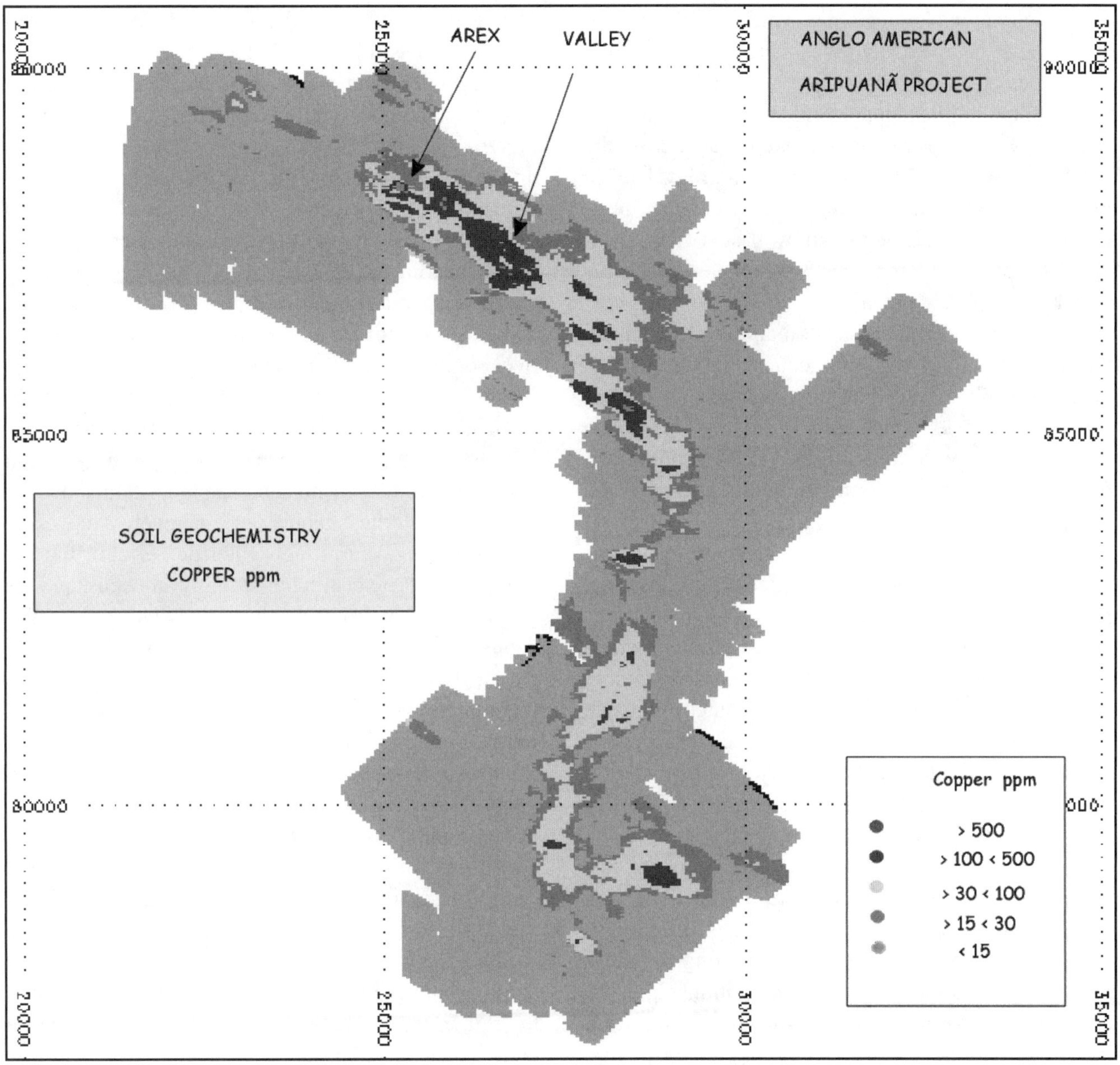

Figure 3. Zinc in soil geochemical map for the Aripuanã project.

mineralization in shallow gold workings, and outcropping lead- and zinc-rich gossan. Since then, two principal mineral prospects have been located, the Arex deposit of Anglo American and the nearby Valley deposit of Karmin Exploration (formerly Ambrex). These, and adjacent prospects and anomalies, are currently being explored in a joint venture between Anglo American and Karmin.

REGIONAL GEOLOGY

The Aripuanã district lies within the Guaporé Craton, the major block of Archean to mid-Proterozoic age rocks which underlies central-northern Brazil south of the Amazon river (Fig.1). The craton is made up of granite-gneiss-granulite terrain (termed the Xingu Complex) with inliers of Archean to Lower Proterozoic age supracrustal rocks, which were deformed, metamorphosed and intruded by acid to mafic plutons in tectonic cycles terminating at about the end of Lower Proterozoic time. Subsequently, there was a major anorogenic magmatic event in which predominantly acid volcanics (Uatuma Group) were erupted extensively across the craton, associated with intrusion of high-level felsic plutons. Continued incipient rifting in mid-Proterozoic time formed shallow basins filled with undeformed clastic and minor carbonate sediments, with basaltic flows and sills.

The town of Aripuanã lies on an elevated plateau underlain by flat-lying rift sequence rocks. These unconformably overlie deformed and metamorphosed supracrustal rocks which outcrop a few km. to the north of the town, forming a WNW-ESE trending belt bounded to the north by gneiss-granite terrain of the Xingu basement complex (Fig. 2). The supracrustal belt can be broadly divided into a southern felsic volcano-sedimentary sequence dominated by tuffaceous rocks, and a northerly bimodal basalt-rhyolite package. Both are intruded by a variety of granite plutons and smaller diorite-gabbro intrusions. A prominent circular granite pluton (Rio Branco) outcrops to the NW of Aripuanã. The metavolcanic sequence wraps around this in outcrop, with known mineralization located in distinctively altered rocks along a NW-SE to N-S trending arc, which then swings back to the east where it is partly covered by the younger sediments. Knowledge of the geology of the Aripuana region is at an early stage, and there is uncertainty regarding the tectono-stratigraphic setting of these metavolcanic rocks, including their relationship to the normally undeformed Uatuma volcanics. Age dating indicates that the metavolcanics and their granitic intrusives are close in age at 1.77 to 1.75 Ga, which is within the range of ages measured for the Uatuma volcanics elsewhere.

Local geology and mineralisation

All of the currently known mineralization lies within mainly tuffaceous rocks which are folded, metamorphosed to greenshist rank, and disrupted by faulting. At the Arex and Valley deposits, the host sequence is interpreted as facing to the SSW. The rocks in the footwall of the mineralised zone are felsic lavas, autoclastic breccias and epiclastic and pyroclastic tuffs, altered and metamorphosed to quartz-sericite schists. In the vicinity of mineralization they are strongly sericitic and chloritic. The hangingwall sequence includes well-bedded fine to lapilli tuffs, aphyric rhyolitic flows, graded turbidites, argillites and calc-silicate rocks. Isoclinal folding is recognised, with sub-vertical penetrative axial plane cleavage, and there is evidence for SSW-vergent thrusting and subsequent shearing on E-W and WNW striking structures.

Broadly stratabound mineralization can be traced by soil geochemistry and intermittent gossan outcrops over some 30 km. of strike (Fig.3). Drilling at several localities along this belt has encountered primary mineralization below the zone of surface weathering, consisting of tabular and lenticular bodies of massive and semi-massive to disseminated sulphides dominated by pyrite, sphalerite, galena and chalcopyrite. The enclosing rocks are variably chloritic, sericitic, biotite-rich, calc-silicate bearing or strongly siliceous, and are interpreted as hydrothermally altered felsic tuffs, tuffaceous sediments, and cherty to calcareous exhalites.

The two principal deposits located to date are both incompletely explored. A preliminary resource estimate of about 12 million tonnes at 6.3 % Zn, 2.2 % Pb has been published by Karmin for Valley, and Anglo American have reported that Arex is of a similar size and grade. It also contains copper-rich zones. There are small occurrences of gold mineralization with disseminated pyrite in strongly sericitic metatuffs adjacent to the base metals mineralization.

The deposits have been interpreted as either volcano-exhalative in origin, or intrusion-related hydrothermal replacements. At Arex in particular, a clear zonal relationship is evident between pyritic zinc-lead mineralization and adjacent copper mineralization with associated magnetite, pyrrhotite and elevated gold values. The consistency of this relationship in folded host rocks points strongly to a volcano-exhalative origin, in which the copper-rich mineralization occupies the original footwall feeder zone underlying sea-floor replacement and exhalative zinc-rich mineralization. The broadly stratabound form, sulphide mineralogy, mineral textures, and the nature of the altered host rocks, are consistent with this interpretation, although there has clearly been disruption, re-crystallization and remobilization during deformation and metamorphism. Elsewhere along the mineralised belt, extensive discordant stringer copper mineralization has been found in a thick felsic tuffaceous unit overlain by massive pyrite lenses carrying weak zinc, further supporting the volcano-exhalative interpretation.

If this genetic interpretation is correct, these are the first VMS-type deposits of significant size to have been found in the Precambrian rocks of Brazil.

THE PALMEIRÓPOLIS DEPOSIT, TOCANTINS STATE, BRAZIL: A TYPICAL METAMORPHOSED VOLCANOGENIC MASSIVE SULPHIDE DEPOSIT

SYLVIA M. ARAUJO
Instituto de Geociências - Universidade de Brasília, Brasília - DF - Brazil -70.910-900
email: sylviaa@unb.br

ABSTRACT

The Palmeirópolis massive sulphide (Zn-Cu-Pb) deposit in south Tocantins State, Brazil, occurs in the lower part of the Proterozoic Palmeirópolis volcano-sedimentary Sequence. The Palmeirópolis Sequence is part of a large bimodal volcano-sedimentary belt located in central Brazil. The deposit consists of four highly deformed massive sulphide lenses with an estimated resource of 4 Mt at 1.23 % Cu, 4.64 % Zn, 0.72 % Pb and 25.1 g/t Ag. The sulphide bodies are underlain by hydrothermal alteration zones consisting mainly of anthophyllite-biotite (cordierite-garnet) rocks, plagioclase-biotite rocks and by sillimanite-quartz rocks. Chemically, the alteration zone rocks with their strong depletion of alkalies and enrichments of magnesium, aluminium and ore metals resemble the chlorite zones that underlain many non-metamorphosed volcanogenic massive sulphide deposits. These rocks are interpreted to be mainly basalts that had undergone hydrothermal alteration during ore deposition and subsequently were metamorphosed to the upper amphibolite facies.

The sulphide ore is characterized by sphalerite, chalcopyrite, pyrrhotite, pyrite, and galena. The sulphides were significantly altered by metamorphic and deformational effects and no remnants of the original texture were observed. The metamorphic and deformational effects include development of triple junction in sphalerite and pyrrhotite, recrystallization of pyrite as euhedral cubic porphyroblasts, deformation of twins in pyrrhotite and curved cleavage traces in galena. The Palmeirópolis ore is characterized by a typical durchbewegung fabric.

The study of the Palmeirópolis volcanogenic massive sulphide deposit, the first one found at the large volcano-sedimentary belt of central Brazil, allows the establishment of important exploration guides to the region.

INTRODUCTION

The Palmeirópolis deposit consists of Zn-Cu sulphide lenses with an estimated geological resource of 4 Mt, having an average grade of 1.23 % Cu, 4.64 % Zn, 0.72 % Pb and 25.1 g/tonne Ag. The deposit, located about 20 km east of the city of Palmeirópolis, Tocantins State, Brazil (Fig. 1), was discovered in 1977 by CPRM (Companhia de Pesquisa e Recursos Minerais) after an airborne geophysical survey (Projeto Aerogeofísico Serra da Mesa). More than 25,000 m of diamond drilling was carried out between 1977 and 1989 and three bodies called C-1, C-2, C-3 and one small prospect, named Cabeceira Verde, have been found (Figueiredo et al., 1981).

Palmeirópolis is a typical example of a volcanogenic massive sulphide (VMS) deposit associated with bimodal tholeiitic volcanic rocks, characterized by a well developed hydrothermal alteration zone underneath the ore bodies. The ore and its host rocks have undergone amphibolite facies regional metamorphism (Araujo et al., 1995). Identification of primary features on VMS deposits that were metamorphosed under high-grade conditions is not straight forward because their textures, structures and mineralogical composition are, in many cases, radically different from the original. The study of the Palmeirópolis deposit allow an evaluation of the mineralogical, chemical and isotopic changes that occurred on the ore and host rocks as an effect of the high-grade metamorphism. Based on these studies, it is possible to suggest exploration guides for VMS deposits within high grade terrains and, particularly, for mineralizations

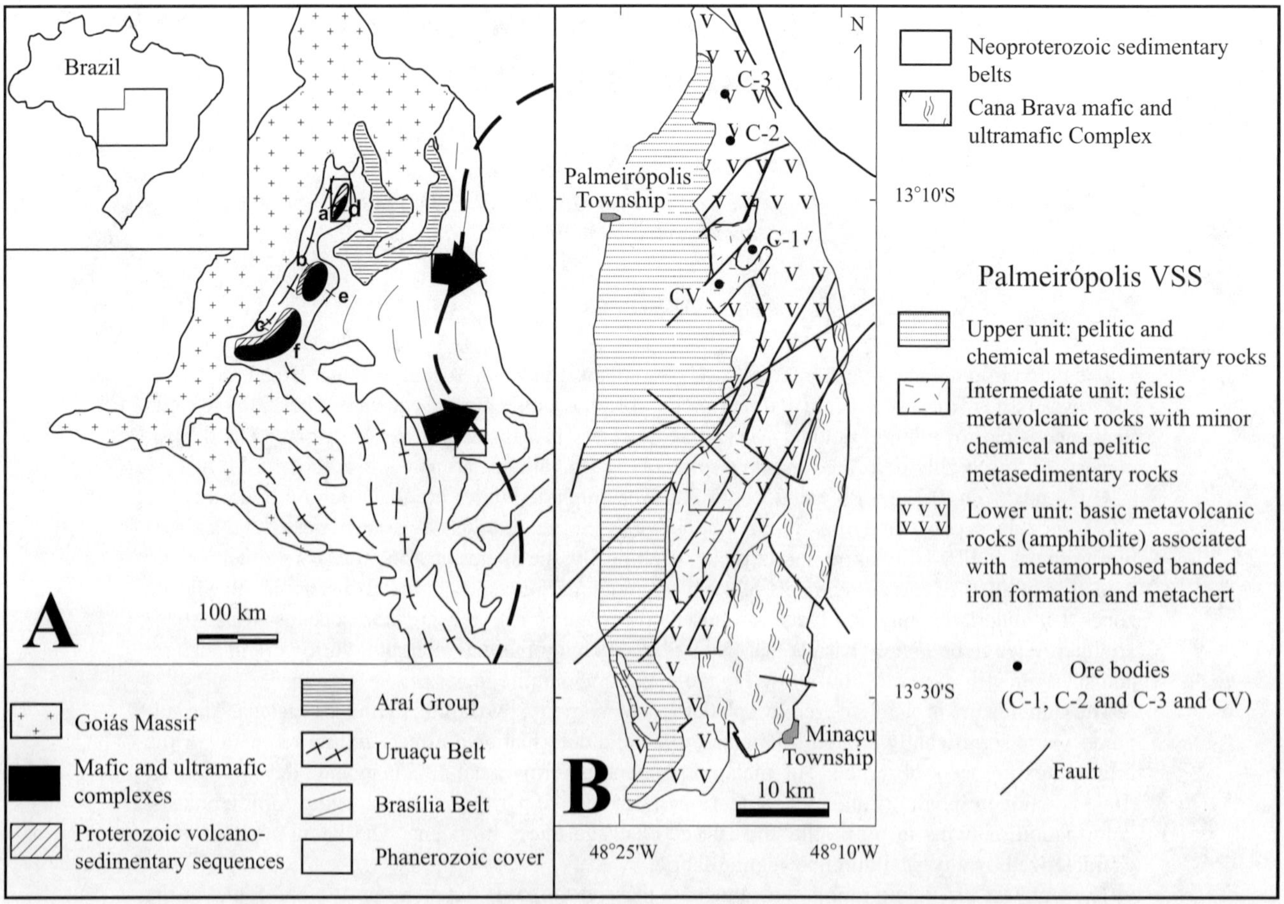

Figure 1. A) Geological sketch map of central Brazil. Heavy line indicates the limit of the São Francisco Craton. Arrows indicate tectonic vergence of supracrustal rocks (a; Palmeirópolis Sequence; b: Indaianópolis Sequence; c: Juscelândia Sequence; d: Cana Brava Complex; e: Niquelândia Complex; f: Barro Alto Complex). B) Simplified geological map of the Palmeirópolis volcano-sedimentary Sequence (VSS) (located by small box in A) with the four ore bodies location. Modified from Araujo et al. (1995).

associated with the volcano-sedimentary sequences that are located at the western border of the large granulitic mafic-ultramafic complexes of central Brazil.

GEOLOGICAL SETTING

The Palmeirópolis deposit is situated within the Palmeirópolis volcano-sedimentary sequence (PVSS), part of a 300 km long volcano-sedimentary belt that includes the southern Indaianópolis and Juscelândia volcano-sedimentary sequences. The belt is located at the western border of the granulitic mafic-ultramafic complexes of central Brazil (Cana Brava, Niquelândia and Barro Alto). Together, the volcano-sedimentary sequences and the mafic-ultramafic complexes form a linear array within Proterozoic fold belts located between the Amazon and São Francisco Cratons. The main geotectonic units present in the region are the Goiás Massif, the Araí Group and Neoproterozoic sedimentary belts, including the Uruaçu and the Brasília Belts (Marini et al., 1984; Fuck et al., 1987) (Fig. 1A).

There is no widely accepted model for the geological setting of the PVSS. Its stratigraphic relationship to the adjacent units is not clear because of limited exposure, faulted contacts and paucity of reliable geochronological data.

The PVSS is a bimodal tholeiitic sequence (Araujo and Nilson, 1988) that has been subdivided into three units (Figueiredo et al., 1981) (Figs. 1B, and 2). The lower unit consists of large volume of fine-grained

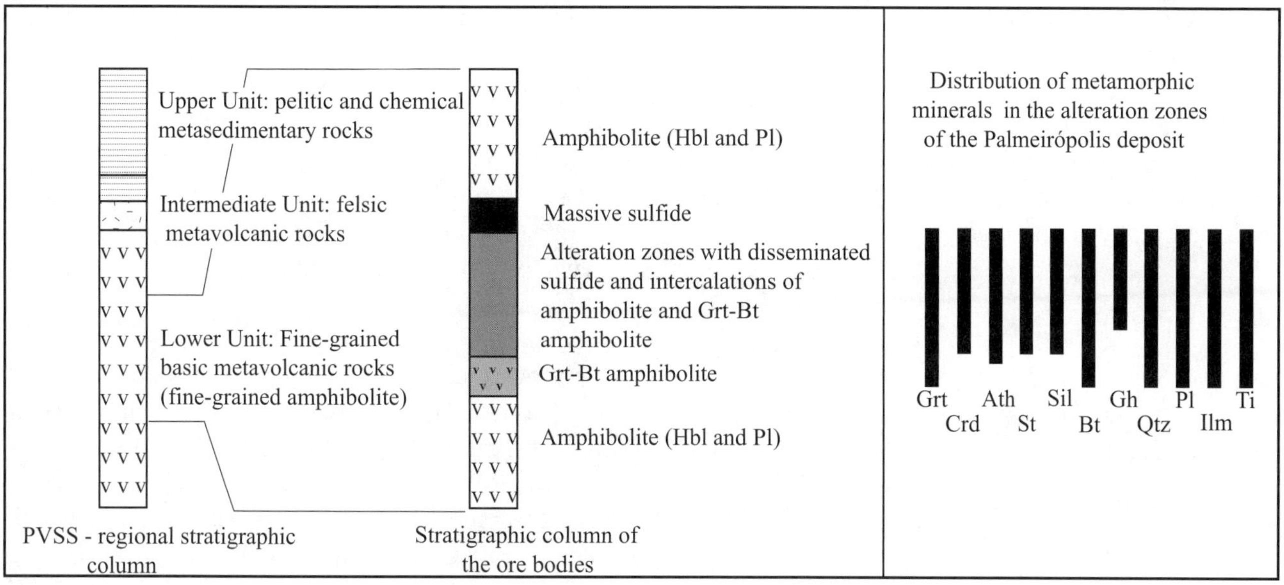

Figure 2. General stratigraphic columns of the Palmeirópolis volcano-sedimentary Sequence (PVSS) and the ore bodies illustrating the mineralogy of the alteration zones. Ath: anthophyllite; Bt: biotite; Crd: cordierite; Gh: gahnite; Grt: garnet; Hbl: hornblende; Ilm: ilmenite; Pl: plagioclase; Qtz: quartz; Sil: sillimanite; St: staurolite; Ti : titanite. Modified from Araujo and Nilson (1988).

amphibolite containing lenses of metamorphosed banded iron formation and chert. This unit represents an extensive episode of submarine basic volcanism associated with initial breakup of continental crust and development of new ocean floor during the Proterozoic (Araujo and Nilson, 1987). Related intrusive activity includes basic and ultrabasic dykes and granitic bodies that cut this unit.

The PVSS intermediate unit contains metamorphosed felsic volcanic to sub-volcanic bodies represented by quartz-biotite-muscovite-plagioclase schist, quartz-biotite-plagioclase schist and quartz-muscovite schist. Metre scale xenoliths of amphibolites are observed within the metamorphosed felsic subvolcanic bodies.

The upper unit of the PVSS contains interbedded pelitic and chemical metasedimentary rocks.

The PVSS was metamorphosed under amphibolite facies conditions. Based on the stability of the mineral associations and on mineral pairs geothermometers, peak metamorphic temperature is estimated to have been 550 to 625ºC and pressure between 2 and 5.5 kbars (Araujo et al., 1995)

Geochronological data based on Rb-Sr systematics suggest a Mesoproterozoic age of ca. 1300 Ma for the PVSS (Girardi et al., 1978; Drago et al., 1981). Pb-Pb dating of galena from the Palmeirópolis deposit suggests an age in the range of 1170 to 1270 Ma (Ralph Thorpe, Geological Survey of Canada, pers. comm.). These data are not conclusive and do not establish the precise age of the PVSS, but they do suggest that the sequence is not older than 1300 Ma.

GEOLOGY OF THE PALMEIRÓPOLIS DEPOSIT

The geology of the Palmeirópolis deposit has been described by Figueiredo et al. (1981), Araujo and Nilson (1988) and Araujo and Scott (1991). The rocks have undergone deformation and metamorphism that obscured many of their original features. Despite this, the main units may be further divided to show a significant internal succession. The stratigraphic column in Figure 2 relates the internal stratigraphy at the deposit to that of the Palmeirópolis volcano-sedimentary sequence.

The C-1, C-2 and C-3 sulphide bodies are hosted by rocks of the lower unit of the Palmeirópolis sequence. These ore bodies are associated with amphibolite and a heterogeneous package of hydrothermally altered rocks, represented mainly by anthophyllite-biotite assemblages with lenses of amphibolite. Metamorphosed felsic subvolcanic bodies, are also present in the vicinity of the C-1 and C-2 ore bodies, but no felsic rock is in contact with ore.

The sulphide bodies are located at the contact between the amphibolite and the alteration zone rocks. From top to the base of the deposit the following stratigraphy is observed:

- typical amphibolite with hornblende and plagioclase
- massive sulphide
- disseminated sulphide in alteration zone assemblages
- garnet-biotite amphibolite
- typical amphibolite with hornblende and plagioclase

The upper contact between the massive sulphide and the amphibolite is sharp. The lower contact between the sulphide body and the alteration zone is gradational over a few centimetres to metres.

The Cabeceira Verde Prospect is associated with felsic rocks of the PVSS intermediate unit. The ore is hosted by quartz-muscovite-K feldspar schists. Sulphide minerals, represented mainly by pyrite, are preferrentially oriented according to the rock foliation.

Host Rocks

Amphibolite

The amphibolite is a homogeneous, dark-green, fine to medium grained, foliated rock with nematoblastic texture (Fig. 3a). Porphyroblastic crystals of hornblende (up to 0.3 cm) and relict phenocrysts of plagioclase (0.2 cm) are also present. Amphibolites with alternating felsic (plagioclase, quartz, garnet) and mafic (hornblende, titanite, ilmenite) layers are observed (Fig. 3b).

Hornblende (60 to 80 % of the total volume) and plagioclase (10 to 25 % of the total volume) are the essential minerals. Biotite, garnet, titanite, ilmenite, epidote, carbonates, quartz, and apatite are always observed. Diopside and scapolite are rare. Pyrite and pyrrhotite are common along the foliation or in fractures. The C-3 sulphide body is related to a large volume of amphibolite that is almost completely chloritized.

The PVSS amphibolite has restricted silica content from 45.7 to 51.3 wt. %, low Al_2O_3 content (11.8 to 16.8 wt. %) and relatively high concentrations of CaO (7.1 to 16.9 wt. %), FeO*(> 11.0 wt. %) and TiO_2 (>0.9 wt. %). Cr values are particularly low and indicate either that the amphibolite has been generated from Cr-poor mantle or that Cr was removed (probably as Cr-spinel) in earlier stages of magma crystallization. The low Ni contents (57 to 128 ppm) suggest derivation from a very fractionated magma (Araujo et al., in press)

Major, minor and trace element chemistry as well as petrographical data indicate two distinct groups of amphibolites. Group I rocks have chemical composition similar to the N-MORB, and their REE patterns are 10 to 20 times the chondrite. Group II is characterized by enrichment of the whole spectrum of incompatible elements in relation to the MORB. The REE chondrite-normalized patterns of the group II amphibolites are flat at 30 to 40 times chondrite values. Group II amphibolites are similar to the rocks associated with the alteration zones of the volcanogenic ore bodies and are interpreted to be products of hydrothermal alteration related to the origin of the deposit. However, based on the evidence of incompatible trace element ratios, it is possible that magmatic differentiation played a role in the generation of the two amphibolite groups.

Felsic schists

The intermediate unit of the PVSS is represented by felsic schists having a very restricted distribution in the vicinity of the Palmeirópolis ore bodies. They are light gray, foliated, with lepido-granoblastic texture and characteristically show relict phenocrysts of K feldspar (Fig. 3c). The matrix of these rocks contains abundant quartz, K-feldspar and muscovite and/or biotite. When the volume of biotite is greater than muscovite, plagioclase is found in place of K-feldspar. Titanite, zircon and pyrite are minor minerals.

The felsic schists are considered to be metamorphosed acid to intermediate volcanic to subvolcanic bodies partially affected by hydrothermal alteration, but this alteration was not pervasive allowing the preservation of primary igneous textures (as relict phenocrysts of feldspar) and causing only minor chemical changes (Araujo and Nilson, 1988; Araujo et al., in press). Metric to submetric amphibolite

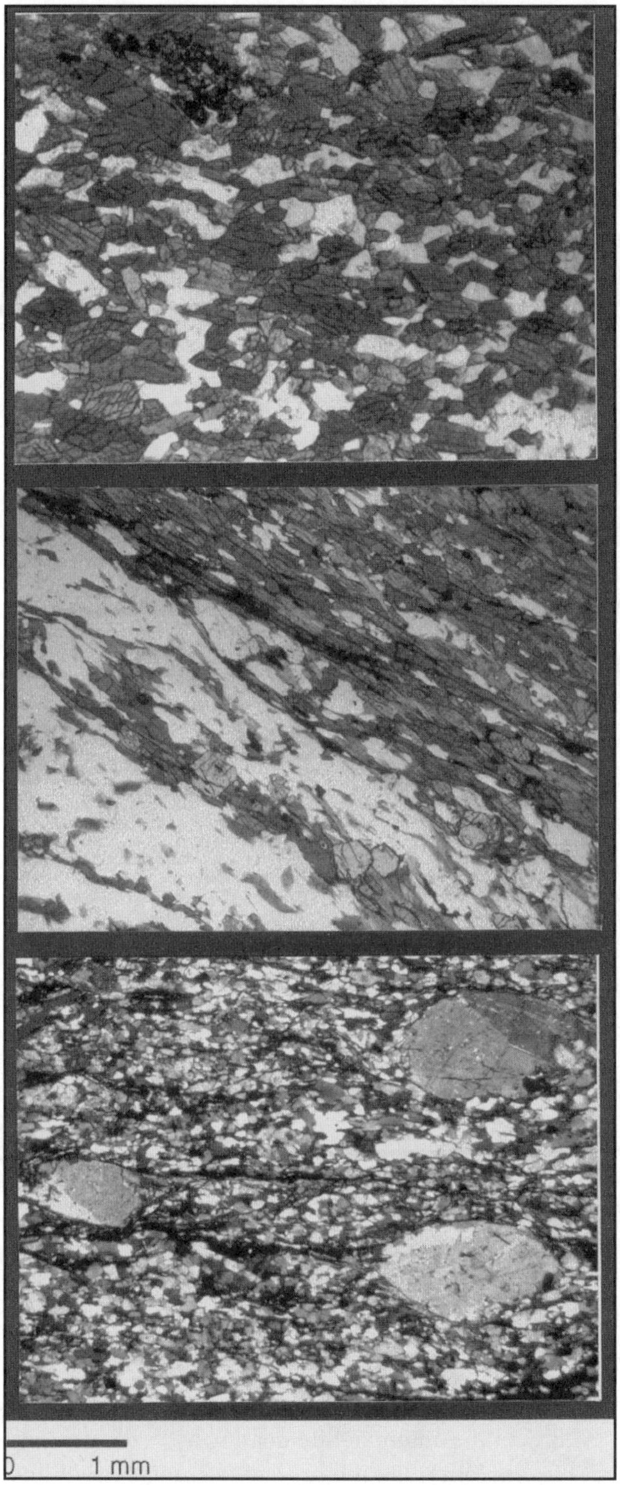

Figure 3. Photomicrographs of the PVSS rocks. A) Typical amphibolite. This rock has a well-developed nematoblastic texture and is composed by hornblende and plagioclase. The darkest areas are small clusters of titanite. Plane-polarized light. B) Banded amphibolite, the mafic bands consist mainly of hornblende, titanite and ilmenite; plagioclase and quartz predominate in the felsic bands. Although garnet can be found either in mafic or felsic bands, they seem preferentially associated with the mafic. Plane-polarized light. C) Felsic schist of the intermediate unit of the PVSS. This rock is well-foliated, with lepidogranoblastic texture and shows relict phenocrystals of K feldspar. Cross-polarized light.

xenoliths are observed within the subvolcanic body associated with the Cabeceira Verde Prospect.

The felsic metavolcanic rocks are distinguished by their unusual high Ta, Hf, Zr, U, Th and REE contents when compared to the amphibolites. Variable levels of MgO (0.60 to 5.37 wt. %) and variable but mainly high levels of K_2O (up to 6.32 wt. %) characterize these rocks. Chemically these rocks range from andesite to rhyolite, but the most acid terms are predominant.

Alteration zone assemblages

Hydrothermally altered rocks containing between 5 and 40 % of sulphide minerals are associated with the three sulphide bodies at the Palmeirópolis deposit. These rocks constitute the primary alteration zone that is typical of massive sulphide deposits (Franklin et al., 1981; Lydon, 1984, 1988). At Palmeirópolis the altered rocks are characterized by anthophyllite-biotite (garnet-cordierite) (Figs. 4A and 4B), plagioclase-biotite (Fig. 4C), and sillimanite-quartz assemblages (Fig. 4D). These rocks do not comprise a homogeneous package. In fact, a marked feature of the Palmeirópolis deposit is the presence of centimetre- to metre-thick bands of typical amphibolite (displaying no hydrothermal alteration effects) within the alteration zone. This amphibolite frequently grades into the anthophyllite-biotite rocks, but sharp contacts are also observed. The hydrothermal alteration that affected the host rocks of the Palmeirópolis deposit is therefore channelized and not pervasive. Even though felsic metavolcanic rocks are located in the vicinity of the C-1 ore body, this rock type was not observed within the C-1 alteration zone, and it is also not associated with the other two ore bodies, C-2 and C-3.

The rocks that comprise the alteration zone are medium- to coarse-grained with large tabular to fibrous radial anthophyllite crystals, and garnet and

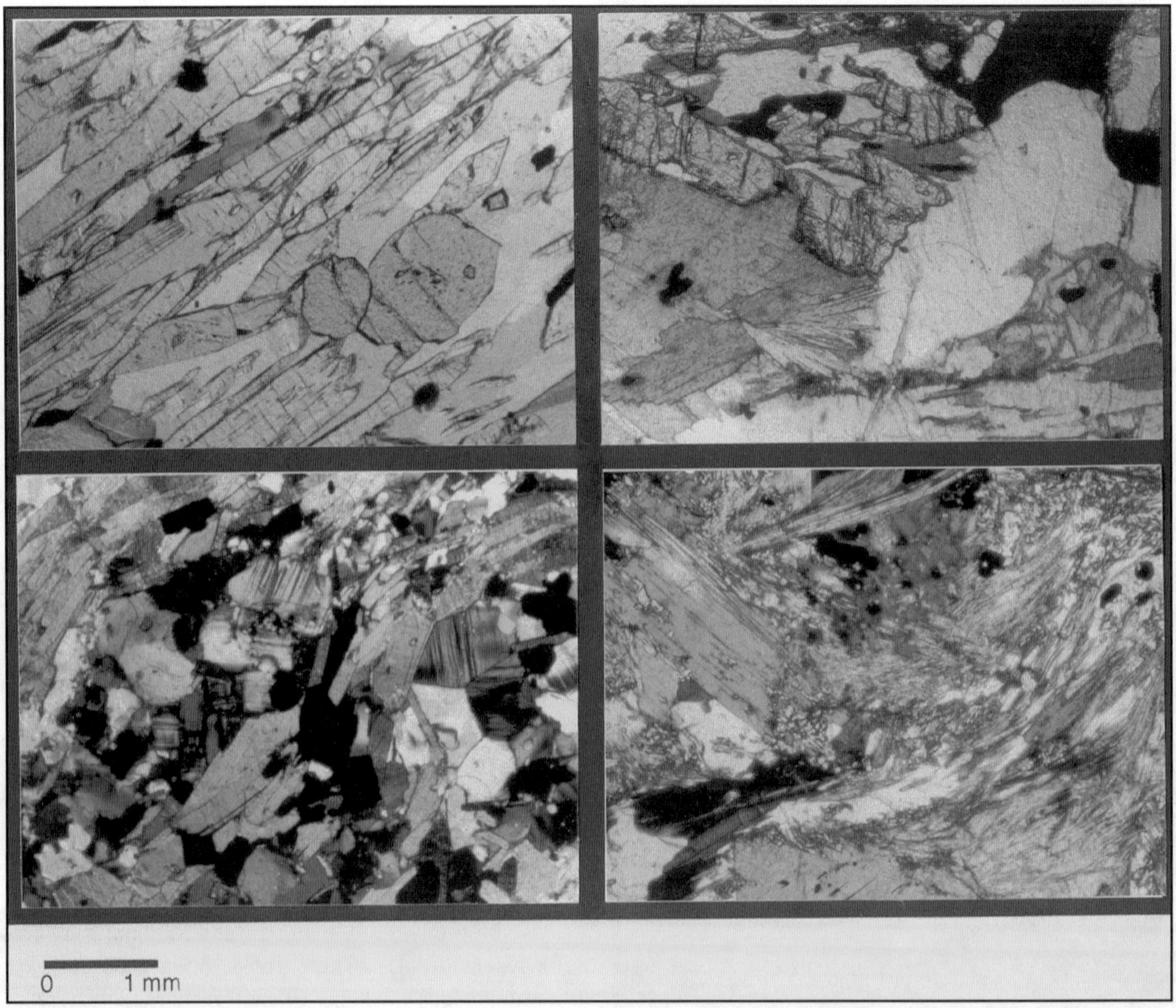

Figure 4. Photomicrographs of the Palmeirópolis deposit alteration zones. A) Anthophyllite-biotite assemblage. Tabular crystals of anthophyllite (Ath) associated with biotite (Bt) define strong foliation, idioblastic to subidioblastic garnet porphyroblasts (Grt) are common. Plane-polarized light. B) Anthophyllite-biotite assemblage. Rock composed by biotite (Bt) , cordierite (Crd), staurolite (St), quartz (Qtz) and sulphides (black). Chlorite (Chl) is retrometamorphic after biotite and cordierite is partially replaced by pinite. Note lacking of foliation. Plane-polarized light. C) Biotite-plagioclase assemblage. This rock shows poorly developed lepidogranoblastic texture and is composed by plagioclase (Pl), quartz (Qtz) and biotite (Bt). Cross-polarized light. D) Quartz-sillimanite assemblage. This rock is composed by biotite (Bt), quartz (Qtz) and sillimanite (Sil). Plane-polarized light.

staurolite porphyroblasts. Quartz, plagioclase (andesine composition), cordierite, staurolite, gahnite, hornblende, diopside, and fibrous sillimanite are commonly present. Apatite, zircon, titanite, rutile are accessory. Gahnite is always present in the sulphide-rich zones. Pyrrhotite, pyrite, sphalerite, chalcopyrite, and galena are always present. Sulphides are more abundant associated with the anthophyllite-bearing assemblages.

The alteration zone has great chemical variability in its major elements. SiO_2 content ranges from 39.7 to 87.8 wt. % and MgO from 0.34 to 16.1 wt. %. Variable CaO and alkalis, and also variable but mainly high Al_2O_3 contents are typical.

Chemically the anthophyllite-biotite rocks in the

Palmeirópolis deposit resemble the chlorite zones that underlie many non-metamorphosed VMS deposits, showing a strong depletion of alkalis and enrichment of magnesium, aluminum and ore metals. Cr, Ni and Sc contents are also high when compared with the other rocks from the alteration zones, and they are the best elements to discriminate among the different alteration zone assemblages (Araujo et al., in press).

The biotite-plagioclase assemblage is characterized by rocks having higher CaO contents than the two other assemblages at the alteration zones. Values for Cr, Ni, Co and Sc are intermediate between values for the anthophyllite-biotite and the sillimanite-quartz assemblages.

The sillimanite-quartz assemblage is characterized by high SiO_2 content, Al_2O_3 content above 6.0 wt. %, and MgO content ranging from 0.34 to 5.88 wt. %. Cr, Ni and Sc values are very low.

When compared to MORB, the three assemblages from the alteration zones are enriched in the LILEs, have lower Sr and higher Th contents. The LILEs content of the anthophyllite-biotite assemblages are compared to the content of the felsic schists. However, Zr, Hf, Sm and Yb contents are lower, and P, Cr, Ni and Sc contents are higher in the anthophyllite -biotite assemblages than in the felsic schists. The HFSEs and the REE contents of the anthophyllite-biotite assemblage resemble that of the trace element enriched amphibolite (Group II). The trace and rare earth element contents of the biotite-plagioclase assemblage and the quartz-sillimanite assemblage are in general comparable to the content of the felsic schists.

Chemically, the Palmeirópolis alteration zones show great variability. They are characteristically enriched in trace and rare earth element, and these enrichments increase from the anthophyllite-biotite through the biotite-plagioclase to the sillimanite-quartz assemblages. The alteration zones at the Palmeirópolis deposit consist of a mixed volcanic unit, comprise by mafic and felsic components, but with a strong predominance of the mafic component. High silica rocks characterize the felsic components.

Oxygen isotopic analyses were carried on samples associated with the Palmeirópolis deposit, this study allows one to evaluate the effects of the metamorphism on the oxygen isotopic signature of the alteration zone (Araujo et al., 1993; 1996b; 1996c). Amphibolite from Palmeirópolis has whole-rock $\delta^{18}O$ values between 5.6 and 7.9‰. The anthophyllite-biotite rocks have similar $\delta^{18}O$ values (5.2 to 7.9‰) and are much higher than those commonly reported for chlorite zones ($\delta^{18}O$ between 2 and 3‰) associated with other VMS deposit . No isotopic distinction was observed between the host rocks (amphibolite) and the alteration zones represented by anthophyllite-biotite assemblages. The different isotope behavior observed in the alteration zones associated with the Palmeirópolis ore bodies when compared to other similar VMS deposits may reflect the small volume of altered rocks present at Palmeirópolis. The small size of the alteration zone at Palmeirópolis, and its intimate intercalation with unaltered host rocks, favor isotopic rehomogenization by means of pervasive fluid flow during the metamorphic event (Araujo et al., 1996c).

Massive Sulphide Bodies

The massive sulphide bodies average 1 to 3 m in thickness, and have a strike length of about 120 m. However, folding and deformation clearly modified their morphology and these can not be considered their original thickness and length.

The contact of the sulphide zones with the hangingwall and the footwall rocks vary from sharp to gradational. In general, the footwall contact is more gradational than the hanging-wall, and it is marked by increase in Cu content and by the conspicuous presence of highly altered rocks (anthophyllite-biotite assemblages). The footwall assemblages are characterized by gahnite (zinc-bearing spinel) and by Zn-rich staurolite (Araujo et al., 1995).

Irregular blocks of country rocks are engulfed locally by sulphides to produce breccias. Folding and shearing, with irregular sulphide injections into wall rocks are also common along the margins of the deposit.

Mineralogy and textures in massive sulphide bodies

The C-1, C-2 and C-3 ore bodies have very similar mineralogy characterized by intimately intermixed pyrrhotite, pyrite, sphalerite, chalcopyrite and minor galena. Arsenopyrite, mackinawite, cubanite, molybdenite, ilmenite, magnetite and titanite are accessory minerals.

Pyrrhotite is the dominant matrix sulphide (Fig. 5A), occurring as a mosaic of grains characterized by triple junctions. Deformed twin lamellae are observed in pyrrhotite grains.

Sphalerite grains, characterized by strong red internal reflections, tend to developed 120 triple junctions.

Chalcopyrite is observed in two distinct textures: (a) as individual crystals and (b) as inclusions within sphalerite. The distribution of chalcopyrite inclusions may vary from randomly dispersed to crystallographically oriented rows of blebs or rods within sphalerite. Presence of inclusion-free sphalerite is also observed, in these cases the border of sphalerite crystals are marked by aligned blebs of chalcopyrite (Fig. 5B). Few crystals of chalcopyrite shows development of laths of cubanite and inclusions of mackinawite.

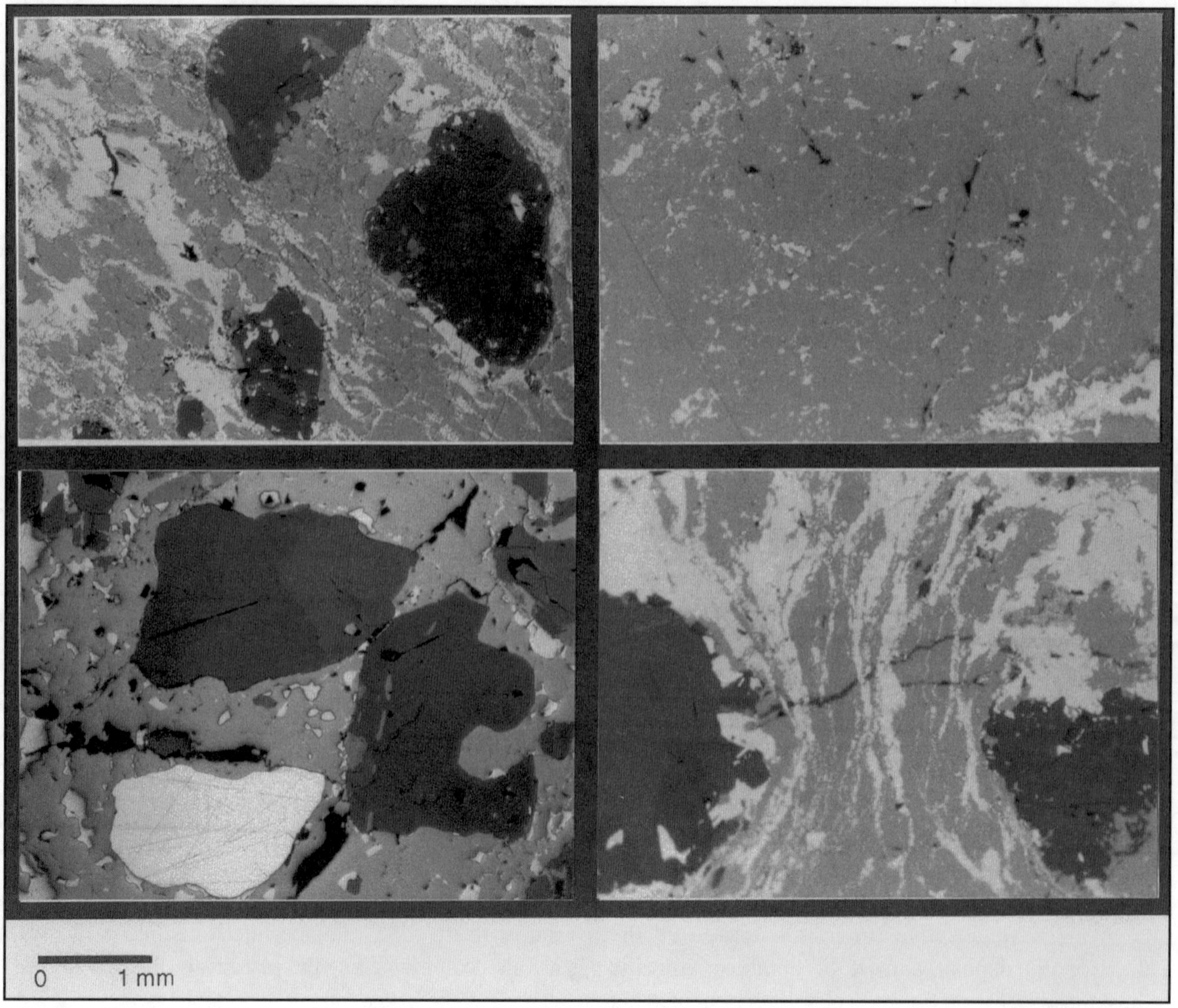

Figure 5. Photomicrographs of the Palmeirópolis ore. A) Palmeirópolis ore composed by sphalerite (sph) and pyrrhotite (po). Plane-polarized light, oil immersion. B) Aligned blebs of chalcopyrite (white) along boundaries of sphalerite grains (sph). Plane-polarized light, oil immersion. C) General aspect of the Palmeirópolis ore, rounded fragments of the host rocks within a sulphide matriz composed mainly by sphalerite (sph). Pyrrhotite (po), pyrite (py) and galena (ga) are also presented. Plane-polarized light, oil immersion. D) "Durchbewegung" texture, showing the sulphide flowage between rounded gangue fragments. Plane-polarized light, oil immersion.

Pyrite tends to recrystallize as euhedral cubic porphyroblasts. These porphyroblasts can be fractured, the fractures are usually sealed by other sulphides, such as galena.

Galena has a erratic distribution in the Palmeirópolis ore bodies. The presence of galena in the C-1 and C-2 ore bodies is constant, but subordinated, the C-3 ore body contains minor galena. Galena from the Palmeirópolis deposit displays curved cleavage traces.

The textures and structures displayed by the Palmeirópolis ore result from the dynamic deformation and heating accompanying the amphibolite facies regional metamorphism.

The C-1 and C-2 ores contain breccias in which pyrrhotite, sphalerite and minor chalcopyrite surround millimetre to centimetre scale subrounded fragments of the host rocks to produce a typical "Durchbewegung" fabric (Figs. 5C and 5D).

The massive sulphide of the C-3 ore body is homogeneous although local banding is observed. This banding is characterized by intercalations of pyrrhotite-rich layers with sphalerite- or chalcopyrite-rich layers. The contact between the banded ore and the massive ore is gradational.

CONCLUSIONS AND APPLICATIONS FOR VMS EXPLORATION AT THE PALMEIRÓPOLIS REGION

A number of small massive sulphide ore bodies occur in rocks from the lower unit of the Palmeirópolis volcano-sedimentary Sequence, Brazil. Host rocks include mainly basic metavolcanic, now amphibolites. The deposit is associated with mineralogically complex hydrothermally altered zones. The alteration zones rocks chemically display enrichment in trace and rare earth element, these enrichments increase from the anthophyllite-biotite through the biotite-plagioclase to the sillimanite-quartz assemblages. The alteration zones at the Palmeirópolis deposit consist of a mixture of mafic and felsic components, but with a strong predominance of the mafic component.

Suggestions for exploration on the Palmeirópolis region were outlined by Araujo et al. (in press) and including:

1. The main targets in the Palmeirópolis volcano sedimentary sequence are the areas close to felsic schists. These felsic bodies may have provided a heat source for the hydrothermal cell and a volatile magmatic phase that produced some of the trace element enrichment associated with the ore bodies, and indicate a hiatus during the building of the volcanic pile.

2. The Palmeirópolis region is characterized by a large volume of amphibolite. Amphibolite (Group II amphibolite) associated with the ore bodies is characteristically enriched in trace elements. An exploration program should focus on the trace element content of the amphibolite, mainly its Zr, Hf and REE content. Amphibolite with high trace element contents should indicate potential areas of mineralization within the Palmeirópolis Sequence (Araujo et al., 1996a). Modern airbone/eletromagnetic surveys may outline the contacts between groupI and group II amphibolite on a regional scale.

3. Given that the Palmeirópolis volcano-sedimentary sequence is only a small part of a major volcano-sedimentary belt, exploration programs should involve the entire belt, including the Juscelândia (Fuck et al., 1981) and Indaianópolis (Danni et al., 1982) volcano-sedimentary sequences. Considering the great similarities among the three sequences (Marini et al., 1984), the same exploration approach may be applied everywhere.

REFERENCES

Araujo, S.M., Fawcett, J.J. and Scott, S.D.. 1995. Metamorphism of hydrothermally altered rocks in a volcanogenic massive sulphide deposit: the Palmeirópolis, Brazil example.Revista Brasileira de Geociências, 25: 173-184.

Araujo, S.M., Gorton, M.P. and Scott, S.D. 1996a. Os anfibolitos enriquecidos em elementos traços da Seqüência vulcano-sedimentar de Palmeirópolis, Tocantins: uma ferramenta na prospecção de metais básicos na região. Congresso Brasileiro de Geologia, 39, Sociedade Brasileira de Geologia, Salvador, Anais , 3: 178-180.

Araujo, S.M., Longstaffe, F.J. and Scott, S.D. 1996b. Effects of the high-grade metamorphism on the oxygen isotope composition of the alteration zones associated with the Palmeirópolis volcanogenic massive sulphide deposit, Tocantins State, Brazil. Congresso Brasileiro de Geologia, 39, Sociedade Brasileira de Geologia, Salvador, Salvador, Anais , 7: 339-342.

Araujo, S.M., Longstaffe, F.J. and Scott, S.D. 1993. Oxygen isotopes and hydrothermal alteration associated with Geco, Canada and Palmeirópolis, Brazil volcanogenic massive sulphide deposits: evidence for isotopic rehomogenization during high-grade metamorphism. Geological association of Canada – Mineralogical Association of Canada Annual Meeting. Program with Abstracts, p. A3.

Araujo, S.M. and Nilson, A.A. 1988. Depósito de zinco, cobre e chumbo de Palmeirópolis, Goiás, Edited by C. Schobbenhauss and C.E.S. Coelho. Ministerio das Minas e Energia-Departamento Nacional da Producão Mineral-Companhia Vale do Rio Doce, Principais Depósitos Minerais do Brasil, v. 3, pp.171-180.

Araujo, S.M. and Nilson, A.A. 1987. Caracterização petroquímica e petrotectônica dos anfibolitos da Sequência vulcano-sedimentar de Palmeiropolis - Goiás. Congresso Brasileiro de Geoquimica, 1, Sociedade Brasileira de Geoquimica, Anais, 1: 335-348.

Araujo, S.M., Scott, S.D. and Longstaffe, F.J. 1996c. Oxygen isotope composition of alteration zones of highly metamorphosed volcanogenic massive sulphide deposits: Geco, Canada and Palmeirópolis, Brazil. Economic Geology, 91: 697-712.

Araujo, S.M. and Scott, S.D. 1991. The Palmeirópolis massive sulphide deposit, Brazil. Geological Association of Canada – Mineralogical Association of Canada. Program with Abstracts, p. A4.

Araujo, S.M., Scott, S.D. and Gorton, M.P. in press. Protoliths of highly metamorphosed, hydrothermally altered rocks of the Palmeirópolis, Brazil volcanogenic massive sulphide deposit. Journal of South America Earth Sciences.

Danni, J. C. M., Fuck, R. A. and Leonardos Jr., O. H. 1982. Archean and Lower Proterozoic Units in Central Brazil. Geol. Rundschau, 71: 291-317.

Drago, V.A.; Pinto, A. do C.; Montalvão, R.M.G. de; Santos, R.O.B. dos; Simões, M.A.; Oliveira, F.C.; Bezerra, P.E.L.; Prado, P.; Fernandes, C.A.C. and Tassinari, C.C.G. 1981. Geologia, in: Projeto RADAMBRASIL. Folha SD.22 Goiás. Rio de Janeiro, p. 27-300.

Figueiredo, J.A.; Leão Neto, R. and Valente, C.R. 1981. Depósitos de sulfetos maciços de Zn, Cu e Pb da região de Palmeirópolis, GO. Simposio de Geologia do Centro Oeste, 1. Ata, Goiânia, Sociedade Brasileira de Geologia - Núcleos Centro-Oeste and Brasília, p. 422-441.

Franklin, J. M., Sangster, D. M., and Lydon, J. W. 1981. Volcanic associated massive sulphide deposits. Economic Geology 75th Anniversary Volume, p. 485-627.

Fuck, R. A., Danni, J. C. M., Winge, M., Andrade, G. F. de, Barreira, C. F., Leonardos, O. H., and Kuyumjian, R. M. 1981. Geologia da região de Goianésia. Simposio de Geologia do Centro Oeste, 1. Ata, Goiânia, Sociedade Brasileira de Geologia - Núcleos Centro-Oeste and Brasília, p. 447-467.

Fuck, R.A.; Pimentel, M.M. and Botelho, N.F. 1987. Granitoid rocks in west-central Brazil: a review. International Symposium on granites and associated mineralizations, Anais, Salvador, SGRM – Sociedade Brasileira de Geologia, p. 53-59.

Girardi, V.A.V.; Kawashita, K.; Basei, M.A.S. and Cordani, U.G. 1978. Algumas considerações sobre a evolução geológica da região de Cana Brava, a partir de dados geocronológicos. Congresso Brasileiro de Geologia, 30, Sociedade Brasileira de Geologia, Recife, Anais , 1: 337-348.

Lydon, J. W. 1984. Volcanogenic massive sulphide deposits, part I: a descriptive model. Geoscience Canada, 11: 195-202.

Lydon, J. W. 1988. Volcanogenic massive sulphide deposits, part II: genetic models. Geoscience Canada, 15: 43-65.

Marini, O.J.; Fuck, R.A.; Danni, J.C.M.; Dardenne, M.A.; Loguercio, S.O.C. and Ramalho, R. 1984. As faixas de dobramentos Brasília, Uruaçu e Paraguai-Araguaia e o Maciço Mediano de Goiás. Coordinator by C. Schobbenhauss. Ministerio das Minas e Energia – Departamento Nacional da Producão Mineral, Geologia do Brasil, pp. 251-303.

THE POTENTIAL FOR VOLCANOGENIC MASSIVE SULPHIDE DEPOSITS IN THE MAGMATIC-ARC-RELATED VOLCANO-SEDIMENTARY BELTS IN AND AROUND THE SÃO FRANCISCO CRATON, BRAZIL

LYDIA MARIA LOBATO

Departamento de Geologia, IGC, Universidade Federal de Minas Gerais, Av. Antônio Carlos 6627, Pampulha, Belo Horizonte, Brazil, 31270.901, lobato@igc.ufmg.br

FRANCISCUS JACOBUS BAARS

Department of Geological Sciences, University of Cape Town; Roots Rock Ltda., Av. Afonso Pena 4343/402, Mangabeiras, Belo Horizonte, Brazil, 30130.008, baarsf@rootsrock.com.br

HARDY JOST

Instituto de Geociências, Universidade de Brasília, Cx. Postal 04465, Campus Universitário, Brasília, Brazil, 70910.900, hjost@tba.com.br

MARIA DA GLÓRIA DA SILVA

Departamento de Geologia, Universidade Federal da Bahia, Rua Caetano Moura 123, Federação, Salvador, Brazil, gloria@ufba.br

JOSÉ CARLOS CUNHA

Companhia Baiana de Pesquisa Mineral, Quarta Avenida 460, Centro Administrativo, Salvador, Brazil, 41745.000, zecunha@cpbm.com.br

SEBASTIÃO GOMES CARVALHO

IGCE, Universidade Estadual de São Paulo, Rua 10 2527, Rio Claro, São Paulo, Brazil, 13500.230, carvalho@rc.unesp.br

ABSTRACT

Few volcanic massive sulphide (VMS) deposits have been discovered in Brazil, despite exploration campaigns during the late 1970's and 1980's, which focussed on mafic-ultramafic, greenstone belt (GB)-type targets. In the light of significant advances in the characterisation of Brazilian geology since then, this article analyses the potential for VMS mineralization in GBs and metavolcano-sedimentary sequences in and around the São Francisco Craton.

For the purpose of this review, a tectonic classification system for VMS deposits is used. It embodies five VMS types, which are dominated by intra-oceanic, oceanic-arc volcanic rocks (Types 1, 3 and 4) and by epi-continental, ocean-continent, continental-margin arc predominantly sedimentary associations (Types 2 and 5). A five-fold classification based on host rock composition closely mirrors the former classification in most aspects. The classification schemes are integrated, suggesting that it is the most appropriate and practical for elaborate analyses of both occurrences and tectono-stratigraphic provinces.

The present analysis of VMS potential adopts a very generic definition for GBs, taking into account all metavolcano-sedimentary sequences that contain evidence for their origin in intra-oceanic or epi-continental back-arc environments and the tectono-stratigraphically associated arc settings. The partial preservation of these rock sequences, within and at the margins of the present-day São Francisco Craton, occurred during collisional tectonic events. Although some of the critical data are available for the São Francisco Craton GBs in the states of Minas Gerais, Goiás, Tocantins, Bahia and Sergipe, adequate, peer review of some of the data is lacking in some cases, which hampers the estimation of their potential for hosting VMS deposits.

The Archean GBs encompass Crixás, Pilar de Goiás, Guarinos, Goiás, Faina, Rio das Velhas, Piumhi, Morro do Ferro, Cuieté Velho, Contendas-Mirante, Tremedal, Mundo Novo, Jacobina, Umburunas, Ibitira-Ubiraçaba, Brumado, Bate-Pé, Guajeru, Licínio de Almeida, Urandi, Riacho da Santana, Boquira Belt, Ibiajara, Paramirim and other small volcano-sedimentary tracts. In the Palaeoproterozoic, the Rio Itapicuru, Rio Capim, Rio Salitre, Barreiro, Colomi, Casa Nova, Almas-Dianópolis, Porto Alegre, Pindorama, Conceição do Tocantins, Mossâmedes, Rio do Peixe, Silvânia, Araí, Dom Silvério greenstone belts are focused. The Mesoproterozoic is represented by the Palmeirópolis, Indaianópolis and Juscelândia volcano-sedimentary belts, and the Neoproterozoic by the Salinas and the Goiás Magmatic Arc belts (Bom Jardim de Goiás, Arenópolis, Iporá-Amorinópolis, Jaupací, Mara Rosa, Chapada and Santa Terezinha). Volcano-sedimentary belts of unknown age embody Riacho dos Machados, Rio Paraúna, Serro - Alvorada de Minas, Pedro Pereira and others.

The identified VMS deposits and showings are concentrated in Archean, Meso- and Neoproterozoic sequences. The ten most important are the Mundo Novo Prospect, Mundo Novo (Bahia State); Ribeirão da Folha, Salinas Formation; Salobro, Riacho dos Machados Group; Cuieté Velho, Cuieté Velho Sequence; Bico de Pedra, Rio das Velhas GB (Quadrilátero Ferrífero); Alpinópolis, Alpinópolis Sequence (all five in Minas Gerais State); Bom Jardim de Goiás, Bom Jardim de Goiás Sequence; Zacarias, Mara Rosa Sequence; Palmeirópolis, Palmeirópolis Sequence; Mina III, Crixás (all four in the State of Goiás). Controversy does exist regarding the volcanogenic nature of some the above deposits.

The Salobro Deposit is mineralised in a sequence of unknown, Precambrian age. The early Meso- and Late-Neoproterozoic sequences also contain abundant evidence of the presence of local heat sources, relevant primary igneous textures, and some of the requisite hydrothermal alteration features. Significantly, the volcano-sedimentary successions are similar to many Phanerozoic VMS-hosting sequences, embodying a variety of nascent rift, back-arc and arc systems in intra-oceanic and especially epi-continental palaeo-environments.

The Archean sequences of Goiás also contain very well preserved sequences with a strong VMS potential. The Rio das Velhas, and Morro do Ferro GBs are, in contrast, pervasively deformed, obliterating much primary evidence of the origin of its volcano-sedimentary sequence. The Archean sequences of Bahia State appear to preserve many primary volcano-sedimentary textures, suggesting a greater potential for economic VMS-grade and -geometry preservation.

In the case of the Archean and Palaeoproterozoic of Bahia State, recent exploration advances demand evaluation for investment prioritisation. The compilation of a whole range of geological and geophysical data, from the different volcano-sedimentary sequences of central and northern São Francisco Craton, confirm, in most cases, the presence of metabasalts and sedimentary rocks. Both of the latter rock sequences commonly reveal an ocean-floor affiliation, an important indicator of the metallogenetic potential for VMS ore deposits. Amongst these, the Mundo Novo, Umburunas, Rio Itapicuru, Rio Salitre and Riacho de Santana GBs stand out as particularly favourable cases.

In other sequences of Bahia, characterised as intra- or epi-continental (Boquira, Licínio de Almeida-Urandi GBs) and even rift-type (Contendas-Mirante) basins, the existence of an oceanic, volcanic substratum is not unequivocally registered in the geochemical fingerprints of the metavolcano-sedimentary rocks. There too, the presence of metacherts, Mn-rich and carbonate metasedimentary rocks and BIFs, amongst others, is conspicuous, suggesting that critical processes of chemical and/or hydrothermal precipitation may have acted. The significance of these rocks should be investigated, case-by-case, in order to distinguish between volcanogenic-exhalative potential (polymetallic, Zn-rich, Type-5 VMS deposits) and sedimentary-rock-exhalative potential (large volume, Au-Cu-poor, polymetallic SEDEX deposits).

In general, the potential for bimodal, mafic-dominated (Type 1), ophiolitic (Type 3) and, perhaps, Besshi (Type 4) VMS deposits is greatest in the Archean GBs (Goiás and Quadrilátero Ferrífero GBs, as well as the Bahia Archean GBs). Significant potential also exists for the bimodal, felsic-dominated (Type 2) VMS deposits in the intermediate and upper sections of those GBs and of the Palaeoproterozoic sequences (including Riacho dos Machados and the numerous Palaeoproterozoic Bahia GBs). The potential for bimodal, siliciclastic (Type 5) VMS deposits in the Archean of Goiás is relatively high, given the importance of sedimentary-rock-dominated, volcano-sedimentary intercalations there. The same may be true for some of the Archean, sedimentary-rock-dominated GBs of Bahia, particularly in the western Gavião Block, the Guanambi-Corretina Block and the Sobradinho Domain.

Beyond the demonstrable Archean potential for VMS deposits, perhaps the most important preliminary conclusion of this contribution is the strong potential for VMS deposits, particularly Types 5 and 2, in the Meso- and Neoproterozoic sequences, borne out by the predominance of many occurrences there. While both Types 3 and 4 VMS deposits appear to occur in the restricted, yet diagnostic, exposures of intra-oceanic rocks, these sequences are overwhelmingly metasedimentary in nature. This leads to two specific problems for the realisation and correct evaluation of this postulated tendency. First, traditional, Precambrian GB-based exploration efforts in Brazil have focussed exclusively on the metavolcanic sequences, in particular in mafic and ultramafic rocks. The present analysis shows this prejudice to be unfounded under the given geological circumstances and the empirical criteria taken from a world-wide database. Second, both the Archean and Proterozoic sequences are generally metamorphosed under all facies conditions, from anchimetamorphic to granulitic. The recognition of, in particular, aluminous and ferromagnesian mineral assemblages and their distinction as either regionally metamorphic or metamorphosed hydrothermal is critical. Both weathering decomposition and the preferred, often precipitated, attribution of an exclusively regionally metamorphic origin to minerals like the alumino-silicate polymorphs, garnet, cordierite and biotite, can seriously hamper field observation.

This problem is illustrated in the case of the Mateus Leme – Pitangui Belt, Rio das Velhas GB, and of the Salinas Group, at São José da Safira. In more felsic-volcanic areas (Type 2, and possibly Type 5 VMS deposits), and particularly in deposits which formed at volcaniclastic-dominant, shallow seawater depths (< ~1500 m), Na depletion and aluminous assemblages (kaolinite, andalusite, kyanite, pyrophyllite, diaspore, chloritoid, corundum) characterise much of the paraconformable hydrothermal alteration associated with these deposits.

In the light of these data, emphasis should be placed on the appropriate characterisation of the potential of Archean and Proterozoic sequences in terms of necessary, VMS-controlling factors. Much, semi-detailed and regional mapping is required, together with urgent sequence stratigraphy and sufficient geochemical fingerprinting. Appropriate definition of existing occurrence types is lacking, and will surely assist objectively in the search for other, economically important VMS deposits.

INTRODUCTION

Volcanogenic massive sulphide (VMS) deposits occur in submarine volcanic rocks of all ages, from the presently forming deposits in modern spreading-ridge, arc and back-arc environments, to deposits in the pre-3.4 Ga volcanic strata of the Pilbara Block in Australia. They are massive (over 60 % sulphide), lenticular accumulations on or near the sea floor in association with volcanic activity. They occur in a wide variety of tectonic regimes and almost all have a close association with at least minor amounts of sedimentary rock. They are a major source of copper, zinc, lead, silver and gold (Franklin et al. 1998).

A number of Archean greenstone belts (GBs) are host to VMS, Cu-Zn ± Pb deposits, which notably also contain subordinate quantities of Au and Ag. A major VMS province occurs in the Superior Province, Canada, and particularly the Abitibi Belt. Important VMS deposits are also known in the Slave Province (see review by Herrington et al. 1997), almost all considered to form a Cu-Zn group. Less important deposits are recorded in many Archean GBs elsewhere in the world (e.g. Canada, Australia, Southern Africa, South America, and China), the paucity of discovered deposits in other Archean terrains being partly a function of exploration effort. Australian examples are reviewed by Barley (1992), with deposits in the Pilbara Craton embodying a small Zn-Pb-Cu group. Franklin et al. (1998) reclassify disparate VMS types into a unified, geotectonic system, which is the basis for the present analysis. Most recently, Barrie & Hannington (1999b) edited a thorough review of VMS deposits and deposit-forming processes.

Few VMS deposits have been discovered in Brazil, despite exploration campaigns during the late

1970's and the 1980's, which focussed on mafic-ultramafic, GB-type targets. In the light of significant advances in the characterisation of Brazilian geology since then, this article analyses the potential for VMS mineralization in GBs and metavolcano-sedimentary sequences in and around the São Francisco Craton. We adopt a very generic definition for GBs, implicit in the compilation presented by de Wit & Ashwal (1997). We refer to all metavolcano-sedimentary sequences that contain evidence for their origin in intra-oceanic or epi-continental back-arc environments and the tectono-stratigraphically associated arc settings.

The foundation for this analysis of the potential for VMS deposits in and around the São Francisco Craton lies in a review description of the critical, genetic characteristics necessary for the their formation and preservation. The available data from the various identified volcano-sedimentary sequences in and around the Craton are compared with this empirical set of criteria in order to establish relative probabilities for VMS occurrences. Thereby, a dynamic system of target valuation is created that can be modified with the discovery of new, critical data.

THE FORMATION OF VMS DEPOSITS

Characteristics and associations

Type examples of GB-hosted VMS deposits occur in the Superior Province. They comprise clusters or "camps" commonly with one or more large or giant deposits in association with numerous smaller deposits. The deposits tend to be associated with specific volcano-stratigraphic horizons marked by felsic volcanism, which are commonly boundaries between contrasting rock types (e.g. andesite and rhyolite) (Lydon 1988, Sawkins 1990, Groves & Barley 1994, Franklin et al. 1998). Orebodies tend to occur at stratigraphic levels where the presence of tuff and chert layers indicates a break in the volcanic activity. Most economic deposits contain in the range of 1 to 10 Mt of ore, with a few in the range 10 to 50 Mt. Typical grades are >1 % Cu and >3 % Zn. Rare examples are larger. The largest is the Kidd Creek Deposit containing 130 Mt ore at 2.7 % Cu and 6.5 % Zn, and lesser Pb at 1.9 % and 16 g/t Ag.

An idealised deposit (Franklin et al. 1998) comprises a lenticular or pod-like body containing more than 60 % massive sulphides, and zoned from a sphalerite, pyrite and/or galena-rich top to a pyrite- and chalcopyrite-rich base. Sedimentary chert or "exhalites" may occur along strike from the massive sulphide bodies. Commonly, a discordant, hydrothermal alteration zone gradationally underlies the massive or near-massive sulphides. This contains chlorite ± quartz ± sericite ± carbonate, as well as chalcopyrite-pyrite stringer mineralization, together interpreted as the zone of fluid discharge. Regionally extensive, semi-conformable alteration zones may be present below the ore zone. At low metamorphic grades, alteration assemblages include sericite-quartz-calcite/dolomite, whereas those at some depth below Noranda-type deposits reflect silicification and spilitisation.

Most of the VMS camps are associated with bimodal volcanic assemblages of submarine, intermediate to felsic flows and pyroclastic rocks, interpreted to represent stratovolcanoes, central volcanic complexes, or large composite cones. Many authors stress a caldera setting, cauldron subsidence and resurgence, and localisation of volcanic vents and alteration pipes along synvolcanic faults. Fewer deposits are associated with komatiite-tholeiite assemblages consisting of various combinations of komatiites, tholeiitic basalts, icelandite, FIII-type rhyolites and calc-alkaline andesite and rhyolite. However, the Kidd Creek Deposit occurs in this latter association.

Such volcanic rocks are believed to have erupted from high-level, subvolcanic, zoned basic-felsic magma chambers that may be represented by the subvolcanic intrusions, which commonly occur one to several kilometres stratigraphically below the VMS deposits. These intrusions are interpreted to be heat, and possibly metal, sources ("heaters") for the VMS deposits, driving convective hydrothermal activity and mineralization (Franklin et al. 1998).

Many of the VMS clusters are associated with felsic volcanic rocks of distinctive trace-element geochemical composition, the so-called FIII-type volcanic rocks of Lesher et al. (1986). Kerrich & Wyman (1997) present a thorough review of the trace-element characterisation of potential VMS-hosting volcano-stratigraphic settings, on the basis of the studies by Campbell et al. (1981, 1982) and Barrie et al. (1993)

at Abitibi & Kuroko, Lesher et al. (1986) in the Superior Province, and Pearce (1996).

The felsic volcanic rocks that host VMS deposits characteristically display flat rare-earth-element-patterns, moderate to pronounced Eu anomalies, low to intermediate La/Yb ratios (0.8 to 9.0) and variable high-field-strength-element (HFSE) contents. Typically, the VMS-hosting volcanic sequences are characterised as having their origin in oceanic rifts, rifted island arcs or calc-alkalic arcs. Continental and alkalic arc settings are concluded to be associated with barren sequences. These geochemical sampling techniques apply to the entire or part of the volcanic sequence. For exploration it is not necessary to sample only the specific, volumetrically insignificant, felsic centres of volcanism that generally host VMS deposits.

Some authors (e.g. Gaskarth & Parslow 1987, Vivallo & Claesson 1987) have generically associated the occurrence of VMS deposits in Proterozoic volcano-sedimentary sequences with the tholeiitic to calc-alkaline transition in the paleo-arc evolution. In an attempt to predict the existence of VMS deposits in often poorly characterised GBs, this generic association may be the best available approximation to volcanic evolution. It may critically direct research and exploration efforts and regional targeting before the more elaborate, trace-element-fingerprinting techniques.

Classification

VMS deposits have been classified on the basis of their composition (e.g. Cu-Zn-Pb triangle, Franklin et al. 1981; Au rich deposits, Poulsen & Hannington 1995), geological setting (e.g. tectonic regime, Barrie & Hannington 1999a) or host rock composition (e.g. Divi et al. 1979). About 80 % of the world's VMS deposits are in arc-related strata, with the remaining 20 % in mid-ocean ridge ophiolitic settings. Some of the latter are rifted marginal basins and others are in preserved mid-ocean ridges.

Franklin et al. (1998) present a tectonic classification system, embodying three types (1, 3 and 4) dominated by volcanic rocks (intra oceanic, oceanic arc) and two (2 and 5) with a significant sedimentary association (epi-continental, ocean-continent, continental-margin arc; Figure 1). A five-fold classification by Barrie & Hannington (1999a), based on host rock composition, closely mirrors that of Franklin et al. (1998) in most aspects. It presents the notion of VMS-deposit classification in a very practical format, in that host-rock lithological packages are used to classify the deposits. It may be considered to be easier to apply, particularly to ancient environments, since it requires only an evaluation of the host lithological package and not of the tectonic environment of rock formation as such. We present the classification schemes in an integrated manner below, suggesting that it is the most appropriate and practical for elaborate analyses of both occurrences and tectono-stratigraphic provinces, as in the present analysis.

Type-1 or bimodal-mafic-type deposits form in arcs above ocean-floor-dominated subduction. They constitute the volcanic, bimodal group, whose stratigraphical pile is basalt-dominated (well over 50 %), with a lesser felsic component (<25 %) resulting in a mafic/felsic ratio of 3:1. The mafic rocks are tholeiitic and locally calc-alkaline, and the felsic rocks have a high SiO_2-content in calc-alkaline rhyolites, suites that are produced through the melting of oceanic crust. Siliciclastic rocks are confined to a few intraflow clastic units, and to proximal epiclastic rocks. Pyroclastic strata are subordinate. Pillow basalts, felsic flows and flow domes are prominent. These deposits are the richest Cu-bearing types and are the most common of all VMS-types, typically known to occur in Late Archean to Palaeoproterozoic GBs, although younger deposits do occur.

Type-2 or bimodal-felsic-type deposits are related to ocean-continent subduction. They are dominated by felsic volcanic rocks (generally 50 to 70 %), comprising calc-alkaline to high-SiO_2 rhyolites. Siliciclastic rocks constitute some 15 % of the host-rock pile, more abundant than in the bimodal-mafic group. Submarine pyroclastic strata dominate. The remaining rocks are calc-alkaline or tholeiite to calc-alkaline mafic rocks, generally andesitic in composition with moderate vesicularity. Hyaloclastite is common. Rocks are both intrusive and volcanic. The Kuroko Deposit is the best-known example of this second most-numerous group, which accounts for the largest volumes of Zn and Ag. While ages are in general similar to those of the bimodal-mafic group, these are most abundant in Phanerozoic systems.

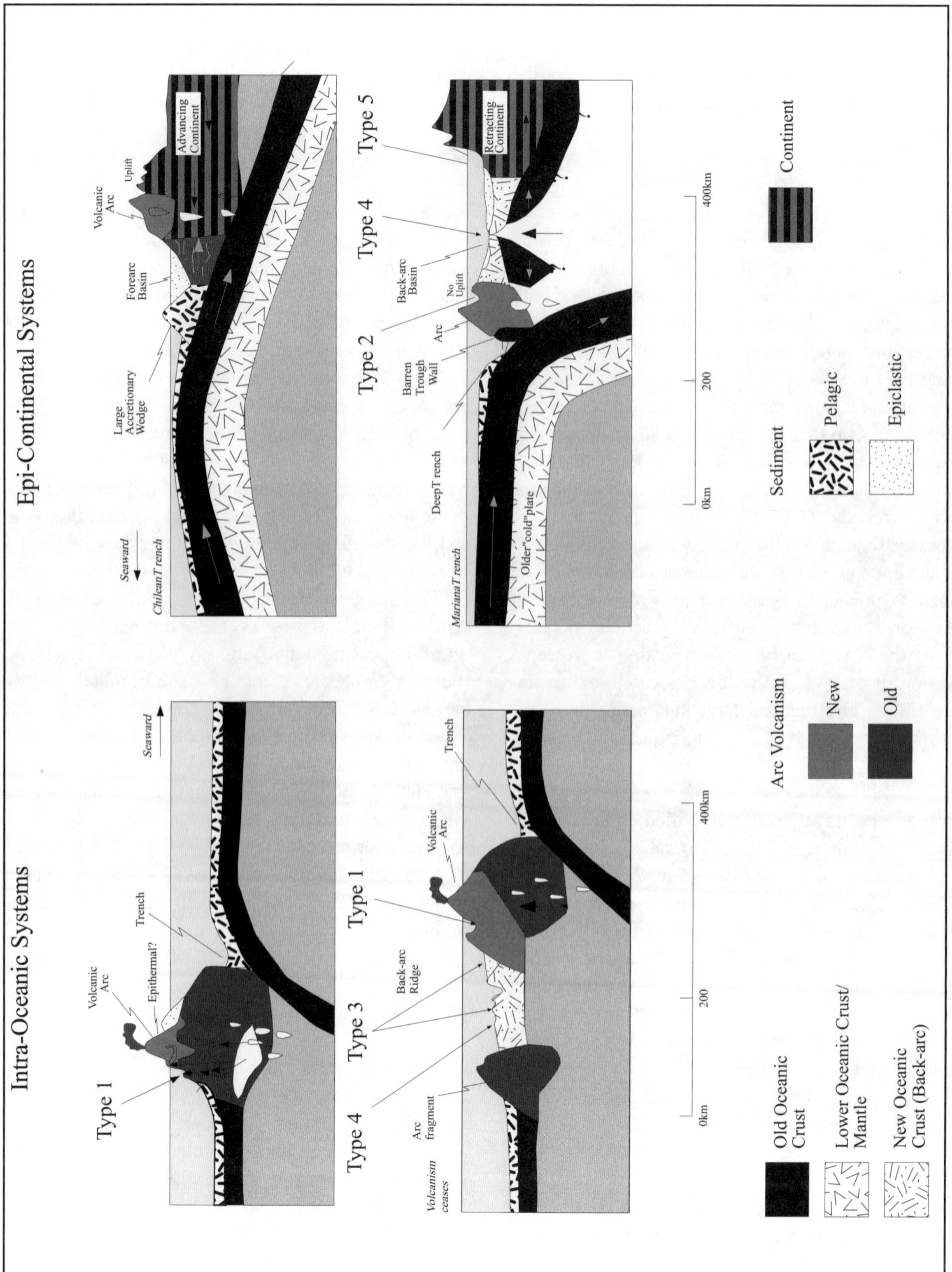

Figure 1. Tectonic distribution of VMS types

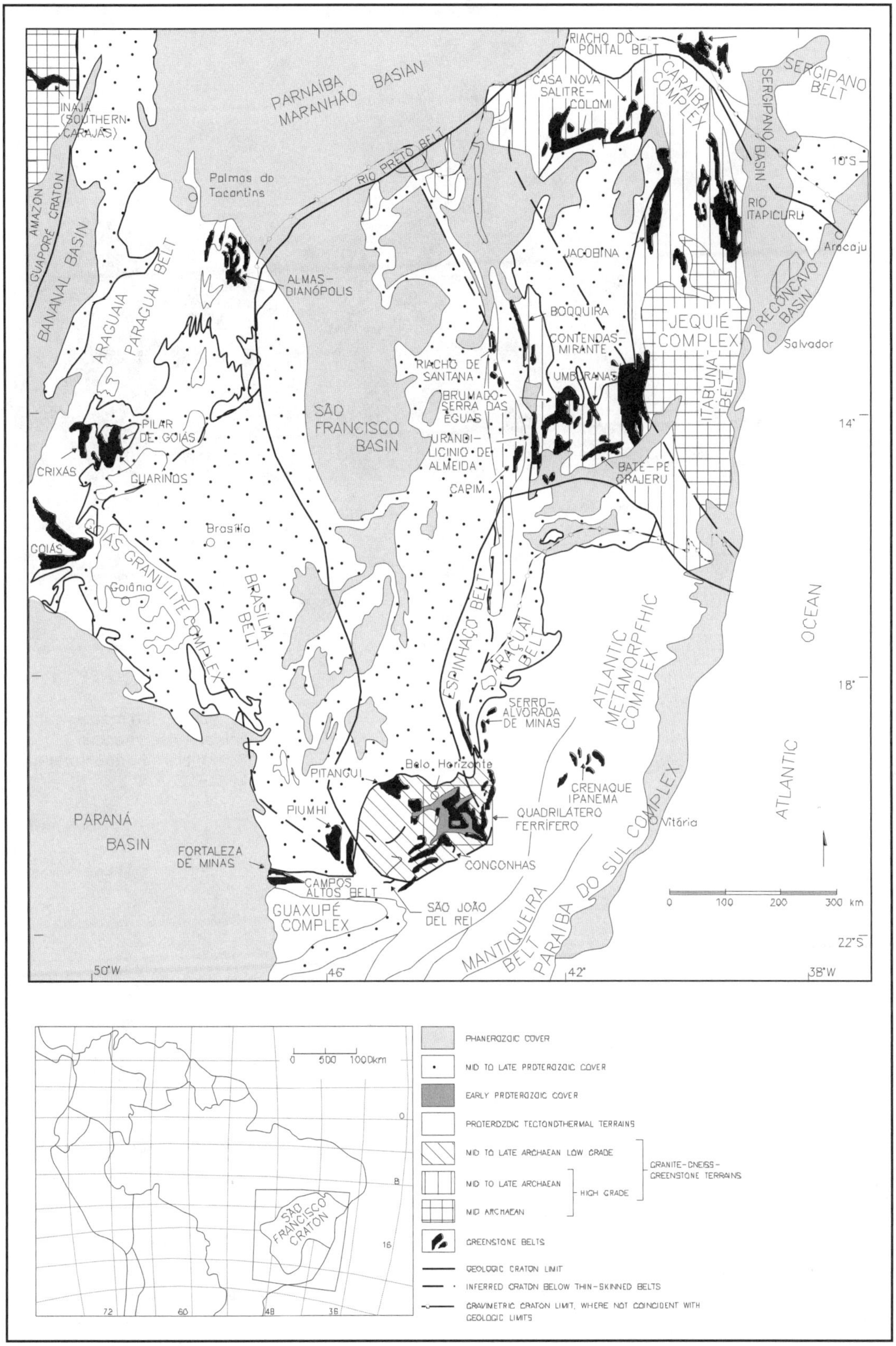

Figure 2. Geological map of the Sao Francisco Craton and its greenstone belts.

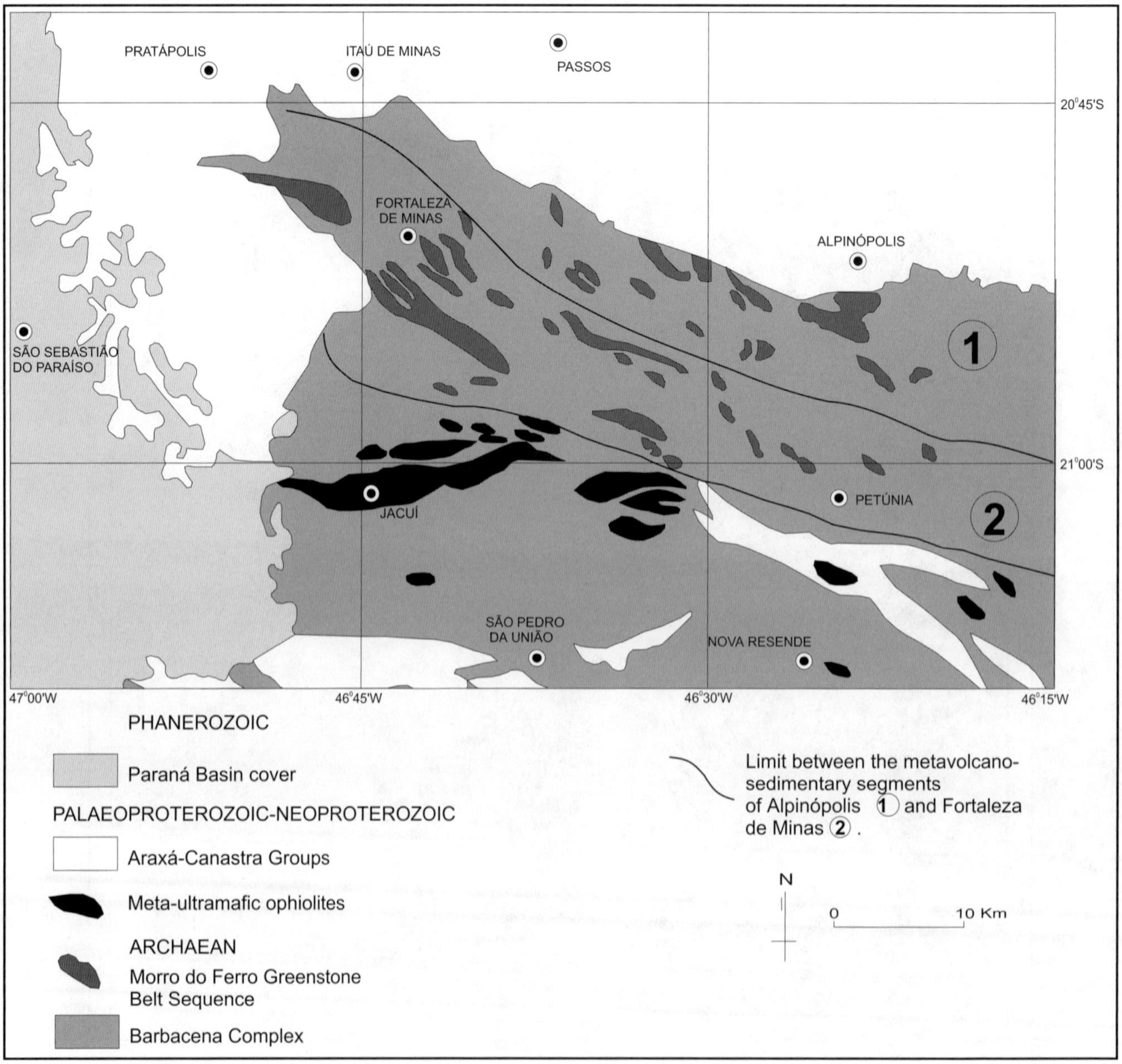

Figure 3. Simplified geological map showing the distribution of the granite-greenstone terranes at the southwest of Minas Gerais State. Modified after Carvalho et al. 1999.

Type-3 or mafic-type deposits are hosted in volcanic ophiolitic sequences, strongly dominated by tholeiites and local boninites (>75 %), with rare or absent felsic volcanic rocks. Host piles have less than 10 % siliciclastic or ultramafic rocks. The deposits most commonly originate at a mid-ocean-ridge, but also form above intra-oceanic subduction zones and at back-arc spreading ridges. The richest in Cu and the poorest in Pb, they are amongst the least abundant of the VMS types. They typically occur in Phanerozoic ophiolites, with a few, giant deposits in the Late Archean (e.g. Kidd-Munro Deposits, Abitibi Subprovince) and the Palaeoproterozoic (e.g. Amiss Group Deposits, Saskatchewan).

Type-4 or mafic-siliciclastic-type deposits occur in basalt-sediment, back-arc sequences with near-equal

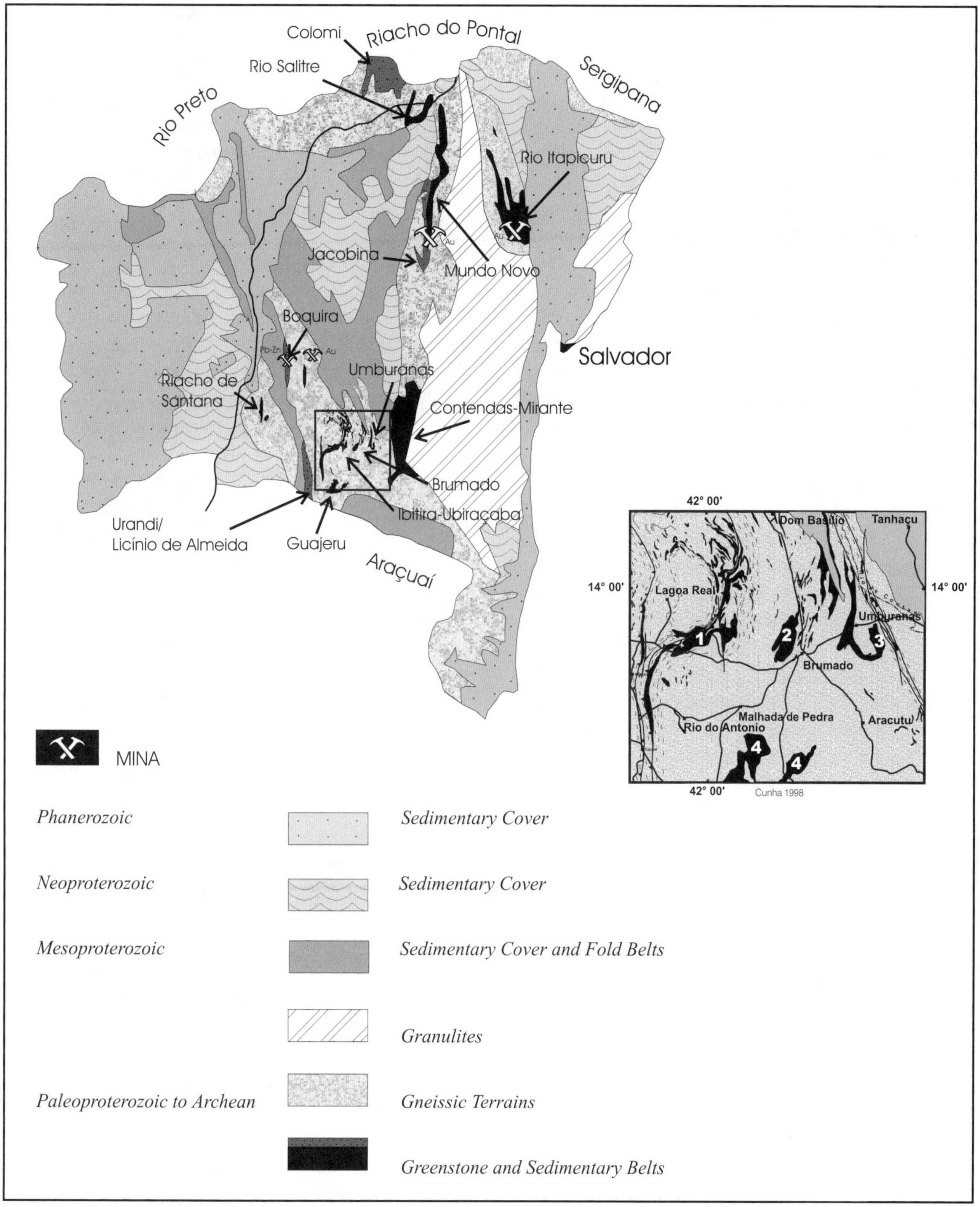

Figure. 4: Geological map of the northeastern São Francisco Craton with the distribution of greenstone belts after da Silva and Cunha (1998)

proportions of mafic volcanic or intrusive rocks and turbiditic siliciclastic sedimentary rocks that may be carbonate bearing. In the Japanese-type examples, deep-water pelites, wackes and subordinate quartzites predominate. Felsic volcanic rocks are rare or absent. These deposits are typically Mesoproterozoic or younger, and are commonly complexely deformed. The Besshi deposits of Japan and the Windy Craggy deposit of British Columbia are examples. They represent the least abundant of all VMS types.

Type 5 or bimodal-siliciclastic-type deposits occur in mature, epi-continental arcs and back-arcs, containing near-equal proportions of mainly felsic volcanic and siliciclastic strata. Felsic volcanic rocks are calc-alkaline while mafic volcanic rocks are tholeiitic and locally alkaline. Hangingwall basalt is absent or minor. Sedimentary and epiclastic rocks comprise up to 80 % of the sequence. Examples are Bathurst (New Brunswick) and the Iberian Pyrite Belt (Portugal), typifying the Phanerozoic host sequences of the deposit group. These deposits have the greatest tonnages, the largest deposit sizes, the lowest Cu contents and the highest Pb contents of all VMS types.

Thirty-four percent of VMS deposits world-wide are Paleozoic. Archean and Proterozoic deposits equally share 29 % of total metal content and together constitute 40 % of all deposits. The median deposit size of each arc-, Besshi- and ophiolite-type, is about 1-1.5 Mt. Type-5 deposits are much larger, on average 4 Mt. lead content is anomalously high in felsic settings. Metal distribution in Phanerozoic mafic volcanic Types 1, 3 and 4 reflects that of MORB. Type-5 metal proportions reflect that of continental crust, although their Ag/Au ratios are usually high. Type-2 deposits are richer in Au, compared with Ag, particularly in the Proterozoic belts.

Criteria: critical elements of a convective system

The body of evidence over the years supports a generalised, convective, hydrothermal model (Franklin et al. 1998). The nine principal elements of such a system are: (i) heat energy: sub-volcanic intrusion; (ii) metal sources; (iii) high temperature reaction zone: convective system; (iv) magmatic source; (v) insulating cap; (vi) fluid conduit; (vii) near surface interaction zone: alteration pipes; (viii) vent sites: depositional mounds; (ix) "distal" fallout and hydrothermal plumes. For mineral exploration, the two most important characteristics are the large-scale, lower, semi-conformable alteration zones, and the palaeo-heat source. These attributes are subtle, requiring careful mapping and petrographic analysis, along with judicious use of analytical and isotopic data to elucidate the petrochemical sequence.

Heat energy

VMS metals precipitate from acid hydrothermal solutions. Low pH is maintained by convective pumping and/or seafloor-fluid temperatures above 375ºC. High geothermal gradient or focussed, intrusive system heat source is required. Types 1 and 3 deposits have well documented sub-volcanic intrusions, as at Noranda. These are up to 60 km^2, multiple intrusions, with no contact aureole. Disseminated, porphyry-like copper sulphides and miarolitic cavities are common. Felsic intrusions are common, though a layered gabbro underlies Matagami. Intrusions associated with Type-2 deposits are similar to those of Type 1. The role of intrusions at Type 3, ophiolite deposits, is unclear, as with Type 4 deposits. Mafic sills may be important. synvolcanic intrusions within sequences of Type 5 deposits are poorly documented.

Igneous petrochemistry

There is a fragile relationship between magma type and the abundance or composition of deposits. Sub-volcanic intrusions and related volcanic rocks have aberrant petrochemical trends, caused by unusually rapid heat removal to the hydrothermal system, assimilation of hydrated country rock, or interaction with seawater. Extensive fractionation may be evident in both major element and REE trends. (i) For Types 1, 2 and 3 sodic dacite and rhyolite dominate the felsic melts. (ii) In Type 5, and possibly 2, more K-rich, continent-derived melts may be evident. These are more volatile-rich and their fluids may resemble epithermal, high-sulphidation fluids. (iii) Type 4 deposits include MORB, but alkalic and within-plate basalt compositions are present as well. (iv) Type 3 deposits are typical in modified, alkalic E-MORB, with LREE- and LLE-enriched, back-arc compositions. Differentiated plagiogranites may occur. (v)

Basalts of Types 1 and 2 are related to nascent-rifted arcs, and Types 3 and 4 to mature back-arcs. (vi) Archean through Cenozoic mafic sequences are LREE-enriched and display Eu negative anomalies, by plagioclase removal or hydrothermal alteration.

Semi-conformable hydrothermal alteration

In basalt-dominated areas (Types 1, 3 and 4), the lower semi-conformable alteration assemblage is albite-epidote-actinolite-quartz. The uppermost alteration of Type 1 deposits is Na-depleted and proximally pervasive. The lower alteration zones are metal-depleted, particularly Cu. Silicification and epidotisation, with loss of Ca and addition of Na (as albite), dominate. Type 3 alteration is similar. In shallow levels at Cyprus, adularia and smectite occur.

Type 2, and possibly 5, alteration displays laterally extensive carbonate alteration (proximal siderite) immediately subjacent to the deposits. Organic-rich strata may occur. Na depletion and Al-rich assemblages (andalusite) dominate. The alteration style resembles that associated with high-sulphidation epithermal deposits. Alternatively, Type-2 alteration is characterised, from top to bottom, by quartz-microcline-biotite through chlorite-quartz-albite to quartz-albite-chlorite-epidote. This is similar to that of older, mafic-dominated systems, where celadonite and K-micas are more common and K-feldspar less so. Type 4 alteration is poorly documented.

The literature is abundant with descriptions of the other, non-critical elements of convective systems, such as discharge-zone alteration. This is beyond the scope of this critical analysis.

Age relationships

The database of Franklin et al. (1998) shows that VMS deposits are by far the most abundant in the Paleozoic Era. They contain even a greater proportion of the base metals than expected from their abundance. Although Paleozoic deposits account for only 34 %, they carry 58 % of the total metal. Archean and Proterozoic deposits have similar metal contents and abundance: 15 % and 14 %; 19 % and 21 %, respectively.

In the recent contribution by Barrie & Hannington (1999a), a through-time distribution of VMS is reviewed. The main periods of mineralization in terms of number of deposits are bracketed between ~2750-2700 Ma – Late Archean; 1900-1800 Ma – Palaeoproterozoic; 500-450 Ma – Cambro-Ordovician; 390-250 Ma – Devonian through Permo-Carboniferous; and 30-0 Ma – Neogene. The abundance of both bimodal-felsic and bimodal-siliciclastic in the Phanerozoic reflects a decrease in the global heat flux with time, with more evolved, felsic arcs in the Phanerozoic.

GREENSTONE BELT-TYPE, VOLCANO-SEDIMENTARY SEQUENCES

Definition of greenstone belt-type volcano-sedimentary sequence

Greenstone belts (GBs) represent some of the earliest records of Earth's lithospheric history, and many also contain substantial ore deposits. De Wit & Ashwal (1995, 1997), on whose analysis this review is based, indicate that only some 40 of the 260 known GBs have been adequately described and quantitatively documented. There is no satisfactory definition of the term GB. It is indiscriminately applied to remnants of ancient (mostly Archean) supracrustal rocks with a variable volume of slightly metamorphosed, hence green, igneous rocks. Because many of these rocks are significantly deformed, these supracrustal assemblages were also frequently referred to in the early part of this century as "schist belts". In fact, definitions of GBs emphasise low-grade assemblages, and the worse exposed and higher-grade areas tell similar but partially obscured stories.

The term "greenstone belt" is inherited from times when most detailed geological maps were published world-wide at scales between 1:100 000 and 1:250 000, requiring the use of regional terms. The study of these terrains principally aimed to separate the granitoids and gneisses from the "green stones". At scales around 1:10 000 to 1:25 000, GBs are shown not to be the simple supracrustal sequences with layer-cake stratigraphy buckled into synclines, that they were depicted to be as late in the early 1980s. Instead, they are thin sheets with large cross-sectional aspect ratios. Many greenstone successions are allochthonous with respect to surrounding sialic crust. They appear at all metamorphic grades, but the most common are those at greenschist and sub-greenschist facies.

GBs are as complex and variable as Phanerozoic orogenic belts, with a multiplicity of tectonic environments. The characterisation of these palaeotectonic environments has become one of the most important objectives of GB research (e.g. Condie 1994). The partial preservation of these rock sequences, within and at the margins of the present-day São Francisco Craton, occurred during collisional tectonic events. As is the case in Brazil, research continues in many cases with only rudimentary knowledge of the cartographic distribution of lithological units. In some cases, the data, even at a regional scale, are sparsely distributed in short, imprecise conference publications, unpublished post-graduate theses, or unpublished company reports. We present some of the critical data for the São Francisco Craton GBs in the states of Minas Gerais, Goiás, Tocantins, Bahia and Sergipe. Adequate, peer review of some of the data is lacking in some cases, which hampers the estimation of their potential for hosting VMS deposits.

GB distribution in the São Francisco Craton

In the context of the foregoing definition of GBs, this contribution lends on classical reviews by de Almeida & Hasui (1984), and Mascarenhas et al. (1984), as well as recent ones by Schrank & da Silva (1993), Pedrosa-Soares et al. (1994), and Baars (1997, 2000 in prep.) in order to define the distribution of GBs in the São Francisco Craton. The first publications emphasise the Archean and Palaeoproterozoic GBs. Of late, it has been possible to classify various other metavolcano-sedimentary sequences as generic GBs, on account of detailed cartography and geochemical characterisation. In this sense, we recognise that the geology of the São Francisco Craton and its marginal mobile belts represent a continuous history of basin generation, ocean formation and closure, ocean-continent and continent-continent collision, cratonic stabilisation, intracratonic subsidence and renewed rifting from the Archean to the Cenozoic. Indeed, the Mesozoic Rocas Verdes Complex, Chile, is proposed to be a short-lived, modern analogue to complex, ancient GBs (Sawkins 1990, p. 6, Stern & de Wit 1997).

Baars (2000 in prep.) suggests that the São Francisco Craton, as it was sculptured by the end of the Neoproterozoic, the Brasiliano Event, is represented by a map distribution similar to that of the precursor Paramirim Craton at the end of the Palaeoproterozoic. This is in spite of long-held claims that the Craton was concentrically and significantly reduced in size by general, cratonward tectonism, especially during the Brasiliano / Pan-African Event. The tectonic processes of this age that affected the São Francisco Craton were essentially diachronous, thin-skinned events with extensive fold-and-thrust belts masking underlying, stable cratonic crust. In terms of GB and volcano-sedimentary-belt distribution, this interpretation is consistent with the distribution of Archean and Palaeoproterozoic GBs within the craton interior and the internal zones of the post-Palaeoproterozoic mobile belts, to the exclusion of younger GBs. In addition, the younger volcano-sedimentary belts are concentrated, coincident with one another and with remnants of ancient GB tracts, in the central and outer zones of the mobile belts that surround the peculiarly shaped Craton. A few, minor, Neoproterozoic remnants are thrust cratonward to allochthonous and rootless positions in the broad inner zones. To the extent that host-rock-formation era has a bearing on VMS potential, these regional observations are very important and will only be enriched by additional, precise geochronological determinations of the GB and volcano-sedimentary sequences in and around the São Francisco Craton.

While the critical heat flow conditions have changed significantly in these periods, from the Archean to the Neoproterozoic / Eopaleozoic, the fundamental litho and asthenospheric processes that control plate tectonism have remained in place. The cyclicity of metallogenesis has reduced its frequency and some of its detailed geochemical characteristics through time. Nevertheless, the essential supply of metal abundance from the mantle to the crust during regional, extensional events has persisted (Sawkins 1990, Barley & Groves 1992).

Volcanogenic massive sulphide exploration in the São Francisco Craton has focused on Archean and Palaeoproterozoic GBs. In the light of (i) the empirical abundance of VMS deposits associated with various geological era, and (ii) the generic association of VMS deposits with arc-related volcano-sedimentary sequences, exploration in and around the São Francisco Craton and its orogenic belts should consider other geological terrains as preliminary targets. The only place for era-based prejudice is that which takes into account the occurrence of VMS deposits world-wide associated with the five main geological era indicated above.

The greenstone belts

This section does not provide an in-depth review of the geology of the GBs object of the study. It aims to provide the reader with the general, critical geological data for each GB that are necessary to characterise the potential for VMS. The descriptions are organised in order of apparent GB age. Despite tectono-metamorphic overprinting, rocks of most belts commonly occur at low strain, such that original structures and textures may be preserved. Thus, igneous or sedimentary terminology is widely used, and the prefix 'meta' is implicitly inferred but, in most places, textually omitted.

Archean

Crixás, Pilar de Goiás, Guarinos, Goiás, Faina

The Archean terranes of the State of Goiás occur within an approximate 50 000-km^2 area of the southern portions of the Goiás Massif. They comprise about 80 % of granite-gneiss complexes ranging in age from 2.9 to 2.4 Ga and linear GBs of 3.2 to 2.9 Ga. The granite-gneiss complexes are made up of gneisses and intrusive bodies, mostly of granodiorite and tonalite, with minor granite. The GBs are typically metamorphosed at low grades, resting allochthonously on the granite-gneiss complexes, having been deformed during several episodes ranging in age from Archean to Neoproterozoic. The limits of the Archean segments are entirely tectonic with rock units assigned to the Palaeo-, Meso-, and Neoproterozoic.

The GB rock assemblages occur in five belts of 40- to 150-km length and, on average, 6 km width. Three belts cluster in the north (Crixás, Guarinos, and Pilar de Goiás) and two 80 km to the south (Goiás and Faina). The first stratigraphic subdivisions of the northern GB were proposed by Danni & Ribeiro (1978) and Sabóia (1979), and of the southern GB by Danni et al. (1981). Work by Jost & Oliveira (1991) and Resende et al. (1998) considerably improved the knowledge about the lithologic compositions, preserved sequences, and their palaeogeographic significance. It has become clear that the five belts evolved with similar lower volcanic sections, giving way to sedimentary sections deposited in contrasting palaeogeographic settings.

The preserved volcanic sections consist of lower komatiites, locally with primary volcanic features such as cumulate and spinifex textures, flow layering, flow breccias, and pillows. Tholeiitic basalts follow, containing relict-pillowed flows, vesicles, varioles, and flow breccias. Metachert and Algoma-type banded iron formation (BIF) occur as sedimentary intercalations.

The preserved sedimentary record in Crixás, Goiás, and in the eastern portion of Guarinos indicates that the prevailing environment was a long-lived euxenic environment, with carbonaceous schists giving way to shallow-water limestone sequences at Crixás and Goiás. These are overlain by rhythmic quartzite-shale sequences (Theodoro 1995, Resende et al. 1998). Sedimentation in the western portion of the Guarinos GB initiated with a complex assemblage of mafic tuffs alternating with proximal turbidites, laterally disposed with respect to the main mafic volcanic pile. Both the basalts and the turbidites are overlain by an 80-m-thick BIF containing, at the base, at least four well preserved exhalative mounds with wide hydrothermal alteration zones and feeders (Resende 1994, Resende & Jost 1995). A thick sequence of carbonaceous schists follows, and is in turn unconformably overlain by a rhythmic quartzite-shale sequence. In the Pilar de Goiás GB, basic volcanism ceased in favour of a 250 mthick, graded shale sequence, chert and upper calc-silicate rocks. Sedimentary rocks in the Faina GB consist of two typical shelf quartzite-shale-carbonate sequences. The lower of these rests on basalts via an erosional unconformity, and is separated from the upper by a regression surface followed by transgression.

Evidence of felsic volcanic activity is rare in these five GBs. To date, there is only secure evidence in the Goiás GB. A lenticular, 300 m thick dacite unit, with minor rhyolitic, pyroclastic rocks, overlies basalts and is laterally interlayered with carbonaceous schists. Chert, locally rich in pyrite and interlayered with carbonaceous schist, occurs as narrow intercalations in the pyroclastic section. There is no evidence of felsic volcanic contribution in the Pilar de Goiás GB. In Crixás, a pumice-rich horizon of carbonaceous schist is evidence of a distal contribution (Theodoro 1995). There are probable ash-falls, represented by a muscovite-rich matrix of BIFs overlying basalts, in the western portion of the Guarinos GB (Resende 1994), and by the pure sericite schist within carbonaceous schists at the east of that GB (Jost et al. 1995). Coincidentally, all these evidences occur within a similar stratigraphic position as the pyroclastic rocks of the Goiás GB. Thus, they may be interpreted as being related to a single, terminal, felsic volcanic event. In the Faina GB, felsic dykes that crosscut the basalts, but do not the overlying sedimentary sequence, may be related to the same event.

Recent U-Pb SHRIMP data (Queiroz et al. 1999) indicate that granitoid complexes adjacent to the Crixás Greenstone Belt have an age of 2842 ± 6 Ma, and were emplaced within the metamorphosed and overturned GB. The komatiites of the Crixás belt yield a Sm-Nd age of 2825 ± 98 Ma (Arndt et al. 1989). However, due to alteration after eruption and mobilisation of the REE, the authors suggest that the volcanic rocks may be older than 3.0 Ga. Uranium-Pb SHRIMP data from titanite (Queiroz et al. 1999) indicate that the granitoids underwent tectonic recycling at about 2.0 Ga. Internal K-Ar and Rb-Sr isochrons, as well as Ar-Ar release data obtained by Fortes et al. (1993, 1997) and Fortes (1996) from samples of schists indicate that thrusting ranges in age from 650 Ma to 500 Ma, and is thus Neoproterozoic in age. These schists are interpreted as metamorphosed hydrothermal alteration zones underlying the massive sulphide bodies and are sampled from high strain zones.

Compiled data shows that the basalts of the five GBs are similar to modern back-arc environment, but differ in their high Sr, Cr, and Ni content. Chondrite-normalised REE vary from flat to slightly enriched in LREE. The felsic volcanic rocks of the Goiás GB have a geochemical nature that may be explained by differentiation from a mantle source. Geochemical data about the sedimentary record of the five belts (Jost et al. 1996, Resende 1998, Resende et al. 1998) indicate a predominantly-mafic source area, with minor felsic contribution. This indicates that neither a continent nor an arc was sufficiently near to feed the depositional sites. A mid-ocean ridge of a back-arc environment is interpreted as the origin for these GBs.

Herein, the authors propose that the Mina III Gold Mine may represent a distal, gold-only VMS deposit. No other VMS deposits have yet been found or described in any of these five gold-rich belts. The scarcity of felsic volcanic rocks, the apparent lack of felsic sub-volcanic intrusions, and the prevalence of basalts suggest that mafic intrusions may have been the heat source to drive hydrothermal systems within the basalt piles. Alteration pipes have been found only in the Guarinos GB (Resende 1994, Resende & Jost 1995), but their depositional result is a thick magnetite-hematite bearing BIF. Controversy persists regarding this proposal, considering that many authors suggest an epigenetic, deformation-related origin (most recently Fortes et al. 1997).

Quadrilátero Ferrífero (or Rio das Velhas) and others

The Quadrilátero Ferrífero (QF) is a metamorphic complex of rock sequences from the Archean and the Palaeoproterozoic, including TTG-batholith domes, folded and thrust into a 80 x 80 km quadrangular format. This entity is known as the Iron Quadrangle for hosting extensive, economic Lake Superior-type iron formations, and sub-economic, Archean, Algoma-type iron formations. Most authors refer to the GB as the Rio das Velhas GB, in view of the typical sequence comprised by the supergroup with the same name, although Baars (1997) preferred the more generic term QF GB. The belt is famous for its lode-gold deposits (e.g. Ladeira 1991, Lobato et al. 1998, Lobato et al. 2000b).

The Rio das Velhas GB (e.g. Zucchetti et al. 1998, Baltazar & Pedreira 1998, Lobato et al. 2000a) is composed of a lower sequence of ultramafic to mafic and intermediate volcanic rocks at the base of the Nova Lima Group, with minor BIFs. These are followed by pelites and BIFs, significant greywackes, turbidites and interbedded, felsic to intermediate pyroclastic rocks. Arenites, argillites, turbidites and calc-silicate rocks, at the top of the Group succeed the cessation of volcanism in the pile. The stratigraphy gives way to the Maquiné Group, which is dominated by clastic, terrigenous sedimentary rocks, represented by quartz schists, quartzites and conglomerates. The Companhia de Pesquisa de Recursos Minerais (see Zucchetti & Baltazar 1998) mapped the GB, refining its stratigraphy (Dorr 1969) and indicating new type localities for some of its units.

Baars (1997) cites evidence for an origin of basal komatiites around 3.19 and 3.22 Ga near Congonhas. Machado et al. (1996) report detrital zircon ages from 3.54 to 3.0 Ga in QF sedimentary rocks, while Machado & Noce (1993) indicate an age of 3029 Ma for a zircon from acid volcanic rocks of the Nova Lima Group. Carneiro (1992) and Noce (1995) present U-Pb age determinations that prove a long, Archean to Palaeoproterozoic history of felsic dome generation and metamorphism in and around the GB, reviewed in Noce et al. (1998). Thermal and isotopic perturbation continued through to the Neoproterozoic.

Compelling data regarding the geochemical nature of the mafic volcanic rocks of the Nova Lima Group (Zucchetti 1998) show that various families of basalts are preserved in the sequence. These data, in addition to evidence for the presence of komatiites (Schorscher et al. 1982) at the ultramafic end of the spectrum and andesites and rhyolites with intermediate and felsic compositions, show that the Rio das Velhas Greenstone Belt contains a wide spectrum of mid-ocean ridge basalt and arc-related rocks. This highlights the need for more detailed mapping and geochemical data to define more clearly the tectonostratigraphic subdivisions within the QF.

In this context, the structural branches of the QF are important clues to deciphering the complexity of this Archean terrane. The GBs at Mateus Leme-Pitanguí in the NW (Romano 1990, 1993), Itapecirica in the W, Itabira-Nova Era (NE), Oliveira-São João del Rei-Barbacena (SW; Ávila 1992), and Congonhas in the S-SE (Seixas 1988, Seixas & Baars 1991, Rosa Seixas et al. 1998, Rosa Seixas et al. 1999a,b) are continuous, structural extensions of the QF (with azimuth directions indicated in paraentheses). Each contains rocks of similar affiliations to those of the Rio das Velhas Supergroup, although commonly in much less deformed states. In general the data are either absent, inconclusive or simply contradictory as to the real stratigraphic correlation between these sequences. In view of this, we adopt an integrated regional vision of the geology of these greenschist and greenstone belts.

Aluminous hydrothermal alteration occurs in tholeiitic basalts of the basal Ouro Fino Unit, Nova Lima Group. These locally display deca- to centimetre-thick bands carrying anthophyllite and cordierite. They are variably schistose, and also contain quartz, plagioclase, Mg-chlorite, phlogopite and accessory garnet, cummingtonite, tourmaline and rutile (da Silva 1998a).

In the north-western Mateus Leme – Pitanguí Belt extension of the Rio das Velhas GB, Romano (1990, 1993) describes extensive hydrothermal alteration over 50 km in length and hectametric width. The alteration is hosted entirely within volcanic and volcaniclastic rocks with characteristic chert intercalations of the Pitangui Group, correlate of the Nova Lima Group. Various spectacular textures and aluminous assemblages are carefully described, and they encompass four types. Nodular peraluminous rocks consist of tubular, elliptic and spheroidal nodules of corundum, with or without kyanite/andalusite, enveloped in pyrophyllite-diaspore-kaolinite haloes. Accessory tourmaline, rutile and chloritoid, and rare barite are present. Massive, fine-grained muscovitites contain subordinate pyrophyllite, tourmaline, kaolinite and rutile. Restricted, coarse-grained quartz-muscovite-kyanite schists contain secondary pyrophyllite, diaspore and kaolinite. Quartz-sericite schists dominate in the extensive hydrothermal alteration zone, and host the other peraluminous rock types. Fine-grained granular-lepidoblastic sericite and embayed, corroded quartz intergrow commonly hosting thin monomineralic chloritoid-kyanite-diaspore-pyrophyllite-tourmaline rocks. Massive pyrophyllite constitutes agalmatolite ore, or lard stone. Romano & Carmo (1992) map and describe proximal peraluminous, sericitic and distal propyllitic alteration zones. Chlorite, carbonate, epidote and sulphide subzones are described by Frizzo et al. (1991), with a transition to keratophyric volcanic rock. Sulphidation is sparsely disseminated in the peraluminous zone, and relatively abundant in the external alteration zones.

Romano (1993) considers these mineral assemblages to be associated with post-volcanic, metasomatic, hydraulic-fracture fluid infiltration and heat flux. This is correlated to a classic epithermal system (Rose & Burt 1979), with the peraluminous zone corresponding to the advanced argillic alteration. Other aluminous minerals, such as ilmonite, garnet, staurolite, amphibole and sillimanite are interpreted to have a metamorphic origin.

The meticulous description by Romano (1993), transcribed here in some detail, serves to highlight the care that is necessary in the geological cartography of apparently exclusively regional metamorphic assemblages. The mineral assemblages in the Mateus Leme – Pitangui Belt may correspond to the high-sulphidation, shallow-water hydrothermal alteration pattern associated with gold-bearing VMS deposits (Hannington et al. 1999, Figure 2). Gold occurrences are in fact present in the Pitangui region.

Piumhi

The small Piumhi GB, at the extreme south-west of the São Francisco Craton, is composed of a basal, komatiite- and tholeiite-bearing unit, the Ribeirão Araras Group, and an overlying, sedimentary-rock-dominated unit, the Paciência Group (Schrank 1982). The allochthonous, chromitite-bearing and spinifex-textured Lavapés Group contains mylonitic rocks that are intensely deformed, with field relationships similar to ophiolite mélange complexes (Schrank & da Silva 1993). Both mafic-ultramafic and felsic magmatism are important throughout the lower two units of the tectono-stratigraphic pile, with numerous examples of differentiated clinopyroxenite sills, and predominantly rhyodacite sills, dykes and domes. Alkaline mugearite and trachyte sills also intrude the package.

Schrank (1982) describes geochemical signatures for a succession of komatiites, komatiitic basalts, tholeiitic MORB, alkaline basalt and Archean-type, calc-alkaline andesites (Jahn & Schrank 1983) in a mafic-dominated volcano-sedimentary pile that was emplaced around 3116 +10/-7 Ma within a sedimentary basin, metamorphosed during a 2.4 Ga thermal event. Schrank & da Silva (1993) further indicate a history of intrusive and tectonic events through 1127, 726 and 635 ± 2 Ma.

Morro do Ferro

The Morro do Ferro GB (Teixeira & Danni 1979, Teixeira et al. 1987, Schrank & da Silva 1993) covers various 3 km wide tracts over a 60 km long belt between Alpinópolis and Fortaleza de Minas, Minas Gerais, to the south of the São Francisco Craton. The granite-greenstone terrains of the south-western Minas Gerais crop out within the framework of the Barbacena Complex (Hasui et al. 1993) represented by isotropic granitoids and varied migmatites. Their volcanic rocks are characterised by dominant komatiitic chemistry and subordinate komatiitic basalt chemistry. Soares et al. (1990), Hasui (1993) and de Carvalho (in prep.) attribute the tectonic emplacement of the GBs to Trans-Amazonian (Ebernian) thrusting and NW-oriented transcurrent fault systems.

The various tracts that constitute this broad belt are lithologically (Teixeira et al. 1987), stratigraphically and metallogenetically (de Carvalho 1990) distinct, characterising two regional segments. In the Fortaleza de Minas segment, tens of mafic-ultramafic volcanic bodies are identified, representing cyclic volcanic flows throughout the stratigraphic column, all less than 20 m thick. The lower unit contains differentiated komatiites, with flow-top and flow-base spinifex, olivine-cumulate, pillow and flow breccia textures, tuffs, chemical and clastic sedimentary rocks, and rare tholeiites. The unit hosts the Fortaleza de Minas (O'Toole) Ni-Cu-Co-PGE-Au Deposit (Brenner et al. 1990) at the base of a serpentinitic peridotite flow, in basal contact with a BIF. De Carvalho et al (1999) shows evidence for the origin of the mineralization from immiscible sulphides in an igneous melt. The upper unit differs in that it is entirely sedimentary rock dominated.

The komatiite-rich Alpinópolis segment displays some distinctive features (Szabó 1989). It comprises numerous, correlatable, volcano-sedimentary bodies, tectonically intercalated within the Barbacena Complex. De Carvalho (1990) describes four suites, viz. the ultrabasic, basic, sedimentary and acid intrusive suites, best exposed at the Ribeirão da Conquista River. The thin ultrabasic suite contains pyroxenitic and serpentinitic volcanic peridotites and komatiitic basalts, with local spinifex and cumulate textures. Basic amphibolites, in place schistose, represent the overlying tholeiitic, Mg-rich basaltic unit. The komatiitic to tholeiitic volcanic rocks are marked by the apparent absence of an calc-alkaline evolution.

Various aluminous and carbonaceous sedimentary schists and ferruginous and/or graphitic quartzites are intercalated with these suites, interpreted to represent tuffs, pelites, marls and ferruginous cherts. At Bom Jesus da Penha, Mg-rich basalts, ultramafic rocks, amphibolites, marls, and pelitic, aluminous and carbonaceous sedimentary rocks are overlain by a succession of pelitic, arkosic and chemical sedimentary rocks, and quartzites with quartz-muscovite schists. Deformed, granitic intrusive bodies, up to 400 m in length, are intercalated in the former rock units. At contacts with ultramafic rocks, centimetric tourmaline crystals, quartz, margarite and corundum develop. The metamorphic, errorchron age of 2918 ± 105 Ma from the enveloping migmatites (Artur et al. 1990) represents a minimum age for the GB.

The Alpinópolis segment is distinct from the Fortaleza de Minas GB in that it displays much fewer peridotitic flows, more tholeiitic basalt flows, thicker cherts, no BIFs, aluminous sedimentary rocks and tuffs. It has a distinct metallogenetic character. Carvalho (1990) integrates geophysical and surface and subsurface geochemical data to identify 16 subeconomically mineralised, sulphide orebodies there, containing Zn, Cu and Ni.

Cuieté Velho

The Cuieté Velho Metavolcano-sedimentary Sequence, Pocrane Complex (Paes et al. 1998, Paes 1999, Paes et al. 2000) near the town of Conselheiro Pena, is part of the northern Mantiqueira Province, in eastern Minas Gerais. Amphibolites, tremolite-actinolite and biotite schists, quartzites and lesser talc schists predominate at the base. Intermediate biotite schists with quartzite lenses, in association with calc-silicate rocks, amphibolite and talc schists grade to quartzites at the top. Unaltered amphibolites and hornblende schists display a MORB, tholeiitic signature, and geochemical characteristics compatible with greenstone-belt, Archean basalts. Tremolite-actinolite schists are interpreted as metamorphosed cumulate rocks. Cogenetic mafic rocks have a Sm-Nd isochron age of 3099 ± 142 Ma, with an ΣNd(T) of +1.1. Other well documented, volcano-sedimentary sequences in the São Francisco Craton have similar geochemical features. Old gold workings in sheared, hydrothermally altered amphibolites occur close to the contact with Neoproterozoic, calc-alkaline granites of the Galiléia Suite (Nalini et al. 1998). A small massive sulphide occurrence is reported (J.H. Grossi Sad, pers. comm.) although inadequately described.

The Cuieté Velho Sequence represents an Archean, greenstone-belt-type fragment. The presence of this tectonic fragment well within the Araçuaí Belt suggests that the São Francisco Paleocontinent extended at least to the proximities of the studied area. This is farther east than previously alluded to. This is corroborated by the sedimentary and metamorphic polarities preserved within the Rio Doce Group, also suggesting a westward continental provenance and tectonic domain (Paes et al.2000)

Contendas-Mirante, Tremedal, Mundo Novo, Jacobina

The Contendas-Jacobina Lineament, with a general N-NE trend and more than 500 km of extension, corresponds to a suture zone preserved at a Palaeoproterozoic continent-continent collision zone. According to Sabaté et al. (1990), the lineament marks the limits between oriental and central crustal domains of the northern São Francisco Craton (the Jequié and Gavião Domains). The Contendas-Mirante Volcano-Sedimentary Belt, the Mundo Novo GB and the Jacobina Group describe the lineament.

The *Contendas-Mirante* Volcano-Sedimentary Belt (Marinho 1991) is predominantly constituted by supracrustal rocks metamorphosed in the greenschist facies, with a progressive increase to the amphibolite facies towards its margins. The metamorphic assemblages parallel two N-S-oriented coaxial fabrics. The package is composed of three lithostratigraphic units.

The Lower Unit comprises tholeiitic mafic and calc-alkaline felsic volcanic rocks, as lava flows and dominant pyroclastic subunits, with intercalations of immature siliciclastic and chemical sedimentary rocks, including marbles, cherts and BIFs. Cunha (1996) recently identified a komatiitic basalt in this unit. Marinho (1991) uses Sm-Nd, Pb-Pb and U-Pb isotopes to determine ages between 3.0 and 3.3 Ga for the volcanic rocks.

The Intermediate Unit is composed of pelitic to psammitic, and epiclastic sedimentary rocks, with subordinate calc-alkaline mafic and minor intermediate volcanic rocks. Lead-Pb age determinations (Marinho 1991) suggest an age of 2.5 Ga for the mafic volcanic rocks. Metamorphic Rb-Sr rehomogenisation occurred at around 2.0 Ga. The Upper Unit is essentially composed of epiclastic sandstones and conglomerates. Nutman et al (1992) use detrital zircons from conglomerate to establish a deposition period between 2.15 and 1.9 Ga, the latter also a Late-Trans-Amazonian granite age. Several Archean and Proterozoic granitoid plutons and some mafic-ultramafic intrusions, including the 2.47 Ga, gabbro-dominated Rio do Jacaré Stratified Sill (Marinho 1991), truncate the entire system. The latter contains four massive, V-rich, PGE-bearing, titano-magnetite orebodies.

Da Silva (1996) suggests that the dominantly pelitic Tremedal Sequence may be a tectonic remnant, to the south, of the Contendas Mirante GB. Aluminous mineral assemblages, reported as regional metamorphic, and fuchsite-bearing rocks may attest to the eventual metallogenic potential.

Marinho (1991) proposes basin formation in continental through oceanic-rift environments for the whole package. Marinho et al. (1994) and da Silva & Cunha (1999) describe how rocks of the Lower Unit are source to many stream-sediment Pb, Zn, Cu, As, Ag and Au anomalies, and persistent, high, native-Zn and -Cu counts in the Contas and Sincord River terraces. Electromagnetic anomalies define expressive bedrock conductors. Several ubiquitous vein-type barite occurrences, with Cu-Pb sulphides, disseminated Zn, a few Au showings, massive pyrite-pyrrhotite bodies suggests a polymetallic sulphide potential.

The *Mundo Novo* GB, first defined by Mascarenhas & da Silva (1994), is located between the towns of Piritiba and Mundo Novo. It is dominated by low-grade metamorphosed basalt lava flows and andesitic to dacitic pyroclastic rocks, associated with greywackes, and chert- and, BIF-derived chemical-exhalative sedimentary rocks. Allochthonous, ultramafic tectonic slices, from the Jacobina Group, occur within the Mundo Novo sedimentary rocks. Late uplift is inferred as a result of basement arching, leading to erosion and rifting, and having created thereby conditions of formation for the Jacobina Group quartz-pebble conglomerates.

Geochronological data indicate GB-formation at the Archean-Palaeoproterozoic transition at around 2.7 - 2.5 Ga. Da Silva (1998b) reports a Sm-Nd model age $T_{(DM)}$ of 2.6 Ga, determined in dacites from the Mundo Novo area.

Common gold garimpos are associated mainly with ultramafic rocks (Silveira & Conceição Filho 1991). Polymetallic base-metal sulphide showings were discovered by Unigeo-Anglo American Corp. at Fazenda Coqueiro, associated with magnetic and geochemical anomalies, and confirmed in drillcore through bimodal volcanic rocks (Mascarenhas & da Silva 1994).

Umburunas, Ibitira-Ubiraçaba, Brumado, Bate-Pé, Guajeru, Licínio de Almeida, Urandi

The Gavião Block, situated in the Brumado region in central-southern Bahia, exhibits vast exposures of the Archean cratonic basement, including the oldest known rocks of Brazil in the crust-derived, 3.35 Ga Boa Vista - Mata Verde Complex (Nutman et al 1996). The latter complex displays $T_{(DM)}$ of 3530 (Wilson 1987, Marinho 1991). The Sete Voltas and Serra dos Pombos Complexes display similar patterns (Martin et al. 1991, Marinho et al. 1993). They are dominantly granite-gneissic and migmatitic terrains, with sedimentary and volcano-sedimentary GB enclaves of the Archean and Palaeoproterozoic.

These decakilometric, curvilinear tracts have distinct lithologic and stratigraphic characteristics within the range of preserved sequences in the Serrinha Block. Here, the first and most spectacular records of komatiitic flows with well-preserved spinifex textures were identified in the northern São Francisco Craton lobe. The most expressive areas were individually characterised with the denominations of Umburanas (Cunha & Fróes, 1994), lbitira-Ubiraqaba, Brumado and Guajeru (Cunha et al. 1994) GBs (as per Barbosa & Dominguez 1996).

The well-documented Umburanas GB consists of three lithostratigraphic units, associated with three distinct volcanic cycles (Cunha & Fróes 1994). The Lower Unit is composed of basal, spinifex-textured komatiites and ultramafic volcanic rocks, and tholeiitic basalts and dacites. Quartzites with conglomeratic horizons, pelitic and chemical sedimentary rocks (BIFs, cherts, carbonates, calc-silicate rocks), and minor intercalations of felsic volcanic rocks. The Intermediate Unit is dominated by felsic volcanic rocks of the third volcanic cycle, with subordinate pyroclastic, epiclastic and mafic-flow correlates. The Upper Unit is constituted essentially of carbonates. The entire sequence is truncated by granitoid intrusions. At least two deformation phases accompany dominant greenschist-facies metamorphic assemblages.

Geochronological data from Sm-Nd, single-zircon Pb-Pb and SHRIMP U-Pb isotope systems indicate ages around 3.0 Ga for the mafic volcanic rocks and quartzites of the Lower Unit of the Umburanas GB, and around 2.7 Ga for the felsic volcanic rocks of the Intermediate Unit (Cunha & Fróes 1994).

The *Ibitira-Ubiriçaba and Brumado* GBs are characterised by sequences with amphibolitic basalt and gabbro, chemical sedimentary rocks (BIFs, marbles, calc-silicate rocks), ultramafic rocks, carbonates, quartzites and calc-silicate quartzites, and felsic volcanic rocks (Moraes et al. 1980, da Silva 1996). The Bate-Pé GB tract also registers greenschist-facies metamorphism, predominantly in quartzites and mica schists. Aluminous minerals, garnet, kyanite and staurolite are present at places (Dias Lima et al. 1981). The age of these GBs is not precisely determined, although their proximity and geological similarity with the better-studied, Archean Umburunas GB is used as evidence in favour of an Archean origin.

The *Guajeru* GB in the southwestern portion of the Gavião Block is constituted, at the base, by tholeiitic basic and komatiitic ultrabasic schists and serpentinites, with quartzite and carbonate intercalations. The intermediate and upper portions of the sequence are dominantly sedimentary with oxide-facies BIFs, fuchsitic quartzites and carbonates.

Active research and mineral exploration developed in the Umburunas, Ibitira-Ubiraçaba, Brumado, Bate-Pé, Guajeru GBs, mainly by the Companhia Baiana de Pesquisa Mineral-CBPM, have resulted in numerous target discoveries of Cu-Zn massive sulphide occurrences, Au, Ni-Cu (PGE) and Cr, the best results to date occurring in the Umburunas GB. Important Cu-occurrences are known in ultramafic and calc-silicate rocks (0.4 to 2.1 % Cu) and Au in sheared felsic volcanic rocks (0.1 to 7.45 g/t Au).

The *Licínio de Almeida and Urandi* Belts are dominantly sedimentary and are located to the west, within the Gavião Block, at the eastern margin of the Espinhaço Range. Souza et al. (1990) define the Licínio de Almeida as a group of low-grade rocks consisting of aluminous schists, and pelitic, calc-silicate and chemical sedimentary rocks, including manganoan BIFs (Rocha et al. 1998), marbles and cherts. Direct correlation with the other GBs of the Gavião Block is difficult. Rocha (1990) interprets the Belt as resulting from an episode of mixed psammitic-pelitic-chemical sedimentation during the Late Archean, without proximal volcanism. Chemical sedimentary rocks in the Urandi Belt have a possible volcanic contribution. Furthermore, amphibolites there are ascribed to amphibolite-facies BIFs, emphasising the sedimentary nature of the Belt. Potential for VMS deposits is restricted to the bimodal-siliciclastic type. The Licínio de Almeida Belt is well known for its significant manganoan-BIF-hosted manganese deposits.

Riacho da Santana

In the Guanambi-Correntina Block at the west of Bahia State, some remnants of GB-type volcano-sedimentary sequences occur, the Riacho de Santana GB being the most expressive example (Silveira & Cunha 1997). This Belt includes three main lithostratigraphic units: (i) the Lower Unit, composed of komatiitic volcanic rocks associated with chemical and detrital sedimentary rocks; (ii) the Intermediate Unit, constituted by mafic and felsic volcanic rocks, and chemical and pelitic sedimentary rocks; and (iii) the Upper Unit, which is essentially represented by mixed siliceous-carbonate platform sedimentary rocks, with basalt intercalations. Local greenschist-facies metamorphic imprint displays lateral variations to the amphibolite facies. Plutons, including the Cara Suja Massif, dykes and sub-volcanic sills have an alkaline affiliation. Sm-Nd and Pb-Pb $T_{(DM)}$ model ages of 2.33 Ga and 2.7 Ga for the basalts and 2.0 Ga for alkaline intrusive rocks, respectively, confirm the Archean origin of the GB (Paim et al. 1999).

Intensive mineral exploration by the CBPM indicates several favourable targets (Silveira & Cunha 1997). These include base-metal massive sulphide and gold targets, all related to hydrothermal alteration features, with the presence of chemical and chemical-exhalative sedimentary rocks, ultramafic, mafic and felsic volcanic rocks, and porphyritic alkaline intrusive rocks. An expressive, 100 m strike-length gossan is reported, associated with a tuff, chert and carbonates package. It is associated with an 800 m IP/R anomaly, with rocks yielding grades of up to 1.3 % Cu and 2 to 5 g Au/t.

Boquira Belt, Ibiajara, Paramirim and others

The Paramirim Block at the west of Bahia State consists of granite-gneisses and migmatites, and volcano-sedimentary to dominantly sedimentary sequences, forming narrow, isolated, N-S tracts. The interpretation of such associations as representatives of discrete volcano-sedimentary sequences, or as fractions of the same, disrupted GB is controversial. The largest strip, with some 64 km length and 3 km width and known as the Boquira Belt, hosts stratabound and/ or stratiform Pb-Zn(-Cd-Ag) ores, including the deposits of the now inactive Boquira Lead Mine. It was first described by Gonçalves (apud Cunha et al. 1994) and Nagell (1970).

Rocha (1985) and Carvalho (1982) describe iron formations of oxide, carbonate and silicate facies, with quartz-magnetite, quartz-hematite, silicate-magnetite and carbon-magnetite subfacies. These rocks are intercalated in quartzites and carbonates. There are no proven records of volcanic rocks, although banded amphibolites of unclear origin are important, particularly at base metal mineralised localities (Fleischer & Espourteille 1998). The record is interpreted as an isolated chemical-sedimentary sequence formed in a Late-Archean, shallow-water epi-continental basin containing anaerobic organisms (Rocha 1985). Banded gneiss intercalations are common, as are chlorite-garnet-biotite schists.

The Pb-Zn(-Cd-Ag) mineralizations in the Boquira Formation (Cassedane 1972, Rocha 1985, Fleischer & Espourteille 1998), best represented at the exhausted Boquira Lead Mine, is closely associated with the amphibolitic, siliceous magnetite BIF subfacies. These are, in turn, hosted by dolomitic carbonates, at places in contact with quartzites by way of epidotite horizons. The steep, concordant tabular and folded orebodies at Boquira produced some 5.6 Mt ore between 1959 and 1985, at weighted average grades of 8.9 % Pb and 1.4 % Zn.

Other volcano-sedimentary linear tracts in the Paramirim Block contain Cu-associated Au mineralizations, as at Baixa Funda in lbiajara. Soares et al. (1990) denominate the Paramirim Belt stretching some 45 km over a narrow band of 1 to 4 km. It contains some volcanic in addition to sedimentary rocks, attesting to a possible GB association.

Palaeoproterozoic

Rio Itapicuru

The major Rio Itapicuru GB (Kishida 1979, da Silva 1987, Schrank & da Silva 1993, Baars 1997) is located in the north-eastern portion of the Serrinha Block, Bahia. Narrow volcano-sedimentary belts and tracts in a classic GB architecture stretching over 100 km envelop N-S-trending, elongate granite and gneiss domes. The GB itself covers some 700 km^2, and is comprised of a lowermost mafic volcanic unit, an intermediate felsic unit and an uppermost sedimentary unit. The mafic rocks are ocean-floor tholeiites, which are overlain by arc calc-alkaline volcanic sequences. Turbiditic sedimentary rocks, with a significant volcanogenic component, and chemical sedimentary rocks, including chert and BIFs top the sequence. This supracrustal association exhibits a greenschist to amphibolite metamorphic imprint. Syn and late-tectonic granites and gabbros intrude the system.

All geochronological data clearly indicate the complete Palaeoproterozoic development of the Rio Itapicuru GB (de Brito Neves et al. 1980, Gaál et al. 1987, da Silva 1992), from basin formation through ocean-continent subduction, orogenesis and late shear-zone gold mineralization, between 2.2 and 1.95 Ga. Negative εNd values for felsic volcanic rocks, an inherited, xenolith-hosted zircon of 2.9 Ga corroborate chemical evidence for crustal contamination during felsic magmatism. Nevertheless, there is still clear evidence for oceanic crustal recycling in the felsic chemical signatures. The latter rocks are associated with 100 Ma older P MORB tholeiites in a bimodal sequence. Da Silva (1992) proposes a fully developed and subducted back-arc and coupled continental volcanic arc geotectonic setting. In that sense, the Rio Itapicuru GB may represent a major, Trans-Amazonian suture zone preserved within the present-day northern São Francisco Craton (da Silva 1987, Sabaté et al. 1990, Barbosa & Dominguez 1996).

Regional thrust and shear structures are known to host significant lode-gold mineralization (e.g. Vieira et al. 1998). Regional metamorphic assemblages indicate greenschist and lower-amphibolite conditions. Hydrothermal alteration beyond the shear-zone-related, Fazenda Brasileiro and Maria Preta Gold Mines (Alves da Silva & Matos 1991) is briefly described at a few places (da Rocha Neto & Pedreira 1994). It is possible that local, aluminous amphibolite-facies assemblages, with sillimanite, kyanite, garnet, cordierite, represent metamorphosed volcanogenic alteration zones, such as at the central, elongate Ambrósio Dome (Matos & Davison 1987; e.g. Fazenda Varginha Gold Prospect, da Rocha Neto & Pedreira 1994). Syn- and late-volcanic intrusive relationships are common throughout the GB sequence (da Silva 1998, Gomes et al. 1998).

Base metal occurrences and geochemical anomalies are known at various sites in the GB. Massive sulphide showings have been reported at at least two CBPM, pelite- and albitic chert-dominated prospects (da Rocha Neto & Pedreira 1994). Extensive Si-K-Ca hydrothermal alteration is associated with Au-Cu at another site. Gomes et al. (1998) provide initial evidence for the undiscovered importance of magmatic hydrothermal mineralization at Lagoa do Gato, 15 km east of Fazenda Brasileiro. The well-documented transition from tholeiitic to calc-alkaline associations and the mineralised margins of the intrusive Teofilândia Dome serve as an important regional guide for VMS potential.

Rio Capim

The dismembered, far-northern extension of the Rio Itapicuru GB, east of the town of Uauá, comprises the Rio Capim GB as defined by Winge & Danni (1980). It encompasses a lower unit of tholeiitic basalts and an upper unit of calc-alkaline felsic volcanic rocks. It is interpreted to represent a remnant of ensialic, back-arc basin fill, metamorphosed in the amphibolite facies, with local retrograde re-equilibration to greenschist-facies assemblages (Winge 1984). The CBPM has identified a number of pyrite-dominated, disseminated sulphide Cu-Zn and Au targets hosted in the felsic section.

Rio Salitre, Barreiro, Colomi, Casa Nova

In the region of the middle São Francisco River, the Sobradinho Domain seems to represent a northwards prolongation of the Serrinha and Paramirim Blocks (Barbosa 1996). Included in this domain are volcano-sedimentary sequences, including the Rio Salitre and Barreiro Complexes (Dalton de Souza et al. 1979) and other sedimentary sequences, with subordinate volcanic rocks, known as Colorni and Casa Nova Complexes. These are located within the framework of the Riacho do Pontal Fold Belt, defined by Dalton de Souza et al. (1979).

Dalton de Souza & Teixeira (1981) describe the Rio Salitre GB as a low-grade volcano-sedimentary sequence, comparable to a greenstone belt. It is composed of ultramafic, mafic and felsic volcanic rocks, with associated psammitic, pelitic and chemical-exhalative sedimentary rocks (Dalton de Souza & Teixeira 1981). Ribeiro & da Silva (1998) define the Rio Salitre volcano-sedimentary sequence, and its associated intrusive rocks, as a granite-greenstone terrain. It shows the presence of tholeiitic to komatiitic ocean-floor basalts, associated with arc-type felsic volcanic rocks and with dominantly volcanogenic chemical-pelitic sedimentary rocks. Whole-rock, Rb-Sr geochronological data indicate Proterozoic ages around 2.0 Ga for the supracrustal rocks of the Sobradinho Domain, and Ri of 0.706. (Dalton de Souza et al. 1979, Brito Neves et al. 1980).

Base-metal and gold mineralizations have been identified in these GBs. A belt with concentrations of massive and disseminated sulphides with a 1600 m strike extension and 20n m width, known as the Sabiá target, has also been discovered. A massive sulphide horizon is hosted by tremolitised calc-silicate rocks of the upper part of the lower volcanogenic portion of the Rio Salitre GB.

Almas-Dianópolis, Porto Alegre, Pindorama, Conceição do Tocantins

Granite-GB terranes of the south-eastern portion of Tocantins State were first described by Costa (1984), who grouped the supracrustal rocks into the Riachão do Ouro Group. The GB of the Almas-Dianópolis region occurs in a number of curvi-linear, NS-trending belts. The three best known are the Almas, Porto Alegre and Dianópolis GBs separated by a variety of gneiss and intrusive complexes. The granitoid complexes have an elliptical plan view and consist of variable proportions of trondhjemite, tonalite, granodiorite, monzogranite, quartz monzodiorite and quartz diorite (Cruz & Kuyumjian 1994).

Rubidium-Sr geochronological data are available only for one tonalite intrusion (Serra do Boqueirão Suite), which yields ages of 2050 ± 276 Ma and 2217 ± 85 Ma (Costa 1984), interpreted as the result of isotopic resetting of Archean rocks. The region also contains several small hornblende-gabbro, pyroxenite, and hornblendite bodies that intrude the GB. The lack of intense internal deformation in the intrusions and the partial overlap of the intrusions by the sedimentary rocks of the Mesoproterozoic Natividade Group, led Cruz & Kuyumjian (1994) to interpret their intrusion during the Late Archean to Early Proterozoic in age. The most detailed studies of the Almas-Dianópolis GB are presented by Cruz (1993), Cruz & Kuyumjian (1994), Kwitko et al. (1995), Kuyumjian & Cruz (1996) and Ferrari & Choudhuri (1999a, b), and of the Conceição do Tocantins GB by Thomsen & Kuyumjian (1994a,b).

Cruz (1993) proposes a stratigraphy for the GBs with two units in complex contact relationships. The Lower Metavolcanic Unit occurs in the western portion of the Almas GB, in the north-western part of the Porto Alegre GB, and throughout the Dianópolis GB. It comprises basalt flows metamorphosed in the greenschist and lower amphibolite facies. Komatiites are restricted to the northern extremity of the Dianópolis GB (Padilha 1984). Hydrothermal alteration of the basalts is common along later shear zones (Silva et al. 1990, Kwitko et al. 1995). A geochemical section across basalts at the Córrego Paiol Gold Mine suggests their tholeiitic to calc-alkaline origin (F.J. Baars et al. unpubl. data). Ferrari & Choudhuri (1999b) confirm the occurrence of tholeiitic, intra-continental basalts and dacites with some calc-alkaline arc rocks. The Upper Metasedimentary Unit occurs in the eastern portions of the Almas GB and in the northern parts of the Porto Alegre GB. It consists of carbonaceous schists with intercalations of oxide-facies BIF, chert, quartzite and minor, felsic volcanic rocks.

Rock types of the Conceição do Tocantins GB are in general similar to those of the Almas-Dianópolis GB. However, the former contains a higher frequency of BIFs. The BIFs of the Conceição do Tocantins are commonly the country rocks to Au-bearing, hydrothermally altered zones (Thomsen & Kuyumjian 1994b).

Mossâmedes

The Mossâmedes Sequence (Simões 1984, Barbosa 1987) occurs as a narrow ENE belt in the vicinities of the town of Mossâmedes, Goiás, overlying shallow-water, greenschist-facies conglomerates, quartzites, and pelites of the Serra Dourada Sequence, corresponding to early-rift deposition. Volcanic rocks of the Mossâmedes Sequence comprise greenschist- to lower amphibolite-facies basalts and andesites. These may contain horizons rich in quartz and epidote, with minor amphibole, locally with more than 50 % epidote, suggesting intense pre-metamorphic hydrothermal alteration of selected volcanic intervals. These rocks are overlain by a succession of dacitic to rhyolitic tuffs and subvolcanic intrusions. The felsic rocks commonly contain intercalations of muscovite schists with variable amounts of kyanite, chlorite, and pyrite, interpreted as metamorphosed synvolcanic hydrothermal alteration products. The top of the volcanic pile is marked by a white, pyrite-bearing chert. The upper section of the sequence is made up mostly of pelites, calcic schists, and carbonaceous phyllites with subordinate felsic pyroclastic rocks. Geochemical data (Barbosa 1987) show that the volcanic rocks are similar to modern, low-K, tholeiitic, arc assemblages. Volcanic rocks of the overlying Mossâmedes Sequence dated by Fuck & Pimentel (1990) yield a Rb-Sr age of 1933 ± 70 Ma and a Sm-Nd model age of 2200 Ma, and by Pimentel et al. (1996) an isochronic Rb-Sr age of 1978 ± 55 Ma.

Rio do Peixe

The Rio do Peixe Sequence (Nascimento 1985) crops out in a wide area between Jaraguá and Pirenópolis, Goiás, associated as thrust slivers with the sedimentary rocks of the Araxá Group. Justo (1994) describes that the sequence overlies granitoids of a Rb-Sr age of 2600 Ma, thereby, interpreting the rocks as Palaeoproterozoic. The sequence registers greenschist- to lower amphibolite-facies metamorphism, and consists of four sub-units (Justo 1994). The lowest sub-unit displays mafic to ultramafic flows and pyroclastic rocks, with minor subvolcanic microgabbro and peridotite intrusions. The mafic association underlies an assemblage of felsic rocks described as tonalitic gneisses overlain by calc-silicate rocks followed by pelites.

Silvânia

The Silvânia Sequence (Lacerda Filho et al. 1991) occurs within a sygmoid-shaped area 1 to 6 km wide and 45 km long near the town of Silvânia, and is in tectonic contact with granulites of the Anápolis-Itauçu Granulite Complex. Detailed investigation of the Sequence by Freitas (1994) led to the identification of large units consisting of basal basalts, locally with igneous textures, followed by quartzites, pelites and carbonaceous schists. Based on lithogeochemical data, the author interprets the amphibolites as derived from low-K tholeiites, with enrichment in Na and K in the more differentiated terms, and as formed in an island-arc environment. The metamorphic mineral assemblages result from high-pressure amphibolite facies, re-equilibrated under greenschist to lower amphibolite facies. Throughout the volcano-sedimentary assemblage, Freitas (1994) and Freitas & Kuyumjian (1995) describe the occurrence of several Al-rich, Au-bearing schists containing kyanite, topaz and diaspore interpreted as syn-tectonic, hydrothermal products of the sequence, which also affected the surrounding A-type granitic to trondhjemitic gneisses.

Araí

The Araí Group, as defined by Araújo & Alves (1979), is interpreted by Schobbenhaus Filho (1993) as the result of syn-rift volcanic activity followed by a post-rift sedimentary sequence, represented by the Arraias and Traíras Formations, respectively. The former consists of quartzites with intercalations of siltite, intra-formational conglomerate, and basaltic, andesitic and dacitic volcanic rocks. The latter is made up of pelites, calc-schists, chlorite schists, and marbles. The sequence underwent greenschist-facies metamorphism and deformation during eastward thrusting. Uranium-Pb radiometric data from zircon crystals of rhyolites of the Arraias Formation yield ages of 2160 Ma and 1774 Ma, respectively for the upper and lower intercepts. For Pimentel et al. (1991), the age of 1774 Ma could reflect the Paranã granitic magmatism.

Dom Silvério

The Dom Silvério Group is a sedimentary-rock-dominated tract recognised to extend over 160 km by 4 km east of the Quadrilátero Ferrífero. The Group is tectonically emplaced within ortho- and paragneisses. Dürkop (1994), Linder (1994) and Dürkop et al. (1997) describe the sequence as consisting of a structurally inferior quartzite sequence and an overlying sequence white-mica-rich quartzite, paragneiss and mica schists.

The Belt is represented by a unit, exposed at the southern portion, of rare ultramafic rocks and an overlying unit of mica schists with quartzite intercalations. Generally, the ultramafic rocks are talc-tremolite-chlorite schists, although an outcrop of harzburgite is also reported (Jordt Evangelista 1992). The schists contain garnet, kyanite, sillimanite, muscovite and staurolite as aluminous minerals (Jordt Evangelista & Roeser 1988, Candia et al. 1995). The precise cartography and characterisation of the Dom Silvério Belt is hampered by the intercalation of the pelitic and psammitic rocks with banded, paragneisses apparently belonging to the basement complex.

In the northern portion, quartzites predominate. Subordinate mica schists, marbles, gondites and calc-silicate rocks are present, displaying a rich variety of mineral assemblages. The diopside and tremolite calc-silicate rocks also display spessartine, while some quartzites contain cummingtonite. The Saúde District manganese deposits are hosted in gondites, various quartzites, in turn associated with many calc-silicate and carbonate rock types. In all rock types, aluminous mineral assemblages are important (Jordt

Evangelista et al. 1990, Dürkop et al. 1997).

The ultramafic rocks are Mg-rich apparently with a komatiitic basalt signature, although this is not unequivocal. Brueckner et al. (1998) report the Sm-Nd $T_{(DM)}$ model age of schists as 2269 Ma and $T_{(CHUR)}$ model age as 2111 Ma, suggesting mantle extraction of the protoliths of the sedimentary rocks between those times. Metamorphic mineral separates clearly indicate that metamorphism occurred at 549 Ma. Jordt Evangelista (1992) conclude that the Dom Silvério Group is a Palaeoproterozoic GB. There are no published polymetallic occurrences there, although the wide lithological and mineralogical varieties attract attention in terms of VMS potential.

Mesoproterozoic

The eastern portions of the Goiás Massif (Queiróz & Jost 1998) contain a north-south trending, 300 km long, east-vergent thrust zone, considered as the western limit of the Brasília Belt (Fuck 1994). The hangingwall of the fault contains the layered mafic-ultramafic Cana Brava, Niquelândia, and Barro Alto Complexes, from north to south. These are metamorphosed in the granulite facies. They consist of dunites, websterites, pyroxenites, gabbros, norites, and anorthosites (Girardi et al. 1978, Danni & Leonardos 1980, Girardi et al. 1986, Correia 1994, Ferreira Filho et al. 1994, Ferreira Filho 1995, Suita 1996, Lima 1997). The layered complexes were intrusively emplaced during the Palaeo- to Mesoproterozoic transition, around 1.60 to 1.56 Ga, and were metamorphosed during the Neoproterozoic (Hasui & Almeida 1970, Tassinari et al. 1981, Fuck et al. 1989, Fugi 1989, Oliveira 1993, Correia 1994, Ferreira Filho et al. 1994, Correia et al. 1997). The footwall of the fault consists of both Archean gneisses and Neoproterozoic sedimentary rocks of the Brasília Belt.

To the west, the complexes are overlain by thick volcano-sedimentary sequences metamorphosed under amphibolite facies and known, from north to south, as the Palmeirópolis, Indaianópolis (or Coitezeiro), and the Juscelândia Sequences. Their stratigraphy and geochemical composition are very similar, perhaps representing parts of a once larger basin. The Juscelândia Sequence apparently contains a more complete volcanic section, initiating with lower, continental rift-type basalts that evolved into MORB equivalents.

Palmeirópolis

The Palmeirópolis Sequence (Ribeiro Filho & Teixeira 1981, Leão Neto & Olivatti 1983, Araújo 1986) is sub-divided into three units. The Lower Unit begins with coarse, banded amphibolites that give place to felsic pyroclastic rocks and greywackes, in turn underlying an assemblage of amphibolite, pelite and quartzite cut by mafic and ultramafic dykes. The Intermediate Unit contains felsic volcanic rocks with minor pelite and BIF. The Upper Unit consists of pelites with minor chert and BIF. The geochemical composition of the amphibolites is similar to that of modern mid-ocean ridge basalts (Araújo 1986, Araújo et al. 1996a). The Palmeirópolis Sequence and associated VMS deposits are detailed by Araújo (2000, this volume).

Indaianópolis

The Indaianópolis (Danni & Leonardos 1980) or Coitezeiro Sequence (Brod 1988) lies to the west of the Niquelândia Complex, the contact being a 3 to 4 km wide, vertical, dextral, strike-slip shear zone, the Rio Traíras Lineament. The Sequence consists of five units (Brod 1988). The lowest unit encompasses pelites with minor carbonate schist, BIF and chert, followed by a thick package of basaltic to andesitic lavas and pyroclastic rocks, locally with vesicles and flow structures. The mafic volcanic rocks underlie sub-volcanic rhyolite bodies, ignimbrites, lapilli-tuffs and, locally, chert. These, in turn, underlie a rhythmic succession of shallow-water pelite and quartzite giving place to alternating carbonaceous schist and magnetite-sericite schist, underlying a chloritoid schist. The top of the sequence consists only of pelites.

The amphibolites of the Coitezeiro Sequence are derived from midocean ridge volcanic rocks (Danni et al. 1982, Araújo et al. 1995). Brod (1988) further demonstrates the geochemical and spatial affiliation of those tholeiitic rocks with the felsic volcanic rocks. Alkaline basalts are, however, similar to the oceanic, intra-plate, Hawaiian basalts.

Juscelândia

The Juscelândia Sequence (Fuck et al. 1981)

consists, from base to top, of fine amphibolites with intercalations of chert, felsic gneisses (including minor amphibolite, calc-silicate rocks), felsic tuffs, and pelites with felsic and mafic volcanic intercalations. Based on lithogeochemical data, Moraes (1992) and Moraes & Fuck (1994) first interpreted the sequence as being similar to the upper portions of ophiolite complexes and formed in a back-arc or intra-arc environment. The geochemical composition of the mafic volcanic rocks is similar to that of volcanism in modern back-arc environment. Calc-alkaline or shoshonitic contributions, that may anchor an arc to the basin, are absent.

Recently, Moraes (1997) describes that the Sequence is made up of a bimodal volcanic association with hypabyssal, felsic intrusions. The geochemical composition of the amphibolites indicates a lower/intermediate section derived from continental rift or plateau basalts, and an upper section from N-MORB basalts. The felsic rocks are metamorphic products of rhyolites, rhyodacites and sub-volcanic, continental rift granites. Apparently, the early volcanism occurred in a continental rift, which evolved to an open-ocean basin system.

Neoproterozoic

The Neoproterozoic metavolcano-sedimentary sequences of the central Brazilian Shield are not traditionally considered to be GBs. Nevertheless, in adopting a generic definition of intra-oceanic and epicontinental, volcano-sedimentary origin, we propose a series of important examples that, in terms of VMS potential, are at least as important as the older counterparts. Two important tectono-stratigraphic systems, apparently containing compatible sequences, are not considered here. These are the Araxá Group to the west, which contains bimodal volcanism and an ophiolite mélange (Strieder 1993), and the Andrelândia Group to the south (Ribeiro et al. 1995, Paciullo et al. 1998).

Salinas

The Salinas Formation is part of the Macaúbas Group at the eastern margin of the São Francisco Craton (Pedrosa-Soares et al. 1992). It represents the submarine, sedimentary-rock-dominated, sand-mud sequence of Neoproterozoic age that incorporates part of the tectono-stratigraphic evolution of the Craton margin, precursor to the West Congo-Araçuaí Orogen. Metasedimentary rocks of varied, micaceous pelites and psammites, with a significant calcareous component, important carbonaceous schists and clastic sedimentary rocks dominate the Formation. Minor volcano-sedimentary facies comprise BIF, chert, graphite and hyper-aluminous schists, and contains tectonic slivers of ultramafic and mafic rocks, which have petrochemical signatures that indicate their origin at a mid-ocean ridge (Pedrosa-Soares et al. 1992, Pedrosa-Soares et al. 1998). The Ribeirão da Folha Facies has N-MORB-type basalts dated at around 816 ± 72 Ma. Pedrosa-Soares & Noce (1998) entrench the debate (Söllner et al. 1991, Costa et al. 1995) on the existence of an extensive, pre-orogenic, ocean basin along the eastern margin of the Craton. They postulate the correlation of the Salinas Formation rocks with other, higher-grade equivalents further south, as well as citing extensive evidence in favour of the presence of a well developed magmatic arc within the Atlantic Metamorphic Belt.

In the São José da Safira area, Minas Gerais State, ultramafic rocks consist of serpentinite with preserved peridotite cores, talc-anthophyllite schists and coarse-grained, diopside-rich bodies with a tremolite matrix. They are closely associated with BIF (magnetic oxide, sulphide and silicate types), muscovite and graphite schists. This rock assemblage is interpreted as an ophiolitic mélange that is intercalated along thrust surfaces with two different sequences. The underlying, older unit is correlated to the Salinas Formation (distal Macaúbas Group). It is composed of quartz-muscovite-biotite schist with garnet, staurolite, kyanite, and/or sillimanite; quartz-garnet-amphibole-rich calc-silicate rock; and sparse amphibolite lenses, respectively derived from metamorphosed deep-sea pelite, marl, and igneous mafic rocks. The overlying, younger sequence consists of orthoquartzite, laminated, hematite and mica quartzite, and is correlated to the Capelinha Formation (Neves & Ferreira 1999).

As a working model, the authors interpret these rocks as remnants of the Adamastor-Brazilide oceanic lithosphere, as described for rocks from the Ribeirão da Folha area. Further geochemical and isotopic investigation is underway to better constrain this assumption.

Goiás Magmatic Arc: Bom Jardim de Goiás, Arenópolis, Iporá-Amorinópolis, Jaupací, Mara Rosa, Chapada, Santa Terezinha

The Goiás Magmatic Arc consists of orthogneisses and metavolcano-sedimentary sequences exposed between Sanclerlândia and Bom Jardim de Goiás (Pimentel & Fuck 1992). It extends northwards to the town of Mara Rosa (Viana et al. 1995) and probably to the northern part of the Goiás Massif, in Porangatu and Porto Nacional. Geochemical and isotopic data of the best known terranes in the south show that the rocks belonging to the Goiás Magmatic Arc formed as intra-oceanic arc, accreted between ca. 930 and 600 Ma (Pimentel & Fuck 1992). The oceanic crust that separated the Amazon and São Francisco-Congo Cratons during the Neoproterozoic is almost entirely obliterated by deformation.

For the purpose of this contribution, the magmatic-arc rock association is subdivided into the Southern and Northern Domains, separated by the remnant of Archean terranes of Goiás. Both segments are made up of calcic and calc-alkaline orthogneisses, volcano-sedimentary sequences, pelite sequences with minor mafic-ultramafic ophiolite slivers, and narrow and long bodies of granitic mylonites. Several late- to post-tectonic granites of ca. 590 and 480 Ma intrude the arc rocks.

The Southern Domain comprises the Bom Jardim de Goiás, Arenópolis, Iporá-Amorinópolis, Jaupací Sequences.

The *Bom Jardim de Goiás Sequence* crops out over ca. 50 km^2 to the south-east of the town of Bom Jardim de Goiás. Seer (1985) divides the sequence into five units metamorphosed under greenschist facies. The lower unit consists of locally pillowed basalt and andesite flows, with subordinate pyroclastic rocks. These underlie a succession of andesitic to dacitic tuffs, containing layers of chert hosting Cu-Au mineralization near a small, dioritic pluton. The sequence follows with sub-aerial rhyolitic tuffs, and minor rhyolitic and andesitic flows. The overlying units are sedimentary. The lowermost unit encompasses polymictic conglomerates, sub-arkoses, greywackes, siltites and rhythmites, derived from the erosion of the volcanic pile, granite and gneisses. The upper unit contains shallow-water quartzites, mica schists and conglomerates.

The *Arenópolis Sequence* is a NNW-trending belt, covering 500 km^2, flanked by calcic orthogneisses, between the towns of Piranhas and Arenópolis. Pimentel (1985) and Pimentel & Fuck (1987) divide the sequence into two major units metamorphosed under greenschist to lower amphibolite facies, and separated by a narrow zone of banded gneisses, locally migmatitic. The western unit contains pelites, marbles, fine amphibolites, quartzites and pyrite-bearing chert. Small, metamorphosed bodies of coarse gabbro, peridotite, pyroxenite, and serpentinised dunite intrude the sequence. The eastern unit contains basalt, commonly pillowed, and andesite flows, followed by dacitic to rhyolitic pyroclastic rocks underlying greywackes, feldspathic schists and quartzites. Geochemical data (Pimentel & Fuck 1987) suggest that the eastern unit derived from an arc volcanic pile while the eastern from an outer arc sequence. Rhyolites of the Arenópolis Sequence yield a Rb-Sr age of 928 ± 8 Ma (Pimentel & Fuck 1992).

The *Iporá-Amorinópolis Sequence* near the town of Iporá, in Goiás, consists of the distinct NS-trending Iporá and NNW-trending Amorinópolis segments. They are some 7 km wide and 10 km long. At Iporá, basalts have minor intercalations of rhyolitic and dacitic tuffs, and pelites, locally with conglomerates. These are metamorphosed in the greenschist to lower amphibolite facies (Rodrigues 1996). Hydrothermal alteration of the volcanic rocks is widespread, and is represented by muscovite schists with variably abundant amounts of magnetite, kyanite, chlorite, and chloritoid (Franco et al. 1994). The Amorinópolis segment contains a predominantly rhyolitic, tuffaceous assemblage, with minor andesitic and basaltic layers, and subordinate pelites, greywackes and conglomerates. To Franco et al. (1994) and Rodrigues & Pimentel (1995), the geochemical composition, the bimodal character, and the paucity of andesite are compatible with the sequence's origin in a mature arc or a marginal basin.

The *Jaupací Sequence* occurs within an NS-trending, greenschist- to lower amphibolite-facies belt extending between Jaupaci and Israelândia, Goiás, limited by gneisses and intrusive granites. The sequence was defined by Amaro (1989) and consists of basalts, which prevail in two NNE-trending zones separated by felsic volcanic rocks. The basalts preserve porphyritic texture and vesicles. They are geochemically similar to modern low-K tholeiites, typical of island-arc environment. The felsic volcanic rocks predominate over the mafic equivalents. They are calc-alkaline, mostly tuffaceous rhyolites and dacites. Small, sub-volcanic granodiorite and granite bodies intrude the SE portion of the sequence. Amaro (1989) considers that propylitisation of volcanic rocks near these plutons may indicate hydrothermal activity during intrusion, and targets to be considered during future exploration. Pimentel & Fuck (1992) suggest that the easterly Jaupaci and Iporá-Amorinópolis Sequences are younger arc rocks than the Arenópolis and Bom Jardim de Goiás Sequences.

The Northern Domain comprises the Mara Rosa, Chapada and Santa Terezinha Sequences.

The *Mara Rosa Sequence* (Ribeiro Filho 1981), occurring between the towns of Mara Rosa and Porangatu, is an assemblage of volcano-sedimentary rocks disposed in NNE-trending narrow belts separated by tonalitic and granodioritic orthogneiss blocks. Arantes et al. (1991) detail the supracrustal sequences, dividing them into three NNE-trending belts. They are metamorphosed under greenschist to lower amphibolite facies. The eastern belt consists of greywackes, mafic and intermediate flows and tuffs, and felsic tuffs. The central belt contains predominantly mafic volcanic rocks, BIFs and manganese formations, carbonaceous schists and minor ultramafic rocks. The western belt comprises lower mafic volcanic rocks, followed by felsic tuffs and a thick package of sedimentary rocks. Geochemical data presented by Viana (1995) indicate that the Mara Rosa Sequence evolved under an ensimatic, juvenile, island-arc environment.

The Posse and Zacarias Gold Deposits occur in the eastern belt at Mara Rosa. Gold at Posse is hosted in a NW-trending and NE-dipping shear zone crosscutting felsic volcaniclastic rocks of the eastern belt (Arantes et al. 1991, Kuyumjian 1999). However, Palermo (1996) interprets the mineralization as syngenetic and hosted by a hydrothermally altered, A-type granite. Felsic volcanic rocks of the Posse Gold Deposit and a tonalite yield zircon U-Pb ages of 862 ± 8 Ma and 856 +13/-7 Ma, respectively, and a titanite recrystallisation age of 632 ± 4 Ma. The Zacarias Deposit occurs in the central belt and is a volcanogenic Au-deposit hosted by a chert with barite occurring within andesitic to basaltic, locally felsic volcanic rocks.

The *Chapada Sequence* occurs to the SSW of the Mara Rosa Sequence. It was originally defined by Machado (1981) as comprising gneisses, migmatites, actinolite, talc and sericite schists, quartzites, carbonaceous schists and BIFs correlated to the Crixás GB. Ribeiro Filho (1981) argues in favour of a Proterozoic age. Kuyumjian (1989) identifies a sedimentary and an amphibolite sequence. The sedimentary rocks encompass quartzites and mica schists with variable amounts of staurolite, kyanite, garnet, and biotite, as well as chert and BIF. The amphibolites comprise mafic volcanic rocks with intercalations of pelite and BIF. Late tonalite, granodiorite, gabbro, hornblendite and pyroxenite intrusions cut the sequences. Kuyumjian (1989) interprets an origin in an immature ocean-island arc that evolved to a back-arc basin. The basalts are similar to modern arc equivalents, while the granitoids are mantle derived, with minor crustal contamination. Viana et al. (1995) argue that the Chapada and Mara Rosa Sequences are geochemically and lithologically similar. The Chapada Cu-Au Deposit occurs within a wide, metamorphosed hydrothermal alteration zone in calc-alkaline basalts and dacites, intimately related to intrusive tonalites and diorites (Kuyumjian 1999).

The *Santa Terezinha Sequence*, of unknown precise age, is situated to the north of the Archean Crixás GB terranes. Souza & Leão Neto (1981) correlate the rocks with the Mara Rosa Sequence, while Machado (1981) interprets it as the top of the Crixás GB. Ribeiro Filho (1981) correlates it to the Mesoproterozoic Juscelândia, Coitezeiro, and Palmeirópolis Sequences. Owing to intense shear deformation, the stratigraphy is very complex. Biondi (1990) describes the most common rocks as chlorite-muscovite-quartz schists, interlayered with minor magnetite-muscovite schists, muscovite quartzite and chlorite-talc schist. The latter hosts one of Brazil's most important emerald deposits within carbonatised, chloritised and sericitised ultramafic rocks. The sequence formed in a turbiditic, deep-marine environment, with episodic felsic and ultramafic volcanism and related exhalative deposits (BIFs and chert).

Unknown age

Riacho dos Machados

The metavolcano-sedimentary Riacho dos Machados Group is part of the Araçuaí Fold Belt at the eastern margin of the São Francisco Craton. It is host to gold mineralization at the recently-closed Riacho dos Machados Mine (da Fonseca 1993). The sequence comprises ultramafic, mafic and acid volcanic rocks intercalated with pelites. The gold is shear zone-hosted and associated principally with a sulphide-bearing, quartz-muscovite schist, derived from the hydrothermal alteration of pelitic and quartz feldspathic schists. Dacitic and mafic/ultramafic rocks are of calc-alkaline and tholeiitic sub-alkaline association, respectively, compatible with their formation in an epi-continental volcanic arc (da Fonseca et al. 1997 and references therein). The pelites have textures and geochemical composition compatible with greywackes. The thrust faults that establish the regional architecture, and which host the gold mineralization, are related to a continental collision of unknown age between the precursor to the São Francisco Craton and the Guanambi-Correntina Block.

A more complex stratigraphy is inferred for less known parts of the volcano-sedimentary sequence to the north and south (Mourão et al. 1997, Noce et al. 1997, de Abreu & Belo de Oliveira 1998). In the extreme north, the Salobro sequence contains chemical sedimentary and acid volcanic rocks that host the eponymous massive sulphide occurrence.

Rio Paraúna, Serro - Alvorada de Minas, Pedro Pereira and others

Various greenstone-type associations are tectonically wedged within the Mesoproterozoic Espinhaço Supergroup and the Archean through Palaeoproterozoic, ortho- and paragneiss Guanhães Complex, off the eastern edge of the São Francisco Craton (Almeida Abreu 1993, Pedrosa-Soares et al. 1994, Baars 1997). Between Serro and Alvorada de Minas, Uhlein (1982) describes a complex, volcano-sedimentary sequence with important stratiform and pod-like chromite concentrations. Fogaça (1982) defines the volcano-sedimentary Rio Paraúna Supergroup near Diamantina. Other gneiss-hosted, tectonic slivers are poorly mapped in a discontinuous arcuate tract west and north of Guanhães town, near the limits of the eponymous tectonic complex (Baars 1997, Grossi Sad et al. 1997). The Pedro Pereira GB is hosted within the Archean Gouveia Complex (Machado et al. 1989).

Unfortunately, relatively little is known about the tectono-stratigraphic details of these narrow sequences, therefore turning impracticable any real evaluation of the potential for VMS mineralization on the basis of the same criteria used for the other GBs under evaluation.

IDENTIFIED VMS DEPOSITS AND SHOWINGS

This section briefly aims to describe the geology of the few known occurrences of VMS, base-metal deposits of the São Francisco Craton. Systematic exploration is lacking and it is notable that each one of the ten occurrences cited below are set in its own, geologically distinct, volcano-sedimentary environment. The contexts range from the Bico de Pedra Deposit hosted in Archean, felsic rocks of the mafic-dominated Nova Lima Group, to the Ribeirão da Folha showings hosted by Neoproterozoic ultramafic diopsidites and cherts of the sedimentary rock predominant Salinas Formation. This fundamentally underpins the assertion that the VMS potential in the selected sites is real, widespread and requires only focussed exploration and research efforts to be realised. Below, the ten known occurrences in the region under study are arranged in geographic, compass order, from north-east through south to north-west.

Mundo Novo Prospect, Mundo Novo, BA

During 1997, the CBPM undertook regional geological investigations of the region around the town of Mundo Novo, in epynomous GB, Bahia State (Mascarenhas & da Silva 1994). Preliminary geochemical and aerial geophysical surveillance, coupled with further detailing suggested an important metal potential for Zn and other base metals. Seven drill holes total 1700 m. One of the latest drilling intercepted a massive layer of about 8 m, averaging 15 % Zn and low Pb, Cu, Ag and Au, at a depth between 369 and 384 m. Another hole also intercepted a massive sulphide zone. It is 28 m thick, revealing an average grade of 7.2 % Zn, including a 9 m thick zone at 11.2 % Zn (CBPM, written communication). Significant polymetallic, VMS potential is inferred.

Ribeirão da Folha, Salinas Formation, MG

The VMS potential of the Salinas Formation is most forcefully founded upon the occurrence of pyrite-dominated, massive sulphide layers associated with chemical sedimentary rocks in the Ribeirão da Folha Facies (Pedrosa-Soares et al. 1992, Pedrosa-Soares 1995) and in the São João da Safira region (Neves & Ferreira 1999), to the south. In the former, disseminated sulphides are widespread, and metric, massive sulphide (pyrite, and less pyrrhotite and chalcopyrite) pods are typical of diopsidites. Field data presented above corroborate further VMS potential in the Salinas Formation, on the basis of metamorphosed hydrothermal alteration assemblages.

Salobro, Riacho dos Machados Group, MG

The Salobro Zn-Pb massive sulphide deposit is hosted by a ferruginous, siliceous horizon of the volcano-sedimentary Salobro Sequence, possible correlate of the Riacho dos Machados Group. De Abreu & Belo de Oliveira (1998) suggest that the deposit may represent a sedimentary-exhalative deposit. Nevertheless it is included here, since the published data are inconclusive with regard to the correct metallogenic classification.

The deposit is located about 15 km west of Porteirinha, Minas Gerais, in the Serra do Coco (Mourão et al. 1997). The base of the sequence is dominated by quartz schists, with varying amounts of amphibole, mica, chlorite and epidote, quartzites, locally conglomeratic, magnetite BIF, and levels rich in graphite and garnet (de Abreu & Belo de Oliveira 1998). The sulphide-rich horizon occurs within amphibole schist, of probable magmatic origin. Pyrrhotite, pyrite, sphalerite and chalcopyrite occur both as massive, centimetric to metric, banded horizons, and as breccia-disseminated ore. Textural evidence indicates that the former post-dates the disseminated mineralization. Quartz-sulphide breccias are also present. De Abreu & Belo de Oliveira (1998) report grades of 3.9 % Zn and 1.1 % Pb. The origin of the deposit is not clearly established or reported to date. Significant aluminous hydrothermal alteration features are described elsewhere, at São João da Safira (see above), in tectonic extensions of the Salinas Formation.

Cuieté Velho, Cuieté Velho Sequence, MG

Massive sulphide layers are reported (J.H. Grossi Sad, pers. comm., Mineração Cuieté Velho 1995) within calc-silicate rocks in abandoned mine adits, in the Cuieté Velho volcano-sedimentary sequence.

Bico de Pedra, Quadrilátero Ferrífero, MG

Borba (1998) describes the Au-Zn-Cu-Pb-Ag mineralization at Bico de Pedra, located in the Dom Bosco Syncline, southern Quadrilátero Ferrífero. It occurs along the sheared contact of the Palaeoproterozoic Itacolomi Group with the Nova Lima Group. The sulphide orebodies are hosted mainly in the trondhjemitic Bico de Pedra Aplite and mafic Nova Lima rocks, invariably close to their contact. Centi- to decimetre-thick orebodies dominate, but individual layers of up to 50 cm as well as a 2 m thick, densely mineralised ore zone have been described.

At deeper levels, gold is associated with Cu, and Zn and Pb are associated at shallower levels. The mineralization is characterised by sulphide-rich, mainly pyritic bands, concordant with the mylonitic foliation. The hydrothermal alteration of the aplite is marked by early sericite (after albite), carbonate and pyrite development, and later sulphidation with pyrite, pyrrhotite, chalcopyrite, and galena. Metallic bismuth occurs in the sulphides. Sphalerite and biotite are typical of the waning stage.

A total of 30,000 tonnes of sulphide ore at 1.45 g Au/t, 0.36 % Cu, 1.53 % Zn, 0.52 % Pb, and 44 g Ag/t are reported. Lyrio et al. (1976) and de Matos (1991) consider the mineralisation to be syngenetic with exhalative volcanism of Archean age. De Matos (1991) indicates that the volcano-sedimentary sequence was deposited in a back-arc environment.

Borba (1998) interprets the mineralization as shear-related, developed from a magmatic hydrothermal fluid during the Trans-Amazonian Event, which is to have been responsible for the trondhjemitic magmatism.

Alpinópolis, Alpinópolis Sequence, MG

Sixteen sulphide orebodies are identified by de Carvalho (1990) in the Alpinópolis GB on account of integrated geophysical, surface and subsurface geochemical, and drillcore geological data at a single one of various prospects in the area. Drilling has intersected massive- and disseminated-sulphide horizons. They constitute extremely deformed orebodies, with variable thicknesses between 1 and 4 m, concordant with the mylonitic foliation. The predominant lithological association of the mineralization is with sedimentary garnet-chlorite and sillimanite-biotite schists, and ferruginous quartzites. Some orebodies occur within ultramafic rocks.

Sulphides are similar independent of host rock association. In order of abundance, the minerals are pyrrhotite, with or without pentlandite solid solutions, pyrite, and minor sphalerite and chalcopyrite. Magnetite, chrome-magnetite, chromite and ilmenite constitute the oxides. The detected mineralizations are subeconomic at up to 0.4 % Zn, 0.3 % Cu and 0.15 % Ni.

De Carvalho (1990) and de Carvalho et al. (1992) suggest that these attenuated sulphide concentrations are distinct from the Ni-rich orebodies of the Fortaleza de Minas GB, registering evidence for their origin in ocean-floor, volcanogenic exhalative systems. They may be modelled, in an idealised GB-section, within the tholeiite to calc-alkaline transition, immediately above the ultrabasic section and below the sedimentary-rock-dominant section. The working hypothesis serves as a basis for further exploratory testing, both with regard to other known sulphide intersections and possible undiscovered orebodies. It would be crucial to investigate the nature of the metamorphic assemblages, in order to detect occult, aluminous hydrothermal alteration assemblages. The nature of the protoliths should be characterised, with a view to defining the nature of the possible VMS target too.

Bom Jardim de Goiás, Bom Jardim de Goiás Sequence, GO

The lower portion of the Bom Jardim de Goiás sequence hosts chalcopyrite-pyrite Cu-Au mineralization in chert layers near a dioritic pluton, within an intermediate to felsic volcanic and pyroclastic pile that overlies basalt. Seer (1985) characterises VMS-type lenticular mineralization with associated hydrothermal alteration.

Zacarias, Mara Rosa Sequence, GO

The Zacarias Gold Deposit occurs in the central belt of the Mara Rosa Sequence. The Au-only mineralization is volcanogenic, hosted in chert occurring within andesitic to basaltic, and locally 860 ± 8 Ma felsic volcanic rocks. The associated, massive barite is ubiquitous. One of the authors (H. Jost) describes the occurrence as a possible distal, Au-only, VMS system.

Palmeirópolis, Palmeirópolis Sequence, GO

The potential for VMS deposits in the three Mesoproterozoic, volcano-sedimentary sequences of Goiás and Tocantins is dictated by the occurrence of a Zn-Pb-Cu deposit with a 7 Mt reserve at Palmeirópolis. This reserve occurs in two orebodies averaging 3.5 % Zn, 0.9 % Pb, and 1.2 % Cu, and 6.7 % Zn, 1.5 % Pb, and 0.4 % Cu, respectively, and excludes a third orebody. The deposit was first announced by Figueiredo et al. (1981), with further description by Marques & Marques (1985), and detailed by Araújo (1986) and Araújo & Nilson (1988). It occurs close to the contact of amphibolites and intermediate to felsic volcanic rocks with the small, plagiogranitic Morro Solto Pluton. The orebodies overly a Cu-rich stringer ore enveloped by alteration haloes. The three orebodies are mineralogically similar and contain pyrrhotite and pyrite with associated sphalerite, chalcopyrite, and galena. The alteration haloes, studied in detail by Araújo et al. (1995, 1996b,c, 1998), are formed by an inner core of anthophyllite-biotite-cordierite-bearing rocks, followed by biotite-cordierite-rich rocks, and an outer rim of sericite-rich rocks (Araújo 2000, this volume).

Mina III, Crixás, GO

The gold-bearing massive sulphide deposit of Mina III was discovered by the end of the 1970's by a joint venture of Inco and Kenecott. Underground production at Mina III began at the end of the 1980's through Mineração Serra Grande S.A., a joint venture between Mineração Morro Velho S.A. (Anglo American Corp.) and INCO. Mina III is situated in the Crixás GB, about 3 km south of the town of Crixás. The authors emphasise the controversy regarding the true classification of the deposit. Many papers suggest an epigenetic, deformation-related origin (most recently, Fortes et al. 1997). The inclusion of the deposit here is aimed at proposing an alternative working model to account for certain descriptive features that are not compatible with the published hypothesis.

According to Yamaoka & Araújo (1988), Mina III contains orebodies that are subdivided into the main Upper and Lower Zones, and the minor Intermediate and Garnet Zones. The Upper Zone is a massive sulphide deposit, containing 5.2 Mt averaging 12.7 g Au/t. The Lower Zone consists of a gold-bearing quartz vein, 0.5 to 5.0 m thick, 500 m long along strike and 1200 m along plunge.

Kuyumjian (1981), Yamaoka et al. (1985), Thomson (1986, 1987, 1991), Yamaoka & Araújo (1988), Thomson & Fyfe (1990), Bettencourt et al. (1991), Fortes (1991, 1996), Magalhães (1991) have addressed the structural controls of the Mina III gold orebodies. There is a consensus that they are controlled by an east-vergent thrust fault. Queiroz (1995) describes the latter fault to be confined to a 5-km wide, WNW-trending transtensional belt of the northern portion of the Crixás GB. At the mine site, the high-strain foliation dips at 255/40, and the lineation-parallel orebodies plunge at 300/38. The local structure is delineated by the metamorphic foliation, and bedding is transposed in the north-westerly plunging, asymmetric Rio Vermelho Antiform (Magalhães 1991) whose axial plane dips at 037/80. Furthermore, the orebodies are contained in strained zones cross-cutting the stratigraphic sequence and metamorphic foliation, entrenching the notion that the mineralization is younger than the metamorphic peak and the structural overturning (Thomson & Fyfe 1990).

The country rocks of the massive sulphide lenses encompass carbonaceous schist, oolitic, laminated (possibly stromatolitic) and massive marble belonging to the Ribeirão das Antas Formation, and basalts of the Rio Vermelho Formation.

The Mina III Upper-Zone Deposit consists of an array of massive sulphide lenses 0.5 to 2.5 m thick, 50 to 200 m long along strike and up to 400 m along plunge. The lenses commonly contain 50 % to 90 % coarse arsenopyrite + pyrrhotite, in variable proportions, and parts contain only arsenopyrite or pyrrhotite. Other minerals are magnetite, ilmenite and chalcopyrite. The gangue is a fine to very fine association of quartz, plagioclase, carbonate, sericite, biotite, white mica, epidote and rutile. Gold occurs as irregular 5 to 10 μm flakes (locally up to tens of millimetres in diameter) as inclusions in arsenopyrite, ilmenite and quartz.

Locally the massive sulphide lenses grade into a dark grey to black, fine schist consisting of pyrrhotite and magnetite, with minor ilmenite, arsenopyrite and chalcopyrite, in a gangue of biotite, chlorite, quartz, sericite, carbonate, plagioclase, tremolite-actinolite, and garnet. In this case, gold is rare and occurs as fine inclusions in arsenopyrite.

The ore locally contains centimetric to decimetric, milky quartz veins, concordant or discordant with the local foliation. Where present within pyrrhotite-rich zones, the veins commonly have coarse arsenopyrite and may bear additional gold.

The massive sulphide lenses are intimately related to a rock assemblage with abundant Al- and Fe-rich minerals. These host rocks are grouped into quartz-chlorite-carbonate-muscovite schists, biotite-rich marbles, muscovite schist, chlorite-muscovite schists, and chlorite-garnet schists, in gradational relationships amongst themselves and the basalts. The schists are interpreted as metamorphosed hydrothermal products of basalt. In general, these schists occur on top of the massive sulphide lenses. Considering that the sequence is overturned, the alteration products were originally underneath the lenses, an important feature to the present interpretation of the origin of the ore.

The quartz-chlorite-carbonate-muscovite schists are light green and consist of fine to medium quartz, chlorite, Fe-dolomite, muscovite, and minor biotite, ilmenite, pyrrhotite, pyrite and arsenopyrite. The biotite marbles are light beige, massive to well foliated, and consist of Fe-dolomite, phlogopite, quartz, and white mica, with minor plagioclase, arsenopyrite, chlorite, and rutile. Their stable C- and O-isotope composition (Fortes 1996) is compatible with their origin as hydrothermal products. Muscovite schists and chlorite-muscovite schists are light-beige to silvery or green, and contain very fine muscovite, locally paragonite, and chlorite, with minor ilmenite, albite-oligoclase, quartz, biotite, chlorite, chloritoid, almandine, tourmaline, arsenopyrite, pyrrhotite, chalcopyrite and hematite. The chlorite-garnet schist (Garnet Ore Zone) is dark-green and contains almandine porphyroblasts up to 5 cm in diameter, and minor quartz, biotite, chloritoid, muscovite, grunerite, Fe-dolomite, plagioclase, epidote, ilmenite, hematite, arsenopyrite, pyrrhotite and chalcopyrite.

Primary fluid inclusions in the quartz of the gangue of the massive sulphide lenses (Fortes 1996) are somewhat complex and contain a variety of components. Isochoric curves of these early fluid inclusions indicate that trapping took place at a wide pressure interval, between 0.2 to 2.5 kbar, at a temperature range of 475° to 350°C. Late fluid inclusions are compositionally simple and ice melting homogenises to liquid between 107° and 222°C.

Yamaoka et al. (1985), and Yamaoka & Araújo (1988) interpret the Mina III orebodies in general as syngenetic, exhalative massive sulphide and chert (quartz vein) with further remobilisation by folding and shearing. Simultaneously, Thomson (1986) proposed that the ore formed by a post-metamorphic metasomatic process related to Neoproterozoic thrusting. From the end of the 1980's on, the literature adopted the epigenetic and thrust-related origin for all the Mina III orebodies, altering only minor details relative to Thomson's (1986) proposal. The prevailing consensus holds therefore that Neoproterozoic thrusting is a common control at all orebodies. Consequently, in recent years, all the Au-orebodies of the Crixás GB have been interpreted under one single thrust-related model, fundamentally directing exploration.

The literature about the gold deposits of the Crixás GB has however failed to account for the Al-Fe-rich, silicate hydrothermal alteration related to the massive sulphide lenses. While it represents a very distinctive feature in these lenses, it contrasts with the typical carbonate alteration associated with Au-rich quartz veins of the Lower Zone of Mina III. Carbonate alteration is also present at other nearby reserves, such as the disseminated ore zones of Mina Nova and Pompex. Peculiar features of the massive sulphide lenses also encompass (i) their composition, with pyrrhotite + arsenopyrite grading into magnetite-rich zones; (ii) their association with altered basalts; (iii) the extensive asymmetric gold-bearing hydrothermal alteration zones (Intermediate and Garnet Ore Zones); (iv) the alteration, in general stratigraphically underlying the sulphide lenses.

These combined features suggest that it may be more appropriate to model the massive sulphide lenses of Mina III as volcanogenic exhalative in origin. Late modification, in particular plunge control, by way of deformation would still hold true, as proposed by Yamaoka et al. (1985). Low base-metal concentrations in the Mina III massive sulphide deposit may be compatible features characteristic of the distal portions of either ophiolite–hosted, Type-3 deposits, or of mafic-siliciclastic, Type-4 deposits, such as those at Besshi, but with particularly low base-metal contents. The hypothesis should be tested on the basis of relative polymetallic concentrations, compared to the natural database of Franklin et al. (1998).

POTENTIAL FOR VMS-TYPE MINERALIZATIONS IN SÃO FRANCISCO GBS & VOLCANO-SEDIMENTARY SEQUENCES

Quantification of potential

The relative potential for the existence of a mineral substance in a given terrane can be semi-quantitatively estimated on the basis of appropriate, critical geological criteria (Adams 1985). The potential for VMS mineralization is estimated as a probability function of geological favourability and target maturity (MacKenzie 1996). From foregoing discussions, it is clear that geological favourability for VMS mineralization comprises evidence for (i) the existence of a heat source (ii) association with a semi-conformable, hydrothermal alteration zone with mineralization (iii) petrochemically appropriate, volcano-sedimentary rock sequence and/or (iv) appropriate age (Franklin et al. 1998, Barrie & Hannington 1999a, Sangster 1998).

Target maturity reflects the existing knowledge base in terms of quality of results and quantity (Adams 1985). The result is a relative measure of the geological potential of each terrane for VMS mineralization. Since the criteria for different VMS deposit types vary (Franklin et al. 1998), the VMS potential of a given terrane for each type varies accordingly. A database is currently being developed to measure these potentials in the volcano-sedimentary sequences of the São Francisco Craton. The preliminary results of this exercise must produce results that are compatible with the qualitative evaluation, presented in this paper, of the compared data for each volcano-sedimentary terrane. Until such time, as the qualitative and quantitative descriptive data presented in this broad overviewed are adequately synthesised into the comparative database, VMS potential can only truly be qualified for the entire São Francisco Craton and its marginal terranes. A semi-quantitative, relative estimate of VMS potentials in the host rocks of the broad study region, therefore, ensues as our next goal.

Qualification of geological potential

The known VMS occurrences in the studied region are concentrated in Archean, Meso- and Neoproterozoic sequences. The Salobro Deposit is mineralised in a sequence of unknown, Precambrian age. The early Meso- and Late-Neoproterozoic sequences also contain abundant evidence of the presence of local heat sources, relevant primary igneous textures, and some of the requisite hydrothermal alteration features. Significantly, the volcano-sedimentary successions are similar to many Phanerozoic VMS-hosting sequences, embodying a variety of nascent rift, back-arc and arc systems in intra-oceanic and especially epi-continental palaeo-environments.

The Archean sequences of Goiás also contain very well preserved sequences with a strong VMS potential. The Rio das Velhas, and Morro do Ferro GBs are, in contrast, pervasively deformed, obliterating much primary evidence of the origin of its volcano-sedimentary sequence. The Archean sequences of Bahia State appear to preserve many primary volcano-sedimentary textures, suggesting a greater potential for economic VMS-grade and -geometry preservation.

In the case of the Archean and Palaeoproterozoic of Bahia State, where recent exploration advances demand evaluation for investment prioritisation, the following broad proposals are made. The compilation of a whole range of geological and geophysical data from the different volcano-sedimentary sequences of central and northern São Francisco Craton confirm, in most cases, the presence of basalts and sedimentary rocks. Both of the latter rock sequences commonly reveal an ocean-floor affiliation, an important indicator of the metallogenic potential for VMS ore deposits. Amongst these, the Mundo Novo, Umburunas, Rio Itapicuru, Rio Salitre and Riacho de Santana GBs stand out as particularly favourable cases.

In other sequences of Bahia, characterised as intra- or epi-continental (Boquira, Licínio de Almeida-Urandi GBs) and even rift-type (Contendas-Mirante) basins, the existence of an oceanic, volcanic substratum is not unequivocally registered in the geochemical fingerprints of the volcano-sedimentary rocks. There too, the presence of cherts, Mn-rich and carbonate sedimentary rocks and BIFs, amongst others, is conspicuous, suggesting that critical processes of chemical and/or hydrothermal precipitation may have acted. The significance of these rocks should be investigated, case-by-case, in order to distinguish between volcanogenic-exhalative potential (polymetallic, Zn-rich, Type-5 VMS deposits) and sedimentary-rock-exhalative potential (large volume, Au-Cu-poor, polymetallic SEDEX deposits).

In general, the potential for bimodal, mafic-dominated (Type 1), ophiolitic (Type 3) and, perhaps, Besshi (Type 4) VMS deposits is greatest in the Archean GBs, such as Goiás and Quadrilátero Ferrífero GBs, as well as the Archean Bahia GBs. Significant potential also exists for the bimodal, felsic-dominated (Type 2) VMS deposits in the intermediate and upper sections of those GBs and of the Palaeoproterozoic sequences, including Riacho dos Machados and the numerous Palaeoproterozoic Bahian GBs. The potential for bimodal, siliciclastic (Type 5) VMS deposits in the Archean of Goiás is relatively high, given the importance of sedimentary-rock-dominated, volcano-sedimentary intercalations there. The same may be true for some of the Archean, sedimentary-rock-dominated GBs of Bahia, particularly in the western Gavião Block, the Guanambi-Corretina Block and the Sobradinho Domain.

Beyond the demonstrable Archean potential for VMS deposits, perhaps the most important preliminary conclusion of this contribution is the strong potential for VMS deposits, particularly Types 5 and 2, in the Meso- and Neoproterozoic sequences, borne out by the predominance of many occurrences there. While both Types 3 and 4 VMS deposits appear to occur in the restricted, yet diagnostic, exposures of intra-oceanic rocks, these sequences are overwhelmingly sedimentary in nature. This leads to two specific problems for the realisation and correct evaluation of this postulated tendency. First, traditional, Precambrian GB-based exploration efforts have focussed exclusively on the volcanic sequences, in particular in mafic and ultramafic rocks. The present analysis shows this prejudice to be unfounded under the given geological circumstances and the empirical criteria taken from a world-wide database. Second, both the Archean and Proterozoic sequences are generally metamorphosed under all facies conditions, from anchimetamorphic to granulitic. The recognition of, in particular, aluminous and ferromagnesian mineral assemblages and their distinction as either regional metamorphic or originally hydrothermal (metamorphosed) is critical. Both weathering decomposition and the preferred, often precipitated, attribution of an exclusively regional metamorphic origin to minerals like the alumino-silicate polymorphs, garnet, cordierite and biotite, can seriously hamper field observation.

This problem is illustrated in the case of the Mateus Leme – Pitangui Belt, Rio das Velhas GB, cited above. Romano's (1993) meticulous description permits the reader to visualise a regional hydrothermal alteration system, be it volcanogenic or post-volcanic. At slightly higher metamorphic grades, the ubiquitous aluminous assemblages and their field relationships would readily be overlooked as reflecting an exclusively regional metamorphic origin. This suggestion remits one, for example, to the case of the Salinas Group, at São José da Safira. Kyanite-muscovite schist occurs in association with anthophyllitic serpentinised, or carbonate-diopsiditic ultramafic slivers, and BIF. Careful analysis shows that the respective kyanite-muscovite, anthophyllite and carbonate-diopside assemblages bear no relationship to the regional Barrovian field metamorphic profile. Teixeira and Kuyumjian (1991) apply the hot-spring alteration model to explain the high-Al alteration assemblage in the Mateus Leme-Pitangui area. They consider the subvolcanic granite at Pará de Minas as the best heat source for this ancient volcanogenic system. The authors relate the presence of gold-antimony mineralizations in the Pitangui region to this system.

As indicated by Hannington et al. (1999), in more felsic-volcanic areas (Type 2, and possibly Type 5 VMS deposits), and particularly in deposits that formed at volcaniclastic-dominant, shallow seawater depths (< ~1500 m), Na depletion and aluminous assemblages (kaolinite, andalusite, kyanite, pyrophyllite, diaspore, chloritoid, corundum) characterise much of the paraconformable hydrothermal alteration associated with these deposits. In the past, shallow-water environments were considered largely non-prospective for VMS, owing to effects of boiling on high-temperature hydrothermal fluids, and the tendency for metals to be deposited in vertically, extensive, sub-sea floor stockworks rather than as massive sulphides on the sea floor. The occurrence of highly cation-depleted aluminium silicates, like in high sulphidation epithermal systems, seem to reflect alteration by acidic hydrothermal fluids generated (i) by phase separation of a boiling hydrothermal fluid; (ii) by alteration at high water/rock ratios of an evolved seawater hydrothermal fluid, or (iii) by possible incorporation of magmatically-generated ore fluids (see Gibson et al. 1999). According to Hannington et al. (1999), where magmatic volatiles are involved the acidic nature of hydrothermal solutions promotes advanced, high-Al, argillic alteration, and the formation of a unique assemblage of Cu-Fe sulphides (e.g. enargite, luzonite, tennantite, bornite-pyrite, covellite), similar to that associated with high-sulphidation epithermal Au-Cu deposits. This gives rise to the application of a 'high-sulphidation' model to some gold-rich, shallow-water VMS (Sillitoe et al. 1996).

In the light of these data, emphasis should be placed on the appropriate characterisation of the potential of Archean and Proterozoic sequences in terms of necessary, VMS-controlling factors. Much, semi-detailed and regional mapping is required, together with urgent sequence stratigraphy and sufficient geochemical fingerprinting. Appropriate definition of existing occurrence types is lacking, and will surely assist objectively in the search for other, economically important VMS deposits.

ACKNOWLEDGEMENTS

This review has been made possible due to continued financial support of Conselho Nacional Científico e Tecnológico-CNPq, PADCT and FAPEMIG. The GAC is thanked for its support of the present volume. Earlier, regionally separate versions of this contribution (Lobato et al. 1998, 1999) were presented at a CAPES-PADCT/ADIMB meeting in Salvador in September 1998 (Misi & da Silva 1998) and published by the Ministério de Minas e Energia/Companhia de Pesquisa de Recursos Minerais/Departamento Nacional da Produção Mineral for a PDAC'99 promotional stand. We thank the CAPES-PADCT organ (LML, MdGdS), as well as the companies Companhia Vale do Rio Doce-Docegeo (FJB) and CBPM (JCC), for their sponsorship of authors' participation in the former event and thereby ultimately stimulating the present analysis. The authors are particularly grateful to and commend the parastatal CBPM for placing much data in the public medium, allowing for more objective evaluations of the geological terranes under its auspices. JCC is indebted to that company for permission to participate in the present effort. SGC performed much of his research with the financial assistance of FAPESP and the permission and logistical assistance of Rio Tinto subsidiary companies, to whom both he is grateful. LML and FJB thank Dr. David Sangster for his inspiring review of an early version of the manuscript referring to the southern portion of the São Francisco Craton and the VMS review. We are grateful to the volume editor Ross Sherlock (SRK Inc.) for his persistence and co-ordination of the present publication, which we hope will provide both new stimulus for investments in base-metal exploration in Latin America, in particular in Brazil's São Francisco Craton, as well as a useful review of VMS-related topics for students and researchers.

REFERENCES

de Abreu, F.R. and Belo de Oliveira, O.A. 1998. Geologia e ocorrências de zinco e chumbo do Prospecto Salobro, Porteirinha, MG. In Anais do 40o Congresso Brasileiro de Geologia, Sociedade Brasileira de Geologia, Núcleo de Minas Gerais, Boletim 15, pp. 140.

Adams, S.S. 1985. Using geological information to develop exploration strategies for epithermal deposits. In Geology and Geochemistry of Epithermal Systems. Edited by B.R. Berger and P.M. Bethke. Society of Economic Geology, Reviews in Economic Geology, Vol. 2, pp. 273-298.

de Almeida, F.F.M. and Hasui Y. (Editors) 1984. O Pré-Cambriano do Brasil. Edgard Blücher, São Paulo.

Almeida Abreu, P.Â. 1993. A evolução geodinâmica da Serra do Espinhaço Meridional, Minas Gerais, Brasil. Ph.D. thesis, Freiburg Universität, Freiburg, Germany.

Alves da Silva, F.C. and Matos, F.M.V. 1991. Economic geology and structural controls of the orebodies from the medium Itapicuru gold district. In Proceedings of Gold '91, the Economics, Geology, Geochemistry and Genesis of Gold Deposits. Edited by E.A. Ladeira. A.A. Balkema, Rotterdam, pp. 629-635.

Amaro, V.E. 1989. Geologia e petrologia da seqüência metavulcânica de Jaupaci - GO e lineamentos associados. M.Sc. dissertation, Universidade de Brasília, Brasília, Brazil.

Arantes, D., Osborne, G.A., Buck, O.S. and Porto C.G. 1991. The Mara Rosa Volcano-Sedimentary Sequence and Associated Gold Mineralization. In Proceedings of Gold '91, the Economics, Geology, Geochemistry and Genesis of Gold Deposits. Edited by E.A. Ladeira. A.A. Balkema, Rotterdam, pp. 221-229.

Araújo, S.M. 1986. Petrologia e mineralizações sulfetadas da seqüência vulcano-sedimentar de Palmeirópolis, GO. M.Sc. dissertation, Universidade de Brasília, Brasília, Brazil.

Araújo, S.M. 2000. The Palmeirópolis Deposit, Tocantins State, Brazil: a typical metamorphosed volcanogenic massive sulfide deposit. In VMS Deposits of Latin America (this volume). Edited by R. Sherlock and A.Logan. Geological Association of Canada, Toronto.

Araújo, V.A. and Alves, A.C. 1979. Projeto Canabrava-Posto Real. Departamento Nacional de Produção Mineral / Companhia de Pesquisa de Recursos Minerais, Goiânia, Relatório Final.

Araújo, S.M. and Nilson, A.A. 1988. Depósito de zinco, cobre e chumbo de Palmeirópolis, Goiás. In Principais Depósitos Minerais do Brasil. Edited by C. Schobbenhaus Filho and C.E.S. Coelho. Ministério de Minas e Energia / Departamento Nacional de Produção Mineral / Companhia Vale do Rio Doce, Vol. 3, pp. 171-180.

Araújo, S.M., Fawcett, J.J. and Scott, S.D. 1995. Metamorphism of hydrothermally altered rocks in a volcanogenic massive sulfide deposit: the Palmeirópolis, Brazil example. Revista Brasileira de Geociências, 25: 173-184.

Araújo, S.M., Gorton, M.P. and Scott, S.D. 1996a. Os anfibolitos enriquecidos em elementos traços da seqüência vulcano-sedimentar de Palmeirópolis, Tocantins: uma ferramenta na prospecção de metais básicos na região. In Anais do 39o Congresso Brasileiro Geologia, Sociedade Brasileira de Geologia, Núcleo de Bahia - Sergipe, Volume 3, pp. 178-180.

Araújo, S.M., Longstaffe, F.J. and Scott, S.D. 1996b. Effects of the high-grade metamorphism on the oxygen isotope composition of the alteration zones associated with the Palmeirópolis volcanogenic massive sulfide deposit, Tocantins State, Brazil. In Anais do 39o Congresso Brasileiro Geologia, Sociedade Brasileira de Geologia, Núcleo de Bahia / Sergipe, Volume 7, pp. 339-342.

Araújo, S.M., Scott, S.D. and Gorton, M.P. 1998. Protoliths of highly metamorphosed, hydrothermally altered rocks of the Palmeirópolis volcanogenic massive sulfide deposit, Brazil. Journal of South American Earth Sciences. In press.

Araújo, S.M., Scott, S.D. and Longstaffe, F.J. 1996c. Oxygen isotope composition of alteration zones of highly metamorphosed volcanogenic massive sulfide deposits: Geco, Canada and Palmeirópolis, Brazil. Economic Geology, 91: 697-712.

Artur, A.C., Wernick, E. and Kawashita, K. 1990. Migmatização policíclica do sul de Minas Gerais e áreas adjacentes do Estado de São Paulo: Caracterização estrutural/petrográfica e dados geocronológicos. In Anais do 36o Congresso Brasileiro de Geologia. Sociedade Brasileira de Geologia, Vol. 6, 2827-2842.

Ávila, C.A. 1992. Geologia, petrografia e geoquímica das rochas intrusivas Pré-Cambrianas (Unidade Metadiorítica Ibitutinga e Unidade Metatrondhjemítica Caburu) nas rochas do Greenstone Belt Barbacena, São João d'el Rei, Minas Gerais. M.Sc. dissertation, Universidade Federal do Rio de Janeiro, Rio de Janeiro, Brazil.

Baars, F.J. 1997. The São Francisco Craton. In Greenstone Belts. Edited by M.J. de Wit and L.D. Ashwal. Clarendon Press, Oxford, Chapt. 5.5, 529-557.

Baars, F.J. 2000 (in prep.). The tectonic evolution of the southern São Francisco Craton: tectonostratigraphic, geochronological and geochemical Aspects. Ph.D. Dissertation. University of Cape Town, Cape Town, South Africa.

Baltazar, O.F. and Pedreira, A.J. 1998. Associações litofaciológicas. In Projeto Rio das Velhas – Mapa Geológico Integrado, Escala 1:100.000, e Texto Explicativo. Edited by M. Zucchetti and O.F. Baltazar. Departamento Nacional de Produção Mineral / Companhia de Pesquisa de Recursos Minerais – Belo Horizonte, CD-ROM, pp. 43-48.

Barbosa, J.S.F. 1996. O embasamento arqueano e proterozóico inferior do Estado da Bahia. In Geologia da Bahia: texto explicativo para o mapa geológico ao milionésimo. Edited by J.S.F. Barbosa and J.M.L. Dominguez. Superintendência de Geologia e Recursos Minerais, Secretaria da Industria, Comércio e Mineração do Estado da Bahia, Salvador.

Barbosa, J.S.M. and Dominguez, J.M.L. 1996. Geologia da Bahia - Texto Explicativo. Superintendência de Geologia e Recursos Minerais do Estado da Bahia, Salvador.

Barbosa, P.A.R. 1987. Geologia e recursos minerais das seqüências supracrustais à leste de Mossâmedes-GO. M.Sc. dissertation, Universidade de Brasília, Brasília, Brazil.

Barley, M.E. 1992. A review of Archean volcanic-hosted massive sulfide and sulfide mineralization in Western Australia. Economic Geology, 87: 855-872.

Barley, M.E. and Groves, D.I. 1992. Supercontinent cycles and the distribution of metal deposits through time. Geology 20, 291-294.

Barrie, C.T. and Hannington, M.D. 1999a. Classification of VMS deposits based on host rock compositions. In Volcanic-associated Massive Deposits: Processes and Examples in Modern and Ancient Settings. Edited by C.T. Barrie and M.D. Hannington. Society of Economic Geologists, Reviews in Economic Geology, Vol. 8, 1-11.

Barrie, C.T. and Hannington, M.D. (Editors) 1999b. Volcanic-associated Massive Deposits: Processes and Examples in Modern and Ancient Settings. Society of Economic Geologists, Reviews in Economic Geology, Vol. 8.

Barrie, C.T., Ludden, N.J. and Green, T.H. 1993. Geochemistry of volcanic rocks associated with Cu-Zn and Ni-Cu deposits in the Abitibi Subprovince. Economic Geology, 88: 1341-1358.

Bettencourt, J.S., Costa, A.R., Souza, L.H. and Matos, T.T. 1991. Controls of gold mineralization in the Córrego Geral Sector, north central section of the Crixás greenstone belt: a preliminary report. In Proceedings of Gold '91, the Economics, Geology, Geochemistry and Genesis of Gold Deposits. Edited by E.A. Ladeira. A.A. Balkema, Rotterdam, pp. 699-703

Biondi, J.C. 1990. Depósitos de esmeralda de Santa Terezinha (GO). Revista Brasileira de Geociências 20: 7-24.

Borba, R.P. 1998. O Magmatismo Ácido e sua Relação com a Mineralização Aurífera de Bico de Pedra, Greenstone Belt Rio das Velhas, Quadrilátero Ferrífero, Minas Gerais. M.Sc. dissertation, Universidade Estadual de Campinas, Campinas, Brazil.

Brenner, T.L., Teixeira, N.A., Oliveira, J.A.L., Franke, N.D. and Thompson, J.F.H. 1990. The O'Toole Nickel Deposit, Morro do Ferro Greenstone Belt, Brazil. Economic Geology, 85: 904-920.

de Brito Neves, B.B., Cordani, U.G. and Torquato, J.R.F. 1980. Evolução geocronológica do Precambriano do Estado da Bahia. In Geologia e Recursos Minerais do Estado da Bahia. Secretaria de Minas e Energia do Estado da Bahia, Coordenação da Produção Mineral, Salavador, Textos Básicos No. 3, pp. 1-125.

Brod, J.A. 1988. Geologia das rochas vulcano-sedimentares da região de Indaianópolis, GO, e lineamentos adjacentes. M.Sc. dissertation, Universidade de Brasília, Brasília., Brazil.

Brueckner, H., Cunningham, W.D. Alkmim, F.F. and Marshak, S. 1998. Implications of new Precambrian Sm-Nd dates from the Quadrilátero Ferrífero and adjacent Araçuaí Orogen. In Abstracts of the 14th International Conference on Basement Tectonics. International Basement Tectonics Association - Universidade Federal de Ouro Preto, 24-25.

Campbell, I.H., Coad, P. and Franklin, J.M. 1982. Rare earth element in volcanic rocks association with Cu-Zn massive sulphide mineralogy: a preliminary report. National Research Council of Canada, Ottawa, Vol. 19, pp. 619-623.

Campbell, I.H., Franklin, J.M., Gorton, M.P., Hart, T.R. and Scott, S.D. 1981. The role of subvolcanic sills in the generation of massive sulfide deposits. Economic Geology 76: 2248-2253.

Carneiro, M.A. 1992. O Complexo Metamórfico Bonfim Setentrional (Quadrilátero Ferrífero, Minas Gerais): litoestratigrafia e evolução geológica de um segmento de crosta continental Arqueana. Ph.D. thesis, Universidade de São Paulo, São Paulo, Brazil.

Carvalho, I.G. 1982. Considerações sobre o quadro geotectônico do distrito de Boquira, estado da Bahia. In Anais do 32o Congresso Brasileiro de Geologia. Sociedade Brasileira de Geologia, Núcleo de Bahia – Sergipe, Vol. 1, pp. 234-245.

de Carvalho, S.G. 1990. Geologia, petrologia e metalogenia da seqüência vulcano-sedimentar de Alpinópolis, Minas Gerais. Ph.D. thesis, Universidade de São Paulo, São Paulo, Brazil.

de Carvalho, S.G. 2000 (in prep.) Structural controls of the deformed and metamorphosed komatiite-associated Fortaleza de Minas Ni-Cu-Co Deposit, Minas Gerais, Brazil.

de Carvalho, S.G., Antônio, M.C. and Brenner, T.L. 1999. A atuação de processos tectono-metamórficos e seus efeitos modificadores na jazida de sulfeto maciço de Fortaleza de Minas: Implicações na tipologia, teores e quimismo do minério. In Anais do 5o Congresso de Geoquímica dos Países de Língua Portuguesa e 7o Congresso Brasileiro de Geoquímica. Sociedade Brasileira de Geoquímica, pp. 246-248.

de Carvalho, S.G., Soares, P.C. and Barbour, A.P. 1992. Mineralizações nos terrenos granito-greenstone de Alpinópolis e Fortaleza de Minas. Universidade Estadual Paulista, Geociências, 11: 19-47.

Cassedane, J.P. 1972. Catalogue déscriptif des gîtes de plomb du Brésil. Ph.D. thesis, Université de Clermont-Ferrand, Clermont-Ferrand, France.

Condie, K.C. (Editor) 1994. Archean Crustal Evolution. Elsevier, Amsterdam, Developments in Precambrian Geology, No. 11.

Correia, C.T. 1994. Petrologia do Complexo Máfico-Ultramáfico de Cana Brava. Ph.D. thesis, Universidade de São Paulo, São Paulo, Brazil.

Correia, C.T., Girardi, V.A.V., Tassinari, C.C.G. and Jost, H. 1997. Rb-Sr and Sm-Nd geochronology of the Cana Brava layered mafic-ultramafic intrusion, Brazil, and considerations regarding its tectonic evolution. Revista Brasileira de Geociências, 27: 163-168.

Costa, A.G., Rosière, C.A., de Moreira, L. and Fichel, D.P. 1995. Caracterização geotectônica do setor setentrional da Faixa Ribeira: Evidência de acresção neoproterozóica no leste de Minas Gerais, Brasil. Geonomos – Universidade Federal de Minas Gerais, 3: 51-68.

Costa, J.B.S. 1984. Aspectos litoestruturais e evolução crustal da região centro-norte de Goiás. Ph.D. thesis, Universidade Federal do Pará, Belém, Brazil.

Cruz, E.L.C.C. 1993. Geologia e mineralizações auríferas do terreno granitóide-greenstone de Almas-Dianópolis, Tocantins. M.Sc. dissertation, Universidade de Brasília, Brasília.

Cruz, E.L.C.C. and Kuyumjian, R.M. 1994. Um possível controle metamórfico para as mineralizações auríferas de Almas-Dianópolis-TO. In Resumos Expandidos do 4o Simpósio de Geologia do Centro-Oeste. Sociedade Brasileira de Geologia, Núcleo do Centro-Oeste, pp. 43-46.

Cunha, J.C.C. 1996 (Restricted). Prospecto Jurema-Oeste / Alvo Boa Sombra: Relatório Interno. Companhia Baiana de Pesquisa Mineral, Salvador.

Cunha, J.C.C. and Fróes, R.J.B. 1994. Komatiitos com textura spinifex do Greenstone Belt de Umburanas, Bahia. Companhia Baiana de Pesquisa Mineral, Série Arquivos Abertos, No. 7.

Cunha, J.C.C., Lopes, O.A.C., Fróes, R.J.B., Oliveira, N.S. and Santana, E.A.N. 1994. Projeto Ibitira-Brumado: Relatório Final. Companhia Baiana de Pesquisa Mineral, Salvador.

Dalton de Souza, J. and Teixeira, L.R. 1981. Prospecto Rio Salitre: Geologia e prospecção geoquímica preliminar no Complexo Rio Salitre: Relatório Final. Companhia de Pesquisa de Recursos Minerais / Secretaria de Minas e Energia do Estado da Bahia, Salvador.

Dalton de Souza, J., Fernandes Filho, J., Guimarães, J.T. and Lopes, J.N. 1979. Projeto Colomi: Geologia da Região do Médio São Francisco: Relatório Final. Companhia de Pesquisa de Recursos Minerais / Departamento Nacional de Produção Mineral, Salvador, Vol. 1.

Danni, J.C.M. and Leonardos Jr., O.H. 1980. Granulite ultrametamorphism and deformation in ancient composite layered intrusion: The Niquelândia Complex, Brazil. In Extended Abstracts of the 26th International Geological Congress. International Union of Geological Sciences, Paris, Vol. 1, pp. 35.

Danni, J.C.M. and Ribeiro C.C. 1978. Caracterização estratigráfica da seqüência vulcano-sedimentar de Pilar de Goiás e de Guarinos, Goiás. In Anais do 30o Congresso Brasileiro de Geologia. Sociedade Brasileira de Geologia, Núcleo do Nordeste, Vol. 2, pp. 582-596.

Danni, J.C.M., Dardenne, M.A. and Fuck, R.A. 1981. Geologia da região de Goiás (GO): O "Greenstone Belt" da Serra Santa Rita e a Seqüência Serra do Cantagalo. In Atas do 1o Simpósio de Geologia do Centro-Oeste. Sociedade Brasileira de Geologia, Núcleo do Centro-Oeste, pp. 265-280.

Danni, J.C.M., Fuck, and Leonardos Jr., O.H. 1982. Archean and Lower Proterozoic units in central Brazil. Geologische Rundschau, 71: 291-317.

Dias Lima, J.A., Oliveira, J.E., Costa, I.V.G., Bomfim, L.F.C., Barral, N.M. and Santos, R.A. 1981. Projeto Aracaju: Relatório de Fase I. Departamento Nacional de Produção Mineral / Companhia de Pesquisa de Recursos Minerais, Brasília.

Divi, S.R., Thorpe, R.I. and Franklin, J.M. 1979. Application of discriminant analysis to evaluate compositional controls of stratiform massive sulfide deposits in Canada.

Mathematical Geology, 11: 391-406.

Dorr II, J.V.N. 1969. Physiographic, stratigraphic and structural development of the Quadrilátero Ferrífero, Minas Gerais. United States Geological Survey, Professional Paper 641-A.

Dürkop, C. 1994. Geologische Feldkartierung und petrologisch-petrographisch–geochemische Unteruchungen an Gesteienen de "Dom Silvério Gruppe" in Minas Gerais, Brasilien. Graduation dissertation, Bonn Universität, Bonn, Germany.

Dürkop, C., Linder, B. and Jordt Evangelista, G.H. 1997. Caracterização petrológica e geoquímica do Grupo Dom Silvério no seu local tipo, região de Dom Silvério, MG. In Anais do 9o Simpósio de Geologia de Minas Gerais. Sociedade Brasileira de Geologia, Núcleo de Minas Gerais, Boletim 14, 105-106.

Ferrari, M.A.D. and Chouhuri, A. 1999a. Tectônica e mineralização aurífera da Mina Córrego do Paiol, Almas – TO. In Anais do 7o Simpósio Nacional de Estudos Tectônicos. Sociedade Brasileira de Geologia, Núcleo de Bahia - Sergipe, pp. 34-36.

Ferrari, M.A.D. and Choudhuri, A. 1999b. Variações químicas nas rochas vulcânicas do greenstone belt de Almas – TO. In Anais do 5o Congresso de Geoquímica dos Países de Língua Portuguesa e 7o Congresso Brasileiro de Geoquímica. Sociedade Brasileira de Geoquímica, pp. 492-494.

Ferreira Filho, C.F. 1995. Petrologia do Complexo Máfico-Ultramáfico Acamadado de Niquelândia: Uma re-interpretação à luz dos novos dados petroquímicos. In Resumos Expandidos do 5o Simpósio Geologia do Centro-Oeste. Sociedade Brasileira de Geologia, Núcleo do Centro-Oeste, 105-107.

Ferreira Filho, C.F., Kamo, S., Fuck, R.A., Krogh, T.E. and Naldrett, A.J. 1994. Zircon and rutile U-Pb geochronology of the Niquelândia layered mafic and ultramafic intrusion, Brazil: constraints for the timing of magmatism and high grade metamorphism. Precambrian Research, 68: 241-255.

Figueiredo, J.A., Leão Neto, R. and Valente, C.R. 1981. Depósitos de sulfetos maciços de Zn, Cu, e Pb da região de Palmeirópolis, GO. In Atas do 1o Simpósio Geologia do Centro-Oeste. Sociedade Brasileira de Geologia, Núcleo do Centro-Oeste, 422-441.

Fleischer, R. and Espourteille, F.E. 1998. The Boquira Lead-Zinc Mine in central Bahia, Brazil. In Base Metal Deposits of Brazil. Edited by M.d.G. da Silva and A. Misi. Ministério de Minas e Energia / Companhia de Pesquisa de Recursos Minerais / Departamento Nacional de Produção Mineral, Belo Horizonte, 44-53.

Fogaça, A.C.C. 1982. Geologia e mineralizações auríferas na região de Costa Sena, MG: Uma abordagem preliminar. Graduation report, Universidade de Brasília, Brasília, Brazil.

da Fonseca, E. 1993 Depósito aurífero de Riacho dos Machados, norte de Minas Gerais: Hidrotermalismo, deformação e mineralização associados. M.Sc. dissertation, Universidade Federal de Minas Gerais, Belo Horizonte, Brazil.

da Fonseca, E., Lobato, L.M. and Baars, F.J. 1997. The petrochemistry of the auriferous, volcanosedimentary Riacho dos Machados Group, central-eastern Brazil: geotectonic implications for shear-hosted gold mineralization. Journal of South American Earth Sciences, 10: 423-443.

Fortes, P.T.F.O. 1991. Geologia do depósito aurífero Mina III, Crixás, Goiás. M.Sc. dissertation, University of Brasília, Brasília, Brazil.

Fortes, P.T.F.O. 1996. Metalogenia dos depósitos auríferos Mina III, Mina Nova e Mina Inglesa, Greenstone Belt de Crixás, Goiás. Ph.D. thesis, University of Brasília, Brasília, Brazil.

Fortes, P.T.F.O., Pimentel, M.M. and Teixeira W. 1993. Geocronologia Rb/Sr das rochas encaixantes do depósito aurífero Mina III and Goiás. In Resumos Expandidos do 4o Congresso Brasileiro de Geoquímica. Sociedade Brasileira de Geoquímica, pp. 250-252.

Fortes, P.T.F.O, Cheilletz, A., Giuliani, G. and Féraud, G. 1997. A Brasiliano age (500 ± 5 Ma) for the Mina III gold deposit, Crixás Greenstone Belt, Central Brazil. International Geology Review, 39: 449-460.

Franco, H.A.F., Campos J.E.G. and Danni J.C.M. 1994. A Seqüência Vulcano-Sedimentar Iporá/Amorinópolis: Uma contribuição. In Anais do 38o Congresso Brasileiro de Geologia. Sociedade Brasileira de Geologia, Vol. 2, 108-109.

Franklin, J.M., Hannington M.D., Jonasson I.R. and Barrie C.T. 1998. Arc-related volcanogenic massive sulphide deposits. In Metallogeny of Volcanic Arcs. Coordinated by D.V. Lefebure. British Columbia Geological Survey, 1998 Cordilleran and Pathways 1998 Conference, Vancouver, Fascicules N1-32.

Freitas, M.E. 1994. Hidrotermalismo na região de Vianópolis, Goiás. M.Sc. dissertation, Universidade de Brasília, Brasília, Brazil.

Freitas, M.E. and Kuyumjian, R.M. 1995. Variação química das micas durante o hidrotermalismo peraluminoso de Vianópolis, GO. Sociedade Brasileira de Geologia, Núcleo do Centro-Oeste, Boletim de Geociências do Centro-Oeste, No. 18, pp. 44-56.

Frizzo, C., Takai, V. and Scarpelli, W. 1991. Auriferous mineralization at Pitangui, Minas Gerais. In Proceedings of GOLD'91: the Economics, Geology, Geochemistry and Genesis of Gold Deposits. Edited by E.A. Ladeira. A.A. Balkema, Rotterdam, pp. 579-583.

Fuck, R.A. 1994. A Faixa Brasília e a compartimentação tectônica na Província Tocantins. In Resumos Expandidos do 4o Simpósio de Geologia do Centro-Oeste. Sociedade Brasileiro de Geologia, Núcleo do Centro-Oeste, pp. 184-187.

Fuck, R.A. and Pimentel, M.M. 1990. Geocronologia de rochas gnáissicas da área de Mossâmedes-Sanclerlândia, Goiás. In Resumos Expandidos do 36o Congresso Brasileira Geologia. Sociedade Brasileira de Geologia, Núcleo do Nordeste, pp. 333.

Fuck, R.A., Danni, J.M.C., Winge, M., Andrade, G.F., Barreira, C.F., Leonardos Jr., O.H. and Kuyumjian, R.M. 1981. Geologia da região de Goianésia. In Atas do 1o

Simpósio de Geologia do Centro-Oeste. Sociedade Brasileira de Geologia, Núcleo do Centro-Oeste, pp. 447-467.

Fuck, R.A., de Brito Neves, B.B., Cordani, U.G. and Kawashita, K. 1989. Geocronologia Rb-Sr no Complexo de Barro Alto, Goiás: Evidências de metamorfismo de alto grau e colisão continental há 1.300 Ma. no Brasil Central. Geochimica Brasiliensis, 3: 125-140.

Fugi, M. 1989. REE Geochemistry and Sm/Nd geocronology of the Cana Brava Complex - Brazil. M.Sc. dissertation, Kobe University, Kobe, Japan.

Gaál, G., Teixeira, J.B.G., d'el Rey Silva, J.L.H. and da Silva, M.da G. 1987. Early Proterozoic crustal evolution and metallogenesis, northwestern Bahia, Brazil. Transcript of a lecture proferred at the International Symposium on Granites and Metallogenesis, Salvador, October 1987. Sociedade Brasileira de Geologia, Núcleo de Bahia – Sergipe.

Gaskarth, J.W. and Parslow, G.R. 1987. Proterozoic volcanism in the Flin Flon greenstone belt, east-central Saskatchewan, Canada. In Geochemistry and Mineralization of Proterozoic Volcanic Suites. Edited by T.C. Pharoah, R.D. Beckinsdale and D. Rickard. Blackwell Scientific Publications, Oxford, pp. 183-200.

Gibson, H., Morton, R.L. and Hudak, G.J. 1999. Submarine volcanic processes, deposits, and environments favorable for the location of volcanic-associated massive sulfide deposits. In Volcanic-associated Massive Deposits: Processes and Examples in Modern and Ancient Settings. Edited by C.T. Barrie and M.D. Hannington. Society of Economic Geologists, Reviews in Economic Geology, Vol. 8, pp. 13-51.

Girardi, V.A.V., Rivalenti, G. and Sinigoi, S. 1986. The petrogenesis of the Niquelândia layered mafic-ultramafic complex, Central Brazil. Journal of Petrology, 27: 715-744.

Girardi, V.A.V., Kawashita, K., Basei, M.A.S. and Cordani, U.G. 1978. Algumas considerações sobre a evolução geológica da região de Cana Brava, a partir de dados geocronológicos. In Anais do 30o Congresso Brasileiro de Geologia. Sociedade Brasileira de Geologia, Núcleo do Nordeste, pp. 337-347.

Gomes, F.C.A., Kwitko, R. and Nascimento, H.S. 1998. Caracterização da seqüência metavulcanossedimentar e alteração associada na região de Lagoa do Gato, Distrito Aurífero de Fazenda Brasileiro – BA. In Anais do 40o Congresso Brasileiro de Geologia. Sociedade Brasileira de Geologia, Núcleo de Minas Gerais, Boletim 15, pp. 125.

Grossi Sad, J.H., Lobato, L.M., Pedrosa-Soares, A.C. and Soares Filho, B.S. (Co-ordinators). 1997. Projeto Espinhaço em CD-ROM (textos e anexos). Companhia Mineradora de Minas Gerais, Belo Horizonte.

Groves, D.I. and Barley, M.E. 1994. Archean Mineralization. In Archean Crustal Evolution. Edited by K.C. Condie. Elsevier, Amsterdam, pp. 461-504.

Hannington, M.D., Poulsen, K.H., Thompson, J.F.H. and Sillitoe, R.H. 1999. Volcanogenic gold in the massive sulfide environment In Volcanic-associated Massive Deposits: Processes and Examples in Modern and Ancient Settings. Edited by C.T. Barrie and M.D. Hannington. Society of Economic Geologists, Reviews in Economic Geology, Vol. 8, pp. 325-356.

Hasui, Y. and de Almeida, F.F.M. 1970. Geocronologia do Centro-Oeste brasileiro. Boletim da Sociedade Brasileira Geologia, 19: 5-26.

Hasui, Y., Haralyi, N.L.E. and Costa, J.B.S. 1993. A megaestruturação pré-cambriana do território brasileiro com base em dados geofísicos e geológicos. Universidade Estadual Paulista, Geociências, 12: 7-31.

Herrington, R.J., Evans, D.M. and Buchanan, D.L. 1997. Metallogenenic aspects. In Greenstone Belts. Edited by M.J. de Wit and L.D. Ashwal. Clarendon Press, Oxford, Chapt. 2.5, 177-219.

Jahn, B.M. and Schrank, A. 1983. REE geochemistry of komatiites and associated rocks from Piumhi, southeastern Brazil. Precambrian Research, 21: 1-20.

Jordt Evangelista, H. 1992. O grupo Dom Silvério, SE de Minas Gerais: Petrografia, metamorfismo, geoquímica e geologia econômica. In Anais do 6o Simpósio de Minas Gerais. Sociedade Brasileira de Geologia, Núcleo de Minas Gerais, Revista da Escola de Minas - Universidade Federal de Ouro Preto, 45: 121-123.

Jordt Evangelista, H. and Roeser, H. 1988. Contribuição à petrologia do Grupo Dom Silvério, sudeste de Minas Gerais. In Anais 35o Congresso Brasileiro de Geologia. Sociedade Brasileira de Geologia, Núcleo do Pará, Vol. 3: 1183-1192.

Jordt-Evangelista, H. & Roeser, H., Carmo, V.E.F. 1990 Sobre o manganês no Distrito de Saúde e suas rochas encaixantes (Grupo Dom Silvério), Minas Gerais REM: Revista Escola de Minas, 43(4):36-43.

Jost, H. and Oliveira, A.M. 1991. Stratigraphy of the greenstone belts, Crixás region, Goiás, central Brazil. Journal of South American Earth Sciences, 4: 201-214.

Jost, H., Theodoro, S.M.C.H., Figueiredo, A.M.G. and Boaventura, G.R. 1996. Propriedades geoquímicas e proveniência de rochas metassedimentares detríticas arqueanas dos greenstone belts de Crixás e Guarinos, Goiás. Revista Brasileira de Geociências, 26: 151-166.

Jost, H., Kuyumjian, R.M., Freitas, A.L.S., Costa, A.L.L., Nascimento, C.T.C., Vasconcelos, F.M., Galotti, L., Martins, M.C.A., Carvalho, M.N. and Condé, V.C. 1995. Geologia da porção norte do Greenstone Belt de Guarinos, GO. Revista Brasileira de Geociências, 25: 51-60.

Justo, L.J.E.C. 1994. Jaraguá, Folha SD.22-Z.O.IV. Companhia de Pesquisa de Recursos Minerais, Programa de Levantamentos Geológicos Básicos do Brasil (PLGB), Brasília.

Kerrich, R., Wyman, D.A. 1997. Review of development in trace element fingerprinting of geodynamic setting and their implications for the mineral exploration. Australian Journal of Earth Sciences, 44: 465-487.

Kishida, A. 1979. Caracterização geológica e geoquímica das seqüências vulcanossedimentares do médio Rio Itapicuru (Bahia). M.Sc. dissertation, Universidade Federal da Bahia, Salvador, Brazil.

Kuyumjian, R. 1999. The magmatic arc of western Goiás: a

promising exploration target. In Base metal deposits of Brazil. Edited by M.d.G. da Silva and A. Misi. Ministério de Minas e Energia / Companhia de Pesquisa de Recursos Minerais / Departamento Nacional de Produção Mineral, Belo Horizonte, 69-83.

Kuyumjian, R.M. 1981. Geologia e mineralizações auríferas dos greenstone belts da faixa Crixás, Goiás. M.Sc. dissertation, Universidade de Brasília, Brasília, Brazil.

Kuyumjian, R.M. 1989. The geochemistry and tectonic significance of amphibolites from the Chapada Sequence, Central Brazil. Ph.D. thesis, Imperial College, University of London, London, United Kingdom.

Kwitko, R., Masotti, F.S., Baars, F.J., de Abreu, F.R., Ferrari, A.J.D., Fuck, R.F., Gomes, R.P., Ribeiro, E., Tallarico, F., Vial, D.S. and Viana, F.H. 1995. Petrografia, alteração hidrotermal e mineralização aurífera da jazida de Córrego Paiol, Almas, Tocantins. In 5o Congresso Brasileiro de Geoquímica. Sociedade Brasileira de Geologia, CD-ROM.

Lacerda Filho, J.V., Marques, V., Scislewiski, G., Jorge, L., Justo, E.C. and de Oliveira, C.C. 1991. Projeto Geologia da Região Centro-Oeste, Folha Carariba. Companhia de Pesquisa de Recursos Minerais, Goiânia.

Ladeira, E.A. 1991. Genesis of gold in the Quadrilátero Ferrífero: a remarkable case of permanency, recycling and inheritance - a tribute to Djalma Guimarães, Pierre Routhier and Hans Ramberg. In Proceedings of GOLD'91: the Economics, Geology, Geochemistry and Genesis of Gold Deposits. Edited by E.A. Ladeira. A.A. Balkema, Rotterdam, pp. 11-30.

Leão Neto, R. and Olivatti, O. 1983. Projeto Palmeirópolis – Relatório de Etapa Preliminar. Departamento Nacional de Produção Mineral / Companhia de Pesquisa de Recursos Minerais, Goiânia.

Lesher, C.M., Goodwin, A.M., Campbell, I.H. and Gorton, M.P. 1986. Trace-element geochemistry of ore-associated and barren, felsic metavolcanic rocks in the Superior Province, Canada. Canadian Journal of Earth Sciences, 23: 222-237.

Lima, T.M. 1997. Geologia, estratigrafia e petrologia da porção sul do Complexo Máfico-Ultramáfico de Cana Brava, Goiás. M.Sc. dissertation, Universidade de Brasília, Brasília, Brazil.

Linder, B. 1994. Geologische Feldkartierung und petrologisch-petrographisch-geochemische Unteruchungen an Gesteienen de "Dom Silvério Gruppe" in Minas Gerais, Brasilien. Graduation dissertation, Bonn Universität, Bonn, Germany.

Lobato, L.M., Vieira, F.W.R., Ribeiro-Rodrigues, L.C., Pereira, L.M.M., Menezes, M., Junqueira, P.A. and Martins Pereira, S.L. 1998. Styles of hydrothermal alteration and gold mineralisations associated with the Nova Lima Group of the Quadrilátero Ferrífero: Part I, description of selected gold deposits. Revista Brasileira de Geociências 28: 339-354.

Lobato, L.M., Baars, F.J. and Jost H. 1999. The potential for VMS deposits in the greenstone belts in and around the southern portion of the São Francisco Craton, Brazil. In Base metal deposits of Brazil. Edited by M.d.G. da Silva and A. Misi. Ministério de Minas e Energia / Companhia de Pesquisa de Recursos Minerais / Departamento Nacional da Produção Mineral.

Lobato L.M., Ribeiro-Rodrigues L.C., Vieira F.W.R. 2000a. The Archaean Rio das Velhas Greenstone Belt in the Quadrilátero Ferrífero region, Minas Gerais, Brazil: II. Geology and genesis of gold deposits. Mineralium Deposita, under review.

Lobato L.M., Ribeiro-Rodrigues L.C., Zucchetti M., Noce C.M., Baltazar O.F., da Silva L.C., Pinto C.P. 2000b. The Archaean Rio das Velhas Greenstone Belt in the Quadrilátero Ferrífero region, Minas Gerais, Brazil:. I. The tectonic, magmatic and structural setting of Brazil's premier gold province. Mineralium Deposita, under review.

Lydon, J.W. 1988. Volcanogenic massive sulphide deposits, Part 2: genetic models. In Geoscience Canada, Ore Deposit Models Series, 1: 43-65.

Lyrio, J.G.G., Leal, E.D.L. and Oliveira, J.A.L. 1976. Pesquisa em Bico de Pedra – Ouro Preto- MG. In Resumos do 29o Congresso Brasileira Geologia. Sociedade Brasileira de Geologia, Núcleo de Minas Gerais, pp. 279-280.

Machado, E.E. 1981. Novas considerações e integração geológica da região de Pilar-Crixás/Mara Rosa-Porangatu. In Atas do 1o Simpósio de Geologia do Centro-Oeste. Sociedade Brasileira de Geologia, Núcleo do Centro-Oeste, pp. 300-318.

Machado, N. and Noce, C.M. 1993. A evolução do setor sul do Cráton do São Francisco entre 3.1 e 0.5 Ga baseada em geocronologia U-Pb. In Anais do 2o Simpósio Cráton São Francisco. Sociedade Brasileira de Geologia, Núcleo de Bahia - Sergipe / Superintendência de Geologia e Recursos Minerais do Estado da Bahia, pp. 100-102.

Machado, N., Schrank, A., Noce, C.M. and Gauthier, G. 1996. Ages of detrital zircon from Archaean-paleoproterozoic sequences: implications for greenstone belt setting and evolution of a Transamazonian foreland basin in the Quadrilátero Ferrífero, SE Brazil. Earth and Planetary Science Letters, 141: 259-276.

Machado, N., Schrank, A., de Abreu, F.R., Knauer, L.G. and Almeida Abreu, P.A. 1989. Resultados preliminares da geocronologia U/Pb na Serra do Espinhaço Meridional. In Anais do 5o Simpósio de Geologia de Minas Gerais. Sociedade Brasileira de Geologia, Núcleo de Minas Gerais, Boletim 10, pp. 171-174.

MacKenzie, B. 1996. Economic Guidelines for Mineral Exploration: Seminar Notes - Agosto 1996. Rio Doce Geologia e Mineração S.A., Rio de Janeiro.

Magalhães, L.F. 1991 Cinturão de cisalhamento de empurrão Córrego Geral - Meia Pataca: Geologia, deformação, alteração hidrotermal e mineralizações auríferas associadas, Crixás, Goiás. M.Sc. dissertation, Universidade de Brasília, Brasília, Brazil.

Marinho, M.M. 1991. La sequence volcano-sedimentaire de Contendas-Mirante et la bordure Occidental du Bloc de Jequié (Craton du São Francisco, Brésil): un exemple de transition Archeen-Proterozoique. Ph.D. thesis, Université de Clermont-Ferrand, Clermont-Ferrand, France.

Marinho, M.M., Barbosa, J.S.F. and Vidal Ph. 1993. O embasamento do Cráton do São Francisco no sudeste da Bahia: Revisão geocronológica. In Anais do 2o Simpósio do Cráton do São Francisco. Sociedade Brasileira de Geologia, Núcleo de Bahia - Sergipe, 12-16.

Marinho, M.M., Galvão, C.F., Nonato, I.F., Luz, D.d.S., Brito, R.S.C., Pedreira, A.J. and Vianna, I.A. 1994. Geologia e potencialidade mineral da borda nordeste da Faixa Contendas-Mirante e do Sill do Rio Jacaré, Bahia. Companhia Baiana de Pesquisa Mineral, Série Arquivos Abertos, No. 6.

Marques, V.J. and Marques, M.T.G. 1985. Ambiência geológico-geotectônica da Seqüência Vulcano-sedimentar de Palmeirópolis (GO): guias e controles das mineralizações. In Atas do 1o Simpósio de Geologia do Centro-Oeste. Sociedade Brasileira de Geologia, Núcleo do Centro-Oeste, Vol. 2: 208-224.

Martin, H., Sabaté, P., Peucat, J.J. and Cunha, J.C. 1991. Comtes Rendues de l'Académie de Sciences de Paris, 313 II: 531-538.

Mascarenhas, J.d.F. and Silva, E.F.A. 1994. Greenstone Belt de Mundo Novo: Caracterização e implicações metalogenéticas e geotectônicas no Cráton do São Francisco. Companhia Baiana de Pesquisa Mineral, Série Arquivos Abertos, Vol. 5, 32p.

Mascarenhas, J.d.F., Pedreira, A.J.d.C.L., Misi, A., Motta, A.C., Sá, J.H.d.S. 1984. Província São Francisco. In O Pré-Cambriano do Brasil Edited by F.F.M. de Almeida and Y. Hasui. Edgard Blücher, São Paulo, Chapt. 4, pp. 46-122.

Matos, F.M.V. and Davison, I. 1987. Basement or intrusion? The Ambrósio Dome, Rio Itapicuru Greenstone Belt, Bahia, Brazil. Revista Brasileira de Geociências, 17: 442-449.

de Matos 1991. Petrogenetische Entwicklung der Schichtgebundenen Au-Fuhrenden Sulfidlagerstatte Bico de Pedra, Minas Gerais - Brasilien. Ph.D. thesis, Ruprecht-Karls Universität., Germany.

Mineração Cuieté Velho Ltda. – MCV 1995. Relatório de Pesquisa para Ouro – 830.200/82: Relatório Final de Pesquisa. Departamento Nacional de Produção Mineral, Delegacia de Minas Gerais, Belo Horizonte.

Misi, A. and da Silva, M.d.G. (Co-ordinators) 1998. Atas do Workshop sobre os Depósitos Minerais Brasileiros de Metais-Base. Agência para o Desenvolvimento Tecnológico da Indústria Mineral Brasileiro / Universidade Fedral da Bahia / Sociedade Brasileira de Geologia, Núcleo de Bahia - Sergipe, Salvador.

Moraes, R., 1992. Metamorfismo e deformação da Seqüência Vulcano-Sedimentar Juscelândia, Goiás, e geoquímica de seus anfibolitos. M.Sc. dissertation, Universidade de Brasília, Brasília, Brazil.

Moraes, R., 1997. Condições e Evolução do Metamorfismo no Complexo Barro Alto e Litogeoquímica do Vulcanismo Bimodal da Seqüência Juscelândia, Goianésia, Goiás. Ph.D. thesis, Universidade de Brasília, Brasília., 378p.

Moraes, R. and Fuck, R.A. 1994. Deformação e metamorfismo das seqüências Juscelândia e Serra da Malacacheta, Complexo de Barro Alto, Goiás. Revista Brasileira de Geociências 24: 189-197.

Moraes, L.C., Martins, A.B.M., Sampaio, A.R., Gil, C.A.A. and Andrade Filho, E.L. 1980. Relatório Final do Projeto Brumado-Caetité: Relatório de Fase I. Departamento Nacional de Produção Mineral / Companhia de Pesquisa de Recursos Minerais, Salvador.

Mourão M.A.A., Grossi Sad, J.H. and da Fonseca, E. 1997. Geologia da Folha Janaúba, Minas Gerais. In Projeto Espinhaço em CD-ROM (textos e anexos). Co-ordinated by J.H. Grossi Sad, L.M. Lobato, A.C. Pedrosa-Soares, B.S. Soares Filho. Companhia Mineradora de Minas Gerais, Belo Horizonte, pp. 9-123.

Nagell, R.H. 1970. A formação Boquira e os depósitos de rninério de churnbo e zinco em Boquira. Ministério de Minas e Energia - Departamento Nacional de Produção Mineral, Recife.

Nalini, Jr. H.A., Bilal, E. and Correia Neves, J.M. 1998. Mineralogical, geochemical and isotopic constraints of Neoproterozoic granitoids (Urucum and Galiléia Suites) eastern Minas Gerais State, Brazil. In Abstracts of the 14th International Conference on Basement Tectonics. International Basement Tectonics Association - Universidade Federal de Ouro Preto, 44-46.

Nascimento, F.S. 1985. Projeto Rochas Vulcanossedimentares Frente Rio do Peixe: Relatório Preliminar de Pesquisa. Metais de Goiás S.A., Goiânia.

Neves, A.C. and Ferreira, J.C.H. 1999. Mapeamento litoestrutural da região de São José da Safira - Minas Gerais. Graduation dissertation, Universidade Federal Minas Gerais, Belo Horizonte, Brazil.

Noce, C.M. 1995. Geocronologia dos eventos magmáticos, sedimentares e metamórficos na região do Quadrilátero Ferrífero, Minas Gerais. Ph.D. thesis, Universidade de São Paulo, São Paulo, Brazil.

Noce, C.M., Teixeira, W. and Machado, N. 1997. Geoquímica dos gnaisses TTGs e granitóides neoarqueanos do Complexo Belo Horizonte, Quadrilátero Ferrífero, Minas Gerais. Revista Brasileira de Geociências, 27: 25-32.

Noce, C.M., Teixeira, W., Carneiro, M.A. and Machado, N. 1998. U-Pb zircon ages and Sm-Nd signatures of basement rocks in the Southern São Francisco Craton: Implications for Archean crustal evolution. In Abstracts of the 14th International Conference on Basement Tectonics. International Basement Tectonics Association - Universidade Federal de Ouro Preto, pp. 152-154.

Nutman, A.P., Cordani, U.G. and Sabaté, P. (1992). Shrimp U-Pb ages of detrital zircons from the mid-Proterozoic Contendas-Mirante Supracrustal belt, São Francisco Craton, Bahia, Brazil. South American Journal of Earth Sciences.

Oliveira, A.M. 1993. Petrografia, estratigrafia, petroquímica e potencialidade para elementos do grupo da platina (EGP) do Complexo de Barro Alto, na região de Goianésia, Goiás. M.Sc. dissertation, Universidade de Brasília, Brasília, Brazil.

Paciullo, F.V.P., Ribeiro, A., Andreis, R.R. and Trouw, R.A.J. 1998. Sedimentary, igneous and thermo-tectonic events in the folded belts at the southern border of the São Francisco Craton, Minas Gerais State, Brazil. In Abstracts of the 14th International Conference on Basement Tectonics. International Basement Tectonics Association - Universidade Federal de Ouro Preto, pp. 66-68.

Padilha A.V. 1984. Formação Córrego dos Boiadeiros - Uma seqüência komatiítica na base do Grupo Nova Lima, Supergrupo Rio das Velhas - Quadrilátero Ferrífero - Minas Gerais. In Anais do 33o Congresso Brasileiro de Geologia. Sociedade Brasileira de Geologia, Núcleo do Rio de Janeiro, pp. 2668-2679.

Paes, V.J.C. 1999. Geologia e Geoquímica de Rochas Metamáficas e Meta-Ultramáficas da Região de Alvarenga-MG e suas Implicações Geotectônicas e Metalogenéticas. M.Sc. dissertation, Universidade Federal de Minas Gerais, Belo Horizonte, Brazil.

Paes, V.J.C., Lobato L.M., Silva, S.L. and Baars, F.J. 1998. Geologia da Quadrícula de Alvarenga, Minas Gerais: Caracterização litológica e estrutural. In Anais do 40o Congresso Brasileiro de Geologia. Sociedade Brasileira de Geologia, Núcleo de Minas Gerais, Boletim 15, pp. 30.

Paes, V.J.C., Lobato, L.M., Pimentel, M.M. and Baars, F.J. 2000. Archean mafic and ultramafic rocks within the Neoproterozoic Araçuaí Orogen at Cuieté Velho, Minas Gerais, Brazil: geotectonic implications. 31st International Congress, Rio de Janeiro, Brazil, in press.

Paim, M.M., Rosa, M.d.L.S., Conceição, H., Barreto Santos, E. and Bastos Leal, L.R. 1999. Litogeoquímica, geoquímica isotópica e implicações para a petrogênese do Maciço Sienítico de Cara Suja – Sudoeste da Bahia. In Anais do 5o Congresso de Geoquímica dos Países de Língua Portuguesa e 7o Congresso Brasileiro de Geoquímica. Sociedade Brasileira de Geoquímica, pp. 569-571.

Palermo, N. 1996. Le gisement aurifére Précambrien de Posse (Goiás, Brésil) dans son cadre géologique. Ph.D. thesis, l'École Nationale Supérieure de Minas de Paris, Paris, France.

Pearce, J.A. 1996. A user's guide to basalt discrimination diagrams. In Trace Element Geochemistry of Volcanic Rocks: Applications for Massive Sulphide Exploration. Edited by D.A. Wyman. Geological Association of Canada, 79-114.

Pedrosa-Soares, A.C. 1995. Potencial aurífero do Vale do Araçuaí, MG: História da exploração, geologia e controle tectono-metamórfico. Ph.D. thesis, Universidade de Brasília, Brasília, Brazil.

Pedrosa-Soares, A.C. and Noce, C.M. 1998. Where is the suture zone of the Neoproterozoic Araçuaí-West Congo Orogen? In Abstracts of the 14th International Conference on Basement Tectonics. International Basement Tectonics Association - Universidade Federal de Ouro Preto, pp. 35-37.

Pedrosa-Soares, A.C., Vidal, Ph., Leonardos Jr., O.H. and de Brito Neves B.B. 1998. Neoproterozoic oceanic remnants in eastern Brazil: further evidence and refutation of an exclusively ensialic evolution for the Araçuaí – West Congo Orogen. Geology 26: 519-522.

Pedrosa-Soares, A.C., Dardenne, M.A., Hasui, Y., de Castro, F.D.C. and de Carvalho, M.V.A. 1994. Nota explicativa dos mapas geológico, metalogenético e de ocorrências minerais do Estado de Minas Gerais, na escala 1:1.000.000. Companhia Mineradora de Minas Gerais, Belo Horizonte.

Pedrosa-Soares, A.C., Noce, C.M., Vidal, Ph., Monteiro, R.L.B.P. and Leonardos Jr., O.H. 1992. Toward a new tectonic model for the Late Proterozoic Araçuaí (SE Brazil) – West Congolian (SW Africa) Belt. Journal of South American Earth Sciences, 6: 33-47.

Pimentel, M.M. 1985. A Seqüência Vulcano-sedimentar de Arenópolis, GO: Petrologia ígnea e metamórfica, contexto geotectônico e considerações metalogenéticas preliminares. M.Sc. dissertation, Universidade de Brasília, Brasília, Brazil.

Pimentel, M.M. and Fuck, R.A. 1987. Origem e evolução das rochas metavulcânicas e metaplutônicas da região de Arenópolis (GO). Revista Brasileira de Geociências 17(1): 2-14.

Pimentel, M.M. and Fuck, R.A. 1992. Neoproterozoic crustal accretion in central Brazil. Geology 20: 375-379.

Pimentel, M.M., Fuck, R.A. and d'el Rey Silva, J.L.H. 1996. Dados Rb-Sr e Sm-Nd da região de Jussara-Goiás-Mossâmedes (GO), e o limite entre terrenos antigos do Maciço de Goiás e o arco magmático de Goiás. Revista Brasileira de Geociências 26: 61-70.

Pimentel, M.M., Heaman, L., Fuck, R.A. and Marini, O.J. 1991. U-Pb zircon geochronology of Precambrian tin-bearing continental-type acid magmatism in central Brazil. Precambrian Research 52: 321-335.

Queiróz, C.L. 1995. Caracterização dos domínios estruturais e da arquitetura do Greenstone Belt de Crixás, Goiás. M.Sc. dissertation, University of Brasília, Brasília, Brazil.

Queiróz, C.L. and Jost, H. 1998. Polycyclic deformation on an Archean crustal segment of the Goiás Massif, Central Brasil. In Abstracts of the 14th International Conference on Basement Tectonics. International Basement Tectonics Association - Universidade Federal de Ouro Preto, pp. 166-169.

Queiróz, C.L., Jost, H. and McNaughton, N.J. 1999. U/Pb-SHRIMP ages of Crixás granite-Greenstone Belt terranes: from Archaean to Neoproterozoic. In Resumos Expandidos do 7o Simposio Nacional de Estudos Tectônicos. Sociedade Brasileira de Geologia, Núcleo de Bahia – Sergipe, pp. 35-37.

Resende, L. 1994. Estratigrafia, petrografia e geoquímica da seqüência sedimentar do Greenstone Belt de Pilar de Goiás, GO. M.Sc. dissertation, Universidade de Brasília, Brasília, Brazil.

Resende, M.G. 1998. Estudo da evolução das supracrustais metassedimentares dos greenstone belts de Goiás e Faina, GO. Ph.D. thesis, Universidade de Brasília, Brasília.

Resende, M.G. and Jost, H. 1995. Petrogênese de formações ferríferas e metahidrotermalitos da Formação Aimbé, Grupo Guarinos (Arqueano), Goiás. Revista Brasileira de Geociências, 25: 41-50.

Resende, M.G., Jost, H., Osborne, G.A. and Mol, A. 1998. The stratigraphy of the Goiás and Faina greenstone belts, Central Brazil: a new proposal. Revista Brasileira de Geociências,

28: 77-94.

Ribeiro Filho, W. 1981. Reavaliação da geologia de Pilar – Mara Rosa. In Atas do 1o Simpósio de Geologia do Centro-Oeste. Sociedade Brasileira de Geologia, Núcleo do Centro-Oeste, pp. 281-299.

Ribeiro Filho, W. and Teixeira, N.A. 1981. Seqüência vulcano-sedimentar da borda oeste dos complexos de Niquelândia e Cana Brava. Sociedade Brasileira de Geologia, Núcleo do Centro-Oeste, Boletim Informativo 10, 157-173.

Ribeiro, A.F. and da Silva, M.d.G. 1998. O Greenstone Belt do Rio Salitre (GBS), Dominio Sobradinho, porção norte-nordeste do Cráton do São Francico, Bahia, e mineralizações associadas. In Anais do 40o Congresso Brasileiro de Geologia. Sociedade Brasileira de Geologia, Núcleo de Minas Gerais, Boletim 15, pp. 65.

Ribeiro, A.F., Andreis, R.R., Trouw, R.A.J., Pacuillo, F.V.P. and Valença, J.G. 1995. Evolução das bacias proterozóicas e o termo-tectonismo brasiliano na margem sul do Cráton São Francisco. Revista Brasileira de Geociências, 25: 235-248.

Rocha, G.M.F. 1985. Caracterização faciológica da formação ferrífera de Boquira, encaixante da mineralização de Pb/Zn. M.Sc. dissertation, Universidade Federal da Bahia, Salvador, Brazil.

Rocha, G.M.F. 1990. Caracterização da fácies ferrífera de Boquira, encaixante da mineralização de chumbo-zinco. In Geologia e Recursos Minerais do Estado da Bahia. Secretaria de Minas e Energia do Estado da Bahia, Coordenação da Produção Mineral, Salvador, Textos Básicos, Vol. 8.

Rocha, G.M.F., de Souza, S.L. Garrido, I.A.d.A. and de Miranda, L.L.F. 1998. Distrito manganesífero de Urandi-Licínio de Almeida, Bahia: geologia e potencialidade econômica. Companhia Baiana de Pesquisa Mineral, Série Arquivos Abertos, No. 12.

da Rocha Neto, M.B. and Pedreira, A.J. 1994. Geologia e recursos minerais do Greenstone Belt do Rio Itapicuru, Bahia. Companhia Baiana de Pesquisa Mineral, Série Arquivos Abertos, No. 4.

Rodrigues, J.B.R. 1996. Geocronologia e geoquímica da seqüência vulcano-sedimentar de Iporá e rochas graníticas associadas. M.Sc. dissertation, Universidade de Brasília, Brasília, Brazil.

Rodrigues, J.B.R. and Pimentel, M.M. 1995. Características geoquímicas e isotópicas de rochas granitóides e metavulcânicas da região de Iporá, GO. In Anais do 5o Simpósio de Geologia do Centro-Oeste. Sociedade Brasileira de Geologia, Núcleo do Centro-Oeste, pp. 123-124.

Romano, A.W. 1990. Évolution tectonique de la région nord-ouest du Quadrilatère Ferrifère – Minas Gerais – Brésil. Ph.D. thesis, Université de Nancy I, Nancy, France.

Romano, A.W. 1993. O Supergrupo Rio das Velhas da Faixa Mateus Leme-Pitangui - parte meridional do Cráton do São Francisco, MG – e seu sistema de alteração hidrotermal. Universidade Federal de Minas Gerais, Geonomos, 1: 16-32.

Romano, A.W. and Carmo, J.C.C. 1992. Estratigrafia e alteração hidrotermal das rochas do supergrupo Rio das Velhas no sinclinório de Pitangui-Pequi. Universidade Federal de Ouro Preto, Revista da Escola de Minas, 45: 115-117.

Rosa Seixas, L.A., Hippert, J, Bardintzeff, J.-M. and Bonin, B. 1998. Tracing the generation of TTD plutonic rocks: Heritage of magma mixing/mingling and fractionation. In Abstracts of the 14th International Conference on Basement Tectonics. International Basement Tectonics Association - Universidade Federal de Ouro Preto, pp. 155-158.

Rosa Seixas, L.A., Hippert, J., Bardintzeff, J.-M. and Bonin B. 1999a. Alteração hidrotermal em komatiitos: Dois casos contrastantes ao sul do Quadrilátero Ferrífero, Minas Gerais, Brasil. In Anais do 5o Congresso de Geoquímica dos Países de Língua Portuguesa e 7o Congresso Brasileiro de Geoquímica. Sociedade Brasileira de Geoquímica, pp. 587-589.

Rosa Seixas, L.A., Hippert, J., Bardintzeff, J.-M., Platevoet, B. and Bonin B. 1999b. Etudes des minéraux riches en terres rares dans les microfractures d'une métakomatüte Archéene de la région de Vargem Alegre, Minas Gerais (Brésil): donées préliminaires. Université de Paris-Sud, Centre d'Orsay, Journée de Doctorands.

Rose, A.W. and Burt, D.M. 1979. Hydrothermal alteration. In Geochemistry of Hydrothermal Ore Deposits. Edited by H.L. Barnes. John Wiley and Sons, New York, pp. 173-235.

Sabaté, P., Cuney, M. and Vidal, Ph. 1990. Expressão estrutural e plutônica de uma colisão Transarnazônica no Cráton do São Francisco (Bahia-Brasil). In Boletim de Resumos do 36o Congresso Brasileiro de Geologia. Sociedade Brasileira de Geologia, Núcleo do Nordeste, pp. 323.

Sabóia, L.A. 1979. Os greenstone belts de Crixás e Goiás, GO. Sociedade Brasileira de Geologia, Núcleo do Centro-Oeste, Boletim Informativo 9, pp. 44-72.

Sangster, D.F. 1998. Volcanic-exhalative massive sulphide deposits. In Base metal deposits of Brazil. Edited by M.d.G. da Silva and A. Misi. Ministério de Minas e Energia / Companhia de Pesquisa de Recursos Minerais / Departamento Nacional de Produção Mineral, Belo Horizonte, pp. 13-15.

Sawkins, F.J. 1990. Metal Deposits in Relation to Plate Tectonics: 2nd edition. Springer-Verlag, New York.

Schobbenhaus Filho, C. 1993. O Proterozóico Médio no Brasil, com ênfase na região centro-oeste: Uma revisão. Ph.D. thesis, Albert Ludwig Universität., Freiburg, Germany.

Schorscher HD, Santana FC, Polônia JC, Moreira JMP (1982) Quadrilátero Ferrífero-Minas Gerais State: Rio das Velhas greenstone belt and Proterozoic rocks. In: International Symposium on Archean and Early Proterozoic Geological Evolution and Metallogenesis, Abstracts and Excursions, Sociedade Brasileira de Geologia, Salvador, pp. 44.

Schrank, A. 1982. Pétrologie des komatiites et des roches associées de la ceinture verte du Massif Précambrien de Piumhi (Minas Gerais – Brésil). Ph.D. thesis, Université du Paris-Sud, Paris, France.

Schrank, A, and da Silva, M.d.G. 1993. Os greenstone-belts do Cráton do São Francisco. In O Cráton do São Francisco. Edited by J.M.L. Dominguez and A. Misi. Sociedade

Brasileira de Geologia, Núcleo de Bahia - Segipe / Superintendência de Geologia e Recursos Minerais do Estado da Bahia / Conselho Nacional de Pesquisa, Salvador, pp. 85-118.

Seer, H.J. 1985. Geologia, deformação e mineralização de cobre no Complexo Vulcano-sedimentar de Bom Jardim de Goiás. M.Sc. dissertation, Universidade de Brasília, Brasília, Brazil.

Seixas, L.A.R. 1988. Geologia e metalotectos de ouro de uma fração do Lineamento Congonhas, MG. M.Sc. dissertation, Universidade de Brasília, Brasília, Brazil.

Seixas, L.A.R. and Baars, F.J. 1991. Características geoquímicas das rochas ultramáficas do Lineamento Congonhas, Minas Gerais, Brasil. In Anais do 1o Congresso de Geoquímica dos Países de Língua Portuguesa e 3o Congresso Brasileiro de Geoquímica, Sociedade Brasileira de Geoquímica, Vol. 1, pp. 185-190.

Sillitoe, R.H., Hannington, M.D. and Thompson, J.F.H. 1996. High-sulfidation deposits in the volcanogenic massive sulfide environment. Economic Geology, 91: 204-212.

Silva, A., de Souza, L.H. and Ferreira, M.C.B. 1990. Alteração hidrotermal da seqüência de rochas do alvo Córrego Paiol e mineralização aurífera associada. In Anais do 30o Congresso Brasileiro de Geologia. Sociedade Brasileira de Geologia, Núcleo do Nordeste, Vol. 3, pp. 1129-1143.

da Silva, L.C. 1998a. Petrologia e geoquímica. In Projeto Rio das Velhas – Mapa Geológico Integrado, Escala 1:100.000, e Texto Explicativo. Edited by M. Zucchetti and O.F. Baltazar. Departamento Nacional de Produção Mineral / Companhia de Pesquisa de Recursos Minerais – Belo Horizonte, CD-ROM, pp. 55-103.

da Silva, M.d.G. 1987. Geochemic, Petrologie und geotektonische Entwicklung eines proterozoischen Grönsteingijrtels: Rio Itapicuru, Bahia, Brasilien. Ph.D thesis, Universität Freiburg, Freiburg.

da Silva, M.d.G. 1992. Evidências isotópicas e geocronológicas de um fenômeno de acrescimento crustal transamazônico no craton do São Francisco, Estado da Bahia. In Anais do 37o Congresso Brasileiro de Geologia. Sociedade Brasileira de Geologia, Núcleo de São Paulo, Vol. 2, pp. 181-182.

da Silva, M.d.G. 1998b. Uma idade modelo Sm-Nd para as vulcânicas félsicas do Greenstone Belt de Mundo Novo (GBMN) e suas implicações. In Anais do 40o Congresso Brasileiro de Geologia. Sociedade Brasileira de Geologia, Núcleo de Minas Gerais, Boletim 15, pp. 51.

Silveira, W.P. and Conceição Filho, V.M. 1991. Avaliação geológica do potencial aurífero do prospect Vargem Comprida, Pindobaçu, Bahia: Relatório. Companhia Baiana de Pesquisa Mineral / Secretaria de Minas e Energia do Estado da Bahia, Salvador.

Silveira, W.P. and Cunha, J.C. 1997. Síntese da geologia do greenstone belt de Riacho de Santana. Companhia Baiana de Pesquisa Mineral / Secretaria de Minas e Energia do Estado da Bahia, Salvador.

Simões, L.S.A. 1984. Geologia do Grupo Araxá na região de Mossâmedes, Goiás, e as ocorrências minerais associadas. M.Sc. dissertation, Universidade de Brasília, Brasília, Brazil.

Soares, P.C., Fiori, A.P. and Carvalho, S.G. 1990a. Tectônica colisional oblíqüa entre o Bloco Paraná e a margem sul do Cráton do São Francisco, no Maciço de Guaxupé. In Anais do 36o Congresso Brasileiro de Geologia. Sociedade Brasileira de Geologia, Núcleo do Nordeste, pp. 2723–2734.

Soares, J.V., Garrido, I.A.A., Oliveira, N.S. and Fróes, R.J.B. 1990b. Projeto Macaúbas: Relatório Final. Companhia Baiana de Pesquisa Mineral / Secretaria de Minas e Energia do Estado da Bahia, Salvador.

Söllner, F., Lammerer, B. and Weber-Diefenbach, K. 1991. Die Krustenentwicklung in der Küstenregion nördlich von Rio de Janeiro/Brasilien. Universität München, Münchner Geologische Hefte, No. 4.

Souza, J.O. and Leão Neto, R. 1981. Mapeamento geológico na área do garimpo de Santa Terezinha de Goiás. Relatorio Ministério de Minas e Energia / Departamento Nacional de Produção Mineral / Companhia de Pesquisa de Recursos Minerais, Goiânia.

de Souza, S.L., de Moraes, A.M.V., Lopes, G.A.C. and Cruz, M.J.M. 1990. Projeto Caetité: Relatório de Fase II. Companhia Baiana de Pesquisa Mineral, Salvador.

Stern, C.R. and de Wit, M.J. 1997. The Rocas Verdes 'Greenstone Belt', southernmost South America. In Greenstone Belts. Edited by M.J. de Wit and L.D. Ashwal. Clarendon Press, Oxford, Chapt. 5.5, pp. 791-801.

Strieder, A.J. 1993. Deformação e metamorfismo na região de Santa Cruz de Goiás: Correlação tectonoestratigráfica e evolução tectônica regional. Ph.D. thesis. Universidade de Brasília, Brasília, Brazil.

Suita, M.T.F. 1996. Metalogenia e geoquímica de platinóides em complexos máfico-ultramáficos do Brasil: Alguns critérios e guias com ênfase no Complexo Máfico-Ultramáfico de Barro Alto (Goiás, Brasil central). Ph.D. thesis. Universidade Federal do Rio Grande do Sul, Porto Alegre, Brazil.

Szabó, G.A.J. 1989. Contexto geológico e petrologia das rochas Meta-Ultramáficas de Alpinópolis, MG. M.Sc. dissertation, Universidade de São Paulo, São Paulo, Brazil.

Tassinari, C.C.G., Siga Jr. O. and Teixeira, W. 1981. Panorama geocronológico do centro-oeste brasileiro: Solução, problemática, sugestões. In Atas do 1o Simpósio de Geologia do Centro-Oeste. Sociedade Brasileira de Geologia, Núcleo do Centro-Oeste, pp. 93-114.

Teixeira, N.A. and Danni, J.C.M. 1979. Geologia da raiz de um greenstone belt na região de Fortaleza de Minas, Minas Gerais. Revista Brasileira de Geociências, 9: 17-26.

Teixeira, N.A. and Kuyumjian R. 1991. The Mateus Leme-Pitangui hydrothermal zone: do they represent a fossil hot spring system in the Rio das Velhas greenstone belt, Central Brazil? In Proceedings of Gold '91, the Economics, Geology, Geochemistry and Genesis of Gold Deposits. Edited by E.A. Ladeira. A.A. Balkema, Rotterdam, pp. 171-177.

Teixeira, N.A., Gaspar, J.C., Brenner, T.L., Cheney, J.T. and Marchetto, C.M.L. 1987. Geologia e implicações geotectônicas do Greenstone Belt do Morro do Ferro (Fortaleza de Minas – MG). Revista Brasileira de Geociências, 17: 209-220.

Theodoro, S.C. 1995. Ambiente de sedimentação da formação Ribeirão das Antas, Grupo Crixás, Goiás. M.Sc. dissertation, Universidade de Brasília, Brasília, Brazil.

Thomsen, F.P.R. and Kuyumjian, R.M. 1994a. As formações ferríferas bandadas da região de Conceição do Tocantins - TO: Caracterização preliminar. In Anais do 38o Congresso Brasileiro de Geologia. Sociedade Brasileira de Geologia, Núcleo de Santa Catarina, Vol. 1, pp. 72-73.

Thomsen, F.P.R. and Kuyumjian, R.M. 1994b. Caracterização geoquímica preliminar das rochas granitóides da Região de Conceição do Norte (TO). In Anais do 4o Simpósio de Geologia do Centro-Oeste. Sociedade Brasileira de Geologia, Núcleo do Centro-Oeste, pp. 26-27.

Thomson, M.L. 1986. Petrology of the Crixás gold deposit, Brazil: Evidence for gold associated with hydrothermal alteration subsequent to metamorphism. In GOLD'86: Proceedings of an International Symposium on the Geology of Gold. Edited by A.J. MacDonald. pp. 284-296.

Thomson, M.L. 1987. The Crixás Gold deposit, Brazil: metamorphism, metasomatism and gold mineralization. Ph.D. thesis. University of Western Ontario, London, Canada.

Thomson, M.L. 1991. Multiphase deformation and metamorphism of the Crixás Greenstone Belts, Goiás, Brazil. Journal of South American Earth Sciences, 4:119-130.

Thomson, M.L. and Fyfe, W.S. 1990. The Crixás gold deposit, Brasil: thrust-related postpeak metamorphism gold mineralization of possible Braziliano Cycle age. Economic Geology, 85: 928-942.

Uhlein, A. 1982. Geologia e mineralização de cromita e itabiritos da região do Serro, MG. M.Sc. dissertation, Universidade de Brasília, Brasília, Brazil.

Viana, M.G. 1995. Geocronologia e geoquímica das rochas ortognáissicas e metavulcânicas da região de Mara Rosa, Norte de Goiás. M.Sc. dissertation, Universidade de Brasília, Brasília, Brazil

Viana, M.G., Pimentel, M.M., Whitehouse, M.J. and Machado, N. 1995. O arco magmático de Mara Rosa, Goiás: Dados geoquímicos e geocronológicos e suas implicações regionais. Revista Brasileira de Geociências, 25: 111-123.

Vieira, M.B., Lobato, L.M., Assis, C.M., Gomes, F.C., Silva, R.A., Nascimento, H.S and Orlandi, P.H. 1998. Contribuição ao estudo da alteração hidrotermal da mina de ouro de Fazenda Brasileiro, Bahia. In Anais do 40o Congresso Brasileiro de Geologia. Sociedade Brasileira de Geologia, Núcleo de Minas Gerais, Boletim 15, pp. 130.

Vivallo, W. and Claesson, L. 1987. Intra-arc rifting and massive sulphide mineralization in an early Proterozoic volcanic arc, Skellefte district, northern Sweden. In Geochemistry and Mineralization of Proterozoic Volcanic Suites. Edited by T.C. Pharoah, R.D. Beckinsdale and D. Rickard. Blackwell Scientific Publications, Oxford, pp. 69-80.

Wilson, N. 1987. Combined Sm-Nd, Pb-Pb and Rb-Sr geochronology and isotope geochemistry in polymetamorphic Precambrian terrains: examples from Bahia, Brazil and Channel Island, U.K. M.Sc. dissertation, Oxford University, Oxford, United Kingdom.

Winge, M. 1984. A seqüência vulcano-sedimentar do Grupo Capim - Bahia. In Geologia e Recursos Minerais do Estado da Bahia. Edited by P.V.S. Viveiros de Sá and F.B. Duarte. Secretaria de Minas e Energia do Estado da Bahia, Coordenação da Produção Mineral, Salvador, Textos Básicos, Vol. 5, pp. 43-103.

Winge, M. and Danni, J.C.M. 1980. Compartimentos geotectônicos pré-brasilianos entre Caratacá e Bedengo, municipio de Uauá, Bahia. In Anais do 31o Congresso Brasileiro Geologia. Sociedade Brasileira de Geologia, Núcleo de Santa Catarina.

de Wit, M.J. and Ashwal, L.D. 1995. Greenstone belts: what are they? South African Journal of Geology 98: 505-520.

de Wit, M.J. and Ashwal, L.D. 1997. Greenstone Belts. Clarendon Press, Oxford.

Yamaoka, N.W. and Araújo, E.M. 1988. Depósitos de Ouro da Mina III, Crixás Goiás. In Principais Depósitos Minerais do Brasil. Edited by C.Schobbenhaus Filho and C.E.S. Coelho. Ministerio de Minas e Energia/Departamento Nacional de Produção Mineral/Companhia Vale do Rio Doce, Vol. 3, pp. 491-498.

Yamaoka, W.N., Araújo, E.M. and Garcia, M.P. 1985. Relatório Final de Pesquisa. Mineração Serra Grande Ltda., Crixás, Goiás.

Zucchetti, M. 1998. Geoquímica dos metabasaltos do grupo Nova Lima, Supergrupo Rio das Velhas, Quadrilátero Ferrífero, Minas Gerais. M.Sc. dissertation, Universidade Federal de Minas Gerais, Belo Horizonte, Brazil.

Zucchetti, M. and Baltazar, O.F. (Editors). 1998. Projeto Rio das Velhas – Mapa Geológico Integrado, Escala 1:100.000, e Texto Explicativo. Departamento Nacional de Produção Mineral / Companhia de Pesquisa de Recursos Minerais – Belo Horizonte, Belo Horizonte, CD-ROM.

Zucchetti, M., Baltazar, O.F. and Raposo, F.O. 1998. Estratigrafia. In Projeto Rio das Velhas – Mapa Geológico Integrado, Escala 1:100.000 e Texto Explicativo. Edited by M. Zucchetti and O.F. Baltazar. Departamento Nacional de Produção Mineral / Companhia de Pesquisa de Recursos Minerais – Belo Horizonte, CD-ROM, pp. 13-42.

THE PAUL ISNARD GOLD-COPPER OCCURRENCE, FRENCH GUIANA: THE FIRST VOLCANOGENIC MASSIVE SULPHIDE OCCURRENCE IN THE GUIANA SHIELD?

James Franklin[1], Carlos Bertoni[2], Michel Boudrie[3], Jean-Paul Bout[3], Declan Costelloe[5], Francis Lillié[4], Laurent Millo[3] and Jean-François Sauvage[3]

[1] Franklin Geosciences Ltd., [2] Golden Star Resources Ltd., [3] Guyanor Ressources S.A, [4] Asarco Guyane Française S.a.r.l., [5] Consultant

Abstract

The Paul Isnard copper-gold occurrence, in Northwestern French Guiana, consists of disseminated and vein sulphide minerals and gold in Early Proterozoic (ca. 2.2 Ga) felsic and mafic volcaniclastic strata and flows. The felsic strata are comprised entirely of pyroclastic ash and lapillistone. The mafic strata are basalt flows and hyaloclastite lenses, with intercalated pelite. The area has been penetratively deformed; the strata are steeply south dipping, and cut by synvolcanic, later bedding-parallel and still later high-angle faults. The felsic rocks are Na-rhyolite and dacite, with trace element contents similar to Types 1 and II (Lesher et al. 1986) arc or back-arc associations. The arc-tholeiitic mafic rocks may have been deposited in a local basin, which was structurally transposed into its present configuration.

The gold and base metals are distributed in a broadly stratiform, but locally crosscutting series of zones, in both the felsic and mafic strata. Gold is associated with disseminated and vein pyrite, with subordinate chalcopyrite and sphalerite. Copper and gold have a close spatial association; zinc (along with anomalous lead) is most abundant at the margins of the gold-copper zone. The strata have been intensely altered; alkali depletion is widespread, with sericite and iron chlorite as the main alteration minerals. The altered rocks are strongly aluminous (excess normative corundum). Near the most Fe-chloritized sections, Na and Ca are enriched.

The Paul Isnard occurrence is probably a sub-seafloor replacement deposit formed as part of a synvolcanic, volcanogenic massive sulphide (VMS) -like hydrothermal system. Deposition was at moderate (~1000 m) water depth, where adiabatic cooling caused copper and gold to precipitate from a convectively driven hydrothermal fluid. Zinc and lead precipitated in the cooler outer parts of the system. Thus the occurrence is likely of the VMS-type, and represents the first such occurrence in the Guiana Shield.

Introduction

Early Proterozoic volcanic arcs are prolific hosts of volcanogenic massive sulphide (VMS) mineralization (Gibson and Franklin 1998). For example, the Trans Hudson volcanic strata in the Canadian Shield contain about five times the base metal value per km^2 as the renowned Archean Abitibi belt! Smaller districts containing volcanic rocks of the same age, such as the Jerome and Wisconsin districts in the USA, and the Skellefte and Bergslagen districts of Sweden, seem to be similarly prolific. In these, and most other VMS-bearing districts, the ore is confined to arc-related volcanic sequences. Both mafic- and felsic dominated sequences are productive, with the former typically more Cu-rich, the latter more Zn, Pb and Au rich.

No VMS deposits have been discovered in the Proterozoic portions of the Guiana Shield. The equivalent (in age, at least) strata in the Birimian of West Africa (Burkina Faso) contain several VMS occurrences, including Perkoa, a zinc-rich deposit containing at least 4 million tonnes of ore. Some important questions in terms of assessing the potential of Early Proterozoic sequences in the Guiana Shield include determining if the volcanic rocks are submarine, if they represent some portion of an arc or back-arc sequence, and if any occurrences of VMS-style mineralization are present. The Paul Isnard occurrence may be the first in this Shield area to have VMS characteristics, and thus indicate potential for this type of deposit. The study presented herein is preliminary, based on field observations augmented by geochemical data. Much additional petrographic and mineralogic work will be required to validate these preliminary interpretations.

PROPERTY LOCATION

The Paul Isnard properties are located in Northwestern French Guiana, South America, approximately 180 km west of the capital city of Cayenne (Fig. 1). They cover an area of 430 square kilometres. The project is accessible by air from Cayenne and also by a 120 km lateritic road from the town of Saint-Laurent-du-Maroni, which has port facilities and can be reached from Cayenne by a 260 km surfaced public road.

The area is covered by dense tropical rain forest

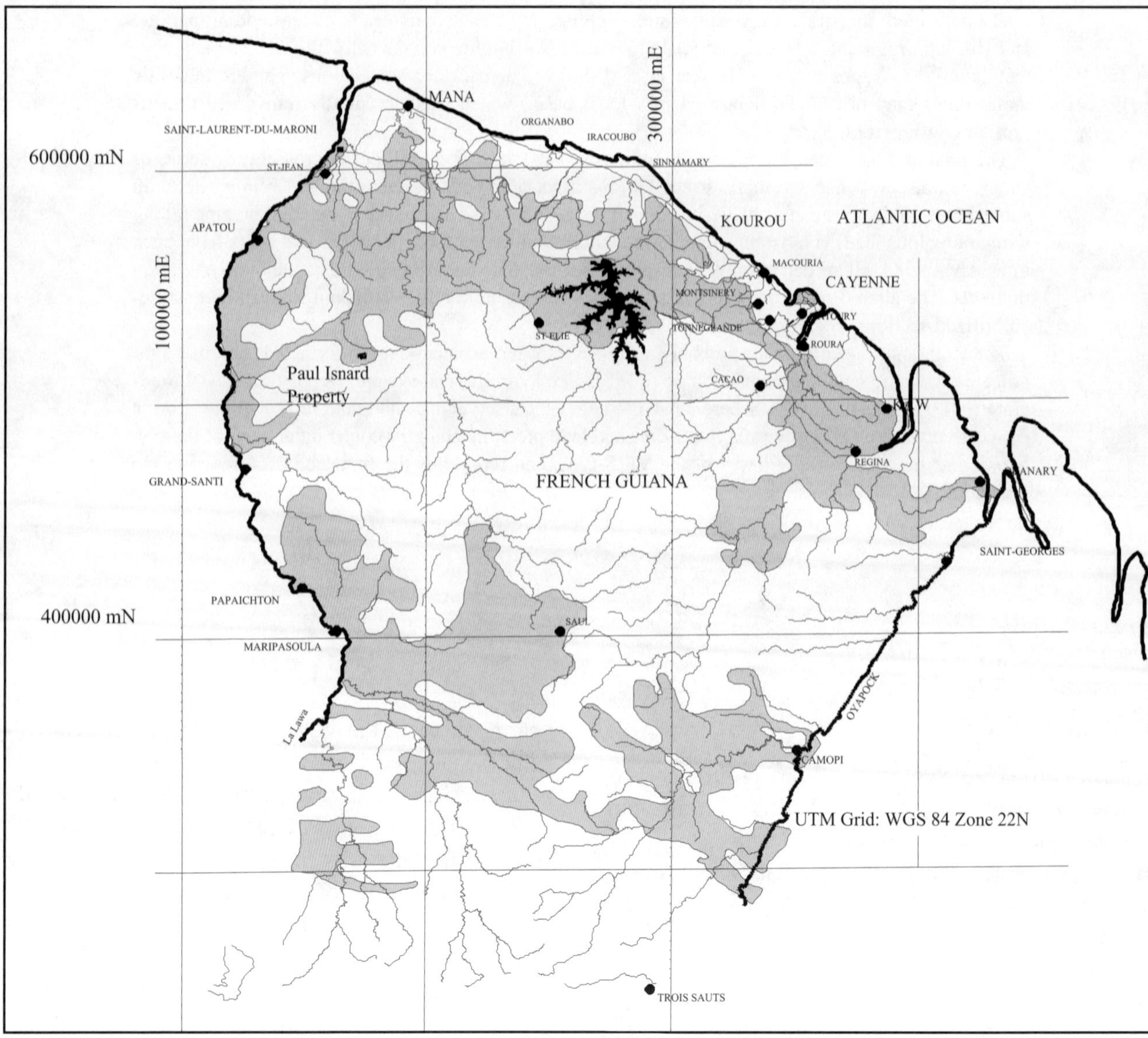

Figure 1. Location of the Paul Isnard prospect in French Guiana. The stippled areas outline the Early Proterozoic greenstone belts.

and dominated by two important massifs: Massif Dekou-Dekou and Massif Lucifer, with elevations of 460 and 540 m above sea level respectively. The climate is equatorial, hot and rainy, with little seasonal variation: annual average minimum and maximum temperatures are 22°C and 32°C respectively. The area receives an annual average of 2.5 m of rainfall.

HISTORY OF EXPLOITATION AND GEOLOGICAL EXPLORATION

This area of French Guiana is one of the major historical gold-producing regions of the country. Artisan miners have exploited surficial gold since the end of last century and in an industrial way since the end of World War II. Guyanor Ressources S.A. acquired the properties in October 1994, through the acquisition of the alluvial mining company Sotrapmag. In April 1997, Sotrapmag terminated one century of alluvial mining. At the end of 1999, Guyanor Ressources S.A. established contracts with small local alluvial mining societies, in order to start alluvial exploitation again.

Geologists from the Government of France have been exploring the Paul Isnard area since 1883, and since 1930 through France's national mining office, Bureau des Mines Guyanais (BMG) and subsequently Bureau de Recherches Géologiques et Minières (BRGM). In 1930 and 1958, the BMG explored using trenches and adits in the quartz vein - associated gold zones (Elysée and Montagne d'Or properties). In 1976, BRGM covered the two greenstone belts in French Guiana with 500 m by 2000 m geochemistry grids for gold and base metals, as part of the French Guiana Mining Inventory. The office continued the exploration between 1977 and 1982 with 250 by 100 m and 100 m by 50 m geochemistry grids for gold in the north and in the east of the area (St Pierre and Dégrad-Neuf zones). In 1985, the BRGM developed an interest in Montagne d'Or zone, or "Golden Mountain", on the northern flank of the Massif Dekou-Dekou. Between 1985 and 1991, several geochemistry grids in the zone showed a large gold anomaly. Presently, Guyanor Ressources, a 71 % owned subsidiary of Golden Star Resources (GSR) holds 100 % of the Paul Isnard property.

Guyanor started exploration in the Montagne d'Or zone in 1994 with an airborne radiometric and magnetic survey. Between 1995 and 1999, 56 diamond drill holes comprising 10,916 m were completed, and 635 m of fresh rock was channel sampled on the numerous outcrops located in the creeks. The entire zone has been surveyed with ground geophysics (IP, magnetic, mise a la masse and in part with ground and down-hole EM surveys). Much of the history of recent exploration is in Millo et al., 1999

GEOLOGY OF THE GUIANA SHIELD

The Paul Isnard project lies within the Precambrian Guiana Shield, which stretches from the mouth of the Amazon River in Brazil to the Orinoco River in Venezuela. The Guiana Shield is composed, in order of age, of Archean formations, Lower Proterozoic greenstone belts, plutonic complexes, Middle Proterozoic continental detrital deposits, and Mesozoic and Cenozoic sedimentary strata (Bardoux et al. 1997).

Archean rocks occur only in Venezuela, with the Imataca complex, dated at 3.4 Ga (see Choubert, 1994 for a review of most of the age data presented herein). Several Lower Proterozoic greenstone belts, each trending ESE-WNW, are present in the Guiana Shield. These include the Pastora Supergroup and Supamo complex in Venezuela, Mazaruni and Barama series in Guiana and the Northern and Southern Paramaca series in French Guiana. These range in age between 2.20 and 2.07 Ga, and are comprised of volcano-sedimentary sequences including ultramafic, mafic, intermediate and felsic components. These supracrustal strata have been deformed by the Transamazonian orogeny at about 2 Ga. Mafic to felsic plutonic complexes intruded the greenstone belts during and just after their formation.

GEOLOGY OF THE PAUL ISNARD AREA

The Paul Isnard area (Fig. 1) is located in the Early Proterozoic greenstone belt that forms part of the northern Paramaca sequence. This distinctive belt is separated from a more southerly belt by a plutonic complex, the Massif Central Guyanais. It extends from the eastern part of Surinam to the eastern border of French Guiana, (Choubert, 1964, Manier, 1992, Milesi et al. 1995, Vanderhaeghe et al. 1998).

L'Ile de Cayenne sequence, dated at 2.144 Ga

(Milesi et al. 1995), is the oldest in French Guiana. It consists of highly metamorphosed rocks, including migmatite, amphibolite and quartzite. This is overlain (stratigraphically) by the Paramaca sequence that has radiometric ages of between 2.20 and 2.07 Ga. The Paramaca sequence formed in extensional continental and subduction related arc- and back-arc environments, and consists of metavolcanic and metasedimentary strata. The relationship between the L'Ile de Cayenne and Paramaca sequences is unclear; and although some authors continue to distinguish them, they seem to have formed during the same events. During the first Transamazonian collisional (compressional) orogenic phase, dated at about 2.10 Ga, the Paramaca sequence was deformed and metamorphosed to upper greenschist to lower amphibolite assemblages. Gabbro (2.15 Ga), diorite (2.11 Ga) and granite (2.10 - 2.08 Ga) intrusions that cut these strata have distinct contact metamorphic haloes.

The Ensemble Détritique Supérieur (EDS), composed of detrital sediments, formed in pull-apart basins located along the northern margin of the Paramaca greenstone belt, along major east-west reverse-sinistral Sillon Nord-Guyanais fault system, during the second Transamazonian orogenic phase. During this transcurrent tectonic event, dated at about 2.08 Ga, all of the strata in the greenstone belt were again deformed and metamorphosed. Much later, some doleritic dykes and associated small gabbro and basaltic intrusions were emplaced during the opening of Atlantic, 196 Ma ago.

The first geological mapping in the Paul Isnard area was done by the BRGM (Choubert, 1964) and has been extensively modified by Guyanor Resources since 1994. This area of Paramaca felsic to mafic metavolcanic and metasedimentary strata has been intruded extensively by gabbro and dioritic plutons. The Paul Isnard volcanic assemblage is bounded by the granite-gneiss complex of the Massif Central Guyanais to the south, east and west, by the L'Ile de Cayenne rocks to the southeast and by the Ensemble Détritique Supérieur (EDS) sedimentary-filled basin to the north. In addition to the reverse-sinistral fault between EDS and Paramaca units in the north, other faults cut the area. These have highly variable trends.

Several gold-bearing occurrences comprise Paul-Isnard project area. The Paramaca units (Montagne d'Or zone in the south, and Dégrad-Neuf zone in the east) contain gold and sulphide mineralization in felsic volcanic rocks. In the Élysee zone in the west gold is associated with quartz veining in granite. The EDS occurrence (Saint Pierre zone) contains gold associated with a faulted contact and with gold-bearing conglomerate, and in some regional faults (BRGM showed the existence of gold mineralization along a NWN-SES fault to the east between Paramaca and dioritic units).

The area has been affected by its equatorial climate, and the rocks are highly weathered. A typical weathered profile in Paul Isnard area consists, from the surface, of colluvium (0 to 1 m deep), massive clay with quartz and saprolite fragments (1 to 3 m deep), mixed lateritic clay - saprolite (mottled zone, 3 to 6 m deep), saprolite zone (15 to 20 m) deep and fresh rock (20 m deep). This extensive lateritic overburden and the dense vegetal cover result in large zones of the area remaining unmapped and under-explored.

STRATIGRAPHY, VOLCANOLOGY AND PETROCHEMISTRY

The Montagne d'Or area (Fig. 2) is a bimodal volcano-sedimentary pile, sheared and metamorphosed to upper greenschist - lower amphibolite assemblages (Schwartz, 1996; Hubé, 1997). The sequence is a steeply dipping south facing homocline with a bedding-parallel E-W foliation. The primarily volcanic and sedimentary strata contain semi-concordant and crosscutting intrusions. The simplified stratigraphic sequence includes a lower mafic unit, overlain by a thick felsic unit, with an upper mafic unit that occurs primarily in the eastern part of the area, and an uppermost sedimentary unit. There are a few outcrops of the volcanic rocks and the upper sedimentary sequence is exposed in stream beds. Most of the information provided below is based on drill core observations. These are augmented by 208 analyses for major and minor elements (XRF and ICP-MS determinations), 471 ICP analyses (hot aqua regia extraction) for base metals, and 9150 ICP analyses for gold. All samples were taken well below the saprolite zone, to avoid any effects of element mobility associated with the weathering. Tables 1 and 2 provide average com-

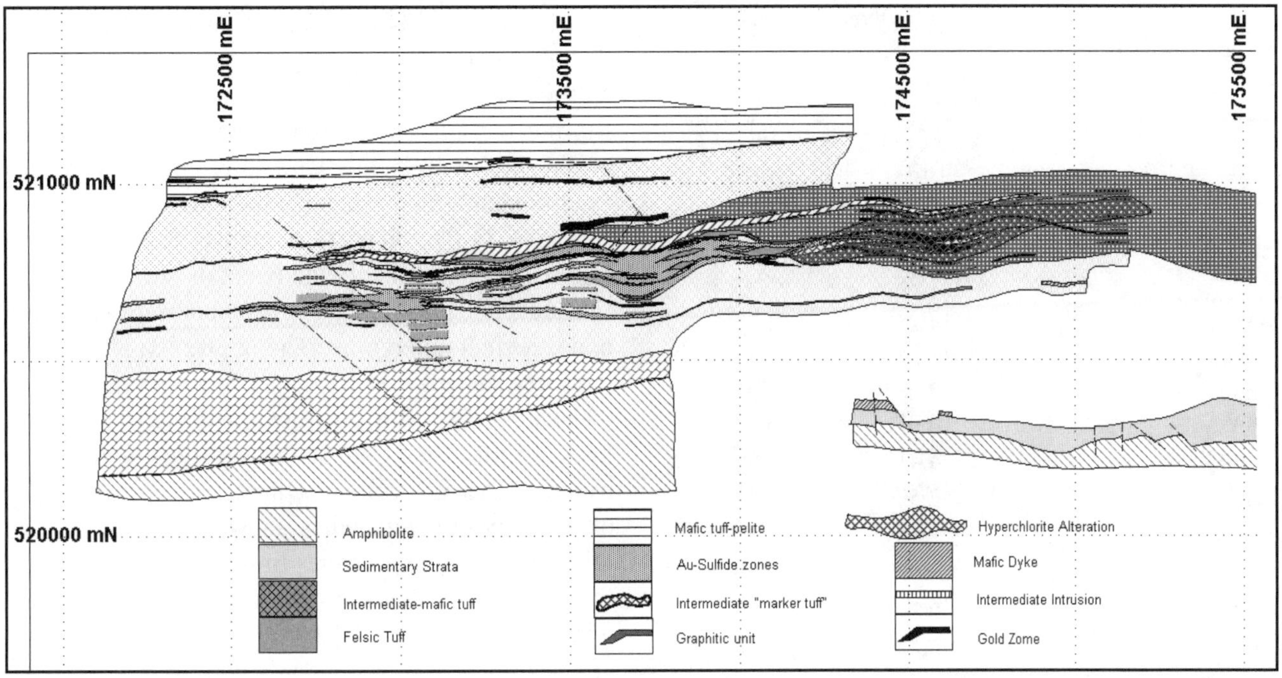

Figure 2. Generalized geology of the Paul Isnard area. The sequence is south – facing. The "tuff-pelite" unit at the north of the sequence is predominantly mafic. The distribution of the sulphide-rich zone is an interpretation based on correlations between drill-holes. Analysis of the data (herein) suggest that the sulphide and gold are distributed in a semi-conformable zone, but that their original distribution may have been controlled by syn-volcanic faults. The distribution of the most significant semi-conformable alteration ("hyperchlorite") is also shown. The geographic positions for this and subsequent diagrams is the Universal Transverse Mercator grid, based on the parameters for WGS84, zone 22N.

positions of each of the major litho-stratigraphic units in the area. Stratigraphic facing is determined on the basis of graded beds in the felsic sequence. The stratigraphic sequence, from north to south in the area is as follows.

Lower mafic unit

The base of the pile is composed of a lower mafic unit, consisting of 1 to 2 m (apparent thickness) of rhythmically bedded mafic tuff, changing upwards to graphitic pelite, which contains pyrrhotite. This unit has not been studied in detail. It contains intercalated mafic sills, some of which contain epidote. The strong sedimentary character in the upper portion of this unit may indicate that it defines the top of an earlier volcanic cycle. The paucity of distinct pillows or epiclastic strata and fine-grained nature of the mafic-derived sedimentary beds suggest that the unit was deposited in a low relief environment.

Felsic Unit

This unit is composed predominantly of distinctly bedded ash flow or water-lain tuff units, and contains some intercalated intermediate (mixed) tuff units. Graded tuff beds indicate a consistent facing direction to the south. The unit is composed of many repeated cycles of coarse to fine ash deposits, which may be subdivided into three "facies", each typical of a portion of a water-lain pyroclastic eruptive sequence. All of the "facies" or members of an eruptive cycle are similar in composition (Table 1). The coarse basal member, generally logged as "felsic lapilli tuff", is composed of well-sorted clasts, typically 1 to 5 cm in diameter (Fig. 3). The lapilli tuff members have very little matrix. The clasts are commonly equant (where not strained) and zoned, with silicified or chloritized outer margins that may be replaced bubble-walls. Most of the lapilli units contain abundant quartz crystals. The basal portions of some lapilli units are locally reversely graded. In addition to those units logged

Table 1. Average compositions of the three members of a felsic pyroclastic ash flow unit.

	Felsic Lapilli Tuff	Felsic Tuff	Felsic "Welded" Tuff
Weight %			
SiO_2	69.24	71.75	66.93
Al_2O_3	14.60	14.25	13.76
CaO	2.53	1.83	1.14
MgO	1.07	0.88	1.21
MnO	0.07	0.07	0.10
$Fe_2O_3{}^T$	4.00	4.41	8.90
K_2O	2.37	2.52	3.06
Na_2O	3.49	2.98	1.90
P_2O_5	0.10	0.06	0.09
TiO_2	0.32	0.27	0.35
LOI	1.97	2.30	3.44
PPM			
Ba	937	968	1009
Cu	37	210	488
Pb	10	31	16
Nd	18	16	17
Ni	12	12	14
Nb	2	7	2
Yb	1	1	1
Y	5	5	7
Zr	101	86	89
Zn	26	56	232

as lapilli tuff, the units noted in the logs as "felsic agglomerate" are probably the coarsest facies of each ash-flow sequence. Such coarse fragments identify the beginning of a new eruption and may indicate proximity to a volcanic centre.

The second "facies" or member comprises the central portion of each ash flow cycle, and is composed of fine to medium-grained ash, locally termed "felsic tuff". Quartz crystals, identical in size to those in the coarser basal units, are scattered throughout most of these. Again, this member is well sorted.

The third "facies" comprises the upper portion of each ash flow, and is composed of very fine ash. These units have an aphanitic groundmass, but contain quartz crystals in about the same abundance as the other units. They are logged as both "felsic welded tuff" and "felsic tuff", but the presence of welding has not yet been petrographically confirmed. These portions of the ash flow have lower silica, Na_2O and CaO contents than the other two zones, and higher MgO, Fe_2O_3(t) and K_2O contents. These chemical differences are probably the result of the higher reactivity of the fine-grained ash to both seawater and hydrothermal alteration. The higher MgO content indicates that the ash was in contact with seawater when it was still hot. Such enrichments in MgO and losses of Na_2O and CaO have been noted in many districts, including Noranda (Dimroth, 1975). A picture of a composite ash bed is shown in Figure 3. The thickness of each bed varies from about 15 cm to over four metres. A few mafic intervals are intercalated with the felsic tuff beds near the top of this unit.

Upper mafic unit

Both mafic intrusions (sills and dykes) and mafic flows are present in this section. The unit consists largely of sheet flows, which may have ponded against a synvolcanic fault. The mafic flows are intercalated with felsic ash flows to the east for a short lateral distance. The flows are usually almost featureless, but include a few vesicle zones and possible hyaloclastite. Pillows, although evident, are not abundant. Vesicles are both quartz and chlorite (after Mg-zeolite?) - filled. Distinct, irregular chloritic fragments adjacent to zones of vesicles identify the hyaloclastite zones. The exceptional homogeneity of other parts of this mafic unit may suggest that it includes some very fine-grained intrusions. The principal constituents of this unit include:

1) Mafic and Intermediate Tuff: Three types of mafic and intermediate tuff are present. The "mafic banded tuff" is comprised of distinctly banded units that occur between flows. The bands are discontinuous, and they probably are a combination of basaltic detritus and deformed hyaloclastite that formed between pillowed flows. They define flow boundaries and are compositionally almost identical to the mafic flows. Other units logged as mafic tuff are composed of intercalated mafic and felsic

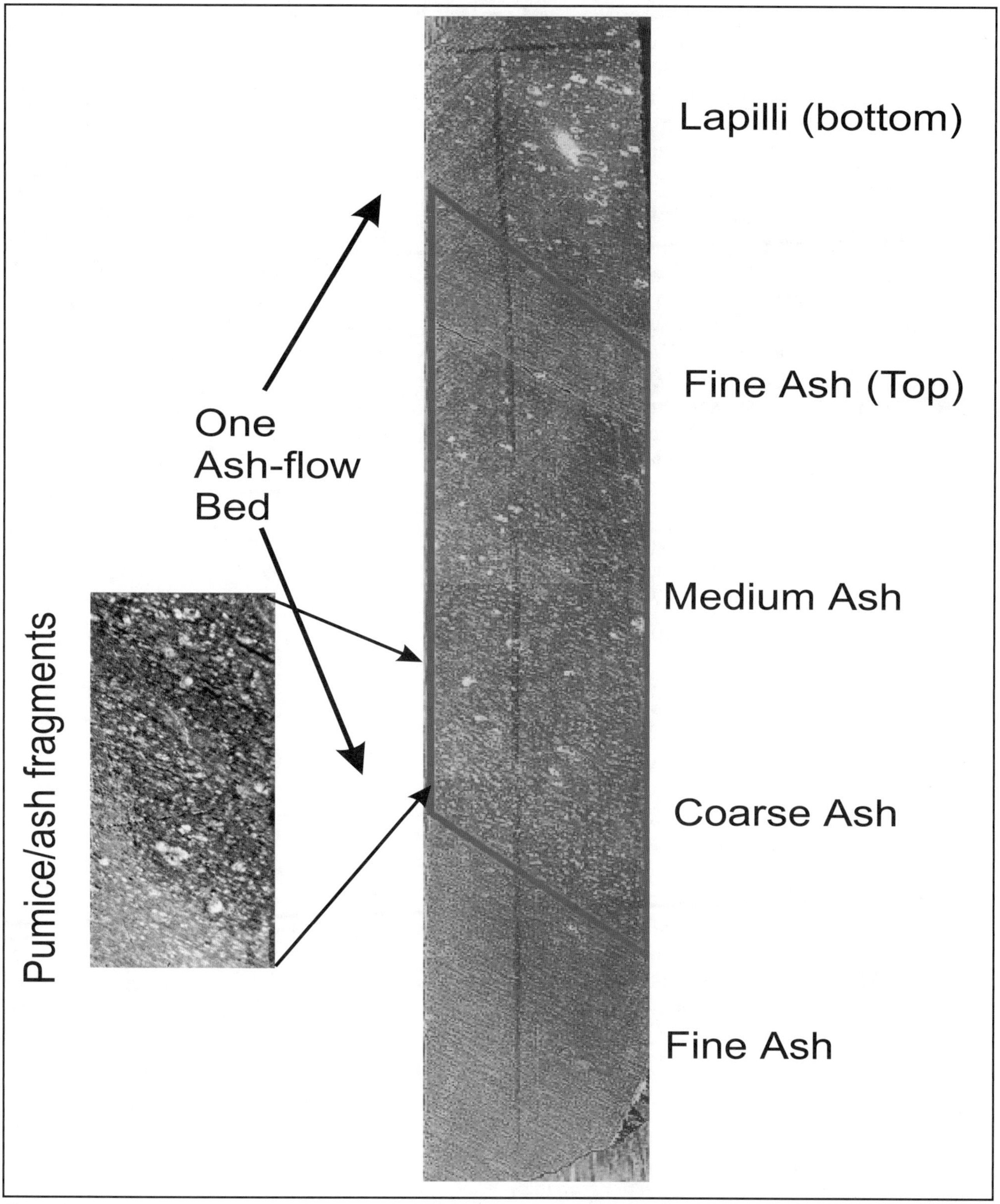

Figure 3. A composite of several contiguous pieces of drill core, illustrating graded ash flow beds with gradational clast sizes. On the left, a close-up of the bottom of ash flow bed with coarse juvenile lapilli supported in a finer matrix. Note also the matrix-supported quartz crystals. This texture represents either the base of a volcanogenic turbidite or debris flow. MO97-27-54.2m

detritus. These are interflow horizons, and mark a pause in volcanic activity. Some are highly deformed, and others display excellent graded beds providing consistent facing indications (all to the south). The mixed tuff layers generally have higher silica contents (51-55 %, Table 2) compared with the mafic flows, and also have lower TiO_2 contents (typically 0.5-0.9 % TiO_2). Many of the mafic tuff units are garnetiferous, reflecting a slight lowering of alkalis and moderate to high Mn contents. Many of these units have unusually high Ni contents and contain disseminated sulphides; their origin discussed below.

2) Mafic Intrusions: The mafic intrusions are all very fine-grained. Locally their contacts are not parallel to schistosity, and all show some strain near their margins. The fine-grained nature of the intrusions and their altered margins also are typical of synvolcanic intrusions. All contacts are deformed, indicating that these dykes were emplaced early in the history of this area. Although no chemical data are available for them, the similarity of their textural and mineralogical attributes to those of the volcanic rocks indicate that they may be synvolcanic, and are petrogenetically related to the upper mafic unit. Their orientation could not be determined, but the positions of all intrusions were plotted (along with the hyperchlorite distribution, discussed below) on a separate plan (Fig. 4). The mafic intrusions show very poor to no lateral continuity. For example, abundant dykes in hole MO98 54 are not evident in the adjacent hole, MO97 32. A similar lack of correlation is observed in holes MO9 38 and 27. This general lack of horizontal continuity may indicate that the dykes were oriented at right angles to the strata.

The "Intermediate Intrusion" is a unique and easily identified unit that is locally sub-parallel to the strata, but actually transects two major units, the felsic unit and upper mafic unit. All sections of this intrusion are remarkably similar in texture and mineralogical composition. The white elongate feldspar relict grains are set in a dark grey groundmass. Albite, epidote and quartz have replaced the feldspar crystals. The groundmass is composed of a fine-grained aggregate of quartz, feldspar, mica and carbonate. The feldspar phenocrysts are typically deformed into subrounded ovoid shapes, and have quartz and carbonate in their pressure shadows. The groundmass biotite is aligned in the foliation plane. The unit forms a series of distinct thin sub concordant sills that post-date volcanism, but predate deformation.

Table 2: Average compositions of mafic rocks in the Paul Isnard area

	Mafic dykes	Mafic flows	Mafic banded tuff	Mafic lava
N	3	12	10	25
SiO_2	55.16	53.54	51.01	49.88
Al_2O_3	13.87	13.20	13.74	13.54
CaO	6.14	6.29	8.38	9.26
MgO	3.76	5.09	4.96	5.92
MnO	0.14	0.17	0.21	0.20
Fe_2O_3T	13.21	13.21	13.68	14.02
K_2O	2.67	1.66	1.12	0.43
Na_2O	1.44	1.78	2.01	2.24
P_2O_5	0.13	0.22	0.12	0.12
TiO_2	0.57	0.94	1.20	1.33
LOI	5.16	3.52	3.15	2.45
PPM				
Ba	786	640	442	139
Cu	627	683	115	153
Pb	27	15	16	32
Nd	18	28	12	11
Ni	40	93	70	82
Nb	3	3	4	4
Yb	1.3	1.8	2.3	2.8
Y	10	16	19	23
Zr	81	89	85	85
Zn	148	194	219	104

Upper sedimentary unit

The sediments were not specifically examined. Their presence towards the southern part of the Paul

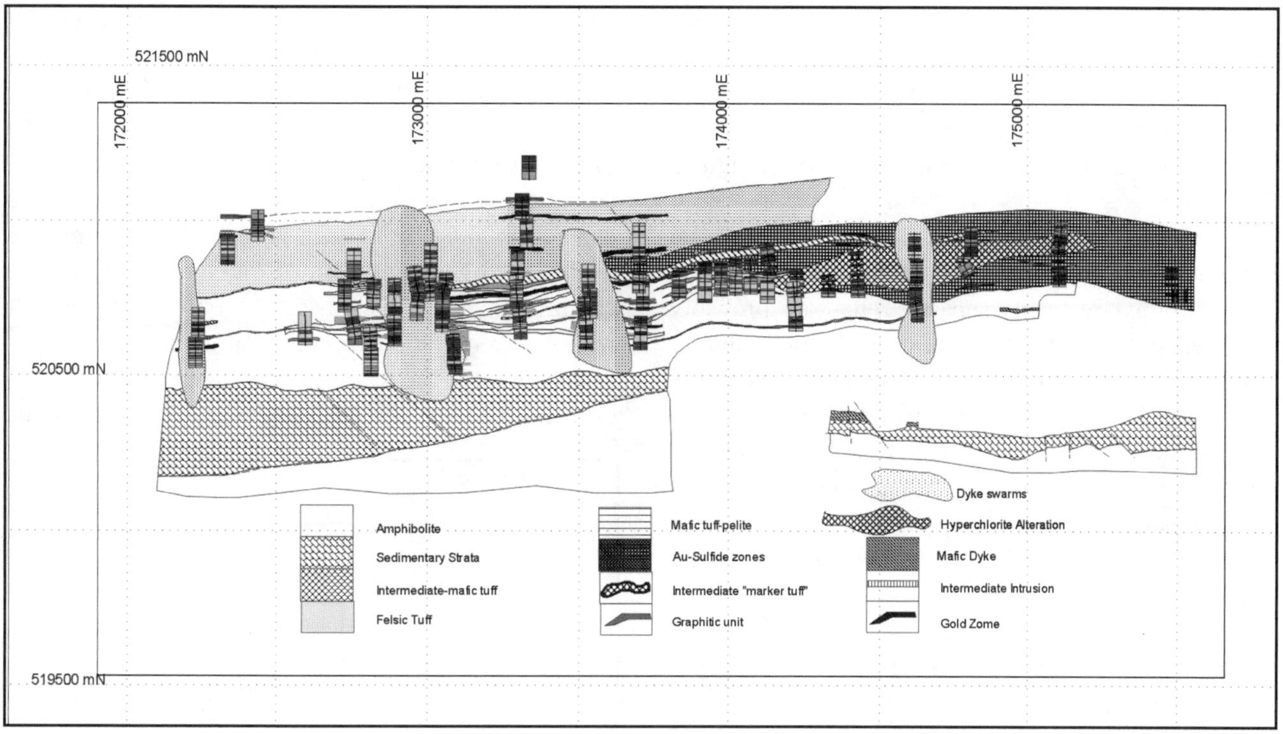

Figure 4. Same area as Figure 2, but showing the distribution of dykes and "hyperchlorite" alteration. The dykes do not correlate from hole to hole, suggesting that they are oriented perpendicular to the strata. These zones are generalized from the core logs.

Isnard property may indicate the waning stage of, or a hiatus in felsic volcanism.

STRUCTURAL FEATURES

Foliation is consistent throughout the area, strikes E-W with dips to the south varying between 70° to 85°. No major folds have been observed in the zone, but very rare centimetre-scale folds have been noted in the drill core. Two major E-W faults exist in the Montagne d'Or zone. The first is located in the north at the top of the lower mafic unit, and is identified by a graphitic layer that is several centimetres thick. No mineralization is associated with this fault. The second is located in the south of the zone and is evident in the airborne geophysical maps; it forms a distinct cliff and separates the sedimentary strata from the amphibolite unit to the south. Near this cliff, mylonite – like fabric has been observed in outcrops. Hubé, (1997) showed a sinistral movement on this fault. This fault contains some pyrite, but no gold. Two other minor structural trends are evident, NW-SE and NE-SW. These directions have been interpreted from creek deviations and some rare fault breccia. They correspond to a later tectonic phase than that which formed the prevalent E-W foliation, and have not offset the strata.

PETROCHEMICAL OBSERVATIONS

To assess the petrochemical attributes of the rocks the major and trace element data were examined statistically and grouped on the basis of immobile element plots and calculated petrogenetic factors. These groups of samples were then compared with the lithotypes assigned in the original core logs, and if the petrochemical data were ambiguous, the core was re-examined. Given that mafic and felsic volcanic and intrusive rocks were already recognized in the area, the objective of this statistical exercise was to see if further division of the lithologies on a chemical basis was possible. The frequency distributions of the least mobile major and trace elements (TiO_2, Y, Zr, Yb, and Nb) and the Rare Earth

Elements (REEs)) were examined. Only the "least altered" samples were used to assign petrochemical parentage; intensely altered samples (see discussion of alteration, below) were excluded.

The results for some of these are shown in Figures 5, 6 and 7.

The probability plots of TiO_2 and Y (Fig. 5) reveal three distinct populations of data. The felsic and mafic groups are totally separated, and are probably petrogenetically unrelated. The origin of the intermediate group of rocks is more problematical, and may be a result (in part) of mixing of the mafic and felsic populations. These are also evident on the TiO_2 vs. Y, Yb, Zr and Ni plots (Fig. 6). The population statistics are summarized in Table 3.

Contoured binary plots of the immobile element data illustrate that the three compositional groups are coherent with respect to SiO_2 (Fig. 6). In these, the mafic rocks all lie very close to the 48 % SiO_2 contour, and the felsic samples form a distinct, well defined linear array (see Zr vs. TiO_2 plot) with about 70 to 74 % SiO_2. Those samples that lie off of this linear trend may be altered, and will be re-examined later.

The "intermediate' samples have one unusual chemical attribute, illustrated in the Ni vs. TiO_2 plot in Figure 6. In establishing a classification system based on chemical composition (above) these samples were usually classified as "intermediate". If the trace element distributions are solely the result of mixing between felsic and mafic end-members, they should lie in the envelope between these groups, shown on the Ni-TiO_2 plot. Many of the "intermediate" samples lie above this envelope (i.e. have unusually high Ni contents). The higher Ni content (in comparison to Mg, for example) may indicate the presence of organically generated sulphides. Ni is typically very abundant in pyrite or pyrrhotite associated with organic-rich rocks (see Pasava et al, 1996 and references therein).

Once the samples were divided into lithological groups, various indices were calculated, and the samples were eventually tested for alteration effects (see discussion of alteration, below). Standard normative calculations and various "alteration indices" were calculated. In addition to using frequency distribution plots of typical "mobile" elements to establish indicators of various types of mineralization, the calculated abundance of normative corundum is an excellent indicator of alteration. Alteration tests are more useful if applied to single lithologies; thus before using them, a few additional tests of the major lithological groups as defined by either logging or chemical classification are needed to be undertaken, in order to ensure the integrity of each group. Also, information on the petrogenetic origin of the various lithologies can provide some insights as to the types of mineralization that might occur in the Paul Isnard area.

In Figure 7, the REE elements are plotted as chondrite normalized "spider" diagrams, for each of the

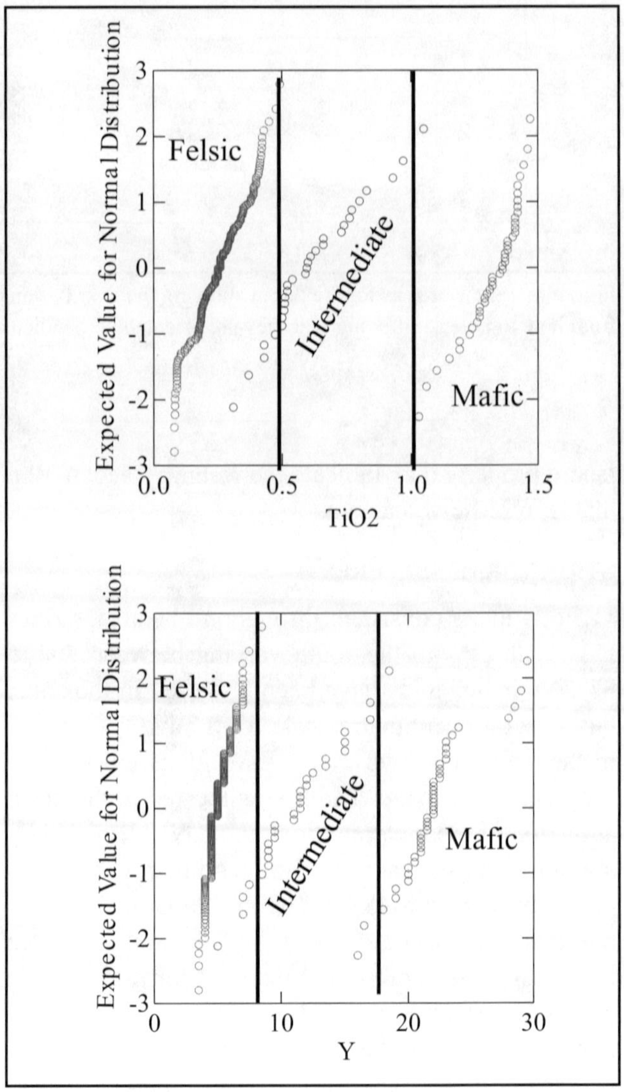

Figure 5. Frequency distributions of TiO_2 and Y for the three lithotypes, separated on the basis of chemical composition

Table 3. Threshold and range values for definition of lithologies on a chemical basis

		TiO_2 (%)	Ni (ppm)	Yb (ppm)	Y (ppm)
Felsic	A	< 0.1	<20	>2.5	>6
	B	0.1-0.2			
	C	0.2-0.4			
Intermediate		0.4-1.3	20-85	0.74-2.5	6-22
Mafic		>1.3	>85	<2.5	<22

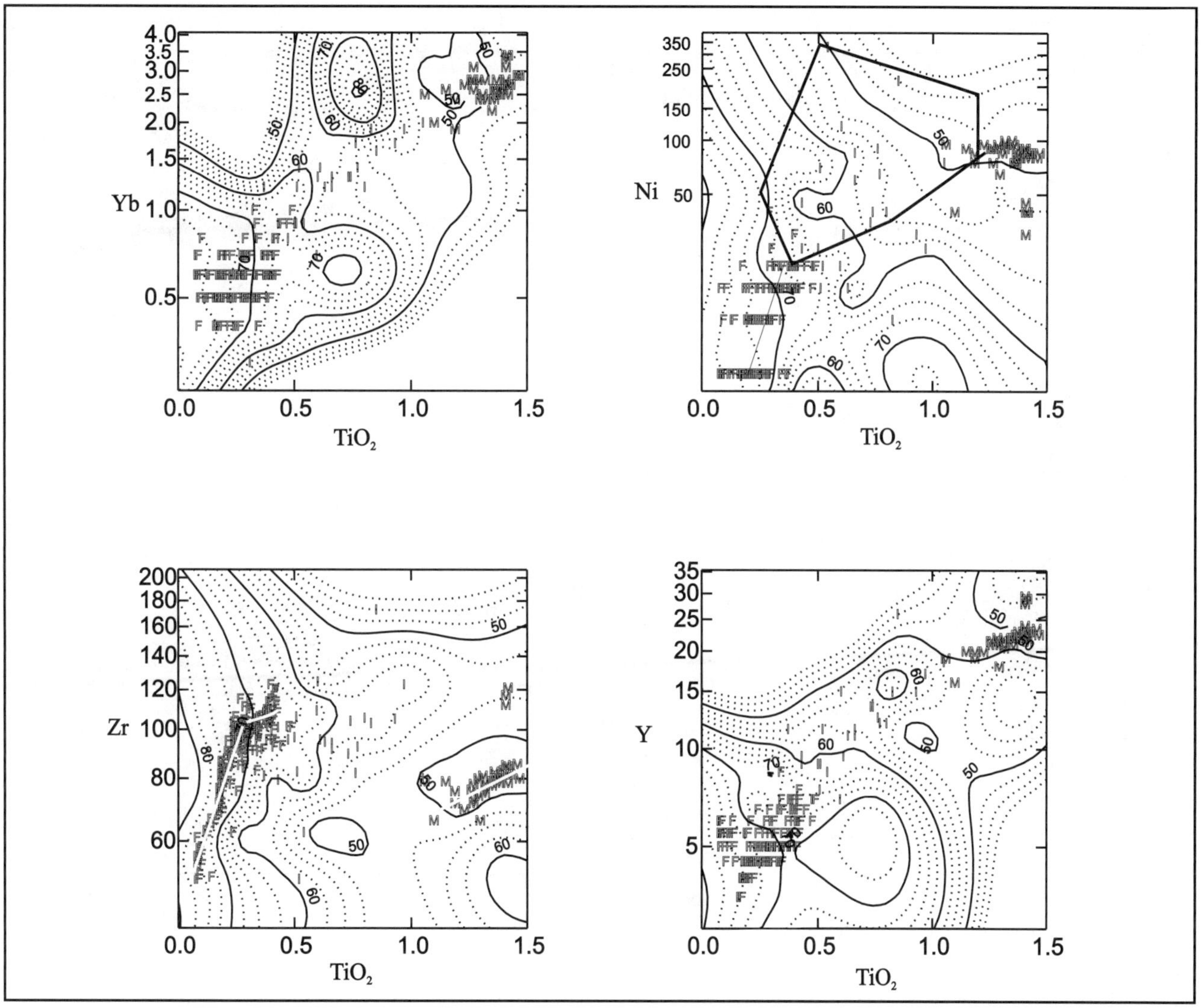

Figure 6. Binary plots of immobile elements, contoured with silica abundance; petrogenetic trends are illustrated on the Zr-TiO_2 plot, and the high Ni samples are outlined in the Ni-TiO_2 plot. Note on the TiO_2-Zr plot that there are two populations of felsic rocks (white lines), and two of mafic rocks.

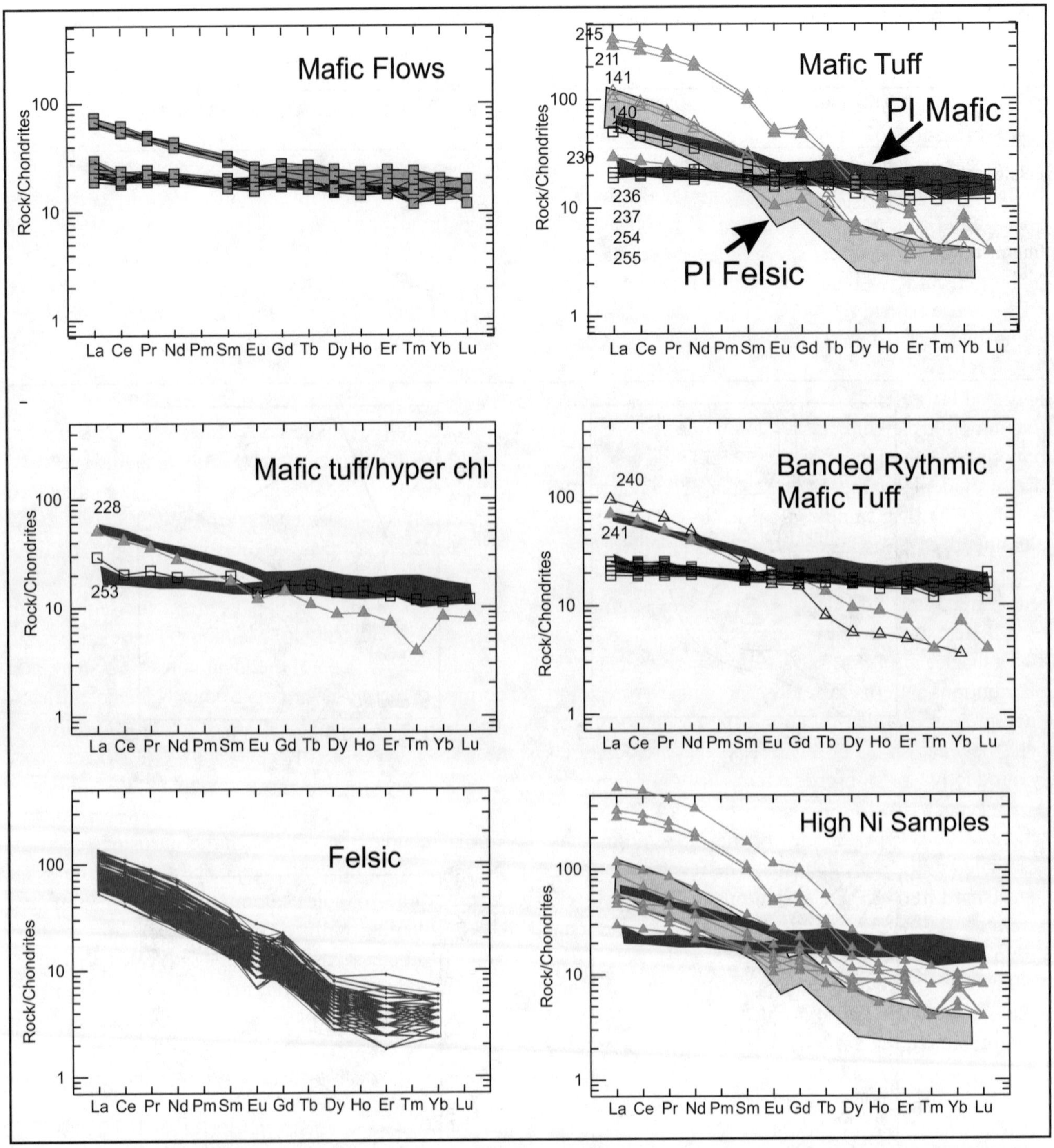

Figure 7. Plots of the REE element distributions of the major lithologies as defined by the PI logs. Note that "felsic" includes the felsic tuff, lapilli tuff and welded felsic tuff groups.

major lithologies plus the "high Ni" group of samples. The REE profiles of the felsic and mafic groups are clearly distinct. The felsic samples all lie in an envelope that is characterized by light-REE enrichment, a steep slope, and a moderately well developed negative Eu anomaly.

The mafic rocks at Paul Isnard form two groups (Fig. 8). Most of the mafic rocks lie in a very narrow envelope, with virtually no change between the light and heavy REE normalized abundances, and are similar to those found in back-arc ocean floors associated with ocean-ocean subduction zones. These are similar to the bulk of the mafic rocks at Snow Lake, and are also similar to many Archean basalt sequences associated with VMS deposits. A second group of basalt samples from Paul Isnard have slightly enriched light REEs, more typical of evolved arcs or back arcs. The melts that formed these LREE-enriched units were possibly contaminated by partial assimilation of hydrated crust. These two groups are also evident in the immobile element classification plots (Fig. 8). The bimodal distribution of mafic compositions is particularly evident on the Y-Zr-Ti plot (c.f. Pearce and Cann, 1973). The samples that lie closest to the calc-alkaline field are those with the light REE enrichment. These basalt samples have high K and Na contents, and may indicate that the mafic magma has assimilated some crustal material.

Lesher et al (1986) have established typical REE distribution patterns for Archean felsic rocks, and have proposed a classification scheme that discriminates between suites of felsic rocks that are potentially productive or non-productive for VMS deposits. Their Type 1 rhyolite group has low VMS potential, whereas their Types 2 and 3 groups are commonly associated with VMS deposits. The felsic rocks from Paul Isnard have REE distributions that most closely resemble the Type I sequence, with a subordinate group in the Type 2 composition (Fig. 9). Bailes and Galley (1996) provided the data for REE distributions associated with the highly productive Early Proterozoic Snow Lake district of Manitoba, and a similar data set was obtained for the Skellefte district of Sweden, another major Early Proterozoic VMS district. The Snow Lake and Skellefte data are also Type II. The Paul Isnard felsic melts are typical of highly evolved arcs (or those with a stronger continental association).

CONCLUDING REMARKS ON THE PETROCHEMISTRY AND VOLCANOLOGY

The felsic rocks form an extensive series of waterlain tuff cycles, each with a coarse, lapilli-dominated base (containing juvenile or primary pyroclastic fragments), a medium to coarse fragment centre and a fine ash top. Alteration and exceptionally good sorting of each ash flow unit are consistent with a subaqueous pyroclastic flow depositional mechanism. Clasts were altered by contact with seawater (Mg-enriched, Si and partially Na depleted), while still hot ash. Pyroclastic eruptions usually form if water depths are less than 2 km, and typically form in moderate (~1000-500 m) water depths, necessary to promote magma vesiculation prior to eruption (see Gibson et al., 1999). Such fragments may be transported away from the eruptive centre and deposited in deeper water. However, the coarse nature of the basal fragments in each cycle at Paul Isnard may indicate proximity to a volcanic vent. The paucity of sedimentary units in this sequence indicates that it was deposited rapidly.

The Paul Isnard felsic rocks have highly fractionated REE compositions, and are most similar to the most evolved rocks in upper part of the sequence in the Snow Lake district of Manitoba. These latter strata formed near the end of the local volcanic history, and formed the uppermost parts of that volcanic edifice.

The mafic rocks consist of massive and pillowed flows, bedded tuff strata and subvolcanic intrusions. Lower mafic unit contains abundant epidote, and may represent the upper portion of a lower semiconformable alteration system. Mafic intrusions occur in both the felsic and mafic sequences, show little or no lateral (hole to hole) continuity, and probably are dyke swarms, filling synvolcanic fault zones. Chloritization at their margins indicates that they were intruded into seawater-saturated strata. In many VMS districts, synvolcanic dykes generally occur in paleo-faults. In the Noranda district and elsewhere the abundance of such dykes defines both caldera boundaries and hydrothermal fluid conduits (Gibson and Watkinson, 1990). The dyke swarms illustrated in Figure 4 may define paleo-fracture zones, which could have been conduits for hydrothermal discharge. The bedded tuff units consist of a variety of lithologies, many of which are of mixed (felsic-mafic) origin.

The Paul Isnard mafic rocks are typical island-arc tholeiites. They display some evidence of melt contamination, suggesting that they resided in a shal-

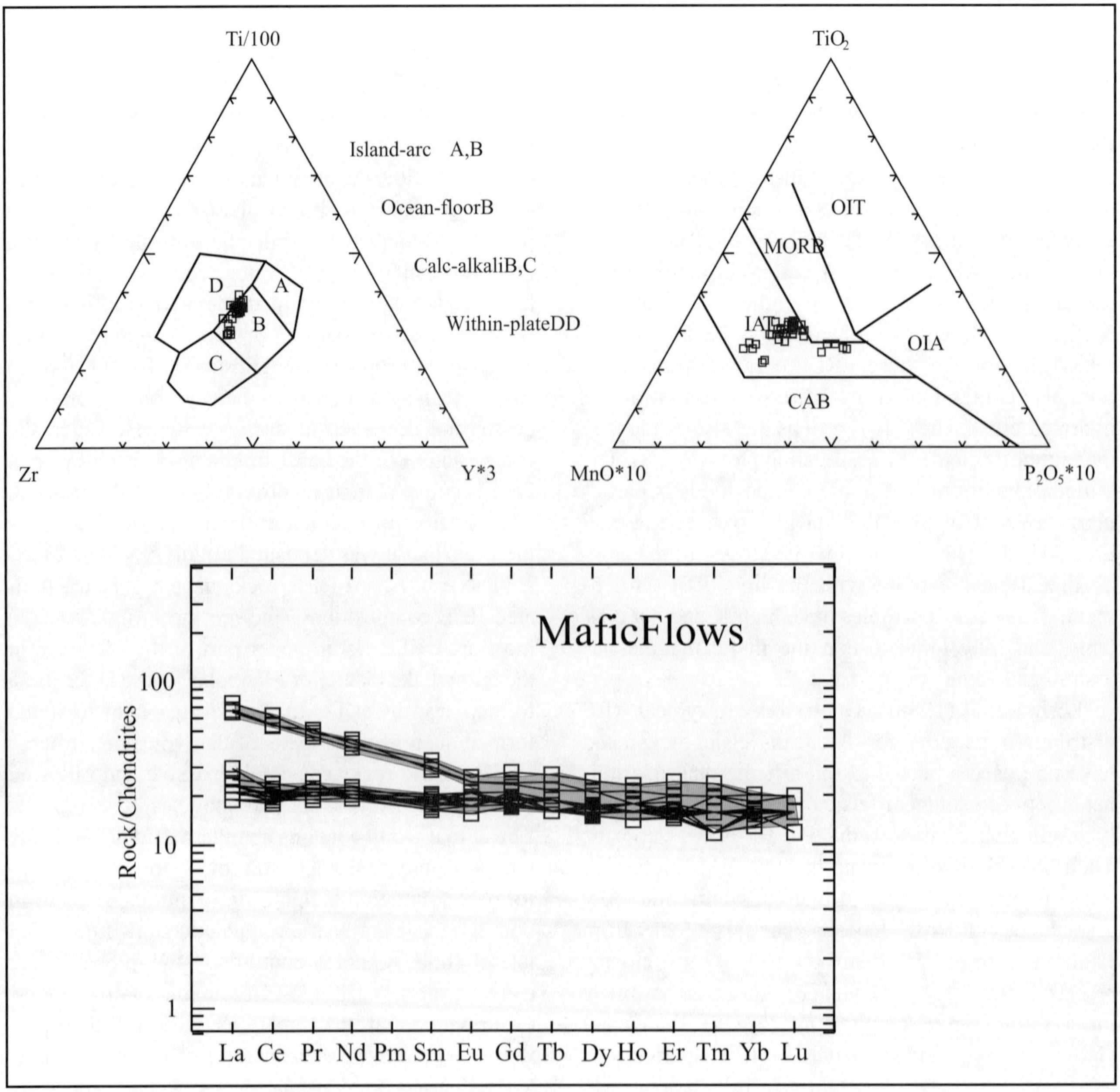

Figure 8. Immobile element and REE plots of the mafic rocks form the PI drill core. Note the bimodal distribution of data in all three plots; the group to the left in the upper two plots corresponds to the samples with light REE enrichment. All of the mafic compositions are island-arc tholeiite.

low subvolcanic magma chamber. Compositional trends such as this are observed in other VMS districts, and may be attributed to very high-T conditions at medial or upper crustal levels. Such conditions are ideal for engendering large-scale hydrothermal circulation, and indicate excellent VMS potential.

The mafic flows may be part of a synvolcanic fault block, with the felsic units deposited in an adjacent basin (see below). The abundance of mafic dykes in the adjacent felsic units adds support to the argument that the western edge of the mafic flow unit is an early fault. Such faults are excellent loci for hydrothermal fluids, and the fact that this western termination coincides with one of the thickest portions of gold-copper

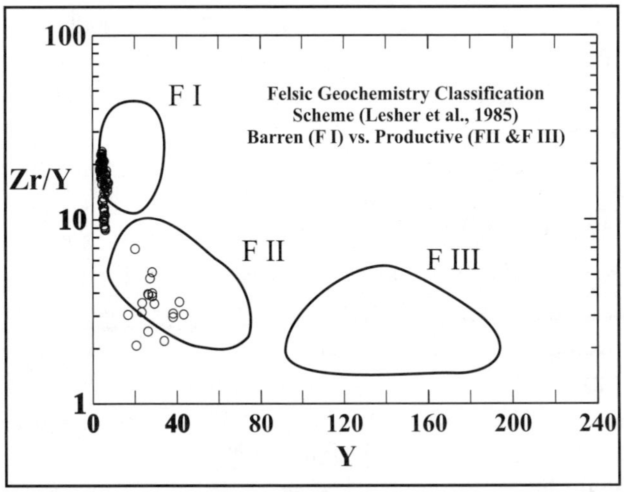

Figure 9. Plot illustrating the Lesher classification system for felsic rocks, plotted with the Paul Isnard samples. Note that they form two groups: Most are "Type 1" and subordinate groups are 'Type 2" compositions.

mineralization may be highly significant.

Alteration

Alteration occurs as two principal types. The most visible type is composed of zones of intense chloritization, termed "hyperchlorite". The second is less prominent "sericitization" associated with some of the more sulphide-rich sections. In addition to the visible alteration, chemical alteration is detected using major and minor element data.

In many sections of core through the gold-rich zones there are some correlations between the locations of hyperchlorite and high gold contents. The strongest gold zones are commonly adjacent to these zones, but in some areas, anomalous gold is unrelated to the hyperchlorite zones. Thus it is important to examine the alteration attributes of high gold zones, as well as those of the hyperchlorite zones.

For most, the wall rocks associated with most hydrothermal ore deposit types (VMS, epithermal, porphyry, skarn mesothermal vein Au and others) the alkali elements (Na, K, Ba, Li) together with Ca and Sr are highly mobile, and alumina is residual. Fe is added (usually as sulphide minerals, but also as silicates) in many deposit types. Copper and zinc are both added in VMS alteration zones as well as to wall rocks of a few other deposit types (skarns, some high sulfidation epithermal deposits). The data were tested for these additions and depletions.

Hyperchlorite zones

These are composed of variably chloritized portions of felsic and mafic volcanic units, as well as some mafic intrusions. They are generally a few metres in core length, and have gradational boundaries. Most contain some disseminated- and vein- sulphide. Hyperchlorite occurs in all lithologies except the "intermediate intrusion" unit. Examples of hyperchlorite alteration are shown in Figure 10. For the most part, this form of alteration occupies a very limited stratigraphic interval, particularly in the eastern part of the area. To the west, where they occur predominantly in the upper mafic unit, these zones are less well defined stratigraphically. In almost all occurrences, hyperchlorite has a close spatial relationship with the widest gold and base metal mineralization. The textural and mineralogical attributes of the hyperchlorite zones seem quite similar in both mafic and felsic settings. However, in order to examine the origin and significance of it more closely, this lithology will be examined separately for each of these two principal host rocks.

In felsic rocks, the edges of the unit are defined by chlorite veining. Here, quartz eyes are preserved, although most of the primary volcanic texture was destroyed. In the central parts of these zones, all primary features are destroyed, and the sulphide content may increase to as much as 50 %. Figure 10 illustrates a typical section through a hyperchlorite zone in felsic rocks. Here, the felsic ash was partially replaced by chlorite at the outer margins of the zone, and completely replaced in the centre of the zone. Remnant felsic clasts are visible at the margins of the hyperchlorite zone, but completely replaced at its centre. This replacement feature is evident in the adjacent more gold-rich zone, as well.

The felsic lapilli tuff section shown in Figure 10 has distinct lithic clasts in the fourth and fifth rows of the drill core. At the beginning of this section (top of picture) the felsic tuff is gradationally chloritized; this may be incipient "hyperchlorite". After this section is a short section of distinctly bedded intermediate (mixed felsic-mafic) tuff or sediment. The following unit is logged as "mafic tuff"; it has sharp contacts with the felsic units both above and below, and is thus either a dyke or a distinct bed. This is followed by a section of graded felsic tuff and lapilli tuff, which is gradually chloritized towards the end of the box. This is the transition into hyperchlorite, and clearly illustrates the "replacement" or alteration nature of the latter.

In order to establish the chemical relationships of this alteration, a section (DDH MO97-40) within the felsic unit that has major and trace element data was examined more closely. This section includes some hyperchlorite, but is logged as including a mafic tuff unit as well as several mafic dykes.

The REE distributions of these samples indicate that they may all belong to the felsic group (Fig. 11). The samples identified as felsic tuff have typical REE patterns, with steep slope (~3), normalized Yb content of less than 5, and slight negative europium anomalies. The samples of "mafic tuff" (211, 215) and "hyperchlorite" (212, 213) are somewhat similar, but have exceptional slopes (7-9) and high normalized Yb (10). This is surprising, considering that most mafic rocks in the Paul Isnard area have flat REE patterns, at about 10x chondrite. This complexity is shown by Sample 211, which is supposed to represent mafic tuff, but has a pattern much more similar to felsic tuff (c.f. Figure 9). Given the length of the sample (1.2 m), it may have included significant amounts of felsic material. Alternatively, some "mafic tuff" units are actually highly chloritized felsic material.

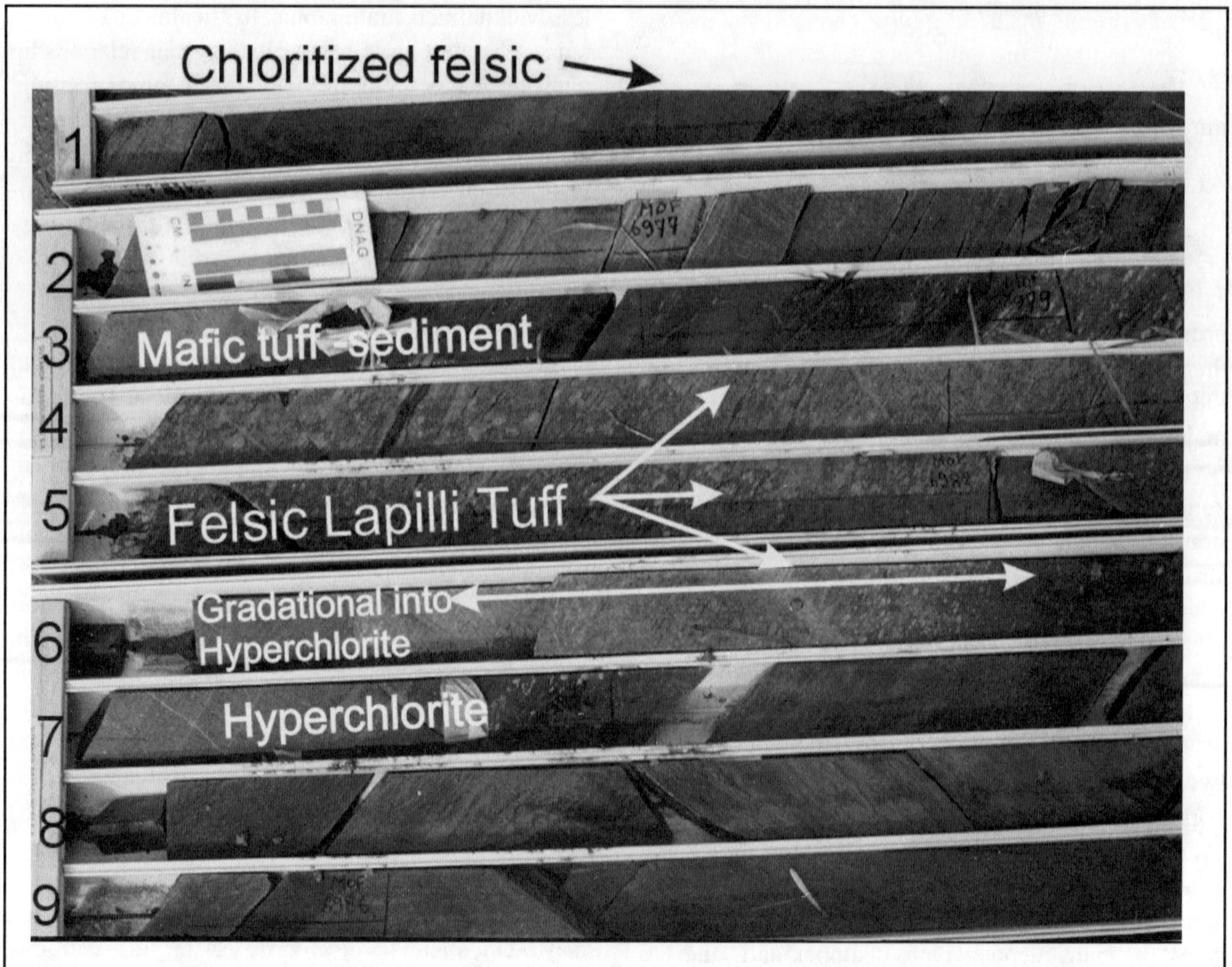

Figure 10. Upper plate: Section of drill core illustrating the gradational nature of the hyperchlorite alteration. This section includes chloritized felsic rocks, a mafic tuff unit, and hyperchlorite. (MO97-40: 182-187).

In order to examine this further, some mass balance tests are applied, using the Grant (1986) isochon method. Samples PIWR 209, 210, 214 and 216 were selected to ensure that the same primary lithology (felsic tuff) is compared. PIWR 214 and 216 are very close to the hyperchlorite zone. The hyperchlorite sample was compared with the mafic tuff samples (211 and 215), as these three have similar REE patterns, TiO_2 and other immobile element contents. All of these comparisons are shown in Figure 12.

As the hyperchlorite zone is approached, the felsic tuff gained Fe_2O_3, K_2O, Cu, Zn and some MnO. It lost CaO, Na_2O and Sr. MgO changes are variable, with a small addition evident in some comparisons. Quartz phenocrysts are preserved through as much as 50 % of the hyperchlorite zones, but in the most intensely altered portions of them, quartz phenocrysts are not evident, and have probably been dissolved.

The gains and losses in the felsic tuff are entirely consistent with alteration associated with high-temperature, metal-rich hydrothermal fluid. The gains in Zn are so large as to be off of the scale used for these diagrams. The copper gains are even larger, and extend well beyond the range of the isochon diagrams.

The down-hole distribution of the key indicator elements in the felsic volcanic rocks (Fig. 13) provides further information on the processes attendant on the formation of the gold zone:

1) The median K_2O content for unaltered felsic rocks is 1.8 % (range = 1.5-2.5 %), for CaO is 2.5 % (range = 2.0-3.0 %), and for Na_2O is 4.5 % (range = 3.8-5 %). Many of the values for K_2O are higher than this in Hole MO97-40. The K_2O - enriched zones are on the stratigraphic hangingwall of the hyperchlorite and gold-rich zones. CaO is locally depleted in the gold-rich zones.
2) The alkali elements are remarkably enriched near the hyperchlorite zone; Na and Ca increase near the centre of the zone, (along with Fe), but decrease to anomalously low contents at its margins.

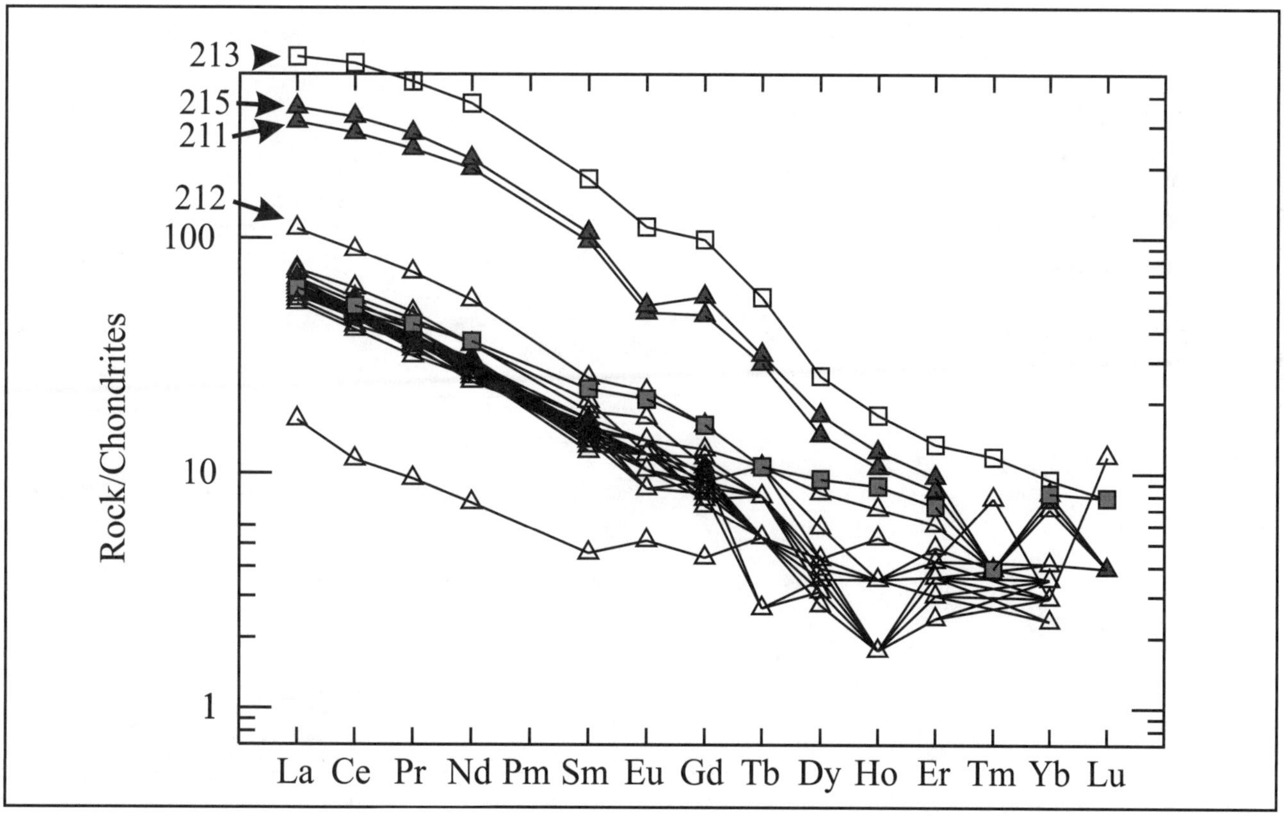

Figure 11. REE distribution patterns in hyperchlorite samples. Numbers to left of data lines are original sample numbers (see text).

3) Copper is enriched in the gold zones, but maximum zinc enrichment is over 50 m away from the gold and hyperchlorite areas. Zinc may be symmetrically enriched about the most gold rich area (adjacent to the hyperchlorite); this distribution is expected if the metals are distributed laterally away from a synvolcanic feeder zone, but this zonation is not consistent with a seafloor depositional site for zinc (or copper). This relationship will be explored more fully later.

Hyperchlorite in the upper mafic sequence:

As noted previously, hyperchlorite zones are more widespread in the upper mafic unit than in the felsic strata. The textural and mineralogical nature of the hyperchlorite is quite similar to that observed in felsic rocks, with each zone gradational into the adjacent basalt. The most intensely chloritized parts have developed a distinct spotted texture, and are probably composed of two types of chlorite. The spots are typically 3 to 8 mm in diameter, and resemble spotted

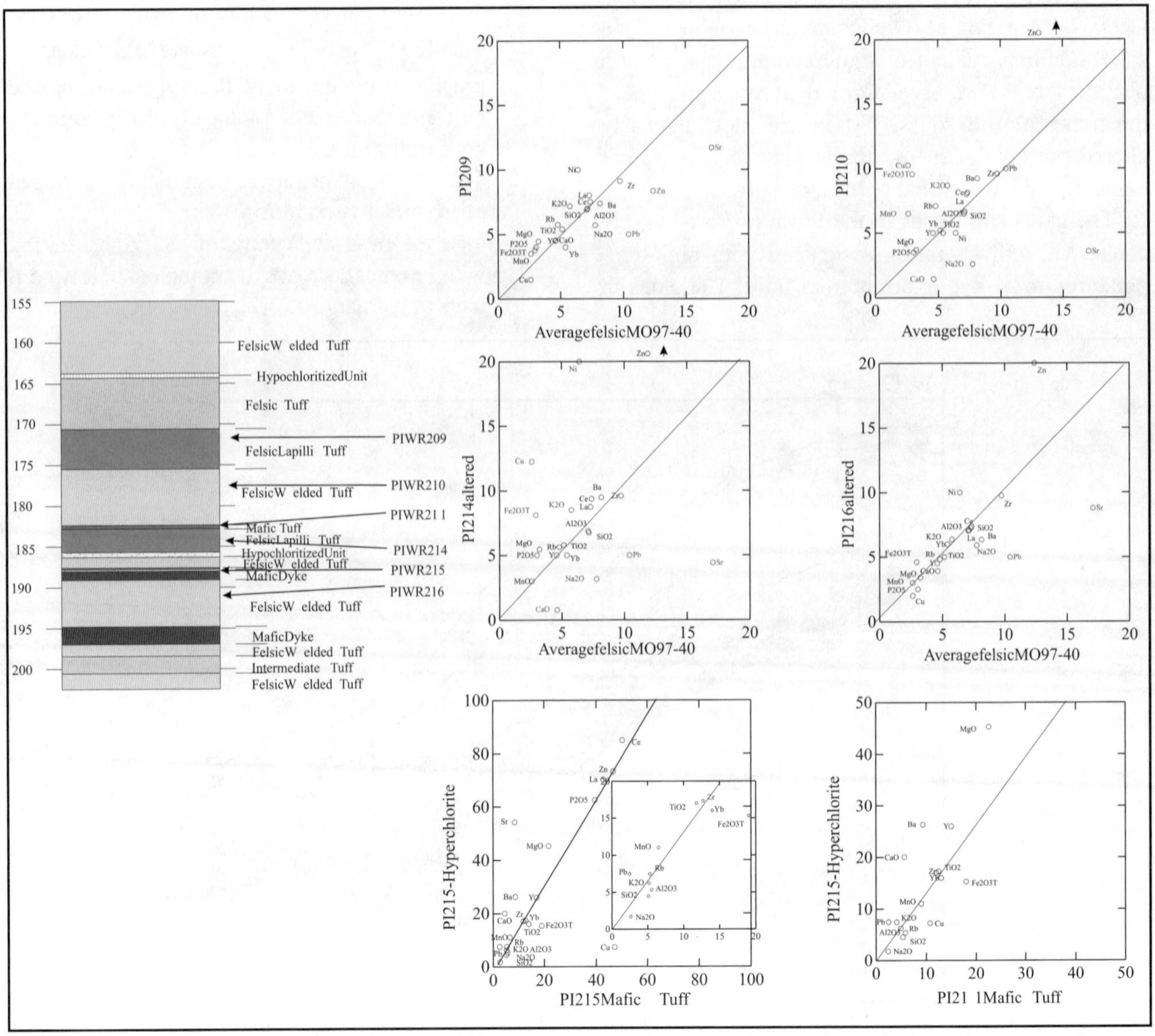

Figure 12. Isochon plots of unaltered and altered felsic rocks, and in chlorite alteration that occurs within or near thin units of mafic rock (MO97-43, lowest two plots). Section at left illustrates the lithological distributions in this hole, and the sample locations.

chlorite alteration observed associated with the Noranda deposits, and elsewhere (Riverin and Hodgson, 1980).

Chemical data from one section of hyperchlorite in mafic rocks (MO97-43) are presented in Figure 14. The chemical changes are similar to those observed in felsic volcanic rocks. The most important change is the addition of iron. Large amounts of zinc and lead were also added, but in the comparisons done here, copper *appears* to have been added only in minor amounts. However, copper has been pervasively added to the entire area, and the lack of an anomalous

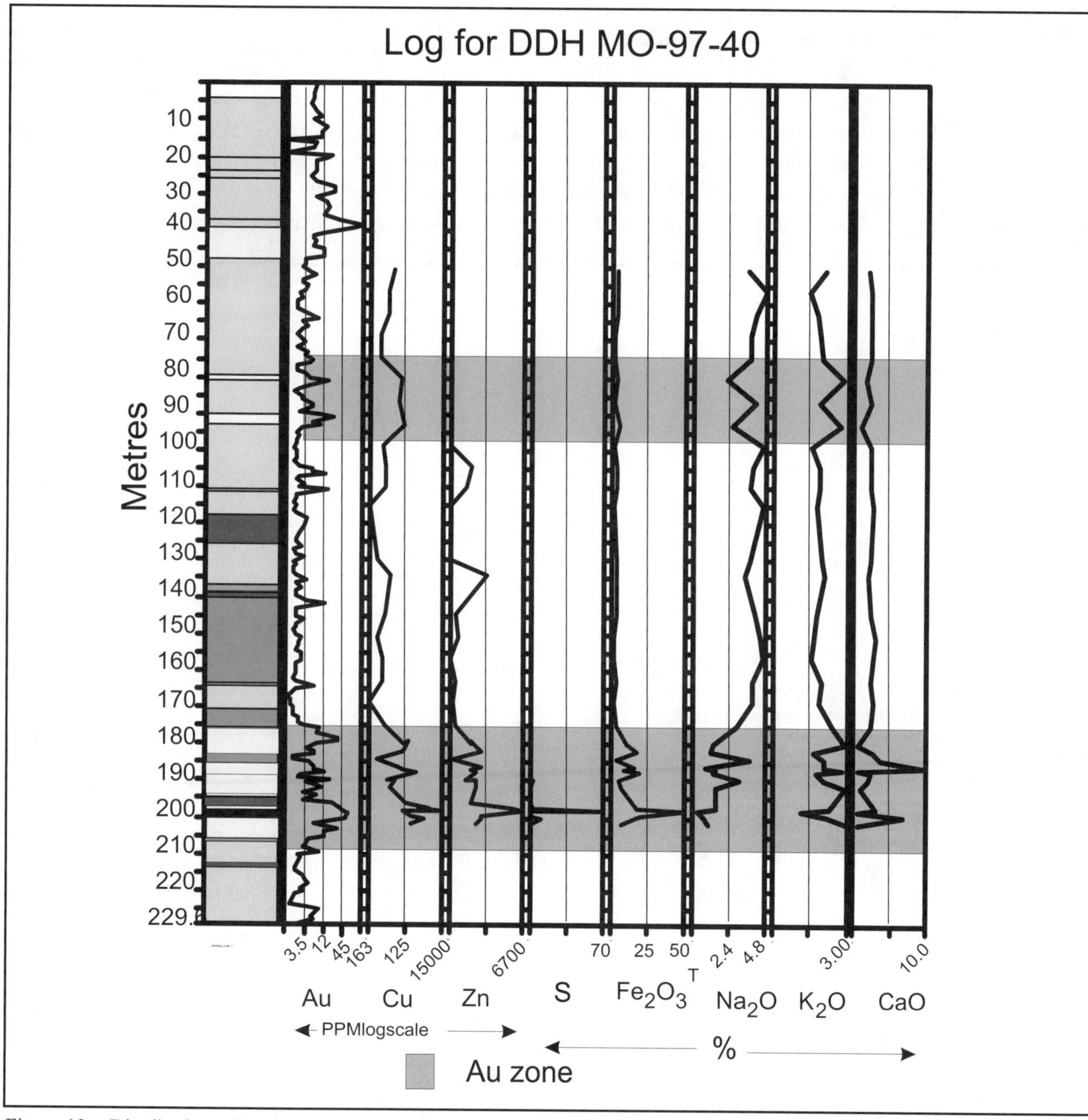

Figure 13. Distribution of base metal, gold and alteration indicator elements in hole MO-97-40. This represents a typical section through a gold-enriched zone, and illustrates the large increases in copper, zinc, iron and sulphur and with gold, and the loss of Na and Ca, and some gain in K, in the mineralized zone

addition may result from the choice of samples (see later discussion). The hyperchlorite zones have lost Na_2O, CaO, Sr, and possibly some MgO. The gains and losses are compatible with alteration from a large volume of Fe-rich hydrothermal fluid that destroyed feldspar.

The origin of this fluid is not entirely clear. A similar form of alteration was noted below the Anderson Lake mine in the Snow Lake district of Manitoba (Walford and Franklin, 1982). The zone at Snow Lake occurs about 150 m below the orebody (probably about 400 m if deformation is removed) and consists of a massive chlorite zone, with only slight enrichment in zinc and copper (a few 100 ppm). The zone at Snow Lake seems to transect the volcanic strata at a very low angle, can be traced for at least 1500 m in the footwall to the deposits, and is gradational upwards (stratigraphically) into the felsic strata that form the footwall to the mines. Alteration in the felsic rocks is dominantly Fe-rich, and is similar to that observed in the Paul Isnard hyperchlorite zones.

Chemical Alteration Associated with Gold Mineralization

As with the hyperchlorite zones, the first approach is to look at the mass balance relations between all elements and gold-rich zones. Two areas are selected, one that represents high gold in mafic rocks (Fig. 15: MO97-43), and one that represents gold enrichment in felsic rocks (Fig. 15: MO97-35). In order to check the

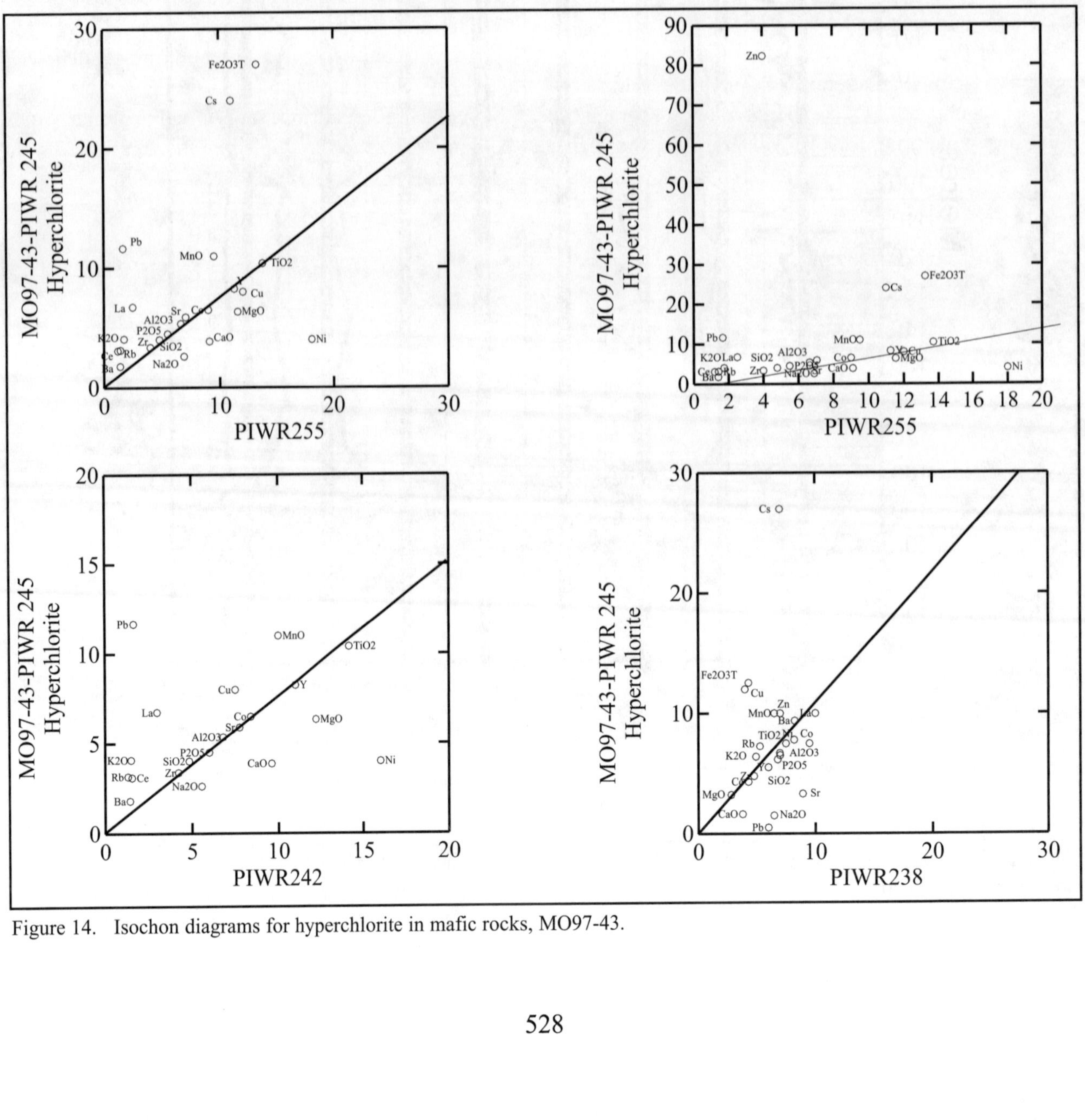

Figure 14. Isochon diagrams for hyperchlorite in mafic rocks, MO97-43.

consistency of the results, a third area (Fig. 16: MO97-32), at the margins of a gold zone, was examined.

Alteration in mafic rocks:

The predominant addition to these rocks (in addition to Au) is Fe (see Figure 16). This is in part due to addition of sulphide, but may also be due to formation of Fe-chlorite. The second-most prominent alteration is addition of K_2O, probably as sericite. Na_2O is strongly depleted in these zones, as well. Zinc, and to a lesser but still prominent extent, lead is enriched in the gold zones, as is copper. Zinc and lead may be the best indicators of mineralization, as they are more specifically enriched in the gold zones.

Alteration in felsic rocks

Three gold-rich sections in DDH MO97-35 were examined (Fig. 16). In the first comparison (uppermost two graphs) an average of three high gold samples was computed and compared with an average of three low-gold samples. The diagram on the right shows very large additions of arsenic, zinc and mercury (in addition to gold). The diagram on the left (details of the lower left corner of the previously described graph) shows that copper, iron and potassium were added, and sodium and calcium are depleted. Sulphides are also enriched (Sulphide %). Rb is enriched, indicating the formation of mica (probably sericite) during alteration, and Sr is strongly depleted, indicating feldspar destruction. The other graphs (Fig. 16) illustrate the same additions and losses, confirming the observations made in the first comparison. In MO97-35 the same changes have occurred, even though the amount of sulphide addition is very small. Here, on the periphery of the gold-enriched zone, Ca and Mg are enriched slightly. Na is not strongly depleted. This combination of changes is compatible with a less intense, seawater-dominated alteration system, in contrast to the alteration associated with the most gold-rich parts of the system.

The alteration attributes observed associated with gold mineralization are typical of those resulting from

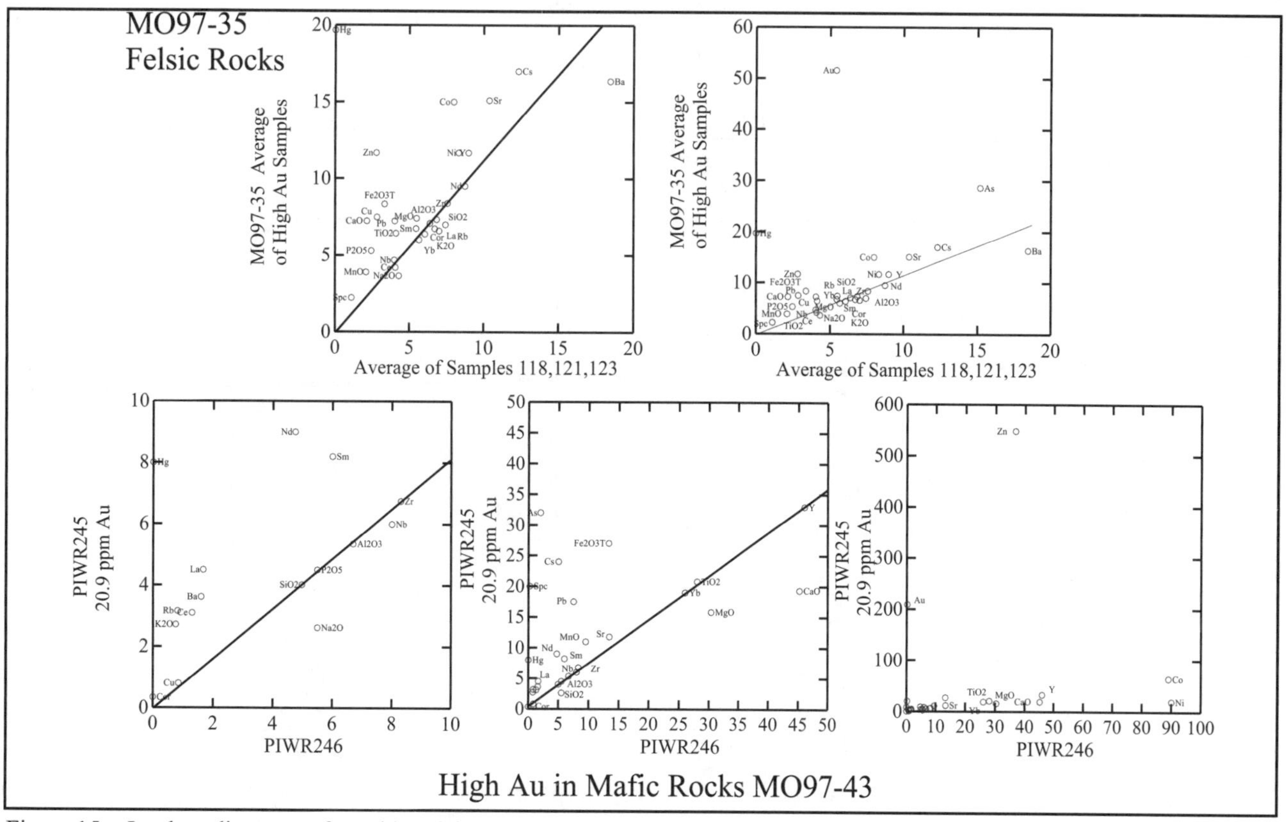

Figure 15. Isochon diagrams of a gold-enriched zone in mafic rocks (MO97-43, lower three graphs) and a zone at the margins of the gold enriched felsic rocks (MO97 35: upper two graphs).

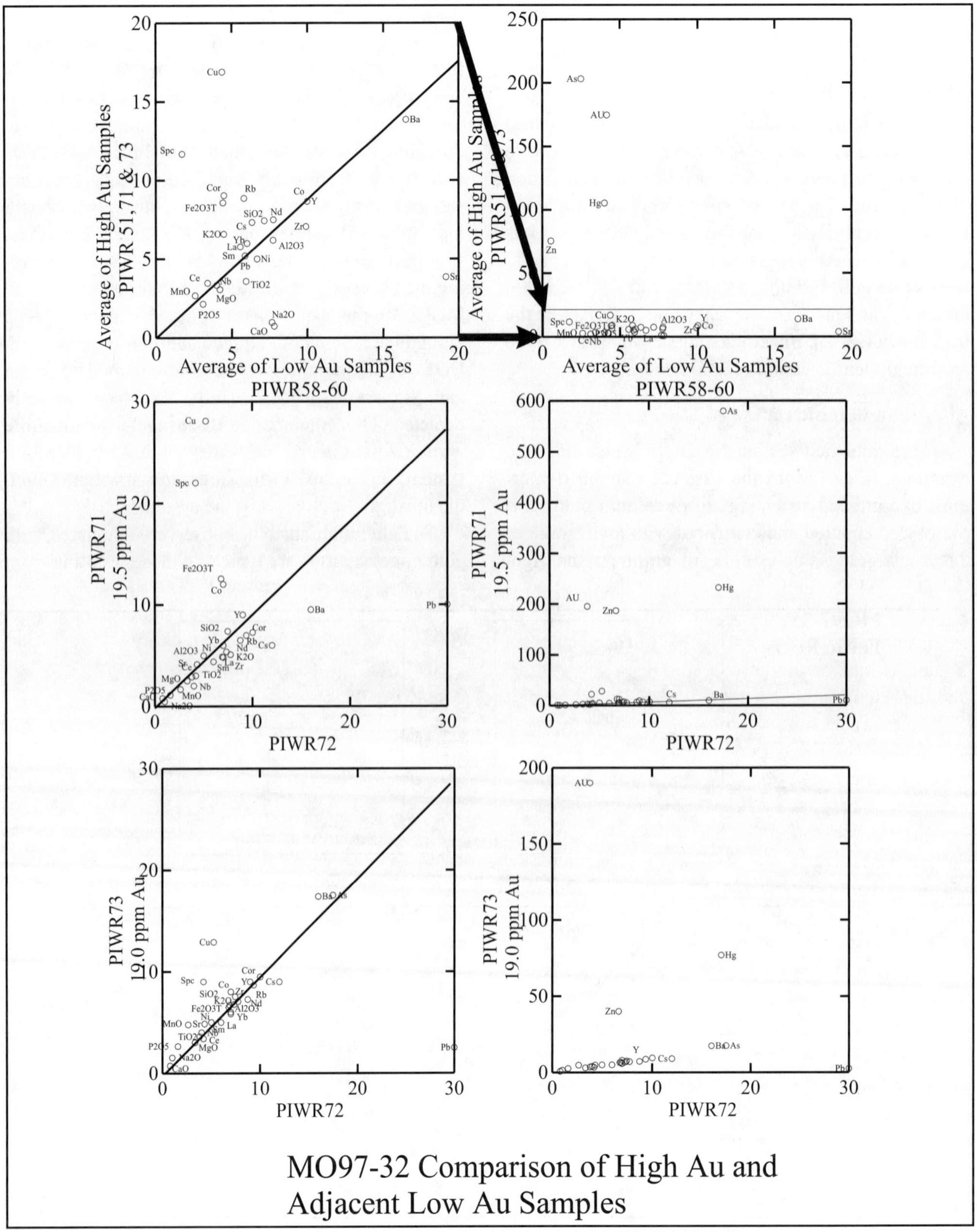

Figure 16. Comparison of high-Au and low Au samples in the felsic rocks of drill hole MO97-32.

high-temperature interaction with a metalliferous, seawater-derived hydrothermal fluid (Franklin, 1996). The abundance of mercury and arsenic may indicate a shallow water depositional environment (c.f. Mattabi, Morton and Franklin, 1987). As there is no gain or loss of Mg in the core zone of the mineralization, there does not seem to have been any involvement of cold seawater in most of the alteration system. However, as Mg is enriched at the margins of the gold-enriched zone (along with CaO), there may have been some heating of trapped seawater, and local precipitation of Mg-clays and possibly anhydrite at the margins of the system. In typical alteration pipes that directly underlie VMS deposits, Mg is added because of the progressive heating of locally down-drawn seawater. Lack of this in the core of the gold-enriched zone indicates that seawater had not penetrated into the centre of that zone. The seawater/rock ratio in the core of the gold-enriched zones at Paul Isnard was therefore very low (c.f. Seyfried and Janecky 1985). This suggests that the mineralization formed sub-seafloor and probably at depths where seawater was unable to penetrate in great quantity.

In summary, the mass balance studies indicate that Fe and K enrichment accompanied gold deposition, and that elements associated with volatile-rich fluids (Hg and As) are also significantly enriched. Only at the margins of the mineralization is there any evidence of locally heated advecting seawater-related alteration. These observations are compatible with a system that was cooling through adiabatic phase separation (i.e. boiling) in the sub-seafloor, precipitating copper and gold in its core, and reacting with both felsic and mafic rocks to form Fe-chlorite and sericite. Cooling must have been occurring at depths sufficient to not engender seawater draw-down, with sufficient permeability to prevent extensive hydrofracturing.

The next step in examining the alteration distribution in the gold-rich zones of the Paul Isnard area is to examine some down-hole distributions. In Figure 17 a series of sections for Hole MO97-35 illustrate the variations in selected major and minor elements, relative to the gold-bearing zone near the end of the hole. These trends confirm the information gained from the isochon plots, and illustrate the magnitude and consistency of chemical alteration trends. All samples are from felsic rocks; there are no hyperchlorite zones in this hole, and only a few mafic dykes. Unfortunately the hole is at the margin of the major gold zone. The data patterns indicate that anomalous copper is distributed over about 100 m from the high gold zones, as is lead. Zinc is not anomalous in this test, but mercury is anomalous over about 150 m. Fe increases substantially over about 150 m away from the high-grade sections, and in many samples K_2O is anomalous for almost 200 m. The distribution of copper and zinc was also examined in Hole MO96-14 (Fig. 18). These data show that anomalous copper and zinc are associated with the gold zones, but not with the hyperchlorite. This adds further to the argument that the hyperchlorite is not directly related to the gold mineralizing event.

The final step is to establish the threshold values that define alteration associated with the gold mineralization. Table 4 is derived from examining the frequency distributions of these elements (not shown). These probability plots for each element generally provide a basis for defining separate anomalous and background populations. Lead and mercury are exceptions; almost all of the values provided for these elements by the analytical method used for this study should be considered anomalous.

Additional Alteration Indicators

One of the more reliable derivative indicators of hydrothermal mineralization is the abundance of normative corundum as an alteration indicator. As feldspar in the groundmass of most volcanic rocks generally was completely replaced, and its cations released to the fluid phase during hydrothermal alteration, excess alumina remained in most altered rocks. This is reflected in the calculated normative corundum content (a good surrogate for measuring excess alumina), which may actually reflect the formation of aluminous clay minerals during alteration. Corundum is generally present in the calculated norm for most submarine volcanic sequences, as most hot volcanic material reacts with seawater, losing some Na and gaining some Mg, a process that generates some excess alumina. Fine-grained tuff tends to react more than coarser-grained fragmental volcanic rocks or flows.

The distribution of normative corundum was

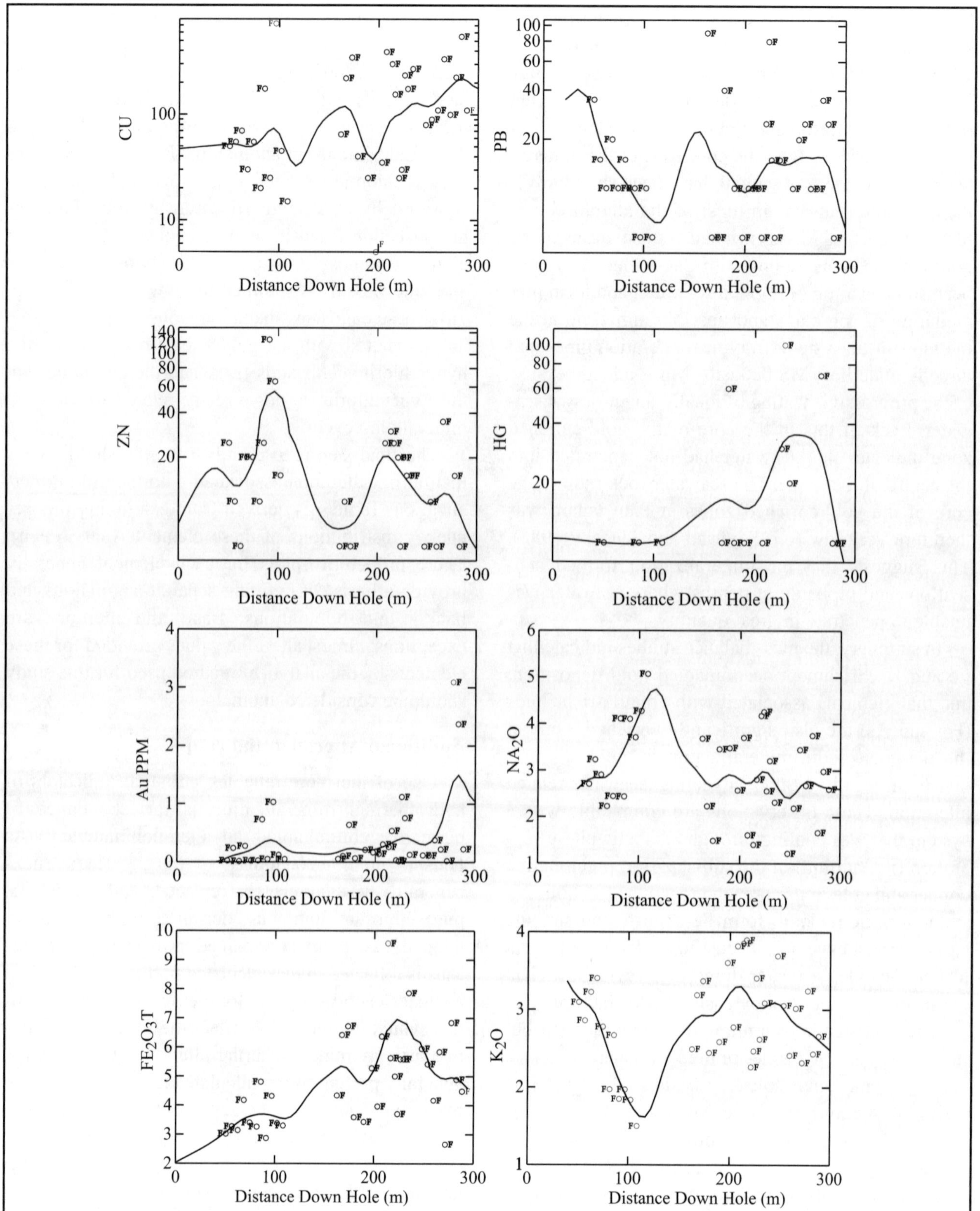

Figure 17. Selected major and minor element distributions in Hole MO97-35. The lines are "best fit" splines through the data, and illustrate the progressive trends down the hole

Table 4. Threshold values for various major and trace elements in felsic volcanic rocks. Values in the indicated ranges are anomalous, and may be used to indicate proximity to Au mineralization.

Element	Threshold	Element	Threshold
Fe_2O_3	>3.9%	Cu	>100ppm
K_2O	>3.3%	Zn	>40ppm
Na_2O	<2%	Pb	>15ppm
CaO	<1.2%	As	>8ppm
		Hg	>50ppb

examined in two ways. Values in excess of 8 % are statistically anomalous and were plotted as zones on a map (Fig. 19). The zone of normative corundum corresponds closely with the distribution of the highest base metal and gold contents; the contoured data indicate that the trend is actually almost N-S, at approximately 90° to strike. Although this treatment of the data is biased by the uneven availability of whole-rock analyses, it may be highly significant in considering the origin and ultimate distribution of the mineralization at Paul Isnard. The trends in distribution of corundum possibly represent the true direction of hydrothermal channels in this part of the system. This trend would be consistent with the presence of a sub-seafloor "pipe" system leading upwards (to the south) towards the paleo-seafloor.

SUMMARY OF ALTERATION STUDIES

The alteration in the Paul Isnard area formed through replacement of all lithologies by Fe-rich chlorite and Fe-sulphides in the hyperchlorite zones. Sulphur and Fe were added to the rocks, as were K, gold and base metals. Na and Ca were concomitantly removed. The precipitation mechanism was likely direct interaction of the hydrothermal fluid with the surrounding rocks, in a fracture system that was orthogonal to the strata. Mg-rich alteration, typical of many VMS environments, is relegated to the periphery of the system, and is probably unimportant as an exploration guide in the Paul Isnard area. Down-draw seawater was unable to reach this portion of the upper crust, probably because it was displaced by upwelling hot hydrothermal fluid.

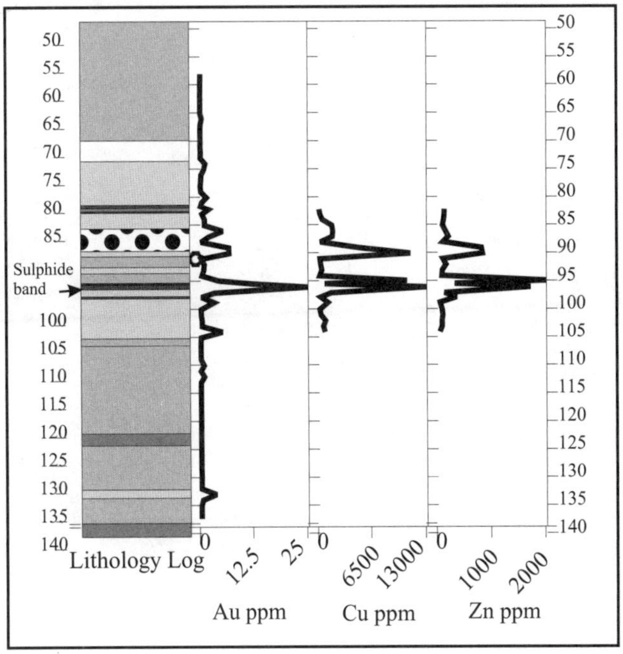

Figure 18. Distribution of gold, copper and zinc in a section of hole. Note that the shading on the log is the same as for Figure 13, the black bands are mafic intrusions, dark gray bands are felsic lapillistone, light gray bands are fine ash, and stippled band is "hyperchlorite" alteration.

BASE METAL AND GOLD DISTRIBUTION

Information regarding the mineralization, available in Schwartz (1996) was augmented in this study by examination of some statistical parameters. Pyrite is the predominant sulphide mineral. It occurs primarily as disseminations, and (more prevalently in the mafic rocks) in veins and stringer-like zones. Massive sulphides have not (yet) been observed. Chalcopyrite is closely associated with the most gold-rich zones, and sphalerite has been observed near the periphery of these zones. Although the property has been explored primarily as a gold prospect, the sulphide zones do contain elevated copper and zinc contents. A resource estimate for gold has been undertaken (Costelloe, 1999 and company files) but not for base metals. Copper and zinc are present in sub-economic amounts, and are significant in considering the genesis of the gold-sulphide zones. In order to provide some indication of the base metal contents of the Paul

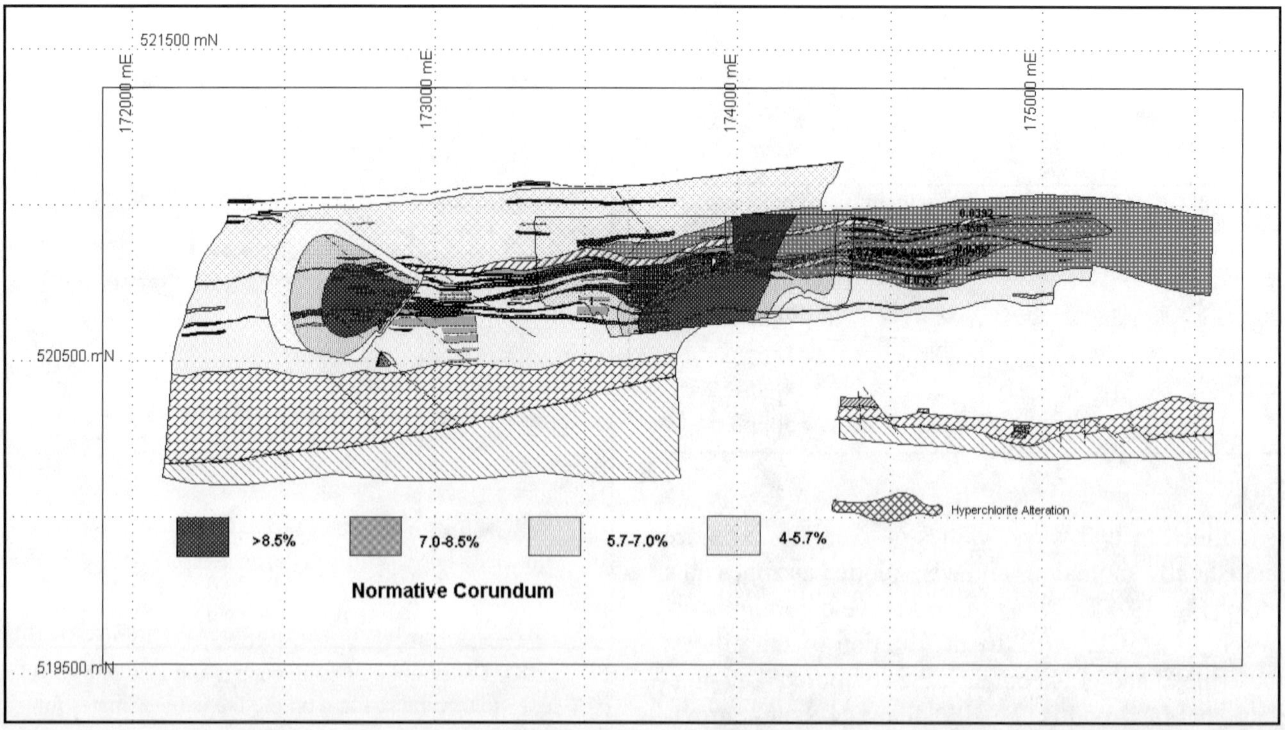

Figure 19. Contour map of normative corundum. Note that the data are constrained by the available drill holes as shown. Two areas of abundant (>7%) normative corundum illustrate the cross-stratal distribution of this alteration indicator. These may represent paleo-discharge zones. Compare with Figure 24 to see the correspondence between the distribution of normative corundum and anomalous zinc and lead.

Isnard area, the available analyses (collected as part of the regional petrochemical study) are examined statistically. The probability distributions of copper, zinc, lead and iron illustrate that the overall base metal contents of the many of the rock samples in the Paul Isnard area are anomalous (Fig. 20) relative to typical metal contents for most volcanic rocks (see Barrie and Hannington, 1999, and references therein). About half of all of the copper contents are above 150 ppm, which typically is a maximum content for mafic volcanic rocks in arc sequences. Similarly, about 20 % of the zinc and lead values exceed 150 and 30 ppm respectively. A substantial number of the samples contain highly anomalous contents (Zn and Cu > 1000 ppm, Pb>30 ppm, Fe_2O_3 >20 %). Clearly, significant amounts of base metals (along with silver, mercury and arsenic) have been added to the Paul Isnard strata.

In an effort to examine key correlations and spatial relationships of the mineralization, all base metal and related data from the ICP (441 samples), gold assay (10349 analyses) and whole rock data (266 samples) sets were combined into a single file and analyzed statistically (Table 5). Base metal values from the ICP data set were used, and it is important to recall that these are obtained by hot aqua regia extraction and therefore representative of the acid-soluble (sulphide, carbonate, limited phyllosilicate) portions of the rock. Sulphur values are visual estimates.

Several observations emerge from this analysis. Generally, few strong correlations are evident. Copper and gold are moderately well correlated, although this correlation is only slightly less strong than that for copper with silver (in contrast to a poor correlation of silver with lead). Silver and gold are also strongly correlated, as are zinc and silver. The Cu-Ag correlation indicates that silver occurs in copper minerals, typical of most Zn-Cu-Pb (Noranda type or bimodal mafic associated) deposits (Franklin et al., 1981). Zinc is not strongly correlated with copper and poorly correlated with gold, indicating that zinc deposition was separated from these other elements. Arsenic is not strongly correlated with any other elements, but antimony has a modest correlation with silver, possibly indicating some sulphosalt presence. Nickel is correlated negatively, or very poorly, with all elements except cobalt. Ni and Co were not part of the Cu-Au mineralization process. Their correlation is related to either a magmatic process, or to the breakdown of organic material in sediments (diagenetic pyrite in graphite-bearing sedimentary strata may contain up to 1 % of Ni and Co). Other correlations were tested to examine the possibility of other genetic models for the Isnard mineralization (not shown); no strong correlation is evident between the base metals and other major or minor elements, including the REEs, U and Th.

No mineralogical or petrographic studies of the sulphide-rich vein systems have been undertaken. As described previously (hyperchlorite zones) all sulphide zones are associated with Fe-rich chlorite alteration; Mg-rich alteration is not associated with them, based on the available data (see discussion of alteration, below). The sulphide veins are intensely deformed and transposed (Fig. 21), and appear to have formed early in the geological history of the area.

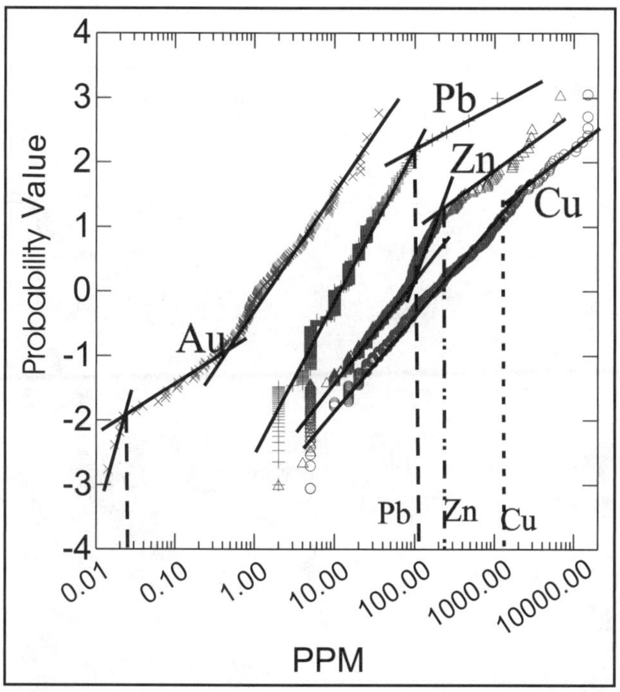

Figure 20. Probability plots for base metals and gold. Note that most elements have at least two populations. Almost all of the gold contents are above typical "background" values for Proterozoic volcanic rocks. Over half of the samples are enriched in copper and zinc, with smaller but distinctive lead enrichment as well.

SPATIAL DISTRIBUTION OF BASE METALS AND GOLD

Contoured abundance data for gold, copper, zinc and lead were plotted on the geological base map for the area. Such plots are dependent on sampling density, which is necessarily confined to the available drill core. The number of data points for gold is extensive, but those for the other metals are more limited. Nevertheless, some interesting patterns emerge (Fig. 22). Although gold appears primarily to be distributed in zones that are parallel to the principal stratigraphic and structural trend, there are distinct discordant zones which cross-cut the strata near the centre of the area. This discordance is more evident of in the contour plots of the base metals. They are not distributed parallel to the strata, but form distinct cross-cutting zones. This may indicate that the entire area is a paleo-discharge zone, with its core (high temperature) represented by copper and gold enrichment, and the margins represented by zinc and lead enrichment.

THE PAUL ISNARD MINERALIZATION: IS IT A PRODUCT OF A VMS SYSTEM?

The sulphide zones formed prior to the first phase of deformation, and may have formed penecontemporaneously with the deposition of the volcanic strata. This observation, combined with the close association of the mineralization with submarine volcanic rocks is consistent with a seafloor or sub seafloor depositional model. The anomalous abundance of copper, zinc, lead and gold, along with anomalous arsenic, antimony and mercury are a typical assemblage associated with a seafloor type hydrothermal system. The distribution of copper, zinc, lead and, to a lesser extent, gold and the most intense alteration indicate that the mineralization was deposited at a high angle to strike, in the sub-seafloor. Thus the base metal and gold zones might be an alteration-pipe style mineralization.

The volcanic rock textures and compositions are indicative of a shallow water depositional environment, and under such conditions, extreme metal sepa-

Table 5. Spearman correlation coefficients for base metals and related elements.

	Cu	Zn	Pb	Sulphur %	Au	Ag	As	Sb	Co	Ni
Cu	1.00									
Zn	0.46	1.00								
Pb	-0.06	0.07	1.00							
Sulphur %	0.59	0.40	-0.04	1.00						
Au	0.72	0.40	-0.06	0.69	1.00					
Ag	0.79	0.68	0.56	0.56	0.70	1.00				
As	0.20	0.12	0.19	0.18	0.15	0.31	1.00			
Sb	0.21	0.28	0.11	0.05	0.17	0.48	0.35	1.00		
Co	0.02	0.51	0.05	0.17	-0.05	0.29	0.14	0.07	1.00	
Ni	0.05	0.45	0.03	0.02	-0.09	0.22	0.00	0.09	0.85	1.00

rations can occur. Examples of this style of mineralization in shallow-water rocks include the Selbaie Mine (Deptuck et al., 1982), and the Headway Coulee occurrence (Osterberg et al., 1987). In these, mineralization is distributed along sub-seafloor fracture-fault systems, which have undergone subsequent transposition during deformation. It is thus worthwhile to consider a mechanism by which copper and gold could be separated from the other VMS constituents.

Figure 23 is used to explain the solubility and boiling constraints on fluids such as were probably present at Paul Isnard. This diagram represents the topology of solubilities of the main metals and gold in a typical VMS system. The major unknown factor in preparing such a diagram is the range of sulphur contents of the hydrothermal fluid. In a boiling system these may vary widely, although if the system that made the Paul Isnard mineralization is typical of those observed on the modern seafloor, the total H_2S content would have been about 0.01m. For a more

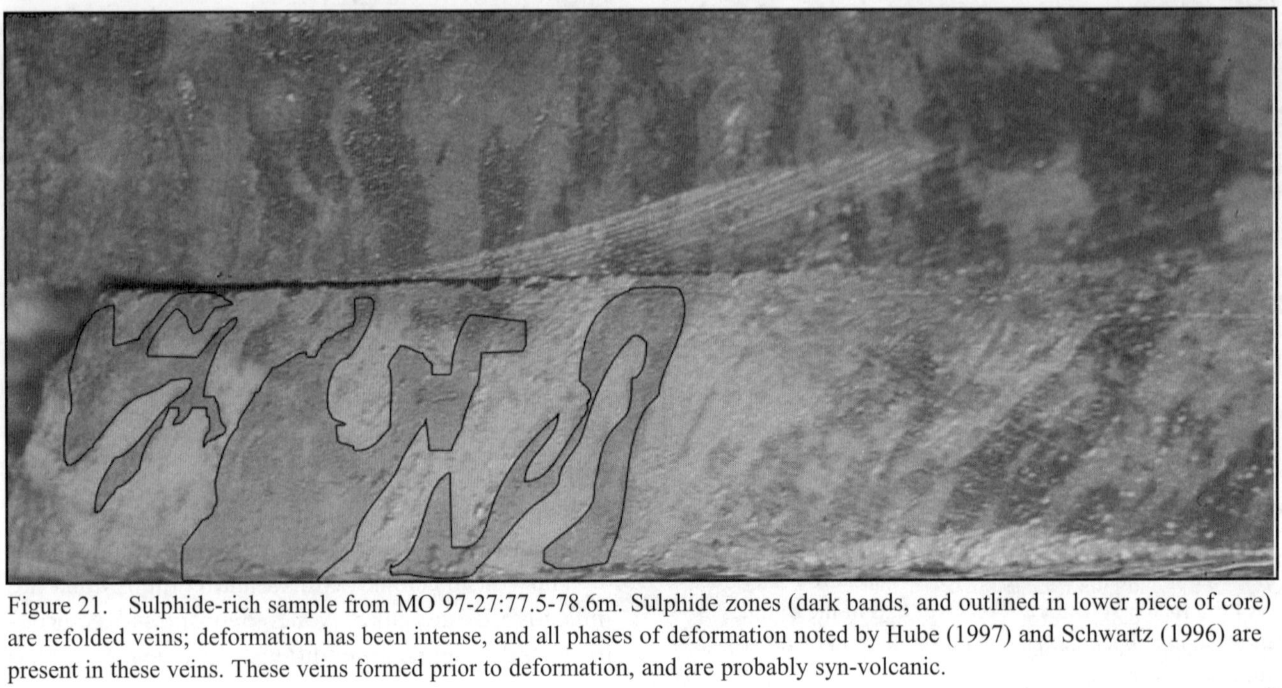

Figure 21. Sulphide-rich sample from MO 97-27:77.5-78.6m. Sulphide zones (dark bands, and outlined in lower piece of core) are refolded veins; deformation has been intense, and all phases of deformation noted by Hube (1997) and Schwartz (1996) are present in these veins. These veins formed prior to deformation, and are probably syn-volcanic.

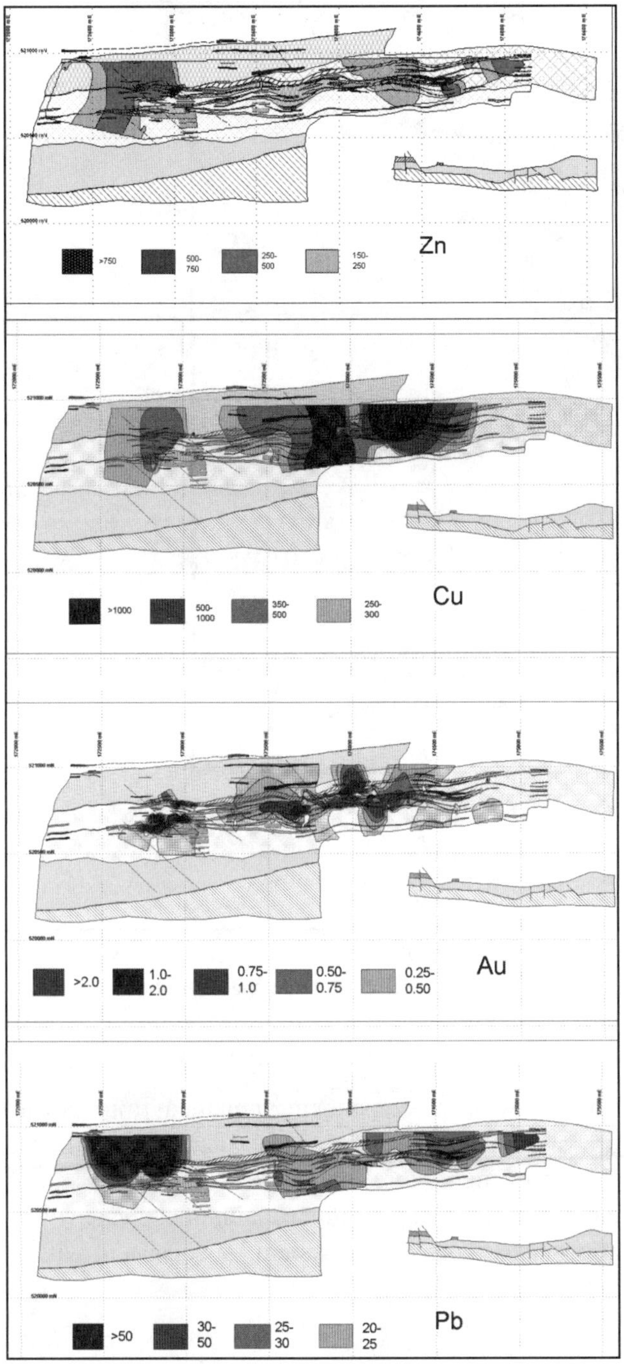

Figure 22. Contour maps of base metals and gold distribution (see Fig. 21 for drill hole locations). Note these all illustrate the cross-stratal distribution of the hydrothermal products. Gold and copper are moderately well correlated, but these elements correlate less well with zinc and lead. The latter are distributed peripherally to the core Cu-Au zone, suggesting a broad lateral zonation consistent with a temperature gradient. The database for gold is comprised of 9150 analyses, and thus is more robust for contouring than that for the base metals (471 samples).

complete review of the geochemical constraints on forming gold-rich VMS deposits, see Hannington et al., 1999. Typical metal contents (as measured in active seafloor vent systems) are 0.08 ppb Au (JMF data, unpublished, based on measurements of vapour-dominated fluids at Axial Seamount), 1-10 ppm Cu and 10-100 ppm Zn (Von Damm, 1990). The base metal contents of ore forming fluids are very sensitive to pH, such that systems forming in felsic dominated back-arc environments have low measured pH values (about 2) compared with the pH of basalt-dominated systems (3-4) (e.g. Fouquet et al., 1993). Boiling tends to increase the pH of the fluid, and decrease the pH of the vapour (Drummond and Ohmoto, 1985). Gold in deep-water (low S activity) systems is generally transported as a chloride complex, and thus precipitates according to the temperature of the fluid. In boiling systems, some of the gold may be transported as a bisulphide complex, particularly if the activity of sulphur is high. These complexes can enhance gold solubility, particularly at low temperatures, and result in a substantial portion of the gold being transported to the seafloor and precipitated, under oxidizing seafloor conditions, in the near-seafloor environment.

From Figure 23 (drawn for the typical range of shallow-water VMS systems) it is evident that all copper will precipitate from a system if the water depth is less than 500 m. In environments that were shallower than 500 m, all copper would precipitate in the subsurface, or by the time a fluid cooled to about 275°C. Also, all of the gold would have precipitated simultaneously if it were transported as a chloride complex. If these conditions were not reached until the fluid emerged from a vent at the seafloor, it is possible that much of the gold would have remained in solution, because of the slow rate at which gold precipitates (a kinetic effect). However, in the case of subsurface cooling, gold would be entirely precipitated at about 300 m below the seafloor, along with copper. Zinc, lead and silver would remain dissolved, and would not precipitate until subjected to radical cooling, either just below the seafloor (at subaerial water depths) or on the seafloor (below 100-200 m water depth).

This subsurface cooling scenario (Fig. 24) would produce precisely the distribution of metals observed in the Paul Isnard area, and would place them in a

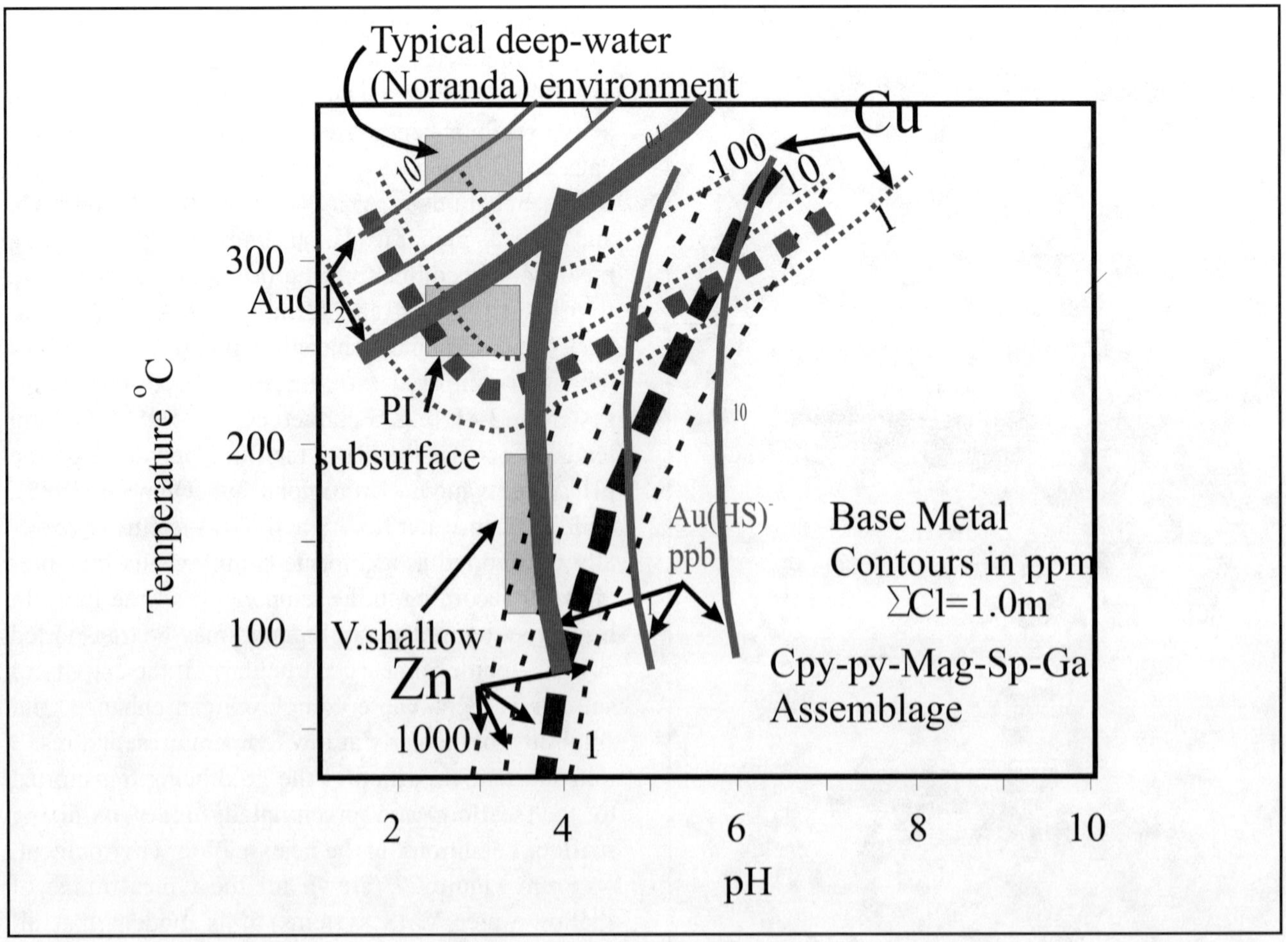

Figure 23. Solubility of copper and zinc (as chloride species) for a typical hydrothermal fluid. Solubility of gold shown as two species; the chloride species is most common in deep water systems, and will co-exist with bisulphide species in boiling systems.

subsurface stringer zone. As a consequence of this, however, there should be significant zinc zone at some stratigraphic level above the copper zone. In the Headway Coulee area, for example, this separation is several hundred metres (Osterberg et al., 1987).

Alteration

The alteration associated with the gold-copper zone is dominated by Fe-chlorite, which can only be produced by interaction of a hot Fe-rich hydrothermal fluid (~300°C) with surrounding rocks. Convective cooling by advecting seawater seems to have been confined to the margins of the system The only Mg enrichment detected in this study is peripheral to the mineralization, indicating that at the margins of the system perhaps some lower-temperature alteration formed, with its constituents obtained from down-drawn cold seawater. The zonal alteration, including Na enrichment (core) and depletion (margin) and K enrichment, with pronounced aluminosilicate alteration in the core of the system, is consistent with a shallow VMS system.

Structural Modification

Explanation of the present distribution of lithologies must take into account the following: The felsic and mafic strata appear to be time equivalent; the transition is sharp between them. Secondly, a few sills transect this contact (the "intermediate intrusion" sills"), but precede most, if not all of the deformation. Thirdly, the area has undergone pervasive deformation with a sense of sinistral shear. Finally, gold-

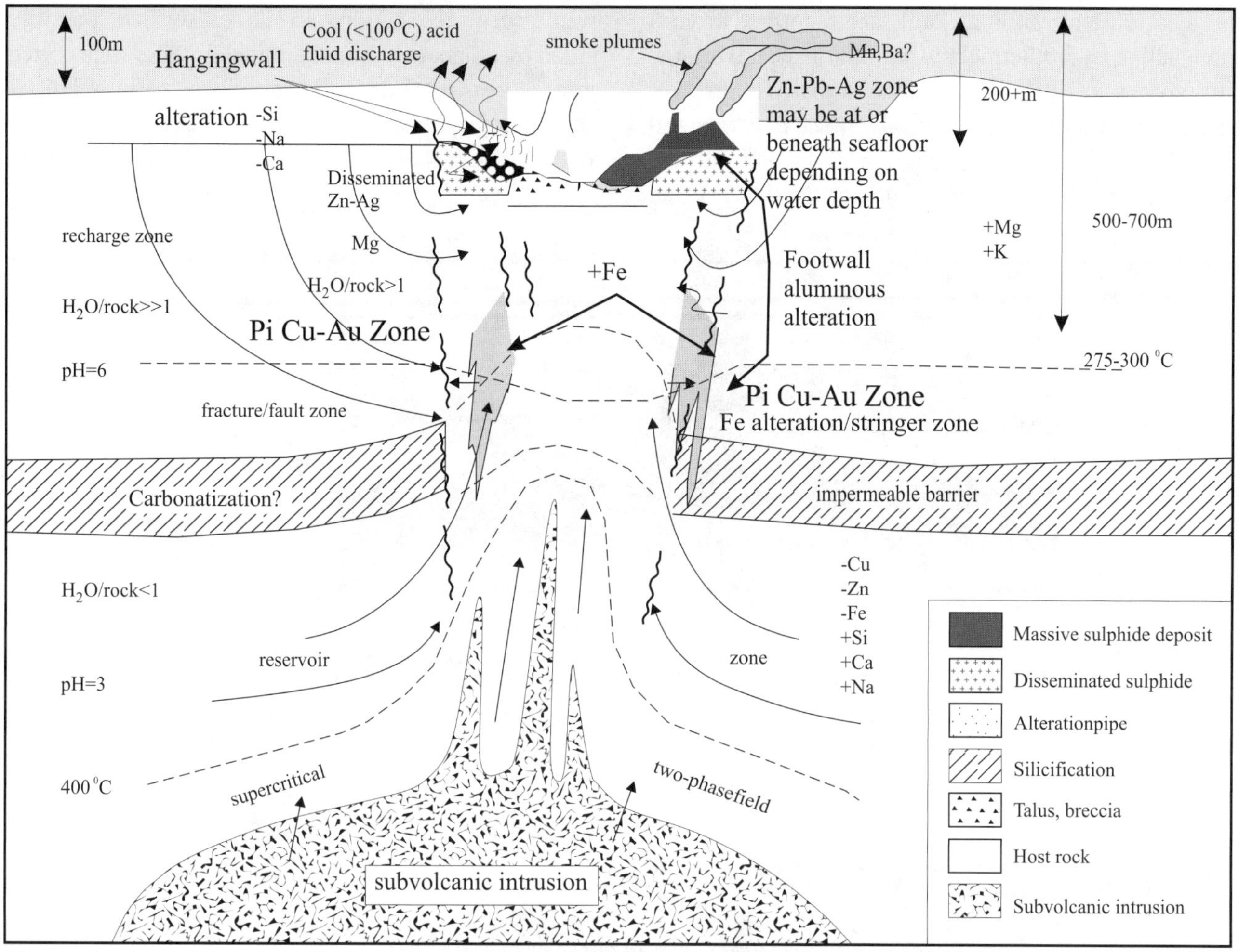

Figure 24. Generalized model for VMS formation (after Franklin, 1996) modified to explain the distribution of Au-Cu mineralization in the Paul Isnard area. Note that many of the features shown in this diagram have not been identified in the PI area.

copper mineralization occurs in both the felsic and mafic strata. One model that can explain these observations is shown in Figure 25. The original depositional site was a back-arc basin, which contained a small pull-apart (rifted) basin that formed in a felsic-dominated sequence, but was filled by basalt. Hydrothermal fluids discharged along rift-boundary faults at the margins of this basin, forming the sub-seafloor copper-gold zones, and presumably a more zinc rich part at a higher stratigraphic elevation. The area subsequently was deformed by sinistral shear (central diagram), forming the resultant geometry illustrated in the lower diagram.

Summary

The Paul Isnard mineralization was precipitated due to subsurface cooling of a hydrothermal system, probably at a combined seawater and rock depth of about 500-600 m. Conductive cooling was probably most important, but boiling may have also occurred. Depending on the water depth at that time, zinc, lead and silver should have precipitated either as a seafloor massive sulphide deposit (if the water depth exceeded 100-200 m) or as a vein and stringer system (shallower than 100-200 m). This deposit might occur a few hundred metres above (to the south of) the gold zone. The strongest alteration (defined by normative corundum, for example- see Figure 19) is in the felsic rocks immediately above the western zinc-enriched zone.

The mineralization at Paul Isnard formed from a convective hydrothermal system that was active during volcanism. It is thus similar to many other synvolcanic VMS-style systems. The metal contents and correlation data are consistent with having formed from a seawater-dominated hydrothermal fluid that was undergoing cooling in the subsurface, possibly aided by adiabatic boiling. All metals were transported in a Cl-bearing fluid, and their close spatial relationship, along with that of anomalous lead, is consistent with a VMS-related origin for the Paul Isnard system.

- Deposition occurred in a back-arc sequence,

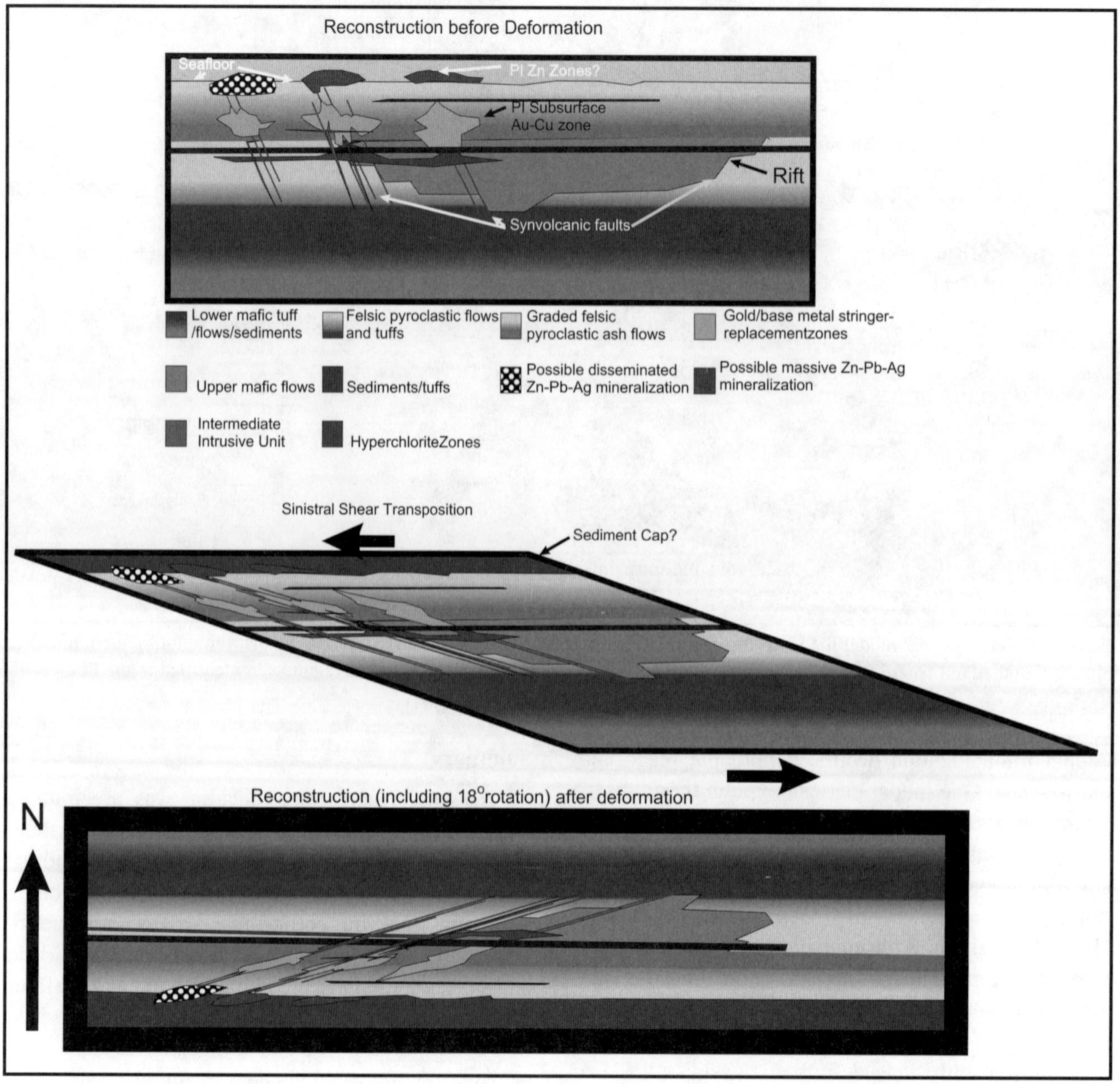

Figure 25. Upper diagram is a reconstruction of the Paul Isnard geology; south is to the top of the diagram. Note that the synvolcanic faults that possibly controlled the emplacement of synvolcanic dykes also became the locus for hydrothermal fluid discharge. The central diagram illustrates the effect of sinistral transpressive deformation. The box indicates the approximate position of the map for the Paul Isnard area. The lower diagram attempts to represent the same model, rotated to the present geographic orientation (stratigraphic top to the south).

and was focussed along synvolcanic faults that also formed the margins of a local pull-apart (rifted) basin. The latter was filled by basalt.

- The gold-copper mineralization intersected thus far formed below the seafloor, and probably at least 300 m, and possibly at about 1000 m below the paleo-ocean bottom. The alteration and sulphides resemble a conventional stringer zone, but all of the alteration is a result of interaction of high temperature mineralizing fluid with the adjacent rocks. Only a small portion of it formed due to advection of cold seawater.
- The overlying volcanic and sedimentary rocks have excellent potential for zinc-lead-silver mineralization. This may occur as vein-disseminated sulphide zones (if the seafloor was under less than 100 m of seawater) or a massive to semi-massive mineralization.
- The entire area underwent sinistral shear and transpressive deformation, structurally thinning and transposition of the strata.
- The volcanic – dominated areas of the Guiana Shield have VMS potential. A combination of geochemical prospecting and geophysical methods that can "see" through saprolite zones might be applied in exploration for additional resources.

REFERENCES

Bardoux, M., Voicu, G. and Lafrance J., 1997.Geological settings of base and precious metal occurrences in Paleoproterozoic terranes of the Guiana Shield. Notes submitted to the NWMA short-course titled: "Geology, geochemistry, geophysics and mineral deposits of the Guiana and West African Shields", 18 p.

Barrie, C.T., and Hannington, M.D. 1999. Classification of volcanic-associated massive sulfide deposits based on host rock compositions. In Volcanic-associated massive sulfide deposits: processes and examples in modern and ancient settings. In Reviews in Economic Geology Volume 8, C.T. Barrie and M.D. Hannington, editors, pp 2-11

Bailes, A.H. and Galley, A.G. 1996. Setting of Paleoproterozoic volcanic-hosted massive base metal sulphide deposits, Snow Lake. In Extech I: A Multidisciplinary approach to massive sulphide research in the Rusty Lake-Snow Lake greenstone belts, Manitoba. Geological Survey of Canada Bulletin 426, G.F. Bonham – Carter, A.G. Galley and G.E.M. Hall, editors, pp105-138.

Choubert, B., 1964. Ages absolus de la Guyane Française (Précambrien Guyanais). C.R. Acad. Sci. Paris, t. 258, p. 631-633.

Costelloe, D. J., 1999. Montagne d'Or zone, Paul Isnard project mineral resource estimation. Guyanor Ressources and Golden Star Resources internal report, 32 p. and appendices.

Deptuk, R., Squair, H., and Wierzbicki, V., 1982. Geology of the Detour zinc-copper deposits, Brouillan Township, Quebec. In Precambrian Sulphide deposits, Special Paper 25, Geological Association of Canada, pp 319-342.

Dimroth, E., 1975. Field trip and field conference on the volcanology and sedimentology of the Rouyn-Noranda area, Aug 4-7, 1975. Quebec Department of Natural Resources, C.P. 277 Rouyn, P.Q., 76p.

Drummond, S.E. and Ohmoto, H., 1985. Chemical evolution and mineral deposition in boiling hydrothermal systems. Economic Geology, vol. 80 p126-147.

Fouquet, Y., Knott, R., Cambon, P., Fallick, A., Rickard, D., and Desbruyeres, D., 1996. Formation of large sulfide mineral deposits along fast spreading ridges: Example from off-axial deposits at 12°43'N on the East Pacific Rise. Earth and Planetary Science Letters, vol. 144, 147-162.

Fouquet, Y., von Stakelberg, U., Charlou, J.L., Erzinger, J., Herzig, P.M., Muhe, R., and Wiedicke, M., 1993. Metallogenesis in back-arc environments: the Lau Basin example. Economic Geology vol. 88, p2154-2181.

Franklin, J.M., Lydon, J.W., and Sangster, D.F., 1981. Volcanic-associated massive sulfide deposits. Economic Geology 75th Anniversary Volume, p. 485-627.

Franklin, J.M. 1999b. Systematic analysis of lithogeochemical data. In "Exploration Tools for Volcanogenic Massive sulphide deposits", short course notes, Mineral Deposits Division of the Geological Association of Canada and the Mineral Deposits Research Unit, Univ. British Columbia, Jan24-25, 1999, 34p.

Franklin, J.M. 1996: Volcanic-associated massive sulfide base metals: in Geology of Canadian Mineral deposit Types, O.R. Eckstrand, W.D. Sinclair, and R.I Thorpe, editors; Geological Survey of Canada, Geology of Canada no. 8, p.158-183.

Gibson, H.L. and Franklin, J.M. 1998. The prolific Early Proterozoic: Bonanza time for volcanogenic massive sulfide deposits; in "The First Age of giant ore Formation: Stratigraphy, Tectonics and Mineralization in the Late Archean and Early Proterozoic", Prospectors and Developers Association Annual Convention, 1998, T.J. Bottrill and P. Sheahan, Editors, pp 115-128.

Gibson, H.L., Morton, R.L. and Hudak, G.J. 1999. Subaqueous volcanism: Environments and controls on VMS mineralization. Economic Geology Review Volume "Volcanic Associated Massive Sulfide Deposits: Processes and Examples in Modern and Ancient Settings, pp13-51.

Gibson, H.L. and Watkinson, D.H 1990. Volcanogenic massive sulphide deposits of the Noranda Cauldron and Shield Volcano, Quebec. In The Northwestern Quebec Polymetallic belt, Canadian Institute of Mining and metallurgy, Special Volume 43, p119-132.

Grant, J.A.:1986. The isochon diagram-a simple solution to Gresens' equation for metasomatic alteration. Economic Geology, vol. 81, no 8, pp1976-1982

Groves, D.I., Barely, M.E., and Ho, S.E., 1988. Nature, genesis and tectonic setting of mesothermal gold mineralization in the Yilgarn Block, Western Australia. In "the geology of gold deposits: the perspective in 1988", Economic geology Monograph 6, p71-85

Hannington, M.D., Poulsen, K.H., Thompson, J.F.H., and Sillitoe, R.H. 1999. Volcanogenic gold in the massive sulfide environment. In Volcanic-associated massive sulfide deposits: processes and examples in modern and ancient settings. In Reviews in Economic Geology Volume 8, C.T. Barrie and M.D. Hannington, editors, pp 325-356.

Hubé, D., 1997. Mise en œuvre des outils géologiques et géophysiques dans le cadre de projets d'exploration d'or primaire. Suivi géologique et géotechniques de sondages carottés. Projets Paul Isnard et Saint Elie; Guyane Française Rapport de stage en entreprise; E.N.S.G. Nancy, 127 p.

Lesher, C.M. Goodwin, A.M., Campbell, I.H., and Gorton, M.P. 1986. Trace element geochemistry of ore associated and barren felsic metavolcanic rocks in the Superior Province, Canada. Canadian Journal of Earth Sciences, vol. 23, p222-237.

Manier, E., 1992. Les conglomérats aurifères de Guyane Française (Protérozoïque Inférieur): dynamique des bassins sédimentaires et contrôle des minéralisations . ENSMP, Mémoires des Sciences de la Terre, n°17, 176 p.

Milési, J.-P., Egal, E., Vernhet, P., Thiéblémont, Y., Cocherie, D., Tegyey, M., Martel-Jantin, B. and Lagny, P., 1995. Les minéralisations du Nord de la Guyane Française dans leur cadre géologique. Chroniques de la Recherche Minière, v. 518, p. 5-58.

Millo, L., Bout, J.-P., Sauvage, J.-F., Suter, N. and Taquet, B., 1999. Paul Isnard and Eau Blanche projects: phase report n°5. Guyanor Ressources internal report, 72 p. and appendices.

Morton, R.L., and Franklin, J.M., 1987. Two-fold classification of Archean volcanic-associated massive sulfide deposits. Economic Geology, v. 82, p. 1057-1063.

Osterberg, S.A., Morton, R.L., and Franklin, J.M.,1987, Hydrothermal Alteration and physical volcanology of Archean rocks in the vicinity of the Headway-Coulee massive sulfide occurrence, Onaman area, Northwestern Ontario. Economic Geology, vol. 82, no.6, p1505-1520.

Pasava, J., Hladikova, J. and Dobes, P. 1996. The origin of Proterozoic metal-rich shales from the Bohemian Massif, Czech Republic. Economic Geology, vol. 91, pp63-79.

Pearce, J.A. and Cann, J.R. 1973. Tectonoc setting of basic volcanic rocks determined using trace element analyses. Earth and Planetary Science Letters vol19 pp290-300.

Riverin, G and Hodgson, C.J. 1980. Wall – rock alteration at the Millenbach Cu-Zn Mine, Noranda, Quebec. Economic Geology vol. 75 p 424-444.

Schwartz, S. 1996. Le prospect de la Montagne d'Or (Guyane Française): modèles tectonométamorphique et métallogénique. Rapport de stage de recherche D.E.A. Université Claude Berbard (Lyon 1), 38 p.

Seyfried, W.E., Jr., and Janecky, D.R., 1985. Heavy metal and sulfur transport during subcritical and supercritical hydrothermal alteration of basalt: Influence of fluid pressure and basalt composition and crystallinity. Geochim. et Cosmochim. Acta, v. 49, p. 2545-2560.

Vanderhaeghe, O., Ledru, P., Thiéblémont, D., Egal, E., Cocherie, A. Tegyey, M., Milési, J.-P. (1998). Contrasting mechanism of crustal growth . Geodynamic evolution of the Paleoproterozoic granite-greenstone belts of French Guiana. Precambrian Research, n° 92, p. 165-193.

Von Damm, K.L. 1990. Seafloor hydrothermal activity: Black smoker chemistry and chimneys: Annual review Earth and Planetary Science, vol. 18. p173-205.

Walford, P.C., and Franklin, J.M.,1982:. The Anderson Lake Mine, Snow Lake. In: R.W. Hutchinson, C.D. Spence and J.M. Franklin, (eds.), "Precambrian Sulphide Deposits", Geological Association of Canada Special Paper 25, p. 481-525.

MINERAL DEPOSITS ASSOCIATED WITH SUBMARINE VOLCANISM OF ARGENTINA

M. Amelia V. Logan
Smithsonian Institution, Department of Mineral Sciences, NHB-119, Washington, D.C. 20560, USA, logan.amelia@nmnh.si.edu

Milka K. de Brodtkorb
CONICET-Universidad de Buenos Aires, Paso 258 –9° A. 1640 Martínez, Argentina, milkabro@gl.fcen.uba.ar

Isidoro B. Schalamuk
Instituto de Recursos Minerales-Universidad Nacional de La Plata, Calle 47 nº522, 1900 La Plata, Argentina, *ischala@museo.fcnym.unlp.edu.ar*

Abstract

The geological and tectonic history of the southern part of South America is complex, and is comprised of several magmatic events and orogenies that have favored the formation of different types of mineral deposits. Ten metallogenic belts that contain deposits associated with submarine volcanism from the Proterozoic to the Jurassic have been recognized in Argentina. Although the Zn-Pb-Ag ± Ba Sedex deposits are the most important from the economic point of view, Cyprus, Kuroko and W volcanogenic type deposits have also been recognized.

One of the oldest metallogenic belt (PRE-ZS1), of Upper Proterozoic age, is comprised of an ophiolitic sequence with associated Cyprus type deposits. Volcanogenic Cyprus type deposits were also formed during the Lower Palezoic (PRE-ZS2 metallogenic belt). The volcanic-exhalative W deposits of the Lower Paleozoic (PRE-PAM1 metallogenic belt) are associated with arc magmatism.

The POS-PAM1 metallogenic belt in NW Argentina hosts the largest known Pb-Zn deposits of the South American Paleozoic. The Aguilar mine, Jujuy, the largest producer of non-ferrous metals in Argentina, has produced more than 25 Mt of ore with an average of 4 % Pb, 6 % Zn and 100 g/t Ag. Pb-Zn-Ag Sedex deposits with Cu-rich proximal zones are hosted by sedimentary rocks of Lower Tremadocian age. The Ordovician intracratonic basin was formed under an extensional regime after the collision of the Arequipa-Antofalla craton to the Brazilian-Río de La Plata craton during the middle Cambrian, and extends northwestward to Peru. Pb-Zn-Ag Sedex deposits were also formed in Proterozoic basins of Patagonia.

In the Ordovician basin of the Precordillera, Zn-Pb-Au-Ag VMS deposits associated with mafic magmatism were formed in a tectonic setting related to an early oceanic rift next to the continent; Ba Sedex deposits were formed in slope sequences (PRE-CUY1 metallogenic belt). Cu-Pb-Zn Kuroko type deposits formed in association with an OIB type magmatism of the Eruptive Puna belt (Arenigian).

During Mesozoic time, accompanying the aperture of the Atlantic Ocean, an extensional regime was established and intracratonic as well as back-arc basins were developed along the periphery of the craton. In the Neuquén basin, Ba Sedex type deposits were formed in association with sequences of Pliensbachian-Toarcian age (POS-SAG1 metallogenic belt). In southernmost South America, Kuroko type deposits associated with silicic volcanism were formed in a Jurassic extensional back-arc basin (POS-AMJ2 metallogenic belt).

Introduction

From the mining perspective, the production of Zn-Pb-Ag from deposits related to submarine volcanism in Argentina represents the entire national production.

Ten metallogenic belts have been recognized, in Argentina, which have deposits associated with submarine volcanism ranging in age from the Proterozoic to the Jurassic (Table 1). In this paper we present the evolution of the metallogenic belts that host mineral deposits associated with submarine volcanism within

Table 1. Metallogenic belts that host mineral deposits associated with submarine volcanism.

Metallogenic Belt	Tectonostratigraphic Unit	Age	Type of deposit
PRE-ZS1	Ophiolites	Proterozoic	Cyprus
PRE-ZS2	Ophiolites	Lower Paleozoic	Cyprus
PRE-PAM1	Metamorphic basement	Upper Proterozoic. -Lower Paleoz	Volcanogenic W
PRE-PAM3	Volcanic Arc	Lower Paleozoic	Kuroko
PRE-PAT1	Metamorphic basement	Proterozoic	Sedex Zn-Pb-Ba-Ag Sedex Ba
PRE-PAT3	Accretionary Prism	Devonian	Sedex Zn-Pb-Ba-Ag
PRE-CUY1	Slope deposits	Lower Paleozoic	Sedex Zn-Pb-Ba-Ag Sedex Ba
POS-PAM1	Intracratonic extensional basin	Lower Paleozoic	Sedex Zn-Pb-Ba-Ag Sedex Ba
POS-AMJ2	Volcanic Arc	Jurassic	Kuroko
POS-SAG1	Intracratonic extensional basin	Jurassic	Sedex Zn-Pb-Ba-Ag Sedex Ba

the framework of the tectonic evolution of the southernmost part of South America. For each belt we describe type deposits as well as the potential to host similar deposits.

The Lower Paleozic POS-PAM1 metallogenic belt (Fig. 1) hosts the largest recognized Paleozoic Pb-Zn deposits in South America, with Mina Aguilar being the largest producer in Argentina (Table 2). Since 1936, Mina Aguilar, Jujuy province, has produced more than 25 Mt of ore with an average of 4 % Pb, 6 % Zn and 100 g/t Ag (Sureda, 1999). Mina Aguilar presently produces an average of 2100 t/day of ore with an average of 5.5 % Pb, 8.2 % Zn and 120 g/t Ag. Reserves are even more significant (Table 2). The largest potential reserves in the district are found in Mina Esperanza (Fig. 7, Table 2) (Sureda., 1999). The development and exploitation of Mina Esperanza, Jujuy, began in 1990 and presently produces 400 t/d.

The Proterozoic PRE-PAT1 metallogenic belt (Fig. 1) hosts the Gonzalito Sedex district (Table 2), which was the third largest producer in Argentina from 1953 to 1979; it produced about 0.8 M t of ore (61,807 t of concentrates of Pb and 12,725 t of concentrates of Zn).

More recently, a district with Kuroko-type massive sulphides in Tierra del Fuego has been identified in the Jurassic POS-AMJ2 metallogenic belt (Table 2). While this district appears very promising, more exploration is required to evaluate the mining potential of the zone.

Tungsten deposits of volcanogenic origin of the Lower Paleozoic PRE-PAM1 metallogenic belt (Fig. 1) represent the largest tungsten reserves of Argentina. These deposits were exploited during Wold War I and II (Table 2) and are currently inactive.

The Cyprus-type deposits of the Proterozoic PRE-ZS1 metallogenic belt (Fig. 1) (Table 2) of Córdoba are small, and were only exploited on a small scale.

Cyprus-type deposits of the Lower Paleozoic PRE-ZS2 metallogenic belt (Fig. 1) include the Salamanca-La Barrera (Mendoza) and Santa Elena (San Juan) deposits (Table 2). Production records exist for the years 1969-1973 of copper minerals that were recovered in the province to produce copper sulphate. Precise production data are not known.

Volcanic-exhalative barite deposits that formed in Lower Paleozoic PRE-CUY1 metallogenic belt and in the Jurassic POS-SAG1 metallogenic belt (Fig. 1) represent a large part of the national production of Ba (Table 2). The most important deposit of the Neuquen basin, Arroyo Nuevo, produced more than 0.2 Mt at 92.4 % $BaSO_4$.

METALLOGENIC BELTS THAT HOST MINERAL DEPOSITS ASSOCIATED WITH SUBMARINE VOLCANISM

The integration of the tectonic settings in a framework of pre-, syn-, and post-accretional processes explains the complex metallogenic history of Argentina (Zappettini, 1999a and b). The metallogenic belts that host deposits associated with submarine volcanism are concentrated in different ages: Proterozoic-Lower Cambrian, Ordovician and Jurassic (Fig. 1, Table 2). In this paper we follow the nomenclature proposed by Nokleberg et al., (1998) for the metallo-

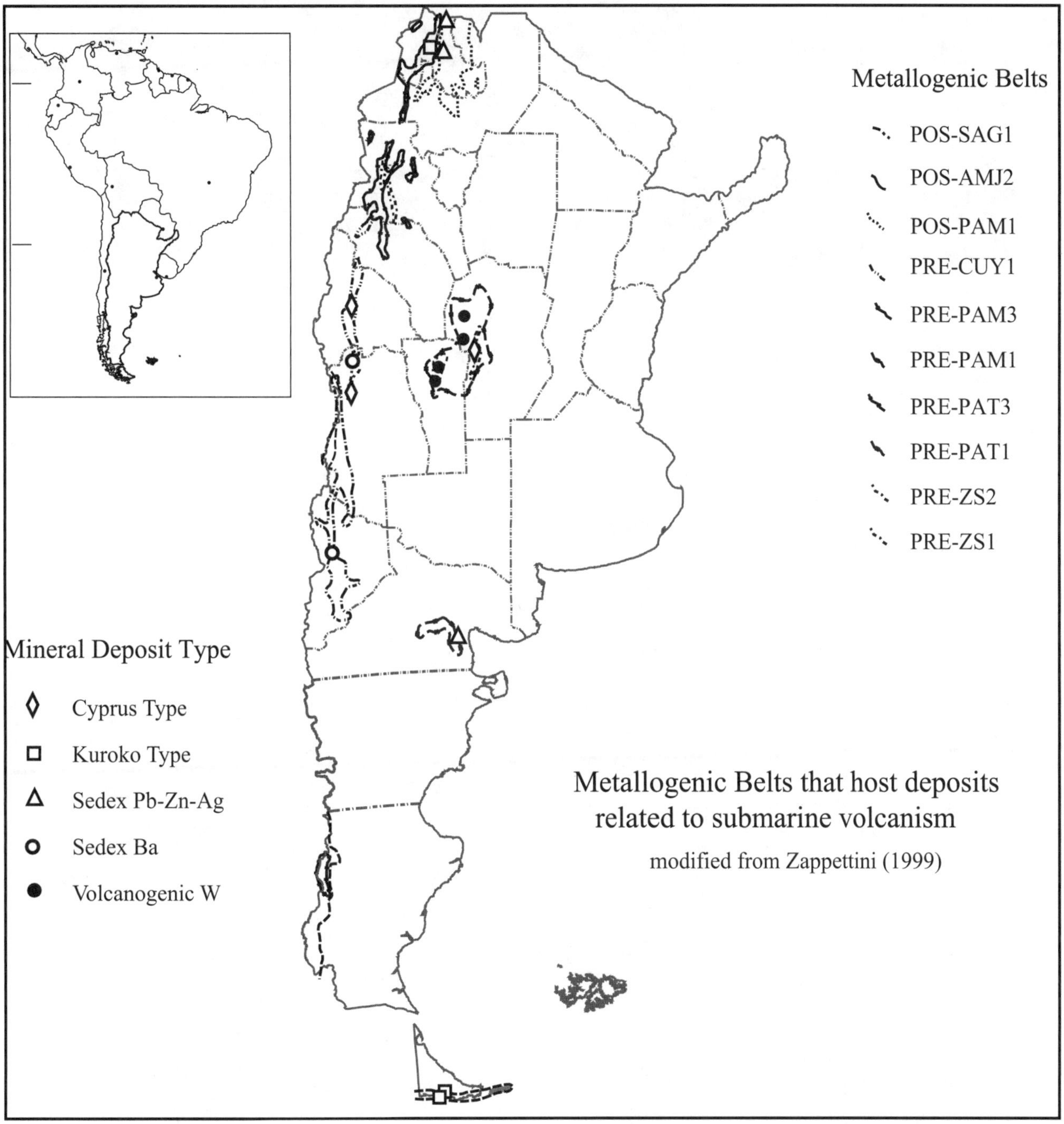

Figure 1. Metallogenic belts that host deposits related to submarine volcanism of Argentina, modified from Zappettini (1999a).

Table 2. Mineral deposits associated with submarine volcanism of Argentina.

Type of deposit	Name	Location	Metallogenic Belt[1]	Tonnage (Mt)	Grades							
					WO_3 (%)	$BaSO_4$ (%)	Ni (%)	Cu (%)	Zn (%)	Pb (%)	Au (ppm)	Ag (ppm)
Cyprus	Tío-Tauro -Tacurú	Córdoba	PRE-ZS1	<0.001				2-7				
	La Salamanca	Mendoza	PRE-ZS2	0.05			0.2	6.5				
	Santa Elena	San Juan	PRE-ZS2	0.5				0.08	3.3	2.1	4.2	87
W Volcanogenic	Altautina	Córdoba	PRE-PAM1									
	Los Guindos	Córdoba	PRE-PAM1									
	La Florida	San Luis	PRE-PAM1	1[2]	0.6-1							
	Pampa de Tamboreo	San Luis	PRE-PAM1									
	Sierra del Morro	San Luis	PRE-PAM1									
Kuroko	Beatriz	Tierra del Fuego	POS-AMJ2	1.5[3]				1.3	2.0		0.16	13.0
	Arroyo Rojo	Tierra del Fuego	POS-AMJ2									
Sedex Pb-Zn-Ag	Aguilar	Jujuy	POS-PAM1	25					15-18	5-15		137-370
	La Colorada	Salta	POS-PAM1	12				0.5	1	1.1		
	Gonzalito	Río Negro	PRE-PAT1	0.5					1.2	8.6		up to 400
Sedex Ba	Arroyo Nuevo	Neuquén	POS-AMJ1	0.5	92.4							
	Canota	Mendoza	PRE-CUY1	0.5								

[1] For ages see Table 1

[2] Tonnage and grades are for all the deposits together

[3] Tonnage and grades are for all the deposits together

genic belts. From the tectonic point of view, Argentina has been divided into five principal terranes (Ramos, 1996): 1, the Río de la Plata craton, 2, Pampia, 3, Cuyania, 4, Chilenia and 5, Patagonia (Fig. 2).

In the following paragraphs, the evolution of the metallogenic belts that developed deposits associated with submarine volcanism is detailed chronologically in a framework of the tectonic evolution of southernmost South America. For each of the belts, type deposits are described as well as the potential for hosting such deposits.

PRE-ZS1 Metallogenic Belt

Tectonic and Metallogenic evolution

The Proterozoic basin of Sierras Pampeanas hosts one of the oldest known metallogenic belt in Argentina, PRE-ZS1, which hosts volcanogenic deposits (Fig. 1). The PRE-ZS1 belt comprises an ophiolitic sequence where Cyprus-type Fe-Cu-Ti-Co and Ni deposits are encountered (Fig. 3). The collision of the Pampia Terrane with the Río de la Plata craton during the upper Proterozoic (750 Ma) as a part of the Brazilian orogen generated a compressional tectonic style and generated an intense penetrative deformation (Ramos, 1992; Mutti, 1992) in the Sierras Pampeanas Orientales overprinting the mineralized bodies. As a result of this collisional event, the obduction of the oceanic crust was produced, along with regional metamorphism that reached amphibolite facies (Di Marco and Mutti, 1992a). The stockwork structures and breccia pipes were deformed and metamorphosed during this event. The amphibolites associated with the deposits show an affinity with ocean ridge basalts in extensional environments (MORB-E) and the deposits of Cu-Fe-Ti-Co-Ni are interpreted to have formed in a submarine setting (Di Marco and Mutti, 1994). During the lower Paleozoic, late to post-tectonic silicic magmatism took place, which only caused very localized changes in the amphibolites (Di Marco and Mutti, 1994).

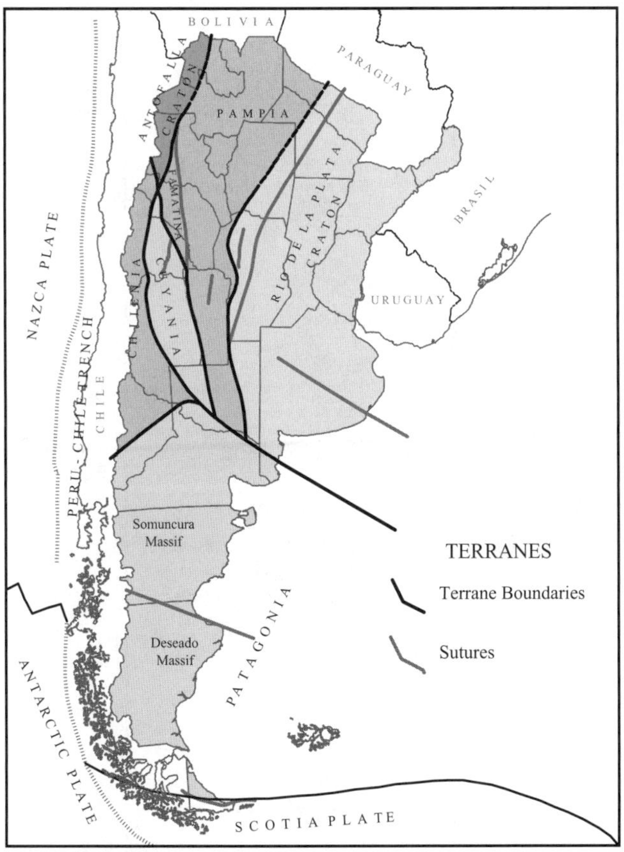

Figure 2. Map of the accreted terranes in Argentina. Modified from Zappettini (1999a); after Ramos (1996, 1988), Kraemer et al. (1995), and Bahlburg and Hervé (1997).

Geology of the deposits

The deposits are hosted in the igneous-metamorphic basement of the Sierras Pampeanas of Precambrian-Lower Paleozoic age (Fig. 3) (Gordillo and Lencinas, 1979). They are characterized by being small, having similar mineralogy, textures and hydrothermal alteration (Di Marco and Mutti, 1994).

The igneous-metamorphic sequence of the Sierras de Córdoba consists of gneisses, schists, amphibolites, marbles, migmatites, mylonites and plutonic rocks. Occasionally, pegmatitic and aplitic veins cross-cut the sequence. The metamorphic grade increases from east to west; from upper greenschist facies (the western flank of the Sierra Chica) to upper amphibolite facies (eastern flank of the Sierra de Comechingones) (Di Marco and Mutti, 1994).

The amphibolites occur as 100-300 m long lenses with a thickness of 10-15 m, and host disseminated or massive-textured ore.

The ore in the Tío, Tacurú and Estrella Gaucha mines consists of magnetite, ilmenite, pyrite, chalcopyrite and hematite; in addition, carrolite and pyrrhotite occur in the Tío and Tauro mines. The alteration assemblages of the host rock consist of:

Tío: quartz-epidote-biotite; Tacurú: quartz-biotite-chlorite and Estrella Gaucha: quartz-epidote-chlorite (Di Marco and Mutti, 1994).

PRE-PAT1 Metallogenic Belt

Tectonic and metallogenic evolution

Patagonia, the last terrane accreted to Gondwana in the upper Paleozoic (Ramos, 1988), hosts the PRE-PAT1 metallogenic belt of Proterozoic age (Fig. 1). During the Proterozoic, an intracratonic rift developed in the Somun Curá terrane with the consequent formation of extensional intracratonic sedimentary basins. In these marginal basins, composed by a platform and deeper clastic facies, sedimentary-exhalative deposits of Pb-Zn-Ag (Fig. 4) developed (Dalla Salda et al., 1999; Aragón et al. (1999). Dolomites and calcites were deposited along the shallow border of the rift, and in deeper waters, around the volcanic centres, clastic sediments and volcaniclastics were deposited. The Pb-Zn-Ag deposits are associated with clastic and chemical sediments, whereas the ocean floor basalts are associated with slope facies (turbidites) in deeper environments. In general, these rocks were deposited in environments of shallow to medium depth on a stable continental margin, far from active plate margins (Dalla Salda et al., 1999). This environment is considered a pre-upper Proterozoic intracontinental rift.

Geology of the deposits

The Gonzalito District is located in the SE of the province of Río Negro (Fig. 4), to the east of the Sierra Pailemán (latitude 41° - 42° S and longitude

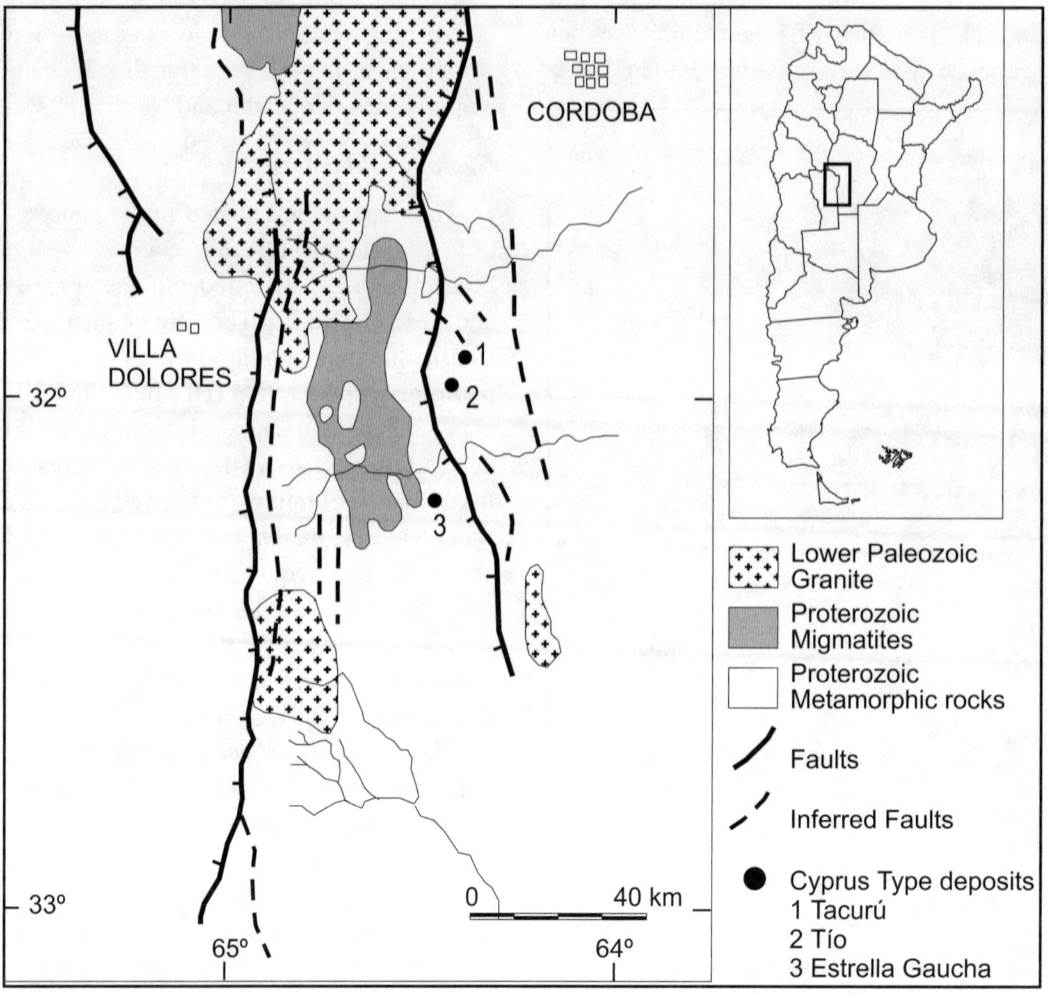

Figure 3. Geology of the Sierra Grande of Córdoba. Modified from Di Marco and Mutti (1994).

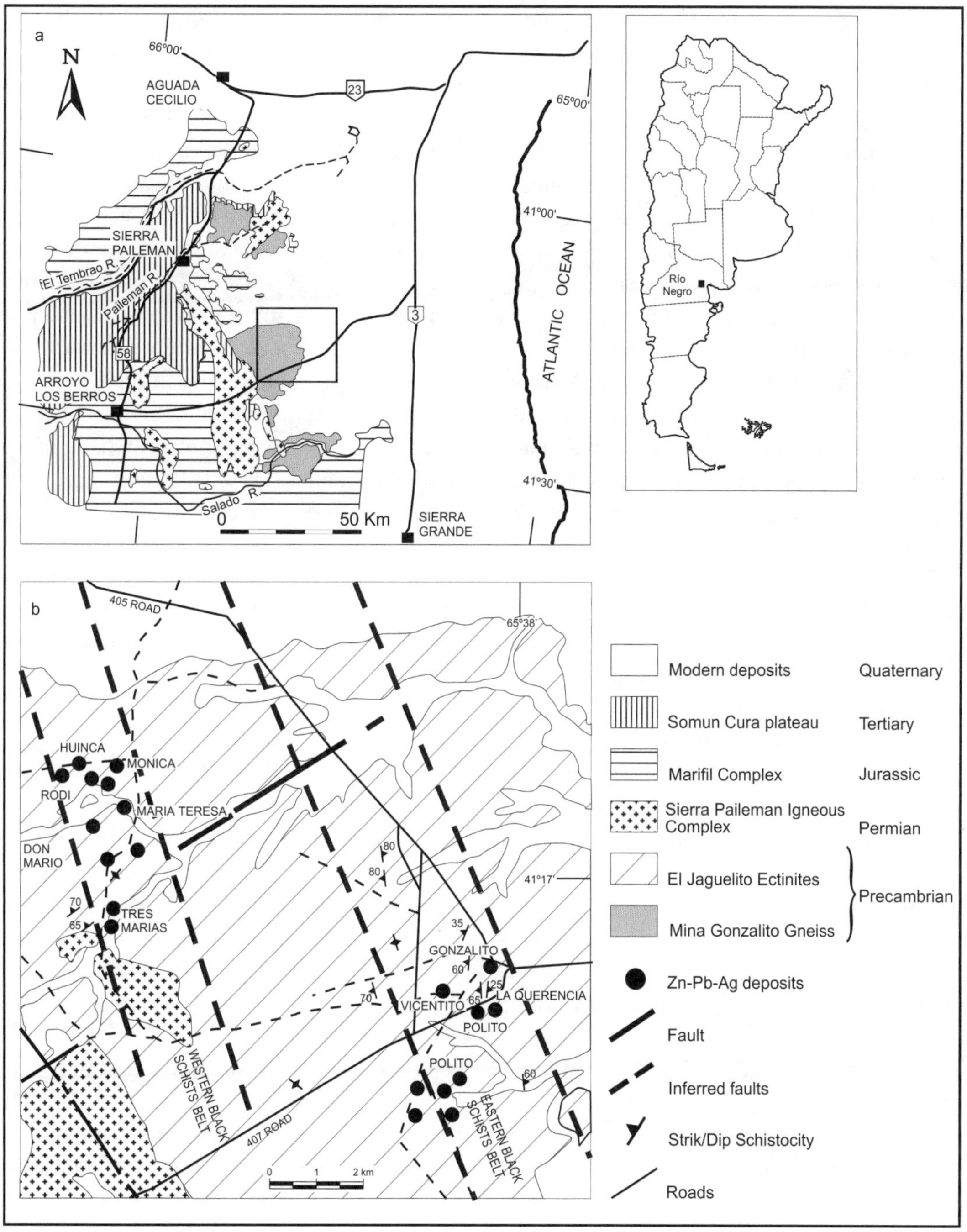

Figure 4a. Geology of Sierra Pailemán, Somun Curá Massif; modified from Aragón et al. (1999); b. Geology of the Gozalito District, modified from Dalla Salda et al. (1999)

65°-66° W). The district consists of sulphide-poor Sedex deposits of Zn-Pb-Ag that formed distal to exhalative sources, and were deformed, metamorphosed and remobilized.

The deposits are located in two belts: the eastern belt includes the mines Gonzalito, Vicentito, La Querencia and Polito; the western belt includes the mines Tres Marías and María Teresa (Fig. 4). Previous studies of the area include Del Mónaco (1971), Zubia (1976), Vallés (1978), De Ferran (1983) and Dalla Salda and Aragón (1994). The regional geology was described by Rosenman (1972), Ramos (1975), Vallés (1978) and Giacosa (1987). The basement consists of the Neoproterozoic Mina Gonzalito Gneiss (ore host rock) and the El Jagüelito ectinites (Ramos, 1975; Linares et al., 1990). The basement complex was intruded initially by Permian plutons (Granito Pailemán) and later by Jurassic lavas and dikes (Marifil Formation). The uppermost units are Cenozoic sediments (Roca Formation) and volcanics (Somun Curá Basalts). Although the metamorphism of Mina Gonzalito Gneiss is Proterozoic, the main deformation and remobilization of the ore are associated with pre-Upper Paleozoic and Pre-Jurassic events. The regional structure is complex, and the change in the strike and dip of the schistosity is related to a complex interference pattern, which shows structural closures and saddles. These structures controlled the redistribution of the ore (Dalla Salda et al., 1999).

The Mina Gonzalito Gneiss in general reached amphibolite facies, although the ore-bearing schists are lower grade (chlorite-garnet schists). The Mina Gonzalito Gneiss is characterized by biotite-, biotite-garnet and occasionally sillimanite gneisses, amphibolites, calc-silicate rocks and synkinematic leucocratic granitoids that are associated with metavolcanics. The ore of the Gonzalito district occurs as disseminated stratabound deposits, however, the highest grade ore occur as lenses of polymetallic massive sulphides that resulted from the remobilization and reconcentration of the latter during Upper Paleozoic and Pre-Jurassic events (Aragón et al., 1999; Dalla Salda et al., 1998). Most of the ore-bearing units are "metalliferous black schists" that bear Zn, Pb, Ag, V and occasionally Au in silicates, oxides, sulphides and carbonates, over thicknesses of 1.2-2.5 m. The ore-bearing metasedimentary sequences are biotite-, amphibolite-, quartz-biotite-muscovite- and quartzo-feldspathic schists. Some marbles, metamarls, amphibolites and quartzo-felsdpathic schists show lower, but still anomalous, metal contents.

The lenses of polymetallic sulphides are foliation parallel, occur as en echelon disks have thicknesses between 0.7 and 1.5 m, and lengths between 30 and 100 m. The mineralogy includes: limonite, manganese oxides, cerussite, anglesite, wulfenite, pyromorphite, galena and vanadinite. Below the level of oxidation (~40 m), the ores consist of galena, sphalerite, pyrite, chalcopyrite, arsenopyrite, marcasite, rhodochrosite and quartz. The best example of remobilized and reconcentrated ore is in the María Teresa mine (Dalla Salda et al., 1999). The metamorphosed sulphides are cross-cut by veins of fluorite in a calc-silicate gangue. The Zn ore consists of Zn-rich chlorites and oxides of Zn, Pb and Mn. In the same sequence, black schists occur with average contents of 17 % Fe and occasionally up to 40.83 %, which is interpreted as an iron formation (Dalla Salda et al., 1999). Some schists are also rich in Mn (Mn>0.8 %). The lenses of massive sulphides have metal contents between 3 and 12 % Zn, Pb and Ag, the strata with disseminated ore have from 1 to 3 % Zn > Pb. The higher values of Zn relative to Pb and S in the strataform ore is, therefore, interpreted to be the result of selective mobilization of Pb as sulphide complexes with its consequent redeposition in structural traps.

PRE-PAM1 Metallogenic Belt

Tectonic evolution of the PRE-PAM1 metallogenic belt

Volcanic-exhalative W deposits of the PRE-PAM1 metallogenic belt (Fig. 1) have a complex geologic history. The PRE-PAM1 metallogenic belt is associated with an arc magmatism that was developed along the western flank of Pampia in a basin generated after the collision of Pampia with the Río de La Plata Craton. During the Lower Cambrian, prior to the accretion of the Cuyania and Antofalla-Arequipa terranes, in a marine basin developed along the western flank of Pampia, a sedimentary sequence (turbidites, sandstones and shales) was deposited, and tholeiitic flood basalts formed, possibly during an initial rifting of the back-arc basin (Brodtkorb and Brodtkorb, 1999). Hydrothermal systems associated with this magmatism generated tungsten deposits (El Morro and Yulto). However, the deposits of La Florida district are associated with silicic volcanism. During the Lower Cambrian, the Antofalla-Arequipa terrane collided with the Pampia terrane (Fig. 2) and produced the deformation and metamorphism of the volcanic-sedimentary sequence (Pampean Orogeny, 580-540

Ma). Nevertheless, the dominant structural style of the region corresponds to deformation during the Famatinian Orogeny (560-360 Ma), which was produced with the collision of the Cuyania terrane with Pampia (Fig. 2) (Ramos et al., 1986; Astini et al., 1996).

Geology of the Deposits

The volcanogenic tungsten deposits are located in Sierra de San Luis, Sierra de Altautina y Sierra Grande de Córdoba (Fig. 5). The geological setting consists of a metamorphic-igneous basement of upper Proterozoic-Lower to middle Paleozoic in age. The dominant rocks are biotitic schists, gneisses, and migmatites, and to a lesser extent anfibolites, limestones, sandstones, which were intruded by pre-, syn- and post-tectonic granites, pegmatites and veins. They occur in two groups that differ in the composition of their associated volcanic rocks as well as in the grade of the superimposed metamorphism. These are: 1) deposits associated with calc-silicate rocks and ortoamphibolites (amphibolite facies), and 2) those associated with silicic metavolcanics, cuarcites, turmalinites and spessartitic cuarcites -coticule- (greenschist facies). The first group occurs in a 300 km long belt along the Sierra grande de Córdoba, Sierra de Altautina (Ametrano, 1996, 1999) and Sierra de San Luis. The mining districts include: Agua de Ramón, Ambul, Zinqui, Los Guindos y Sierra de Altautina (Córdoba), and El Morro, Yulto, San Felipe, Sierra de la Estanzuela, Villa de Praga (San Luis) (Fig. 5). The second group occurs in two low-grade metamorphic belts in the Sierra de San Luis and the districts are: Valle de Pancanta, La Florida, Los Cocos, Pampa de Tamboreo, La Teodolina, El Araucano-La Higuera y Santo Domingo (Fig. 5).

Due to their economic importance, El Morro and Yulto, San Luis, will be described as the type deposit for the first group and La Florida, San Luis, as the type deposit of the second group.

The El Morro Oeste district is localized in a zone 40 km long from N to S in the Sierra de San Luis (Fig. 5). These deposits have been the focus of numerous studies, such as Smith and González Stegemann (1947), Monchablón (1956), Brodtkorb and Brodtkorb (1977, 1980, 1999), Llambías and Malvicini (1982), Delakowitz (1987) and Delakowitz et al. (1991). The largest producers were: El Morro No. 1, La Providencia, El Peje, Los Rodeos and Lucifer.

The geology of the zone includes schists and biotite gneisses; marbles, orthoamphibolites and calc-silicate rocks; pegmatoids of metamorphic origin; synkinematic and postkinematic pegmatites and veins of quartz and tourmaline. The folding of the metamorphic strata is the result of a prolonged and intense pre-Devonian metamorphic event.

The scheelite deposits are stratabound, occur in 6-10 m thick layers, and are closely related to the cal-silicate-rich rocks and the ortoamphibolites (Brodtkorb and Brodtkorb, 1999). The top of the amphibolites shows epidote/clinozoicite, interpreted as submarine hydrothermal alteration. The belts of calc-silicate rocks show a banded structure and consist of hornblende, tremolite-actinolite, epidote and lessor amounts of plagioclase, chlorite and calcite; and quartz, talc, biotite, muscovite, diopside, zircon, apatite, titanite, scheelite, fluorite, sphalerite, pyrite, chalcopyrite, pyrrhotite, magnetite and ilmenite as accessory minerals. The scheelite grains are xenoblastic (0.4-1 mm in size), have variable contents of MoO_4 and are oriented parallel to the schistosity. Tectonization produced significant remobilization, and led to very high concentrations of scheelite along tectonic planes and fold hinges (Brodtkorb and Brodtkorb, 1999). The genesis of these deposits is interpreted to be the result of hydrothermal processes associated with submarine tholeiitic volcanism (Delakowitz et al., 1991; Brodtkorb and Brodtkorb, 1999).

The La Florida mine district (Fig. 5) was one of the four large producers that operated during the First World War and continued to operate intermittently until the 1970s. The geology of the zone includes phyllites and biotite schists with intercalations of quartzites and metavolcanics (Brodtkorb et al., 1985; 1999; Hack et al., 1991). The phyllites consist of muscovite, biotite or chlorite, and quartz; and as accessories, garnet chlorite, andalusite, epidote, zoicite, tourmaline, calcite and pyrite. The quartzites contain plagioclase and zoicite, muscovite and microcline; and as accessories, tourmaline, garnet, chlorite, epidote, zircon and apatite. Disseminated scheelite is associated with metavolcanics. The metavolcanics can be traced for 6 km. The rock consists of phenocrysts of quartz and microcline in a fine-grained matrix of quartz, albite and minor microcline; the accessory minerals are zoicite, garnet, epidote, clinozoicite, apatite, sericite, biotite, scheelite, monazite, ilmenite and hematite. These deposits are well known for their pervasive silicification and tourmalinization (Brodtkorb et al., 1999b).The present structure is due to the Famatinian orogeny. Post-mineralization tectonics produced displacements and divided the deposit into three blocks. Metamorphic remobilization

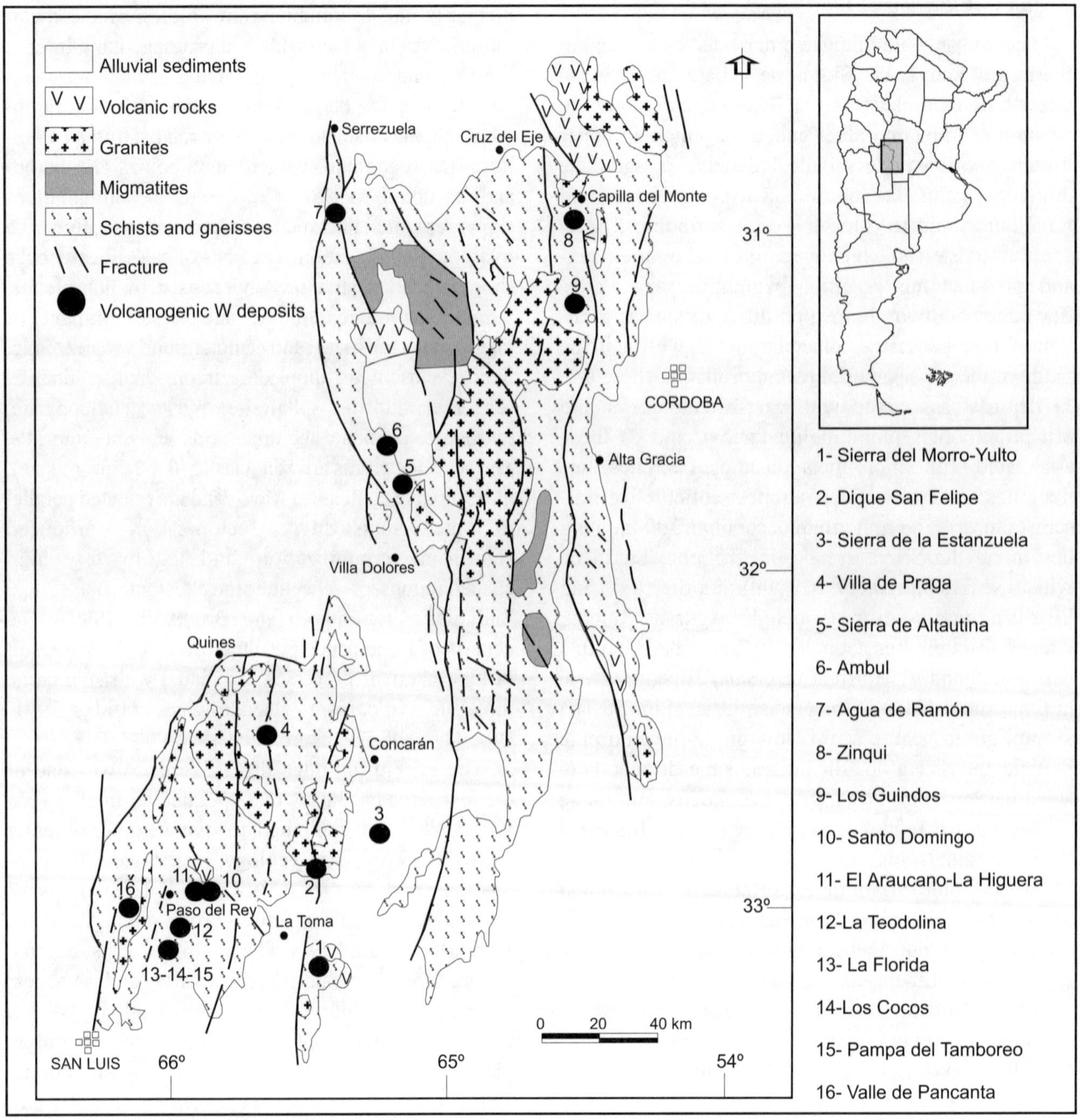

Figure 5. Geology of Sierra de San Luis (San Luis province) and Sierra de Ambul (Córdoba province). Modified from Brodtkorb and Brodtkorb (1999) and Brodtkorb et al. (1999).

form veins of quartz and quartz-tourmaline with outer zones that contain course grained scheelite that provided economic concentrations.

POS-PAM1 Metallogenic Belt

Tectonic Evolution of the POS-PAM1 Belt

The POS-PAM1 metallogenic belt (Fig. 1) hosts the largest known Pb-Zn deposits in the Paleozoic of South America. During the upper Proterozoic, the western margin of Gondwana developed as a deep marine basin that later closed due to a collision of the Arequipa-Antofalla Craton with the Brazilian-Río de La Plata (Pampia terrane) craton in the middle Cambrian (Aceñolaza and Toselli, 1976; Ramos, 1988). After this collision, the Ordovician basin developed between the two cratons in response to the rifting that prevailed until the Middle Ordovician (Ramos, 1988). The Ordovician basin of northwestern Argentina forms part of the intracratonic extensional basin that extends from Peru to northern Argentina (12°-26° south latitude) (Aceñolaza and Toselli, 1976; Coira et al., 1982; Ramos, 1988) (Fig. 6). South of 26° south latitude, the regime was predominantly compressional. This basin was filled with a sedimentary sequence with intercalations of alkaline basalts (OIB type) from the Middle Cambrian to the Tremadocian (Rapela et al., 1992). The sedimentary sequence begins with conglomerates and sandstones of the Middle Cambrian Mesón Group, which lie discordantly on basement and grade upward into pelitic facies, suggesting rapid subsidence. During the Tremadocian, more than 3200 m of shales were deposited (Harrington and Leanza, 1957); locally anoxic conditions are observed in the Sierra de Zenta, Sierra de Aguilar and Sierra de Santa Victoria (Pérez et al., 1998). Sedex Pb-Zn-Ag deposits with proximal sectors rich in Cu (Aguilar, Jujuy; La Colorada, Salta) occur in sedimentary rocks of the lower Ordovician (Sureda and Martín, 1990; Zappettini, 1999a). During the Arenigian, the closing of the Ordovician basin began and the Eruptive Belt of La Puna, a bimodal magmatic arc that generated two belts developed (Coira, 1992). The eastern belt consists of mafic (OIB) and intermediate rocks that are associated with Cu-Pb-Zn Kuroko-type deposits (Escaya Range, Cochinoca, Jujuy); the western belt consists of tholeiitic basalts with enriched mid-oceanic rift basalts (E-MORB) (Coira, 1992; Rapela, 1992). In both the eastern and western belts, the volcanic rocks evolved over time to a calc-alkaline series, indicating, that during the Arenigian the tectonic environment changed from an extensional to a compressional regime, developing a magmatic arc and incipient closing of the Ordovician basin (Ramos, 1988). The sandstones, claystones and black shales of the Arenigian reach 1450 m of thickness (Harrington and Leanza, 1957). The best-known deposit in sedimentary rocks of the Arenigian is La Colorada (Table 2). The Puna Turbidite Complex (Bahlburg et al., 1990) consists of a sequence of 4000 m of laminated shales interbedded with Llanvirnian, Llandeilian and Caradocian sandstones. Syngenetic pyrite, cherts, limestones and silicic volcanics are common in these units (Sierra de Lina, Sierra de

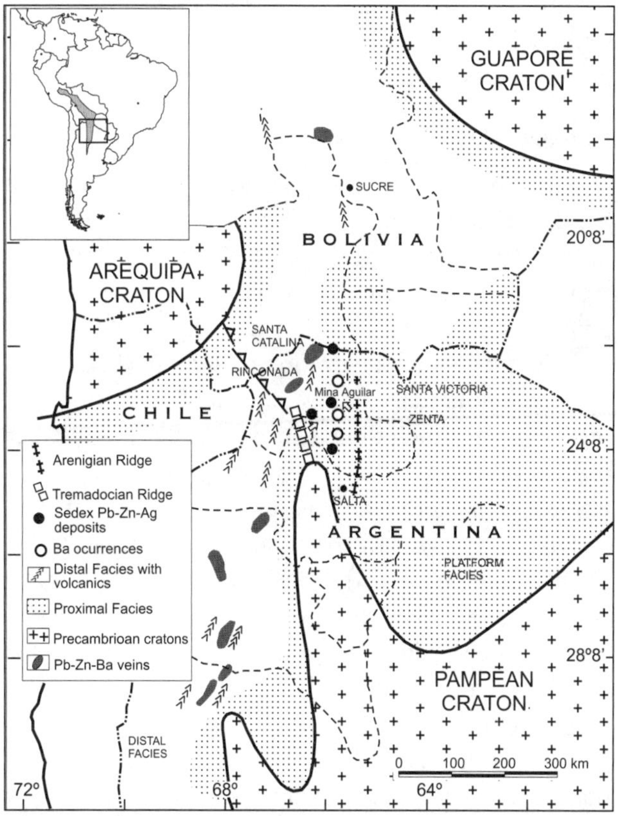

Figure 6. Geology of the Ordovician basin, NW Argentina. Modified from Sureda (1999).

Guayayaos and Cordón Gallegos) (Pérez et al., 1998). By early Cardocian time the closing of the Ordovician basin by the collision of the Arequipa-Antofalla Craton as part of Laurentia (Dalziel, 1997) against the Río de La Plata-Brazilian Craton was accompanied by folding and metamorphism of the Ordovician sedimentary rocks (the Ocloyic orogeny).

The anomalous contents of Zn, Pb, Cu and Ba-Mn found in the sedimentary rocks of the Ordovician basin (in the Cambrian of Nazareno, the Arenigian of Quichagua, and the Llandeilian of Gallegos (Pérez et al., 1998) and their correlation with the biostratigraphy indicate that the Zn-Pb Sedex deposits and the bands of syngenetic sulphides are not limited to the Tremadocian (Pérez et al., 1998). Rather, they are related to the extensional regime that dominated from the Middle Cambrian to the Middle Ordovician. Therefore, the favourable environment for the development of Sedex type deposits, in intracontinental basins during the Tremadocian and in back-arc basins during the Arenigian to Caradocian, make the Ordovician basin of NW Argentina a world-class target for the exploration of Sedex deposits.

Geology of the Deposits

The Pb, Zn and Ag deposits of the Aguilar mine are described in the following paragraphs as an example of the Sedex deposits of the Tremadocian. The Aguilar mine is located in the Sierra de Aguilar, Jujuy Province, at 23°12' of south latitude and 65°42' of west longitude, at an elevation of 4450 m (Fig. 7).

The Aguilar deposit has been the focus of numerous studies, including: Brown (1941), Spencer (1950), Ahlfeld (1955), Brown (1962), Linares (1968), Stipanicic and Linares (1969), Halpern and Latorre (1973), Linares and Latorre (1975), Brodtkorb et al. (1978), Sureda and Amstutz (1981), Alonso et al. (1982), Martín et al. (1986, 1987), Sureda and Martín (1990a,b), and Sureda (1999).

The Sierra de Aguilar is an anticline that consists mostly of marine sedimentary rocks of the Lower and Middle Ordovician (Fig. 8). Large reverse faults delineate a horst. The principal structures strike N-S and correspond to the Andean orogeny. The orebodies are found on the western limb. The Aguilar and Abra Laite granitic plutons were emplaced during the Cretaceous. Radiometric dating by K/Ar and Rb/Sr yield an average age of 118 ±15 M.a. for the Aguilar granite (Linares and Latorre, 1975) (Fig. 7).

Ordovician strata in the Sierra de Aguilar begins with sedimentary rocks in a shallow marine to marine deltaic environment with anoxic facies in a transgressive regime that is assigned to the lower Tremadocian by the presence of Dictyonema sp. (Despensa Formation, Alonso et al., 1982) (Fig. 8) The Lampazar Formation (Harrington and Leanza, 1957; Martín et al., 1986) is composed of a succession of fossiliferous black shales and fine sandstones. It is intercalated with the Padrioc Formation.

The Padrioc Formation (Aceñolaza and Toselli, 1976; Alonso et al., 1982) contains the important exhalative deposits of this metallogenic province (Sureda and Martín, 1990) and is composed of arkosic sandstones and coarse-grained calcareous sandstones with intercalations of limestones, cherts, intraformational conglomerates and black, fossiliferous shales. Upward and laterally are the shales and fine dark sandstones of the Lampazar Formation.

The Cardonal Formation comprises a succession of greenish gray sandstones with lessor interbeds of dark shales that only contain a few small mineralized bodies (Sureda and Martín, 1990a). The Acoite Formation (Harrington and Leanza, 1957) comprises a thick succession (3000 m) of turbidites and green and gray shales interbedded with dark limestones and sandstones of the lower to middle Arenigian. The maroon sandstones and shales of the Sepulturas Formation indicate a change in the source areas of the region, and represent the Guandacol orogeny.

The ore of the Aguilar mine consists of 10 stratiform bodies located in a 200 m thick section in the upper part of the Cuarcitas Aguilar Formation (Spencer, 1950; Alonso et al., 1982). The average dimensions of the orebodies vary between 150 and 1000 m in length, 50 and 300 m in width, and 5 to 80 m in thickness. These mineralized units extend along two km inside the contact metamorphic aureole of the Aguilar Granite, at the southeastern extreme of the outcropping pluton. The Cuarcitas Aguilar (K) Formation consists of metaquartzites, slates and hornfels that resulted from the contact metamorphism caused by the intrusion of the Aguilar Granite.

Outside of the metamorphic aurole, sulphides show primary textures suggesting syngenetic deposition of the sulphides interstratified in thin laminae with cherts, siltstones, barite and claystones (Fig. 9). Framboidal pyrite is common in the sediments and in many cases is still preserved in the contact metamorphic aureole where it is progressively replaced by a recrystallized pyrite.

The primary mineralogy of the ore consists mainly of marmatite, galena and pyrite, with minor pyrrhotite, greigite, chalcopyrite, tetrahedrite-tennantite, pyrargyrite, alabandite, arsenopyrite, magnetite, marcasite and molybdenite. Wurtzite, bournonite, boulangerite, cubanite, jamesonite,

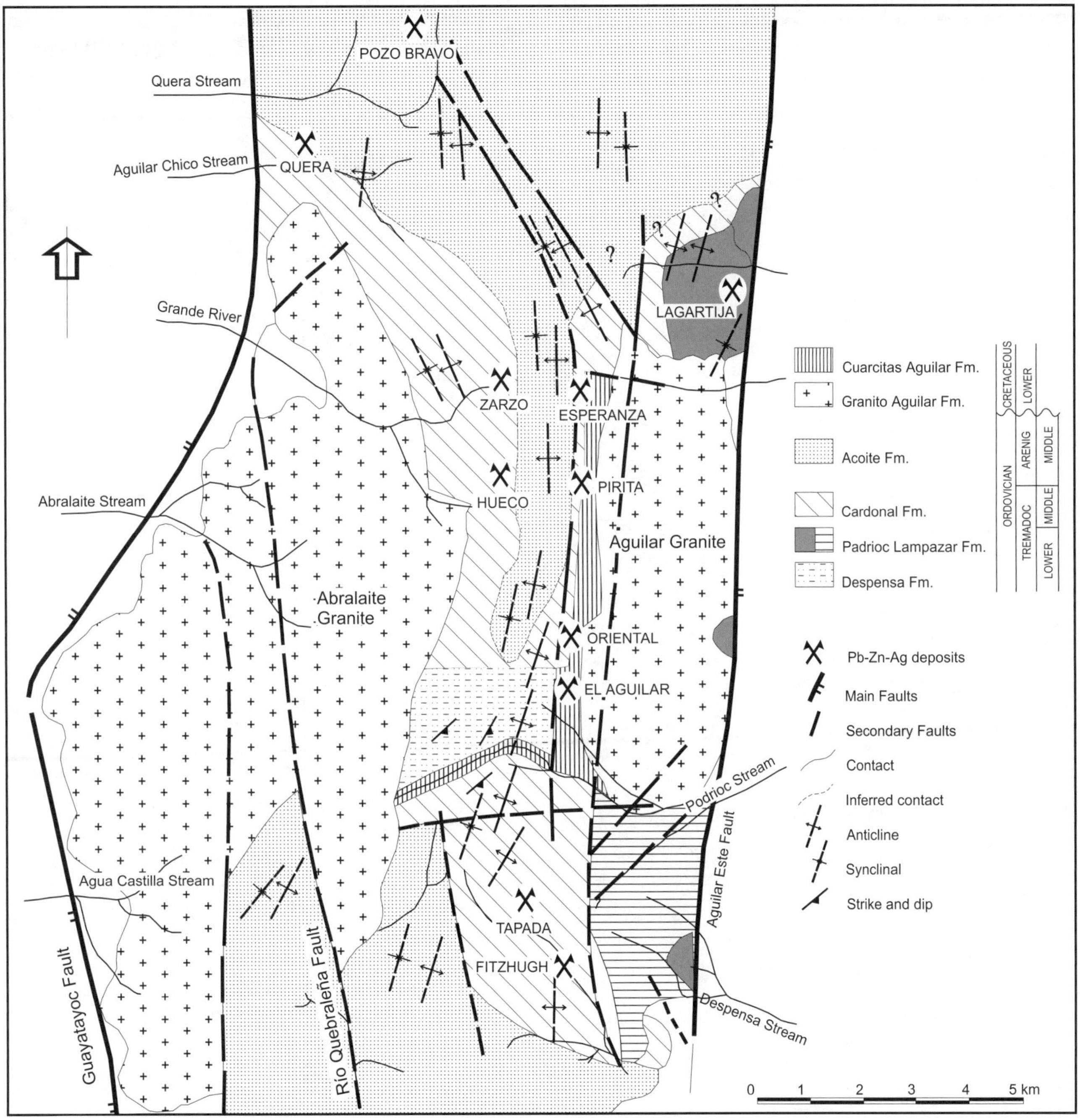

Figure 7. Geology of the Sierra Aguilar District, Jujuy province. Modified from Sureda (1999).

semseyite, gudmundite, stannite, isostannite, mackinawite, breithauptite, ullmannite, and native gold, silver and antimony are present as accessory minerals (Brodtkorb et al., 1978). Of these last accessory minerals, several have been formed by post-depositional processes such as metamorphism and metasomatism.

The ore shows different types of structures, the most common being brecchiated, banded and disseminated (Sureda and Martín, 1990b). The banded structure grades into bands of massive sulphides. The banded structure of the ore is concordant with the stratification of the original rock (Fig. 9). The disseminated structure is present toward the base of the mineralized bodies, and consists of marmatite and galena with subordinate pyrite and pyrrhotite.

Below the ores, there are secondary structures that were formed by remobilization or metasomatism during the intrusion of the Aguilar granite. Geochemical studies indicated that the emplacement of the Cretaceous granites introduced As, B, Be, Mo, Zr and Ti (Martín et al., 1988; Sureda and Martín, 1990a).

The synsedimentary paragenesis of sulphides

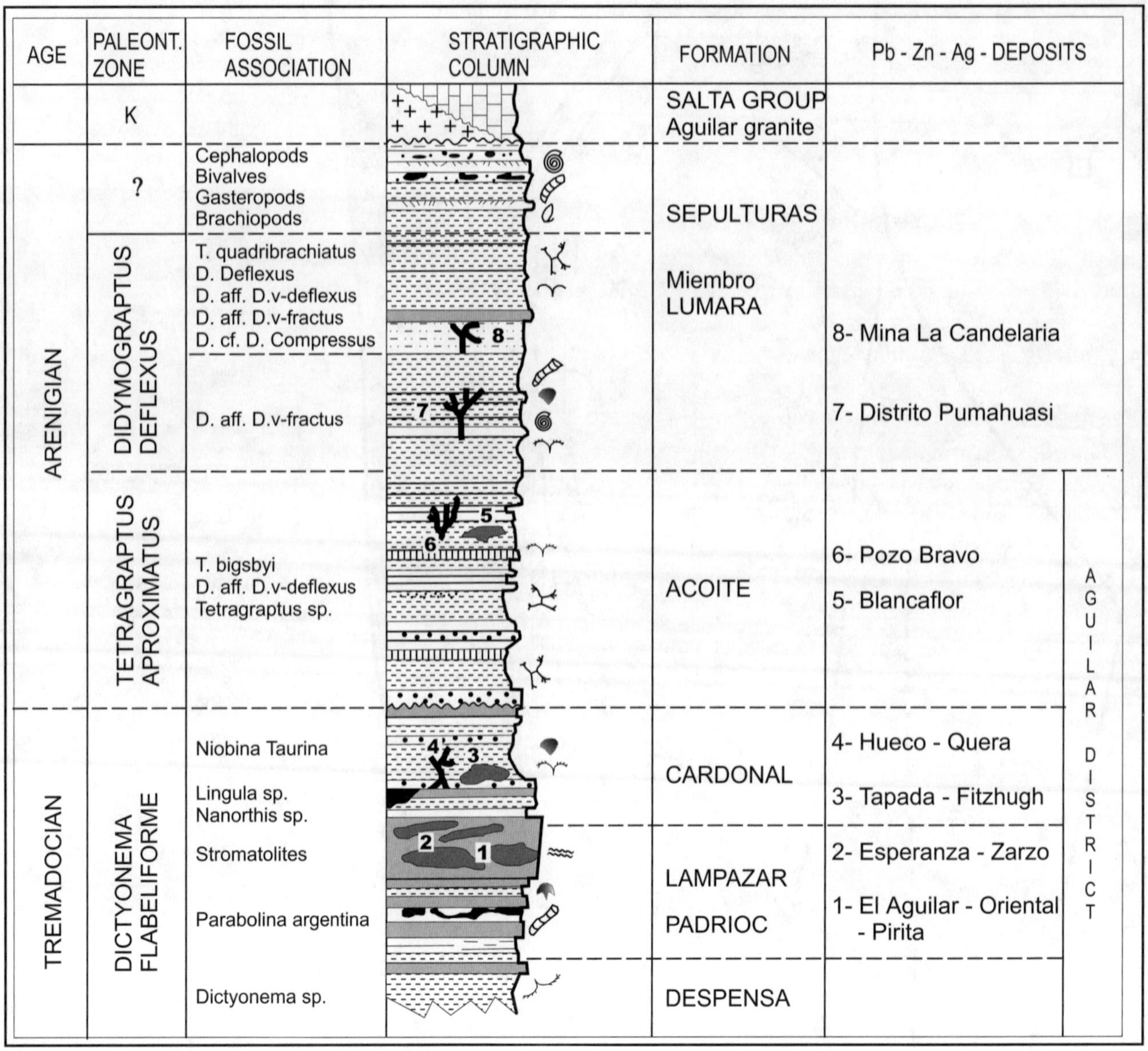

Figure 8. Stratigraphic column of the Sierra Aguilar District and location of the Pb-Zn-Ag deposits. Modified from Sureda (1999).

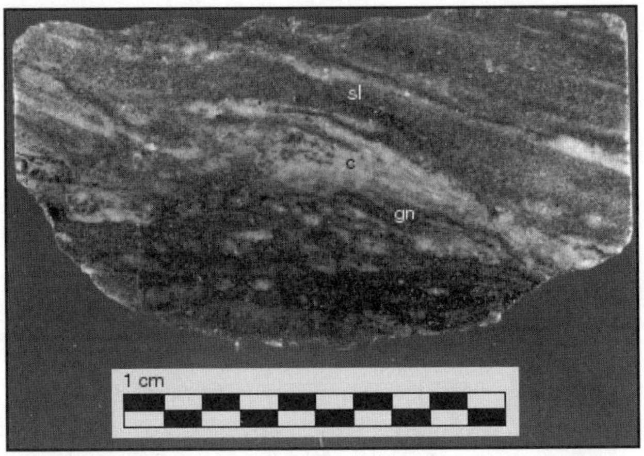

Figure 9. Banded structure in non-metamorphosed ore of the Aguilar District. Alternating layers of galena (gn), sphalerite (sl), carbonates (c) and sediments.

recrystallized as a coarse granular texture (Brodtkorb et al., 1978). The degree of recrystallization varied depending on the metamorphic grade. The ages of the ore calculated (Stipanicic and Linares, 1969) on the basis of lead isotopes (Brown, 1962) in galena are 351 ± 20 m.a. (Russell-Farquhar-Stanton method) and 428 ± 25 m.a. (Holmes-Houterman method). The ages that are somewhat younger than that of sedimentation are attributed to contamination of lead during the Andean orogeny (Sureda and Martín, 1990a).

Isotopic analysis of 40 samples (37 galenas and 3 sphalerites) indicated an average value for $\delta^{34}S$ of +18.3‰, suggesting bacteriological reduction of sulphur from seawater (Linares, 1968).

$^{87}Sr/^{86}Sr$ dates of barites from various deposits of the Quiaqueña metallogenic province show values that are very similar to Ordovician volcanic rocks and suggest an endogenous origin for the Sr and Ba (Barbieri et al., 1987).

PRE-ZS2 Metallogenic Belt

Tectonic Evolution of the PRE-ZS2 Belt

The PRE-ZS2 metallogenic belt (Fig. 1) includes Cyprus-type deposits (Salamanca-Barrera, Mendoza and Santa Elena, San Juan) associated with a sequence of dismembered ophiolites. This ophiolitic sequence represents the suture at a continental scale resulting from the collision of the allochthonous terrane Chilenia (Fig. 2) from the west with the margin of Gondwana toward the Upper Devonian (Haller and Ramos et al., 1984). This suture had been previously recognized by Criado Roque et al. (1981).The Famatinian ophiolites, so called for having developed during the Famatinian orogeny (Aceñolaza and Toselli 1976), extend in a discontinuous belt from 28° south latitude to 33° south latitude and crop out in the western sector of the Precordillera.

Although later tectonics played an important role, the Famatinian opholites are interpreted as the result of an oblique or transverse collision of discontinuous ridges with the continental margin. This collision would have generated strong compression in the fore-arc region at the end of the Ordovician-beginning of the Silurian (Ramos et al., 1984). The collision was the most intense in the southern region, resulting in the greatest structural uplift; the deepest crustal levels and greatest dynamic metamorphism are evidenced here (Haller and Ramos, 1984).

The gabbroic and peridotitic rocks of the eastern end of the Cordillera Frontal are also part of this group (Villar, 1969, 1970; Villar et al., 1982). The Eopaleozoic rocks of the Precordillera Occidental forms a nearly complete ophiolitic sequence in which ultramafic rocks, gabbros and pillow lavas can be recognized. The different members are found separated into different blocks, the product of the intense Famatinian orogeny. The best-developed ultramafic complex is found in the southernmost portion, and is composed of dunites, harzburgites and wehrlites (Villar, 1969; 1979); Villar et al., 1982; Zardini, 1958; 1960 a and b). The grade of serpentinization of the rocks varies from incipient to advanced. Cyprus-type copper deposits are associated with these serpentinites toward the north of the Mendoza River, as are the Cu, Ni, Co and Cr deposits of Novillo Muerto (Villar et al., 1982) and the Salamanca mine. In the Cortaderas range, there are outcrops of ultramafic bodies composed of serpentinized harzburgites and pyroxenites. Gabbroic rocks in the area of Cortaderas are made up of lenticular bodies of microgabbros emplaced concordantly with the stratification (Cucchi, 1972; Villar, 1998). In the area of Los Gateados, Cordillera Frontal of Mendoza, the gabbros occur in contact with the ultramafic rocks and from their chemical characteristics, they can be classified as ocean floor gabbros, principally N-MORB tending toward E-MORB (Villar, 1998). These gabbros correspond to an environment related to an oceanic rift formed in the Eopaleozoic during early stages of the accretion of Chilenia (Villar, 1998).

The upper section of the ophiolites is composed of pillow lavas intruded by small bodies of gabbro and some ultramafic rocks (Haller and Ramos, 1984); locally they are overlain by pelagic deposits, represented by chert layers and finely banded limestones (Quartino et al., 1971). These lavas are associated with massive sulphide deposits such as Santa Elena, San Juan.

The basalts of the Precordillera (upper levels of the Famatinian ophiolites) are highly evolved; they are characterized by a high content of TiO_2 and enrichment in the lighter rare earth elements similar to oceanic tholeiites. They present similarities with poorly evolved back-arc basins and with a ridge segment of transitional and plume type (anomalous ocean ridges), such as the Reykyanes ridge south of Iceland (Kay et al., 1984). One possible model would be an early oceanic rift near the continental margin (Kay et al., 1984).

Geology of the Deposits

The PRE-ZS2 metallogenic belt has sulphide deposits associated with the serpentinites (Salamanca-La Barrera, Mendoza) and basalts in the upper member of the ophiolites (Santa Elena, San Juan) (Table 2).

The Salamanca-La Barrera mines are located in the Cordón del Portillo and have been known since 1852 (Angelelli, 1984). Previous work includes González Stegemann (1949), Brodtkorb (1971).

The geology of the area of the Salamanca mine includes schists, serpentines, orthoamphibolites, and seams of kersantite and quartz. The serpentine bodies are located in micaceous, amphibolitic, chloritic, talc-bearing, garnetiferous and quartzitic schists of Paleozoic age, which also enclose lenticular bodies of dolomitic limestone and actinolite. The serpentine bodies are up to 900 m long by 100 m thick, and resulted from the alteration of peridotites. The Salamanca deposit is formed by a series of lenticular bodies of various dimensions (up to 200 m long) that are located in shear zones within the serpentine. Surrounding the mineralized bodies, there is a zone with disseminated pyrrhotite that contains 0.2-0.5 % Cu. Toward the North of Salamanca thicker serpentinite bodies, which contain the La Barrera and La Luisa deposits, are found. The ore from both Salamanca and La Barrera consists primarily of pyrrhotite (50-70 %) and chalcopyrite (10-20 %), and in lesser proportion, marmatite and cobalt-pentlandite (Brodtkorb, 1971). Supergene minerals include limonite, malachite, hematite, azurite, rare native copper, cuprite and chalcosite. To the east of the Salamanca mine, a Paleozoic granodiorite crops out.

Associated with the basaltic magmatism of the upper levels of the ophiolite, Zn-Pb-Au- Ag Cyprus-type deposits were formed (Santa Elena, San Juan; Méndez et al. 1995; Zappettini and Brodtkorb, 2000).

The Santa Elena mine (Table 2) is located in the Sierra de Alcaparrosa, on the western flank of the Precordillera (31°20' South Latitude and 69°25' West Longitude). The geology of the zone consists of Precambrian leptometamorphic rocks, and Ordovician, Silurian, Devonian and Carboniferous shales, siltstones and sandstones. The sulphides are found associated with basalts that are intercalated with sedimentary rocks of the Ordovician Alcaparrosa Fm. The mineralogy of the ore consists of auriferous pyrite, marcasite, sphalerite, minor chalcopyrite, and arsenopyrite in a gangue of quartz and carbonates. The oxidation zone reaches a thickness of 25 m and consists primarily of hydrated ferric sulphates, which were the focus of exploitation.

In distal facies (slope sequences) of the Ordovician-Silurian basin, exhalative barium deposits were formed (Canota, Mendoza). The barite deposits of Canota are located in the east-central sector of the Precordillera morphostructural unit (Etcheverry et al, 1983, Brodtkorb et al. 1988, Etcheverry and Brodtkorb, 1999) (68°50' and 32°33'/36') at about 1000 m elevation (Fig. 10).

In a belt about 7 km long, various deposits are located, such as the La Victoria and Pirucha mines, the Ramoncito and Don Manuel occurrences in the NE, and the Eugenio José and Vicente occurrences in the SW. The production of La Pirucha was 30,000 t and that of La Victoria, 60,000 t, with reserves of 50-70,000 t.

The stratabound barite deposits are associated with Ordovician shales (Caradocian graptofauna) of the Villavicencio Fm. The Villavicencio Fm. is made up of gray and black shales, with subordinate layers of limestone that outcrop in a belt 4 km long and up to 100 m wide.

The barite occurs as nodules, lenses and in small disseminated crystals in the shales. The nodules have an ellipsoidal to sub-spheroidal form, and they are most commonly 15 to 20 cm long (Etcheverry and Brodtkorb, 1999). The barite is black due to its organic matter content, and its specific weight is low - between 3.97 and 4.15 - due to the significant quantity of clays that remained trapped during the diagenetic formation of the nodules and lenses. The results of chemical analyses show low levels of SrO and CaO and a negative Eu anomaly characteristic of barites of marine origin. Isotopic analysis of $^{87}Sr/^{86}Sr$ performed on various nodules gave average values of 0.70885 ± 3, indicating an origin from Ordovician seawater, while some of the crystals show values of 0.71125 ± 2 (Brodtkorb et al., 1988; Brodtkorb et al., 1990). Analyses of $\delta^{34}S$ show different compositions. One type shows a border-nucleus-border variation of 33.4‰ – 39.9‰ - 27.3‰ and the other, 39.4‰ - 61.0‰- 34.8‰. The heterogeneity of the isotopic distribution shows that the environment was changing during the formation of the nodule. Likewise, the high value of $\delta^{34}S$ suggests bacterially mediated sulphate reduction. The nodular and lentiform textures are considered to be of diagenetic origin, whereas the crystals are believed to be of late diagenetic origin (Etcheverry and Brodtkorb, 1999).

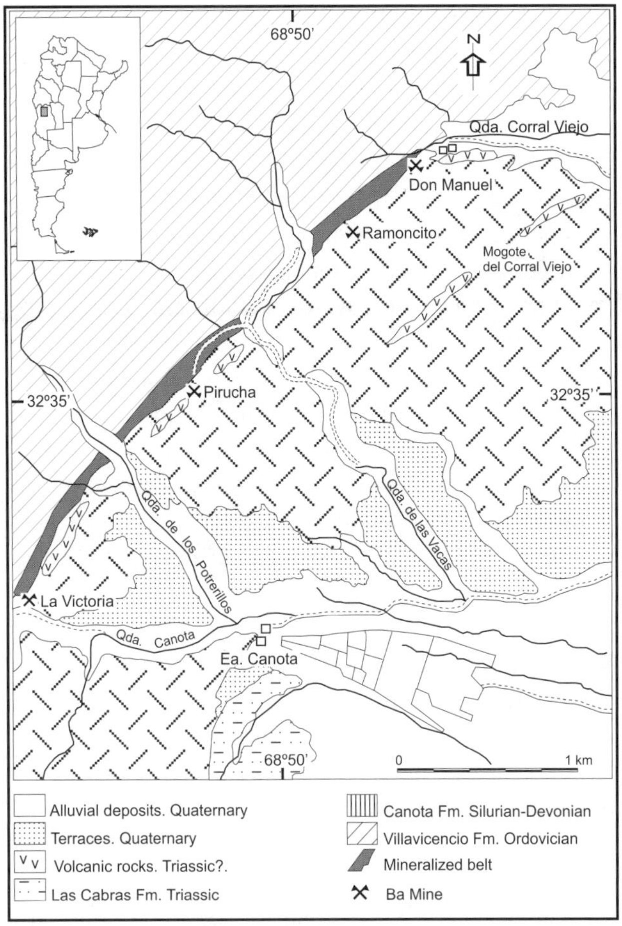

Figure 10. Geology of the Canota District, Mendoza province. Modified from Etcheverry and Brodtkorb (1999).

POS-SAG1 and POS-AMJ2 Metallogic Belts

Tectonic Evolution of the POS-SAG1 and POS-AMJ2 Metallogenic Belts

During the Upper Triassic, accompanying the opening of the Atlantic Ocean, an extensional regime developed that generated intracratonic and backarc basins along the periphery of the craton. Two Mesozoic metallogenic belts are of interest, which from N to S are: POS-SAG1 and POS-AMJ2 (Fig.1).

The POS-SAG1 belt is comprised of the Neuquén basin - an extensive sedimentary basin located between 34 and 40° south latitude (to the east of the Cordillera Principal) which was formed under an extensional regime during the Upper Triassic to Lower Jurassic. It is a sialic backarc basin that developed on Precambrian (?) - Paleozoic to Triassic basement composed of igneous, sedimentary and metamorphic rocks. Thick clastic and volcanic sequences that were deposited in a half-graben with discontinuous depocenters were deposited from the Jurassic to the Cretaceous. Sedex Ba deposits (Arroyo Nuevo, Neuquén, Fig. 11) were formed in association with sequences of Pliensbachian-Toarcian age (Brodtkorb and Etcheverry, 1994; Leanza et al., 1990).

The POS-AMJ2 metallogenic belt is associated

with an extensional backarc basin that developed during the Jurassic in the southernmost part of South America. The formation of the graben was accompanied by extensive volumes of pyroclastic rocks and the intrusion of ryolithic domes, mafic lavas and, over less extensive areas, intermediate lavas. The lowermost strata consists of the Lemaire Fm., a thick volcanic sequence that is intercalated with a sedimentary sequence, overlain by the sediment dominated Yahgán Fm. The volcanic-sedimentary sequence is Upper Triassic to Cretaceous in age (Ametrano et al., 2000). The backarc basin closed in the Upper Cretaceous-Tertiary with the development of a magmatic arc represented by granitic-syenodioritic-dioritic intrusive rocks (Ametrano et al., 2000). The present structure of the Andes of Tierra del Fuego is the result of the Andean orogeny (Cingolani, 1989).

The POS-AMJ2 metallogenic belt, which contains Kuroko-type volcanogenic deposits (mina Beatriz, Arroyo Rojo, Fin del Mundo), formed in association with silicic volcanism. The massive sulphide deposits were formed in small basins on the flanks of the rhyolite domes (Broili et al., 2000).

Geology of the Deposits

Although no VMS deposits have been found in the SAG1 metallogenic belt, the occurrence of Sedex Ba deposits and of iron and manganese formations in the Chachil Formation (Leanza et al., 1990) suggests a potential environment for Sedex deposits. In association with marine fossils of Pliensbachian-Toarcian age, and submarine lava flows that represent the beginning of marine deposition in the Neuquen basin, (de la Cruz and Suárez, 1997) Sedex Ba deposits (Arroyo Nuevo) were formed.

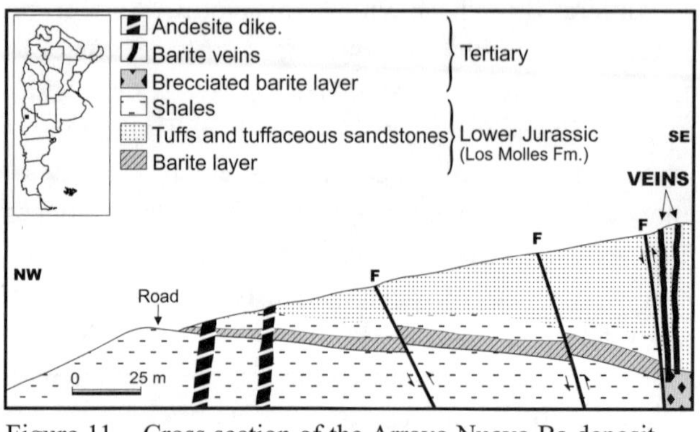

Figure 11. Cross section of the Arroyo Nuevo Ba deposit, Neuquén province.

The VMS deposits of the POS-AMJ2 metallogenic belt occur in two parallel belts striking E-W - the Cordillera Alvear to the north and the Cordillera Sorondo to the south (Broili et al., 2000). The massive sulphide deposits are hosted in Jurassic rhyolites of the Lemaire Formation (Fig. 12). The deposits consist of pyrite (pyrrhotite), sphalerite, galena, and chalcopyrite and occur massive, disseminated and as veinlets. The deposits of the Alvear Range have pyrrhotite, whereas those of the Cordillera Sorondo have only pyrite. The district has more than ten prospects. The most well known prospect is Arroyo Rojo in the Río Encajonado mineral belt. Ametrano et al. (2000) have interpreted that the Beatriz and the Arroyo Rojo deposits represent different portions of a VMS system, the former being a basal portion with a stringer area and the latter a cuspate section.

For more details on the geology of these deposits, the reader is referred to Ametrano et al., (2000) and Broili et al., (2000). The occurrence of other VMS deposits within the same belt in Chile such as Cutter Cove and La Serena (Vivallo, 2000) and the many prospects on the Argentine side encourage further exploration within this belt.

CONCLUDING REMARKS

Argentina hosts many mineral deposits and occurrences associated with submarine volcanism. In particular, the largest concentrations of metals have been correlated with major tectonic events such as the collision of the Arequipa-Antofalla craton with the Brazilian-Río de La Plata craton, and the opening of the Atlantic Ocean.

Historically, the greatest mining potential has been related to the Sedex deposits of the Ordovician basin in Northwestern Argentina (POS-PAM1 metallogenic belt). This basin continues to be one of the most interesting regions in the country for exploration from the metallogenic point of view. Further exploration could greatly increase the potential for the discovery of new Sedex deposits such as Aguilar (Pb-Zn-Ag) and La Colorada (Cu-Zn-Pb). In addition, there are thick sedimentary sequences with volcanic intercalations of Lower Paleozoic age within this metallogenic belt

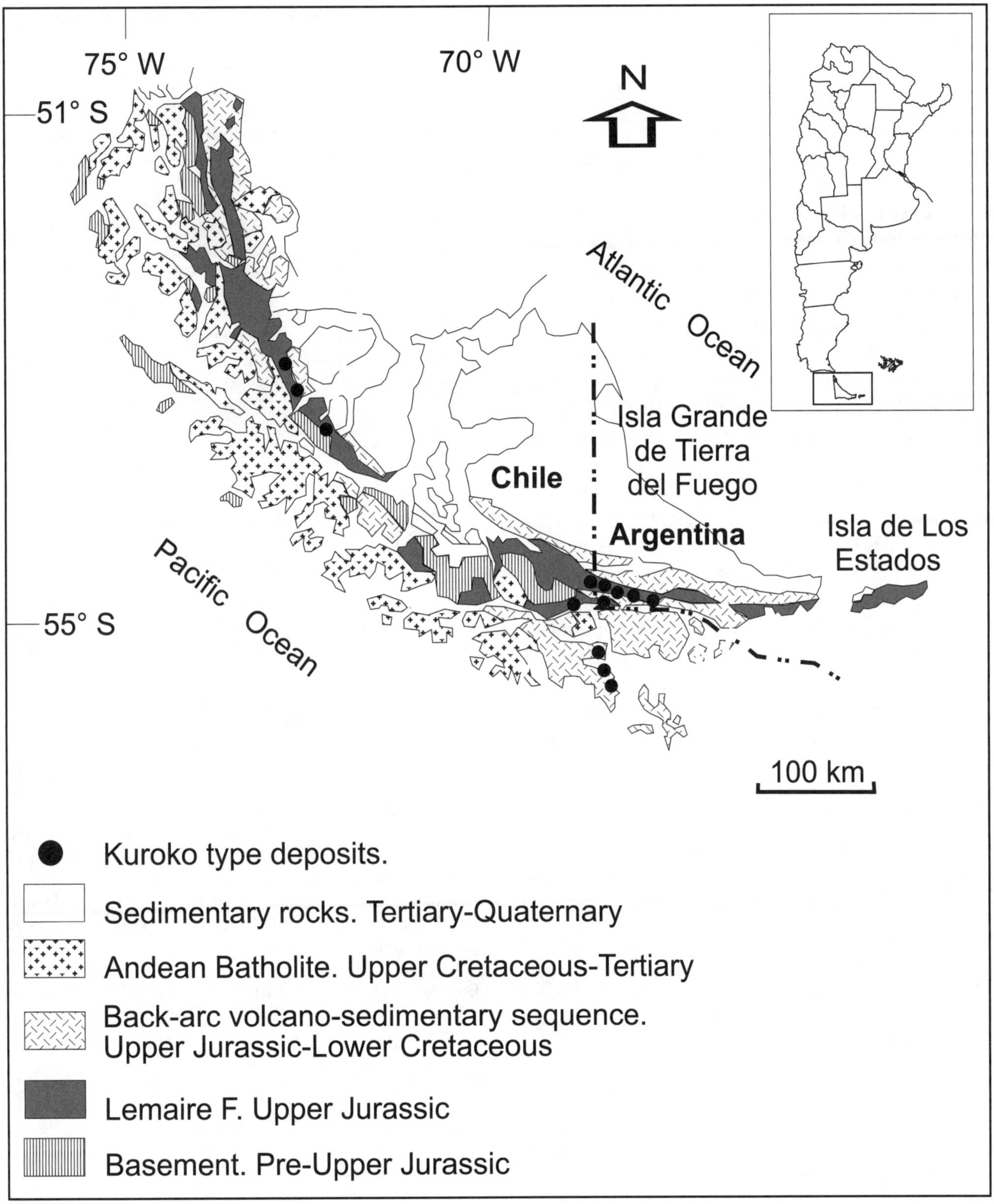

Figure 12. Geology of the Andes of Tierra del Fuego and location of Jurassic VMS deposits. Modified from Ametrano et al. (2000), after Dalziel (1981).

that cover vast surfaces in the provinces of La Rioja and San Juan. Such sequences also have a potential for hosting Sedex deposits.

The recent identificacation of the Gonzalito district in the province of Río Negro as a Sedex type deposits opened up a new regional approach for the exploration of VMS deposits in the North-Patagonian Massif.

The potential for finding economic VMS deposits in the POS-AMJ2 metallogenic belt in the southernmost part of Argentina is very high. The occurrence of similar geological environments to those in Chile that host large VMS deposits such as El Toqui and El Cobre encourages the exploration for VMS deposits in the province of Chubut (Lago La Plata, Lago Fontana).

The POS-AMJ1 and POS-SAG1 metallogenic belts that cover the provinces of Neuquén and Mendoza have a high potential to increase the SO_4Ba reserves of volcanic-exhalative origin and may have economic VMS deposits.

The PRE-PAM1 metallogenic belt is a very favourable region to find new volcanogenic tungsten deposits in the provinces of Córdoba and San Luis.

Summarizing, the diversity of tectonostratigraphic terranes in Argentina makes the country a vast region with favourable geological and tectonic settings for the development of VMS deposits. Therefore, further exploration has promising expectations to find prospects of economic interest.

ACKNOWLEDGEMENTS

The authors would like to thank Eduardo Zappettini from the Servicio Geológico Minero Argentino, Víctor Ramos from the Universidad de Buenos Aires, and Silvia Ametrano and Ricardo Etcheverry from the Universidad Nacional de La Plata for valuable discussions, Adriana González for drawing the figures and Ross Sherlock for his useful review of the manuscript.

REFERENCES

Aceñolaza, F.G. and Toselli, A.J., 1976. Consideraciones estratigráficas y tectonicas sobre el Paleozoico Inferior del Noroeste Argentino. 2° Cong. Latinoamericano de Geol. Actas 5, 2, 755-763.

Ahlfeld, F.,1955. Geologie der Blei-Zinklagerstätte Aguilar, Argentinien. Zeit. Erzb. Met., 8 (12),1-6.

Alonso, R.N., Malanca, S. and Sureda, R.J., 1982. Consideraciones sobre el Ordovícico en la Sierra de Aguilar, Jujuy, Argentina. Inst. Cien. Geol. Rev., (5), 15-37, San Salvador de Jujuy.

Ametrano, S., Etcheverry, R., Echeveste, H., Godeas, M. and Zubia, M., 2000. VMS district of Tierra del Fuego, Argentina. In R.L. Sherlock and M.A.V. Logan, (eds), Volcanogenic Massive Sulfide Deposits of Latin America. Mineral Deposit Division, Geol. Assoc. of Canada.

Ametrano, S., 1996. Los yacimientos de scheelita de la Sierra de Altautina, provincia de Córdoba. Unpub. thesis Universidad Nacional de La Plata, Argentina, p. 317. La Plata.

Ametrano, S., 1999. El distrito scheelítico de la Sierra de Altautina, provincia de Córdoba. In E.Zappettini (ed), Recursos Minerales de la república Argentina . Instituto de Geología y Recursos Minerales SEGEMAR, Anales 35, pages, Buenos Aires.

Angelelli, V., 1984. Yacimientos metalíferos de la República Argentina. Comisión de Investigaciones Científicas de la provincia de Buenos Aires, p. 704. La Plata.

Aragón, E., Dalla Salda, L. and López de Luchi, M., 1999. The metalliferous black schists from Gonzalito, Río Negro. 14° Congreso Geol. Arg. Actas 2, 279-282.

Astini, R.A., Benedetto, J.L. and Vaccari, N. E., 1996. The early Paleozoic evolution of the Argentine Precordillera as rifted, drifted and collided terrane: A geodynamic model. Geol. Soc. of America Bull., 107, 253-273.

Bahlburg, H. y F. Hervé, 1997. Geodynamic evolution and tectonostratigraphic terranes of northwestern Argentina and northern Chile. Geological Society of America, 109 (7), 869-884.

Barbieri, M., Sureda, R.J. and Argañaráz, P., 1987. Datos isotópicos preliminares $^{87}Sr/^{86}Sr$ sobre baritinas del tramo central de la provincia metalogénica Quiqueña (Paleozoico Inferior, República Argentina. 10° Cong. Geol. Arg., Simposio Procesos Metalogénicos, Serie Correlación Geológica, 3, 109-122. San Miguel de Tucumán.

Brodtkorb, M.K. de, 1971. El yacimiento Salamanca, ejemplo de depósito hidrotermal de Cu-Ni, República Argentina. 1° Cong. Ibero-Am. Geol. Econ. Madrid. A 4-1, 1001-1009.

Brodtkorb, M.K. de, Pezzutti, N. Brodtkorb, A., Schalamuk, I.B., Danderfer, J.C., and Danieli, J.C., 1992. Volcanitas de la F. Chachil en el Cerro Atravesada, prov. del Neuquén. Asoc. Geol. Arg. Rev., 47 (3), 263-264.

Brodtkorb, M. K. de and Brodtkorb, A., 1977. Stratabound scheelite deposits in the Precambrian basement of San Luis, Argentina. In Klemm and Schmider (eds), Time and stratabound ore deposits. Springer Verlag.

Brodtkorb, M. K. de and Brodtkorb, A., 1980. Especulaciones sobre un origen singenético-sedimentario de la scheelita presente en las metamorfitas del nordeste de la provincia de San Luis. 6° Cong. Geol. Arg., 3, 37-50.

Brodtkorb, M. K. and Brodtkorb, A., 1999. Yacimientos de scheelita asociados a anfibolitas y rocas calcosilicáticas, San Luis. In E. Zappettini (ed), Recursos Minerales de la República Argentina, Instituto de Geología y Recursos Minerales SEGEMAR, Anales 35, 257-269, Buenos Aires.

Brodtkorb, M.K. de and Etcheverry, R., 1994. Diferentes modelos de depósitos de baritina y celestina de la Cuenca Neuquina, Argentina. 7° Cong. Geol. Chil, 2, pp794-798.

Brodtkorb, M. K. de, Fernández, R., Pezzutti, N. and Brodtkorb, A., 1999 Yacimientos de wolframio asociados a metavolcanitas y metasedimentitas, San Luis. In: E. Zappettini (ed), Recursos Minerales de la República Argentina, Instituto de Geología y Recursos Minerales SEGEMAR, Anales 35, 323-335, Buenos Aires.

Brodtkorb., M.K. de, Lanfranco, J.J. and Sureda, R.J., 1978. Asociaciones minerales y litología del yacimiento Aguilar, provincia de Jujuy, República Argentina. Asoc. Geol. Arg. Rev., 33 (4), 277-298.

Brodtkorb, M.K. de, Pezzutti, N.E., and Brodtkorb, A., 1985. La franja con mineralización scheelítica entre el dique La Florida y Paso del Rey, provincia de San Luis. Asociación Geológica Argentina, Revista, 40(1-2), 51-59.

Brodtkorb, M.K. de, Schalamuk, I.B., Barbieri, M., Puchelt, H., Ametrano, S., Fernández, R. and Etcheverry, R., 1988. Nodular barite deposits of Canota, Argentina. Proceding 7. IAGOD Symposium, 275-286. Swiss.

Brodtkorb, M.K. de, Schalamuk, I.B., Ametrano, S., Fernández, R. and Etcheverry, R., 1990. The barite deposits of Canota, Argentina. In: Fontbote,l., Amstutz,G.C., Cardozo,M., Cedillo, E. and Frutos, J. (eds), Stratabound ore deposits in the Andes. Special publication of the Society for Geology Applied to Mineral Deposits. 8, 193-197. Springer Verlag.

Broili, C., Klohn, M. and Hodder, R.W., 2000. Exploration, geology and mineral deposits of the Fin del Mundo VMS project, Tierra del Fuego, Argentina. In R.L. Sherlock and M.A.V. Logan, (eds.), Volcanogenic Massive Sulfide Deposits of Latin America. Mineral Deposit Division, Geological Association of Canada, 567-591.

Brown, J.S., 1941. Factors of composition and porosity in lead –zinc replacements of metamorphosed limestone. Am. Inst. Min. Met., 144, 250-263.

Brown, J.S., 1962. Ore lead isotopes. Econ. Geol., 57, 673-720.

Cingolani, C., 1989. Southern South America Geotraverse; Tierra del Fuego-Diego Ramírez Islands. Intern. Geol. Cong., Abstracts. 28, 1, 1296-1297.

Coira, B., Davidson, J., Mpodozis, C. and Ramos, V., 1982. Tectonic and magmatic evolution of the Andes of northern Argentina and Chile. Earth Sci. Rev., 18, 303-332.

Criado Roque, P., Mombrú, C. and Ramos, V.A., 1981. Estructura e interpretación tectónica. Geología y recursos naturales de la provincia de San Luis. Relatorio 8° Cong. Geol. Arg., 155-192. Buenos Aires.

Cucchi, R.J., 1972. Geología y estructura de la Sierra de Cortaderas, San Juan-Mendoza, República Argentina. Asoc. Geol. Arg. Rev. 27 (2), 229-248.

Dalla Salda, L. and Aragón, E., 1994. Yacimientos polideformados de Pb, Ag y Zn; Distrito Gonzalito. 7° Congreso Geológico Chileno, 2, 786-790.

Dalla Salda, L., Aragón, E., López de Luchi, M., Benialgo, A. and Di lello, C., 1998. Gonzalito: a Zn-Pb-Ag-V-(Au) Sedex deposit in northeastern Patagonia. 10° Cong. Latinoamericano de Geol. y 6° Cong. Nac. de Geol. Econ., 3, 11. (abstract).

Dalla Salda, L., Aragón, E., López de Luchi, M., Benialgo, A. and Pezzotti, C., 1999. Geology and tectonic setting of Gonzalito mining district, Río Negro. 14° Cong. Geol. Arg., 2, 283-286.

Dalziel, I.W.D., 1981. Back-arc basin in the southern Andes: a review and critical reappraisal. Phil. Transactions of the Royal Society of London, A300, 319-335.

Dalziel, I.W.D.,1997. Neoproterozoic-Paleozoic geography and tectonics; review, hypothesis, environmental speculation. Geol. Soc. of Am. Bull.109, (1), 16-42.

De Ferran, A., 1983. Desarrollo de algunos recursos minerales de la provincia d Río Negro: Ideas y sugerencias. OEA, Unpub. report, Pcia de Río Negro.

De la Cruz, R. and Suárez,M., 1997. El Jurásico de la cuenca de Neuquén en Lonquimay, Chile; Formación Nacientes del Biobio (38°-39° S). Rev. Geol. de Chile. 24, 1, 3-24.

Delakowitz, B., 1987. Geologish-geochemisch- lagerstättenkundliche Untersuchungen zur Genese von Wolframvorkomen in der Sierra del Morro Oeste, Provinz San Luis, Argentinien. Doctoral thesis from the University of Munich, Germany, p. 199.

Delakowitz, B., Höll, R., Brodtkorb, M.K. de and Brodtkorb, A., 1991. Geología y génesis de los yacimientos de scheelita en la Sierra del Morro Oeste, provincia de San Luis. In M. K. de Brodtkorb (ed.), Geología de yacimientos de wolframio de las provincias de San Luis y Córdoba. Publicación del Instituto de Recursos Minerales. Universidad Nacional de La Plata, 1, 49-96, La Plata.

Del Mónaco, A., 1971. Geología económica de los niveles 110 y 140 de la mina Gonzalito (provincia de Río Negro). Asoc. Geol. Arg., Rev., 26, (1), 57-66.

Di Marco, A. and Mutti, D., 1992. Mina Tío en la Pcia. De Córdoba: Aspectos geoquímicos y ambiente de formación. 1° Jorn. De Min., Petrol. y Metal. De Rocas Ultrabásicas, Inst. Rec. Min., 2, 91-98, La Plata.

Di Marco, A. and Mutti, D., 1994. Los depósitos de Cu-Fe y elementos metálicos en anfibolitas de la Sierra Sur de Córdoba, Argentina. 5° Cong. Nac. De Geol. Econom., 174-180.

Etcheverry, R. and Brodtkorb, M.K. de, 1999. El distrito barítico de Canota. In Zappettini, E. (ed), Recursos Minerales de la República Argentina. Instituto de Geología y Recursos Minerales SEGEMAR, Anales 35, 730-732, Buenos Aires.

Etcheverry, R., Fernández, R., Schalamuk, I. and Brodtkorb, M.K. de, 1983. El distritto barítico de Canota, Provincia de Mendoza. 2° Cong. Nac. Geol. Econ., 2, 669-682.

Giacosa, R., 1987. Caracterización de un sector del basamento metamórfico-migmático en el extremo sudoriental del Macizo Nordpatagónico, Pcia. De Río Negro. 10° Cong. Geol. Arg., Actas 3, 51-54.

González Stegmann, E.M., 1949. Exploración "Salamanca-La Barrera", Dpto. Tupungato, pcia. de Mendoza. 1946-1948. Dirección de Fab. Mil. Buenos Aires (unpublished report).

Gordillo, C. and Lencinas, A. 1979. Sierras Pampeanas de

Córdoba y San Luis. 2° Simp. de Geol. Reg. Arg., Actas I, 577-650, Córdoba.

Hack, M., Brodtkorb, M.K. de, Höll, R. and Brodtkorb, A., 1991. Geología y consideraciones genéticas de los yacimientos scheelíticos entre el dique La Florida y Pampa del Tamboreo, provincia de San Luis. In Brodtkorb, M.K. de (ed.), Geología de wolframio de las provincias de San Luis y Córdoba, Argentina. Publicación del Instituto de Recursos Minerales, Universidad Nacional de La Plata, 1, 113-152.

Haller, J. and Ramos, V., 1984. Las ofiolitas famatinianas (Eopaleozoico) de las provincias de San Juan y Mendoza. 9° Cong. Geol. Arg., 2, 66-83. S. C. de Bariloche.

Halpern, M. and Latorre, C.O., 1973. Estudio geocronológico inicial de rocas del noroeste de la República Argentina. Asoc. Geol. Arg. Rev., 28, (2), 195-205.

Harrington, H.J. and Leanza, A.F., 1957. Ordovician trilobites of Argentina. Department of Geology, University of Kansas, Special Publication 1, p. 259.

Höll, R., 1982. Argentinien. Erkundung von Wolframlagersttätten in den Provinzen Córdoba und San Luis. Bericht der Deutschen Gesellschaft für Technische Zusammenarbeit (GTZ), p. 77.

Kay, S.M., Ramos, V.A. and Kay, R.W., 1984. Elementos mayoritarios y trazas de las vulcanitas ordovícicas de la Precordillera occidental: basaltos de rift oceánico temprano (?) próximo al margen continental. 9° Congreso Geológico Argentino, 2, 48-65. S. C. de Bariloche.

Leanza, H., Brodtkorb, M.K. de, Brodtkorb, A. and Danieli, J.C., 1990. La Formación Chachil (Liásico) y sus niveles manganesíferos en el área del Cerro Atravesada, prov. del Neuquén. Argentina. 3° Cong. Nac. de Geol. Econ., Actas, 3, 171-186. Olavarría.

Linares, E., 1968. Geología isotópica del azufre del yacimiento Aguilar, provincia de Jujuy. 3° Jorn. de Geol. Arg., Actas, 2, 191-199.

Linares, E. and Latorre, C.O., 1975. La edad del granito Aguilar, provincia de Jujuy, Argentina. 2° Cong. Ibero-Americano de Geol. Econ., 1, 91-98.

Linares, E., Ostera, H. and Párica, C., 1990. Edades radimétricas del basamento cristalino de Mina Gonzalito y Valcheta, Río Negro. 11° Cong. Geol. Arg., 2, 251-255.

Llambías, E.J. and Malvicini, L., 1982. Geología de los yacimientos de tungsteno de las Sierras del Morro, Los Morrillos y Yulto, provincia de San Luis. Asoc. Geol. Arg., Rev., 37, 100-143.

Martín, J.L., Malanca, S. and Sureda R.J., 1986. Nuevos hallazgos paleontológicos en el Ordovícico de de la Sierra de Aguilar, Jujuy, Argentina. Implicancias estratigráficas y consideraciones geológicas. 8° Cong. Geol. Bol., Bodas de Plata SGB.

Martín, J.L., Malanca, S. and Sureda, R.J., 1987. La fauna graptolítica de la Sierra de Aguilar, Jujuy, Argentina. Algunos comentarios sobre las formaciones ordovícicas. 4° Cong. Latinoamericano de Paleontología, Actas, 2, 599-619. Santa Cruz.

Méndez, V., Zanettini, J.C. and Zappettini, E.O., 1995. Geología y metalogénesis del orógeno andino central, República Argentina. Dirección Nacional del Servicio Geol. Anales 23. Buenos Aires.

Monchablón, A., 1956. Yacimientos de wolframio de la provincia de San Luis. Dirección Nacional de Geología y Minería. Buenos Aires. Unpub. report.

Mutti, D., 1992. Las rocas ultrabásicas-básicas de la Pcia. De Córdoba: interpretaciones geoquímicas e implicancias geotectónicas. I Jorn. de Min. , Petrol. y Metalog. de rocas ultrabásicas, Inst. Rec. Min., 2, 411-432, La Plata.

Nokleberg, W.J., West, T.D., Dawson, K.M., Shpikerman, V.I., Buntzen, T.K., Parfenov, L.M., Monger, J.W. H., Ratkin, V.V., Baranov, B.V., Byalovzhesky, S.G., Diggles, M.F., Eremin, R.A., Fujita, K., Gordey, S.P., Gorodinskiy, M.E., Goryachev, N.A., Feeney, T.D., Frolov, Y.F., Grantz, A., Khanchuck, A.I., Koch, R.D., Natalin, B.A., Natapov, L.M., Norton, I.O., Patton, W.W., Plafker, G., Pozdeev, A.I., Rozenblum, I.S., Scholl, D.W., Sokolov, S.D., Sosuneov, G.M., Stone, D.B., Tabor, R.W., Tsukanovy, N.V., Vallier, T.L., 1998. Summary terrane, mineral deposit and metallogenic belt maps of the Russian Far East, Alaska and the Canadian Cordillera (CD-ROM), United States Geological Survey Open-File Report 98-136.

Palma, M., 1989. La evolución tectosedimentaria durante el ciclo gondwánico en la región extraandina de la provincia de Santa Cruz. Reunión sobre Geotransectas de América del Sur, Mar del Plata, 102-105. Montevideo.

Pérez, W.A., Lencina, R. and Peralta, E.H., 1998. Sedex potential of the Ordovician basin, NW Argentina. 10° Cong. Latinoamericano de Geol. y 6° Cong. de Geol. Econ., 3, 381-386.

Quartino, B., Zardini, R.A. and Amos, A.J., 1971. Estudio y exploración geológica de la región Barreal-Calingasta. Asoc. Geol. Arg., Mon., 1, 15+, 1-184. Buenos Aires.

Ramos, V., 1975. Geología del sector oriental del macizo Nordpatagónico entre Aguada Capitán y la Mina Gonzalito, Provincia de Río Negro. Asoc. Geol Arg., Rev., 30, (3), 274-285.

Ramos, V., 1988. Late Proterozoic-Early Paleozoic of South America- a collisional History. Episodes 11, 168-174.

Ramos, V., 1992. Los ambientes tectónicos de los distritos wolframíferos de las Sas. Pampeanas. Inst. Rec. Min., 1, 185-196, La Plata.

Ramos, V., 1996. Evolución tectónica de la Plataforma Continental. In V. A. Ramos and M. A. Turic (Eds.), Geología y Recursos Naturales de la Plataforma Continental Argentina. 13° Cong. Geol. Arg. y 3° Cong. de Exploración de Hidrocarburos, Relatorio 21, 385-404, Buenos Aires.

Ramos, V., Jordan, T., Allmendinger, R., Mpodozis, C., Kay, S., Cortés, J. and Palma, M., 1986. Paleozoic terranes of the central Argentine-Chilean Andes. Tectonics, 5, 855-880.

Rapela, C.W., Coira, B., Toselli, A. and Saavedra, J., 1992. The lower paleozoic magmatism of southwestern Gondwana and the evolution of the Famatinian orogen. International Geology Review, 34, 1081-1142.

Rosenman, H.L., 1972. Geología de la región del Arroyo Los Berros (vertiente oriental de la Sierra de Somuncurá), Pcia. de Río Negro, Argentina. Asoc. Geol. Arg., Rev., 27, (1),

117-137.

Smith, W.C. and González Stegmann, E., 1947. Tungsten investigations in the Republic of Argentina, 1942-43. Bulletin of the US Geological Survey, 954-A, 2-12.

Spencer, F.N., 1950. The geology of the Aguilar lead-zinc mine, Argentine. Econ. Geol., 45 (5), 405-433. Lancaster.

Stipanicic, P. and Linares, I., 1969. Edades radimétricas determinadas para la República Argentina y su significado geológico. Acad. Nac. Ciencias, Rep. Argen.. Bol. 47, (1), 51-96.

Suárez, M. and de la Cruz, R., 1997. Volcanismo pliniano del Lias durante los inicios de la cuenca de Neuquén, Cordillera del Viento, Neuquén, Argentina. 8° Cong. Geol. Chileno, 1, 266-270.

Sureda, R.J., 1999. Los yacimientos Sedex de plomo y zinc en la sierra de Aguilar, Jujuy. In E. Zappettini, (ed), Recursos Minerales de la República Argentina, Instituto de Geología y Recursos Minerales SEGEMAR, Anales 35, 459-485, Buenos Aires.

Sureda, R.J. and Amstutz, G.C., 1981. Neue Untersuchungen über die schichgebundenen Pb-Zn-Lagerstätten in der Sierra de Aguilar Provinz Jujuy, Argentinien. Zbl. Geol. Paläont., 1 (3/4): 494-504. Stuttgart.

Sureda, R.J. and Martín, J.L., 1990a. El Aguilar mine: an Ordovician sediment-hosted stratiform lead-zinc deposit in the Central Andes. In Fontbote, L. et al. (ed), Stratabound deposits in the Andes, Springer Verlag, Special Publication, 8, 161-174.

Sureda, R.J. and Martín, J.L., 1990b. Mina El Aguilar, provincia de Jujuy, Rep. Argentina. Un depósito SEDEX ordovícico, con metamorfismo de contacto sobreimpuesto, en la provincia metalogénica quiaqueña. Contribuciones al conocimiento de la mineralogía y geología económica de la República Argentina. Asociación Argentina de Geólogos Economistas, Publicación Especial. Homenaje al prof. Ing. Victorio Angelelli, Buenos Aires, 78-91.

Vallés, J., 1978. Los yacimientos minerales ubicados al oeste de la Mina Gonzalito, Departamento San Antonio y Valcheta, Río Negro. Asoc. Geol. Arg., Rev., 33, (4), 325-334.

Varela, R., Cingolani, C., Sato, A., Dalla Salda, L., Brito Neves, B.B., Basei, M., Siga, O. and Teixeira, W., 1997. Proterozoic and Paleozoic evolution of Atlantic area of North-Patagonian Massif, Argentine. South American Symposium on Isotope Geology, Brazil, 326-328.

ssVillar, L.M., 1969. El complejo ultrabásico de Novillo Muerto, Cordillera Frontal, provincia de Mendoza, Rep. Argentina. Asoc. Geol. Arg., Rev., 24, (3), 223-238. Buenos Aires.

Villar, L.M., 1970. Petrogénesis del complejo ultrabásico de Novillo Muerto, Cordillera Frontal, Mendoza. Rep. Argentina. Asoc. Geol. Arg. Rev. 25, 1, 87-89. Buenos Aires.

Villar, L.M., 1998. Los gabros de fondo oceánico de la ofiolita de Cordillera Frontal de Mendoza, Argentina. 10° Cong. Latinoamericano de Geol. y 6° Cong. Nac. de Geol. Econ., 2, 405-410.

Villar, L.M., Donnari, E. and Meyer, H., 1982. Reconsideraciones geológicas sobre el complejo ultrabásico de Novillo Muerto y su mineralización asociada, Cordillera Frontal, Mendoza, Argentina. 5° Cong. Latinoamericano de Geol., 2, 173-184. Buenos Aires.

Vivallo,W., 2000. Los depósitos de sulfuros macizos de origen volcánico-exhalativo en Chile. In R.L. Sherlock and M.A.V. Logan, (eds.), Volcanogenic Massive Sulfide Deposits of Latin America. Mineral Deposit Division, Geological Association of Canada.

Zappettini, E. (ed)., 1999. Mapa metalogenético de la República Argentina (Versión preliminar). Instituto de Geología y Recursos Minerales (SEGEMAR), Anales 32/D.

Zappettini, E. (ed)., 1999b. Recursos Minerales de la República Argentina. Instituto de Geología y Recursos Minerales SEGEMAR, Anales 35, Buenos Aires.

Zappettini, E.O. and Brodtkorb, M.K. de, 2000. The VMS Santa Elena deposit, San Juan province, Argentina. In Volcanogenic Massive Sulfide Deposits of Latin America, R.L. Sherlock and M.A.V. Logan, eds. Mineral Deposit Division, Geol. Assoc. of Canada.

Zardini, R. A., 1958. Serpentinitas del Río Las Tunas, Cuchilla de Yalguaraz, Mendoza. Asoc. Geol. Arg., Rev. 13, (1-2), 67-86. Buenos Aires.

Zardini, R.A., 1960a. Serpentinitas de la Mina "La Mendocina". Uspallata-Mendoza. Asoc. Geol. Arg., Rev., 15,(1-2), 43-51. Buenos Aires.

Zardini, R. A., 1960b. Esquisto talco-actinolítico en la mina "Sol de Mayo", Mendoza. Asoc. Geol. Arg., Rev., 15, (3-4), 181-189. Buenos Aires.

Zubia, M., 1976. Informe preliminar Proyecto 15 BD-Area 13 A, Mosaico 4166IV-BI. Dirección Nacional de Geología y Minería. Unpub. report, 12 p. Buenos Aires.

EXPLORATION, GEOLOGY, AND MINERAL DEPOSITS OF THE FIN DEL MUNDO VMS PROJECT, TIERRA DEL FUEGO, ARGENTINA

CHRIS BROILI
Consulting Geologist, 2622 E. Snead, Spokane, WA 99223 U.S.A.

MEL KLOHN
Yamana Resources Inc., 9 N Post St., Suite 555, Spokane, WA 99201 U.S.A.

ROBERT W. HODDER
20 Mayfair Drive, London, Ontario N6A 2M6 CANADA

ABSTRACT

The Fin Del Mundo project, located at the southernmost end of South America in the Cordillera Fueguina of Tierra Del Fuego, Argentina, is a newly recognized polymetallic volcanogenic massive sulphide (VMS) district, the southernmost such district known in the world. Work by several companies, including Yamana, Noranda and Westmin, have outlined two mineralized belts within parallel east-west trending mountain ranges, the Alvear Range on the north and the Sorondo Range on the south.

Sulphide occurrences are hosted by Jurassic aged rhyolitic volcanic rocks of the Lemaire/Alvear sequence. Within the most explored part of the district, the Sorondo Range, this sequence is comprised of a thick section of shale overlain by an equivalent thickness of mafic and silicic volcanic flows and domes with volcaniclastics. These rocks have been folded and thrusted toward the north-northeast, and metamorphosed to a greenschist facies.

Massive sulphide accumulations formed syngenetically in small basins upon and along the flanks of rhyolite domes. The sulphides are predominantly pyrite in the Sorondo Range and pyrite-pyrrhotite in the Alvear range. Base and precious metals occur within sphalerite, galena and chalcopyrite as massive, disseminated, and stringer sulphide zones. The sulphide minerals have been ductily deformed during subsequent folding, thrusting and metamorphism of the host rocks.

The geology, alteration, and sulphide concentrations are similar in many respects to the well-known Kuroko type VMS deposits, with some similarities to the Noranda polymetallic VMS district in Quebec, the Bathurst District of New Brunswick, the Mount Read Volcanics of west Tasmania, and to the Iberian Pyrite Belt of Portugal and Spain.

Reconnaissance in the Cordillera Fueguina of Tierra del Fuego island, from the Chilean border to its eastern tip, has determined the most promising area lies in its western third. Reconnaissance work consists of regional stream sediment geochemical sampling, mapping, and an extensive airborne geophysical survey.

Detailed exploration has focused primarily upon the Rio Encajonado mineral belt in the Sorondo Range, between the Sargent and Gregores prospects. The most explored occurrence, Arroyo Rojo, has several generations of detailed geologic mapping, sampling, ground geophysics, and seven drill holes. These data suggest a VMS target remains at Arroyo Rojo. Drilling at two of the other showings was inconclusive in one case and negative in the other. There are many other prospects, including Gregores and Rio Hambre, which have favorable exploration potential, and numerous geophysical and geochemical anomalies have yet to be evaluated.

INTRODUCTION

The Fin del Mundo polymetallic VMS Project is located in the southernmost Andes at 55 degrees south latitude on the south coast of the island of Tierra del Fuego, Argentina (Fig. 1). The closest town, Ushuaia, population 40,000, is a busy deep-water port on the Beagle Channel and terminus of Route 3, Argentina's major north-south highway. Known as the southernmost city in the world, Ushuaia is serviced by a major natural gas pipeline and a new, modern airport that provides daily jet service to Buenos Aires and other destinations. With a climate very similar to coastal British Columbia and southeast Alaska, the region has become a popular tourist destination, offering winter skiing, proximity to Tierra del Fuego National Park (northwest of Ushuaia, adjacent to the Chilean border), and an embarkation point for tours to Antarctica.

Favorable host rocks for massive sulphide deposits are within the Cordillera Fueguina along the north side of the Beagle Channel, a few kilometres northeast of Ushuaia. This Cordillera consists of two mountain ranges, 60 km wide by 300 km long, trending east-southeast to west-northwest. These ranges are separated by Tierra Major Valley, a wide U-shaped glaciated valley traversed in part by Route 3 (Fig. 2). The Sorondo Range, in the south, contains the Rio Encajonado mineral belt and the Alvear Range, in the north, hosts the Rio Hambre mineral belt (Fig. 3). Mount Alvear in the Alvear Range is the highest peak at 1,490 m above sea level.

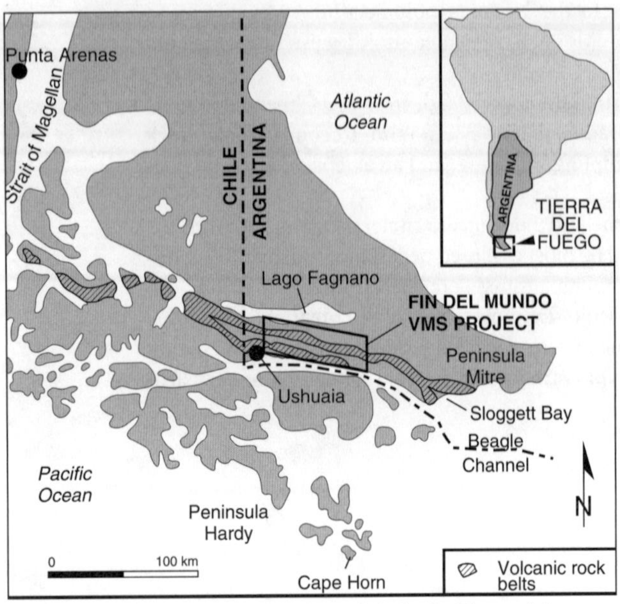

Figure 1. Location of volcanic rock belts in Tierra del Fuego, Argentina and Chile.

At lower elevations, the region is covered by dense deciduous forests, but above 600 m the landscape is mostly bare rock, with glacially scoured mountain scarps and serrate ridges. Small glaciers persist in cirques on south facing valley headwalls of several higher peaks. Although the Rio Encajonado mineral belt is close to tidewater and only eight kilometres from Ushuaia, the massive sulphide occurrences are difficult to reach.

EXPLORATION

Early activity includes some exploitation of pyrite by the original indigenous people of the area (Bridges, 1948) and mining of beach sand for gold near Sloggett Bay (Fig. 1). The first recognized massive sulphide in the region was the Beatriz mine, one bay west of Ushuaia within Tierra del Fuego National Park. At the Beatriz prospect, a 30 m long adit explores a small lens of polymetallic sulphides (Zubia et. al., 1989). Host rocks are sandstones and shales intercalated with felsic volcanics. Specimens found on the dump of the now-caved workings consist of massive to semi-massive, coarse-grained pyrite, marcasite, chalcopyrite, galena, and sphalerite in cherty gangue.

The region's mining and exploration activity is summarized in Table1. Minera Aguilar first recognized the economic significance of polymetallic massive sulphide occurrences in the Rio Encajonado belt in the 1970s during regional reconnaissance exploration for base metals. Subsequent regional mapping in the Sorondo Range noted several extensive colour anomalies and gossan zones in a belt of sericitic felsic volcanic rocks of the Jurassic-age "Alvear Formation." Regional rock and stream silt sampling identified several significant copper, lead, and zinc anomalies hosted by these volcanic rocks.

Follow up work in 1980 discovered a small nunatak containing a lens of polymetallic massive sulphides exposed near the flank of a headwall glacier perched in a hanging valley near the source of the west branch of Rio Encajonado. Minera Aguilar followed up with ground geophysical surveys and identified two strong Turam, SP, and IP anomalies. The exploration program was terminated soon afterward, and this pioneering massive sulphide discovery – later named "Arroyo Rojo"– remained largely neglected until its "rediscovery" by Polimet/Yamana (Fig. 3).

Early in 1994, Compania Minera Polimet, a subsidiary of Yamana Resources Inc., investigated reports of geology with sulphide occurrences in the Fin del Mundo region which sounded akin to polymetallic volcanogenic massive sulphide (VMS) deposits. Polimet applied for cateos (exploration claims) covering approximately 100,000 hectares in the Sorondo and Alvear Ranges, and initiated reconnaissance prospecting and mapping. Geologists found the headwall glacier at the Arroyo Rojo massive sulphide occurrence had progressively retreated in the 14 years since the original discovery and many large new outcrops were now visible. A conspicuous large colour anomaly marked a belt of felsic volcanic rocks and within this belt were several important new showings of massive sulphides.

The subsequent exploration history of the VMS district is somewhat checkered. Yamana consummated joint venture agreements first with Noranda Mining and Exploration and later with Westmin Resources Ltd. Both companies, experienced in evaluating VMS systems, dropped their earn-in interest despite what the authors interpret as encouraging results. All this work is summarized in Table 1.

Yamana's first partner labored for one and a half field seasons during 1995 and 1996. They recognized seven new prospects including Rio Hambre, Rio Cafe and Gregores (Fig. 3). During the latter part of the 1996 field season, after the joint venture agreement was terminated, Yamana discovered another new

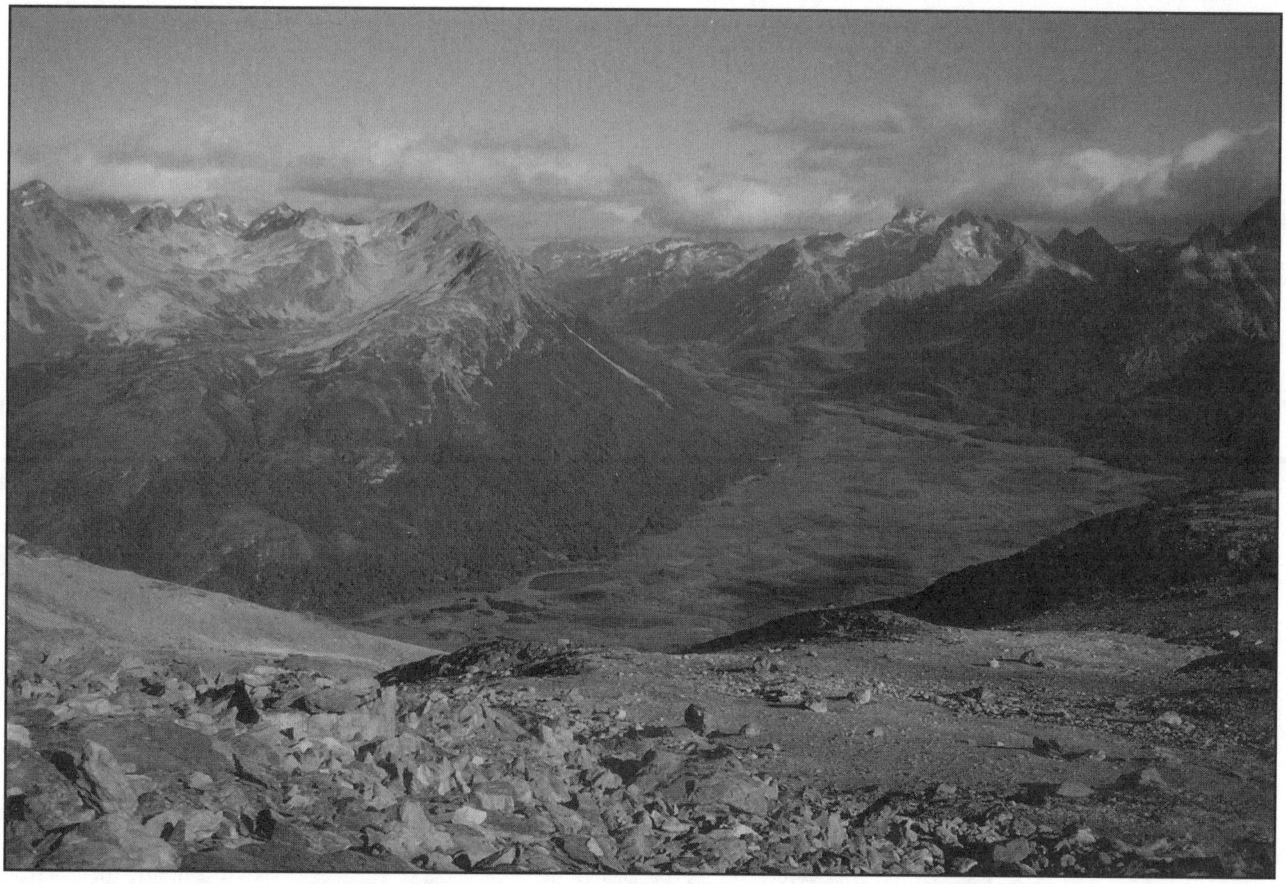

Figure 2. Photo looking west from Sargent prospect, Fin del Mundo project, Tierra del Fuego, Argentina. Tierra Major Valley in centre, flanked by the Alvear Range on the right (north) and the Sorondo Range on the left (south).

sulphide occurrence, Sargent, while giving tours to prospective new partners. Yamana's second partner worked for one field season during 1997. They recognized several new banded sulphide occurrences, including Lago Guanaco, Cerro Portillo, Xerxes, and Desolado (Fig. 3). In addition 18 diamond core holes were drilled on three of the prospects. After this second partner also terminated their interest, Yamana continued a limited field program during the 1998 field season.

REGIONAL GEOLOGY

The metamorphic basement of Tierra del Fuego is a collage of cratonic blocks accreted together during the Paleozoic construction of supercontinent Gondwanaland (Dalziel et. al., 1987; Ramos, 1988). In late Triassic time the South Atlantic Ocean began to open and southern South America broke along several grabens. Voluminous outpourings of felsic pyroclastic rocks, intrusion of felsic domes, mafic lavas, and lesser lavas of intermediate composition accompanied extension and graben development throughout the Jurassic. Along the present site of the Beagle Channel these rocks are submarine in origin and are hosts to the polymetallic VMS deposits of the Rio Encajonado and Rio Hambre belts. To the north and east, within the continent, these same rocks, minus the chemical sediment, are subaerial and constitute the volcanic massifs of central Patagonia where they are hosts to low sulfidation epithermal precious metals deposits.

Stratigraphy

The base of the layered rock sequence, the Lapataia Formation, is exposed in the Sorondo Range and consists of phyllite, schist and gneiss in the amphibolite facies of regional metamorphism. These rocks are exposed at tidewater in Bahia Lapataia where the border of Argentina and Chile intersects the

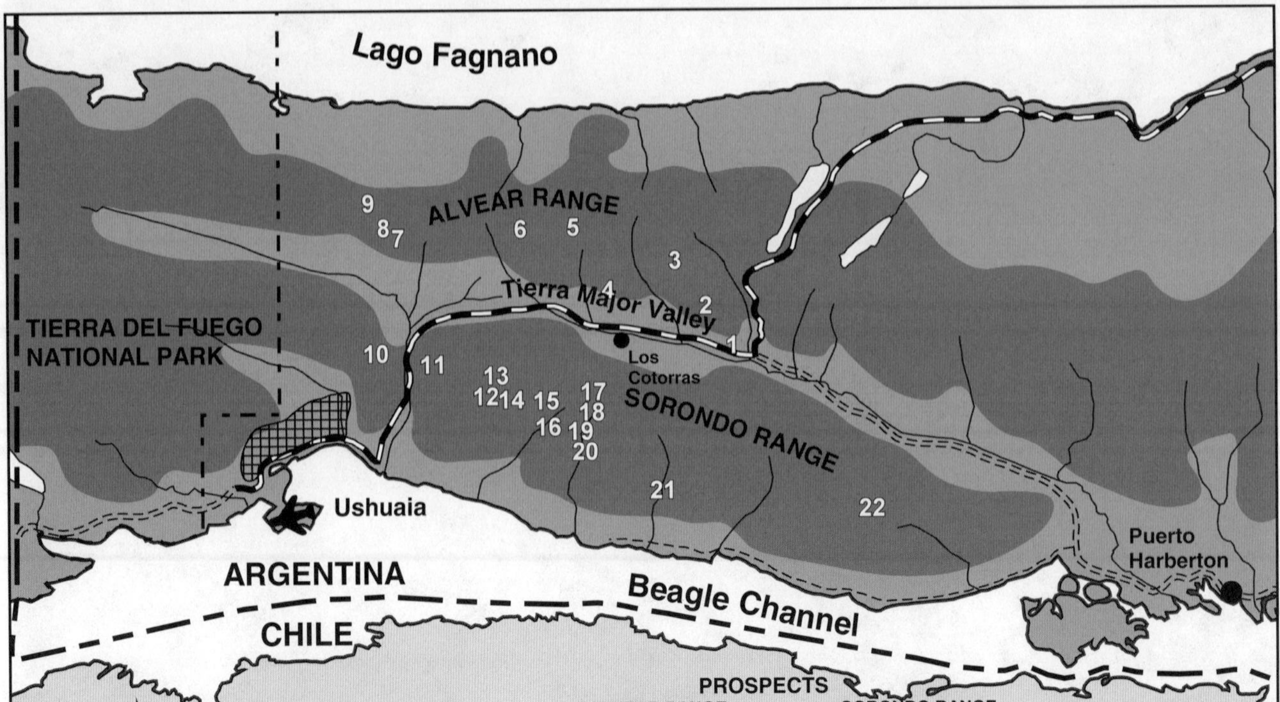

Figure 3. Location of prospects on the Fin del Mundo project, Tierra del Fuego, Argentina.

Beagle Channel (Fig. 3). The Lapataia Formation is considered to be upper Paleozoic to lower Mesozoic in age, based on correlation with isotopically dated rocks of comparable composition exposed farther north. Additionally, rocks of the Lapataia Formation have both foliation and folds that are broken by a cleavage that is deemed main-phase Andean orogeny (Bruhn, 1979, Ametrano et al., this volume).

The Lapataia Formation is unconformably overlain along the Beagle Channel by a thick sequence of subaqueous siliciclastic and pyroclastic rocks and lava flows in the greenschist facies of

Table 1. Mining and exploration history summary.

Year	Operator	Location	Work & Results
< 1800	Yahgan & Alacaloof natives	Beatriz & an island in the Strait of Magellan	mined pyrite for starting fires
1890's	Julius Popper	Sloggett Bay	large dredge mined gold from beach sand; recovered approx. 20,000 oz. gold
1950's	unknown	Beatriz mine	tunnel driven searching for base metals in a massive sulfide
1970's	Minera Aguilar	Sorondo Range	regional mapping and stream sediment geochemistry
1980's	Minera Aguilar	Rio Encajonado	discovered part of Arroyo Rojo showing on a nunatak; followed with SP, IP & Turam surveys; strong anomaly reported
1994	Minera Polimet	Arroyo Rojo	discovered main VMS showing, followed with sampling & mapping
1994	Minera Polimet	Sorondo & Alvear Ranges	reconnoitered region, identified favorable rock float at Rio Hambre & at base of the NW flank of Mt Olivia; acquired land
1995	Noranda	Sorondo & Alvear Ranges	reconnoitered region, geological mapping, stream sed. sampling; discovered 6 new targets including Rio Hambre
1995	Noranda	Arroyo Rojo	sawed channel samples, re-mapped geology; ground geo physics identified weak Max-Min EM anomaly
1995	Noranda	Rio Hambre	discovered, sampled & mapped geology; identified ground geophysical anomaly
1996	Noranda	Sorondo & Alvear Ranges	regional recon. & stream-sed sampling; discovered Gregores showing; completed 2200 line-km airborne helicopter EM survey at 250 m spacing; identified 21 first-order, 60 second-order, & 25 third-order anomalies
1996	Yamana	Sorondo & Alvear Ranges	regional recon. & pan concentrate sampling; discovered Sargent showing
1996	Yamana	Harberton to Peninsula Mitre	regional recon. stream sed. & pan concentrate sampling; area was gold enriched but geology unfavorable for VMS
1997	Westmin	Sorondo & Alvear Ranges	regional recon. & stream sed. sampling; airborne anomalies reclassified & followed up; discovered several new sulfide prospects including Lago Guanaco
1997	Westmin	Sorondo Range	detailed mapping; deciphered stratigraphy, lithofacies & structure
1997	Westmin	Arroyo Rojo, Sargent & Lago Guanco	drilled 18 core holes: Arroyo Rojo (7 holes, 1,585 m), Sargent (8 holes, 1,398 m), Lago Guanaco (3 holes, 507 m)
1998	Yamana	Arroyo Rojo	re-evaluated drill results, found non-assayed core with 3% Zn at bottom of AR-7; recovered additional pcs. of lost AR-1 core with up to 21.4 % Pb, 10.8 % Zn, and 95.4 g/t Ag

regional metamorphism. These rocks, the Serie Tobifera, grade into compositionally and temporally similar, but subaerial, volcanic products northward across Tierra del Fuego and into Patagonia. The region's explorationists have referred to the sequence of volcanic rocks and enclosing marine clastic sedimentary rocks of the Sorondo and Alvear Ranges collectively as the Alvear Formation, although the felsic volcanic rocks that are most abundant toward the base of the section are also separately known as the Lemaire Formation (Borrello, 1972; Caminos et. al., 1981). In this report, this will be referred to as the Lemaire/Alvear sequence.

The Lemaire/Alvear sequence is upper Jurassic in age, based on a few isotopic age determinations and stratigraphic relationships. In the Sorondo Range, specifically in the Rio Encajonado mineral belt, the sequence is up to 5,500 m thick and consists of five mappable entities (Fig. 4). From base to top these are: 1) shale, 3,000 m; 2) lower basaltic andesite hyaloclastite flows and sills, 500 m; 3) volcaniclastic resedimented rhyolite and epiclastic rocks, 500 m; 4) massive to brecciated rhyolite in domes, mounds, and lobe flows, 1,000 m; and 5) uppermost andesite hyaloclastite, 200 to 500 m. The polymetallic VMS occurrences of the Rio Encajonado and Rio Hambre belts cluster on and about massive to brecciated rhyolite domes, mounds, and lobe flows within the massive rhyolite (unit 4).

Subaqueous clastic sedimentary rocks and volcanic rocks of the Lemaire/Alvear sequence are overlain by and are provenance for shale and greywacke of the Cretaceous Yahgan Formation. The Yahgan clastic rocks, which accumulated in a marginal basin, are in turn locally intruded and succeeded by rocks of the Tortuga ophiolite complex of upper Jurassic to lower Cretaceous age (Dalziel et. al., 1974). These rocks reflect the maximum extension along rifts in the marginal basin.

All of the aforementioned rocks are intruded by Cretaceous to Tertiary calc-alkaline plutons of the Patagonian batholith, the south tip of the Andean Cordillera. For the most part, these intrusions crop out on islands south of the Beagle Channel and only sparingly in the Sorondo and Alvear ranges. The stratigraphic section is topped by the Cretaceous to Tertiary-age Hardy Formation, comprised of coarse clastic rocks and mafic lavas which flank plutons and grade downward and laterally into greywacke of the Yahgan Formation.

Structure

Observable structure in the region is mostly attributed to the Andean orogeny. It can be both intense and complex (Bruhn, 1979). Through-going regional structure, dominated by northwest-striking thrusts, normal faults, folds, and cleavage, appears to be contemporaneous and parallel to the original long axis of the marginal basin. The structure developed as part of a north-northeast to south-southwest compressional regime, with horizontal shortening directed toward the continent. The felsic volcanic section appears to

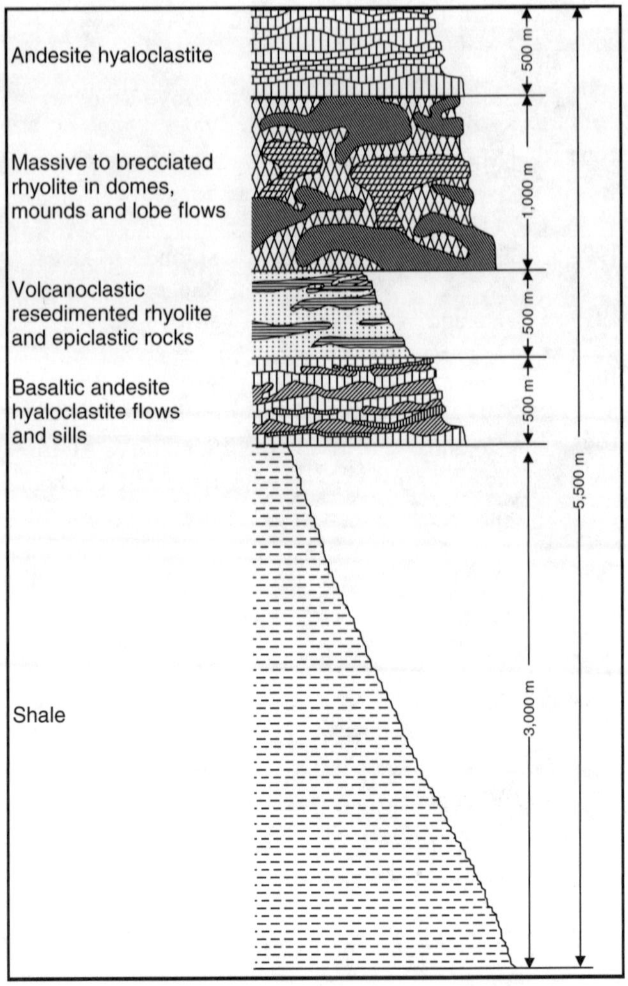

Figure 4. Generalized stratigraphy of the Lemaire/Alvear sequence in the Sorondo Range.

have undergone total shortening on the order of 100 percent in northward verging thrusts and folds (Gibson, 1997).

Exact location of thrust faults is problematic, and correlation of rock sequences across faults is difficult, suggesting large offsets. In the Sorondo Range sedimentary rocks of the younger Yahgan Formation have been mapped as thrust over older volcanic rocks of the Lemaire/Alvear sequence, a structural relationship which implies that the entire section along this contact could be overturned (Lencinas, 1994; Hodder and Terry, 1997). It is also suggested that Tierra Major Valley follows the strike of a major thrust that separates the Sorondo and Alvear ranges and repeats the same stratigraphic sequence in these two ranges (Darch, 1995; Lencinas, 1996; Ametrano et. al., this volume) (Fig. 5).

Folding in the Yahgan Formation is disharmonic with respect to folding in the underlying Lemaire/Alvear sequence (Bruhn, 1979). In general, folds in Yahgan Formation shale and greywacke are tighter, more common, more continuous, and much more conspicuous as compared to those of the Lemaire/Alvear volcanic rocks. In the Sorondo Range, bedding in sedimentary rocks is transposed by slaty cleavage. In the Alvear Range, however, bedding and slaty cleavage both dip south and are essentially parallel. Volcanic rocks are commonly schistose and have aligned chlorite and white mica.

Late penetrative foliation dominates in volcanic rocks of the Lemaire/Alvear sequence. Slaty cleavage crosses contacts between rock types, although at a regional scale it parallels primary layering and major thrusts. Original bedding, difficult to see because of subsequent folding and deformation, is best preserved in shale and mudstone, but it can also be seen in epiclastic rocks, rhyolitic flows, and as flow banding in some of the more massive rhyolites. Mapping indicates that the region's massive sulphide accumulations are along original bedding and layering, not along the later cleavage.

In the Sorondo Range, some overturned anticlines within the Lemaire/Alvear sequence have cores of massive and brecciated rhyolite. The principal massive sulphide occurrences are associated with five rhyolite domes aligned in anticlines along a ten-kilometre belt extending from Sargent to Gregores. This belt strikes west-northwest with an axial plane cleavage inclined 60 degrees to the southwest. Rhyolite domes are interpreted as forming along a prominent rift in a marginal basin. This structural style is comparable to the west side of the Noranda polymetallic VMS district in Quebec where lenses of massive sulphide are within an eight-kilometre long alignment of rhyolite domes. Along this trend, the Millenbach, Amulet, Old Waite, Norbec, and Vauze mines are at approximately the same stratigraphic level, occurring either in topographic depressions upon the domes or in small basins on flanks or between domes (Hodder and Terry, 1997).

GEOLOGY OF THE MINERAL BELTS

In the Rio Encajonado and Rio Hambre belts, VMS prospects are mainly restricted to two principal volcano-sedimentary sequences: 1) on and about rhyolite domes, which probably are along a rifted edge of the marginal basin into which the Lemaire/Alvear sequence was deposited; and 2) strata-bound within volcaniclastic rocks of the Lemaire/Alvear sequence, above basaltic andesite flows and sills but below the horizon of rhyolite domes.

Lithofacies

The Lemaire/Alvear sequence has been most thoroughly mapped in the central part of the Rio Encajonado belt from the Sargent prospect to the Gregores prospect (Fig. 6). The sequence is approximately 50 percent shale, 20 percent basaltic andesite flows, sills, and hyaloclastite, and 30 percent felsic volcanic rocks. Shale is variable in composition and can be subdivided into a northerly siliceous component in the Alvear Range and a southerly more carbonaceous component in the Sorondo Range. The shales probably represent first-order extensional basin fill upon and through which the volcanic rocks were deposited. Flows of basaltic andesite are locally pillowed and commonly amygdaloidal. Hyaloclastite is commonly resedimented. Major definable lithofacies in felsic volcanic rocks are massive rhyolite, rhyolite breccia, and volcaniclastic resedimented rhyolite, all described in more detail below. Epiclastic rocks, the products of deposition in small basins, are intercalated throughout the section. These rocks are moderately well sorted, with polymictic clasts of rhyolite, basaltic andesite, and shale. Clasts retain much of their original textures that, together with the presence of ubiquitous chert representing submarine chemical sediment, are evidence of sub-marine deposition.

The three major lithofacies of the felsic volcanic section are as follows:

1) Massive rhyolite facies – represents original extrusive lava or hypabyssal intrusive rock. It is in large part non-foliated, locally with strong colour banding. It typically contains several percent fine-grained disseminated sulphide minerals, resulting in rusty-orange surfaces on joints and fractures. It is aphyric to porphyritic with quartz eyes and feldspar phenocrysts.
2) Rhyolite breccia facies – largely autoclastic in origin and commonly occurring marginal to massive rhyolite domes. It contains monomictic rhyolite clasts of variable size with jigsaw texture or variable degrees of comminution.
3) Resedimented volcaniclastic rhyolite facies – mainly a crystal-rich sandstone with variable amounts and sizes of lithic and pumiceous fragments. It contains slightly sorted rhyolite clasts, many of which are foliated.

Mineralization and alteration

The majority, and most extensively explored, base metal massive sulphide occurrences are in the Rio Encajonado belt, with fewer and less explored occurrences within the Rio Hambre belt. The occurrences are closely associated with domes of massive to brecciated rhyolite lithofacies of the Lemaire/Alvear sequence and are interpreted to be sulphide concentrations formed in structural depressions upon and flanking the domes (Fig. 7). Examples of three important sites of massive sulphide concentration are as follows:

1) Arroyo Rojo-Lago Guanaco – lenses and clasts of massive sulphide in a depression, or puddle, upon a rhyolite dome complex. This is overlain by rhyolite breccia and hyaloclastite. Footwall rhyolite is veined with quartz and sulphide minerals.
2) Sargent – sulphide minerals, dispersed in layers and massive in clasts, are concentrated within a small basin on the edge of a large composite rhyolite dome that transgresses and lobes over shale.

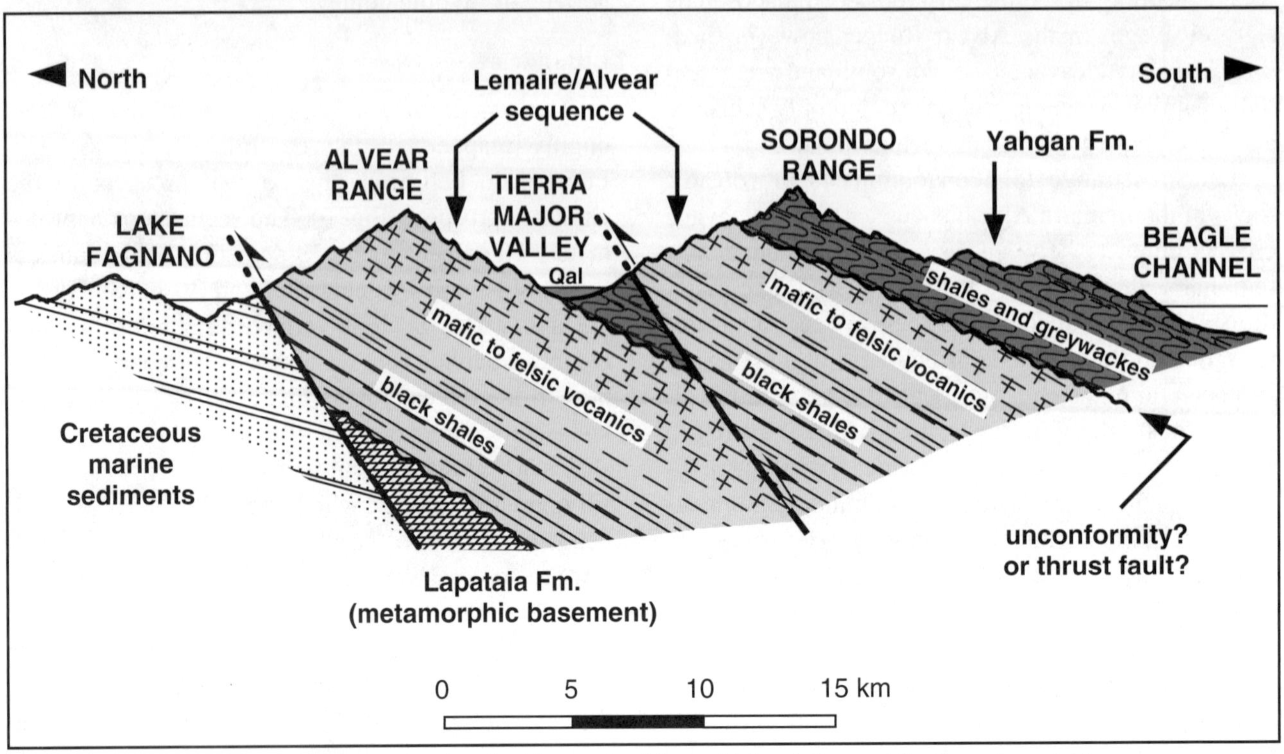

Figure 5. Diagrammatic regional cross-section (looking east) of Tierra Major Valley and the Sorondo and Alvear.

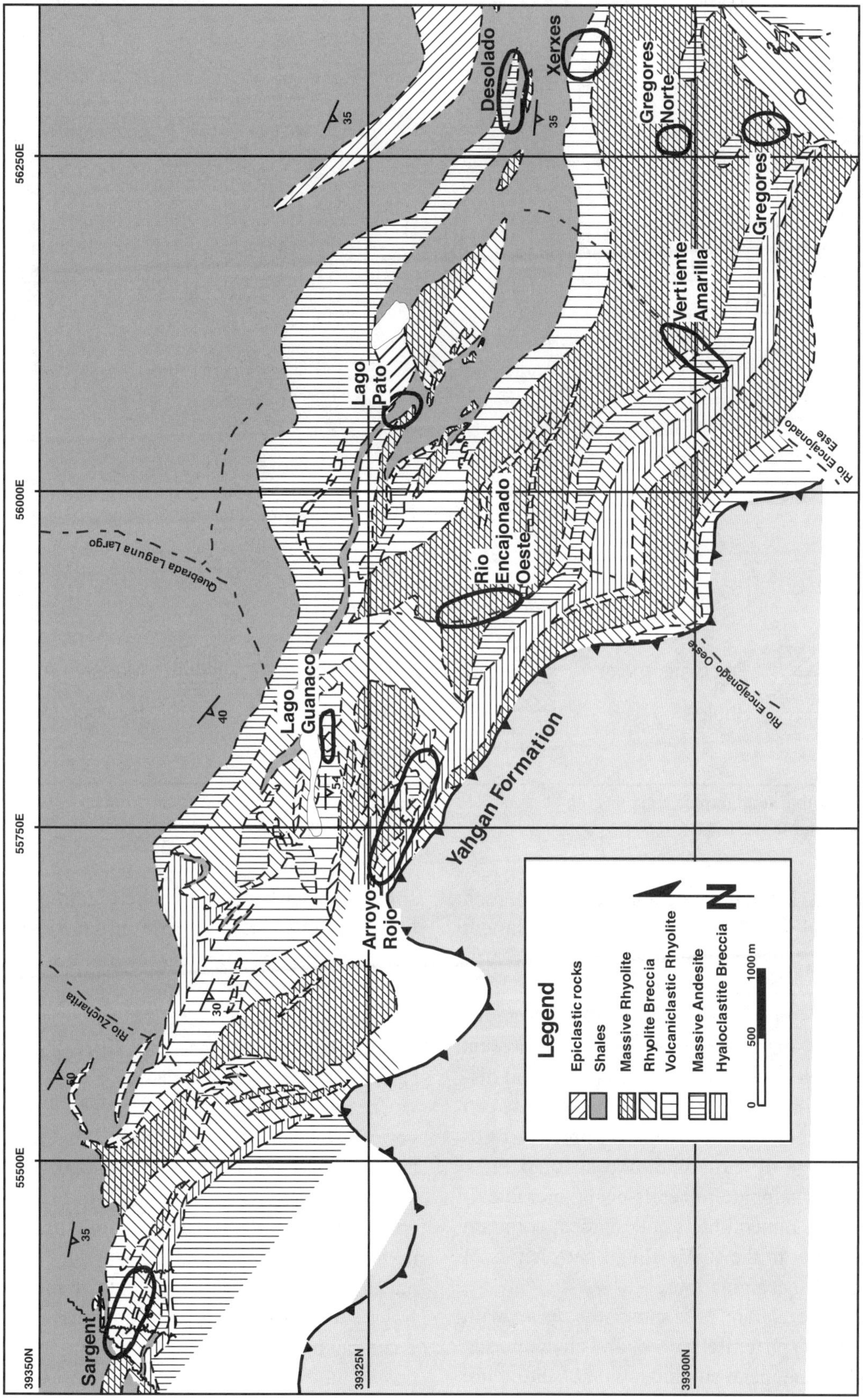

Figure 6. Regional geology and lithofacies interpretation of the central Rio Encajonado mineral belt, Sorondo Range (after D.A. Terry and R.W. Hodder, 1997).

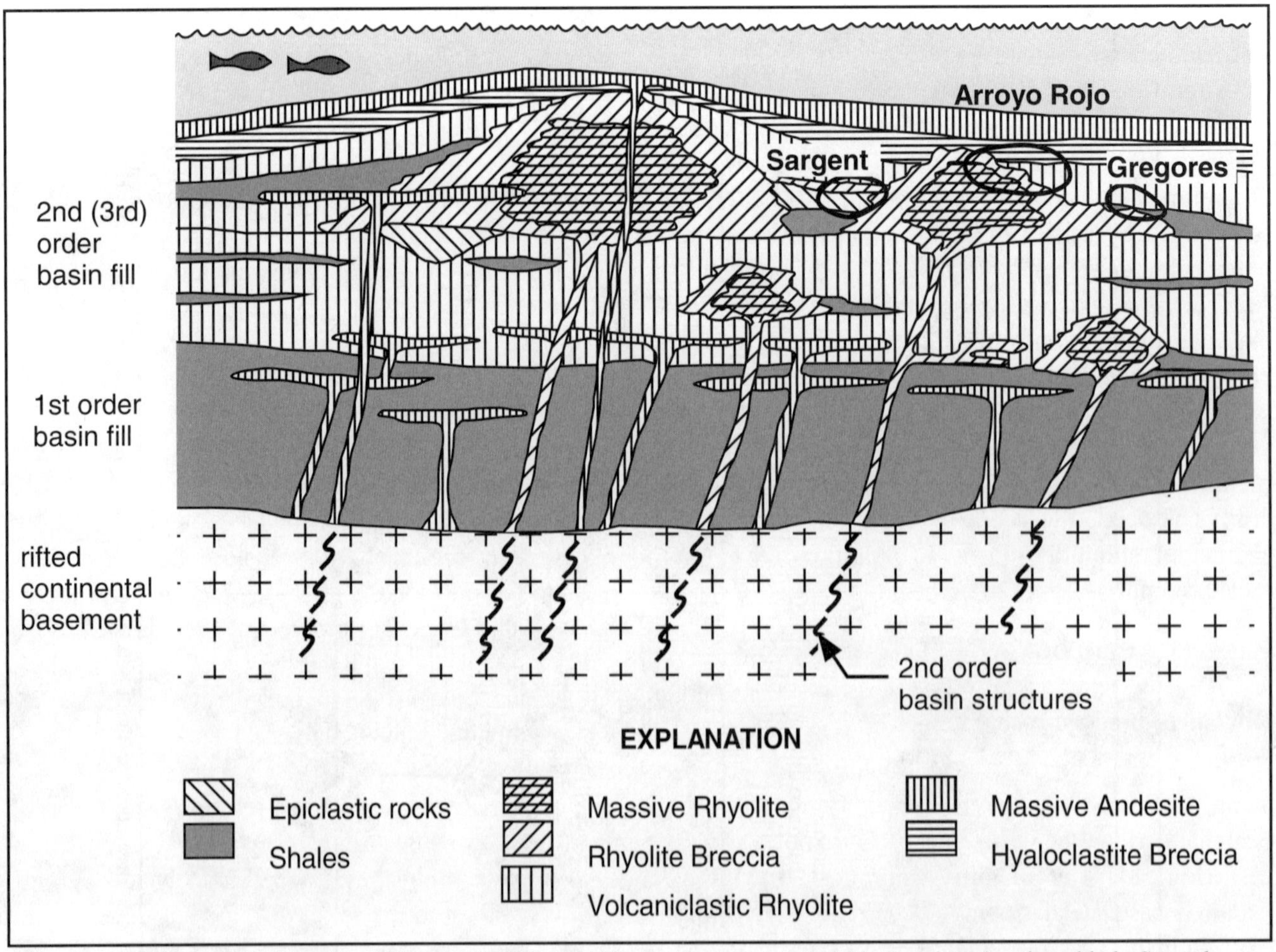

Figure 7. Interpretive stratigraphic column of the Lemaire/Alvear sequence, central Rio Encajonado mineral belt, Sorondo (after D.A. Terry and R.W. Hodder, 1997).

3) Gregores – sulphide minerals in chert-rich rock interpreted as interflow chemical sediment deposited between lobe flows of rhyolite protruding from coalescing rhyolite domes.

Examples of some lesser sulphide concentrations are disseminated sulphide minerals in rhyolite breccia at Xerxes and Rio Encajonado Oeste, layered and disseminated sulphide minerals at the contact between shale and fragmental rhyolite at Rio Hambre, and sulphides at the edge of a rhyolite dike at Lago Pato. Stringer veins of sulphide minerals occur sporadically throughout the mineral belts but are most common in close proximity to the footwall and peripheries of massive sulphide accumulations.

Sulphide minerals are predominantly pyrite with lesser amounts of sphalerite, galena, and chalcopyrite. Exceptionally, base metal sulphide minerals are more abundant than pyrite, as at Gregores. Pyrrhotite is locally as abundant as pyrite in the Rio Hambre belt but is only a minor constituent in sulphide occurrences of the Rio Encajonado belt. Anomalous amounts of arsenic with or without gold are present in several occurrences in Rio Encajonado belt and arsenopyrite is locally present.

In massive occurrences, sulphide minerals are very fine to medium grained with rhythmically interlayered and nodular ferruginous chert. The sulphides may be layered, brecciated, or foliated with textures compatible with shearing, ductile deformation, or mylonitization. Layers have individual bands of galena, or more rarely chalcopyrite, containing augen-like fragments of sphalerite. The bands are commonly 4 to 7 centimetres wide but can be as thin as 0.5 centimetres (Fig. 8). Banded galena is usually very fine grained whereas much of the sphalerite is recrystallized and coarse grained.

Alteration is fairly extensive but commonly obscured by regional greenschist facies metamorphism and foliation, typical of low-rank metamorphic environments. In general, massive sulphide bodies are surrounded by a halo of semi-massive and disseminated sulphide minerals enclosed by silicic and chloritic rock that extends for several metres away from massive sulphide. Surrounding this is a much broader zone of sericitic rock, which is the most common, widespread, and readily recognizable form of alteration in the Fin del Mundo mineral belts. Sericitic rocks may be strongly foliated to schistose and almost always associated with one to five percent finely disseminated sulphide minerals. Sulphide-rich clasts locally comprise 15 to 20 percent of the rock.

PROSPECT GEOLOGY

Rio Encajonado mineral belt

The Rio Encajonado mineral belt extends 30 kms along the Sorondo Range, from near Tierra del Fuego National Park on the west to near Rio Remolino on the east (Fig. 3). The majority and most extensively explored base metal sulphide occurrences are in this belt, with the most important occurrences in the ten kilometre segment extending from Sargent to Gregores.

Arroyo Rojo

Arroyo Rojo is the principal polymetallic VMS occurrence within felsic volcanic rocks of the Lemaire/Alvear sequence, Sorondo Range. Found in the 1980s near the headwaters of a tributary to Rio Encajonado Oeste, the discovery outcrop is above timberline, at 840 m elevation, on a north-facing slope at the upper end of an east trending hanging valley. At the time of initial discovery, a small glacier covered all but a 5 m by 0.5 m part of the sulphide concentration. By the time of "rediscovery" in 1994, the glacier had receded and exposed 200 m of pinching-and-swelling sulphide bodies up to 5 metres wide. Mapping and sampling at Arroyo Rojo outlined a 200 m long zone of discontinuous massive sulphides up to 3.5 m wide with 2.2 percent copper, 3.9 percent lead, 14.5 percent zinc, 1.1 grams/tonne gold, and 140 grams/tonne silver. This work established Arroyo Rojo as a drill target and affirmed the Rio Encajonado mineral belt as geologically favorable for the discovery of polymetallic VMS deposits.

Creek boulders below the exposure are intensely stained with jarosite and iron oxides, and ferricrete is locally conspicuous in glacial outwash down the valley. An orange-red crust of iron oxide patina several millimetres thick coats sulphide-rich rocks and adjacent outcrops (Fig. 8).

The Arroyo Rojo massive sulphide occurrences are on top of a rhyolite dome that appears to occupy the axis of a local anticline (Hodder, 1996; Hodder and Terry, 1997). Sulphide concentrations and enclosing rocks strike east, parallel to the hanging valley, and dip an average 70 degrees to the south. The rocks from base to top are: 1) amygdaloidal andesite flows from 25 to 100 m thick, 2) rhyolite and shale breccia, with block-sized clasts, that underlies the principal sulphide lenses and contains disseminated pyrite, 3) pumice breccia that is the immediate basal part of massive sulphide and consists of vesicular bombs to lapilli-sized and ash-sized particles, and 4) felsic to dacitic crystal lapilli tuff to hyaloclastite breccia that overlies massive sulphide. The latter is approximately 150 m thick and is overlain to the south of the main massive sulphide outcrop by an epiclastic sequence that forms the base of the Yahgan Formation (Darch, 1995).

There are two concordant massive sulphide lenses exposed along strike. They consist of a 70 m long upper (western) lens and 35 m long lower (eastern) lens, which are separated by about 100 m of slightly sulfidic and largely concealed outcrop (Fig. 9a & b). The lenses are from 2 to 4 m thick and consist of banded massive sulphides, mainly pyrite with 10 to 30 percent sphalerite and irregular concentrations of galena and chalcopyrite. The basal part of the massive sulphide concentration is predominantly fine-grained banded pyrite and sphalerite, with coarse local sphalerite up to 3 mm; the upper part contains fine-grained banded chalcopyrite in addition to pyrite and sphalerite (Fig. 8). Galena is common, although difficult to recognize. Microscope study indicates that some chalcopyrite and galena occur in veinlets, many of which are traceable back to massive to semi-massive sulphide layers, from which they apparently have been

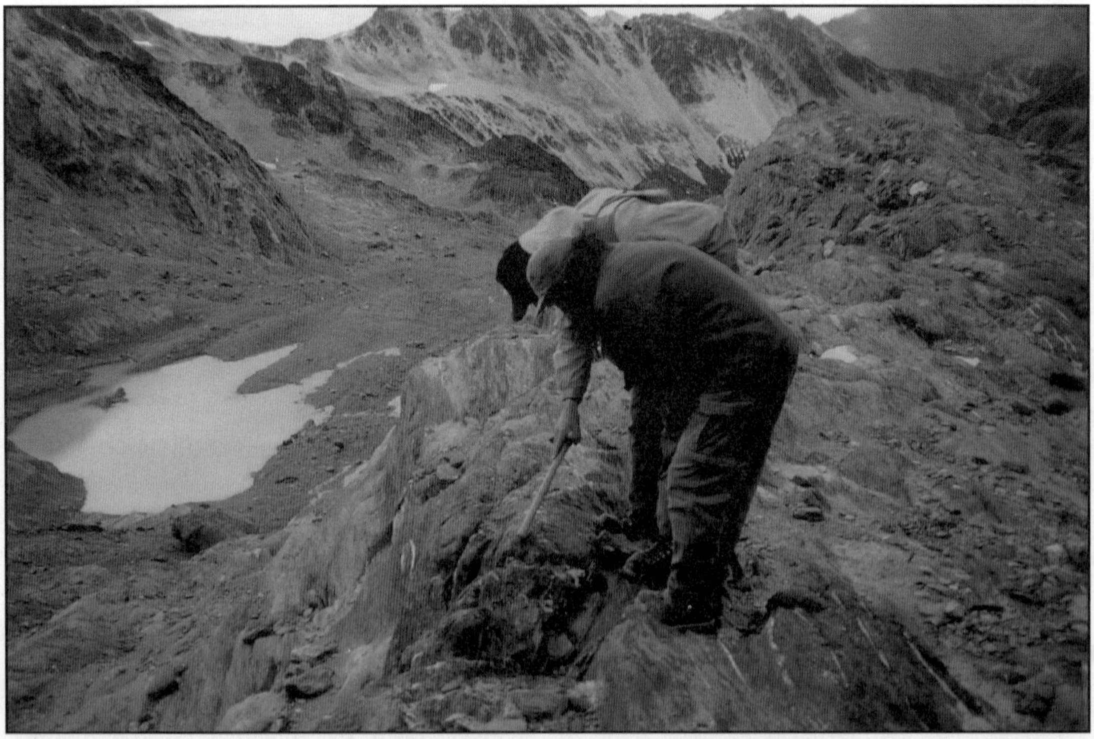

Figure 8a. Overview of Arroyo Rojo upper massive sulphide lens, looking east.

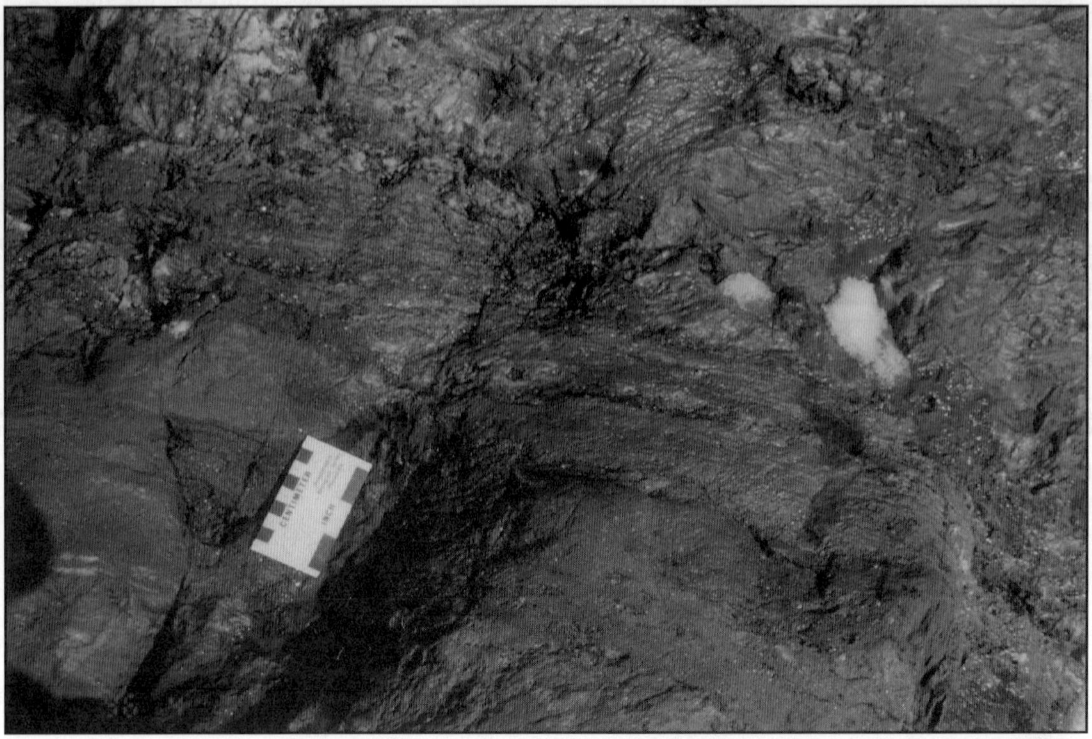

Figure 8b. Massive sulphide outcrop, Arroyo Rojo upper lens. Banded pyrite-sphalerite-galena. Note iron oxide patina which obscures exposure.

remobilized (Boggs, 1994).

Sulphide concentrations have a siliceous gangue and locally contain quartz veinlets and boudinaged augen-like clots of quartz (Fig. 10). Petrographic study shows the siliceous material is fine-grained recrystallized chert. The chert, locally carbonaceous and interlaminated with fine-grained pyrite, is interpreted as a subaqueous chemical sediment (Siems, 1994).

Massive sulphide lenses are surrounded by a 5 m wide envelope of pervasively silicic and slightly chloritic rock containing disseminated and stringer sphalerite, galena and chalcopyrite. This envelope is in turn surrounded by a much broader zone of sericitic schistose rock containing up to 20 percent disseminated pyrite. This outboard sericitic zone covers an area at least 75 m by 400 m in plan.

Samples in a series of sawn channels were taken across the massive sulphide outcrops in 1995 by Darch (1995). The best channel was across the east end of the upper lens with a 4.4 m interval of 18.9 percent zinc, 3.9 percent lead, 0.8 percent copper, 50.9 grams/tonne silver, and 0.9 grams/tonne gold (Fig. 9a and 9b).

During 1997 six core holes were drilled to test the two exposed massive sulphide lenses along 245 m of strike, to a vertical depth of 200 m (Fig. 9a and 9b). The sulphide lenses are very near and closely follow the south wall of the valley, dipping steeply beneath a high, sheer bluff which forms the south valley wall. This location makes it very difficult to position exploration drill holes on the down-dip, hangingwall side of the zone. As a result, all six holes were drilled from the footwall side at very shallow angles to dip (Fig. 11). However, because the holes are inclined close to the orientation of numerous bedding plane features such as faults and chloritic slips, this procedure makes drilling difficult and hinders stratigraphic interpretations. Nevertheless, drilling confirmed massive

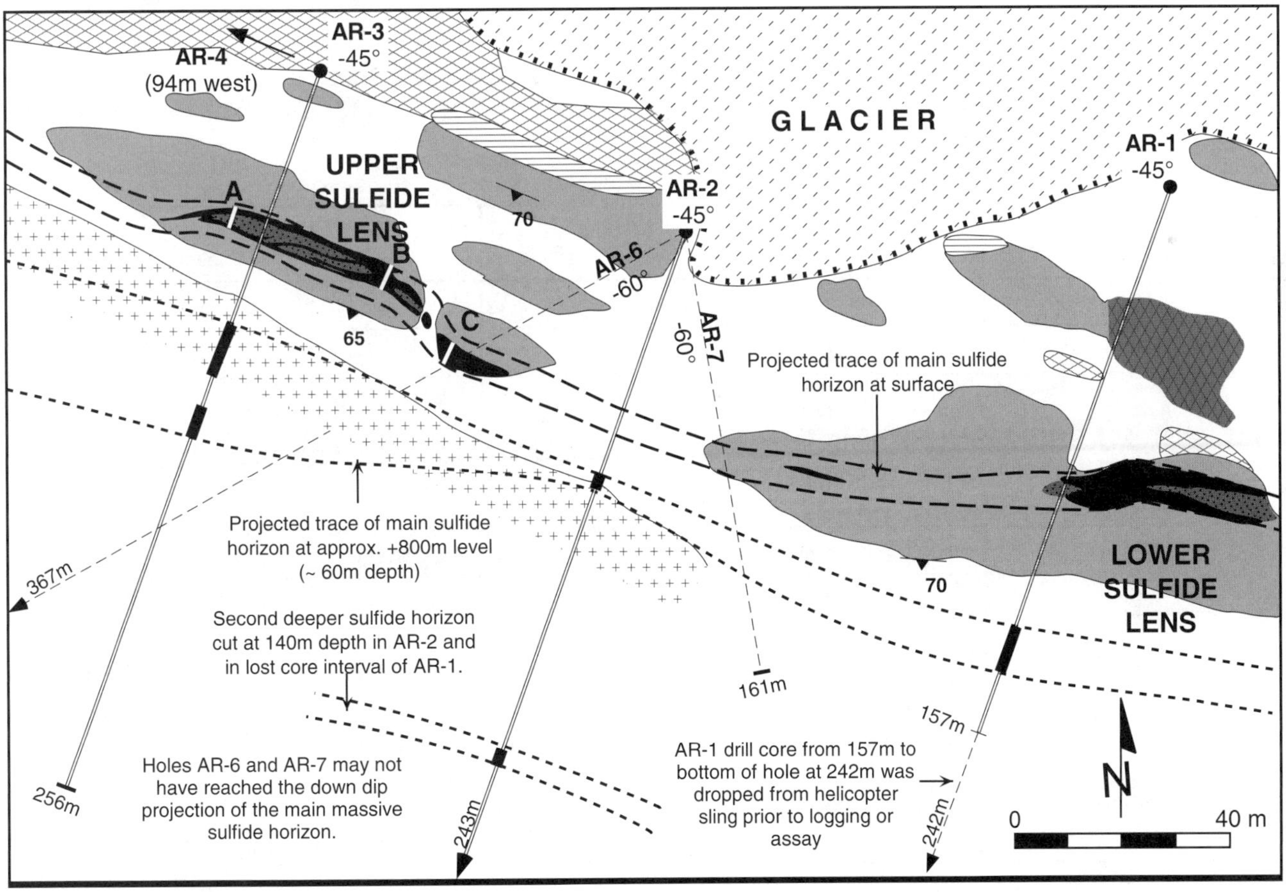

Figure 9a. Geological sketch map of the Arroyo Rojo massive sulphide horizon with drill hole traces projected vertically to the surface. Explanation and assay summaries are given in Fig. 9b.

sulphide lenses are more continuous to depth than along the surface, supporting the earlier interpretation from the ground geophysical survey.

Drill results are summarized in table form in Table 2. The drilling did not intercept a thick interval of high grade massive sulphide, although the authors believe that results overall are encouraging. The best drill intercept is 18.6 m (true thickness) of 1.0 percent copper, 1.4 percent lead, 3.0 percent zinc, and 26 grams/tonne silver (Fig.10). Another hole appears to have stopped in 3 to 5 percent sphalerite in very sericitic and chloritic rhyolite, possibly in footwall just before the massive sulphide horizon (Gibson, 1998). The Arroyo Rojo massive sulphide occurrence remains open at depth, along strike to the east, and possibly along strike to the west (Gibson, 1998). A

EXPLANATION OF MAP UNITS & SYMBOLS

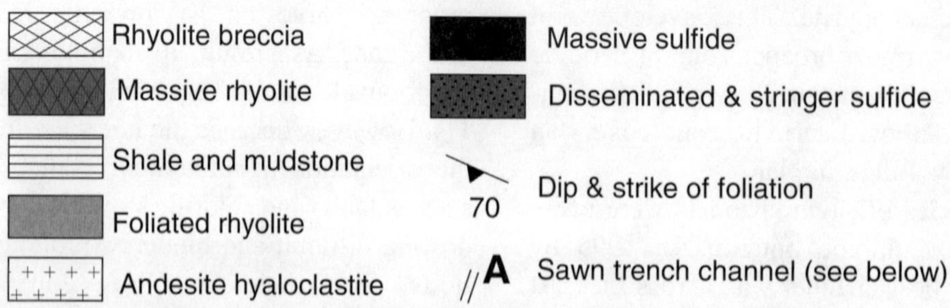

RESULTS OF SURFACE CHANNEL SAMPLES ACROSS ARROYO ROJO MASSIVE SULFIDE OUTCROPS

Sawn trench	Width meters	Cu %	Pb %	Zn %	Ag ppm
A	1.0	—	2.4	—	—
	1.7	1.0	0.9	2.2	22.1
B	3.7	0.7	1.9	11.5	42.4
C	4.4	0.8	3.9	18.9	50.9

MASSIVE SULFIDE INTERCEPTS IN ARROYO ROJO DRILL HOLES

Hole number	Depth meters	True thick. meters	Cu %	Pb %	Zn %	Au ppb	Ag ppm
AR-1	121.3	3.25	0.09	1.54	2.89	42	9
AR-2	42.3	15.40	0.30	0.90	2.30	90	13
	includes	0.75	0.20	2.30	8.75	124	21
	136.0	9.13	0.10	3.50	2.40	30	16
	includes	1.80	0.10	11.60	5.60	50	51
AR-3	63.0	18.57	1.00	1.40	3.00	80	26
	includes	3.66	2.20	3.70	9.40	60	65

Figure 9b. Explanation and assay summaries for Arroyo Rojo sketch map of Figure 9a.

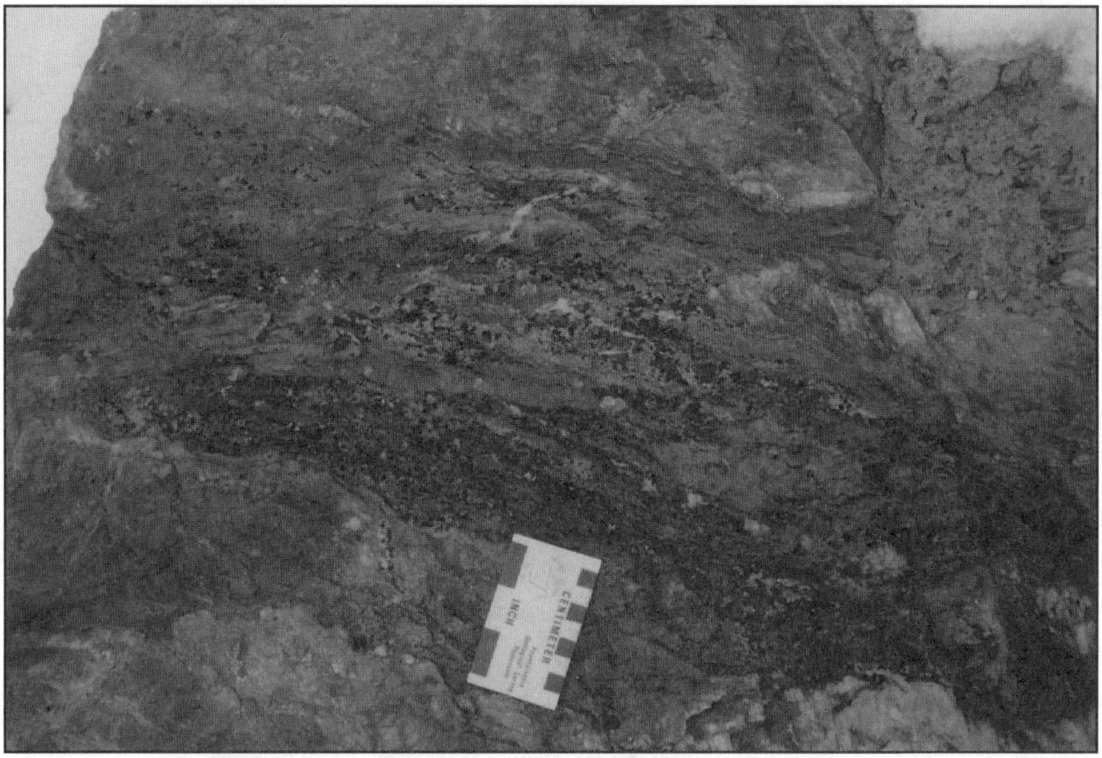

Figure 10a. Massive sulphide outcrop, Arroyo Rojo upper lens. Banded massive pyrite-sphalerite-galena, with dark bands of coarse sphalerite and silica augens.

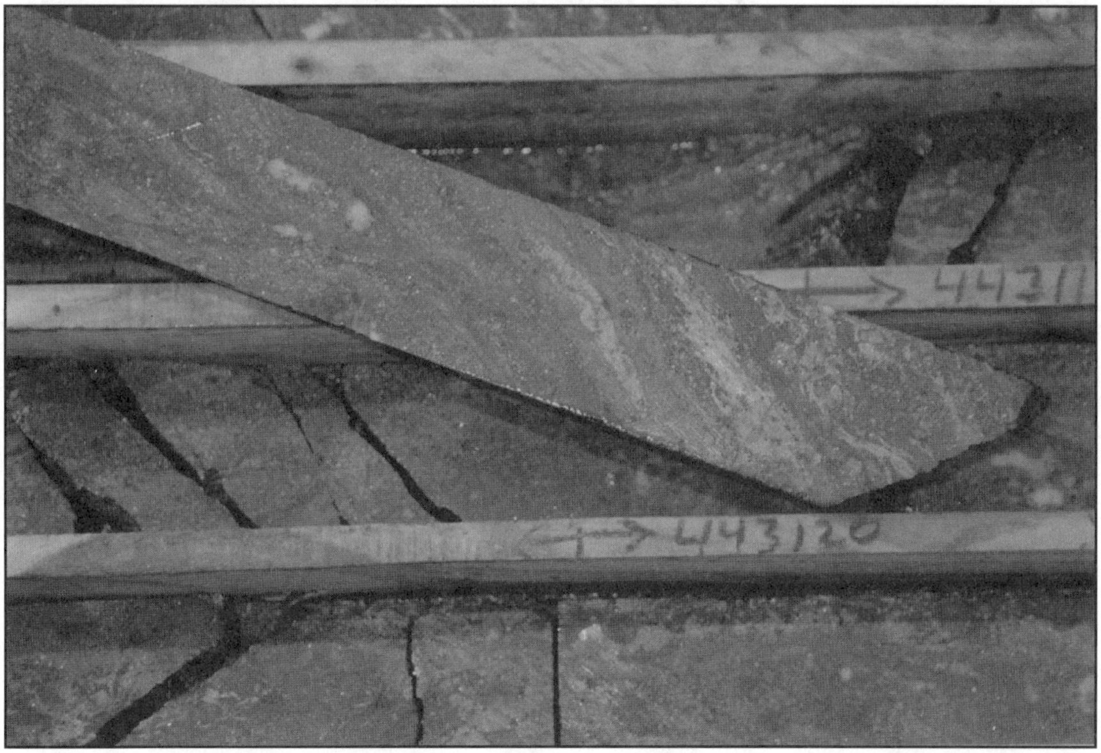

Figure 10b. Drill core from 83 m depth, Arroyo Rojo Hole 3. Banded massive pyrite-sphalerite-galena-chalcopyrite with silica augens.

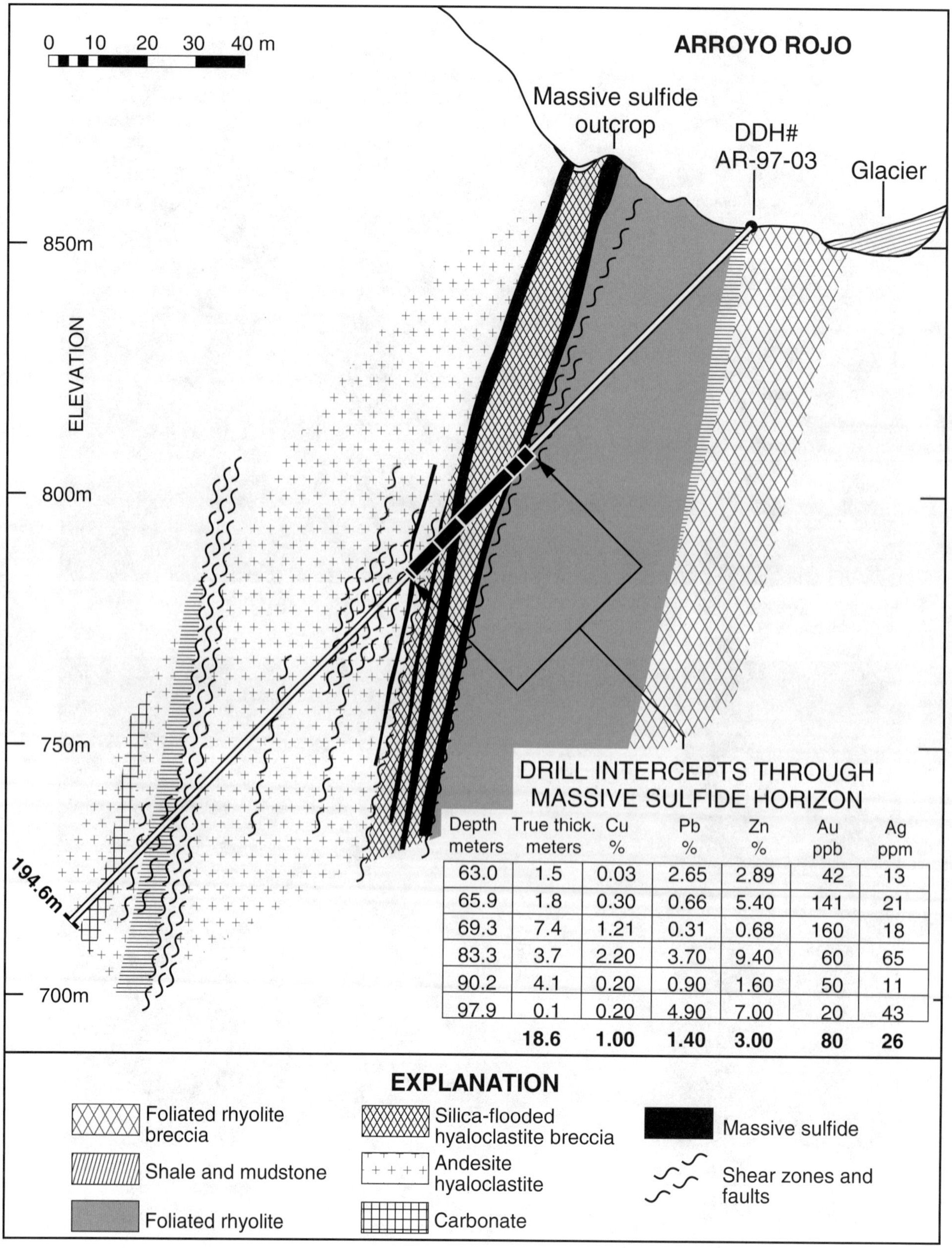

DRILL INTERCEPTS THROUGH MASSIVE SULFIDE HORIZON

Depth meters	True thick. meters	Cu %	Pb %	Zn %	Au ppb	Ag ppm
63.0	1.5	0.03	2.65	2.89	42	13
65.9	1.8	0.30	0.66	5.40	141	21
69.3	7.4	1.21	0.31	0.68	160	18
83.3	3.7	2.20	3.70	9.40	60	65
90.2	4.1	0.20	0.90	1.60	50	11
97.9	0.1	0.20	4.90	7.00	20	43
	18.6	**1.00**	**1.40**	**3.00**	**80**	**26**

Figure 11. Cross-section of Arroyo Rojo Hole 3, looking west.

geophysical anomaly coincident with the Arroyo Rojo horizon, one kilometre east of the main showing, has yet to be drilled.

Sargent

The northwest side of Mount Olivia was first recognized as a prospect in 1994 because of altered float boulders found at the base of the mountain where Route 3 enters Tierra Major Valley from the south. The Sargent occurrence is at 800 m elevation at the top of a northwest facing valley above timberline, directly up slope from a stream sediment copper anomaly (>90 ppm copper) found during 1995. A chalcopyrite-bearing outcrop, 13 m by 25 m, was discovered by the 1996 follow up program. The discovery outcrop strikes west-northwest and dips 50 degrees south (Fig. 12). The Sargent sulphide concentration consists of multiple thin massive sulphide zones with up to 7.5 percent copper over a width of 0.25 m.

The suite of rock types at Sargent is similar to those at Arroyo Rojo and appears to be at approximately the same stratigraphic level. The base is a shale overlain by felsic volcanic rocks, including sericitic massive rhyolite and its brecciated and resedimented clasts. Rhyolite breccia is foliated. The entire felsic volcanic sequence is approximately 400 m thick

Table 2. Drill hole summary.

Prospect	Drill Hole	Depth	Results
Arroyo Rojo	AR-1	242.4	2 massive sulfide zones; upper = 3.25 m (true thickness) @ 1.5 % Pb & 2.9 % Zn; core from deeper zone dropped from helicopter sling prior to assay; select pcs. from 15 to 23 cm long contain up to 21.4 % Pb and 10.8 % Zn, possibly corr. with deeper zone in AR-2
Arroyo Rojo	AR-2	242.6	0.75 m (true thickness) @ 2.3 % Pb plus 8.7 % Zn, plus deeper zone with 1.8 m (true thickness) @ 11.6 % Pb 5.6 % Zn
Arroyo Rojo	AR-3	194.6	18.6 m (true thickness) @ 1.0 % Cu, 1.4 % Pb, 3.0 % Zn, and 26 g/t Ag, including 3.7 m @ 2.2 % Cu, 3.7 % Pb, 9.4 % Zn, and 65 g/t Ag
Arroyo Rojo	AR-4	256.0	no significant intercepts; reinterpretation suggests sulfide horizon possibly offset by left lateral fault and hole may have been prematurely abandoned in footwall rocks (Gibson, 1998)
Arroyo Rojo	AR-5	120.5	prospect hole tested another sulfide showing1 km east of main showing; no significant intercepts
Arroyo Rojo	AR-6	367.5	no significant intercepts; steep hole collared at AR-2 site; reinterpretation suggests hole possibly remained entirely within footwall rocks (Gibson, 1998)
Arroyo Rojo	AR-7	163.2	collared at AR-2 site; ended in 3 to 5 % sphalerite in sericitic & chloritic rhyolite, possibly in footwall just before the massive sulfide (Gibson, 1998)
Sargent	SAR-8	259.1	beneath discovery outcrop; 0.2 m (true thickness) @ 4.9 % Pb and 7.7 % Zn
Sargent	SAR-9	262.0	beneath discovery outctop; 12.7 m (true thickness) @ 0.8 % Cu and 0.2 % Zn
Sargent	SAR-10	227.2	70 m W of discovery outcrop; did not intersect the key horizon
Sargent	SAR-11	27.4	225 m E of discovery otc.; no significant intercepts
Sargent	SAR-12	242.5	225 m E of discovery outcrop; intersected 2 thin massive sulfide layers with best 0.3 m (true thickness) @ 1.0 % Cu, 10.0 % Pb, 27.5 % Zn, and 277 g/t Ag
Sargent	SAR-13	242.5	225 m E of discovery outcrop; stopped short of target depth
Sargent	SAR-14	80.8	70 m W of discovery outcrop; stopped short of target depth
Sargent	SAR-15	56.4	70 m W of discovery outcrop; stopped short of target depth
Lago Guanaco	LG-16	218.1	beneath high grade surface show, intersected stringers with pyrite, galena, & sphalerite
Lago Guanaco	LG-17	71.7	abandoned at shallow depth short of target horizon
Lago Guanaco	LG-18	212.0	450 m E of discovery outcrop; intersected 34 m of quartz vein stockwork in rhyolite, only minor sulfides (pyrite >> sphalerite > galena > chalcopyrite)

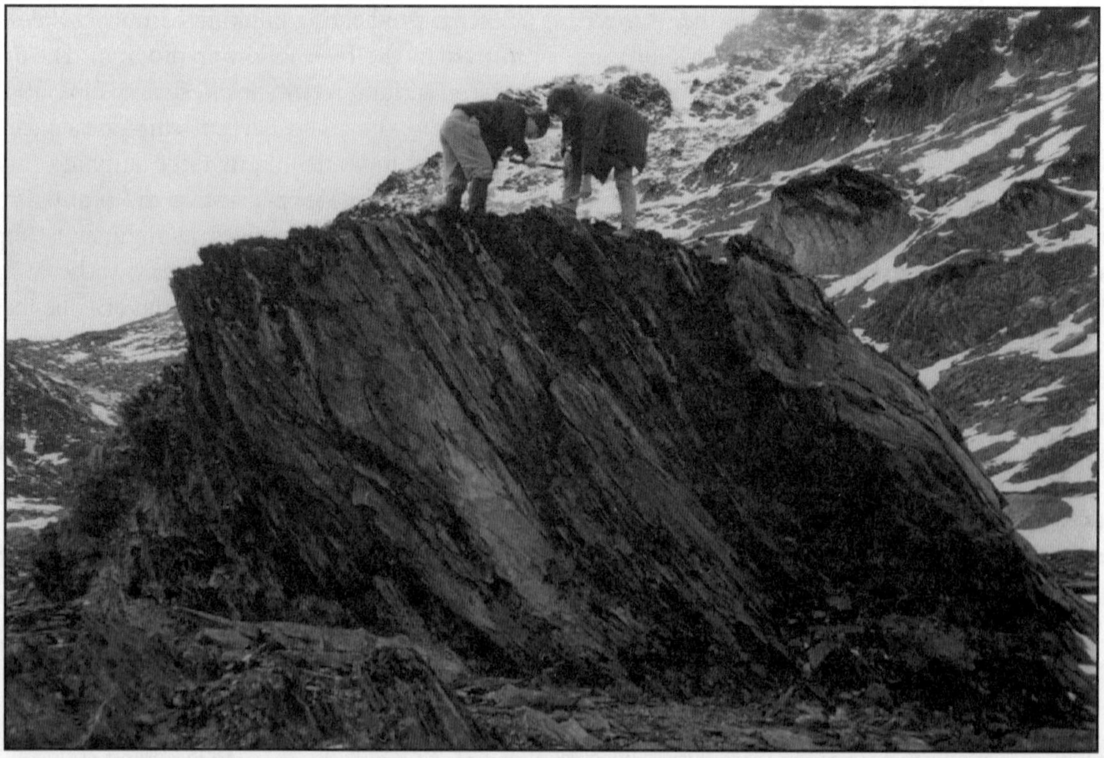

Figure 12a. Discovery outcrop, Sargent prospect, looking east. South-dipping foliated sericitic rhyolite with numerous bands of massive chalcopyrite-pyrite.

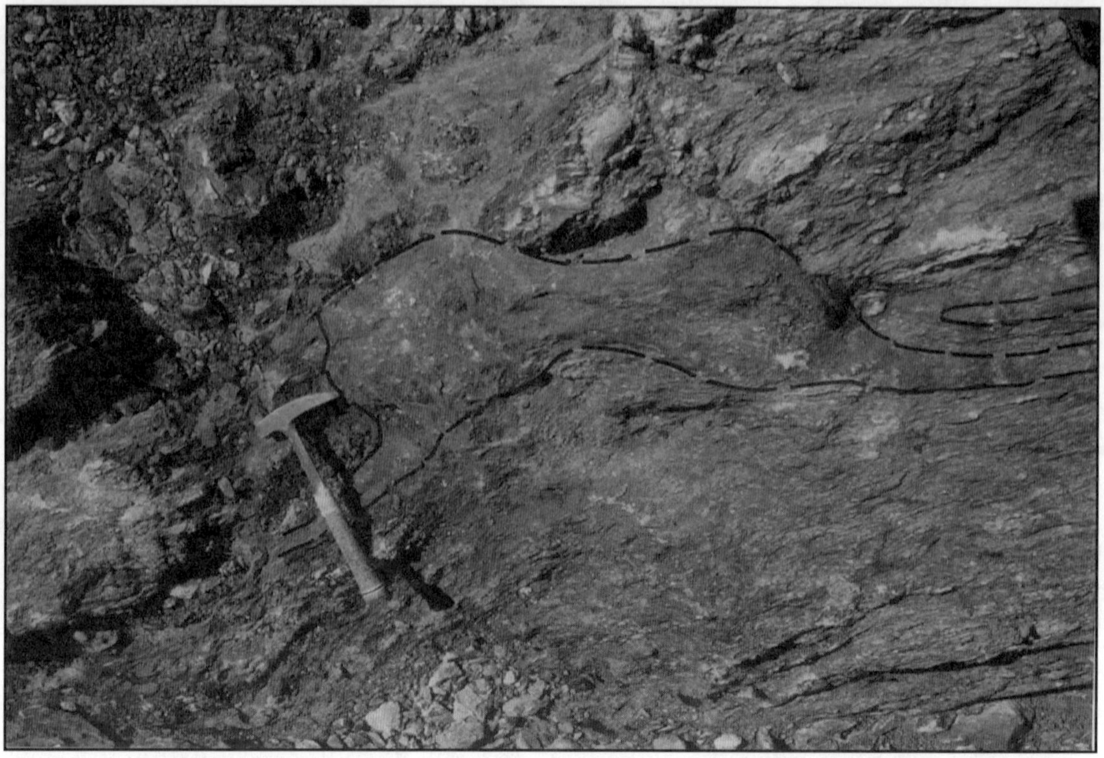

Figure 12b. Outcrop at Sargent prospect with deformed lens of massive chalcopyrite-pyrite in foliated and brecciated sericitic and chloritic rhyolite.

and is intercalated with a green hyaloclastic rhyolite, and overlain by massive rhyolite breccia which is in turn overlain by andesite flows and andesite hyaloclastite breccias.

Sulphide-hosting rocks appear to be along the axis of a local anticline with sulphide concentrations on the flank of a rhyolite dome (Hodder, 1996; Hodder and Terry, 1997). A 6 m wide zone of foliated sericitic rhyolite in the discovery outcrop contains massive to semi-massive sulphide lenses and stringers conformable to foliation. The sulphide zone consists of three thin (4 to 7-centimetres thick) bands of massive chalcopyrite and pyrite. Bands are surrounded by a halo of semi-massive and disseminated sulphide minerals averaging about 10 percent of the rock. An envelope outside of the most sericitic and sulfidic rock consists of dark green-black chlorite rich rock with lesser sericite. Chlorite and sericite tend to replace feldspars. Small quartz veins are common in the rhyolite. The occurrence is interpreted to be a footwall stockwork alteration zone attenuated by regional foliation (Rockingham, 1997).

Eight holes were collared on the Sargent prospect, although only five were successful in reaching target depths because of drilling difficulties caused by complex faulting and shearing. All drill holes intersected significant alteration and several holes intersected prominent stringers of base metal sulphides or thin bands of massive sulphides (Rockingham, 1997).

The drill results are summarized in Table 2. Some holes intersected significant amounts of base metals and alteration in sericitic foliated rhyolite with footwall stringer sulphides, and two holes intersected significant but thin layers of massive base metal sulphides. Other holes were not successful in reaching target depth.

Gregores

The Gregores prospect is above timberline in a rugged hanging valley near Diente de Tiburon, approximately 5.5 km east of Arroyo Rojo. This was identified as an area of interest in 1995 by Darch (1995) from stream sediment samples containing up to 5,526 ppm lead, 1,600 ppm zinc and 44.6 grams/tonne silver. The massive sulphide occurrence was found a year later by following a trail of inconspicuous base metal sulphide-bearing cobbles, devoid of pyrite, up slope to their source.

The suite of rock types is similar to that at Arroyo Rojo and appears to occur at the same approximate stratigraphic level. Gregores, Arroyo Rojo, and Sargent all lie along the axis of a small anticline (Hodder, 1996). The massive sulphide at Gregores is between the lobes of massive flow banded aphyric rhyolite domes and occurs as a flat lying lens between massive rhyolite and rhyolite breccia. The base of the lens is marked by chert and shaly chert.

The Gregores massive sulphide lens, exposed on the face of a steep cliff on the south wall of the hanging valley, is at least 40 m long and from 0.2 to 0.5 m thick. A composite sample collected along the lens contains 29.9 percent lead, 19.9 percent zinc, 750 grams/tonne silver, and 0.58 grams/tonne gold. Sulphide minerals are non-banded fine-grained "steel" galena interspersed with fine-grained sphalerite. Pyrite is sparse to absent, accounting for the general lack of iron-staining and associated wall rock colour anomalies that typically serve as useful prospecting guides elsewhere along the Rio Encajonado belt.

Alteration consists of sericite and added quartz in felsic volcaniclastic rocks. In addition, black chlorite veinlets with minor pyrite are strata-bound with the massive sulphide and dispersed with sericite in rhyolite (Hodder, 1996).

The hanging valley at Gregores has a number of sulphide showings in addition to the aforementioned massive sulphide showing on the cliff face. Stringer-type veins of galena and sphalerite occur in boulders in the creek bottom downstream from the massive sulphide lens. Samples from these boulders contain up to 1.5 percent zinc, 0.9 percent lead and 19.6 grams/tonne silver. During 1997, additional massive galena cobbles were found in glacial till high on the cirque wall 300 m north of the main showing. No outcrop source for this new find has yet been located.

Lago Guanaco

The Lago Guanaco area was identified late in 1996 in an east trending hanging valley about one kilometre north of Arroyo Rojo. It is at 670 m elevation, above timberline, and is stratigraphically lower than the Arroyo Rojo massive sulphide lens. The initial selected sample contained 3.0 percent copper, 11.3 percent lead, 22.6 percent zinc and 147 grams/tonne silver.

The Lago Guanaco prospect is interpreted to be surface stringer and disseminated pyrite with or without sphalerite, galena, and chalcopyrite in a foliated rhyolite breccia in contact with shale. Most sulphide minerals appear to be concentrated along late structures, foliation, and cleavage associated with thrusting (Hodder and Terry, 1997). Samples from hand dug trenches along the trend contain up to 3.0 percent copper, 11.3 percent lead, 22.6 percent zinc, and 147 grams/tonne silver.

The results of three diamond core holes drilled in 1997 were not encouraging. These results are summarized in Table 2.

Other occurrences in the Rio Encajonado belt

The nine other prospects within the belt are shown in Figure 3 and have had a limited amount of work done on them. Most of this work is reported by Rockingham (1997).

Cerro Portillo - Cerro Portillo, west of Sargent across the valley from Route 3 where it enters Tierra Major Valley from the south, consists of chloritic rhyolite in the same stratigraphic sequence as Sargent. Minor stringer veins of chalcopyrite, malachite, and bismuthinite occur sporadically along strike for a few hundred metres, with select samples up to 0.3 percent copper, 1.5 percent zinc, and 0.15 percent lead. Soil sampling has found a number of isolated base metal anomalies.

Rio Encajonado Oeste (Lago Guanaco Muerte) - Stream sediment samples along Rio Encajonado, 1.5 km east and on strike with Arroyo Rojo, consistently have elevated abundance of base metals with locally up to 6,641 ppm lead and 1,060 ppm zinc. Numerous occurrences of stringer sphalerite, galena, chalcopyrite, and pyrite have been found in boulders and outcrops of massive and foliated rhyolite in this area. Additionally, several centimetre-thick layers of massive sphalerite were uncovered in a trench up slope from a local iron seep. Soil sampling substantiates and extends these occurrences and discloses another anomaly in an area covered by till. The limited showings found in the prospect area to date are probably not sufficient to explain the extensive silt sample geochemical anomalies. The Genie-EM survey in 1995 indicates the area is crossed by a conductor, possibly corresponding with a slightly graphitic black shale horizon (Darch 1995).

Xerxes - Select samples collected from a quartz-veined foliated sericitic rhyolite, on the east side of Rio Encajonado Este, 4.5 km east of Arroyo Rojo, contain up to 0.3 percent copper, 11.7 percent zinc, >1,000 ppm lead, and 46 grams/tonne silver. Rhyolite pinches out laterally against unaltered andesite. The volcanic rocks are both overlain and underlain by black argillites, with the underlying argillite capped by a distinctive chert. Follow up soil sampling at 25 m spacing on lines 50 m apart produced a weak multi-element anomaly (copper, lead, and zinc) coincident with the area of the main showing and three single station anomalies from within the rhyolite. Conductors found by a 1995 ground geophysical survey have been attributed to graphitic shale horizons, although the results are not definitive (Darch, 1995).

Gregores Norte - A single rock sample from the northwest side of Diente de Tiburon, upstream from stream sediment anomalies, contains 0.41 grams/tonne gold, 38.7 grams/tonne silver, 11,300 ppm arsenic, and 662 ppm antimony. The host rock is a quartz-veined massive rhyolite containing disseminated arsenopyrite and galena. The rhyolite is within black shales and confined to a narrow ridge at the base of the large Gregores rhyolite dome.

Desolado - Two grab samples from a prominent orange iron seep in a forested area with little outcrop are very anomalous in zinc, copper, manganese, and nickel. Ferricrete boulders have been found above and east of the seep, and small amounts of chalcopyrite occur in shale exposed above timberline on strike with the seep. A grid of 160 soil samples around the seep found elevated gold values but only sparse amounts of base metals.

Vertiente Amarilla - Very anomalous amounts of lead (>1,000 ppm) are in silt samples from a large groundwater spring on the west side of Rio Encajonado Este. The spring is depositing a white non-calcareous material of unknown composition. Soil sampling above the spring identified one spot lead anomaly of 143 ppm.

Lago Pato - A select rock sample has 2.8 percent copper from the slickensided contact between a massive andesite and a rhyolite dike. Sulphides are localized to the contact, which is interpreted to be a thrust fault.

Rio Almanza - Stream sediment samples from the upper reaches of Rio Almanza have elevated amounts of gold. Near the head of the creek, an orange-coloured ridge is topped by massive and foliated domal sericitic rhyolite, locally brecciated with goethite-coated fractures (Lencinas, 1995). Ferricrete boulders are present and oxidized pyrite fragments are found in resedimented rhyolite along the ridge. Rock sampling has found elevated amounts of base metals but has been unable to identify a source for the gold. The anomaly remains unexplained.

Red Sore - A prominent red carbonate groundwater spring along Rio Remolino is upstream from the highest arsenic value (843 ppm) encountered in Darch's (1995) regional stream silt sampling program. The spring deposits are not anomalous in any metals. The arsenic anomaly remains unexplained.

Rio Hambre mineral belt

The Rio Hambre mineral belt extends 30 km along the Alvear Range north of Tierra Major Valley, from near Tierra del Fuego National Park on the west to Rio Hambre on the east. The occurrences are associated with shale-dominated rock sequences and commonly contain almost as much pyrrhotite as pyrite.

Rio Hambre prospect

Rio Hambre is the only occurrence in the Alvear Range with extensive detailed follow up work. The prospect was first recognized in 1994 from sulphide-bearing float boulders along Route 3 where it enters Tierra Major Valley from the north. The occurrence is below timberline and readily accessible by road, but exploration is difficult because of thick vegetation and deep soils.

Stringers and disseminations of sphalerite, galena, pyrite, and minor chalcopyrite are found in boulders and sparse outcrops. Rocks are sericitic schists and graphitic black shales, intercalated with rhyolites and small amounts of pink ferruginous and manganiferous chert. A select sample from one outcrop contains 8.9 percent zinc and 1.0 percent lead.

An irregular 800 m by 2,100 m soil sampling grid was used to define base metal anomalies at the prospect. A total 286 soil samples were collected, with results outlining separate large zinc and lead anomalies. The zinc anomaly (>100 ppm) is 600 m long and trends northwest, the lead anomaly (>60 ppm) is 800 m long and trends north. Individual samples contain up to 921 ppm lead, 437 ppm zinc, 301 ppm copper, 3.4 ppm silver, and 552 ppm arsenic (Darch, 1995).

A follow up Genie-EM and ground magnetic survey conducted during 1995 defines a weakly conductive trend along the southwest edge of the soil grid, following the contact of felsic volcanic rocks with underlying andesites, approximately parallel to Route 3. The conductor is attributed to a narrow graphitic black shale interflow horizon, but the interpretation is complicated by a gas pipeline that crosses the west end of the grid area. The conductive trend is coincident with base metal soil geochemical anomalies and with sulphide-bearing boulders and outcroppings. Darch (1995) concluded that a drill target had been defined. Subsequent in-fill sampling in 1997 affirmed the soil geochemical anomalies, however uncertainty remains whether a drill target has actually been defined (Rockingham, 1997).

Other occurrences in the Rio Hambre belt

The eight other prospects within the belt are shown in Figure 3 and have had a limited amount of work done on them. Most of this work is reported by Rockingham (1997).

Rio Amarillo - A rock sample with 1.79 grams/tonne gold and 9.5 grams/tonne silver was taken from an area of prominent colour anomalies and ferricrete. The rocks are sericitic rhyolite breccia. Subsequent soil and silt sampling confirm elevated gold values, with 268 ppb gold and 178 ppm arsenic in a silt sample from the mouth of a creek below the original rock sample.

Rio Cafe - Rocks are black shale and basaltic andesite, locally pillowed and locally veined with quartz carbonate and patches of mariposite. Fine grained disseminated pyrite-pyrrhotite and thin bands of semi-massive sulphides occur at andesite-shale contacts, and the hillside above a zinc stream sediment anomaly contains ferricrete boulders. Reconnaissance soil samples have up to 3.07 grams/tonne gold, 426 ppm zinc, and 80 ppm lead.

Rio Tristen/Lago Verde - Stringer pyrite and pyrrhotite with small amounts of chalcopyrite are present in a sequence of sericitic and chloritic volcaniclastic rhyolites intercalated with basaltic andesites. One cherty area, approximately 20 m thick and 1 km long, averages 10 percent sulphide with lenses of up to 30 percent pyrite and thin bands of mariposite-bearing massive pyrite (Adams, 1996).

Las Cotorras - Stream sediment and soil samples from an area of sulphide-rich black shales are elevated in zinc and nickel contents, although rock samples have only background concentrations of base metals. The sediment and soil anomalies are reproducible in repeat sampling, but a clear-cut target has yet to be defined.

Bob's Knob - A sample of massive to foliated, siliceous fragmental rhyolite, with local brecciation, quartz veins, and iron-staining, contained 3.64 grams/tonne gold and 8.6 grams/tonne silver. The anomalous sample could not be repeated in the field.

Rio Hambre West - Float from outcrops of orange-stained shale and local foliated resedimented chloritic and sericitic rhyolite contains semi-massive pyrite with minor chalcopyrite and pyrrhotite.

Sombra Grande - Veinlets with traces of chalcopyrite and pyrrhotite occur in foliated rhyolite breccia in a sequence of rhyolite, ladder-veined rhyolite breccia, hyaloclastite and andesite.

Lago Mani - Minor disseminated pyrite and pods of semi-massive pyrite occur in shales intercalated with massive fragmental and foliated schist near a rhyolite dome. Soil sampling failed to identify anomalous amounts of base metal.

GEOCHEMISTRY AND GEOPHYSICS

Because of the temperate climate, chemical weathering of sulphides in Tierra del Fuego may be minimal and fresh sulphides commonly occur within millimetres of the surface of rock. However, in some areas of sulphide concentrations, ferricrete has formed in nearby alluvium and iron-rich patina extensively covers rock exposures. These observations suggest that metals in the Fin del Mundo project can be either mechanically transported or chemically dispersed, thus making it difficult to confidently interpret stream sediment, soil, or pan concentrate geochemical anomalies.

Regional geochemical sampling during the 1995 and early 1996 campaigns found anomalies clustered in several major areas, identifying almost all important sulphide occurrences subsequently found in the Rio Encajonado and Rio Hambre belts. Figure 13 summarizes and identifies subtle geochemical differences between the two belts, with first order arsenic and lead anomalies mainly restricted to streams draining the Rio Encajonado belt and first order barium, cadmium, cobalt, and nickel anomalies restricted to streams in the Rio Hambre belt (Broili and Klohn, 1996). Reinterpretation during 1997 of the earlier stream silt geochemistry results, using different statistical thresholds, found new anomalies (Rockingham, 1997). The results of the various geochemical programs is summarized in Table 1.

Airborne and ground geophysical surveys have been utilized in the district's exploration programs, as summarized in Table 1. At Arroyo Rojo, Turam, SP and IP ground surveys during the early 1980s reportedly identified two distinct anomalies, which were later confirmed by an EM survey in 1995-96. The conductive body appears continuous over a 200 to 250 m strike with a thickness of 1 to 5 m, suggesting the two massive sulphide lenses are connected at shallow depth. Additionally, a non-drilled EM conductor was identified along strike and east of the exposed massive sulphide lenses.

An airborne geophysical survey during 1996 identified many preliminary anomalies (Kendle, 1996). Subsequent work during 1997 found none of the area's massive sulphide concentrations directly related to strong EM conductors, although conductors were commonly present in nearby areas. Many of the geophysical anomalies identified in the original airborne survey have yet to be field checked.

DISCUSSION

Stratiform and strata-bound massive sulphide concentrations in Tierra del Fuego are upon or flank rhyolite domes which intrude a thick section of volcaniclastic and epiclastic rocks that fill a pre-arc marginal extensional basin. These rocks, succeeded by an ophiolite complex emplaced at the height of extension, are overlain by clastic rocks cascading from a rising outboard arc and compressed as that arc closed and deformed the basin. The environment of deposition might be compared to deposits such as those within the Cambrian Mount Read Volcanics of west Tasmania, interpreted by Large et al (1987) and McPhie and Allen (1992) as polymetallic massive sulphide lenses deposited from hydrothermal circulation along early rift faults.

Darch (1995) believed that geology, alteration, and sulphide concentrations in the Fin del Mundo region are similar in many respects to Kuroko type polymetallic VMS deposits. Some of the similarities include geologic age, island-arc environment, a peak in bimodal volcanism, sulphide accumulations in local rhyolite domes in an andesitic (eruptive breccia) pyroclastic sequence, and significant content of precious metals.

Hodder and Terry (1997) noted the similarities in structural style of the ten kilometre long central Rio Encajonado mineral belt to the west side of the Noranda polymetallic VMS district in Quebec. Here, massive sulphide lenses are within an eight kilometre long alignment of rhyolite domes, with several mines at approximately the same stratigraphic level in topographic depressions upon the domes or in small basins between the domes, similar to the Sargent, Arroyo Rojo, Gregores, and other sulphide occurrences in the Rio Encajonado belt.

A recent reclassification of VMS deposits proposed by Barrie and Hannington (1999) includes a bimodal-siliciclastic type that appears to more closely match the general nature and setting of the Fin del Mundo massive sulphide occurrences, although the rocks in Tierra del Fuego have a smaller proportion of volcanic rocks compared to siliciclastic rocks than is

		RIO ENCAJONADO BELT					RIO HAMBRE BELT				
Element	**Threshold in ppm**	**AR**	**S**	**G**	**RE**	**RS**	**RH**	**RC**	**RT**	**LC**	**RA**
As	> 200			●	●	●					
Pb	> 250	●		●	●						
Pb	> 80	●	●	●	●		●				●
Ag	> 1.6		●	●	●		●	●		●	
Cu	> 90	●	●	●				●		●	
Mn	>3,000	●	●		●		●	●		●	●
Zn	> 750	●						●		●	
Zn	> 450	●		●			●	●		●	●
Ba	>1,200							●	●		
Cd	> 6							●	●		●
Co	> 40							●	●		
Ni	> 100							●		●	

Location:

AR - Arroyo Rojo S - Sargent G - Gregores RE - Rio Encajonado Este
RS - Red Sore RH - Rio Hambre RC - Rio Cafe RT - Rio Tristen
LC - Los Catorras RA - Rio Amarillo

Figure 13. Stream sediment geochemical anomaly clusters from Noranda data.

typical for the bimodal-siliciclastic environment. The felsic volcanic rocks of this environment are generally calc-alkaline, possibly derived by partial melting of sedimentary sources, and mafic rocks are generally tholeiitic or slightly alkaline (Barrie and Hannington, 1999). Although this classification has not been verified by chemical analyses of the Fin del Mundo volcanic rocks, subaerial volcanic rocks of comparable age and setting in adjacent Patagonia (Rapela and Pankhurst, 1992) are indeed respectively calc-alkaline and tholeiitic to slightly alkaline. Further, the evidence is compelling that the marginal basin developed on continental crust (Dalziel et al, 1987).

The type examples of the bimodal siliciclastic type VMS deposits are the Iberian Pyrite Belt of Portugal and Spain, and the Bathurst District of New Brunswick, Canada (Barrie and Hannington, 1999). Bimodal-siliciclastic type VMS deposits have the largest tonnages, the largest average deposit size, the least copper, and largest lead content of the five VMS deposit types chartered by Barrie and Hannington.

SUMMARY

Massive sulphide concentrations found to date in Tierra del Fuego are mostly stratiform and stratabound in depressions upon and flanking a line of rhyolite domes. These domes are part of the Jurassic age Lemaire/Alvear sequence and intrude a thick section of silicic volcaniclastic and epiclastic rocks enclosing less voluminous basalt flows and sills. The volcanic rocks are underlain by marine shales of the Lemaire/Alvear sequence and overlain by marine shales of the Cretaceous age Yahgan Formation. The rocks are deformed by folds, thrust faults and normal faults which developed as part of a north-northeast compressional event.

Polymetallic sulphide occurrences are widespread along the Rio Encajonado and Rio Hambre mineral belts. Sulphides occur as disseminations, stringers, and semi-massive to massive lenses of pyrite, pyrrhotite, sphalerite, galena, and chalcopyrite with accessory silica, and they are enclosed by sericitically and chloritically altered volcanic rocks. The massive sulphide lenses are syngenetic and formed coevally with submarine felsic volcanism. The Rio Encajonado occurrences contain almost no pyrrhotite and are associated with arsenic and lead geochemical anomalies. The occurrences in the Rio Hambre belt, enclosed by rock sequences with an abundance of shale, contain abundant pyrrhotite together with pyrite and are associated with barium, cadmium, nickel, and cobalt geochemical anomalies.

The density, distribution, and similar character of occurrences suggests that this area should properly be considered a district – the Fin del Mundo District. Geologically, the district has many similarities to southeast Alaska, but the Fin del Mundo District is still in its exploration infancy. Two of the three drilled prospects merit further drilling, and non-drilled targets remain at other prospects. Many geochemical and geophysical anomalies have yet to be examined in field. Although exploration is difficult and the season is short in Tierra del Fuego, it is no more so than in southeast Alaska, and the reward/risk ratio is comparable.

ACKNOWLEDGEMENTS

The authors thank Yamana Resources Inc. for allowing the publication of this paper and acknowledge the many contributions by Dr. Andres Lencinas, the region's principal exploration pioneer. The data were gathered by many field geologists employed by Minera Polimet, Yamana Resources Inc., Noranda Mining and Exploration Inc., Noranda Exploracion Chile Ltda., and Westmin Resources Ltd., with proprietary project reports by Wayne Darch and Chris Rockingham proving especially useful. These and many others, too numerous to mention, deserve a great debt of gratitude for their valiant efforts in this new VMS district located at the "End of the World

REFERENCES

Adams, G. 1996. General Geology and sulfide occurrences, Upper Rio Tristen Area, Alvear Volcanic Belt, Fin del Mundo Project, Tierra del Fuego. Yamana Resources Inc., unpublished report, 4 p.

Ametrano, S., Etcheverry, R., Echeveste, H., Godeas, M., and Zubia, M. 2000. Distrito VMS de Tierra del Fuego, Argentina. In press, 15 p.

Barrie, C.T. and Hannington, M.D. 1999. Classification of Volcanic-Associated Massive Sulfide Deposits Based on Host-Rock Composition. In Volcanic-Associated Massive Sulfide Deposits: Processes and Examples in Modern and Ancient Settings. Edited by C.T. Barrie and M.D. Harrington. Reviews in Economic Geology, Vol. 8, pp. 1-11.

Boggs, R.C. 1994. Polished thin section examination of sections #1, #2, and #3. Compania Minera Polimet, S.A., unpublished report, 17 p.

Borrello, A.V. 1972. Cordillera Fueguina. En Geologia Regional Argentina. Edited by Leanza. Academia Nacional de Ciencias, pp. 741-753.

Bridges, E.L. 1988. Uttermost Part of the Earth: Indians of Tierra del Fuego. Reprint by Dover Publications, Inc., Mineola New York, 556 p.

Broili, C. and Klohn, M. L. 1996. Summary Pamphlet, Fin Del Mundo Project, Tierra Del Fuego, Argentina. Compania Minera Polimet, S.A. unpublished report, 35 p.

Bruhn, R.L. 1979. Rock structures formed during back-arc basin deformation in the Andes of Tierra del Fuego. Geological Society of America, Bulletin, Pt. 1, v. 90, pp. 998-1012.

Caminos, R., Haller, M., Lapido, O., Page, R., and Ramos, V. 1981. Reconocimiento geologico de los Andes Fueguinos, Territorio Nacional de Tierra del Fuego. Actas 8 Congreso Geologico Argentino, 3, pp. 754-786.

Dalziel, I.W.D. deWit, M.J., and Palmer, K.F. 1974. Fossil marginal basin in the southern Andes. Nature, v. 250, pp. 291-294.

Dalziel, I.W.D., Storey, B.C., Garrett, S.W., Grunow, A.M., Herrod, L.D.B., and Pankhurst, R.J. 1987. Extensional Tectonics and Fragmentation of Gondwanaland. In Continental Extensional Tectonics. Edited by M.P. Coward, J.F. Dewey, and P.L. Hancock. Geological Society of London, Special Publication 28, pp. 433-441.

Darch, W. 1995. Summary of Exploration activities on the Fin Del Mundo Project Area, Province of Tierra Del Fuego, Republic of Argentina, January - April, 1995. Noranda Mining and Exploration Inc., unpublished report, 31 p.

Gibson, K. 1997. A structural summary of the Encajonado Volcanic Belt in the vicinity of Arroyo Rojo and Sargent volcanogenic massive sulfide occurrences, Tierra del Fuego, Argentina. Westmin Resources Limited, unpublished report, 22 p.

Gibson, K. 1998. Summary of Exploration, Fin Del Mundo Project, Province of Tierra Del Fuego, Republic of Argentina, November 1997 to April 1998. Compania Minera Polimet, S.A., unpublished report, 28 p.

Hodder, R. W. 1996. Preliminary review of rock types and setting, Sargent, Arroyo Rojo, and Gregores Prospects of el Fin Del Mundo Project. Westmin Resources Limited, unpublished report, 51 p.

Hodder, R.W. and Terry, D.A. 1997. A second overview of sulfide mineral concentrations in volcanic rock lithofacies at El Fin del Mundo Project, Tierra del Fuego, Argentina. Westmin Resources Ltd., Private report of March 6, 16 p.

Kendle, F. R. 1996. Summary of Exploration Activities on the Fin Del Mundo Project Area, Province of Tierra Del Fuego, Republic of Argentina, January - February 1996. Noranda Exploracion Chile Ltda., unpublished report, 6 p.

Large, R.R., Herrmann, W., and Corbett, K.D. 1987. Base metal exploration of the Mount Read Volcanics, Western Tasmania: Pt. 1. Geology and exploration, Elliott Bay. Economic Geology, v. 82, pp. 267-290.

Lencinas, A. 1994. Tierra del Fuego. Compania Minera Polimet, S.A, unpublished report, 20 p.

Lencinas, A., Kromer, R. and Sanchez, V. 1996. Final Report on Tierra del Fuego Geochemistry and Geology, March 1996. Compania Minera Polimet, unpublished report, 13 p.

McPhie, J., and Allen, R.L. 1992. Facies architecture of mineralized submarine volcanic sequences: Cambrian Mount Read Volcanics, Western Tasmania. Economic Geology, v. 87, pp. 587-596

Ramos, V.A. 1988. Late Proterozoic-early Paleozoic of South America - A collisional history. Episodes, v. 11, no. 3, pp. 168-174

Rapela, C.W., and Pankhurst, R.J. 1992. The granites of northern Patagonia and the Gastre Fault System in relation to the break-up of Gondwana. In Magmatism and the causes of continental break-up. Edited by B.C. Storey, T. Alabaster, and R.J. Pankhurst. Geological Society of London, Special Publication 68, pp. 209-220.

Rockingham, C. J. 1997. Summary of Exploration, Fin Del Mundo Project, Province of Tierra Del Fuego, Republic of Argentina, November 1996 to April 1997. Westmin Resources Limited unpublished report, 47 p.

Siems, P.L. 1994. Final report on the petrography of the Tierra del Fuego property. Compania Minera Polimet, S.A., unpublished report, 35 p.

Zubia, M., Godeas, M., and Ametrano, S. 1989. Area mina Beatriz, Territorio Nacional de Tierra del Fuego, Republica Argentina: una manifestacion de metales de base estratoligada y sinenetica. Edited by M. Brodtkorb and I. Schalamuk. Proyecto 242 IGCP, Simposios sobre el Cretacico de America Latina, Actas, C, pp. 15-44

VMS DISTRICT OF TIERRA DEL FUEGO, ARGENTINA

SILVIA AMETRANO*, RICARDO ETCHEVERRY*, HORACIO ECHEVESTE*, MARTA GODEAS** AND MARIO ZUBIA**

(*) Instituto de Recursos Minerales, Universidad Nacional de La Plata, Calle 47 n° 522. 1900 La Plata, Argentina
E-mail: inremi@museo.fcnym.unlp.edu.ar

(**) Servicio Geológico Minero Argentino (SEGEMAR), J. A. Roca 651. 1322 Buenos Aires, Argentina
E-mail: mgodea@secind.mecon.gov.ar

ABSTRACT

In Tierra del Fuego, a large back-arc basin was developed during the Mesozoic, with polymetallic mineral occurrences (Pb, Zn, Cu, Ag-Au). These occurrences consist of massive bodies, stockworks and also disseminations of iron sulphides occasionally accompanied by base metal sulphides. The occurrences are hosted in marine metasedimentary rocks and in syn-sedimentary silicic intrusions. The exploration and research carried out in the last few years indicates that these deposits are volcanogenic massive sulphide-type (VMS) with overprinted metamorphism. The deposits in Tierra del Fuego are associated with a bimodal magmatism (bimodal-siliciclastic – type).

Bulk chemical analysis of the massive ores and the chemical composition of the individual sulphides suggest that the deposits of the Beatriz mine and Arroyo Rojo prospect represent different portions of a VMS system, the former being a basal portion with a stringer area, and the latter a cuspate section. The action of late cupriferous fluids is demonstrated in the Beatriz mine by abundant chalcopyrite blebs in sphalerite and replacements of cobaltite by chalcopyrite. The absence of barite and the presence of pyrrhotite and magnetite indicate a euxinic depositional environment. Values of $\delta^{34}S$ from massive ores are within the ranges of magmatic sulphide; however, the $\delta^{34}S$ values of pyrite-rich cherts may indicate an additional seawater sulphur contribution.

Several points encourage exploration in Tierra del Fuego: a) the occurrence of several areas with colour anomalies; b) the evidence of other minor hydrothermal episodes at different stratigraphic levels of the volcano-sedimentary sequence; c) the occurrence in Chile, within the same belt, of economically viable deposits, and others still under exploration, indicate a defined metallogeny; the disseminated and stockwork occurrences are not separated of VMS model, but could be part of the already defined schemes for the most important districts.

INTRODUCTION

In Tierra del Fuego, a large back-arc basin was developed during the Mesozoic (Fig. 1a, b), with polymetallic mineral occurrences (Pb, Zn, Cu, Ag-Au; Ametrano et al., 1998). These occurrences consist of massive sulphide bodies, stockworks and disseminations of iron sulphides occasionally accompanied by local enrichment of base metals. The occurrences in the back-arc basin are hosted in marine metasedimentary rocks and in synsedimentary intrusions of rhyolitic volcanics (Fig. 1c). In the past few years there have been surveys and exploration that permit us to tentatively classify these deposits as volcanogenic massive sulphide-type (VMS). Regarding geological data in the area, it has not been surveyed in detail and logistical facilities in this area of the Andes of Tierra del Fuego are very scarce.

The purpose of this paper is to give the results obtained up to now in the area between 54°30' and 55° south latitude and 67°30' and 68°40' west longitude, within the environment of the Tierra del Fuego mountain range. The occurrences are located in the Sorondo and Alvear ranges (Fig. 2).

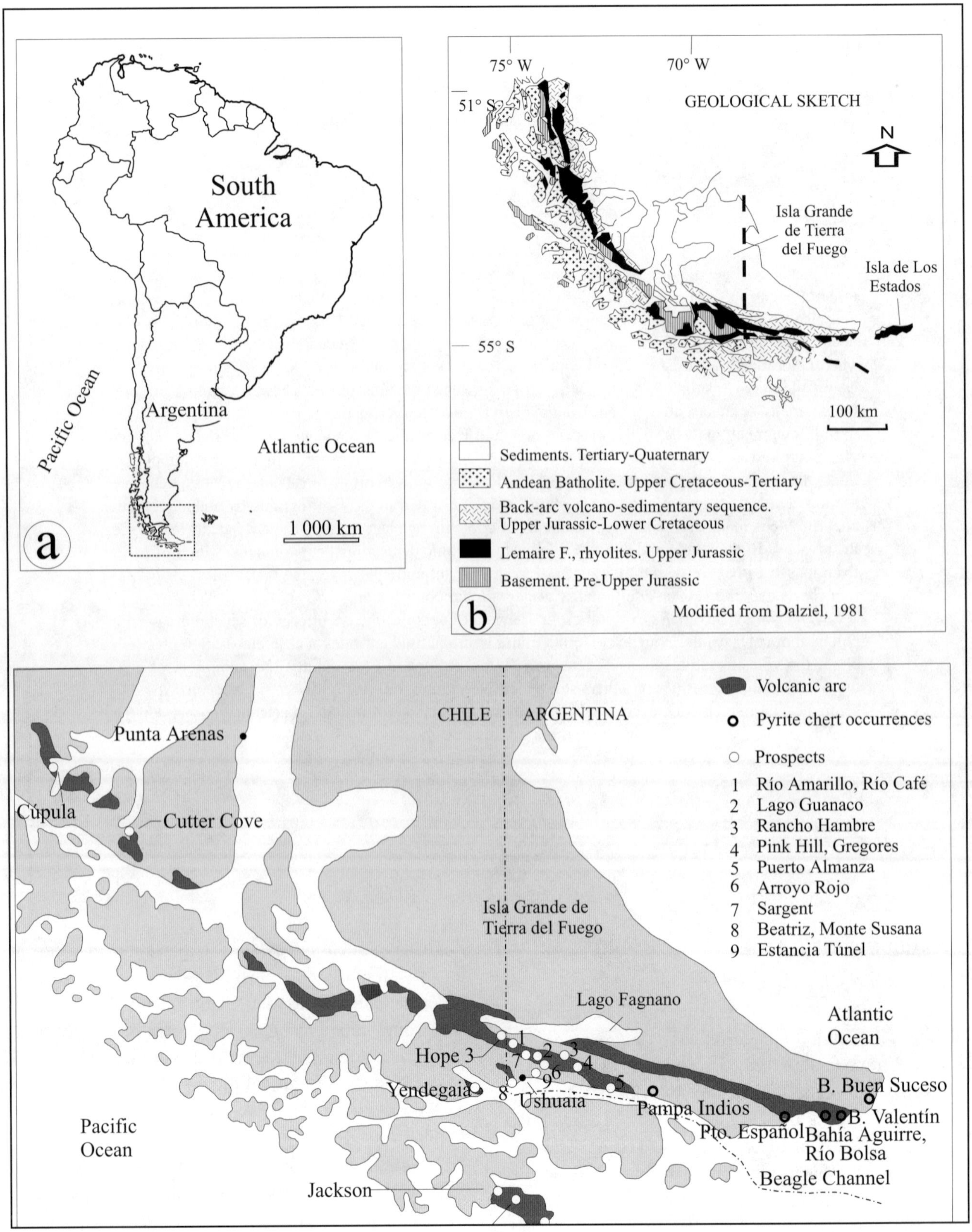

Figure 1. Location and geology of principal polymetallic occurrences.

The only exploitation carried out so far has been placer mining of auriferous sand and gravel placers located in the eastern area of the Beagle channel. This placer mining started at the end of the 19th century and exhausted the placers in a short time. The first record of metalliferous deposits in the region comes from Popper (in Kittl, 1931), who evaluated the auriferous placers at Sloggett bay, which produced approximately 20,000 ounces of gold.

Kranck (1932) presented a systematic study of both sides of Beagle channel, where he surveyed different mountain areas and found base metal sulphides (sphalerite, galena, chalcopyrite and pyrite) in the area. In this paper there are brief references to the occurrences located at Yendegaia bay, the east coast of Roca lake and San Juan bay.

Surveys carried out during the eighties by the Argentine Geological Mining Survey (Servicio Geológico Minero Argentino, SEGEMAR) in the Andes of Tierra del Fuego (Caminos et al., 1981) provided a better geological knowledge of the region and discovered several colour anomalies (Los Castores creek, Remolino river – Túnel, Sloggett bay, Aguirre bay, Fig. 2). A survey, a mineralogical description and the first metallogenic description of Beatriz mine, near Ensenada bay in the Beagle channel in Tierra del Fuego National Park (Fig. 2), was carried out by Zubia et al. (1989 a, b). The polymetallic occurrence associated with this mine was the object of small scale underground exploration, which is believed to have taken place more than 30 years ago.

In the middle 1990's, Yamana Resources Inc. (current owner of the prospects included in the prospection called "Fin del Mundo") formed two separate joint ventures with companies which were successively operators of the project (Broili et al., 2000). From the work carried out by this group up to 1997, several locations with sulphide occurrences were found, namely Sargent, Arroyo Rojo, Gregores, etc. (Fig. 1c). The companies carried out prospecting and exploration tasks, which consisted of airborne electromagnetic profiles, detailed geological works, geochemical sampling (stream sediments and rock chips) and drilling programs on selected targets.

According to Yamana Resources (1998), 18 drill holes were completed, mostly at Arroyo Rojo and Sargent. This company controls other locations with potential polymetallic mineralization (VMS-type) and a precious metal epithermal-type prospect in Chilean territory, associated with Jurassic volcanics (Fig. 1c).

GEOLOGICAL SETTING

The geological environment (Figs. 1b and 2) is characterized by a deformed metamorphic basement represented by accreted prisms, of Upper Paleozoic age. In the southern part of South America, in Tierra del Fuego, during Jurassic time there was an extensional episode (Dalziel et al., 1974; Bruhn et al., 1978) which formed a back-arc basin. During its evolution, a thick silicic volcanic unit was deposited (Lemaire Formation), which was interbedded with marine sedimentary rocks. These sedimentary rocks correspond in their lower levels to high energy environments that evolved towards deeper environment facies represented by pelites and shales during periods of no silicic volcanic activity. Fossils (ammonites, belemnites and inoceramides) found in Chile within black slates, interlayered with volcanics in the Mesozoic sequence, date the unit as Upper Jurassic (Fuenzalida and Covacevich, 1988). These sedimentary rocks with some rhyodacitic volcanic rocks correspond to the Yahgán Formation (Kranck, 1932).

Later, when conditions were suitable for attenuation and fracturing, there was an overflow of basaltic dikes and bodies, which are best exposed in the back-arc basin (Dalziel et al., 1987).

In Argentina, the basement crops out only along the border with Chile (Fig. 2) and is known as the Lapataia Formation. The sedimentary and volcanic rocks of the back-arc basin were later affected by low grade metamorphism and deformed. The intercalation of the rhyolitic volcanic episode (Tuffaceous Series, Thomas, 1949; Lemaire Formation, Borrello, 1969 and 1972) in the volcanic-sedimentary sequence of the back-arc is well exposed in other locations in the Andes (Fig. 1b). The age of the main units of this basin is Upper Triassic to Cretaceous. Dark to greenish mafic rocks, also metamorphosed and located at Paso Garibaldi and other places, represent the rift period according to Dalziel (1981); to the west, in Chile, they are called Rocas Verdes (Dalziel et al., 1974) and other authors suggest they are related to the

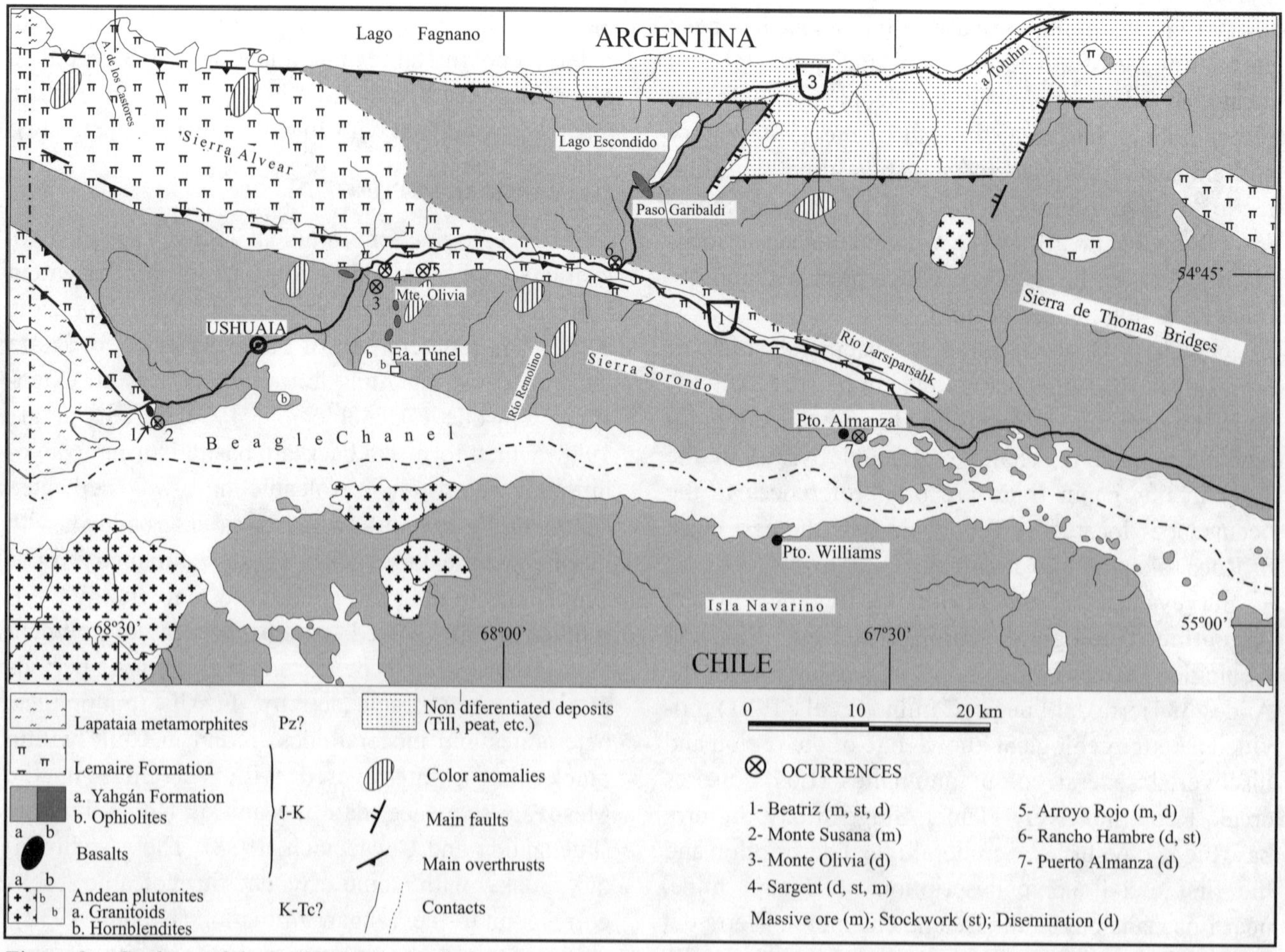

Figure 2. Geology of the study area (compiled after Caminos at al., 1981; Kranck, 1932; Quartino et al., 1989 y Suarez et al., 1985b).

Tortuga Complex.

The evolution was completed with a magmatic arc of plutonic rocks of Late Cretaceous to Tertiary age, when the basin was closed. These rocks form stocks and domes of various compositions (granite - syenodiorite - diorite - hornblendite).

The current tectonic configuration is due to the Andean orogeny, whose compressional effects appear in different tectonic plates, and are limited by reverse faults which are characteristic of the Andes of Tierra del Fuego (Fig. 2). According to Cingolani (1989), during Tertiary time there was a migration of the magmatic arc and a progressive deformation at depth, thus resulting in strike-slip faults and thrust structures along a folded belt with frequent shearing effects. Finally, the region was bisected by transcurrent faults. During the Quaternary, there was a development of alluvial and glacial deposits, as well as large peat plains.

District geology

The geologic setting of the study areas consists of the following stratigraphic units (Fig. 2) : Lapataia metamorphics, Yahgán Formation, Lemaire Formation, ultramafic rocks, and basalts near the Beatriz mine. Lapataia metamorphics (phyllites, schists and gneisses) are basement rocks of Upper Paleozoic age (?) that were metamorphosed to amphibolite facies.

The massive volcanic-sedimentary succession of the back-arc basin is in angular discordance. The silicic volcanic and pyroclastic rocks deposited mainly in a marine environment, belonging to the Lemaire

Formation of Upper Jurassic age, are frequently observed as interdigitations within metasediments of the Yahgán Formation, can be seen at the foot of Mount Susana (Plate 1a, b), and suggest a "wet intrusion". A similar setting has been observed by Pesce et al. (1996) to the east of Arroyo Rojo, in the Termas del Río Valdez area. In other regions the relationships between the metasediments of the Yahgán Formation and the volcanic rocks of the Lemaire Formation is unclear. However, it is assumed that the primary contact of the rhyolitic volcanics is evident in the mentioned sites and it is of sedimentary type. Exposures of this volcanism are common to the east up to the Isla de los Estados (Fig. 1b).

Lithology

The volcanics have undergone low-grade regional metamorphism. They have a blastoporphyritic texture as the result of a complete recrystallization of the matrix. The matrix is an aggregate, sometimes lepidogranoblastic, mainly constituted by quartz and sericite/muscovite, with scarce chlorite, plagioclase, and occasionally stilpnomelane. The relic phenocrysts are quartz, alkaline feldspar and plagioclase. Quartz displays a strong cataclasis, pressure shadows, fluxion, undulatory extinction and punctual and train inclusions. The quartz-sericite matrix is commonly layered and lenticular. Epidote, sphene and prehnite are observed as metamorphic minerals; igneous accessory minerals are apatite and zircon. Pyrite is common, and is even very abundant in automorphic crystals and also as pyritospheres where they are usually rotated and accompanied by pressure shadows. Both mineralogical and chemical compositions (Fig. 5) indicate the rocks are rhyolites, rhyodacites and dacites. The amount of sericite and pyrite is variable, but increases in abundance together. Siliceous veins are usually abundant. The metamorphism superimposed upon the volcanics has obliterated the hydrothermal alteration textures, except for pyritization. In regions of the large rhyolitic domes of the Alvear range, some microscopic textural features suggest an ignimbritic facies. The foliation in the metavolcanic rocks may be very conspicuous.

Trace element data (Fig. 5) indicated that the rocks belong to a volcanic arc. Furthermore, the REE distribution pattern (Fig. 5) suggests that these rhyolites formed in an evolved volcanic arc. The variation in the MgO content in these rocks indicates alteration due to interaction with marine water (Fig. 5). Lentz (1996) pointed out that values higher than 0.5 % MgO correspond to submarine volcanics, and lower values to subaerial volcanics.

Accordingly, and with transitional passages and interdigitations, there is a succession of sedimentary rocks, rhyodacitic pyroclastics, and ignimbrites of Lower Cretaceous age, corresponding to the Yahgán Formation. The sequence was intensely deformed and was affected by low-grade metamorphism (prehnite-pumpellyite facies). The sedimentary rocks have similar characteristics to those of peat-bearing rocks. They are slates, phyllites and sandstones; considerably thick black slates with abundant recrystallized pyrite, relict framboidal pyrite and graphite are common. Silica veins are abundant; their thickness is variable, and they are concordant with the foliation and slaty cleavage.

Quartino et al. (1989) informally named the entire lithological group as "Deformed Complex of the Andes of Tierra del Fuego", to refer to the leptometamorphic and eruptive sequence deformed by folding.

To the south of the Beagle channel, in Chile, an ophiolitic complex has been recognized (massive basalts, dolerites and gabbros); it is partly below the peats of the Yahgán Formation and was called Complejo Tortuga by Suárez et al. (1985a). Kranck (1932), Katz (1972) and Bruhn and Dalziel (1977) have already mentioned these rocks in the Andes of Tierra del Fuego. In the district area, between Mount Olivia and Lake Escondido, there are outcroppings of dark to greenish eruptive rocks that Quartino et al. (1989) assigned to a tholeiitic to calc-alkaline range, partly intrusive and with spilitic characteristics. Relatively serpentinized ultramafic rocks crop out from Estancia Túnel up to Ushuaia Bay, as well as metamorphosed basalts on national road N° 3. Haller and Delpino (1989) considered these lithologies as testimonies of a dismembered ophiolite. On the other hand, Acevedo (1996) and Olivero et al. (1997) considered the quartz diorites and hornblendites from Estancia Túnel as post-tectonic Andean plutonites.

Structure and deformation

The dominating structure is defined as an intense folding to the NE following the formation of an anticlinorium. Andean compressional effects generated several tectonic layers bounded by reverse faults (Fig. 2) that affected the back-arc basin sequences. Dynamic metamorphism caused foliation folding at different scales; boudinage and shearing were also generated. The sequence has a dominant east-west strike and monoclinally dips towards the south. The dominant foliation is parallel to the primary bedding.

METALLIC OCCURRENCES AT TIERRA DEL FUEGO

In addition to the gold placers that once attracted Popper (in Kittl, 1931), other types of occurrences have been determined in the southern part of Tierra del Fuego province, some of them large (Fig. 2). The surveyed deposits correspond to three different types: massive, stockworks, and disseminated. The lack of mining exploitation hinders a clear understanding of the relationship between the geometric types that are described in the following section.

Massive deposits

Polymetallic lenticular bodies where the sulphides represent more than the 60 % and their geometry is controlled by deformational episodes occur in Arroyo Rojo, Sargent and Beatriz mine (Fig.2).

The grain size of the massive sulphide deposits is variable (from very fine to coarse), with pyrite being the sulphide with the greatest response to metamorphic recrystallization. They are hosted in metavolcanic bodies of the Lemaire Formation or in metasediments of the Yahgán Formation that are proximal to rhyolitic bodies.

Mineralogy is simple with banded textures that show the effects of the superimposed metamorphism. Pyrite, sphalerite, chalcopyrite and galena are the most abundant minerals. Pyrrhotite and cobaltite are less abundant, and as accessory minerals marcasite, arsenopyrite, magnetite, tetrahedrite and seleniferous bournonite are found. As secondary minerals, only covellite, malachite, azurite and "limonites" have been identified. The scarce gangue consists of quartz and some calcite.

Macroscopically, textures are characterized by a marked banding of variable grain size, from very fine to coarse, with rare disharmonic folds. Important metamorphic effects observed under the microscope in the massive sulphide include: recrystallization of pyrite into poikilitic megacrystals, annealed texture integrated by sphalerite/chalcopyrite or sphalerite/galena, and peripheral redistribution of chalcopyrite blebs in recrystallized sphalerite grains. Deformational processes are evident through: rotation of pyrite and sphalerite porphyroblasts, pyrite cracking, chalcopyrite fluxion and filling of pyrite fractures and "pressure shadows" around sulphide porphyroblasts (Plate 2).

In addition, there are other occurrences of massive deposits containing only pyrite, linked to a chert host in black shales of the Yahgán Formation. These consist of recrystallized idiomorphic pyrite , medium grain size and high sulphide concentration (50-60 % pyrite vs. 40 % SiO_2), as well as abundant relict partially recrystallized pyritospheres.

Stockwork deposits

These consist of veinlets (maximum 3 to 5 cm thick) hosted both within metasediments and in metarhyolites, along foliation planes or in tensional structures. They are polymetallic, with a simple mineralogy, silica gangue and very scarce carbonate. The most abundant sulphides are chalcopyrite, pyrite and sphalerite; galena is not so abundant, and cobaltite appears as an accessory mineral. Their dimensions are variable; in the case of those hosted in metavolcanics, they constitute in some locations intricate networks.

Disseminated sulphides

Sulphide disseminations occur in metarhyolites and metasedimentary rocks, being more common in black slates. Some concentrated disseminations occur near massive ores, and all are adjacent to rhyolite domes. The disseminations have homogeneous distribution, with fine to coarse grain sizes. Recrystallized pyrite, with a great tendency to automorphism, and relict pyritospheres are very common To a lesser extent pyrrhotite is present. Sphalerite and chalcopyrite were found only in the dissemination at Puerto Almanza.

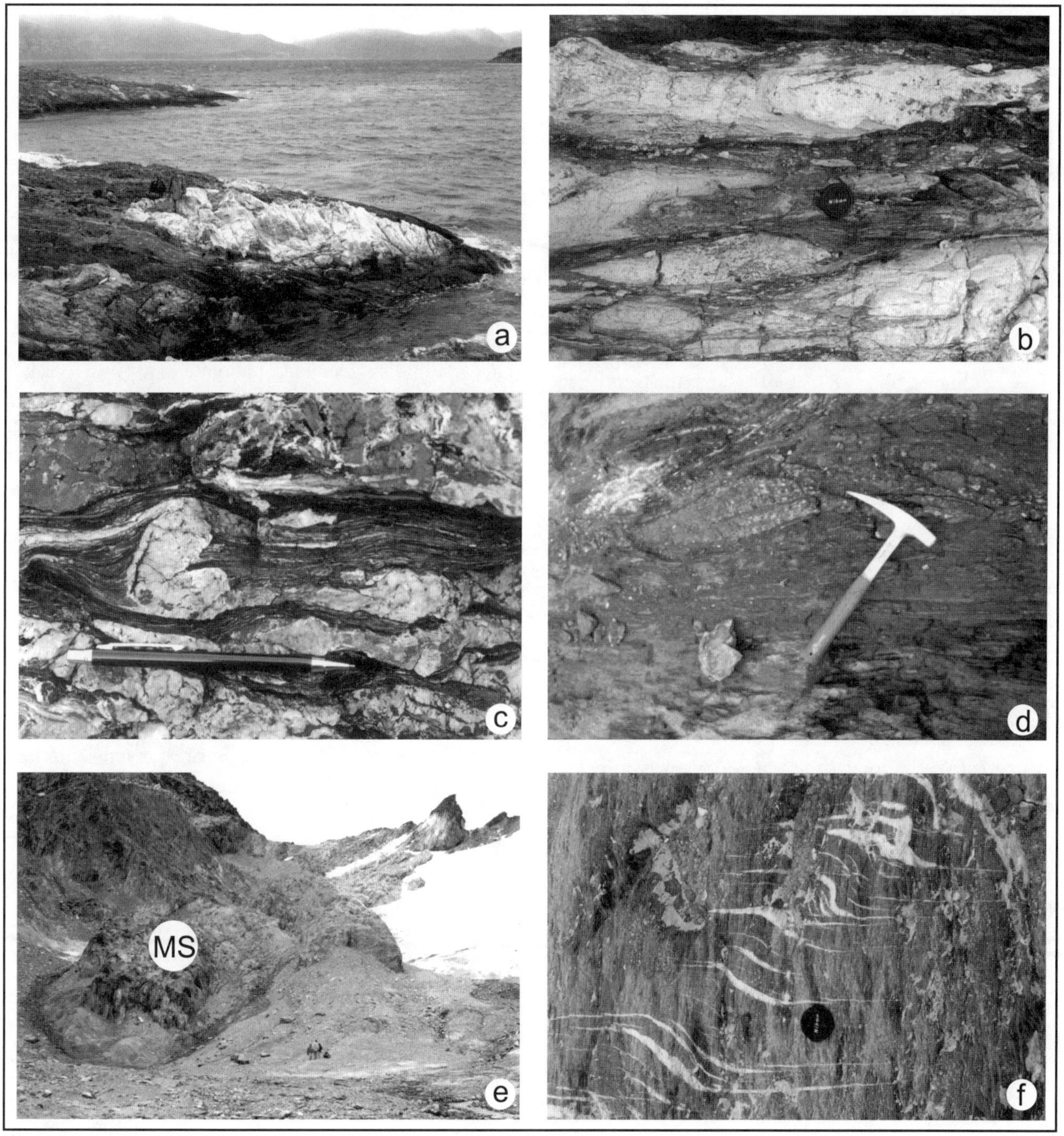

Plate 1 – Field pictures
a) Beatriz mine area, by the coast of Beagle channel. Rhyolites, “wet intrusion” within metasediments (Yahgán Fm.); b) Idem a. Rhyolites (clear) interbedded with metasediments (Yahgán Fm.); c) Monte Susana, close to the coast of the Beagle Channel. Deformed pyritic chert (white and/or clear) within black slates (black); d) Idem e. “Boudinage” in pyritic chert within black slates; e) Arroyo Rojo Prospect. Glacial cirque, outcrops of rhyolites and a massive sulfide lens; f) Idem e. Deformed carbonate veinlets (after a shear zone pattern) within foliated chloritic rhyolites,

STUDY LOCALITIES

Beatriz mine – Mount Susana

Beatriz mine and Mount Susana are located within Tierra del Fuego National Park (Fig. 3). The geology of the area consists of sedimentary rocks of the Yahgán Formation with abundant interdigitations of the Lemaire Formation rhyolites. The deformation generated only rhyolite lenticulation (boudinage?) at different scales (Plate 1 – a, b). However, the cores of the major rhyolitic bodies are faulted with clearly observable scarps. This region is part of an overthrust plate (Zubia et al., 1989 a, b) where the sequence monoclinally dips southwards. Locally, the whole group is sometimes affected by axial plane cleavage. Foliation is parallel to bedding planes.

The Yahgán Formation here consists of interstratified beds of metasedimentary rocks (wackes, siltstones, shales) and rhyodacitic metapyroclastites that were metamorphosed to greenschist facies. To the east, higher in the sequence, they are mainly facies of black shales. The rhyolite of the Lemaire Formation is slightly porphyritic; the matrix is generally recrystallized.The Yahgán Formation shows no thermal aureole along the contact with the Lemaire Formation. As was already mentioned, the whole group is affected by greenschist facies and deformation metamorphism.

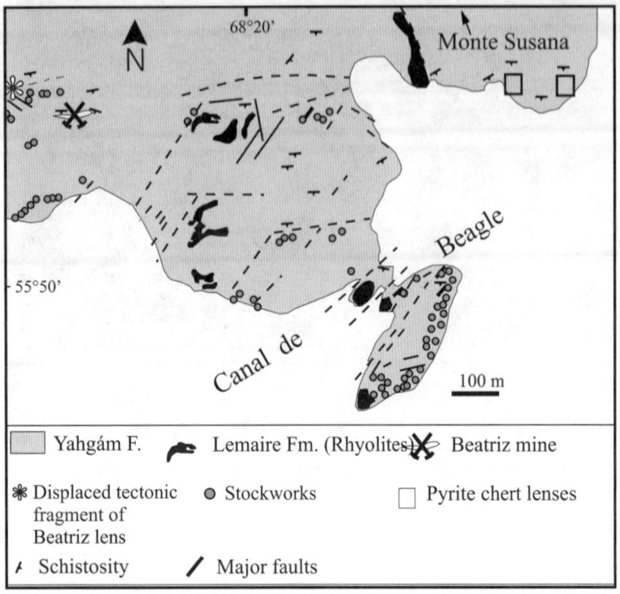

Figure 3. Geological sketch Beatriz-Susana Mount area (simplified after Zubia et al. 1989)

The Beatriz mine, a small occurrence of polymetallic massive sulphides, is located at 54°51'30" SL and 68°27'33" WL; even though this occurrence does not crop out, it can be observed in a prospecting undercut. The geology, petrology and mineralogy were described by Zubia et al. (1989a), and the chemical composition of the sulphides by Ametrano and Paar (1996) The Beatriz mine is a stratiform deposit consisting of a small subconcordant lens with a length of 5 m and a maximum thickness of 0.8 m; its western end is dismembered into veinlets along 12 m due to the deformation. In addition to this, the lens presents a fault displacement of about 300 m (Fig. 3). This lens is hosted in metasandstones and metawackes of the Yahgán Formation, at 200 m of rhyolitic intrusions interdigitated with it. The silicification and abundant pyritization in the wall rock is somewhat obscured by the metamorphism. Siliceous veins are important as a consequence of the metamorphism and deformation. The ore mineralogy consists of chalcopyrite, sphalerite, galena and pyrite as the main components, and pyrrhotite, cobaltite, arsenopyrite, marcasite, magnetite and tetrahedrite as minor or accessory components. The gangue is quartz and scarce calcite.

The texture of the sulphide ore presents marked compositional banding (chalcopyrite – sphalerite) subparallel to the regional foliation. The grain size is very fine (5-10 microns) with relict sedimentary characteristics such as disharmonic folding. Microscopic metamorphic features consist of recrystallized pyrite (poikilitic megacrystals), annealed texture (chalcopyrite/sphalerite), and peripheral redistribution of chalcopyrite blebs in recrystallized sphalerite. The deformation effects include the rotation of pyrite accompanied by "pressure shadows" constituted by the rest of the sulphide mass, also cracking and later filling of the fracture by chalcopyrite. The frequent presence of cobaltite in cubic crystals has textural relations that suggest that this mineral was one of the first to be formed, with an almost stoichiometric chemical composition (42 wt. % As, 32 wt. % Co, 3.3 wt. % Fe, 0.5 wt. % Ni; Ametrano and Paar, 1996). These cobaltite crystals very have often their cores replaced by chalcopyrite, thus resulting in "atoll" crystals (Plate 2, a).

At the Beatriz mine, ore grades vary greatly (Zubia

et al., 1989a). The results obtained from a sampling of fourteen channels, cutting the lens and the wall rock, are the following:

Table 1. Grades of the Beatriz mine, sampling in channels (Zubia et al., 1989a).

	Thickness	Cu % min - max	Pb % min - max	Zn % min - max	Ag g/t min - max	Au g/t min - max
Beatriz	1 m	0.02 - 4.73	0.02 – 4	0.03 – 19	5 – 175	Traces

In an area of approximately 1 km^2 near the Beatriz mine, a stockwork deposit is hosted in foliation planes and tensional structures of the metasedimentary rocks of the Yahgán Formation and in rhyolites of the Lemaire Formation, sometimes in an anastomosing pattern. The area corresponds to that with less vegetation due to its proximity to the coast of the Beagle channel. These veinlets present a variable thickness between 0.5 and 5 cm, and lengths that may reach 10 m. The gangue is almost exclusively quartz and its main components are chalcopyrite and pyrite; minor and secondary elements are sphalerite, galena, cobaltite, covellite, malachite and azurite. The texture is typically that of open space filling. Cobaltite in these veinlets usually presents the same kind of replacement in its core by chalcopyrite resulting in "atoll" crystals.

Sulphide dissemination is present in all of the mapped area (Fig. 3), and consists of pyrite, framboidal pyrrhotite and graphite, in concentrations of 0.1 % or less. Geophysical studies carried out in the area, by IP and magnetometry, as well as soil geochemistry (Zubia et al., 1989a) showed sector anomalies (Fig. 3).

To the east, on the coast of the Beagle channel and at the foot of Mount Susana (Fig. 3), the Yahgán Formation consists mainly of black slates with abundant concordant intercalations of a pyritic chert. These intercalations are distributed within the 15 m thickness of the slates, and extend along strike for more than 1 km. The deformation affecting the rocks, such as microfolding and boudinage, are very evident in this pyritic chert (Plate 1-c, d) due to its differential behavior as compared with that of the slates. More than 50 % of the pyritic chert is recrystallized pyrite with a great tendency to automorphism, as well as pyritospheres. The coastal outcropping, which lacks vegetation, reveals the strong limonitic oxidation accompanying the pyritic chert. Chemical data suggest that this chert is an exhalite.

Mount Olivia

On the western slope of Mount Olivia, adjacent to national route 3, the Yahgán Formation metasedimentary rocks crop out with abundant intercalated beds of black slates. In several of these beds there are disseminated sulphides comprising 30 to 60 % of the rock. These concentrations are hosted in beds parallel to foliation and/or bedding. Their thickness may be up to 0.30 cm and their lengths follow the strike for up to 10 m. The only sulphide is medium to coarse grained pyrite that forms alternating beds of recrystallized pyrite and framboidal pyrite (Plate 2d). Limonitic oxidation is not well developed because of the small exposures the lower elevations, which are forested.

Sargent

This locality is on the northwest slope of Mount Olivia (Fig. 2). The occurrence is hosted in a rhyolitic body exposed within a glacial cirque located above the forest. The exposed rock is mainly reddish in the areas with greater pyritization. A (tectonic?) contact with black slates of theYahgán Formation can be observed in the region. In the cirque, there are outcroppings of metarhyolites with scarce and small intercalations of phyllites and dark slates. The relationship between these lithologies and the dominant rhyolitic body cannot be established due to the glacial denudation that has taken place. Nevertheless, foliation of the outcropping metasedimentary rocks is parallel to the rhyolite contacts. The rhyolites are coarse-

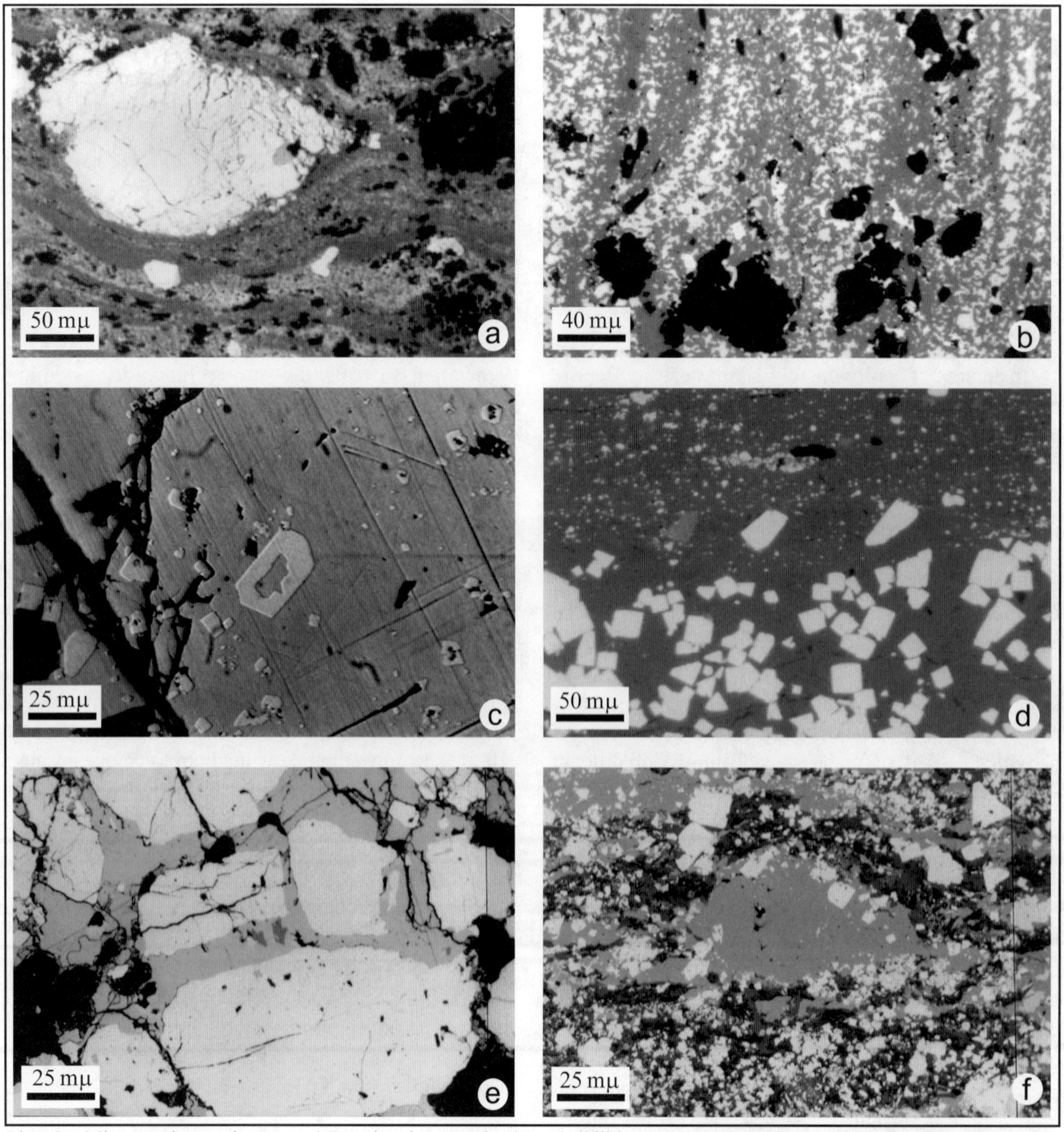

Plate 2 – Microscopic ore pictures a) Beatriz mine, massive lens. Poikilitic pyrite porphyroblasts with chalcopyrite inclusions, fractures filled with chalcopyrite, rotation of crystals and "pressure shadows" of fine grained sulphides (chalcopyrite + sphalerite, annealed texture). Quartz (black); b)Beatriz mine, massive lens. Annealed texture, sphalerite (dark grey) and chalcopyrite (light grey). Pyrite grains (white) and quartz (black); c) Beatriz mine, massive lens. Idiomorphic cobaltite crystals with cores replaced by chalcopyrite in coarse grained chalcopyrite; d) Mount Olivia. Black slate level with high concentration of disseminated pyrite. Upper part: fine grained framboidal pyrite. Down: idiomorphic pyrite e) Sargent, massive sulphide level. Recrystallized and fractured pyrite (clear). Chalcopyrite (medium) filling pyrite fractures with scarse sphalerite (dark grey). Black: rhyolite; f) Arroyo Rojo, massive sulphide lens. Pseudomylonitized sulphides with deformed sphalerite pophyroblasts accompained by pressure shadows (medium grey, big grain in the centre of picture). Abundant cubic pyrite disseminated (white), fine grained framboidal pyrite (upper right). Dark: rhyolite grained, have marked foliation, blastoporphyritic textures and a recrystallized matrix because of regional low-grade metamorphism (with abundant microscopic sericite, chlorite and prehnite replacement). Percentage dissemination of pyrite in rhyolites is variable and is generally associated with sericite. The beds of theYahgán Formation in contact with the rhyolite to the south are pyrite rich black slates, similar to those described along the west slope of Mount Olivia.

A 20 cm thick massive sulphide bed within the rhyolites is intercalated with thin slates, phyllites and chert and consists of recrystallized intensely fractured coarse-grained pyrite (Plate 2e). Pyrite fractures have been sealed by chalcopyrite accompanied by scarce sphalerite. The gangue consists of metarhyolite fragments and scarce quartz. Adjacent to this massive sulphide bed there are veinlets (up to 0.5 cm thick) that consist of galena, sphalerite and pyrite in quartz gangue.

Exploration by Yamana Resources Inc. (1998) indicates two drill intercepts with results in the following table:

Table 2. Intercepts in the Sargent drill holes (Yamana Resources Inc., 1998)

	Thickness	Cu %	Pb %	Zn %
Sargent S 97/12	0.30 m	1	10	27.5
Sargent S 97/9	1.3 m	3.9	-	-

Arroyo Rojo

The Arroyo Rojo massive sulphide deposit is located in an area of difficult access, to the southeast of the Sargent prospect (Fig. 2). At the headwaters of Rojo creek, and in a cirque, is a section of the Lemaire Formation, with a strikingly reddish colour formed by sulphide oxidation. To the south is the contact with the metasedimentary Yahgán Formation. There is no vegetation where a lens of massive sulphide crops out (Plate 1e) along 100 m with a maximum thickness of up to 6 m. This lens is hosted in the metarhyolites and is parallel to the regional foliation (Fig. 4). The metarhyolites are mainly blastoporphyritic with a recrystallized matrix due to greenschist facies metamorphism resulting in an abundance of quartz, sericite and chlorite. Deformation effects displayed by the phenocrysts include rotation and formation of "pressure shadows". Epidote and prehnite are common and minor carbonates and pyritization are abundant. The deformation has generated shearing structures (Plate 1f).

The shape of the massive sulphide lens, and its fragmentation into an upper or western portion and a lower or eastern portion, are due to the deformation. The contacts between the lens and the rhyolites consist of transitional zones of about 50 centimetres. In fact, the boundaries of the massive sulphide lens are defined by an increase of coarse recrystallized pyrite (up to 0.5 cm) in the rhyolite and occur as bands parallel to foliation. In the middle of the massive sulphide lens, large sphalerite porphyroblasts (0.5 to 1 cm) are more abundant than pyrite, forming a massive sulphide in which the gangue is mainly the rhyolite.

Sulphide textures are mainly mylonitic with a predominance of sphalerite lensoidal porphyroblasts. In comparison with the Beatriz mine, Arroyo Rojo contains minor chalcopyrite; sulphide grains are coarser and the carbonatic and siliceous gangue is minor or absent. The sulphides' gross banding has a simple mineralogy composed by sphalerite, galena and pyrite and minor chalcopyrite. Tetrahedrite and seleniferous bournonite are accessory minerals. Framboidal pyrite is very common. Microscopic textures are similar to those described for the Beatriz mine, showing metamorphism and deformation effects such as recrystallization of pyrite and sphalerite, annealed texture (sphalerite/galena), peripheral redistribution of chalcopyrite blebs in recrystallized sphalerite, lenticulation of the sphalerite porphyroblasts, "pressure shadows", etc. (Plate 2f). No cobalt-bearing minerals have been found.

Figure 4, reproduced from Yamana Resources Inc. (1998), indicates the intercept values obtained in drill holes 3, 4 and 5 carried out by Westmin. These drill holes have more zinc and less copper than the Beatriz mine.

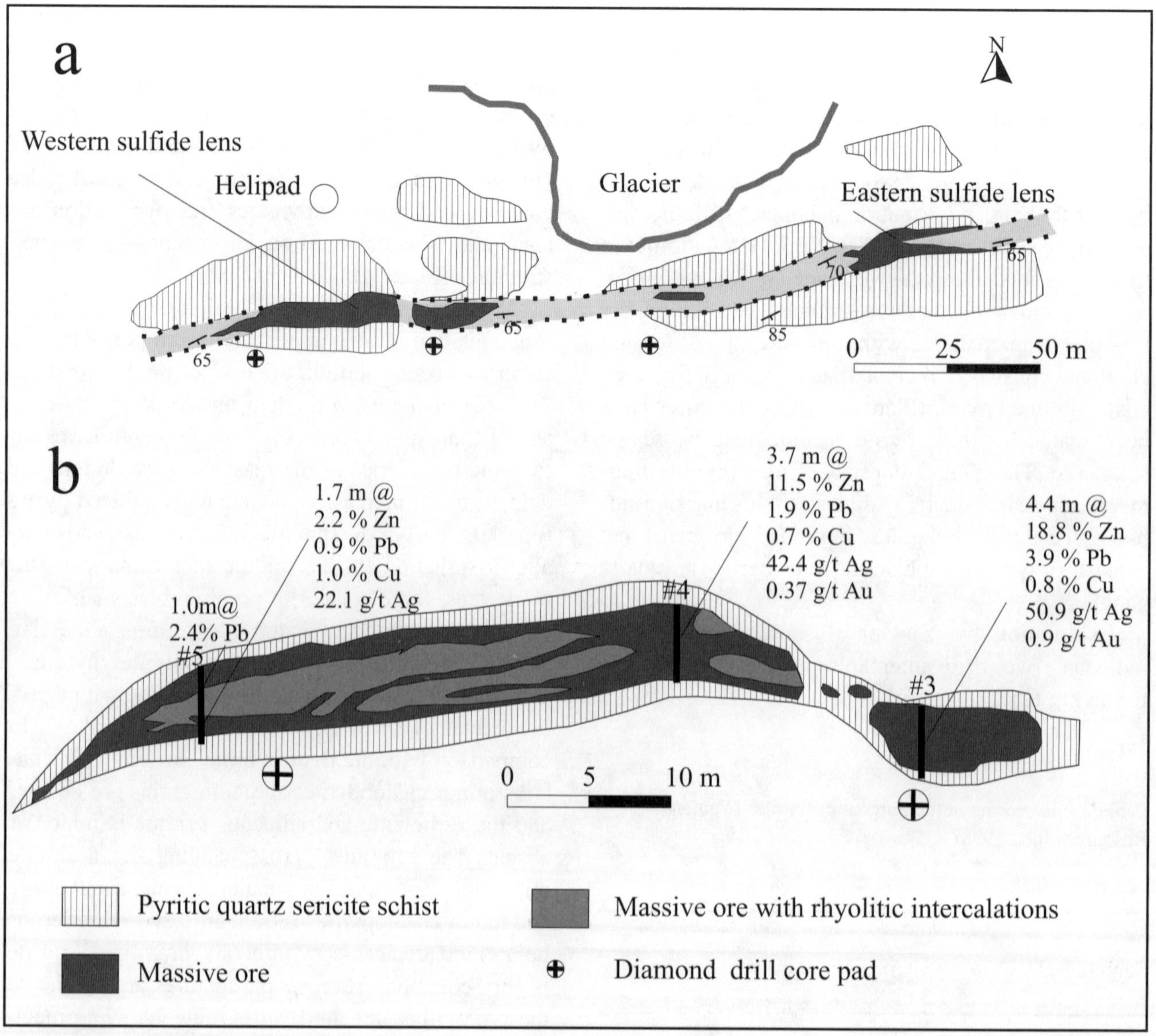

Figure 4. a- Geological sketch of massive sulfiide lenses in Arroyo Rojo. b- Detail of the western sulphide lens. (After Yamana Resources Inc., 1998).

Rancho Hambre

In Rancho Grande (Fig. 2) Lemaire Formation metarhyolites and metarhyodacites and dark slates of theYahgán Formation occur conformably. Foliation is present in both units with a general east-west strike. The metavolcanic rocks are blastoporphyritic, with a recrystallized matrix due to regional low grade metamorphism; phenocrysts present deformation effects such as fracturing, tearing, granulation, "pressure shadows", rotation, crumbly extinction, microfaults, etc. The matrix has recrystallized sericite and chlorite. Dissemination of automorphic pyrite or pyritospheres reaches 1% in the form of generally oxidized, isolated crystals or oriented lenticular groups following the general foliation. Both in the slates and in the volcanics there are veinlets hosted in tensional structures or in foliation planes, consisting of carbonates, quartz and/or very scarce gypsum.

The sulphides observed in this locality are parse

and in thin short stockwork veinlets (maximum 0.5 cm thick). In addition to this, there is very fine grained disseminated pyrite in the metavolcanic-metasedimentary sequence. The veinlets contain quartz and/or carbonate gangue and pyrite as the most abundant components with subordinate sphalerite, galena and chalcopyrite. The microscopic texture corresponds to open space filling.

Puerto Almanza

This locality is on the coast of the Beagle channel (Fig. 2). There is an outcropping section of the Yahgán Formation along some 40 m, with 15 m thickness with a deep reddish tinting, which consists of gray and purple slates, with some intercalated beds of metagraywackes. The dominant foliation trends east-west and deformation appears as local fracturing, microfractures and microlenticulation of its components.

The reddish tinting is due to the presence of oxidized pyrite hosted in the metasedimentary rocks. The dissemination follows the foliation planes, conforming at millimetric levels. Fine grained, automorphic pyrite is dominant, although there are also abundant beds of pyritospheres. In some of these beds, pyrite and pyrrhotite are abundant, whereas sphalerite, galena and chalcopyrite are minor constituents. The sulphides show a deformation caused by crushing, which makes them elongated following the foliation. Coarser-grained sulphides are hosted in quartz-carbonate veinlets within foliation planes.

Other localities

While the area of this survey goes up to Puerto Almanza in the east, Acevedo and Radoszta (1987) recognized pyritic occurrences up to Buen Suceso bay in Le Maire strait (Fig. 1c), always with a spatial connection with the volcanic rocks of the Lemaire Formation.

GEOCHEMICAL AND ISOTOPIC STUDIES

Geochemistry

In addition to chemical analyses of rhyolites (ICP, XRF, NA), evaluations of metal contents (NA, AA, ICP) have been carried out on chips of the pyritic chert, as well as REE analysis (Intertek T.S., Vancouver). Several electronic microprobe analyses were carried out (Universidad de Oviedo, Spain and University of Salzburg, Austria) for the most abundant sulphides. Table. 3 shows all data plotted in Figure 5.

The REE pattern of the pyritic chert is similar to that of the rhyolites (Fig. 5). In addition to this, a triangular diagram (Cu+Co+Ni / Fe / Mn) to discriminate hydrogen rich sediments from hydrothermal alteration (Bonatti, 1975, Fig. 5) indicates that the two analyzed samples of the pyritic chert from Mount Susana (obtained by "chipping") belong to the hydrothermal field.

The trace metal contents of the massive sulphides (Beatriz mine and Arroyo Rojo) when compared with the pyritic chert (Fig. 5), are similar; however, Cu, Zn and Pb are not.

It should be mentioned that zinc contents for the pyritic chert fluctuate between 100 and 700 ppm for the analysis of 3 samples. Thus, the pyritic cherts represent in the Yahgán Formation another expression of a hydrothermal episode with a high silica and pyrite content that, in addition, are hosted in similar levels to that of the rhyolitic bodies (Ametrano and Paar, 1996).

As can be seen in Figure 5 concerning the Beatriz and Arroyo Rojo sulphides, Beatriz has higher contents of Co, Cu, As, Se, Bi and Ag. Cobalt is contained both in cobaltite and pyrite. On the other hand, Arroyo Rojo contains more lead and zinc, and chalcopyrite is subordinate. The metal contents in Beatriz are similar to those found for late Cu-rich basal portions (Bi, Se, Co) of VMS systems. In contrast, Arroyo Rojo shows a dominant Pb-Zn composition which is consistent with an early of the most widely accepted VMS model (Marcoux et al., 1996; Eldridge et al. 1983; Large, 1992).

Figure 5 shows a chart of cadmium contents of sphalerite vs. their mole % in FeS. A slight increase in FeS content can be observed in sphalerite from stockworks at Beatriz, Sargent and Rancho Hambre as compared with the massive sulphides of Beatriz and Arroyo Rojo, not surpassing 10 mole %, as it is the case in the Iberian Belt (Marcoux et al., 1996). Relating to cadmium, all the sphalerites are below the range of epithermal sphalerite established by Bortnikov (1995) - between 0.5 and 2 weight %.

Galena on the charts in Figure 5 clearly shows the

Table. 3 - Chemical data

Chemical data of rhyolites: B and S (Mount Susana), OL (monte Olivia), RH (Rancho Hambre), Sg (Sargent), AR (Arroyo Rojo) - weight % oxides

	SiO_2	TiO_2	Al_2O_3	Fe_2O_3	FeO	MnO	MgO	CaO	Na_2O	K_2O
RH4	82.33	0.09	8.67	1.59	0.32	0	0.08	0.05	1.67	5.18
S1	81.75	0.06	10.77	0.5	0.39	0	0.07	0.11	6.3	0.07
AR1	78.69	0.14	10.14	1.42	1.11	0.04	1.72	3.37	2.13	1.2
OL1	81.18	0.1	10.41	1.24	0.45	0.01	0.46	5.5	0.04	0.61
RH3	75.41	0.14	12.06	1.99	1.08	0.02	0.93	0.33	1.76	6.27
Sg9	81.75	0.09	4.09	6.53	3.86	0.09	3.42	0.03	0.05	0.06
AR2t	70.55	0.99	12.12	5.81	1	0.05	4.77	0.6	0	3.94
B12	79.28	0.07	11.22	1.13	0.45	0	0.09	0.08	3.27	4.4

	P_2O_5	LOI	Sc	Rb	Ba	Sr	Nb	Zr	Ti	Y
RH4	0.01	0.69	0	103	1338	30	7	109	538	12
S1	0	0.25	4	3	22	80	8.9	100	357	17
AR1	0.04	3.44	4	46	290	227	9.1	192	852	69
OL1	0	1.33	4	27	36	517	7	171	600	34
RH3	0.01	1.01	76	143	669	43	7.9	161	833	33
Sg9	0.04	2.78	3	2	0	0	4.9	74	532	12
AR2t	0.16	5.33	34	146	1910	21	4.2	88	5957	14
B12	0	0.63	6	93	3098	86	10	107	420	16

	Th	U	La	Ce	Nd	Sm	Eu	Tb	Yb	Lu
RH4	9.47	2.99	20.94	42.87	16.95	2.59	0.3	0.5	1	0.2
S1	9.92	2.97	12.89	29.75	13.88	2.68	0.2	0.1	1.98	0
AR1	12.19	3.05	16.25	35.55	21.33	5.08	0.81	1.02	5.08	0
OL1	10.01	3	31.02	65.04	30.02	5.7	0.9	0.4	3	0
RH3	12.91	3.97	43.71	87.42	37.75	6.66	1.09	0.99	2.98	0.5
Sg9	3.94	1.97	1.97	3.94	6.89	0.69	0.2	0.39	0.98	0
AR2t	1.57	0.1	5.23	18.83	5.23	2.41	0.73	0.1	1.05	0
B12	12	3	26.01	55.02	18.01	3.6	0.6	0	2	0.3

Chemical data of pyritic exhalites and massive ores of Arroyo Rojo and Beatriz mine - elements ppm (Au ppb)

	Cr	Ni	Co	Cu	Pb	Zn	Mo	Ag	Au	Hg
EP1	146	38	5	73	32	100	34	4.2	38	0.498
EP2	529	101	15	129	68	685	6	2.4	14	0.098
EP3	180		7			148	54	5	56	2
AR1	100	82	9	5000	22300	63000	11	93	492	
MB4		49	120	10500	5547	20291		267	68	

	As	Se	Sb	Te	Bi
EP1	164		18		
EP2	336		1		
EP3	250	30	35		
AR1	231	350	94	1	122
MB4	426	932	30.5	1	523

fluctuating silver contents at the Beatriz mine. Also, the Beatriz mine has higher silver contents than the massive sulphide at Arroyo Rojo. Likewise, selenium and bismuth have higher contents in Beatriz sulphides than Arroyo Rojo. The correlation of Bi/Ag is very good for galena. In every case, stockwork galena has intermediate values.

We conducted more than 100 electron microprobe analyses of pyrites whose results support the following conclusions:

- pyrite of Arroyo Rojo has a higher zinc content (up to 1.5 weight %), demonstrating this abundance made it possible for zinc to enter the pyrite structure;
- gold contents are variable, and the higher contents are accompanied by an arsenic increase;
- the highest gold (0.10 and 0.37 weight %) and arsenic (0.06 and 0.21 weight %) contents were found in disseminated pyrite of Mount Olivia;
- framboidal pyrites have higher arsenic values than the other pyrites, the recrystallization of these framboidal pyrites has been accompanied by a lossarsenic;
- gold was detected, although in lower concentrations than at Mount Olivia, in pyrite of the Estancia Túnel, Rancho Hambre, Sargent dissemination and Sargent chalcopyrite of the massive sulphide.

Lead isotopes

Isotopic analyses of lead were carried out at the University of Carleton, Canada. Two samples of galena from the massive sulphide layers were analyzed, one from Arroyo Rojo and the other from Beatriz (Table. 4).

In comparison with the Stacey-Kramers (1975) average crustal evolution curve, both samples are within the curve error and indicate ages of less than 100 Ma, but this age could be influenced by the metamorphism that affected the sulphides. If this happened, lead in sulphides can include the original lead plus lead introduced to the system during the metamorphism. Also, a small amount of introduced lead could have affected the results, due to uranium caught in pyrite. However, no uranium was found in the concentrate and it should not be considered a major factor. Finally, the lead has a crustal source and the age should be that of metamorphism but the opening of the system adds doubts on it.

Table 4. Isotopic Pb values in 2 samples.

Galena	$^{208}Pb/^{204}Pb$	$^{207}Pb/^{204}Pb$	$^{206}Pb/^{204}Pb$
Beatriz	38.501	15.652	18.504
A.Rojo	38.505	15.645	18.645

*2 sigma = $\pm$ 0.012, 0.014, 0.048 Standard = NBS 981
**Data correction by fractionating + 0.13 % / atomic mass unit according to NBS 981.

Table 5. Results of S isotopes

Mineral	$\delta^{34}S$ ‰
Py Beatriz	0.61
Py A.Rojo	1.60
Sph. Beatriz	-0.35
Sph.A.Rojo	0.79
Py chert Susana M.	7.88

Sulphur Isotopes

Sulphur isotopes were analyzed at the Service of Stable Isotopes of the Universidad de Salamanca, Spain. Two pyrite samples and two sphalerite samples from massive sulphide layers were studied (Beatriz and Arroyo Rojo), as well as pyrite from the pyritic chert at Mount Susana. The standard used was NBS 123.

Values of massive sulphide are within the ranges of magmatic sulphide, more precisely of massive sulphides or hydrothermal processes. On the other hand, sulphur from the pyritic chert at Mount Susana could indicate a complementary contribution of seawater sulphur (Rollinson, 1993).

With pyrite-sphalerite pairs of the massive sulphide, Ohmoto and Ray's (1979) method was applied to calculate temperatures. These calculated temperatures may be related to the metamorphism.

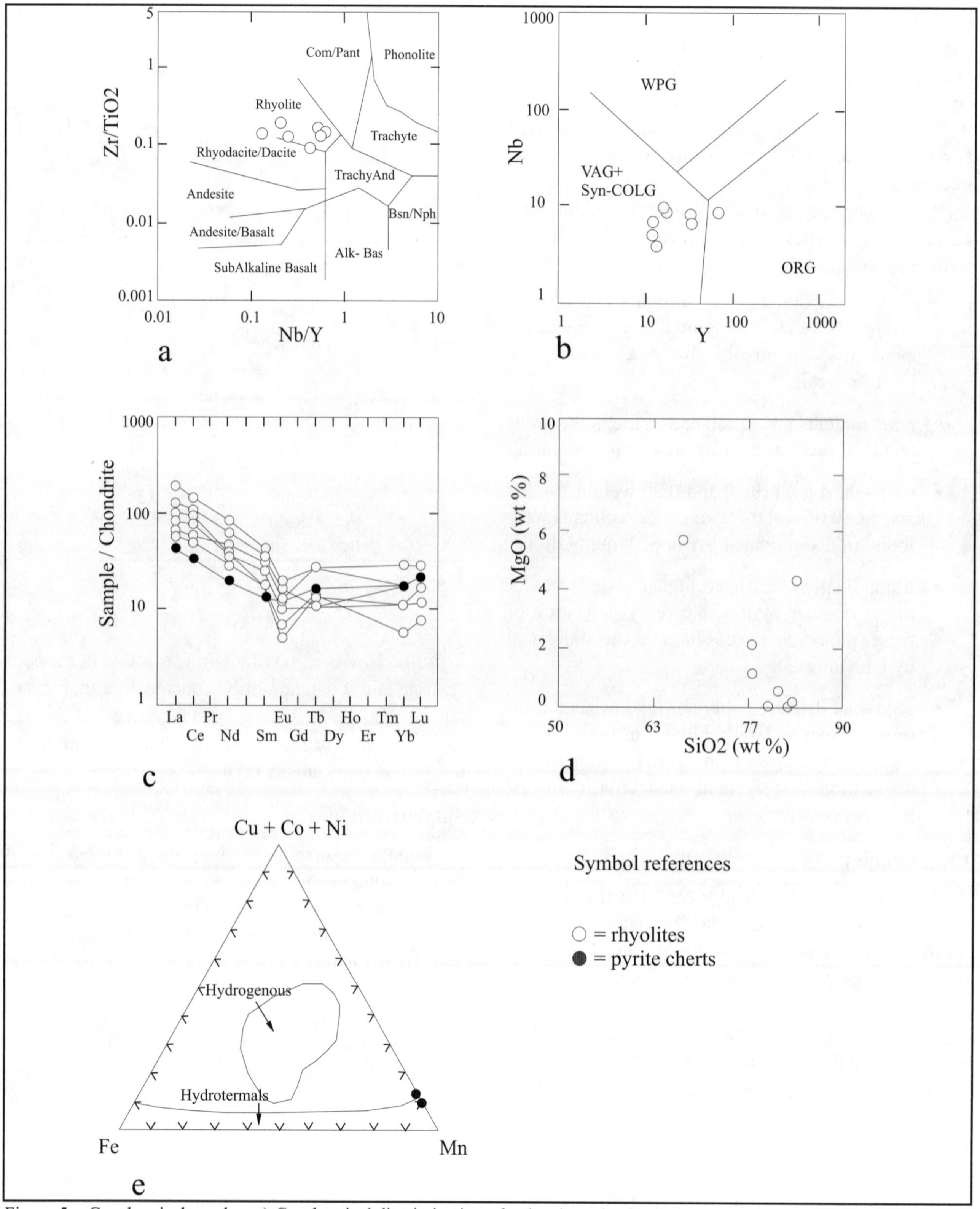

Figure 5. Geochemical graphs. a) Geochemical discrimination of volcanic rock of Winchester and Floyd, (1977); b) Discrimination diagram of the tectonic setting of Pearce et al., (1984); c) Chondrite normalized REE distribution; d) MgO vs SiO_2 relation.; e)- Cu+Co+Ni – Mn – Fe diagram, fields after Bonatti (1975);

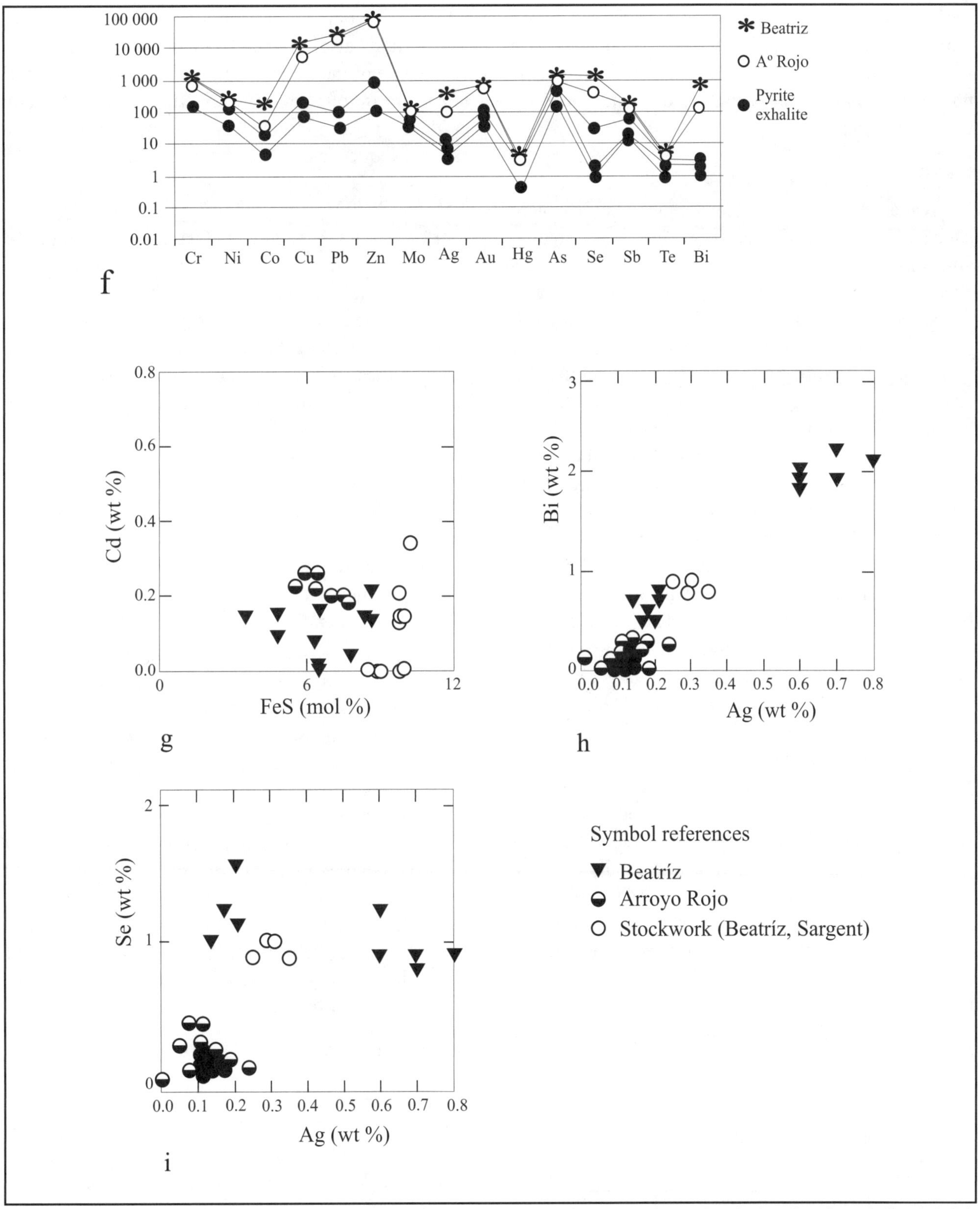

Figure 5 (Continued) f) Metal contents of massive sulphides ores (Arrroyo Rojo and Beatriz mine) and pyrite exhalites; g) Cd vs FeS in sphalerites; h) Bi vs Ag in galenas; i) Se vs Ag in galenas.

The higher recrystallization observed in the granulometry of Arroyo Rojo ore could be related to a somewhat higher temperature reached by metamorphism in this area; thus these are unusual values for this kind of deposits.

GENETIC MODEL

Available data and the geological environment suggest the model of deposits related to submarine volcanism of the massive sulphide - type, with overprinted metamorphism. However, many detailed volcanism studies need to be carried out to distinguish the areas with submarine characteristics from those which might be subaerial. This could be useful when prospecting.

Barrie and Hannington (1997) classify the VMS into 5 types, according to the hosting lithological environment. According to current knowledge of the region, occurrences at Tierra del Fuego would be bimodal-siliciclastic - type (approx. 50 % of silicic volcanics and 50 % of siliciclastics). Franklin et al. (1998) considers this type to be located in arc and back-arc tectonic environments. The latter authors have established a correlation between the deposit volume and the age. Those VMS with larger volumes correspond to Paleozoic, whereas Mesozoic or Cenozoic VMS are smaller.

Canadian Archean massive sulphide deposits, Kuroko deposits in Japan, Australian VMS and the Iberian pyritic belt have permitted a model definition establishing that the upper part of these systems is comprised of massive sulphide (essentially Pb-Zn), and underlying them are Cu-rich massive sulphides and/or a stringer area. On the other hand, studies of Marcoux et al. (1996) agree with those of Eldrige et al.(1983) and the VMS model of Large (1992): Cobalt sulfarsenides were formed at the beginning of VMS genesis, bismuth-bearing mineral phases being deposited during the last episode of copper fluids, which also contained bismuth (tellurium, selenium). These fluids also produced a chalcopyrite precipitate at the base of the initial sulphide mass, thus constituting a cupriferous zone ("interaction zone", Marcoux et al., 1996) forming chalcopyrite blebs in sphalerite as a consequence of replacement processes.

Table. 6. Temperatures calculated with Ohmoto and Ray's (1979) method, using $\delta^{34}S$ of the pair py/sph.

Massive ore Beatriz	247° C – 292° C
Massive ore A. Rojo	293° C - 342.5° C

CONCLUSIONS

Based on the chemical data obtained from the massive sulphides so far, and on the chemical composition of their sulphides, it can be assumed that Beatriz mine and Arroyo Rojo are fragments of the model, the former being a basal portion with a stringer area, and the latter a cuspate section. The action of late cupriferous fluids is demonstrated in the Beatriz mine by abundant chalcopyrite blebs in sphalerite and replacement of cobaltite by chalcopyrite. Absence of barite and presence of pyrrhotite and magnetite are in agreement with an euxinic environment. Fragmentation of the deposits would be coherent with the structure of the tectonic plates of the Andes of Tierra del Fuego.

Some considerations should be noted for the district:

1) Several areas with colour anomalies (Fig. 2) encourage the continuation of prospecting, despite difficult access to the area.
2) The volcano-sedimentary group of the back-arc basin has had other minor hydrothermal episodes, such as those represented by the surveyed pyritic chert.
3) The existence in Chile, within the same arc, of economically viable deposits, and others still being surveyed, indicate a defined metallotect.
4) The disseminated and stockwork occurrences are not a separate VMS model, but are part of the already defined schemes for the most important districts.

ACKNOWLEDGMENTS

Acknowledgments to the Consejo Nacional de Investigaciones Científicas y Técnicas (Conicet, PIA n°6803/96) and to the Servicio Geológico Minero Argentino (SEGEMAR) for their economical support to carry out this survey; to Prof. Dr. W. H. Paar for the great quantity of microprobe analysis; to Yamana Resources Inc. for allowing access to their properties;

to Westmin for their logistic support during field work; to Dr. Donald Sangster for the valuable discussions and the contacts facilitated for isotope studies, and to Dr. Milka K. de Brodtkorb for her support and suggestions.

References

Acevedo, R. D., 1996. Los mecanismos sustitutivos y los factores de evolución en los anfíboles de la Hornblendita Ushuaia, Tierra del Fuego. Revista de la Asociación Geológica Argentina, 51 (1): 69-77.

Acevedo R. D. y A. P. Radoszta, 1987. Manifestaciones piríticas y anomalías metálicas en la costa sur de Tierra del Fuego, Rep. Argentina. X Congreso Geológico Argentino, Actas, 2: 227-230.

Ametrano S. y Paar W., 1996. La composición química de los sulfuros de mina Beatriz, Tierra del Fuego: un aporte para su interpretación metalogenética. XIII Congreso Geológico Argentino y III Congreso de Exploración de Hidrocarburos, Actas, 3: 159-172.

Ametrano S. y Paar W., 1996. Cobaltita en la manifestación de sulfuros masivos, Area mina Beatriz, Prov. Tierra del Fuego. III Reunión de Mineralogía y Metalogenia. Universidad Nacional de La Plata. Publicaciones Inremi N° 5: 55-61.

Ametrano S., Zubia M., Etcheverry R., Godeas M. y Echeveste H., 1998. Depósitos polimetálicos de sulfuros masivos metamorfizados en los Andes Fueguinos. Provincia de Tierra del fuego, Argentina. X Congreso Latinoamericano de Geología y VI Congreso Nacional de Geología Económica, Actas, 3: 148.

Barrie T., y M.D. Hannington (eds.), 1997. Volcanic-associated massive sulphide deposits: Processes and examples in modern and ancient settings. Geological Association of Canada. Society of Economic Geologists. Short Course, Ottawa, Canada, 418.

Bonatti E., 1975. Metallogenesis at oceanic spreading centers. Ann. Review of Earth & Planetary Sciences, 3: 401-413.

Borrello A.V., 1969. Los geosinclinales de la Argentina. Dirección Nacional de Geología y Minería. Anales 14: 188 pp.

Borrello A.V., 1972. Cordillera Fueguina. En Geología Regional Argentina (editor Leanza). Academia Nacional de Ciencias: 741-753. Córdoba, Argentina.

Bortnikov N.S., Dobrovol´skaya M.G., Genkin A.D., Naumov V.B. y V.V. Shapenko. 1995. Sphalerite-galena Geothermometers: Distribution of Cadmium, Manganese, and Fractionation of Sulfur Isotopes. Economic Geology, 90: 155-180.

Broili, C., Klohn, M. and Hodder, R.W., 2000. Exploration, geology and mineral deposits of the Fin del Mundo VMS project, Tierra del Fuego, Argentina. In R.L. Sherlock and M.A.V. Logan, (eds.), Volcanogenic Massive Sulfide Deposits of Latin America. Mineral Deposit Division, Geological Association of Canada, 567-591.

Bruhn R.L. y Dalziel I., 1977. Destruction of the early cretaceous marginal basin in the Andes of Tierra del Fuego. En Talwani M. y Pitman W. (Edits.): Island Arcs, Deep Sea Trenches and Back Arc Basins. American Geophysical Union, 1: 395-405.

Bruhn R.L., Stern C. Y M. J. De Wit, 1978. Field and geochemical data bearing on the development of a Mesozoic, volcano-tectonic rift zone and back-arc basin in the Southernmost South America. Earth & Planetary Sciences Letters, 41: 32-46.

Caminos R., Haller M., Lapido O., Lizuain A., Page R. y Ramos V., 1981. Reconocimiento geológico de los Andes Fueguinos. Territorio Nacional de Tierra del Fuego. 8° Congreso Geológico Argentino, Actas, 3: 754-786.

Cingolani C., 1989. Transect: Tierra del Fuego – Diego Ramirez Islands (Argentina-Chile). Reunión sobre Geotransectas de América del Sur, Actas: 9-13. Mar del Plata, Argentina.

Dalziel I.W.D., De Wit M.J. y K.F. Palmer, 1974. Fossil marginal basin in the southern Andes. Nature, 250: 291.

Dalziel I.W.D., 1981. Back-arc basin in the southern Andes: a review and critical reappraisal. Phil. Transactions of the Royal Society of London, A300: 319-335.

Dalziel, I.W.D., Storey, B.C., Garrett, S.W., Grunow, A.M., Herrod, L.D. y R, J. Pankhurst, 1987. Extensional tectonics and the fragmentation of Gondwanaland. En: Continental Extensional Tectonics, Coward, Dewey y Hancock (ed.). Blackwell Scientific Publications, 637 pp.

Eldridge C.S., Barton P.B. y H. Ohmoto, 1983. Mineral textures and their bearing on formation of the kuroko orebodies. Economic Geology. Monograph 5: 241-281.

Franklin J.M., Hannington M.D., Jonason I.R. y C.T. Barrie, 1998. Arc-related volcanogenic massive sulphide deposits. In: Metallogeny of volcanic arcs, British Columbia Geological Survey, Short Course Notes, open File 1998-5, Section B.

Fuenzalida R. y Covacevich C., 1988. Volcanismo y bioestratigrafía del Jurásico superior y Cretácico inferior en Cordillera Patagónica, Región de Magallanes, Chile. 5° Congreso Geológico Chileno, Actas, 3: 159-183.

Haller M. y Delpino D., 1989. Una ofiolita desmembrada en la Isla Grande de Tierra del Fuego. Reunión sobre Geotransectas de América del Sur. Actas: 160-164. Mar del Plata, Argentina.

Katz H.R., 1972. Plate tectonics and orogenic belts in the south-east Pacific. Nature, 237: 331-332.

Kranck E.H., 1932. Geological investigations in the Cordillera of Tierra del Fuego. Acta Geographica, 4(2): 1-231.

Kittl E., 1931. Los yacimientos auríferos de la República Argentina, su génesis y su posición geológica. Revista Minera, III, 6.

Large R., 1992. Australian Volcanic-Hosted Massive Sulfide Deposits: Features, Styles, and Genetic Models. Economic Geology, 97: 471-510.

- Lentz D. R., 1996. Trace-Element Systematics of Felsic Volcanic Rocks Associated with Massive-Sulphide Deposits in the Bathurst Mining Camp. En: D. A. Wyman (Ed.), Trace Element Geochemistry of Volcanic Rocks: Applications for

Massive Sulphide Ecploration. Geological Association of Canada, Short Course Notes Volume 12. Winnipeg.

Marcoux E., Moëlo Y. y M. Leistel. 1996. Bismuth and cobalt minerals as indicators of stringer zones to massive sulphide deposits. Iberian Pyrite Belt. Mineralium Deposita, 31: 1-26.

Ohmoto H. y R. O. Rye, 1979. Isotopes of sulfur and carbon. In: Barnes H.L. (ed.), Geochemistry of hydrothermal ore deposits: 509-567. Wiley, New York.

Olivero E., Acevedo R. y Martinioni D., 1997. Geología del Mesozoico de bahía Ensenada, Tierra del Fuego. Asociación Geológica Argentina. Revista, 52 (2): 169-179.

Pearce J.A., Harris N.B.W. and Tindle A.G., 1984. Trace element discrimination diagrams for the tectonic interpretation of granitic rocks. Journalof Petrology, v.25: 956-983.

Pesce A., Page S. y N. Rubinstein, 1996. Características petrográficas y eruptivas de la Formación Lemaire, en el área de las Termas del Río Valdez, Tierra del Fuego. XIII Congreso Geológico Argentino y III Congreso sobre Exploración de Hidrocarburos, Actas, 5: 251-256.

Quartino B.J., Acevedo R.D. y Scalabrini Ortiz J., 1989. Rocas eruptivas volcanógena entre Monte Olivia y Paso Garibaldi, Isla Grande de Tierra del Fuego. Asociación Geológica Argentina, Revista, 44 (1-4): 328-335.

Rollinson H. R., 1993. Using Geochemical Data. Longman Scientific & Technical, New York.

Stacey J.S. y J.D. Kramers, 1975. Approximation of Terrestrial Lead Isotope Evolution by Two Stage Model. Earth & Planetary Sciences Letters, 26: 207-221.Suárez M., Hervé M. y Puig. A., 1985 a. Hoja Isla Hoste e islas adyacentes. XII Región. Servicio Nacional de Geología y Minería, Carta Geológica de Chile, 65.

Suárez M., Puig A. y Hervé M., 1985 b. Depósitos de un abanico submarino de Tras-Arco del Mesozoico superior: Formación Yahgán, Islas Hoste y Navarino. IV Congreso Geológico Chileno (Antofagasta), Actas, 1: 534-545.

Thomas E.R., 1949. Geology and petroleum exploration in Magallanes Province, Chile. Bulletin American Association Petroleum Geology, 33-9: 1157.

YAMANA Resources Inc., 1998. Proyecto "Fin del Mundo", Tierra del Fuego, Argentina. Reporte, 4.

Winchester J.A. and Floyd P.A., 1977. Geochemical discrimination of different magma series and their differentiation products using inmobile elements. Chemical Geology, v.20: 325-343.

Zubia M., Godeas M. y Ametrano S., 1989 a. Area mina Beatriz, Territorio Nacional de Tierra del Fuego, República Argentina: una manifestación de metales de base estratoligada y singenética. En Brodtkorb M. y Schalamuk I. (Ed.). Proyecto 242 IGCP, Simposios sobre el Cretácico de América Latina, Actas, C: 15-44. Buenos Aires.

Zubia M., Godeas M. y Ametrano S., 1989 b. Un episodio metalogenético en la Isla Grande de Tierra del Fuego. Reunión sobre Geotransectas de América del Sur, Actas: 213-217. Mar del Plata, Argentina.

THE VMS SANTA ELENA DEPOSIT, SAN JUAN PROVINCE, ARGENTINA

EDUARDO O.ZAPPETTINI
Instituto de Geología y Recursos Minerales – SEGEMAR. Avda. Julio A.Roca 651. 1067 Buenos Aires. Argentina.
E-mail: ezappe@secind.mecon.ar

MILKA K. DE BRODTKORB
CONICET- Universidad de Buenos Aires. Paso 258 –9 A. 1640 Martinez. Argentina. E-mail: milkabro@gl.fcen.uba.ar

ABSTRACT

The Santa Elena deposit is located near the city of Calingasta, province of San Juan, Argentina, on the western side of the Precordillera. The region is characterized by a sequence of turbidites and shales in part associated with basalts locally with pillowed lavas, of Ordovician age. The orebodies are related to the basaltic sequence. The primary sulphide ore has been explored with small underground workings. The mineral association consists of pyrite, marcasite, pyrrhotite, sphalerite, chalcopyrite, arsenopyrite and galena with sulfosalt inclusions, associated to quartz and carbonates. Grades are 1.84 % Pb, 2.51 % Zn, 0.08 % Cu, 83g/t Ag and 4.51g/t Au. The deposit was exploited in the oxidation zone for iron sulphates. Isotopic compositions of pyrite and galena were determined. The $\delta^{34}S$ in pyrite gives +0.2 ‰ ± 0.5 and $\delta^{34}S$ in galena +1.5 ‰ ± 0.5 values. It is considered that this VMS deposit is related to hydrothermal facies associated to the basic magmatism of ordovician age.

INTRODUCTION

The Santa Elena deposit is located in the northern bank of Alcaparrosa river close to km 128 of the national road N° 20, in the Calingasta Department, province of San Juan. The road is now closed, so the deposit can be reached through the Uspallata Valley from Mendoza City. The coordinates of the deposit are 31°20´ South Latitude and 69°25´ West Longitude.

REGIONAL GEOLOGY

The deposit is located in the western side of the Precordillera. The region is characterized by a sequence of turbidites and shales (Don Polo and Alcaparrosa Formations) locally associated with basalts, locally with pillowed lavas (Fig. 1). The sequence is overlain by Silurian shales (Calingasta Formation) and Devonian shales, siltstone, sandstones and conglomerates (El Planchón Formation), Carboniferous sandstones and conglomerates (Del Ratón Formation) and lower Permian sandstones and conglomerates (Del Salto Formation) (Furque and Caballé, 1986).

The whole assemblege is intruded by Permian rhyodacitic-monzonitic subvolcanic stocks that carry a minor Cu-Mo porphyry-type mineralization, dated 267 ± 4 Ma (Sillitoe, 1977). The igneous event is ascribed to the Meso-Choiyoi Intrusive Phase (Caballé, 1986).

The immediate stratigraphy near Santa Elena deposit consists of sedimentary and volcanic sequences (Alcaparrosa Formation) intruded by subvolcanic porphyries. In the Alcaparrosa valley the sedimentary sequence is characterized by gray shales, green limolites, in thin layers, interbedded with psamitic layers. This sequence comprises a very important basic magmatism that includes hypabisal diabase dykes and sills, and submarine pillowed lava flows, known as the Santa Elena Basalts (Meissl and Maidana, 1983).

The pillow lava layers are up to 30 m thick. Along the national road N° 20, there are outcrops of typical lava flows with pillows with diameters between 0.3 and 1 m. The strike of layers varies between N 45°W and N 30°E, with low angle dips (locally up to vertical angles). They are chemically alkaline tholeiitic

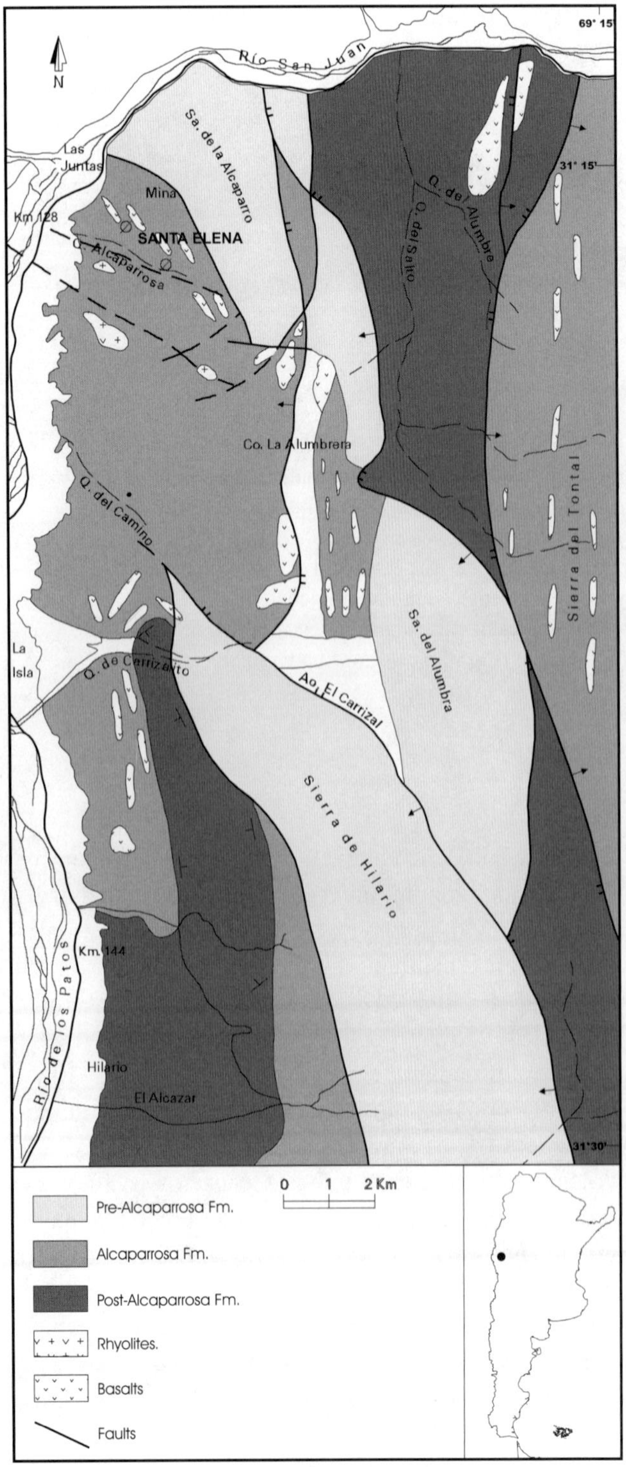

Figure.1 Geology of the Sierra de Alcaparrosa, San Juan (modified from Furque and Caballé, 1986).

basalts. Quartino (1971) recognized associated spillites.

The hypabisal dykes have a typical diabassic structure, formed by basic plagioclase, partly replaced by chlorite and sericite, and locally surrounded by clinopyroxene with ophitic to subophitic structures. As a consequence of alteration, outcrops have red to brownish-red colours.

Kay et al. (1984) made trace element analyses of the basalts, demonstrating an affinity with back arc basin setting, suggesting that their genesis is related with an early oceanic rift close to the continent (Ramos et al., 1984). The presence of chert layers associated with thin layers of limestone is characteristic in Alcaparrosa Formation, close to the top and overlaying lava flows (Quartino et al., 1971; Haller and Ramos, 1984).

MINERALIZATION

The orebodies are emplaced in the basaltic sequence. Meissl and Maidana (1983) have recognized three main mineralized sectors: Alcaparrosa structure, with N 80°W strike, and 60°SSW dip, 260 m length and 6.5 m thick; Alta structure, with N 60° E strike and 63°SE dip, 150 m length; and Diagonal structure, with N 15°E to N 35°E strike and 35°ESE dip, 320 length and 1 to 1.5 m thick (Fig. 2). Other minor orebodies in the region are located 1.8 km SE of Santa Elena (Nira mine and Don Daniel, Quartino et al., 1971).

The Santa Elena was discovered at the beginning of the century and developed for its iron sulphates mineralization. In 1938 the primary sulphide ore was recognized (Stappenbeck, 1910; Angelelli and Trelles, 1938).

The deposit has been exploited in the oxidation zone for iron sulphates. The mine produced 7,000 tonnes at 25 % FeO grade between 1941 and 1974 (Angelelli, 1984). In 1938 Angelelli and Trelles (1938) determined up to 9,500 tonnes of iron oxides resources. Iron sulphates were exploited superficially from trenches. The main work is an 145 m length by 8 m wide open pit, with a 20 m deep shaft in its central part and a 2 m length gallery (Angelelli, 1984). The primary sulphide ore was explored with underground works (shafts and galleries). Grades determined are 1.84 % Pb, 2.51 % Zn, 0.08 % Cu, 83 g/t

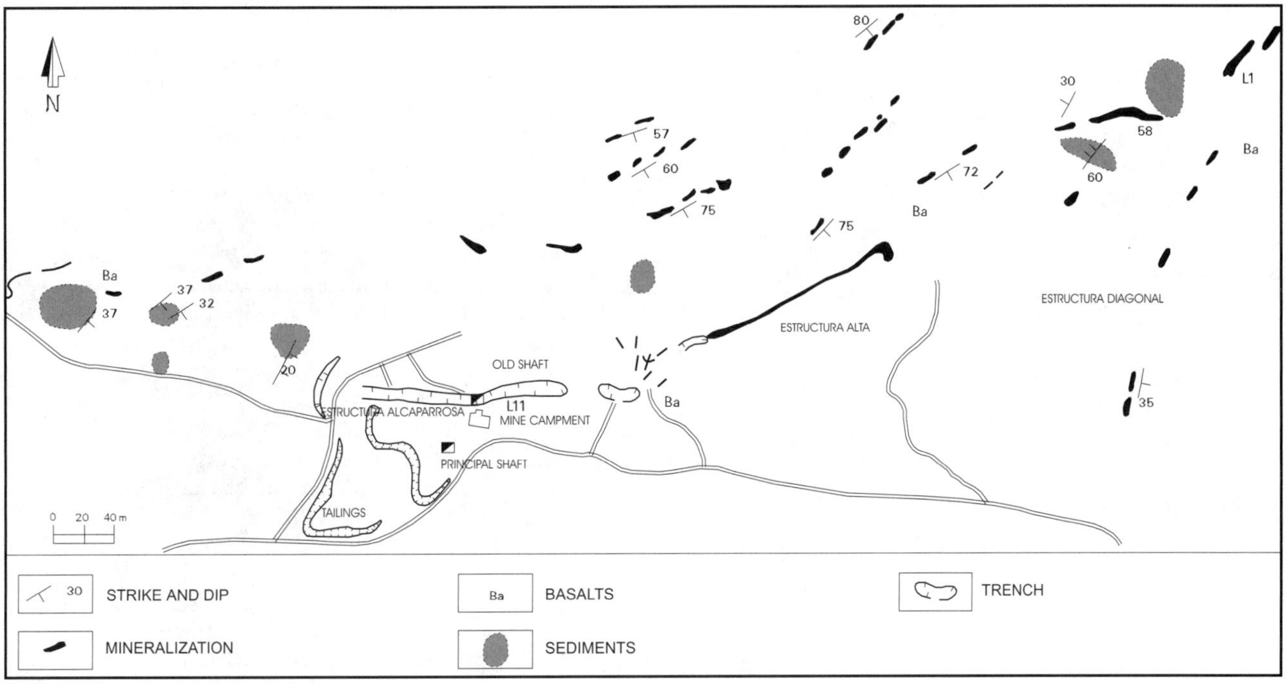

Figure.2 Geology of the Santa Elena mine (modified from Meissl and Maidana, 1983).

Ag and 4.51 g/t Au (Meissl and Maidana, 1983).

MINERALOGY AND ISOTOPIC STUDIES

The primary mineral association consists of pyrite, marcasite, pyrrhotite, sphalerite, chalcopyrite, arsenopyrite and galena with sulphosalt inclusions. Disseminated pyrite, that carries gold, is always present, frequently in relation with basalts. Sphalerite appears in two generations, occurs with chalcopyrite inclusions and is cross cut by arsenopyrite. Marcasite is very frequent and associated with pyrite. Galena, less abundant, is argentiferous. Chalcopyrite is partly altered to chalcocite and covelline. The gangue minerals are quartz, two generations of carbonates and minor amorphous silica and ankerite.

Supergene minerals are hematite, melnikovite, chalcosine, digenite, natroalunite, goethite, kieserite, scorodite, goslarite, epsomite and a series of iron sulphates such as jarosite, ferropalidite, copiapite, sarmientite, amarantite, fibroferrite and botryogen as the most frequent, and in lesser amounts calingastite, slavikite, coquimbite, rozenite, bianchite, kirovite, butlerite and parabutlerite (Angelelli and Trelles, 1938; Toubes-Spinelli, 1982, 1983; Meissl and Maidana, 1983).

The basalts present variable propylititic, pyritic, carbonatic and sericitic alteration.

Isotopic composition of pyrite and galena has been determined. The δS^{34} in pyrite gives +0.2‰ ± 0.5 and δS^{34} in galena +1.5‰ ± 0.5, values that indicate an igneous source.

Lead isotopic ratios in galena are $^{206}Pb/^{204}Pb$: 18.345; $^{207}Pb/^{204}Pb$: 15.586 and $^{208}Pb/^{204}Pb$: 38.086. These values are close to those obtained from Proterozoic rocks of the Precordillera (Abbruzzi et al., 1983). The $^{207}Pb/^{204}Pb$ value is somewhat higher and could indicate a heterogenic mantelic reservoir contaminated by magma-crust interaction.

GENETIC MODEL

The genesis of this deposit requires more detailed studies. Haller and Ramos (1984) relate the mineralization with the ophiolitic sequence and Mendez et al. (1995) associate the mineralization with exhalative submarine events.

We consider that this volcanogenic massive sulphide (VMS) is related to hydrothermal facies associated with a basic magmatism. The presence of disseminated pyrite in the basaltic flows (partly extrusive pillowed lavas) silicified and carbonatized, the presence of chert in the upper sedimentary layers that overlyes the stockwork, and the characteristic mineral paragenesis that appears as lenses, disseminations and stockwork veinlets are consistent with this model.

The presence of a "yellow belt", 6 km length and 1.5 km wide, indicates the importance of the hydrothermal alteration process. The genetic link between the mineralization and the oceanic basalts is confirmed by means of isotopic data.

References

Abbruzzi, J., Kay, S.M. and Bickford, M.E. 1993. Implication for the nature of the Precordilleran basement from Precambrian xenoliths in Miocene volcanic rocks, San Juan Province, Argentina. 12° Congreso Geológico Argentino y 2° Congreso de Exploración de Hidrocarburos. 3, 331-339. Mendoza.

Angelelli, V. 1984. Yacimientos metalíferos de la República Argentina. Comisión de Investigaciones de la Provincia de Buenos Aires, p. 704. La Plata

Angelleli, V. and Trelles, R.A. 1938. Las alumbreras de Rodeo y Barreal y los sulfatos de hierro de Alcaparrosa, provincia de San Juan. Obras Sanitarias de la Nación, Boletín No.2, 8-10, 139-158. Buenos Aires.

Caballé, M. F. 1986. Estudio geológico del sector oriental de la Cordillera Frontal, entre los ríos Manrique y Calingasta (provincia de San Juan). Ph.D. Thesis. University of La Plata. Argentina.

Furque G., and Caballé, M.F. 1986. Descripción geológica de la Hoja 20b- Calingasta, provincia de San Juan. SEGEMAR, unpublished report. Buenos Aires.

Haller M. and Ramos, V.A. 1984. Las ofiolitas famatinianas (eopaleozoico) de las provincias de San Juan y Mendoza. 9° Congreso Geológico Argentino, Actas 2, 66-83. San Carlos de Bariloche.

Kay S.M., Ramos V.A. and Kay R.W. 1984. Elementos mayoritarios y trazas de las vulcanitas ordovícicas de la Precordillera occidental: basaltos de rift oceánico temprano?próximo al margen continental. 9°Congreso Geológico Argentino, 2, 48-65. San Carlos de Bariloche.

Meissl E.F. and Maidana M.R. 1983. Mina Santa Elena. La Alcaparrosa, Calingasta, provincia de San Juan, República Argentina. 2° Congreso Nacional de Geología Económica. Actas 2, pp.551-566. San Juan.

Mendez, V. Zanettini, J.C. and Zappettini, E.O. 1995. Geología y metalogénesis del orógeno andino central, República Argentina. Dirección Nacional del Servicio Geológico. Anales 23. Buenos Aires

Quartino B.J., Zardini A.R. and Amos A.J. 1971. Estudio y exploración geológica de la región Barreal-Calingasta. Provincia de San Juan. República Argentina. Asociación Geológica Argentina. Monografía 1, 1-184. Buenos Aires.

Sillitoe R. H.1977. Permo-carboniferous upper Cretaceous and Miocene Porphyry Copper type mineralization in the Argentina Andes. Economic Geology 72, 1, 99-109.

Stappenbeck R. 1910. La Precordillera de San Juan y Mendoza. Ministerio de Agricultura. Sección Geología, Mineralogía y Minería. Anales 4, 3, 3-179. Buenos Aires.

Toubes-Spinelli R.O.1982. Aluminocopiapita zincífera de la mina Santa Elena, Quebrada de la Alcaparrosa, provincia de San Juan. Revista de la Asociación de Mineralogía, Petrografía y Sedimentología, 13 (1-2), 25-28.Buenos Aires.

Toubes-Spinelli R.O. 1983. Primera mención de kirovita para la República Argentina. Revista de la Asociación de Mineralogía, Petrografía y Sedimentología, 14 (1-2), 3-6. Buenos Aires.

VOLCANIC-EXHALATIVE MASSIVE SULPHIDE DEPOSITS IN CHILE

WALDO VIVALLO
Servicio Nacional de Geología y Minería, Avda Santa María 0104, Santiago, Chile

ABSTRACT

Volcanogenic massive sulphide deposits in Chile are found in Paleozoic metamorphic rocks and Jurassic-Lower Cretaceous volcanic sedimentary sequences. The Paleozoic metamorphic rocks, comprise an accretion prism and contain small Cu and Cu-Zn deposits that have not been economically attractive, particularly south of the 38°S. These are stratiform deposits are hosted by metamorphosed and deformed volcanic-sedimentary sequences. The most important are Tirúa (38°25'), Pirén (39°55'), Mina Silva (46°34'), Manto Rosillo (46°33'), La Serena (52°47') and Cutter Cove (53°21'). The volcanic-sedimentary sequences, that formed in a back-arc basins of the Jurassic-Lower Cretaceous, host the most important massive sulphide type deposits (Cu, Zn-Cu, Zn-Pb-Cu) in Chile, from an economic standpoint. Punta del Cobre (27°30'S) and El Toqui (45°) are the better known districts. However, the genesis of these deposits is still controversial.

INTRODUCTION

Chile is the largest producer of copper in the world, with an annual production of 3.76 million tonnes of fine copper (National Service of Geology and Mining, 1998). In addition, Chile also produces molybdenum, gold, rhenium, lithium and nitrates. In general, almost all of the copper, molybdenum and rhenium production comes from the exploitation of world class porphyry copper deposits, which together with epithermal gold and silver deposits and the Kiruna-type iron deposits, are the foundation of the metal mining industry in Chile.

The abundance and economic importance of the porphyry copper and epithermal deposits have overshadowed the exploration and development of other deposit types. The Pb and Zn production of Chile was less than 16,000 tonnes in 1998 (National Service of Geology and Mining, 1998) and its economic value is marginal when compared to the value of the copper, gold, silver and iron production. Most of the Pb and Zn production comes from the exploitation of the Zn-Cu-Pb-Au-Ag deposits in the El Toqui district, located in the southern region of the country (Fig. 1).

In general, most of the metal deposits known in the country are epigenetic and associated with intrusive magmatism and subaerial volcanic activity and have been well studied and documented. Deposits associated with marine volcanic environments are rare and have received limited attention in the geologic literature. Some references for the metamorphic Paleozoic sequences of Chile's Southern Coastal Cordillera include Alvárez, 1970; Alfaro, 1982, Collao and Alfaro, 1982; Alfaro and Collao, 1990; Collao et al, 1990; Schira et al, 1990; and for the Upper Jurassic-Lower Cretaceous sequence include Camus, 1980; Wellmer et al, 1983 (Fig. 1). However, the genetic affiliation of deposits associated with the Jurassic-Lower Cretaceous volcanic sedimentary sequences is controversial (Marschik, 1996; Townley, 1996).

TECTONIC AND GEOLOGICAL FRAMEWORK

The geological evolution of the Chilean Andes is well summarized in Aguirre (1985) and Mpodozis and Ramos (1990) with metallogeny addressed by Ruiz et al (1965) Frutos et al (1985), Oyarzún (1985) and Ruiz and Peebles (1988).

Chile presently forms an active continental shelf, where an oceanic plate is subducted under the continental crust (e.g. Dewey and Bird, 1970); Aguirre, 1985; Mpodozis and Ramos 1990). However, the existence of a subduction system is recognized clearly only after the Jurassic. This represents a break that allows us to separate the Andean orogenesis into two major periods. The first includes the Paleozoic and

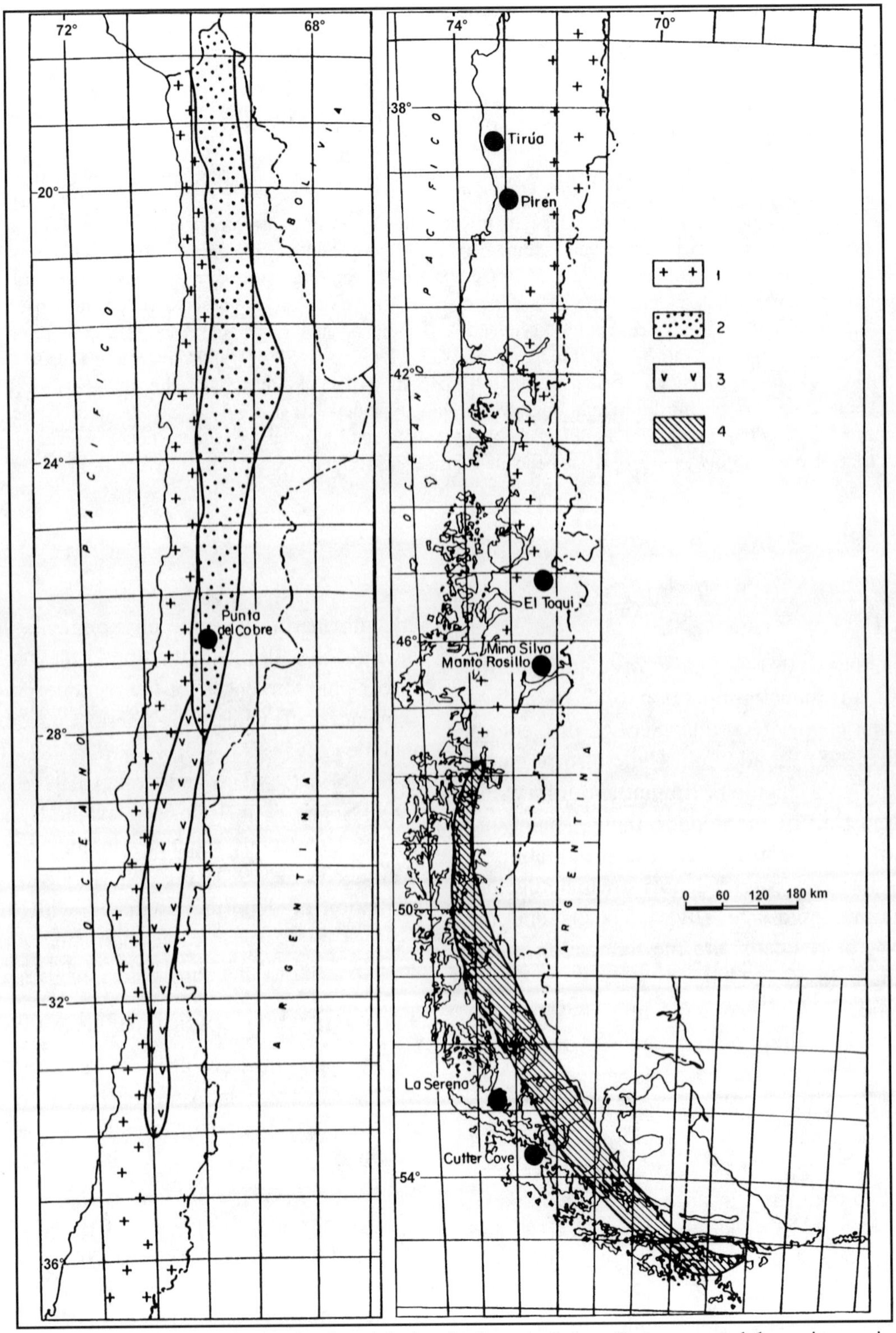

Figure 1. Distribution in the back-arc basins developed during the Jurassic-Lower Cretaceous and the main massive sulphide districts and deposits in Chile. 1, Approximate position of the magmatic arc 2, Tarapacá basin filed with volcanic sequences at the base and carbonated sedimentary rocks at the top 3, Ensialic basin of central Chile with mainly volcanic fill 4, Marginal greenstone basin containing an ophiolitic sequence. Based in Mpodozis and Ramos (1990), Davidson and Mopdozis (1991).

most of the Triassic; while the second, also known as the Andean cycle, corresponds to a geological evolution of the margin under the geodynamic conditions of active subduction, similar to the present configuration (Mpodozis and Ramos 1990; Davidson and Mpodozis, 1991).

The Paleozoic cycle is characterized by successive accretion of allochthonous blocks on the western border of Gondwana. These include, at the north, Precambrian rocks belonging to the Arequipa massive (Mpodozis and Ramos, 1990), while south of the 25°S an accretion prism developed consisting of metasedimentary and metavolcanic blocks of rocks, distributed along the present Coastal Cordillera, parallel to the current coast line (Hervé et al, 1981). The chemical composition of the metavolcanic rocks located south of 34°S show affinity with ocean ridge tholeiitic basalts (e.g. Hervé et al, 1976; Godoy, 1979; Vivallo et al, 1988; Shira et al, 1990). Most of these sequences were affected by low to medium grade metamorphism during the Carboniferous (González Bonorino and Aguirre, 1970; Aguirre, 1985; Kato, 1976; 1985). A magmatic arc represented by calc-alkaline granitoids of the Carboniferous-Permian extends on a north-south direction, almost continuously, from 27 to 45°S (Davidson and Mpodozis, 1991). Acid and granitoid volcanic rocks from the Permian Triassic age belonging to a major magmatic province (Choiyoi) cover and intrude the magmatic Carboniferous Permian arc (Davidson and Mpodozis, 1991). Petrologic evidence indicates that the rocks in this magmatic province originated in an extensional tectonic environment (Kay et al, 1989).

The evolution of the continental margin during the Mesozoic and Cenozoic has been controlled by the existence of an east dipping subduction system. During the Jurassic and Lower Cretaceous, the continental margin was characterized by the development of a series of magmatic arcs and associated back-arc basins, controlled by extension and subsidence, both developed under a Mariana type subduction system (Davidson and Mpodozis, 1991). In general, the magmatic arc is represented by volcanic and plutonic rocks which are distributed in belts with a north-south direction, while the back-arc basins consist of marine sedimentary rocks local accumulations of volcanic rocks (Aguirre, 1985; Mpodozis and Ramos, 1990). From the Upper Cretaceous onwards, in response to regional tectonics, a compressive tectonic system was established (Davidson and Mpodozis, 1991), which closed the back-arc basins leaving the presence of a magmatic arc as the predominant feature.

The back-arc basins of the Jurassic-Lower Cretaceous (Fig. 1) present different characteristics. The marginal greenstone basin (Stern et al., 1976; Dalziel, 1981), located approximately between 51°30'S and 55°S, is characterized by the development of an ophiolitic sequence with the characteristics of the ocean floor. In central Chile an ensialic basin was developed with mostly volcanic fill (Aberg et al, 1984). In the Copiapó area, the rocks at the base of this basin are basaltic andesite volcanic rocks which grades upward into carbonate sedimentary marine sequences.

VOLCANOGENIC MASSIVE SULPHIDE DEPOSITS

Paleozoic

The Coastal Cordillera, at latitude 38° and 42°S, consists mainly of, polymetamorphic and polydeformed Paleozoic rocks. The mineralogical and chemical composition of these rocks indicates that originally they were pelitic and psammitic sediments with interbeds of tholeiitic basalts and ultramafic serpentinized rocks (e.g. Alfaro, 1980). This sequence has been interpreted as part of a dismembered ophiolitic complex which was developed in an ocean ridge environment (Hervé et al., 1976; Aguirre, 1985; Frutos and Alfaro, 1987) or marginal basin (Vivallo et al., 1988; Schira et al., 1990). Locally, small Cu and Zn massive sulphide bodies have been identified associated with metabasalts, which have been interpreted to be exhalative origin (Table 1). The deposits are stratiform and lenticular consisting of pyrite, chalcopyrite, sphalerite, pyrrhotite, with quartz and muscovite as the gangue minerals. Both the sulphide bodies as well as the country rock are deformed and recrystallized (e.g. Schira et al 1990). The nature of the country rock, the stratiform character of the sulphide bodies, together with their mineralogy and textures, suggest that the formation was due to a submarine volcanic environment prior to the metamorphism.

Table 1. Cu, Zn-Cu y Zn-Pb-Cu deposits and showings of probable volcanic-exhalative origin in Chile.

Name	Shape	Ore	Host rock	Resources	Reference
Jurassic-Lower Cretaceous Deposits					
Punta del Cobre District	Veins, Breccia Stratiform	Cu, Au, Zn	Andesite, Dacite	›40 Mt 1-2% Cu, 0,2-0,5 g/t Au , 7 g/t Ag	Camus (1980) Marschik (1996)
El Toqui District	Stratiform Veins	Zn, Pb, Cu, Au, Ag	Limestone, volcanic andesitic rock	10 Mt 8%Zn, 1,5%Pb, 0,6%Cu ,1,5g/t Au, 50g/t Ag	Wellmer et al. (1983) Townley (1996)
Paleozoic Deposits and Showings					
Tirúa	Stratiform	Cu, Zn	Metasedimentary rocks and metabasalt	Small	Collao y Alfaro (1982)
Pirén	Stratiform	Cu, Zn	Metasedimentary rocks and metabasalt	Small	Schira et al. (1990)
Mina Silva	Stratiform	Pb, Zn, Ag	Marble	›100.000t 20% Zn, 20%Pb 800 g/t Ag	Townley (1996)
Manto Rosillo	Stratiform	Zn, Pb, Cu Ag	Phyllite, marble	15.000t 12-40% Zn, 16% Pb 12%Cu, 380g/t Ag	Schneider y Tolosa (1990)
La Serena	Stratiform	Cu	Schist, Metabasalt	Small	Ruiz y Peebles (1988)
Cutter Cove	Stratiform	Cu	Schist, metabasalt	Small	Thomas (1973)

The most important and better known Cu-Zn deposits in this section are Tirúa and Pirén (Table 1, Figure 1). Both deposits correspond to small, and currently uneconomic, massive sulphide bodies associated with metabasalts. The Tirúa deposit consists of massive pyrite-chalcopyrite-sphalerite lenticular bodies hosted in metabasalts. The sulphide bodies have an average thickness of 0.5 m and are about 20 m long and have a strike length of about 150 m (Alvárez, 1970) parallel to the foliation. Seven sulphide intervals were detected in Pirén (Schira et al., 1990), with thickness under 30 cm with unknown lateral extent. The sulphide bodies occur interbedded in a sequence of metasedimentary and metavolcanic rocks. The country rock is not obviously altered, however, Schira et al., (1990) suggests that the local presence of tourmaline is the result of hydrothermal activity. The sulphide bodies contain pyrite, pyrrhotite, chalcopyrite and sphalerite, which show the effect of the recrystallization and deformation produced by the regional metamorphism.

A second group of Pb-Zn-Cu or Zn-Cu massive sulphide deposits are hosted in Paleozoic rocks south of 46°S (Table 1, Fig. 1). The most significant are Manto Rosillo and Mina Silva. Manto Rosillo (Ruiz and Peebles, 1985, Camus 1985; Schneider and Toloza, 1990) consists of stratiform Pb-Zn-Cu massive bodies located in the contact between the phyllites and marble. The contacts with the country rock are abrupt and the orebody is highly folded. The deposit is stratiform with a thickness ranging from 0.5 to 1.5 m, strike length of 250 m and 30 to 40 m width. The deposit shows a vertical zoning with the sphalerite-rich base and an upper interval dominated by pyrite. Present in minor amounts are chalcopyrite, galena, tennantite and tetrahedrite (Ruiz and Peebles, 1988). Microthermometry of fluid inclusions in sphalerite (Toloza, 1987) indicate homogenization temperatures in the range of 417 to 478°C, while the fluid inclusions in calcite associated with sulphides (Townley, 1996) homogenize to a liquid phase in the range of 200 to 290°C with an average salinity of 7 % NaCl eq. The isotopic composition of the S in the sulphides suggests a magmatic origin of this element (Schneider and Toloza 1990).

The Silva Mine (Ruiz and Peebles, 1988) consists of massive sulphide bodies hosted in limestone. Individually, the lenses have average thickness of 10 to 15 m and 30 to 50 m long and are connected by discontinuous veinlets (Roeschmann, 1981). The orebody contains pyrite, arsenopyrite, sphalerite, galena, tetrahedrite and chalcopyrite. Between 1947 and 1962 the production was 40,000 tonnes of Pb and 20,000 tonnes of Zn with grades reaching up to 25 % Zn and 400 g/t Ag (Ruiz and Peebles, 1988). Primary fluid inclusions in calcite intergrown with sulphides have homogenization temperatures in the range of 200 to 250°C and salinity between 6-8 % NaCl eq.

The genesis of these deposits is unclear. Ruiz and Peebles (1988), based in the stratiform character of the massive sulphide bodies and the simple mineralogy of the ore body, suggest an exhalative volcanic origin for both deposits. However, Roeschmann (1981) and Schneider and Tolosa (1990), due to the presence of some discordant structures with the country rock and the proximity to plutonic intrusive bodies, suggest that they formed by metasomatic replacement, genetically associated to the intrusives. On the basis of similar arguments, Townley (1996) interpreted that both deposits are skarns, with an early event of high temperature (>400°C) followed by another at a lower temperature (>300°C). However, the calc-silicate mineralogy of the skarn type deposits, is not recognized.

Cutter Cove (Thomas, 1973), Ancón Sin Salida and La Serena (Ruiz and Peebles, 1988) (Fig. 1), are small polymetallic massive sulphide deposits of presumed volcanic-exhalative origin. These deposits are located in Paleozoic volcanic-sedimentary sequences which extend south of 52°S latitude. The deposits are located on or close to the contact between metabasalts and pelitic schists. Forsythe and Mpodozis (1983) mention the presence of Mn and Fe oxide stratiform deposits associated with Paleozoic pillow basalts in the Madre de Dios Archipelago (50°30'S) in Magallanes.

Upper Jurassic-Lower Cretaceous

Economically the most important stratabound massive sulphide type deposits, of probable volcanogenic origin, are located in Upper Jurassic – Lower Cretaceous volcanic sedimentary sequences. These deposits are concentrated in the mining districts of Punta del Cobre and El Toqui, in the north and south of the country respectively (Fig. 1). Both are located in back-arc volcanic sedimentary sequences (Aguirre, 1985) associated to the development of the magmatic Jurassic-Lower Cretaceous arc (Mpodozis and Ramos, 1990).

The most important district from an economic standpoint is Punta del Cobre (Fig. 2), in the Copiapó region (27° 0' S). The production of this district, from 1800 to 1982, was in the order of 5 million tonnes of ore grading 4.8 % Cu (Camus, 1985). In 1997 the annual production of the district exceeded 2 million tonnes, with an average grade of 1.5 % Cu (Flores, 1996; Díaz et al, 1998). The copper deposits of this district are located in a subhorizontal sequence of predominantly volcanic rocks of the Upper Jurassic to Lower Cretaceous period (Punta del Cobre Formation). This sequence (Fig. 3) consists of basal andesitic rocks on which dacitic domes formed (known locally as "albitófiros"). Epiclastic breccia (basal breccia), conglomerates, ferruginous chert and finely laminated lutites cover the dome and the lower lava discordantly (Camus, 1980). The upper part of the sequence consists of basalts and andesites interbedded with marine sedimentary rocks (Grupo Chañarcillo). The sequence is intruded on the west (Fig. 2) by plutons of granodioritic to dioritic composition (119 and 116 Ma; Arevalo, 1995), which generated an extensive contact metamorphic aureole. The deposits of the district are located mainly in the dacitic domes (albitóforo) and correspond to veins, breccia stacks and stratabound deposits (Fig. 3).

The veins are vertical and intersected the lower part of the sequence and occasionally the basal breccia. Thickness ranges from a few centimetres up to approximately 60 m with strike lengths up to 600 m and vertical extension of 300 m. The mineralization is massive with the development of stockwork veinlets towards both sides of the vein. The main minerals are chalcopyrite with variable quantities of magnetite, specularite, pyrite, pyrrhotite, and lesser sphalerite (2 % Zn). The alteration of the country rock includes silicification, potassic alteration (potassium feldspar, biotite) and actinolite in depth.

Generally, the breccia bodies (Camus, 1985) are tabular and hosted in the domes (albitófiros) with a maximum depth of 150 m with widths ranging from 1 to 60 m. The width decreases in depth and the bodies tend to be wedge shaped. Chalcopyrite is the main mineral in the orebody with variable quantities of pyrite, specularite, quartz and calcite, cementing the breccia. The stratabound deposits occur as lenticular stratiform bodies, with thickness ranging between 1 and 35 m (Marschik, 1996) and lateral extension of a few hundred meters.

The stratabound bodies (Camus, 1985) are restricted

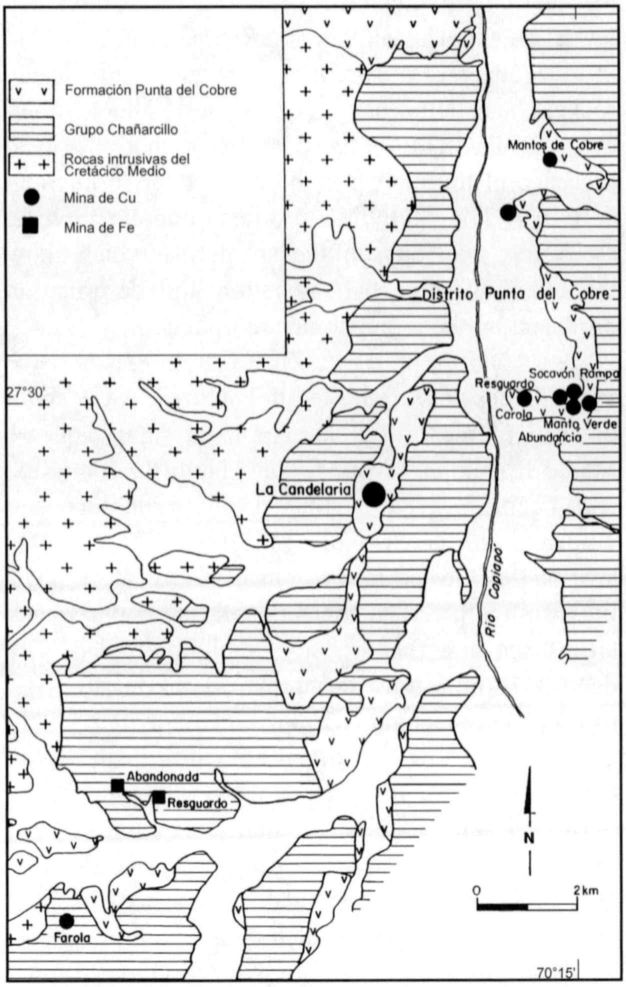

Figure 2. Distribution of the sulphide deposits in the Punta del Cobre district, the "La Candelaria" deposit is located in the centre-west of the district. Towards the south, the stratiform iron (Abandonada) and copper (Resguardo) deposits of the Las Pintadas mining district. Modified by Marschik (1996).

to the contact zone between the volcanic part (albotófiro) and the sedimentary part (basal breccia) of the Punta de Cobre Formation. Mineralization is hosted in a matrix of breccia containing angular clasts of volcanic rocks of the lower units, chert and calcareous rocks. Chalcopyrite is the principal mineral in the orebody and is accompanied by pyrite, specularite and quartz. Towards the wall of the mineralized bodies, the sulphides are replaced by specularite and, locally, can grade laterally to mineralized bodies with specularite in the orebodies.

Regionally, the rocks that are hosted in the sulphide deposits have been affected by an intense sodium metasomatism, producing albitization in the volcanic rocks. A potassic alteration event, with biotite and potash feldspar, is superimposed on the sodium alteration (Marschik, 1996).

Immediately south of the Punta del Cobre district, forming part of the same geological environment, is the Las Pintadas mining district (Fig. 2). This district contains stratiform iron deposits hosted in sedimentary rocks in the basal section of the Chañarcillo Group. It has been suggested that these deposits are volcanic-exhalative in origin (Espinoza 1986, 1990). In the southern part of the district and hosted in volcanic rocks of the Punta del Cobre Formation are stratabound copper deposits of which the Farola mine is the most important. This deposit corresponds to a stratiform body of massive sulphides 10 m thick, 2,000 m long and 140 m wide, with grades of 1.5 % Cu, 0.4 g/t Au and 50 g/t Ag and proven reserves of 1 million tonnes (Lledó, 1998). The minerals in the lower part of the deposit, occur in veinlets and disseminated, while in the top part are massive, stratiform, and locally banded (Lledó, 1998). Chalcopyrite is the main mineral of the body, accompanied by variable quantities of pyrite, pyrrhotite, magnetite and hematite. The alteration assemblage of the country rock includes albite, biotite, actinolite, garnet, chlorite and scapolite.

Camus (1980), on the basis of the spatial and stratigraphic relations of the different types of sulphide deposits (breccia, veins, stratiform) and the volcanic-submarine environment (Segerstrom and Ruiz, 1962; Ortiz et al, 1966; Von Osten, 1967, Lino, 1984; Arévalo, 1995, Lledó, 1998) suggested a common volcanic exhalative origin for deposits of the Punta del Cobre district. Lledó (1997) described the presence of chalcopyrite concretions in the Providencia mine, located immediately north in the Punta del Cobre district and the same geological environment, which are interpreted as being of syngenetic origin.

Marschik (1996) based on the age of the potassic alteration (114 Ma), the presence of batholithic intrusives of a similar age, and the mineralogy of the orebody, suggested an epigenetic origin for the deposits of the district, associated with the emplacement of intrusives and proposed that they represented a transition between the magnetite-apatite Kiruna type deposits and the porphyry copper deposits.

At the La Candelaria mine, Cu-Fe-Au deposits are stratabound and hosted in volcanic rocks of the lower part of the Punta del Cobre Formation (Fig. 3). The sulphides are disseminated, in veins and occasionally stratiform bodies, particularly towards the periphery. The mineralogy of the orebody is similar to that of other deposits in the Punta del Cobre district, with chalcopyrite as the main mineral accompanied by magnetite, hematite, pyrite, pyrrhotite and gold. The proximity of this deposit to other deposits in the district, together with a similar geological environment and mineralogy of the orebody, suggest that they are probably related. However, Ryan et al (1995) suggest that La Candelaria deposit represents a metamorphosed porphyry copper deposit.

The El Toqui district is located approximately 1,700 km south of Santiago, in the Aisén region. This deposit has the most important Zn and Pb resources in Chile. Annual production is on the order of 16,000 tonnes of Zn and 190 kg of gold. The estimated reserves of the district are about 10 million tonnes with an average grade of 8 % Zn, 0.6 % Cu, 1.5 % Pb, 1.5 g/t Au and 50 g/t Ag (Townley, 1996). The deposits are hosted in a volcanic-sedimentary sequence (Fig. 4) consisting of Upper Jurassic-Lower Cretaceous andesitic lavas (Ibañez Formation) overlain by Lower Cretaceous marine sedimentary rocks (Coyhaique Formation). The sequence is intruded by small felsic bodies. The Zn-Pb veins are housed in the volcanic rocks, while the stratiform Zn and Zn-Pb-Cu deposits are restricted to three intervals hosted by calcareous lithologies of the volcanic-sedimentary

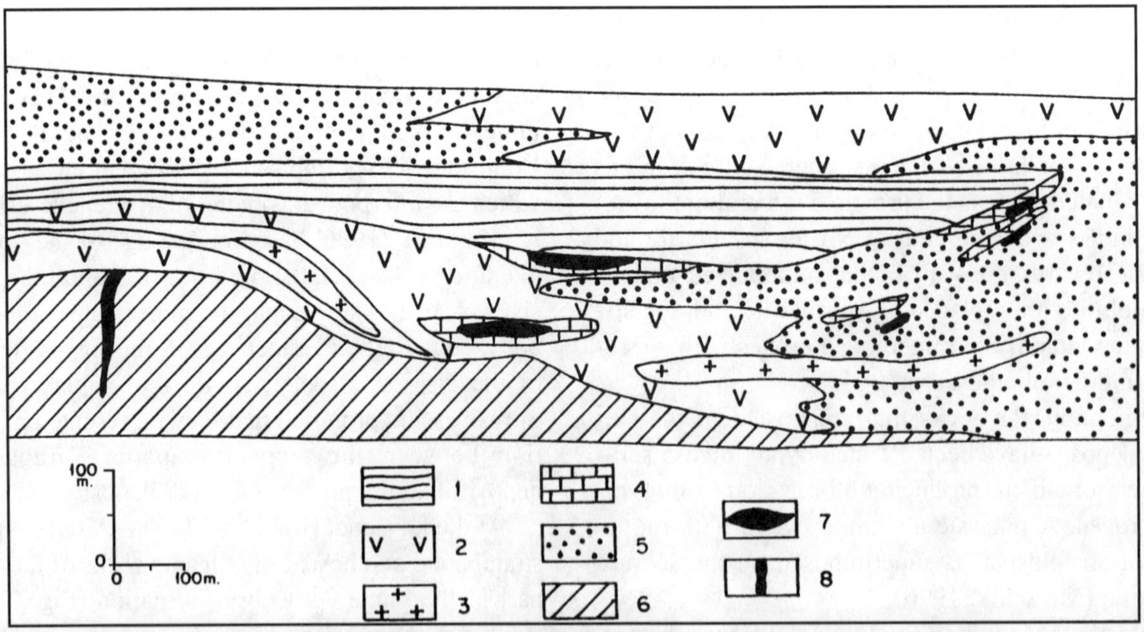

Figure 3. Schematic section showing the stratigraphy and location of the different types of deposit in the Punta del Cobre district. (1) Carbonated rocks of the Chañarcillo (Lower Cretaceous). Units 2 to 5 correspond to the units of the Punta del Cobre Formation (Upper Jurassic, Lower Cretaceous). (2) Top lava, (3) Sedimentary unit, includes basal breccia and lutites with interbedding of chert, (4) Dome (Albitofiro), (5) Lower lava (6) Stratiform deposit, (7) Vein (8) Mineralized breccia. Modified by Camus (1985).

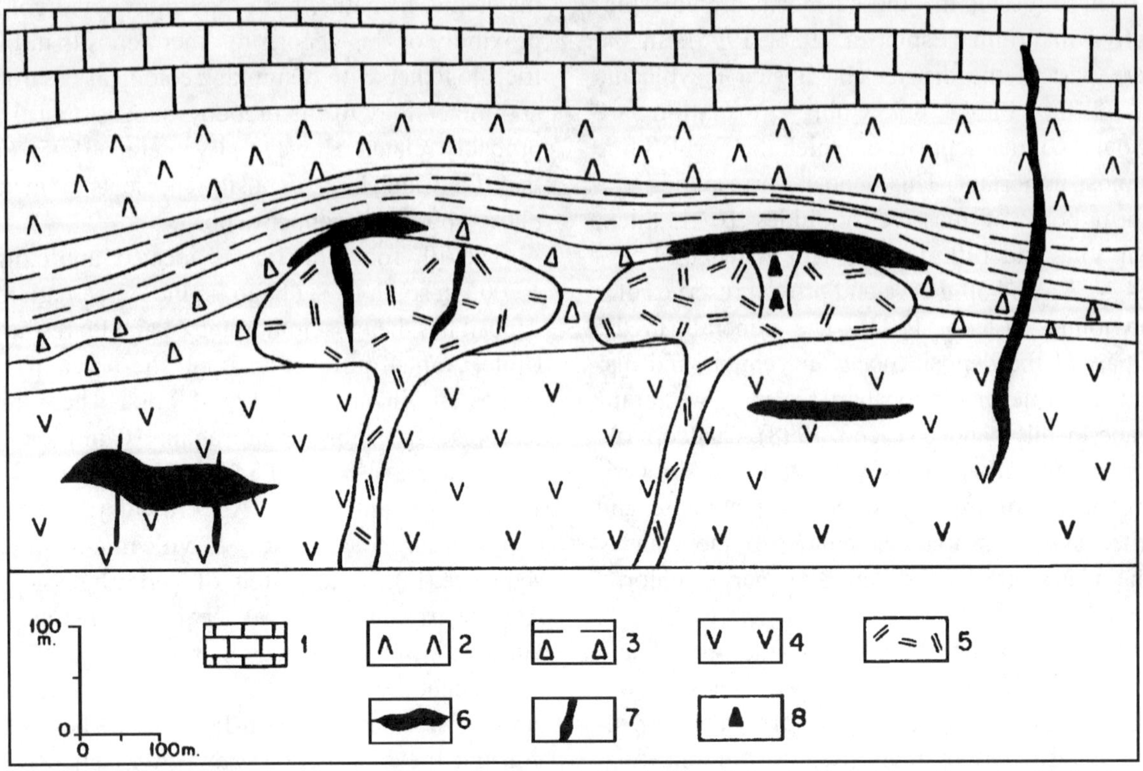

Figure 4. Schematic section showing the stratigraphy and distribution of the stratiform deposits and veins in El Toqui mining district. (1) Lutite, (2) Andesitic tuff, (3) lode, mantle, (4) Limestone (5) Rhyolitic tuff, (6) Altered rhyolitic tuff, (7) Zn-Pb-Cu stratiform deposit, (8) Pb-Zn Vein. Modified from Camus (1985)

sequence (Wellmer et al., 1983). The calcareous lithologies have local calc-silicate assemblages (pyroxene-garnet-epidote) suggesting contact metamorphism. The mineralogy of the orebody includes sphalerite, galena, chalcopyrite, pyrite, pyrrhotite, arsenopyrte, tetrahedrite and gold, replacing marine fossils and hosted in a limestone matrix, with horizons up to 20 m thick. Based on the volcanic sedimentary environment in which the orebody is located, the identification of volcanic centres and the presence of vein and stratiform deposits Wellmer et al (1983) suggest a volcanic-exhalative origin for the mineralization of the district. However, Townley (1996), based on fluid inclusions and radiometric dating of the rocks affected by sericitic alteration associated with the mineralization (106-100 Ma) suggests an affinity with skarn type deposits.

(Translation. Original submitted in Spanish).

ACKNOWLEDGEMENTS

The author would like to express his gratitude to the National Service of Geology and Mining for allowing him the facilities required for the preparation of this work. The opinions included in this paper, are the opinions of this author and do not represent an official position of the Service. This work benefited from the valuable comments of A. Logan. The Figures were drawn by L. Southerland.

REFERENCES

Aberg, G.; Aguirre, L.; Levi, B. 1984. Spreading subsidence and generation of ensialic marginal basin: An example from the Early Cretaceous of central Chile. Marginal basin geology. Edited by B.P. Kokelaar and M.F. Howells. Geological Society of London, Special Publication N° 16, p. 185-193.

Aguirre, L. 1985. The southern Andes. The Pacific Ocean. Edited by A.E.M. Nairm and F.G. Stheli. Plenum Press, New York, Ocean basins and trenches, Vol. 17, p. 265-376.

Alfaro, G. 1980. Antecedentes preliminares sobre la composición y génesis de las cromitas de la Cabaña (Cautín). Geological Magazine of Chile, N° 11, p.29-41.

Alfaro, G. 1982. Distribución de la mineralización en la Cordillera de la Costa entre los 38° y 40° Lat. Sur. III Geological Congress of Chile, Proceedings, Vol. 2, p. E38-E59.

Alfaro, G. and Collao, S. 1990. Massive sulphides in the greenstone belt of south-central Chile, an overview. Stratabound ore deposits of the Andes. Edited by L. Fontboté, G.C. Amstutz, M. Cardozo, E. Cedillo, J. Frutos. Society of Geology Applied to Mineral Deposits, Special Publication N° 8, p. 199-208.

Arévalo, C., 1995. Mapa geológico de la Hoja Copiapó, Región de Atacama. Servicio Nacional de Geología y Minería, Work paper N° 8, 1 map at scale 1:100.000, Santiago, Chile.

Alvárez, O. 1970. Estudio geológico de los yacimientos de hierro de la Cordillera de Nahuelbuta, Provincias de Arauco, Malleco y Cautín. Thesis, Universidad de Chile, 162 p. Santiago, Chile.

Camus, F. 1980. Posible modelo genético para los yacimientos de cobre del distrito minero Punta del Cobre. Geologial Magazine of Chile, N° 11, p. 51-76.

Camus, F. 1985. Los yacimientos estratoligados de Cu, Pb-Zn y Ag de Chile. Geología y recursos minerales de Chile. Edited by J. Frutos, R. Oyarzún and M.Pincheira. Editorial, Universidad de Concepción, Tome II, p. 538-635. Concepción.

Collao, S. and Alfaro, G. 1982. Mineralización sulfurada de hierro, cobre y zinc de la Cordillera de la Costa del sur de Chile. Chile's Geological Magazine N° 15, p. 41-47.

Collao, S., Alfaro, G. and Hayashi, K. 1990. Banded iron formations and massive sulfide orebodies, south-central Chile: geologic and isotopic aspects. Stratabound ore deposits of the Andes. Edited by L. Fontboté, G.C. Amstutz, M. Cardozo, E. Cedillo, J. Frutos. Society of Geology Applied to Mineral Deposits, Special Publication N° 8, p.209-219.

Dalziel, I.W.D. 1981. Back-arc extension in the southern Andes: a review and critical reappraisal. Philosophical Transsaction of the Royal Society of London, Vol. A, N° 300, p. 319-335.

Davidson, J. and Mpodozis, C. 1991. Regional geologic setting of epithermal gold deposits, Chile. Economic Geology, p. 1174-1186.

Díaz, A., Lledó, H. y Vivallo, W. 1998. Yacimientos metalíferos de la Hoja Los Loros, Región de Atacama. Servicio Nacional de Geología y Minería, Mineral Resources Map N° 2, 25p. Santiago, Chile.

Dewey, J. and Bird, J. 1970. Mountain belts and the new global tectonics. Journal of Geophysical Research, Vol. 75, p. 2625-2647.

Espinoza, S. 1986. Sobre el origen volcánico-sedimentario de los mantos ferruginosos Bandurrias y Manolete, al sur de Copiapó. Chile's Geological Magazine, Vol. 13, p. 33-40.

Espinoza, S. 1990. The Atacama-Coquimbo ferriferous belt, northern Chile. Stratabound ore deposits of the Andes. Edited by L. Fontboté, G.C. Amstutz, M. Cardozo, E. Cedillo, J. Frutos. Society of Geology Applied to Mineral Deposits, Special Publication N° 8, p. 353-364.

Flores, P. 1996. Geología de la mina Santos, Comuna de Tierra Amarilla, III región Atacama, Chile. Thesis, Universidad Católica del Norte, Antofagasta, Chile.

Forsythe, R. And Mpodozis, C. 1983. Geología del basamento pre-Jurásico Superior en el Achipielago Madre de Dios, Magallanes, Chile. Servicio Nacional de Geología y Minería, Newsletter N° 39, 63p. Santiago, Chile.

Frutos, J., Oyarzún, R. y Pincheira, M. 1985. Geología y recursos minerales de Chile, Vol. II, p. 442-923. Editorial,

Universidad de Concepción, Concepción.

Frutos, J. and Alfaro, G. 1987. Metallogenic and tectonic characteristics of the Paleozoic ophiolitic belt of the southern Chile Coastal Cordillera. Geologische Rundschau, Vol. 76, p.343-356.

Gelcich, S.; Espinoza, C. y Vivallo, W. 1998. Yacimientos metalíferos de las Hojas Chañaral y Diego de Almagro, Región de Atacama. Servicio Nacional de Geología y Minería, Mineral Resources Map N° 3, 17 p. Santiago, Chile.

Godoy, E. 1979. Metabasitas del basamento metamórfico chileno. Nuevos datos geoquímicos. II Geological Congress of Chile, Proceedings, Vol. III, p. E133-E148.

González Bonorino, F. and Aguirre, L. 1970. Metamorphic facies series of the crystalline basement of Chile. Geologische Rundschau, Vol. 59, p. 979-994.

Hervé, F., Godoy, E., del Campo, M. y Ojeda, J.M. 1976. Las metabasitas de Chile central y austral. I Geological Congress of Chile, Proceedings, Vol. II, p. F175-F187.

Hervé, F., Davidson, J., Godoy, E., Mpodozis, C. and Covacevich, V. 1981. The Late paleozoic in Chile: Stratigraphy, structure and possible tectonic framework. Anais de Academia Brasileira de Ciencias, Vol. 53, p. 361-373.

Kato, T. 1976. The relationship between low-grade metamorphism and tectonics in the Coast Range of central Chile. Ph. D. thesis, University of California L.A., Los Angeles U.S.A.

Kato, T. 1985. Pre-andean orogenesis in the Coast Range of central Chile. Geological Society of America, Bulletin, Vol. 96, p. 918-924.

Kay, S., Ramos, V.A., Mpodozis, C. and Sruoaga, P. 1989. Late Paleozoic to Jurassic silicic magmatism at the Gondwana margin: Analogy to the Middle Proterozoic in North America? Geology, Vol. 17, p. 324-328.

Lino, S. 1984. Geología de la mina Agustina, Comuna de Tierra Amarilla, Provincia de Copiapó, Región de Atacama. Thesis, Universidad Católica del Norte, 161 p.Antofagasta Chile.

Lledó, H. 1997. Hallazgo de ooides de calcopirita en la mina Providencia, implicancias metalogénicas, Copiapó, III Región. VIII Geological Congress of Chile, Proceedings, Vol. 2, p. 1043-1047.

Lledó, H. 1998. Metalogénesis de los cuadrángulos Copiapó, Cerro Chamonate y Nantoco, III Región, Chile. Tesis, Universidad de Chile, 204 p. Santiago Chile.

Marschik, R. 1996. Cretaceous Cu(-Fe) mineralization in the Punta del Cobre belt, northern Chile. Ph. D. thesis, University of Geneva, 191 p. Geneva, Switzerland.

Mpodozis, C. and Ramos, V.A. 1990. The Andes of Chile and Argentina. Earth Sciences Series, Circum-Pacific Council for Energy and Mineral Resources, Vol. 11, p. 59-90.

Ortiz, F., Araya, R., Franquesa, F., Moraga, A. y Zentilli, M. 1966. Informe geológico del distrito minero de Punta del Cobre, Provincia de Atacama. Instituto de Investigaciones Geológicas, Publicaciones Especiales N° 1, 4 Vols., 91 maps at scale 1:500. Santiago, Chile

Oyarzún, J. 1985. La métallogénie andine: cadre géologique, pétrologique et géochimique, et essai d'interpretation. Sc D Thesis, Universite Paris (Orsay). France.

Oyarzún, R., Clemmey, H. and Collao, S.1986. Geologic and metallogenic aspects concerning the Nahuelbuta mountains banded iron formation, Chile. Mineralium Deposita, Vol 21, p. 244-250.

Pincheira, M. and Fontboté, L. 1990. La Negra-Coquimbana manganiferous district, southern Atacama desert, Chile. In Stratabound ore deposits of the Andes. Edited by L. Fontboté, G.C. Amstutz, M. Cardozo, E. Cedillo, J. Frutos. Society of Geology Applied to Mineral Deposits, Special Publication N° 8, p. 365-378.

Pincheira, M., Frutos, J., Hernández, L. y Zamarreño, J. 1994. Antecedentes mineralógico-texturales en la mineralización estratoligada del distrito Punta del Cobre, Chile. VII Geological Congress of Chile, Proceedings, Vol. 2. P. 873-877.

Roeschmann, C. 1981. Estudio geológico minero zona Lago General Carrera, XI Región. Unpublished report, CORFO, AMI 81/23, Santiago, Chile.

Ruiz, C., Aguirre, L., Corvalán, J., Klohn, C., Klohn, E. y Levi, B. 1965. Geología y yacimientos metalíferos de Chile. 305 p. Editorial Universitaria, Santiago.

Ruiz, C. and Peebles, F. 1988. Geología, distribución y génesis de los yacimientos metalíferos chilenos. 334 p. Editorial Universitaria, Santiago.

Ryan, P., Lawrence, A., Jenkins, R., Matthews, J., Zamora, J.C., Marino, E. and Urqueta, I. 1995. The Candelaria copper-gold deposit, Chile. In Porphyry copper deposits of the American Cordillera. Edited by F.W. Pierce and J.G.Bhon. Arizona Geological Society Digest, Vol. 20, p. 625-645.

Servicio Nacional de Geología y Minería, 1998. Chile Mining Industry Yearbook, 144 p. Santiago, Chile.

SERNAGEOMIN-BRGM. 1995. Carta metalogénica Xa Región Sur, Chile. Servicio Nacional de Geología y Minería-Bureau de Recherches Geologiques et Minieres. Registered report IR 95-05, 4 Tomes, 10 Vols. Santiago, Chile.

Schira, W., Amstutz, G.C. and Fontboté, L. 1990. The Pirén Alto Cu-(Zn) massive sulfide occurrence in south-central Chile – A kieslager-type mineralization in a paleozoic ensialic mature marginal basin setting. In Stratabound ore deposits of the Andes. Edited by L. Fontboté, G.C. Amstutz, M. Cardozo, E. Cedillo, J. Frutos. Society of Geology Applied to Mineral Deposits, Special Publication N° 8, p. 229-251.

Schneider, A. and Tolosa, R.1990. The Mining district of the General Carrera lake and the Rosillo Manto deposit, Aysén Province, southern Chile. In Stratabound ore deposits of the Andes. Edited by L. Fontboté, G.C. Amstutz, M. Cardozo, E. Cedillo, J. Frutos. Society of Geology Applied to Mineral Deposits, Special Publication N° 8, p.485-494.

Segerstrom, K. y Ruiz, C. 1962. Cuadrángulo Copiapó, Provincia de Atacama. Instituto de Investigaciones Geológicas. Geological map of Chile, Vol. III, N° 1, 115 p. Santiago Chile.

Stern, C., De Wit, M.J. and Lawrence, Jr. 1976. Igneous and metamorphic processes associated with the formation of

Chilean ophiolites and their implication for ocean floor metamorphism, seismic layering and magnetism. Journal of Geophysical Research, Vol. 81, N° 23, p. 261-272.

Thomas, A. 1973. Geología y perspectivas económicas del yacimiento Cutter Cove, Provincia de Magallanes. Informe Inédito, ENAMI, Santiago, Chile.

Tolosa, R. 1987. Geología y génesis del manto de cinc Rosillo, Aysén, Lago General Carrera. Tesis, Universidad de Chile, 183 p. Santiago, Chile

Townley, B. 1996. Ore deposits, tectonics and metallogenesis of the continental Aysen region, Chile. Ph. D. Thesis, Queen's University, 246 p. Kingston, Canada.

Vivallo, W.; Alfaro, G.; Díaz, L. 1988. Los metabasaltos de la serie occidental de la Cordillera de la Costa, entre los 38°-41° latitud sur: evidencias geoquímicas de cuenca marginal durante el Paleozoico. VII Latin American Geological Congress, Vol. 1, p. 260-273.

Von Osten, G. 1967. Geología general y prospección geofísica del área de Punta del Cobre entre Tierra amarilla y Punta bateas. Tesis, Universidad de Chile, 143 p. Santiago, Chile.

Wellmer, F.W., Reeve, E.J., Wentzlau, E. and Westenberger, H. 1983. Geology and the ore deposits of the Toqui district, Aysen, Chile. Economic Geology, p.1119-1143.

PALEOZOIC MASSIVE SULPHIDE OREBODIES OF THE NAHUELBUTA AND QUEULE MOUNTAINS, SOUTH-CENTRAL CHILE: RESULTS OF GEOTHERMOBAROMETRY AND SULPHUR ISOTOPE STUDIES

Santiago Collao
Departamento Ciencias de la Tierra, Universidad de Concepción, Casilla 160-C, Concepción, CHILE.

Guillermo Alfaro
Instituto de Geología Economica Aplicada, Universidad de Concepción, Casilla 160-C, Concepción, CHILE

Abstract

Volcanic massive sulphide deposits (VMS) occur as scattered outcrops along a NNW-SSE belt in Paleozoic metamorphic rocks of the Coastal Cordillera of Southern Central Chile. Stratigraphically the ores are hosted by green schists which are the dominant rock of the Tirúa Unit.

The massive sulphide deposits outcrop (from N-S) at: Tirúa (Mina Vieja), Casa de Piedra, Hueñaliben, Trovolhue and Pirén localities. The mineralogy of the deposits is dominated by pyrite, pyrrhotite, chalcopyrite and sphalerite and includes lesser quantities of bornite, magnetite, hematite, arsenopyrite, molybdenite, rutile, galena, argentite, chalcocite, covellite, mackinawite and marcasite.

Textural and structural evidence indicate that the ore minerals were formed contemporaneously with the protolith of the green schists, which are interpreted to be recrystallized tholeiitic basalts. A volcanogenic origin for these deposits is suggested by the sulphur isotopic composition found in the pyrite of the massive sulphides (mean of $\delta^{34}S = +3.14‰$), which compared with sulphur isotope data of various other genetic types of deposits, indicates a relationship closer to magmatic and hydrothermal ore mineralization. Mean sulphur isotope values suggest that the mineralization at Casa de Piedra and Hueñaliben (mean of $\delta^{34}S = +0.5‰$) was closer to the hydrothermal centre while that at Tirúa (mean of $\delta^{34}S = +5.9‰$) and Pirén (mean of $\delta\ ^{34}S = +3.5‰$) was more peripheral.

Studies were performed on fluid inclusions in quartz contained in the mineralization and green schists at Tirúa, Casa de Piedra and Pirén. The homogenization temperature in liquid-rich inclusions from the mineralization is similar to that inclusions hosted in the green schists. The wide range of the homogenization temperature (196° to 451°C) may be due to greenschist facies and subsequent retrograde metamorphism.

The presence of an assemblage of albite, epidote, chlorite, calcite, quartz and actinolite suggest that the metabasic host rocks have undergone regional greenschist sub-greenschist facies metamorphism. Sphalerite compositions suggest a pressure range of 3.5 to 9.0 kbars, which is commensurate with the regional metamorphic facies.

The sulphur isotope data presented here is consistent with values derived from a magmatic source and overlap those of modern hydrothermal vent fluids in spreading ridges in basaltic rocks to suggest a volcanic origin for these VMS deposits. Fluid inclusion and sphalerite geobarometric data indicates that successive metamorphic episodes affected massive sulphides and country rocks.

Introduction.

The Paleozoic volcanic massive sulphide mineralization (VMS) (Fig. 1), except for the Mina Vieja de Tirúa, was found between 1978 and 1982 (Collao et al. 1980; Collao and Alfaro 1982; Alfaro and Collao 1990). The more significant sulphide deposits are Mina Vieja de Tirúa and Pirén Alto with orebodies composed of more than 60 % sulphide minerals. The main orebody in Mina Vieja has a maximum thicknesses of 0.5 m and can be followed for 15 m in the direction of the schistosity. At Pirén Alto seven massive sulphide beds with thickness between 0.1 to 0.3

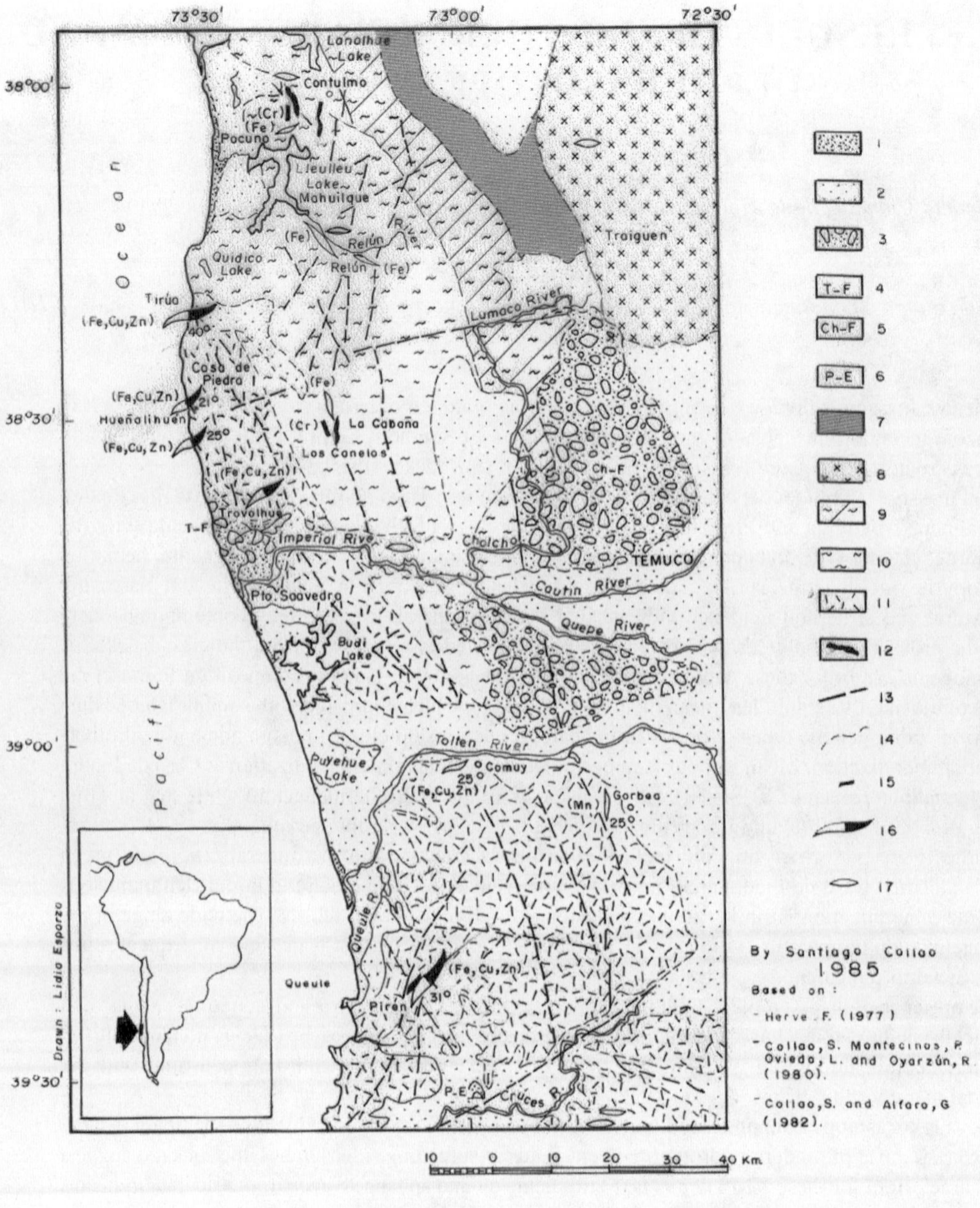

Fig. 1. Geologic map of the Nahuelbuta and Queule Mountains. *Quaternary:* **1** Sandstones, dunes; **2** Sandstones and gravels. *Tertiary:* **3** Sandstones, shales, sillstones, conglomerates belonging to the **4** Tubul Formation (marine); **5** Cholchol Formation (continental); and **6** Pupunahue Strata (continental). *Triassic:* **7** Sandstones and shales. *Paleozoic:* **8** Granitoids; **9** Metapelites and metagraywackes (Eastern Unit); **10** micaschists, metacherts, Fe-bearing metacherts (Nahuelbuta Unit); **11** greenschists, micaschists and metacherts (Tirua Unit); **12** serpentinite bodies; **13** fault; **14** inferred contact; **15** podiform Cr deposits; **16** orebodies, stratabound type; **17** placer deposits (Au)

m are intercalated in the greenschists and oriented along the trend of the schistosity. The other orebodies (Casa de Piedra, Trovolhue, and Hueñalihuén) are smaller. The sulphide mineralization is mainly composed of pyrite, chalcopyrite, sphalerite, and pyrrhotite. The major and minor element contents of the massive sulphide deposits (47 analysis) are: 0.4 % - 1.7 % Cu, 0.1 % - 1.2 % Zn, 0.1 % - 1.2 % Zn, 10 % - 47 % Fe, 29 –115 ppm Ni, 14 – 78 ppm Co, 5 - 470 ppm Pb, 0.08 - 27 ppm Mo, 6 – 92 ppm Ag and 0.04 – 0.05 ppm Au. Mining has not been recorded in this area. Some ore extraction occurred at Mina Vieja de Tirúa early in this century. The whole belt is considered a potential ore source.

Based on petrologic, geochemical and field relationships, the VMS deposits have been interpreted as formed by volcanic-exhalative activity (Collao and Alfaro 1982; Collao 1986; Collao et al. 1990). To explain the conditions of formation of these deposits sulphur isotopic analyses were carried out on pyrite and fluid inclusions determinations were done on samples from Mina Vieja de Tirúa, Casa de Piedra, and Pirén outcrops.

ANALYTICAL METHODS

The isotope analyses on pyrite from the VMS deposits were done at the Department of Geology of the University of Tasmania, Australia and at the Institute of Mineralogy, Petrology and Economic Geology of Tohoku University, Japan (preliminary data in Collao et al. 1990). Additional analyses included in this paper were done at the Research and Reactor Centre of the Scottish University, U.K and GEA Institute, at Concepción University, Chile.

The pyrite samples were treated according to Sasaki et al. (1979). The SO_2 content was obtained by the method of Robinson and Kusakabe (1975) and analyzed on a MM 903 (VG Isogas), Micromass 602 D and on a Sira II-VG Isotech mass spectrometer.

All the microthermometry measurements (n=242) of fluid inclusions were obtained on a Linkam TH 600 type heating and freezing stage (Shepherd, 1981) and carried out in the Institute of Mineralogy, Petrology and Economic Geology of Tohoku University, Japan and in the Department of Earth Sciences, Concepción University, Chile.

Analyses for the geobarometric study on sphalerites were done on an microprobe (EPMA) at the Institute of Mineralogy, Petrology and Economic Geology of Tohoku University, Japan. The geobarometry data presented here was taken from Collao et al. 1986.

REGIONAL GEOLOGICAL SETTING

The massive sulphide deposits occur in Paleozoic metamorphic rocks belonging to the central southern part of the Crystalline Basement of Chile along the coastal cordillera (Fig. 1). The Paleozoic basement is unconformably overlain by marine and continental rocks of Mesozoic and Cenozoic ages (Fig. 1). Plutonic rocks of about 320 Ma (Hervé et al. 1976) outcrop towards the NE margin of the studied area.

Aguirre et al. (1972) divided the Crystalline Basement into two units named the Western and Eastern Series. The Eastern Series is characterized by intercalated metapelites and metagraywackes while mica schists, quartzites, greenschists, metabasalts and serpentinites characterize the Western Series. Both series were affected by deformation and greenschist facies metamorphism. All of the mineralization (VMS; banded iron formation and Cr pods) is contained in the Western Series. In this study the Western Series has been subdivided into two regionally mappable units named the Tirúa and Nahuelbuta (Fig. 1). The Tirúa Unit, is constituted mainly of geenschists (metabasites) with serpentinite bodies and less frequently micaschists and metacherts. In the East, the Nahuelbuta Unit is characterized mainly by grey micaschists (metapelites and metagraywackes, Collao and Montecinos 1996), metacherts, iron metacherts (BIF, Oyarzún et al., 1984) and serpentinites with some Cr pods (Fig. 1).

Massive sulphide mineralization contained in the Tirúa Unit is described below.

The Tirúa Unit and Massive Sulphide Mineralization

The Tirúa Unit is located in the western part of the coastal cordillera comprising the Nahuelbuta and Queule Mountains, which widen towards the South to 70 km at Queule (Fig. 1). The unit is characterized by green schists (dominant) with intercalations of mica schists. Rare occurrences of metacherts intercalated within the green schists and serpentinite outcrop near Pirén.

Based on geochemistry, the green schists have been interpreted as basic metavolcanic rocks of tholeiitic affinity (Godoy 1979; Hervé 1977; Collao et al. 1980).

The Tirúa Unit has been less tectonically deformed than the Nahuelbuta Unit. The penetrative foliation (S2), which is the main regional structural feature affecting both units, has a general strike varying between ENE to NE, dipping 20 – 40º toward SE.

Massive sulphide (Fe, Cu, Zn) mineralization in lens-shaped bodies outcrops along the NNW-SSE fringe of the Tirúa Unit. This massive sulphide mineralization is found in five sectors of the coastal cordillera, south of the village of Tirúa. Individual occurrences listed from North to South are: Tirúa (Mina Vieja), Casa de Piedra, Hueñalihuén, Trovolhue, and Pirén (Fig. 1). The Mina Vieja of Tirúa is the largest deposit and is composed of a main lenticular body with four smaller beds having a general attitude of N 80ºE /40ºSE. The lens-shaped body has a maximum thickness of 0.5 m and can be followed for 15 m along the S2 foliation direction.

In Casa de Piedra and Hueñalihuén the mineralization strikes N 32-36ºE and dips 21-25ºSE. Further south the most important sulphide occurrence is located at Pirén Alto. The ores occur as seven tabular sheets having a general strike of 40ºE and dipping 33ºSE. The ore lenses have a thickness varying between 0.1 to 0.3 m. Laterally they can be followed only for 20 m due to a cover of soil and vegetation.

SULPHIDE MINERALIZATION AND MINERALOGY OF THE HOST ROCKS

The sulphide mineralization consist mostly of pyrite, with lesser amounts of chalcopyrite, sphalerite, and pyrrhotite (Fig. 2A). The ratio of pyrite / chalcopyrite is variable, but always exceeds 5:1. Sphalerite, chalcopyrite and pyrrhotite occur between the grains of pyrite (Fig. 2A) and less frequently form inclusions in pyrite (Figs. 3B, 4A). The sphalerite and pyrrhotite content is lower than the chalcopyrite content, with the exception of some smaller beds at Tirúa and Casa de Piedra mineralizations where sphalerite exceeds the chalcopyrite content. In both deposits minor minerals include bornite, mackinawite, galena, arsenopyrite, molybdenite, chalcocite, covellite, marcasite and magnetite. Argentite has been detected only in Mina Vieja de Tirúa where sphalerite mineralization in some smaller beds tends to exceed chalcopyrite, content. At Pirén and Hueñaliuén deposits the ore mineralization is dominated by pyrite within a matrix of chalcopyrite, pyrrhotite, and minor sphalerite (Fig 2A). Accesories are bornite, mackinawite, and molybdenite. At Pirén deposit other sulphides present as secondary minerals in varying amounts are marcasite, digenite, chalcocite, and covelline. At Trovolhue deposit most of sulphur mineralization as instertitial matrix between pyrite grains has been replaced by limonite (Fig. 2B).

In the metavolcanic rocks major silicate minerals include albite, epidote, chlorite and quartz (Fig. 3A). Other minor minerals include actinolite, muscovite, sphene, calcite and rutile. This mineral assemblage corresponds to that of Miyashiro (1994) for greenschist facies metabasites, which includes actinolite + chlorite + epidote + albite (+ quartz + muscovite + sphene + calcite + opaque minerals). It is also similar to the Type III.1 greenschist metabasite classification proposed by Graham et al. (1983) which is composed of epidote + chlorite + calcite + quartz + albite (with or without sphene, calcite, rutile, muscovite and biotite).

GEOBAROMETRY

The sphalerite geobarometer has been widely and successfully applied to metamorphosed ores (Hutchison and Scott, 1980; Scott, 1983). Compositions of sphalerite inclusions in pyrite represent preserved high pressure-temperature equilibria isolated from further reaction during subsequent retrograde conditions by the relatively inert encapsulating pyrite, may provide reliable estimates of peak pressure (Scott, 1983). It has been possible to apply the sphalerite geobarometer to the Mina Vieja de Tirúa and Pirén Alto deposits because metamorphic sulphide assemblages include intergrown sphalerite, pyrite, pyrrhotite (hexagonal pyrrhotite, according X ray analyses). Sphalerite in equilibrium with pyrrhotite (Fig. 3B) and pyrrhotite, chalcopyrite (Fig. 4A) encapsulated in pyrite crystals can provide pressure information in metamorphic terrains (Scott and

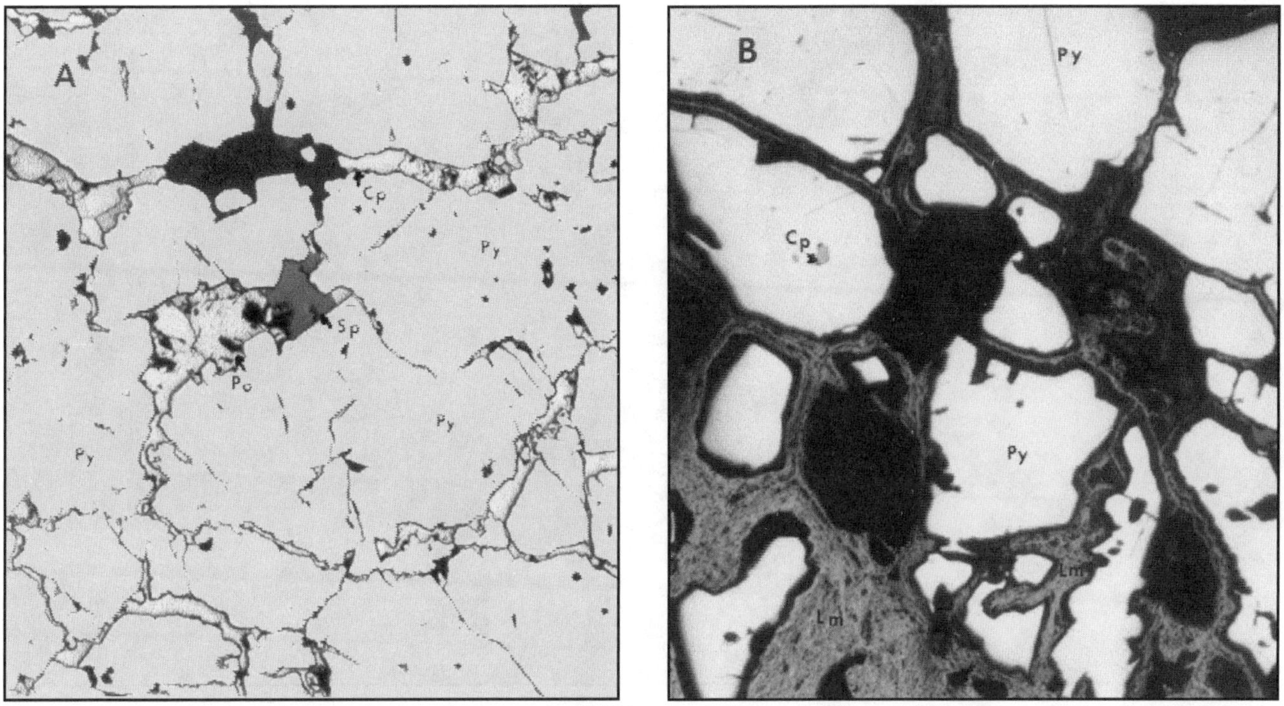

Figure. 2. Photomicrographs of typical occurrences of sulphide mineralization in VMS of Nahuelbuta and Queule Mountains. A. Chalcopyrite (Cp)-pyrrhotite (Po)- sphalerite (Sp) of filling intergranular between pyrite (Py) grains at Pirén Alto orebody. B. Limonite (Lm) and silicate minerals (SM) of filling intergranular between pyrite (Py) grains at Trovolhue orebody. Reflected, polarized light. Magnification x 12.

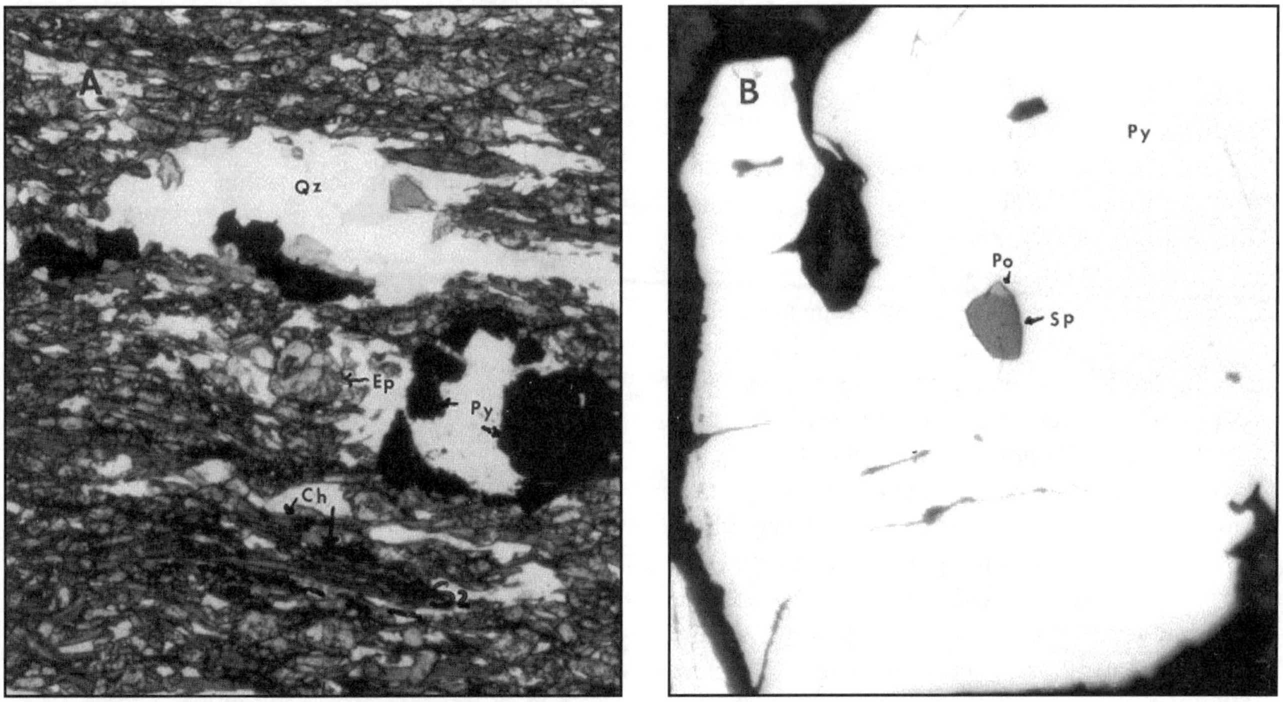

Figure. 3. Photomicrographs of typical occurrences of silicate and sulphide mineralization in VMS of Nahuelbuta and Queule Mountains. A. Epidote (Ep), chlorite (Ch), quartz (Qz) and pyrite (Py) grains in small bands arranged in the attitude of S2 -penetrative foliation planes. Casa de Piedra greenschist rock. Transmited, polarized light. Magnification x 12. B. Inclusion of sphalerite (Sp) -pyrrhotite (Po) within pyrite (Py) grain at Tirúa orebody. Reflected, polarized light. Magnification x 66.

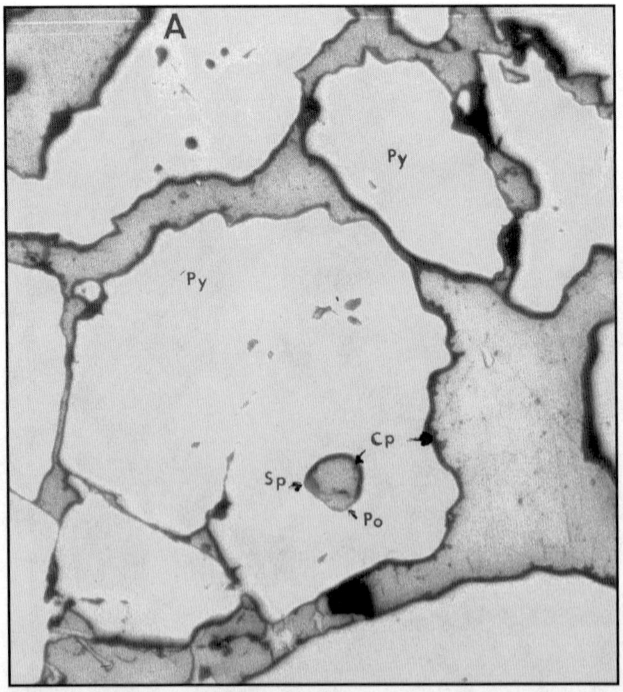

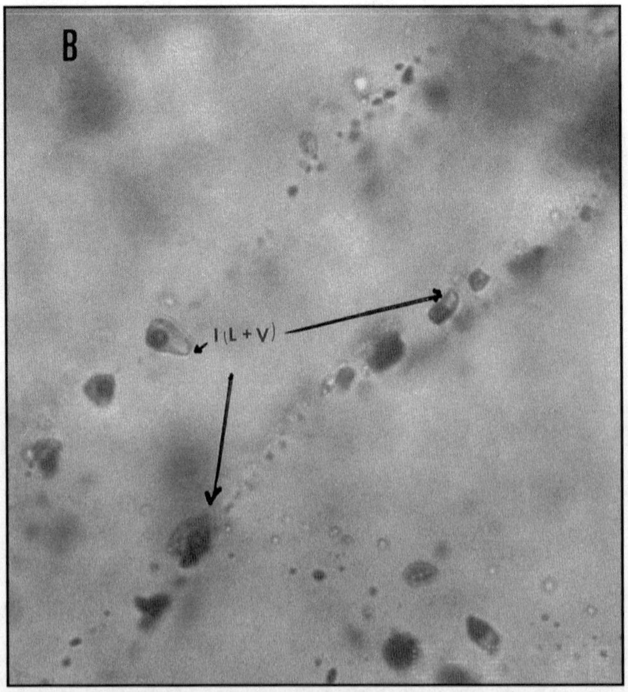

Figure. 4. Photomicrographs with occurrences of sulphide mineralization and fluid inclusions in VMS of Nahuelbuta and Queule Mountains. A. Inclusion with chalcopyrite (Cp) -pyrrhotite (Po)- sphalerite (Sp) withing pyrite (Py) grain at Pirén Alto orebody. Reflected, polarized light. Magnification x33. B. Fluid inclusions type I (fluid-rich variety) trapped in quartz (Qz). Fluid inclusions are distributed as planar pseudosecondary groups. Casa de Piedra orebody. Transmited, polarized light. Magnification x120.

Barnes 1971; Scott 1973; Lusk and Ford 1978; Scott 1983) (Fig. 5).

The sphalerite from the metamorphosed ores shows high values of FeS (11.0 % to 15.7 % molar), indicating that the mineralization experienced a wide pressure range (Table 1). At Pirén Alto the interpreted pressure varies between 3.5 (sphalerite in equilibium with pyrrhotite + chalcopyrite) to 9.0 kbar (sphalerite in equilibium with pyrrhotite) and in Tirúa deposit between 5.8 to 6.2 kbar. The sphalerite geobarometric data matches well with values of 5 kbar to 6 kbar obtained from the chemistry of Ca-Na amphiboles belonging to the greenschist silicate phase (Collao et al. 1986) according to a previous study by Oyarzún (1982) which adopts the method employed by Brown (1976). However, this pressure is slighly higher compared to the pressure given by Schira (1990) for this silicate association, which was estimated at less than 4 kbar in the Pirén area.

FLUID INCLUSION THERMOMETRY

Most fluid inclusions in the quartz grains from the massive sulphide mineralization and greenschist rocks are of a spheroidal or elongated shape. They occur in bands of quartz grains following the penetrative schistosity (Fig. 3A). All the fluid inclusions trapped in quartz correspond to the fluid- rich variety (type I, according to classification of Roedder, 1984) with a small vapor bubble (5 to 20 % of the volume of the inclusion) (Fig. 4B). The inclusions are generally under 15 mm in diameter and are uncommon. Fluid inclusions are distributed as planar clusters (Fig. 4B) and less frequently as small groups or isolated inclusions towards the central part of quartz grains. The isolated inclusions yield higher temperature estimates than the planar groups. The homogenization temperature of fluid inclusions in the massive sulphide ores and from the surrounding greeschist rocks are similar in terms of range, mode, and mean peak values, which range between 196° to 451°C (Table 2, Figs. 6, 7).

Table 1. Composition and mole % FeS in sphalerites from massive sulphides of Nahuelbuta and Queule Mountains, South Central Chile

Deposit	Sample	Wt%							Sphalerite (mole % FeS) in different touching assemblages								Pressure (kb)	
									Encasulated within pyrita						As a matrix			
		Fe	Zn	S	Cu	Cd	In	Mn	Sp+Po	Sp+Po+Cpy	Sp+Cpy	Sp+Cpy+Bo	Sp (*)	Near to	Sp+Po+Cpy	Sp+Cpy	A	B
TIRUA	C-3$_1$	7,7	58,1	33,5	0,4					13,3							6,2	6,3
	C-3$_4$	7,8	58,8	33,8	0,4					13,3							6,2	6,3
	C-3$_5$	8,0	58,0	33,4	0,2	0,5				13,8							5,8	5,9
	C-3$_2$	7,8	57,4	33,3	0,7					13,5							6,0	6,1
	C-3$_3$	7,5	58,1	34,0	0,6					13,0							6,6	6,7
	C-3'$_1$	4,2	63,3	33,1							7,3							
	C-3'$_2$	4,0	62,8	33,6				0,1			7,0							
CASA DE PIEDRA	C-8$_1$	2,8	65,1	33,1									4,7	Gal, Bo+ Cpy				
	C-8$_2$	2,4	64,4	32,4									4,1					
	C-8$_3$	2,6	64,6	32,7									4,4					
	C-8$_4$	2,0	65,0	32,6									3,5					
	C-8$_5$	1,6	65,8	32,7								2,8						
	C-8'$_1$	2,8	63,9	33,1									4,8	Bo+ Cpy				
	C-8'$_2$	2,6	64,0	33,2									4,6					
	C-8'$_3$	2,5	64,0	33,2									4,4					
PIRÉN ALTO – Orebody 7	H-7$_1$	8,8	57,4	33,5						15,2							4,4	4,4
	H-7$_2$	8,5	57,4	33,6				0,1		14,7							4,8	4,9
	H-7'$_1$	7,4	58,4	33,3	0,9			0,2		12,7							6,9	7,0
	H-7'$_2$	7,6	58,2	33,7	0,7					13,1							6,4	6,6
	H-7'$_3$	8,1	59,1	33,2						13,8							5,7	5,8
	H-7'$_4$	7,6	59,3	33,1		0,2				13,1							6,4	6,6
	H-7'$_5$	8,1	57,9	33,4	0,3			0,1		13,9							5,6	5,7
PIRÉN ALTO – Orebody 6	H-6$_1$	7,3	59,0	33,8				0,2		12,6							7,0	7,1
	H-6$_2$	6,4	60,1	33,7					11,1								8,7	8,8
	H-63	6,4	60,6	33,1					11,0								8,9	9,0
	H-64	6,3	61,1	33,1									10,7	Po, Cpy				
	H-65	6,7	59,7	33,4	0,2			0,3					11,6					
	H-66	6,8	60,4	33,1									11,6					
	H																	
	H-6'1	7,0	59,1	33,4					12,2									
	H-6'2	7,3	58,6	33,1		0,4			12,7									
	H-6'3	6,8	59,4	32,8				0,3					11,7					
	H-6'4	6,6	60,1	33,0									11,4	Po				
	H-6'5	6,6	59,5	33,2		0,2							11,5					
PIRÉN ALTO – Orebody 4	H-41	7,2	59,5	33,4	0,4				12,3								7,4	7,5
	H-42	7,5	57,9	32,9	0,3	0,4	0,4	0,4	12,9								6,6	6,7
	H-4'1	9,0	57,0	33,8						15,7							3,9	3,9
	H-4'2	8,8	56,9	33,5	0,6					15,2							4,4	4,4
	H-4'3	8,9	57,2	33,5	0,2					15,4							4,2	4,2
PIRÉN ALTO – Orb. 3	H-31	5,7	60,5	33,4									9,9	Po+ Cpy.				
	H-32	5,4	60,4	33,3	0,4								9,5					
	H-33	5,8	60,8	33,6									10,0					
PIRÉN ALTO – Orb. 2	H-21	8,6	57,9	33,5	0,3								14,7	Cpy+ Po				
	H-22	8,5	58,1	33,1	0,6								14,5					
PIRÉN ALTO – Orebody 1	H-Im1	7,7	58,4	33,5	0,4										13,4		6,2	6,3
	H-Im$_2$	7,8	58,8	33,6											13,5		6,1	6,2
	H-Im$_3$	6,9	59,0	33,6											12,0		7,7	7,8
	H-Im$_4$	7,5	59,2	33,6											12,9		6,6	6,7
	H-Im$_5$	7,6	58,9	33,9	0,4										13,1		6,5	6,6
	H-Im$_6$	7,2	58,8	33,8	0,4										12,5		7,1	7,2
	H-Im$_7$	7,6	58,4	33,8	0,5										13,1		6,4	6,5
	H-Im$_8$	7,3	59,3	33,6											12,6		7,0	7,1
	H-Im$_9$	7,2	58,8	32,2	0,6		0,5								12,4		7,2	7,3
	H-Im$_{10}$	7,8	58,5	33,4											13,5		6,0	6,1
	H-Im$_{11}$	7,9	58,3	33,6			0,7								13,6		5,9	6,0
	H-Im$_{12}$	7,8	57,6	33,6	0,5			0,6		13,8					13,5		6,0	6,1
	H-Ib$_1$	8,0	57,2	33,4	0,6												5,7	5,8
PIRÉN ALTO – Green schist	C-05$_1$	3,2	63,3	32,4	0,8											5,5		
	C-05$_2$	1,7	65,3	32,5	0,3											3,0		
	C-05$_3$	1,7	68,4	32,5	0,6											3,0		
	C-05$_4$	1,7	65,2	32,9												2,9		
	C-05$_5$	1,4	65,2	33,0												2,5		
	C-05$_6$	1,4	64,8	33,1		0,4												

(*) Others minerals near sphalerite (Sp) into the same pyrite grain. Bo: bornite; Cpy: chalcopyrite; Gal: galena; Po: pyrrhotite; Calculated pressure according: A) Hutchison and Scott (1981); B) Lusk and Ford (1978). Sphalerite geobarometric data, from Collao et al. (1986).

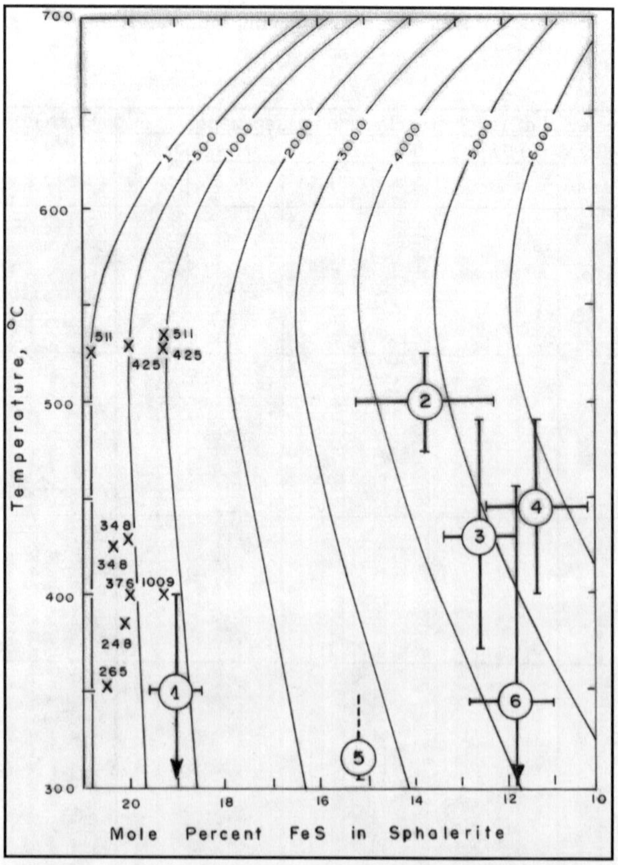

Figure. 5. Composition of sphalerite coexisting with pyrite and hexagonal pyrrhotite as a function of temperature and pressure (in bars) based in Lusk and Ford (1978). Crosses represent experimental points by Scott and Barnes (1971). Circles represent conditions at (1) Central and southern Bolivia, (2) Balmat, New York, (3) Highland - Surprise Mine, Coeur D' Alene, Idaho, (4) Quemont Mine, Noranda, Quebec, (5) Nairne Pyritic Formation, South Australia, and (6) VMS deposits of Nahuelbuta and Queule Mountains, South Central, Chile. Based in Scott and Barnes (1971).

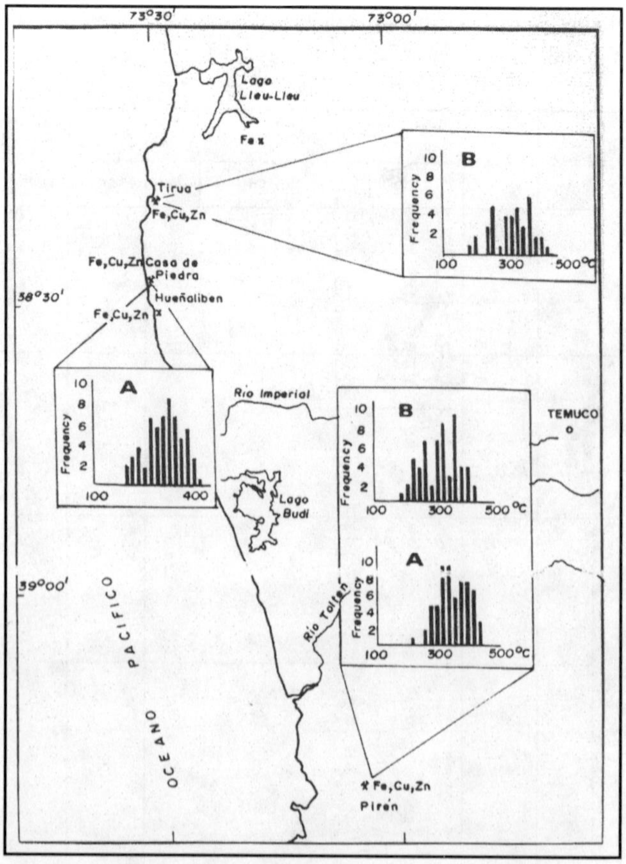

Figure. 6. Homogenization temperature in fluid inclusions in quartz from massive sulphide ores (A) and greenschist rocks (B), South-Central Chile.

The results of freezing measurements in some of the bigger fluid inclusions give estimated salinities between 2.9 to 14.6 weight percent of NaCl equivalent for the massive sulphide ores. Estimated salinities of inclusions in surrounding greenschist rock fall into the low to moderate range of the sulphide ores (Table 2).

The homogenization temperature data was plotted as frequency-temperature histograms (Figs. 6, 7) and is summarized in Table 2. The data shows a certain similitude with respect to the mode and occurrence of the secondary peaks between deposits and to the surrounding greenschist rocks; peaks occur at 390°C, 400°C and 410°C. These peaks mark higher temperature populations in secondary fluid inclusions generated during the metamorphism, which could represent prograde higher grade metamorphic conditions. On the other hand the mode or secondary peaks at 350°C, near the mean of values may represent another important thermometric event of high to moderate temperature, which is observed for each deposit. Peaks around 290 °C and 270 °C (Table 2; Figs. 7, 8) may represent inclusions that formed during a retro-

Table 2. Summary of microthermotric data in massive sulphide ores and surrounding greenschist rocks, from Nahuelbuta and Queule Mountains, South-Central Chile.

Rock and ore deposit	Homogenization Temperature (°C)					Salinity (Wt % of Na Cl)		
	Data Mean	Range	Mode	Secondary peaks	(n)	Data (n)	Range	Mean
Greenschist from Mina Vieja, Tirúa	39	196-445	390	270,350	332	5	2.9-10.8	6.3
Orebody of Casa de Piedra	62	201-446	350	290,410	334	7	3.3-12.2	6.6
Greenschist from Pirén	60	210-450	390	290,350	338	4	5.3-14.6	9.5
Orebody of Pirén	65	228-451	350	400	363			

Fig. 7. Homogenization temperatures are similar in mode and have coincident secondary peaks from the different ores and greenschist rocks as result of metamorphism.

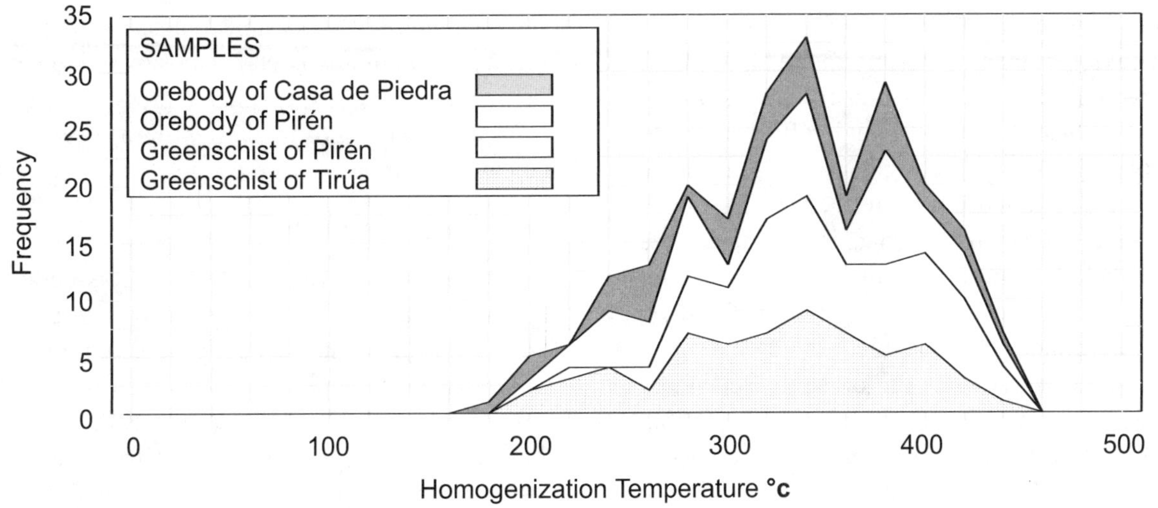

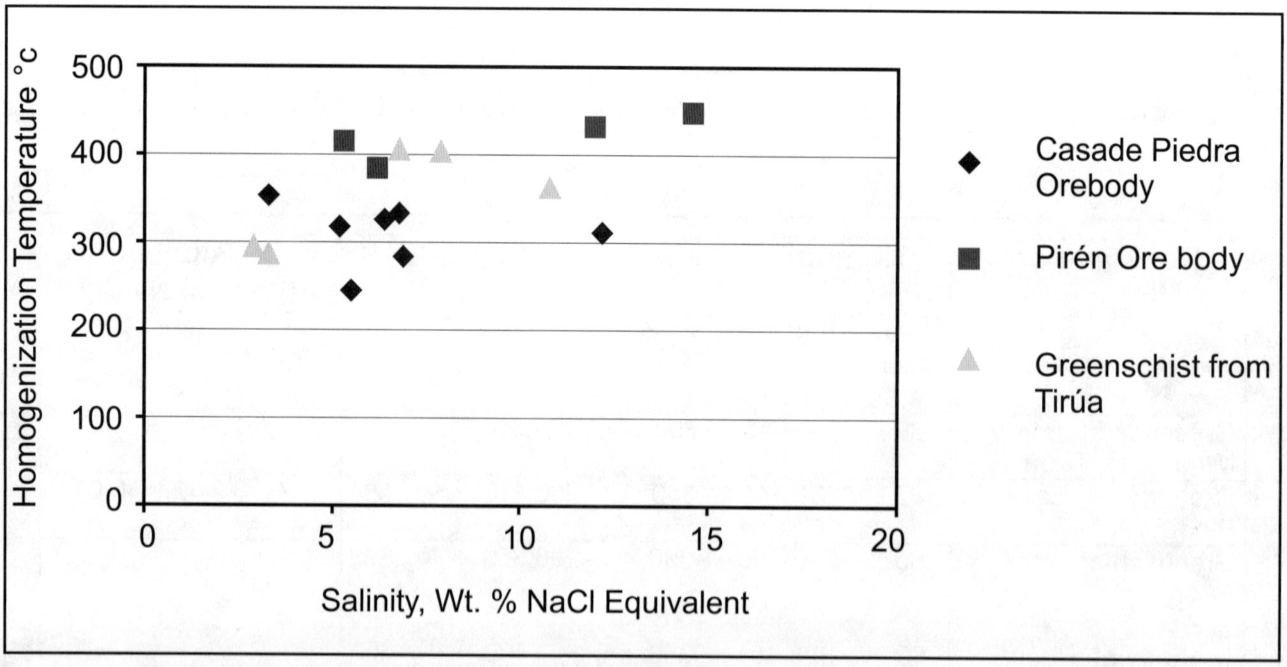

Figure 8. Homogenization termperature versus salinity in fluid inclusions in quartz from some massive sulphide deposits and greenschist rocks, South-Central Chile.

grade metamorphic event or by secondary processes. This population is largely contained in the planar groups of fluid inclusions; those inclusions found in small groups towards the central part of quartz crystals, which are interpreted as primary inclusions and tend to show higher temperatures.

In the diagram of homogenization temperature versus salinity (Fig. 8) most values of lower salinity (less than 7.5 equivalent wt % Na Cl) show a wide range of homogenization temperatures and few values of moderate salinity tend to be higher temperature. In general, such wide variation could reflect a consequence of prograde and retrograde of metamorphic processes as suggested by Touret (1981). However, some of the higher homogenization temperatures could also be due to necking, which produces greater variability in homogenization temperature (Roedder, 1967. All the fluid inclusions of this study may give evidence about metamorphism or some secondary deformational event postmetamorphism. According Crawford (1981) the fluid inclusions in metamorphic rocks, provides information about the composition of fluid phase present during the metamorphism, its evolution during metamorphic mineral growth, and the pressure and temperature conditions of metamorphism.

If the thermo-barometric data are plotted on the metamorphic diagram by Bucher and Frey (1994) it becomes clear that it is equivalent to greenschist and subgreenschist facies conditions (Fig. 9). It is consistent with the mineralogic assemblage indication of the metabasite greenschist facies according Miyashiro (1994). Estimated temperatures using fluid inclusions should be higher if it is possible to determine trapping temperature conditions (trend with arrow indication in the diagram). On the other hand, pressure could be less if is considered information of Shira, 1990 (trend is indicated with arrow in the diagram).

SULPHUR ISOTOPE STUDIES.

Pyrite for sulphur isotope analysis was collected by picking the coarse fraction, which was ground (50 to 100 mesh) and subsequently selected under a stereoscopic microscope.The results are expressed in the conventional $\delta^{34}S$ (CDT) ‰ (Table 3).

The sulphur isotope data in pyrite from the VMS deposits of Nahuelbuta and Queule Mountains show $\delta^{34}S$ values always positive having a range between + 0.1 to + 6.5‰ with a mean of $\delta^{34}S$ = + 3.14‰ (stan-

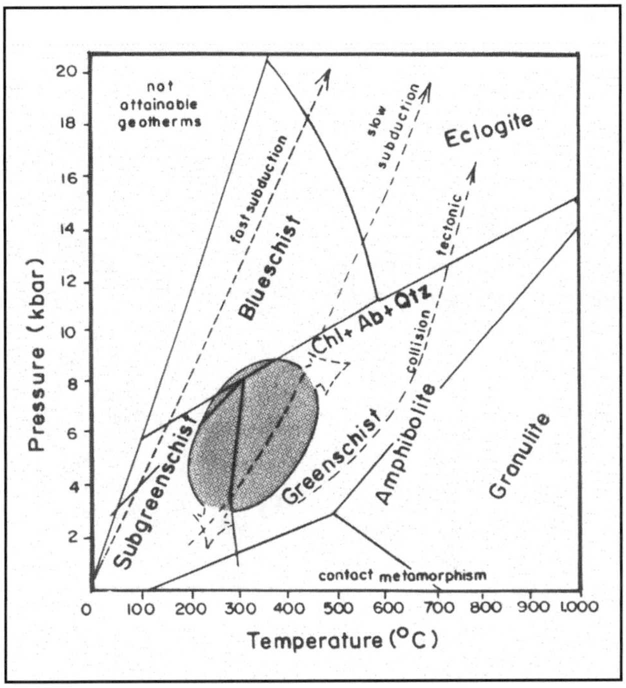

Figure 9. Estimated P-T fields in the greenschist and subgreenschist facies for Chilean massive sulphide deposits. Termperature data is from fluid inclusions. Pressure data is mainly from sphalerite geobarometer. Diagram from Bucher and Frey, 1994.

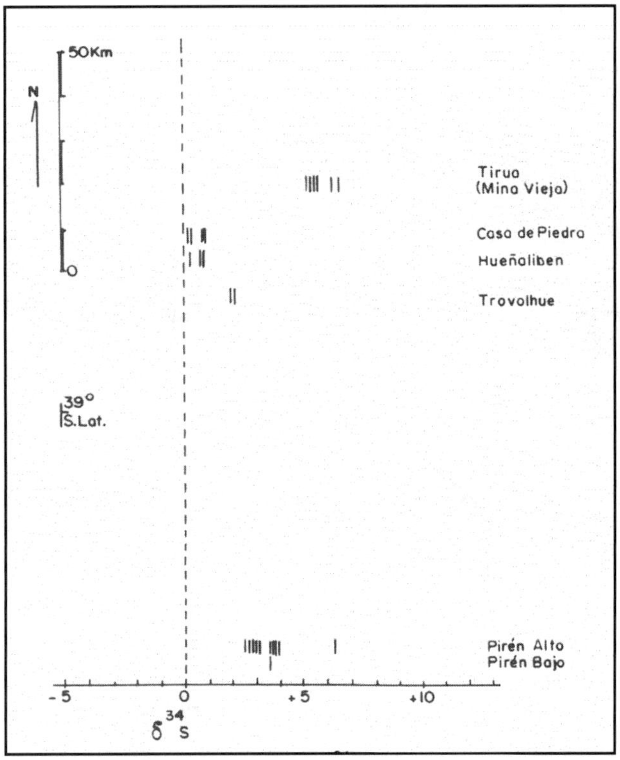

Figure 10. δ ^{34}S in pyrite from massive sulphide deposits, South-Central Chile

dard deviation: 2.1). Compared with sulphur isotope information from various genetic types of deposits (Nielsen 1979), the results are similar to other magmatic and volcanogenic hydrothermal ore deposits. The lower mean value of sulphur isotope ratios from the Casa de Piedra and Hueñaliben deposits (mean of $\delta^{34}S$ = + 0.5‰) suggests that they were more proximal to a hydrothermal vent, than the deposits of Tirúa (mean of $\delta^{34}S$ = + 5.9‰) and Pirén (mean of $\delta^{34}S$ = + 3.5‰) (Fig. 10). Based on the interpretations of sulphur isotope data of the Raul Mine, Perú, by Ripley and Ohomoto (1977), it can be suggested that the magmatic source of mineralizing fluids was more proximal to the massive sulphide ores of Casa de Piedra and Hueñaliben, than those of Tirúa and Pirén.

DISCUSSION AND CONCLUSION

Field and laboratory evidence, such as the well preserved pillow structures in metabasalts, the sulphide mineralogy and the sulphur isotope content of pyrite suggest a submarine volcanic origin for the massive sulphide deposits in the Nahuelbuta and Queule Mountains (Collao et al. 1980; Alfaro et al. 1983; Collao and Alfaro 1982; Alfaro and Collao 1990; Collao et al. 1990). The $\delta^{34}S$ values of pyrite from the massive sulphide ores are similar to those of a magmatic source (Nielsen 1979), seems to most probable. Based on the interpretations of sulphur isotope data of the Raul Mine, Perú, by Ripley and Ohomoto (1977), it can be suggested that the magmatic source of mineralizing fluids was more proximal to the massive sulphide ores of Casa de Piedra and Hueñaliben (mean of values of $\delta^{34}S$ = + 0.5‰), than those of Tirúa (mean of $\delta^{34}S$ = + 5.9‰) and Pirén (mean of $\delta^{34}S$ = + 3.5‰). The $\delta^{34}S$ values are compared with sulphur isotopes analyses in pyrite from the banded iron formation at Mahuilque (mean of – 2.7 $\delta^{34}S$‰, Collao et al. 1990) located to the East of

Table 3. Sulphur isotopic analyses of pyrite from massive sulphide deposits in the Nahuelbuta and Queule Mountains, South-

Outcrop	Data (n)	$\delta^{34}S$ ‰ Range	Mean
Tirúa, Mina Vieja	7	+5.5 - +6.5	+5.9
Casa de Piedra	4	+0.1 - +1.0	+0.5
Hueñaliben	3	+0.3 - +0.7	+0.5
Trovolhue	2	+2.0 - +2.2	+2.1
Pirén Alto y Bajo	11	+2.4 - +6.3	+3.5

the Tirúa unit (Fig. 1) the mineralizing fluids could have been a late stage or a part of distal environment (in the sense of Plimer, 1978). After that, metamorphic processes were prevalent to generate mineral assemblages of greenschist facies for metabasites, as described by Miyashiro 1994, which include actinolite + chlorite + epidote + albite (+ quartz + muscovite + sphene + calcite + opaque minerals).

The homogenization temperature of fluid inclusions in quartz from the different suphide depotits and surrounding greenschist metavolcanic rocks is similar on a regional scale (Figs. 6, 7; Table 2) and varies between 196°C to 452°C. The salinty composition of the fluid inclusions (in the range of 2.9 to14.6 weight percent of NaCl equivalent) is also similar. In general, the trend could be reflecting a consequence of prograde and retrograde of metamorphic processes affecting the metabasites in several events, rearranging the minerals of the greenschist facies.

Sphalerite geobarometry suggests a wide pressure range between 3.5 to 9.0 kbar. Thermobarometric data from fluid inclusions and sphalerite analyses is commensurate with greenschist and subgreenschist P-T conditions, which modified the mineralogy of the mineralization and the host metavolcanic rocks.

References

Aguirre, L.Hervé, F. and Godoy, E. 1972: Distribution of metamorphic facies in Chile: an outline – Kristallynikum, Prague. 9: 7-14.

Alfaro, G. and Collao, S. 1990. Massive sulfides in the Greenstone Belt of South-Central Chile. An overview. In Stratabound ore deposits in the Andes. Edited by Fontboté, L. Amstutz, G.C. Cardozo, M. Cedillo, E. and Frutos, J. Springer Verlag, Berlin, Germany, pp. 199-208.

Brown, P.E. 1876. The crossite content of Ca-amphibole as guide to pressure of metamorphism. Journal of Petrology.18: 53-72.

Bucher, K. and Frey, M. 1994. Petrogenesis of metamorphic rocks.Springer-Verlag, Berlin. 318 p.

Collao, S. and Alfaro, G. 1990. Banded iron formation and massive sulfide orebodies, South-Central Chile: Geologic and isotopic aspects. In Stratabound ore deposits in the Andes. Edited by Fontboté, L. Amstutz, G.C. Cardozo, M. Cedillo, E. and Frutos, J. Springer Verlag, Berlin, Germany, pp. 211-219.

Collao, S. and Alfaro, G. 1982. Mineralización sulfurada de hierro, cobre y zinc en la Cordillera de la Costa, Sur de Chile. Revista Geológica de Chile. 15: 41-47.

Collao, S. Kojima, S. and Oyarzún, R. 1986. Geobarometría en los sulfuros macizos de la franja metamórfica de esquistos verdes, Chile Central-Sur. Revista Geológica de Chile. 28/29: 3-16.

Collao, S. and Montecinos, D. 1996. El origen de las mineralizaciones de hierro y manganeso del basamento metamórfico del Centro-Sur de Chile. Estudos Tecnológicos. Acta Geologica Leopoldensia, Brasil. 43: 167-180.

Collao, S. Montecinos, P. Oviedo, L. and Oyarzún, R. 1980. Estudio genético de las mineralizaciones de hierro de

Mahuilque.Unpublished report. Dpto. Geociencias. Universidad de Concepción, Chile.

Crawford, M. L. 1981. Fluid inclusions in metamorphic rocks - low and medium grade. In a short course in fluid inclusions: Aplicattions to petrology. Edited by Hollister, L.S and Crawford, M.L. Mineralogical Association of Canada. 6: 157-181.

Godoy, E. 1979. Metabasitas del basamento metamórfico chileno, nuevos datos geoquímicos. Actas II Congreso Geológico Chileno.Arica, Chile. 3: 133-148.

Graham, C. M. Greig, K. M. Sheppard, S. M. and Turi, B. 1983. Genesis and mobility of the H2O-CO2 fluid phase during regional greenschist and epidote amphibolite facies metamorphism: a petrological and stable isotope study in the Scottish Dalradian. J. Geol. Soc. London. 140: 577-599.

Hervé, F. 1977. Petrology of the crystalline basement of the Nahuelbuta Mountains, south-central Chile. In: Comparative studies on the geology of the circum-pacific orogenic belt in Japan and Chile. Edited by Ishikawa, T. and Aguirre, L. Japanese Society of Promotion of Science, Tokyo, Japan, pp. 1-52.

Hutchison, M.N., and Scott, S.D. 1980. Sphalerite geobarometry applied to metamorphosed sulfide ores of the Swedish Caledonides and U. S. Appalachians: Noerges Geol. Undersokelse, no. 360, p. 59-72.

Lusk, J. F. and Ford, C.E. 1978. Experimental extension of the sphalerite geobarometer to 10 kbar. American. Mineralogist. 63: 516-519.

Miyashiro, A. 1994. Metamorphic petrology. UCL Press, London, U.K. 404 p.

Nielsen, H. 1979. Sulfur isotopes in lectures in isotope geology. Jager E, Hunziker (eds). Springer, Berlin, Heidelberg, New York., 283-312.

Oyarzún, R. 1982. Geology and geochemistry of the Banded iron Formation in the Nahuelbuta Mountains, Chile. Ph.D. Thesis, Earth Sci. Dept. The University of Leeds. 226 p.

Oyarzún, R. Clemmey, H. and Collao, S. 1984. Chemical characteristics of the Nahuelbuta Mountains banded iron formation, southern Central Chile.Jour. Jpn Assoc Min Petrol Econ Geol. 79: 146-156.

Plimer, I. 1978. Proximal and distal strata-bound ore deposits. Min. Deposita. 13: 345-353.

Ripley, E. M. and Ohomoto, H. 1977. Mineralogic, sulfur isotope, and fluid inclusions studies of the strata-bound copper deposits at the Raúl Mine, Perú. Econ. Geol. 72: 1017-1041.

Robinson, B.R. and Kusakabe, M. 1975. Quantitative preparation of sulfur dioxide for d 34S/ 32S analyses, from sulfides by combustion with cuprous oxide.Anal Chem. 47: 1179-1181.

Roedder, E. 1967. Fluid inclusions as Samples of Ore Fluids. In Geochemistry of Hydrothermal Ore Deposits. Edited by Hubert Lloyd Barnes. The pennsylvania State University. U.S.A. 12: 515-574.

Roedder, E. 1984. Fluid inclusions. Reviews in Mineralogy. Mineralogical Society of America. Edited by P. Ribbe.12: 644 p

Scott, S.D. 1973. Experimental calibration of the sphalerite geobarometer. Economic Geology. 68, N° 4: 466-474.

Scott, S.D. 1983. Chemical behavior of sphalerite and arsenopyrite in hydrothermal and metamorphic environments. Mineralogical Magazine. 47: N° 344: 427-435.

Scott, S.D. and Barnes, H. L. 1971. Sphalerite geothermometry and geobarometry. Economic Geology. 66, N° 4: 653-669.

Schira, W. Amstutz, G.C. and Fontboté, L. 1990. The Pirén Alto Cu-(Zn) massive sulfide occurrence in south-central Chile – a Kieslager-type mineralization in a Paleozoic ensialic mature marginal basin setting. In Stratabound Ore Deposits in the Andes Edited by Fontboté, L. Amstutz, G.C. Cardozo, M. Cedillo, E. and Frutos, J. Springer Verlag, Berlin, Germany, pp. 211-219.

Shepherd,T.J.1981. Temperature-programmable heating-freezing stage for microthermometric analysis of fluid inclusions. Economic Geology. 76: 1244-1247.

Touret, J. 1981. Fluid inclusions in high grade metamorphic rocks. In a short course in fluid inclusions: Aplicattions to petrology. Edited by Hollister, L.S and Crawford, M.L. Mineralogical Association of Canada. 6: 182-208.